Handbook of Nonprescription Drugs

10th EDITION

Notices

The inclusion in this book of any drug in respect to which patent or trademark rights may exist shall not be deemed, and is not intended as a grant of or authority to exercise, any right or privilege protected by such patent or trademark. All such rights or trademarks are vested in the patent or trademark owner, and no other person may exercise the same without express permission, authority, or license secured from such patent or trademark owner.

The listing of selected brand names is intended only for ease of reference. The listed brand names are a representative sampling of drug products, not a comprehensive listing. The inclusion of a brand name does not mean the editors or publisher has any particular knowledge that the brand listed has properties different from other brands of the same drug, nor should its inclusion be interpreted as an endorsement by the editors or publisher. Similarly, the fact that a particular brand has not been included does not indicate the product has been judged to be in any way unsatisfactory or unacceptable.

The convention followed in this book to identify brand names of drugs and other products is to use initial capital letters (when appropriate) and/or trademarks. Nonproprietary, generic, or common names of such articles are cited without initial capitalization or trademarks.

The nature of drug information is that it is constantly evolving because of ongoing research and clinical experience and is often subject to interpretation. Although great care has been taken to ensure the accuracy of the information presented herein, the reader is advised that the authors, editors, reviewers, contributors, and publisher cannot be held responsible for the continued currency of the information or for any errors or omissions in this book or for any consequences arising therefrom. Readers are advised that decisions regarding drug therapy must be based on the independent judgment of the clinician, changing information about a drug, (e.g., as reflected in the literature and manufacturer's most current product information), and changing medical practices.

The editors, authors, and contributors have written this book in their private capacities. No official support or endorsement by any federal or state agency or pharmaceutical company is intended or inferred.

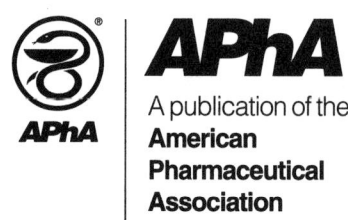

A publication of the
American Pharmaceutical Association

Handbook of Nonprescription Drugs

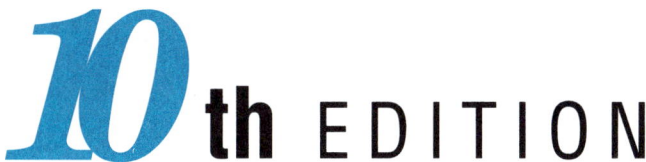th EDITION

Published by
AMERICAN PHARMACEUTICAL ASSOCIATION

*The National Professional Society of Pharmacists
2215 Constitution Avenue, NW
Washington, DC 20037*

Timothy R. Covington, Pharm.D.
Pharmaceutical Editor

Laura C. Lawson
Managing Editor

Linda L. Young
Assistant Managing Editor

Susan C. Kendall
Editorial Coordinator

William B. Mason
Design and Production Artist

James V. McGinnis
Manager of Art and Production

James P. Caro
Senior Director, Division of Programming and Publications

Database Development: Benjamin J. Bluml, Cygnus Systems Development Inc.

Product Table Research: Jennifer L. Brown, Stacy Ferguson, Jaspconia G. Florence

Database Entry: Jaspconia G. Florence, Azadeh S. Kaider

Desktop Publishing Consultant: Thomas J. Piwowar & Associates, Inc.

Editorial Services: EEI

Anatomic Drawings: Walter Hilmers, Jr., and Judith M. Guenther, with Alexa L. Chun

Color Illustration Contributors: Jean A. Borger, Richard C. Childers, Stanley Cullen, Alfred C. Griffin (deceased), Harold L. Hammond, R. Gary Sibbald

Printing: Quebecor America Book Group

Library of Congress Catalog Number 86-640099
ISSN 0889-7816
ISBN 0-917330-63-3

© Copyright 1993, American Pharmaceutical Association, 2215 Constitution Avenue, NW, Washington, DC 20037
© 1967, 1969, 1971, 1973, 1977, 1979, 1982, 1986, 1990

No portion of this publication may be reproduced, stored in a retrieval system, or transmitted in any form or by any means now known or by any future method without prior written permission from the publisher. Requests to reproduce or use data or information from this text should be sent to *Handbook of Nonprescription Drugs*, American Pharmaceutical Association, 2215 Constitution Avenue, NW, Washington, DC 20037. A nominal fee may be assessed for processing of such requests.

Although many individual items of information contained herein may be found in other sources, the material as presented in this format is unique and available nowhere else. The compilation and arrangement of the information in a convenient and readily accessible format represent an extensive amount of staff resources, judgment, effort, and time, and contribute to the originality of the text. The book is fully copyrighted.

The editors and publisher are not responsible for any inaccuracy of quotation or for any false or misleading implication that may arise due to others' use of material in this edition, or due to the quotation of material from editions no longer official.

Contents

Advisory Panel, Authors & Reviewers xi
Preface xxiii
Introduction xxv

1 **The Self-Care Movement** 1
Gary A. Holt and Edwin L. Hall

2 **Patient Assessment and Consultation** 11
Wendy Klein-Schwartz and J. Michael Hoopes

3 **FDA's Review of OTC Drugs** 21
William E. Gilbertson

4 **In-Home Testing and Monitoring Products** 39
Susan M. Meyer
    Electronic Oscillometric Blood Pressure Monitor
      Product Table 639
    Fecal Occult Blood Test Kits Table 641
    Ovulation Prediction Test Kits Table 642
    Pregnancy Test Kits Table 643

5 **Internal Analgesic Products** 49
W. Kent Van Tyle
    Internal Analgesic Product Table 644

6 **Antipyretic Drug Products** 65
Thomas E. Lackner
    Antipyretic Product Table 657

7 **Menstrual Products** 77
Leslie A. Shimp
    Menstrual Product Table 666

8 Cold, Cough, and Allergy Products — 89
Bobby G. Bryant and Thomas P. Lombardi
   Cold, Cough, Allergy Product Table   670
   Topical Decongestant Product Table   704
   Miscellaneous Nasal Product Table   707
   Lozenge Product Table   708

9 Asthma Products — 117
H. William Kelly and Mary Beth O'Connell
   Asthma Inhalant Product Table   711
   Asthma Oral Combination Product Table   712

10 Sleep Aid and Stimulant Products — 135
M. Lynn Crismon and Donna M. Jermain
   Sleep Aid Product Table   713
   Stimulant Product Table   715

11 Antacid Products — 147
Julianne B. Pinson and C. Wayne Weart
   Antacid Product Table   716

12 Emetic and Antiemetic Products — 181
Gary M. Oderda and Jenifer C. Jennings
   Appendix: Major Poison Control Centers   192
   Antiemetic Product Table   722

13 Antidiarrheal Products — 199
R. Leon Longe
   Antidiarrheal Product Table   723

14 Anthelmintic Products — 213
Kathryn K. Bucci
   Anthelmintic Product Table   726

15 Laxative Products — 219
Clarence E. Curry, Jr., and Demetris Tatum-Butler
   Laxative Product Table   727

16 Diabetes Care Products and Monitoring Devices — 237
John R. White, Jr., and R. Keith Campbell

    Appendix 1: Diabetes Information Sources   275
    Appendix 2: Sugar-Free Preparations by
      Therapeutic Category   277

    Insulin Preparations Product Table   739
    Insulin Syringes and Related Products Table   742
    Blood Sugar–Elevating Products Table   744
    Diabetes Monitoring Products Table   746
    Miscellaneous Diabetes Products Table   750

17 Nutritional Products — 283
Loyd V. Allen, Jr.

    Food Supplement Product Table   751
    Iron Product Table   755
    Calcium Product Table   758
    Multiple Vitamin Product Table   762

18 Infant Formula Products — 313
Rosalie Sagraves, Claudia Kamper, and Judi Doerr

    Formula Products for Infants and Children Product Table   790

19 Weight Control Products — 339
Glenn D. Appelt

    Appetite Suppressant Product Table   796

20 Ophthalmic Products — 351
Jimmy D. Bartlett and Mark W. Swanson

    Artificial Tear Product Table   797
    Ophthalmic Decongestant Product Table   799
    Eye Wash Product Table   801

21 Contact Lens Products — 367
Janet P. Engle

    Hard and Rigid Gas-Permeable Lens Product Table   802
    Soft Lens Product Table   804

22 Otic Products — 389
Keith O. Miller

    Otic Product Table   808

23 Oral Health Products — 407
Arlene A. Flynn

    Dentifrice Product Table   809
    Artificial Saliva Product Table   813
    Oral Rinse Product Table   814
    Denture Cleanser Product Table   815
    Denture Adhesive Product Table   816
    Mouth Pain, Cold Sore, Canker Sore Product Table   817

24 Ostomy and Wound Care Products — 433
Michael L. Kleinberg and Moya J. Vazquez

    Appendix: Major Manufacturers of Ostomy Products and Accessories   450

    Ostomy Product Table   820

25 Contraceptive Methods and Products — 453
Louise Parent-Stevens and Roberta S. Carrier

    Appendix 1: Family Planning Information   466
    Appendix 2: AIDS Information Resources   467

    Spermicide Product Table   822
    Condom Product Table   823

26 Hemorrhoidal Products — 469
Benjamin Hodes

    Hemorrhoidal Product Table   825

27 Personal Care Products — 479
Donald R. Miller and Mary Kuzel

    Personal Care Product Table   828

28 Topical Anti-Infective Products — 493
Dennis P. West and Susan V. Maddux

    Topical Anti-Infective Product Table   831

29 Acne Products — 511
Joye Ann Billow

    Appendix: Acne Information Sources   520

    Acne Product Table   836

30 Dermatologic Products — 521
Joye Ann Billow

    Dermatitis and Psoriasis Product Table   840
    Dry Skin Product Table   844
    Dandruff and Seborrhea Product Table   850

31 Diaper Rash and Prickly Heat Products — 543
Gary H. Smith
   Diaper Rash and Prickly Heat Product Table 854

32 External Analgesic Products — 551
Arthur I. Jacknowitz
   External Analgesic Product Table 855

33 Burn and Sunburn Products — 563
Robert H. Moore III
   Burn and Sunburn Product Table 859

34 Sunscreen and Suntan Products — 575
Edward M. DeSimone II
   Sunscreen and Suntan Product Table 862

35 Poison Ivy and Poison Oak Products — 589
Henry Wormser
   Poison Ivy and Poison Oak Product Table 867

36 Insect Sting and Bite Products — 597
Farid Sadik
   Insect Sting and Bite Product Table 873
   Pediculicide Product Table 875
   Insect Repellent Product Table 876

37 Foot Care Products — 609
Nicholas G. Popovich
   Callus, Corn, Wart Product Table 877
   Athlete's Foot Product Table 879

About the Product Tables — 637

Product Table Section — 635 - 880

Color Plates — Following page 452

Product Table Index — 881

General Index — 883 - 914

About APhA — 915

Advisory Panel, Authors & Reviewers

Advisory Panel

William L. Blockstein, Ph.D.
Professor Emeritus, School of Pharmacy, University of Wisconsin–Madison, Madison, Wisconsin

L. N. "Red" Camp, III, B.S. Pharmacy
Pharmacist, Camp Pharmacy, Titusville, Florida

Bernadette Eichelberger, Pharm.D.
Clinical Pharmacy Coordinator, Kaiser Permanente, Washington, DC

Janet P. Engle, Pharm.D.
Assistant Dean, College of Pharmacy, University of Illinois at Chicago, Chicago, Illinois

Edward G. Feldmann, Ph.D.
Pharmaceutical Consultant Services, Falls Church, Virginia

Benjamin J. Gruda, B.S. Pharmacy, R.Ph.
Pharmacist, Fays Drugs, Potsdam, New York

Kenneth W. Lem, Pharm.D.
Associate Dean for Educational Affairs, Lecturer in Clinical Pharmacy, School of Pharmacy, University of California, San Francisco, California

1 The Self-Care Movement

Authors

Gary A. Holt, R.Ph., M.Ed., Ph.D.
Assistant Professor of Pharmacy Practice, School of Pharmacy, Samford University, Birmingham, Alabama

Edwin L. Hall, Ph.D.
Professor of Pharmacy Administration, School of Pharmacy, Samford University, Birmingham, Alabama

Reviewers

Peter P. Lamy, Ph.D., Sc.D.
Director, The Center for the Study of Pharmacy and Therapeutics for the Elderly, School of Pharmacy, University of Maryland, Baltimore, Maryland

Richard P. Penna, Pharm.D.
Associate Executive Director, American Association of Colleges of Pharmacy, Alexandria, Virginia

Dorothy L. Smith, Pharm.D.
President, Consumer Health Information Corporation, McLean, Virginia

2 Patient Assessment and Consultation

Authors

Wendy Klein-Schwartz, Pharm.D.
Associate Professor of Pharmacy Practice, School of Pharmacy, University of Maryland, Baltimore, Maryland

J. Michael Hoopes, Pharm.D.
Vice President, Drug Counter Pharmacies, Gaithersburg, Maryland

Reviewers

Danial E. Baker, Pharm.D.
Director, Drug Information Center, College of Pharmacy, Washington State University at Spokane, Spokane, Washington

Virginia J. Galizia, Ph.D.
Associate Clinical Professor, College of Pharmacy and Allied Health Professions, St. John's University, Jamaica, New York

William C. Gong, Pharm.D.
Associate Professor of Clinical Pharmacy, School of Pharmacy, University of Southern California, Los Angeles, California

Daniel A. Hussar, Ph.D.
Remington Professor of Pharmacy, Philadelphia College of Pharmacy and Science, Philadelphia, Pennsylvania

Michael Montagne, Ph.D.
Director, Center for Drug Education, Associate Professor of Social Pharmacy, College of Pharmacy and Allied Health Professions, Northeastern University, Boston, Massachusetts

Gilbert N. Weise, B.S. Pharmacy, F.A.C.P.
Pharmacist, Weise Pharmacy, Jacksonville, Florida

3 FDA's Review of OTC Drugs

Author

William E. Gilbertson, Pharm.D.
Director, Division of OTC Drug Evaluation, Food and Drug Administration, Rockville, Maryland

Reviewers

David B. Brushwood, J.D.
Professor of Pharmacy Health Care Administration, College of Pharmacy, University of Florida, Gainesville, Florida

Joseph L. Fink III, B.S. Pharmacy, J.D.
Associate Vice Chancellor for Academic Affairs, University of Kentucky, Lexington, Kentucky

Jesse C. Vivian, J.D.
Associate Professor, College of Pharmacy and Allied Health Professions, Wayne State University, Detroit, Michigan

Gary L. Yingling, Esquire
Partner, McKenna & Cuneo, Washington, DC

4 In-Home Testing and Monitoring Products

Author

Susan M. Meyer, Ph.D.
Director of Academic Affairs, American Association of Colleges of Pharmacy, Alexandria, Virginia

Reviewers

Wesley G. Byerly, Pharm.D.
Director, Drug Information Service, North Carolina Baptist Hospital, Winston–Salem, North Carolina

Stephen M. Caiola, M.S.
Associate Professor of Pharmacy Practice, School of Pharmacy, University of North Carolina, Chapel Hill, North Carolina

Betsy A. Carlisle, Pharm.D.
Clinical Assistant Professor, University of Texas at Austin, Austin, Texas

Diane Nykamp, Pharm.D.
Associate Professor of Pharmacy Practice, Southern School of Pharmacy, Mercer University, Atlanta, Georgia

Captain Wynn W. Waite, Pharm.D.
Chief, Inpatient and Clinical Pharmacy Services, United States Air Force, Scott AFB, Illinois

5 Internal Analgesic Products

Author

W. Kent Van Tyle, Ph.D.
Professor of Pharmacology, College of Pharmacy, Butler University, Indianapolis, Indiana

Reviewers

Ann B. Amerson, Pharm.D.
Professor, College of Pharmacy, University of Kentucky, Lexington, Kentucky

Joseph Greensher, M.D., F.A.A.P.
Medical Director and Associate Chairman, Professor of Pediatrics, Department of Pediatrics, Winthrop–University Hospital, Mineola, New York

Peter J. S. Koo, Pharm.D.
Pharmacist Specialist, Pain Management, Associate Clinical Professor of Pharmacy, University of California, San Francisco, California

Arthur G. Lipman, Pharm.D.
Professor of Clinical Pharmacy, College of Pharmacy, University of Utah, Salt Lake City, Utah

James K. Marttila, Pharm.D., M.B.A.
Pharmacy Director, Mayo Pharmacy System, Mayo Foundation for Medical Education and Research, Rochester, Minnesota

6 Antipyretic Drug Products

Author

Thomas E. Lackner, Pharm.D., F.A.S.C.P
Vice President of Consulting—Midwest, Pharmacy Corporation of America, Minneapolis, Minnesota

Reviewers

Richard D. Leff, Pharm.D., F.C.C.P.
Associate Professor of Pediatrics and Pharmacy Director, Pediatric Pharmacology, University of Kansas Medical Center, Kansas City, Kansas

Larry M. Lopez, Pharm.D., F.C.C.P.
Associate Professor of Pharmacy, College of Pharmacy, University of Florida, Gainesville, Florida

Robert L. Snively, B.S. Pharmacy
Consultant Pharmacist, Edgehill Pharmacy, Georgetown, Delaware

W. Kent Van Tyle, Ph.D.
Professor of Pharmacology, College of Pharmacy, Butler University, Indianapolis, Indiana

Donald B. Wiest, Pharm.D.
Associate Professor of Pharmacy, College of Pharmacy, Medical University of South Carolina, Charleston, South Carolina

7 Menstrual Products

Author

Leslie A. Shimp, Pharm.D., M.S.
Associate Professor of Pharmacy, College of Pharmacy, The University of Michigan, Ann Arbor, Michigan

Reviewers

Charma A. Konnor, Pharm.D.
Director, Division of Drug Quality Evaluation, Food and Drug Administration, Rockville, Maryland

Connie Lee Barnes, Pharm.D.
Assistant Professor, School of Pharmacy, Campbell University, Buies Creek, North Carolina

Constance A. McKenzie, Pharm.D.
Director, Drug Information, School of Pharmacy, Campbell University, Buies Creek, North Carolina

Rosalie Sagraves, Pharm.D.
Associate Professor of Pharmacy Practice, Adjunct Associate Professor of Pediatrics, College of Pharmacy, University of Oklahoma Health Sciences Center, Oklahoma City, Oklahoma

Geralynn B. Smith, M.S.
Assistant Professor, College of Pharmacy and Allied Health Professions, Wayne State University, Detroit, Michigan

8 Cold, Cough, and Allergy Products

Authors

Bobby G. Bryant, Pharm.D.
Associate Professor, Albany College of Pharmacy, Union University, Albany, New York

Thomas P. Lombardi, Pharm.D.
Clinical Pharmacy Coordinator, Department of Pharmacy, St. Peter's Hospital, Albany, New York

Reviewers

Jeffrey C. Delafuente, M.S.
Associate Professor and Associate Chairman, College of Pharmacy, University of Florida, Gainesville, Florida

Alex Gringauz, R.Ph., Ph.D.
Professor of Medicinal Chemistry, Arnold & Marie Schwartz College of Pharmacy and Health Sciences, Long Island University, Brooklyn, New York

H. Won Jun, Ph.D.
Professor of Pharmaceutics, College of Pharmacy, The University of Georgia, Athens, Georgia

Raymond W. Roberts, Pharm.D.
Director, Home Infusion Services, FoxMeyer Corporation, Carrollton, Texas

Karen J. Tietze, Pharm.D.
Associate Professor of Clinical Pharmacy, Philadelphia College of Pharmacy and Science, Philadelphia, Pennsylvania

9 Asthma Products

Authors

H. William Kelly, Pharm.D.
Professor of Pharmacy, College of Pharmacy, University of New Mexico, Albuquerque, New Mexico

Mary Beth O'Connell, Pharm.D.
Associate Professor, College of Pharmacy, University of Minnesota, Minneapolis, Minnesota

Reviewers

Sandra M. Gawchik, D.O.
Co-Director, Division of Allergy & Immunology, Crozer Chester Medical Center, Chester, Pennsylvania

Pamela A. Simon, Pharm.D.
Clinical Assistant Professor, College of Pharmacy, University of Illinois at Chicago, Chicago, Illinois

Craig S. Stern, Pharm.D.
President, ProPharma Pharmaceutical Consultants, Northridge, California

Mark Stiling, R.Ph., Pharm.D.
Clinical Pharmacy Coordinator, Ireland Army Community Hospital, Fort Knox, Kentucky

10 Sleep Aid and Stimulant Products

Authors

M. Lynn Crismon, Pharm.D.
Professor and Head, Clinical Division at Austin, College of Pharmacy, University of Texas at Austin, Austin, Texas

Donna M. Jermain, Pharm.D.
Clinical Pharmacist, Assistant Professor, Scott and White Hospital, Texas A&M University, Temple, Texas

Reviewers

Kenneth Bachmann, Ph.D., F.C.P.
Professor of Pharmacology, College of Pharmacy, The University of Toledo, Toledo, Ohio

Patricia A. Camazzola, Pharm.D.
Director, Department of Pharmacy, Huron Valley Hospital, Milford, Michigan

Alice L. Paysinger, Pharm.D.
Assistant Professor of Clinical Pharmacy Practice, School of Pharmacy, The University of Mississippi, University, Mississippi

Barbara G. Wells, Pharm.D.
Associate Professor and Vice Chair, College of Pharmacy, University of Tennessee, Memphis, Tennessee

Michael Z. Wincor, Pharm.D.
Assistant Professor of Clinical Pharmacy, Psychiatry and the Behavioral Sciences, Schools of Pharmacy and Medicine, University of Southern California, Los Angeles, California

11 Antacid Products

Authors

Julianne B. Pinson, Pharm. D.
Assistant Professor of Pharmacy Practice, School of Pharmacy, Campbell University, Reynolds Health Center, Winston–Salem, North Carolina

C. Wayne Weart, Pharm.D.
Professor of Community Pharmacy Practice, Associate Professor of Family Medicine, Medical University of South Carolina, Charleston, South Carolina

Reviewers

Stephen M. Caiola, M.S.
Associate Professor of Pharmacy Practice, School of Pharmacy, University of North Carolina, Chapel Hill, North Carolina

Bruce C. Carlstedt, Ph.D.
Associate Professor of Clinical Pharmacy, School of Pharmacy and Pharmacal Sciences, Purdue University, West Lafayette, Indiana

Bruce D. Clayton, Pharm.D.
Associate Dean, Professor of Pharmacy Practice, College of Pharmacy, Butler University, Indianapolis, Indiana

Roy C. Parish, Pharm.D.
Assistant Professor, College of Pharmacy, The University of Georgia, Athens, Georgia

Pamela A. Simon, Pharm.D.
Clinical Assistant Professor, College of Pharmacy, University of Illinois at Chicago, Chicago, Illinois

12 Emetic and Antiemetic Products

Authors

Gary M. Oderda, Pharm.D., M.P.H.
Professor and Chairman, Department of Pharmacy Practice, College of Pharmacy, University of Utah, Salt Lake City, Utah

Jenifer C. Jennings, Pharm.D.
Assistant Professor of Clinical Pharmacy, Department of Pharmacy Practice, College of Pharmacy, University of Utah, Salt Lake City, Utah

Reviewers

Betsy A. Carlisle, Pharm.D.
Clinical Assistant Professor, University of Texas at Austin, Austin, Texas

William D. King, R.Ph., M.P.H., Dr.P.H.
Associate Professor of Pediatrics, School of Medicine, University of Alabama–Birmingham, Birmingham, Alabama

Alan H. Lau, Pharm.D.
Associate Professor and Research Coordinator, College of Pharmacy, University of Illinois at Chicago, Chicago, Illinois

Anthony J. Silvagni, D.O., Pharm.D.
Professor of General Practice and Clinical Pharmacology, College of Osteopathic Medicine, University of Health Science, Kansas City, Missouri

Anthony R. Temple, M.D.
Executive Director, Medical, McNeil Consumer Products Company, Fort Washington, Pennsylvania

13 Antidiarrheal Products

Author

R. Leon Longe, Pharm.D.
Professor, College of Pharmacy, The University of Georgia, Athens, Georgia

Reviewers

Mark L. Britton, Pharm.D.
Clinical Pharmacy Coordinator, Department of Veterans Affairs Medical Center, Oklahoma City, Oklahoma

Joseph T. DiPiro, Pharm.D.
Professor of Pharmacy, University of Georgia, Augusta, Georgia

Herbert L. DuPont, M.D.
Mary W. Kelsey Professor and Director, Center for Infectious Diseases, School of Public Health, The University of Texas Medical School, Houston, Texas

Wayne A. Kradjan, Pharm.D.
Associate Dean, School of Pharmacy, University of Washington, Seattle, Washington

John J. Piecoro, Jr., Pharm.D., M.S.
Professor, Division of Pharmacy Practice and Science, College of Pharmacy, University of Kentucky, Lexington, Kentucky

14 Anthelmintic Products

Author

Kathryn K. Bucci, Pharm.D.
Assistant Clinical Professor in Community and Family Medicine, Duke University, Durham, North Carolina

Reviewers

J. Fred Bennes, B.S. Pharmacy
Director of Pharmacy Services, The Health Care Plan, Inc., Buffalo, New York

Donald O. Fedder, B.S.P., M.P.H., Dr.P.H.
Professor and Director of Community Pharmacy Programs, School of Pharmacy, University of Maryland, Baltimore, Maryland

Robert A. Mangione, M.S.
Assistant Dean of Pharmacy Student Affairs, Clinical Professor of Pharmacy, College of Pharmacy and Allied Health Professions, St. John's University, Jamaica, New York

David E. Stewart, Pharm.D.
Vice President, Stewart's Pharmacy, Inc., McMinnville, Tennessee

15 Laxative Products

Authors

Clarence E. Curry, Jr., Pharm.D.
Associate Professor of Pharmacy Practice, College of Pharmacy and Pharmacal Sciences, Howard University, Washington, DC

Demetris Tatum-Butler, Pharm.D.
Clinical Pharmacy Coordinator, Greater Laurel–Beltsville Hospital, Laurel, Maryland

Reviewers

R. Randolph Beckner, Pharm.D., M.H.A.
Manager, Quality Assurance Department of Pharmacy, Barnes Hospital, St. Louis, Missouri

Eddie L. Boyd, Pharm.D., M.S.
Associate Dean, College of Pharmacy, Xavier University of Louisiana, New Orleans, Louisiana

Anthony T. Buatti, B.S. Pharmacy, M.B.A.
Assistant Professor of Health Care Administration, College of Pharmacy and Allied Health Professions, St. John's University, Jamaica, New York

Janice A. Gaska, Pharm.D.
Adjunct Associate Professor of Clinical Pharmacy, Philadelphia College of Pharmacy and Science, Philadelphia, Pennsylvania

Katheryn W. Russi, M.P.A.
Director, Division of Pharmacy Practice, College of Pharmacy, Drake University, Des Moines, Iowa

16 Diabetes Care Products and Monitoring Devices

Authors

John R. White, Jr., Pharm.D.
Assistant Professor of Pharmacy Practice, College of Pharmacy, Washington State University at Spokane, Spokane, Washington

R. Keith Campbell, M.B.A., C.D.E.
Associate Dean, Professor of Pharmacy Practice, College of Pharmacy, Washington State University, Pullman, Washington

Reviewers

Charles Y. McCall, Pharm.D.
Associate Professor, College of Pharmacy, The University of Georgia, Athens, Georgia

David A. Sclar, B.S. Pharmacy, Ph.D.
Assistant Professor of Health Care Administration, College of Pharmacy, Washington State University, Pullman, Washington

Kenneth A. Skau, Ph.D.
Associate Professor of Pharmacology, College of Pharmacy, University of Cincinnati—Medical Center, Cincinnati, Ohio

Condit F. Steil, Pharm.D., C.D.E.
Clinical and Consultant Pharmacist, Pharmacy Corner, Ashland, Kentucky

Michael S. Torre, B.S. Pharmacy, M.Sc.
Clinical Professor of Pharmacy and Chairman, Department of Clinical Pharmacy Practice, College of

Pharmacy and Allied Health Professions, St. John's University, Jamaica, New York

17 Nutritional Products

Author

Loyd V. Allen, Jr., Ph.D.
Professor & Head, Pharmaceutics, College of Pharmacy, University of Oklahoma, Oklahoma City, Oklahoma

Reviewers

Carl J. Malanga, Ph.D.
Associate Dean for Academic Affairs and Administration, School of Pharmacy, West Virginia University Health Sciences Center, Morgantown, West Virginia

Merlin V. Nelson, Pharm.D.
Department of Pharmacy Practice, College of Pharmacy and Allied Health Professions, Wayne State University, Detroit, Michigan

Gail H. Rosen, Pharm.D.
Director, Nutrition Support Services, Department of Pharmacy Services, University of Maryland Medical System, Baltimore, Maryland

J. Ken Walters, Jr., Pharm.D.
Director of Pharmacy, Sheppard Pratt Hospital, Baltimore, Maryland

18 Infant Formula Products

Authors

Rosalie Sagraves, Pharm.D.
Associate Professor of Pharmacy Practice, Adjunct Associate Professor of Pediatrics, College of Pharmacy, University of Oklahoma Health Sciences Center, Oklahoma City, Oklahoma

Claudia Kamper, Pharm.D.
Assistant Professor, College of Pharmacy, University of Oklahoma, Oklahoma City, Oklahoma

Judi Doerr, R.D., L.D.
Pediatric Clinical Dietitian, Children's Hospital of Oklahoma, Oklahoma City, Oklahoma

Reviewers

F. James Grogan, Pharm.D.
Clinical Pharmacist, IVT_x, St. Louis, Missouri

Cynthia S. Kirman, Pharm.D.
Drug Information Specialist, Clinical Pharmacy Services, Value R_x Pharmacy Program, Bloomfield Hills, Michigan

Donna F. Veal, Pharm.D.
Assistant Professor, School of Pharmacy, Samford University, Birmingham, Alabama

Paul C. Walker, Pharm.D.
Adjunct Assistant Professor, College of Pharmacy and Allied Health Professions, Wayne State University, Detroit, Michigan

19 Weight Control Products

Author

Glenn D. Appelt, Ph.D., R.Ph., F.A.C.A.
Pharmacology Consultant, Boulder Beach Consulting Group, Gulf Shores, Alabama

Reviewers

Robert L. Beamer, Ph.D.
Professor of Medicinal Chemistry and Biochemistry, College of Pharmacy, University of South Carolina, Columbia, South Carolina

Patricia A. Camazzola, Pharm.D.
Director, Department of Pharmacy, Huron Valley Hospital, Milford, Michigan

William S. Lackey, B.S. Pharmacy
Retired Pharmacist, Past President of A.C.A., Tucson, Arizona

Nancy A. Letassy, Pharm.D.
Assistant Professor of Pharmacy Practice, College of Pharmacy, University of Oklahoma, Oklahoma City, Oklahoma

Leon Shargel, Ph.D.
Director of Pharmacokinetics, Chelsea Laboratories, Inc., West Hempstead, New York

20 Ophthalmic Products

Authors

Jimmy D. Bartlett, O.D., D.O.S.
Associate Professor of Optometry, School of Optometry, University of Alabama at Birmingham, Birmingham, Alabama

Mark W. Swanson, O.D.
Assistant Professor, Department of Optometry, University of Alabama at Birmingham, Birmingham, Alabama

Reviewers

Chris Bapatla, Ph.D.
Assistant Director, Pharmacy Sciences, Alcon Laboratories, Inc., Fort Worth, Texas

Alexander F. Demetro, Pharm.D.
Pharmacist, Westwood Prescriptionists, San Jose, California
Richard G. Fiscella, R.Ph., M.P.H.
Assistant Professor of Pharmacy Practice, College of Pharmacy, University of Illinois at Chicago, Chicago, Illinois
Ralph W. Trottier, Ph.D., J.D.
Professor and Attorney at Law, Morehouse School of Medicine, Atlanta, Georgia
John R. Yuen, Pharm.D.
Nuclear Pharmacist, Syncor International Corporation, Los Angeles, California

21 Contact Lens Products

Author

Janet P. Engle, Pharm.D.
Assistant Dean and Clinical Associate Professor of Pharmacy Practice, College of Pharmacy, University of Illinois at Chicago, Chicago, Illinois

Reviewers

William J. Benjamin, O.D., Ph.D.
Associate Professor, School of Optometry, University of Alabama at Birmingham, Birmingham, Alabama
Timothy Lesar, Pharm.D.
Assistant Director of Pharmacy, Albany Medical Center, Albany, New York
Thomas F. Patton, Ph.D.
Director, Pharmaceutical R&D, Merck & Co., Inc., Rahway, New Jersey
Captain Wynn W. Waite, Pharm.D.
Chief, Inpatient and Clinical Pharmacy Services, United States Air Force, Scott AFB, Illinois
John R. Yuen, Pharm.D.
Nuclear Pharmacist, Syncor International Corporation, Los Angeles, California

22 Otic Products

Author

Keith O. Miller, Pharm.D.
Pharmacy Department, Wadley Regional Medical Center, Texarcana, Texas

Reviewers

Carl F. Emswiller, Jr., B.S. Pharmacy
Pharmacist, Emswiller Pharmacy, Leesburg, Virginia
E. Paul Larrat, Ph.D.
Assistant Professor of Epidemiology, College of Pharmacy, University of Rhode Island, Kingston, Rhode Island
Michael S. Maddux, Pharm.D.
Assistant Dean for Clinical Development, St. Louis College of Pharmacy, St. Louis, Missouri
Dennis Richmond, M.D.
Lafayette Family Physicians, Lafayette, Indiana
Ralph W. Trottier, Ph.D., J.D.
Professor and Attorney at Law, Morehouse School of Medicine, Atlanta, Georgia

23 Oral Health Products

Author

Arlene A. Flynn, B.S. Pharmacy, B.S. Biology, M.Ed.
Assistant to the Dean, College of Pharmacy, University of Illinois at Chicago, Chicago, Illinois

Reviewers

Paul L. Doering, M.S.
Professor of Pharmacy Practice, College of Pharmacy, University of Florida, Gainesville, Florida
Lowell S. Lakritz, D.D.S.
Private Practitioner, General Dentistry, Madison, Wisconsin
Roger H. Scholle, D.D.S.
Editor, Illinois State Dental Society, Springfield, Illinois
Carl Stone, D.D.S., M.A.
Associate Professor, School of Dentistry, University of Detroit Mercy, Detroit, Michigan
Kenneth W. Witte, Pharm.D.
Clinical Assistant Professor, Department of Pharmacy Practice, College of Pharmacy, University of Illinois at Chicago, Chicago, Illinois

24 Ostomy and Wound Care Products

Authors

Michael L. Kleinberg, M.S., F.A.S.H.P.
Director of Professional Services, Immunex Corporation, Seattle, Washington

Moya J. Vazquez, R.N., M.B.A
Product Manager, Immunex Corporation, Seattle, Washington

Reviewers

George B. Browning, B.S. Pharmacy
President, Medical Arts Pharmacy, Inc., Melbourne, Florida

Mary M. Losey, M.S.
Director, Office of Student Services, School of Pharmacy and Pharmacal Sciences, Purdue University, West Lafayette, Indiana

Gary Schmidt, B.S. Pharmacy
Clinical Instructor, University of Wisconsin–Madison, Madison, Wisconsin

Joan Lerner Selekof, R.N., B.S.N., C.E.T.N.
Enterostomal Therapy Nurse, University of Maryland Medical System, Baltimore, Maryland

25 Contraceptive Methods and Products

Authors

Louise Parent-Stevens, Pharm.D.
Clinical Assistant Professor, College of Pharmacy, University of Illinois at Chicago, Chicago, Illinois

Roberta S. Carrier, Pharm.D.
Assistant Professor, School of Pharmacy, University of Wisconsin–Madison, Madison, Wisconsin

Reviewers

Sandra H. Hak, Pharm.D.
President, ProPharma, Ltd., Germantown, Tennessee

David L. Lourwood, Pharm.D.
Clinical Assistant Professor of Pharmacy Practice, College of Pharmacy, University of Illinois at Chicago, Chicago, Illinois

Daniel R. Mishell, Jr., M.D.
Lyle G. McNeile Professor and Chairman, Department of Obstetrics and Gynecology, School of Medicine, University of Southern California, Los Angeles, California

Timothy D. Moore, M.S., R.Ph.
Senior Director and Clinical Professor, Department of Pharmacy, The Ohio State University Hospitals, Columbus, Ohio

Ronald J. Ruggiero, Pharm.D.
Associate Clinical Professor, School of Pharmacy, University of California, San Francisco, California

26 Hemorrhoidal Products

Author

Benjamin Hodes, Ph.D.
Professor of Pharmaceutics and University Director, Division of Continuing Education, Duquesne University, Pittsburgh, Pennsylvania

Reviewers

Thomas D. DeCillis, B.S. Pharmacy
Pharmacist Director (Retired), U.S. Public Health Service, North Port, Florida

Ross L. Egger, M.D.
Medical Director, St. John's Health Care Corporation, St. Johns Hospital, Anderson, Indiana

Anthony Palmieri III, Ph.D.
Director, Intellectual Property, The Upjohn Company, Kalamazoo, Michigan

Quentin M. Srnka, Pharm.D., M.B.A.
Director, Center for Pharmacy Management and Research, College of Pharmacy, University of Tennessee, Memphis, Tennessee

Larry N. Swanson, Pharm.D.
Professor and Chairman, Department of Pharmacy Practice, School of Pharmacy, Campbell University, Buies Creek, North Carolina

27 Personal Care Products

Authors

Donald R. Miller, Pharm.D.
Associate Professor of Pharmacy Practice, College of Pharmacy, North Dakota State University, Fargo, North Dakota

Mary Kuzel, Pharm.D.
Assistant Clinical Professor of Pharmacy Practice, North Dakota State University, Fargo, North Dakota

Reviewers

Linda C. Hogan, M.S.
Director of Licensing, Marion Merrell Dow Inc., Kansas City, Missouri

Alan W. Hopefl, Pharm.D.
Associate Professor of Pharmacy Practice, St. Louis College of Pharmacy, St. Louis, Missouri

Lawrence A. Lemchen, R.Ph.
Clinical Consultant Pharmacist, Pharmacy Corporation of America, Seattle, Washington

Geralynn B. Smith, M.S.
Assistant Professor, College of Pharmacy and Allied Health Professions, Wayne State University, Detroit, Michigan

Linda Gore Sutherland, M.B.A., R.Ph.
Coordinator, Drug Information, School of Pharmacy, University of Wyoming, Laramie, Wyoming

28 Topical Anti-Infective Products

Authors

Dennis P. West, Ph.D., F.C.C.P.
Vice-President, Scientific Affairs, GenDerm Corporation, Lincolnshire, Illinois

Susan V. Maddux, Pharm.D.
Clinical Pharmacy Coordinator, Group Health Plan, St. Louis, Missouri

Reviewers

Miriam P. Calhoun, B.S.
Consultant, Pharmaceutical Regulatory Affairs, Food and Drug Administration (Retired), Potomac, Maryland

Robert J. Cluxton, Pharm.D.
Associate Professor, College of Pharmacy, University of Cincinnati—Medical Center, Cincinnati, Ohio

Howard Maibach, M.D.
Professor of Dermatology, Dermatology Department, University of California Hospital, San Francisco, California

Karen I. Plaisance, Pharm.D.
Associate Professor, School of Pharmacy, University of Maryland, Baltimore, Maryland

Marilyn K. Speedie, Ph.D.
Professor, School of Pharmacy, University of Maryland, Baltimore, Maryland

29 Acne Products

Author

Joye Ann Billow, Ph.D.
Professor of Pharmaceutical Sciences, College of Pharmacy, South Dakota State University, Brookings, South Dakota

Reviewers

Darrell F. Bennett, B.S. Pharmacy, R.Ph.
Pharmacist, California Poly Health Center, California Polytechnic State University, San Luis Obispo, California

Mary E. Gross, Pharm.D.
Associate Professor of Clinical Pharmacy–Geriatric Pharmacy, College of Pharmacy and Health Science, Drake University, Des Moines, Iowa

Henry A. Palmer, Ph.D.
Clinical Professor, School of Pharmacy, The University of Connecticut, Storrs, Connecticut

Charles D. Ponte, R.Ph., Pharm.D., C.D.E.
Professor of Clinical Pharmacy and Family Medicine, School of Pharmacy, West Virginia University Health Sciences Center, Morgantown, West Virginia

J. Richard Wuest, Pharm.D., R.Ph.
Professor of Clinical Pharmacy, University of Cincinnati—Medical Center, Cincinnati, Ohio

30 Dermatologic Products

Author

Joye Ann Billow, Ph.D.
Professor of Pharmaceutical Sciences, College of Pharmacy, South Dakota State University, Brookings, South Dakota

Reviewers

J. Fred Bennes, B.S. Pharmacy
Director of Pharmacy Services, The Health Care Plan, Inc., Buffalo, New York

Emery W. Brunett, Ph.D.
School of Pharmacy, University of Wyoming, Laramie, Wyoming

George E. Francisco, Pharm.D.
Associate Professor and Associate Dean, College of Pharmacy, The University of Georgia, Athens, Georgia

Anthony J. Lamonica, B.S. Pharmacy
President, Prescription Shoppe, Inc.-ACA, Everett, Massachusetts

31 Diaper Rash and Prickly Heat Products

Author

Gary H. Smith, Pharm.D.
Professor of Pharmacy Practice, College of Pharmacy, The University of Arizona, Tucson, Arizona

Reviewers

Timothy J. Boehmer, B.S. Pharmacy
Staff Pharmacist, Providence Hospital, Anchorage, Alaska

John A. Bosso, Pharm.D., F.C.C.P.
Professor and Vice Chair for Research, Hospital Pharmacy Practice and Administration, Medical University of South Carolina, Charleston, South Carolina

Miriam P. Calhoun, B.S.
Consultant, Pharmaceutical Regulatory Affairs, Food and Drug Administration (Retired), Potomac, Maryland

Debra Ricciatti-Sibbald, M.S.
President, Debary Dermatologicals, Mississaugua, Ontario

Paul C. Walker, Pharm.D.
Adjunct Assistant Professor, College of Pharmacy and Allied Health Professions, Wayne State University, Detroit, Michigan

32 External Analgesic Products

Author

Arthur I. Jacknowitz, Pharm.D.
Professor and Chairman, Department of Clinical Pharmacy, School of Pharmacy, West Virginia University Health Sciences Center, Morgantown, West Virginia

Reviewers

Martin D. Higbee, Pharm.D.
Associate Professor, College of Pharmacy, The University of Arizona, Tucson, Arizona

Phillip R. Oppenheimer, Pharm.D.
Associate Dean, School of Pharmacy, University of Southern California, Los Angeles, California

W. Steven Pray, Ph.D.
Professor of Pharmaceutics, School of Pharmacy, Southwestern Oklahoma State University, Weatherford, Oklahoma

Martha M. Rumore, Pharm.D., J.D.
Associate Professor, Pharmacy Administration, Arnold & Marie Schwartz College of Pharmacy and Health Sciences, Long Island University, Brooklyn, New York

Craig S. Stern, Pharm.D.
President, ProPharma Pharmaceutical Consultants, Northridge, California

33 Burn and Sunburn Products

Author

Robert H. Moore III, Ph.D.
Professor of Pharmacology, School of Pharmacy, Samford University, Birmingham, Alabama

Reviewers

Robert W. Bennett, M.S.
Associate Professor of Clinical Pharmacy, Department of Pharmacy Practice, School of Pharmacy and Pharmacal Sciences, Purdue University, West Lafayette, Indiana

Julie Rivkin Berman, Pharm.D.
Clinical Specialist—Burn Unit, Detroit Receiving Hospital and University Health Center, Detroit, Michigan

Miriam P. Calhoun, B.S.
Consultant, Pharmaceutical Regulatory Affairs, Food and Drug Administration (Retired), Potomac, Maryland

Walter T. Gloor, Ph.D.
Adjunct Professor, School of Pharmacy and Allied Health Professions, Creighton University, Omaha, Nebraska

Katheryn W. Russi, M.P.A.
Director, Division of Pharmacy Practice, College of Pharmacy, Drake University, Des Moines, Iowa

34 Sunscreen and Suntan Products

Author

Edward M. DeSimone II, Ph.D.
Associate Professor of Administration and Social Sciences, Assistant Dean for Academic Affairs, School of Pharmacy and Allied Health Professions, Creighton University, Omaha, Nebraska

Reviewers

Julie Rivkin Berman, Pharm.D.
Clinical Specialist—Burn Unit, Detroit Receiving Hospital and University Health Center, Detroit, Michigan

Martin J. Jinks, Pharm.D.
Professor and Chair, Pharmacy Practice Department, College of Pharmacy, Washington State University, Pullman, Washington

Linda K. McCoy, Pharm.D.
Manager of Clinical Pharmacy Services, Good Samaritan Regional Medical Center, Phoenix, Arizona
Katheryn W. Russi, M.P.A.
Director, Division of Pharmacy Practice, College of Pharmacy, Drake University, Des Moines, Iowa
Stewart B. Siskin, Pharm.D.
Associate Director, Clinical Research, Bristol–Myers Squibb Company Pharmaceutical Research Institute, Buffalo, New York

35 Poison Ivy and Poison Oak Products

Author

Henry Wormser, Ph.D.
Professor of Pharmaceutical Chemistry, College of Pharmacy and Allied Health Professions, Wayne State University, Detroit, Michigan

Reviewers

David C. Beck, M.D.
Clinical Assistant Professor of Dermatology, School of Medicine, Indiana University, West Lafayette, Indiana
Jerry D. Karbeling, B.S. Pharmacy
Community Pharmacist, Big Creek Pharmacy, Polk City, Iowa
Kenneth R. Keefner. Ph.D., R.Ph.
Associate Professor, School of Pharmacy and Allied Health Professions, Creighton University, Omaha, Nebraska
Robert B. Sause, Ph.D.
Associate Professor, College of Pharmacy and Allied Health Professions, St. John's University, Jamaica, New York
Joel L. Zatz, Ph.D.
Professor of Pharmaceutics, College of Pharmacy, Rutgers University, The State University of New Jersey, Piscataway, New Jersey

36 Insect Sting and Bite Products

Author

Farid Sadik, Ph.D.
Professor and Associate Dean, College of Pharmacy, University of South Carolina, Columbia, South Carolina

Reviewers

Virginia J. Galizia, Ph.D.
Associate Clinical Professor, College of Pharmacy and Allied Health Professions, St. John's University, Jamaica, New York
Howard Maibach, M.D.
Professor of Dermatology, Dermatology Department, University of California Hospital, San Francisco, California
James R. Morse, M.S.
Assistant Professor, College of Pharmacy, The University of Arizona, Tucson, Arizona
Victor A. Padron, R.Ph., Ph.D.
Associate Professor of Pharmacy Practice, School of Pharmacy and Allied Health Professions, Creighton University, Omaha, Nebraska
Robert B. Sause, Ph.D.
Associate Professor, College of Pharmacy and Allied Health Professions, St. John's University, Jamaica, New York

37 Foot Care Products

Author

Nicholas G. Popovich, Ph.D.
Professor and Head, Department of Pharmacy Practice, School of Pharmacy and Pharmacal Sciences, Purdue University, West Lafayette, Indiana

Reviewers

Donald O. Fedder, B.S.P., M.P.H., Dr.P.H.
Professor and Director of Community Pharmacy Programs, School of Pharmacy, University of Maryland, Baltimore, Maryland
Thomas J. Holmes, Jr., Ph.D.
Associate Professor, School of Pharmacy, Campbell University, Buies Creek, North Carolina
Edward R. Hommel, D.P.M.
Clinical Assistant Professor, Department of Family Medicine, School of Medicine, University of Wisconsin–Madison, Madison, Wisconsin
Damien Howell, M.S., P.T.
Damien Howell Physical Therapy, Richmond, Virginia

Preface

The goals of the American Pharmaceutical Association include advancing standards of pharmacy practice; fostering safe, effective, appropriate, and economical nonprescription drug use; and expanding professional practice prerogatives of pharmacists. These goals are assisted substantially by publication of the *Handbook of Nonprescription Drugs*. The 10th Edition of the *Handbook* has refined and updated the world's most comprehensive drug information database dealing exclusively with nonprescription drugs. Conscientious use of the *Handbook* by pharmacists and pharmacy students will foster optimal pharmacotherapy, advance the evolution of pharmaceutical care, and serve the public health.

In an era of health care reform and cost containment, numerous issues concerning quality and cost of health care present opportunities to pharmacists. One of these areas is management of self-limiting conditions with nonprescription drugs. Consumers want and need more information on the appropriate use of these agents. New strategies and initiatives are needed to optimize self-care with nonprescription pharmaceuticals. The pharmacist is the most qualified and appropriate *learned intermediary* to help the patient with optimal use of nonprescription drugs.

Pharmacists are strategically positioned in health care to assess patient needs, recognize conditions that are self-treatable with nonprescription drugs, and advise and counsel patients. If self-care with a nonprescription drug is appropriate, the pharmacist is generally available and well qualified to:

- Help in product selection;
- Assess patient risk factors;
- Counsel patients regarding proper use;
- Monitor for drug allergies or hypersensitivities, adverse drug reactions, and drug–drug interactions;
- Monitor response to therapy;
- Assess clinical outcomes;
- Discourage use of fraudulent or quack remedies;
- Assess the ability of a nonprescription drug to mask symptoms of a serious medical condition;
- Prevent delays in seeking medical attention by referring the patient to a physician.

Nonprescription drug sales at the wholesale level were approximately $12 billion in 1991 and $13.2 billion in 1992. Sales are projected to increase 8–10% per year and, by 1996, could increase by $4–5 billion. Factors fostering such sales growth are the projected reclassification of numerous prescription drugs to nonprescription status, the availability and positive public perception of the pharmacist, the emerging growth of the self-care movement, and the ever increasing safety and efficacy of the nation's supply of nonprescription drugs due in large part to the FDA-coordinated OTC Drug Review.

The pharmacist's clinical competency relative to the provision of cognitive informational services to patients on safe, appropriate, effective, and economical nonprescription drug use is vital. The 10th Edition of the *Handbook of Nonprescription Drugs* is the greatest single tool available to enhance professional competence and expand patient services in the domain of nonprescription pharmacotherapy. The American Pharmaceutical Association is pleased to offer this valued resource and pledges an ongoing commitment to further expansion and refinement of this publication.

John A. Gans, Pharm.D.
Executive Vice-President
American Pharmaceutical Association

Introduction

By today's standards the first edition of the *Handbook of Nonprescription Drugs* was modest indeed. Early editions did, however, reflect the vision of the leadership of the American Pharmaceutical Association regarding the potential of the profession to serve the consumer in this increasingly important sector of health care.

No publication enjoys the privilege of multiple editions unless it provides value, currency, comprehensiveness, and utility. The *Handbook* has evolved as a flagship publication of APhA and is one of the great books in American pharmacy. This definitive work is recognized worldwide as the authority in nonprescription pharmacotherapy. Accordingly, the *Handbook* is a valuable resource for pharmacists who face the challenges of advising their patients on self-care every day.

The Self-Care Movement

Many Americans are strongly committed to a higher degree of ownership of decisions about their personal health. An informed partnership between patients and providers of health care is appropriate. More than 400 relatively minor, self-limited conditions can be treated with nonprescription drugs. Additional groups of nonprescription agents are available for contact lens care, conception control, dental health, and feminine hygiene. Also, home diagnostics and monitoring products are emerging as useful adjuncts to health maintenance.

Approximately 70% of consumers self-medicate regularly, and an estimated 40% of the U.S. population use at least one nonprescription drug within any given 48-hour period. Approximately 30% of all drug expenditures are for nonprescription drugs. Further, an estimated 60% of all purchased medication units are nonprescription drugs.

Sales of nonprescription pharmaceuticals are increasing 8–10% a year. These purchases, which amounted to more than $13 billion in 1992, may reach $18 billion by 1995 or 1996 and could exceed $34 billion a year by the year 2000. Nevertheless, nonprescription drug expenditures account for less than 2% of the total annual U.S. health care expenditure.

Drug Reclassification: Rx to OTC

The "Rx-to-OTC switch" process has been in place since the 1951 Durham-Humphrey Amendments to the Federal Food, Drug and Cosmetic Act. In 1992 the FDA appointed the Over-the-Counter Drugs Advisory Committee to provide focus, expertise, and direction on Rx-to-OTC switch issues. Since 1976 more than 50 prescription drugs have been granted nonprescription status by the FDA. More than 50 additional prescription drugs, representing 10 pharmacologic classes, have been identified by the Nonprescription Drug Manufacturers Association (NDMA) as prospective Rx-to-OTC switch candidates.

Nationwide savings due to nonprescription drug availability are estimated to be more than $20 billion a year, and these savings are rising. The NDMA estimates that nonprescription 1% hydrocortisone saved patients $144 million during its first year of availability. The savings resulted from reduced physician visits, fewer sick days, and a decreased need for more costly prescription alternatives. The availability of certain nonprescription cough and cold medications that were formerly prescription-only is estimated to save consumers approximately $1 billion a year.

Both self-care and Rx-to-OTC switching are gaining momentum. Some factors fueling this momentum include:

- The safety and efficacy of nonprescription drugs;
- Patients' desire for a higher degree of ownership in their health care;
- The aging of America;
- Rapidly escalating health care costs;
- A commitment to health care reform that encourages cost containment without compromising quality;
- No significant third-party fiscal constraints on the use of nonprescription drugs;
- Escalating research and development costs to bring new prescription drugs to market;
- Increasing generic competition with legend prescription drugs;
- Potential savings associated with the prudent use of nonprescription drugs.

The Pharmacist as a Learned Intermediary

Self-care that includes the use of nonprescription drugs should not be a random process in which the patient acts alone or in an information vacuum. Effective self-care requires highly informative, readable, and understandable package labeling and patient education materials that foster safe, appropriate, and effective nonprescription drug use. Equally necessary is public access to a qualified, learned intermediary to assist in nonprescription drug selection, use, and monitoring.

The public health can be greatly served by the pharmacist as that intermediary in nonprescription drug selection and use. The pharmacist is the only health professional who receives formal, university-level education and training in nonprescription drug pharmacotherapy. This training is supported by in-depth instruction in pathophysiology, pharmaceutics, medicinal chemistry, and pharmacology. The pharmacist's knowledge is enhanced by drug information databases. Further, the pharmacist has a strategic position in the community as a drug-information expert who is readily available to the public and as a provider of nonprescription drugs. This tremendous health resource should not be undervalued or overlooked.

The pharmacist is uniquely qualified to help patients use nonprescription drugs safely, appropriately, effectively, and economically. The 10th Edition of the *Handbook* is designed to help pharmacists:

- Conduct a patient assessment;
- Recognize problems that are self-treatable with nonprescription drugs;
- Differentiate self-treatable conditions from those requiring medical intervention;
- Advise and counsel patients on the proper course of action (no treatment, self-treatment, or referral to a physician or other caregiver).

If self-care with a nonprescription drug is appropriate, the pharmacist is strategically positioned to:

- Assist in product selection;
- Assess patient risk factors;
- Counsel patients regarding proper use;
- Maintain a patient drug profile that includes nonprescription drugs;
- Monitor for drug allergies or hypersensitivities;
- Monitor for adverse drug reactions;
- Monitor for drug–drug interactions;
- Monitor for response to therapy;
- Monitor for symptoms of drug overuse and dependency;
- Discourage use of fraudulent and "quack" remedies;
- Assess the potential of nonprescription drugs to mask symptoms of a more serious condition;
- Prevent delays in seeking appropriate medical attention.

Consumers want and need more information on nonprescription drug therapy. However, the public's ability to comprehend and apply manufacturer-supplied product information is highly stratified. Further, package labeling has limitations because of the uniqueness of many clinical situations. New strategies and initiatives in optimizing self-treatment with nonprescription drugs need to include the pharmacist.

About the 10th Edition

The 10th Edition of the *Handbook of Nonprescription Drugs* builds on the success of prior editions and the high-quality work of numerous editors, authors, and reviewers. This edition has retained the most valued and acclaimed features of past editions while sharpening the applied, clinical focus of the book. The primary goal of this edition is to present information in a manner that enhances the delivery of pharmaceutical care.

There has been an explosion of information covering nonprescription drugs. The *Handbook* is designed to serve as the *best single* compendium to promote rational drug therapy and optimize therapeutic outcomes in the use of nonprescription drugs, while minimizing therapeutic misadventures. Authors, reviewers, and editors have worked diligently to provide information that encourages analysis and evaluation by health practitioners and that fosters the best clinical judgment possible.

With this edition, the *Handbook* has entered a third generation of sophistication in content, utility, and value. Major improvements in the 10th Edition include:

- Eighteen new authors, selected for their expertise in the chapter subject matter;
- Chapter text that has been significantly updated to reflect contemporary thought and recent FDA actions, including Rx-to-OTC switches;
- Inclusion in each chapter of information on special populations, such as pediatric, geriatric, and pregnant patients;
- Greater standardization of the format of all chapters;
- In response to reader input, a book that is about 20% shorter, achieved primarily through tight design, an increase in cross-referencing among chapters, and the most rigorous copy editing in several editions;
- Also in response to reader feedback, a book that is considerably lighter but no less sturdy, achieved through use of a high-quality paperback binding;
- The most current product tables ever published in the *Handbook*, produced for the first time from an electronic database;
- A new index to product table names, added to make product tables more accessible;
- Product tables gathered in the second half of the book for easier access by readers to both tables and text;
- Product table updates that will be issued periodically;
- Product tables that have been thoroughly reviewed, with headings and information significantly revised to reflect changing FDA rulings and new formulations;
- In the product tables, the addition of "flags," such as "sugar-free," and "gluten-free," to help pharmacists locate products that meet special needs;
- Development of a separate *Case Studies Workbook* as a companion to the *Handbook*: each of the seven sections in the *Workbook* contains three case studies and 30 continuing education (CE) questions, offering a total of 21 case studies for use in pharmacy schools and 21 hours of CE credit for pharmacists.

In our effort to standardize chapter content, authors focused on the following types of information:

- Assessment criteria;
- Pharmacoepidemiology of the condition;
- Etiology of the condition;
- Anatomy and physiology of the affected area;
- Pathophysiology of the affected system;
- Signs and symptoms of the condition;
- Drugs indicated to treat the condition;
- Contraindications to drug use;
- Warnings and precautions relative to drug use;
- Adverse effect profile of drugs;
- Drug–drug interactions and potential clinical consequences;
- Special considerations regarding use of a particular drug in a pediatric or geriatric patient;
- Product selection guidelines;
- Administration and dosage guidelines;
- Guidelines for patient education and counseling.

We are pleased with the progress made regarding consistency of chapter content. Our commitment is to continue to enhance the quality and value of the *Handbook* as an applied clinical tool that can be used to enhance rational pharmacotherapy with nonprescription drugs.

To say that chapter content in this edition is peer-reviewed is an understatement. The practitioner and academic communities of pharmacy, medicine, dentistry, optometry, nursing, and other professional groups represented the primary quality assurance input for each chapter. No fewer than five external reviewers per chapter ensure the quality, validity, currency, and comprehensiveness for which the *Handbook* is known.

Acknowledgments

An editorial project of the magnitude of developing a new *Handbook* edition involves and, in fact, requires the active participation, commitment, and loyalty of scores of individuals. To extend group acknowledgments to authors, coauthors, reviewers, editorial staff, production staff, graphic artists, and consultants seems too impersonal, yet to mention all individually is beyond our space limitations.

Nonetheless, special recognition is due the 52 authors and coauthors. These individuals are the true content experts. Their professional competence, intellect, loyalty, and commitment to this project deserve our highest professional gratitude. The authors and coauthors manifested a passion to advance the standards of pharmacy practice, serve health practitioners, and contribute to the public health. Our debt of gratitude to them is great; our thanks is deep and profound. Their gift to the profession and the public has meaning and value beyond words.

To our 156 reviewers, we also express sincere gratitude. In an era of emphasis upon quality, the reviewers served as the primary quality assurance group for the 10th Edition. The reviewers suggested highly significant refinements to *Handbook* chapters.

The seven-member advisory panel, which set the course for the 10th Edition, also deserves heartfelt thanks. These individuals launched the project of editing and producing this edition. The panel epitomized the values of group thinking, professional maturity, experience, and variety of creative thought. When the splinters and fragments of deliberations were collected, the 10th Edition had a clear direction and focus.

The leadership and support of John A. Gans and James P. Caro for the 10th Edition are gratefully acknowledged. The assistance of Edward G. Feldmann, Ph.D., as consultant and information resource on this project is recognized and greatly appreciated, as is his leadership on the 9th and prior editions. A very profound thanks also to William L. Blockstein, Ph.D., pharmaceutical editor for the 9th Edition, who set an extraordinary standard for excellence.

Deep appreciation goes to pharmaceutical manufacturers and distributors of nonprescription drugs who validated product information and provided additional data on new and reformulated products. Many manufacturers, especially those of large product lines, invested literally weeks of work in updating the table information. They, and the book's readers, are rewarded with the most current product tables ever produced. The manufacturers' patience and responsiveness helped immeasurably in developing our computerized database. With the database, the process of updating is now ongoing rather than episodic, and we look forward to continuing and expanding our working relationship with industry.

A cadre of three very special staff members of APhA have earned particular recognition. Their professional competency, commitment, and work ethic are reflected in the 10th Edition.

Susan C. Kendall, Editorial Coordinator, coordinated the flow of editorial material among authors, reviewers, and editors. With tact, consideration, and persuasion, she shepherded the text through its initial phases. In addition, Ms. Kendall accomplished the task of updating the product tables: a Herculean effort requiring mastery of an entirely new computer database and establishing and maintaining contact with over 400 pharmaceutical manufacturers regarding more than 4,400 individual product entries.

Linda L. Young, Assistant Managing Editor, assisted with literally every stage of this project. Her experience in preparing the 9th Edition and her editorial expertise increased the quality of every aspect of the book. In addition, Ms. Young single-handedly managed the preparation of chapter text, front matter, and back matter for publication. She set the schedule and selected and managed the work of word processors, copy editors, proofreaders, and indexers. She was the final quality check and authority on all editing. She worked closely with authors regarding copy editing and reconciled the often conflicting demands of space, time, and budget. Throughout, she helped to maintain the accuracy and quality that are crucial to the book.

Laura C. Lawson, Managing Editor, deserves our highest expression of thanks. Ms. Lawson was truly the cement that held this editorial project together through her tremendous energy, work ethic, organizational skills, editorial ability, computer literacy, human resource management skills, competency, and professionalism. I am pleased to have had the opportunity to work closely with such an individual in the development of a product in which we all can take a measure of satisfaction.

To serve as the pharmaceutical editor of one of the premier publications in American pharmacy has been an honor and a privilege. To all my professional colleagues in this enterprise, I offer my thanks for your cooperation and contribution. To the American Pharmaceutical Association and its membership, you presented me an opportunity and challenge; I have done my best to fulfill your faith and trust in me. To my wife, Betsy, and our two daughters, Courtney and Abby, thank you for your patience and sacrifice when I have been distracted or unavailable at times due to this project.

The 10th Edition of the *Handbook* is complete. Although I am very pleased with the end-product, I remain committed to the idea that we can always improve the book. To that end, work on the 11th Edition has already begun: the paradigm shift toward self-care with nonprescription drugs requires no less in our efforts to serve the profession and the public.

Timothy R. Covington, Pharm.D.
Pharmaceutical Editor

CHAPTER 1

The Self-Care Movement

Gary A. Holt and Edwin L. Hall

A Cultural Perspective

Americans are increasingly interested in self-care, as evidenced by research that suggests that self-treatment and self-care practices are widespread. Health care professionals have a corresponding interest in understanding this important trend, which must be viewed within the context of American culture.

Sick-Role Options

Once people decide that something is wrong (e.g., pain, discomfort, or other symptoms have developed), they usually adopt a sick role for which certain options are available. One might postulate an illness experience model that considers these options (Table 1). Prospective patients can tolerate the problem or turn to one of the domains of health care in our society: popular, folk, or professional. Each domain has its own system, social roles, interaction settings, and institutions. The popular domain (i.e., self-care) is the most common option involved in initial responses to illness episodes. Even when a decision is eventually made to enter the folk or professional domains, decisions still occur in the popular domain, usually within the context of the family.

Sick-role options often result in negotiations and transactions between the patient and health care providers. These transactions generally involve the participants' beliefs, attitudes, values, expectations, and goals. When practitioners and patients disagree, clinical management and patient counseling can become more difficult. For example, parents may ask the pharmacist to recommend cold products that are inappropriate for infants or small children. Even when the pharmacist makes a physician referral, the parents may insist on using the inappropriate products instead.

Various social and cultural factors also influence the options selected. For example, people who have grown up in rural cultures where medical care is inaccessible may have a much greater tolerance for pain, discomfort, and illness in general. In recent times, the practitioner–patient interaction has changed. In the traditional active–passive model, the patient was not an active participant in care[1] but was instead expected to follow the practitioner's advice without question. However, increasing numbers of contemporary patients are demanding equal power and mutually satisfying relationships with practitioners. As patients become more involved in their own health care, they may seek out practitioners who are willing to accommodate their increased participation in the process.

Self-Care

Self-care has been defined as a process in which individuals function in their own behalf regarding health promotion; health decision making; and the prevention, detection, and treatment of diseases or other health problems. This definition emphasizes that the individual is an active participant in the decision-making process and is the subject rather than the object of health care decisions.[2]

Self-care practices include anything that individuals do in their own behalf that they believe will promote or improve health status. This can include health maintenance activities, disease prevention, both traditional and nontraditional medical practices, and folk or popular remedies. It can also include practices that ultimately prove *not* to be in an individual's best health interests.

The self-care movement encourages consumers to develop skills and knowledge in both illness and wellness. Self-care involves more than just those things people do for themselves; it also includes the things people do for each other. This social network can include family and friends as well as self-help groups of various kinds. However, self-care practices, including self-medication, should not be viewed as a substitute for supervised medical treatment when professional intervention is indicated.

Self-Medication

Although self-medication is one self-care practice, not all self-care involves medication. In a general way, self-medication may be viewed as the use of any nonprescription drug for the treatment or prevention of health-related problems with or without professional assistance. Theoretically, this could include poor or even hazardous self-care decisions. Nonprescription products are usually used without medical supervision, even though consultations with health professionals are often involved. The Nonprescription Drug Manufacturers Association (NDMA) emphasizes that self-medication decisions should involve the informed, appropriate, and responsible use of nonprescription products. The NDMA further states that responsible self-medicating does not include the use of prescription drugs without medical supervision (e.g., those drugs obtained from family or friends or left over from a previous illness).[3]

Studies indicate that the average American experiences one potentially self-treatable health problem every 3 days and that about 90% of people report being "a little under the weather" at some time during each month.[4] People appear more likely to self-treat when they perceive their illness to be not serious or not amenable to

TABLE 1	An illness experience model that considers self-care options

Problem is perceived by the patient
Illness experience options
   Do not treat
   Treat
      Popular domain (self, family, social network)
         Self-treatment:
            Home remedy (e.g., alcoholic beverages, honey, lemon, baking soda, onions, hot or cold water)
            Nonprescription products
            Prescription medications already at home
      Folk domain (nonprofessional healers)
         Naturopathic healers
         Herbalists
         Acupressure therapists
      Professional domain
         Traditional medical care
Outcome

Information extracted from:
Health Care Practices and Perceptions—A Consumer Survey of Self-Medication. Pub No HHR–72792. Washington, DC: Harry Heller Research Corp; Feb 1984.
Wolinsky FD. *The Sociology of Health: Principles, Professions and Issues.* 2nd ed. Boston: Little, Brown and Co; 1988: 122–60.

professional medical intervention.[1] Tables 2 and 3 summarize common consumer complaints that are often self-treated. Self-medication practices are learned early and extend throughout life. One study found that 75% of children under age 2 had been given a nonprescription drug at least once. Mothers have been found to keep as many as 16 nonprescription medications on hand for use with their children; the average number was 5.5.[5] In another study, 54% of ambulatory elderly patients indicated that they had nonprescription medications at home that were not being used, while 38% were currently using a nonprescription product of some kind. Furthermore, many people supplement prescription medications with self-prescribed products.[6]

Nonprescription Drugs

Generally speaking, nonprescription drugs are defined as drugs that are considered to be safe and effective for consumers to use without professional supervision, provided the required label directions and warnings are followed.[7] (They are also known as over-the-counter (OTC) products.) Historically, nonprescription drugs have also been referred to as *patent* or *proprietary medicines.* Both of these terms are considered obsolete because of the regulations that now govern the sale of nonprescription products as well as the negative connotations associated with the patent medicines of the late 1800s and early 1900s. Use of the term *proprietary* has also been questioned because consumers are no longer considered to be the sole target audience of these products. Some nonprescription products are promoted to physicians and other health professionals more heavily than they are to the public.

It is not definitively known how many nonprescription products are available to Americans. However, 300,000 is the figure quoted most often. (See Chapter 3, "FDA's Review of OTC Drugs.")

Historically, nonprescription medications have been promoted for treating the symptoms of minor, self-limiting conditions (e.g., headaches or colds). Many contemporary nonprescription products are also used to effect cures (e.g., of fungal infections), to prevent a disease or disorder (e.g., motion sickness), or to manage chronic conditions (e.g., diabetes) once a diagnosis has been made by a health professional.

Cultural Trends: Factors That Influence Self-Care

Table 4 summarizes some of the many factors that are thought to influence self-care practices, cultural attitudes, and policies. This table reflects beliefs of both consumers and health professionals, and includes important considerations regarding self-care and self-medication, realistic clinical roles for self-care products, appropriate consumer counseling efforts, and the development of realistic therapeutic expectations and objectives.

Consumer Attitudes and Beliefs

Consumer attitudes and beliefs affect health decisions, such as which domain to use for care. For example, changing values, beliefs in prevention, overall health and fitness, and individual acceptance of a personal responsibility for health can affect consumer willingness to use self-care products. The degree to which the individual perceives a condition to be serious can affect how that individual will react to illness.[8]

Some concern has been expressed that self-care practices could reduce the demand for high-quality care or the support for efforts to improve and expand needed professional services. For example, trends in self-medication might become an excuse for not providing professional services to the poor or other groups.

Demands for self-care products appear to be deeply rooted in the American culture. Threats to cherished cultural values such as independence and freedom of action are deeply resented. At least one study has suggested that the use of nonprescription medications may be viewed as a means for coping with stress and exerting control over life.[9] Thus, nonprescription products may be valued as a symbol of this independence.

Consumers recognize that they are an integral component of the U.S. health care system, and they continue to look for self-care opportunities, including self-medication. The importance of self-medication may be increasing because of a greater social emphasis on individual responsibility for health and because of social trends that discourage dependence on professional intervention.[10] In fact, consumers often lament that health care providers have too much control, restricting access to desired medications and related products. In reality, health care professionals have a legitimate obligation to help ensure public health.[1]

Consumers may self-medicate to avoid contact with health professionals. When consumers become dissatisfied with the care that has been provided, they may question the ability of the professional domain to satisfy their needs.[11] At least one study has indicated that individuals with the greatest trust in physicians and traditional medicine were least likely to purchase questionable products on their own,[12] whereas another indicates that elderly persons who are skeptical of medical care are more likely to use nonprescription products.[9]

There is some evidence that some consumer fears, anxieties, and suspicions are justified. Health scholars have

TABLE 2 Summary of commonly occurring consumer complaints in a two-week period

Category	% reporting a complaint
Digestive	40
Eye/ear/mouth	44
Feminine	27
General well-being	53
Pain	57
Respiratory	49
Skin	67

Most common specific complaints	% reporting the complaint
Common cold	19
Headaches	21
Minor cuts/scratches	19
Minor eye problems	22
Minor fatigue	20
Muscle aches and pains	25
Overweight	28
Upset stomach/indigestion	25

Adapted from *Health Care Practices and Perceptions—A Consumer Survey of Self-Medication*. Pub No HHR–72792. Washington, DC: Harry Heller Research Corp; Feb 1984.

TABLE 3 Examples of problems that are considered amenable to varying levels of self-medication therapy and nonprescription products

Aches and pains (minor functional)	Glucose testing (blood)
Acne	Glucose testing (urine)
Albumin testing (urine)	Halitosis
Allergic rhinitis	Head lice
Anemia	Headache
Athlete's foot	Heartburn
Bacterial infections (superficial, uncomplicated, topical)	Hemorrhoids
	Insect bites and stings
Blood pressure monitoring	Insomnia
Boils	Jock itch
Burns (minor thermal)	Ketone testing (blood)
Calluses	Ketone testing (urine)
Canker Sores	
Cold Sores	Mineral deficiency
Colds	Motion sickness
Constipation	Nasal congestion
Contact dermatitis (e.g., poison ivy, poison oak)	Nausea/vomiting
	Occult blood in feces
Contact lens care	Ovulation prediction
Contraception	Periodontal disease
Corns	pH (urine)
Cough	Pharyngitis
Cuts (superficial)	Pinworm
Dandruff	PMS
Dental care	Pregnancy testing
Dental plaque indicator	Prickly heat
Diabetes mellitus (e.g., insulin and diabetic supplies)	Scrapes (topical)
	Sprains
Diaper rash	Strains
Diarrhea (e.g., traveler's)	Sunburn
	Swimmer's ear
Dry skin	Vaginal candidae infection
Dysmenorrhea	
Dyspepsia	Vitamin deficiency
Feminine hygiene	Warts
Fever	Xerostomia
Flatulence	

Reprinted from Covington TR. *Overview of Nonprescription Drug Therapy and the Self-Care Movement*. Paper presented at the 139th Annual Meeting of the American Pharmaceutical Association in San Diego; March 14, 1992.

TABLE 4 Factors likely to influence the pattern and extent of self-medicating and self-care attitudes and practices

Consumer attitudes and beliefs

Perceived seriousness of disease

Levels of acceptance by health professionals and consumers

Changing values

Growing beliefs in prevention and planning for health and health care

Increased emphasis on overall health and fitness

Individual acceptance of a personal responsibility for health

Growing public frustrations with, and suspicions of, the medical industry and its institutions, and estrangement from health care providers

Consumer education and sophistication

Educational level and sophistication of the public

Quality and quantity of information and communication available to consumers

Quality and quantity of communication between patients and health professionals

Availability of pharmacists and other health professionals with useful, free information

Educational materials available to the consumer through the lay press, media, and other sources

Patterns, quality, and types of advertising

Language and information provided on package labeling and package inserts

Demographic characteristics

Aging population

Gender differences

Accessibility/availability considerations

Distribution and availability of health care professionals and health services (including home health services)

Products

Range and types of products permitted for nonprescription sale

Development and availability of new products and new technology, including those designed to meet new needs

Competition

Packaging

Safety

Efficacy

Economy

Increasing health care costs

Standards of living and the economy

Convenience

Alternate approaches to health

Acceptance and acknowledgment of self-care as a response to disease

Alternate health care approaches (e.g., naturalism, herbalism, holism)

---

questioned the safety and efficacy of many traditional health care practices, raised concerns about the competency of some practitioners, expressed concerns about iatrogenesis, and reflected social frustrations with the traditional health care system.[13]

Other sources of anxiety may exist as well. Patients may be embarrassed about being examined by health professionals or about discussing personal matters. This latter concern is of particular interest to the pharmacist because patient–practitioner interactions often take place in locations (e.g., the dispensing counter or product aisles) where they can be overheard by other patrons. (See Chapter 2, "Patient Assessment and Consultation.")

Patients may fear what they might be told by health professionals. For example, children are often afraid they will be given injections. Adults may fear that the diagnosis or therapy may alter their normal lifestyles; elderly people may fear loss of independence and institutionalization.[14] Additionally, perceptions of illness may vary depending on cultural orientation.[15] Adults may dislike being associated with certain conditions or may actually desire others.

Consumer Education/Sophistication

It appears that many consumers are taking a more active role in their own health care, particularly through self-education. As of 1979, an estimated 5,000 self-help books were available to the American public.[16] A bookstore representative indicated that the sales of traditional medical books increased by 39% from 1989 to 1990.[17] These statistics attest to the popularity of independent study regarding health matters, particularly in times of economic difficulty. One study has indicated that consumer knowledge about drug products is relatively more accurate than it is about other products.[18] And it appears that many consumers also read medication labels more carefully now.[19] As a result, they may be more willing to acknowledge the limitations of self-care and make appropriate lifestyle changes.[4]

Historically, consumers have tended to gather bits and pieces of information from health professionals, advertisements, friends, relatives, books, magazines, and various other sources.[4,20] The accuracy of available medical and health information can vary considerably, depending on both the source and the ability of the consumer to interpret the information that has been obtained. For example, a survey of 1,233 Americans indicated that 35% use the *Physicians' Desk Reference* (*PDR*) for information.[20] Even though the *PDR* is not written for consumers, it can be found in most major bookstores. It is important to realize, however, that being informed does not necessarily mean being enlightened. People can have information without having understanding (e.g., inappropriate use of medical references), which can lead to poor self-care decisions.

While many consumers have become more informed, others harbor misinformation and inaccurate beliefs regarding medications, therapy, and health care in general. Misinformation and inaccurate beliefs can result in unrealistic expectations and the use of inappropriate self-care. For example, consumers may expect cold products to "cure" a cold. Others may believe a daily bowel movement is essential for good health. When consumers are misinformed, they may select inappropriate products for their needs, or they may use appropriate products incorrectly. A study that examined how mothers selected and used nonprescription products to treat their children's symptoms indicated disapproval by experts regarding how the children were medicated.[5]

All medications can be misused or abused. The term *abuse* most correctly denotes misuse associated with social or cultural disapproval. For example, a medication may be taken too often or not often enough, too large or too small a dose may be taken, doses may be omitted, therapy may be discontinued prematurely, or products may be stored improperly. The more familiar concept of abuse usually involves deliberate recklessness, attempts to derive pleasurable sensations, and escape behaviors.

Generally speaking, consumers lack the background needed to diagnose most clinical conditions accurately. People prefer problems that are simple, easy to comprehend, and readily amenable to self-care efforts.[21] Because one disease can mimic another, potentially serious conditions may be misdiagnosed. Consumers must learn to acknowledge the limits of their abilities to self-diagnose and self-treat, as well as the risks of exceeding those limits.

Self-care practices, and especially self-diagnosis, can be affected by the tendency of many consumers to view symptoms as being temporary. Thus, they may delay seeking professional help to see how the condition evolves. Similarly, the use of nonprescription products can mask symptoms that would normally be good diagnostic indicators or a warning that a more serious problem is developing.

Self-care decisions, including self-diagnosis and the willingness to seek out professional help, are influenced by various factors (Table 5). These factors represent individual experiences with various diseases and health professionals, perceptions of seriousness and inconvenience, and the consumer tendencies discussed above.

The degree of consumer sophistication, education, and ability and willingness to interpret and use label information is important in determining the appropriateness of self-care. For example, studies have suggested that less educated people are more likely to treat problems, more likely to contact a professional, and more likely to take prescription medications already in the home. Well-educated individuals are more likely to purchase the brands recommended by a pharmacist.[22] This may occur because they have greater self-confidence in their own judgment or a greater appreciation for the pharmacist's expertise.[4,22] Well-educated individuals also tend to be younger. Less educated individuals may report more chronic problems with aging and be more isolated, both of which conditions can contribute to self-care orientations.[4,9]

Education, per se, may not prevent consumers from making inappropriate health care decisions. At least one study has indicated that college graduates seem more likely than those without a degree to use questionable treatments.[12] In another study, individuals with more education were found to make the same types of interpretation errors regarding common label instructions as people with less education. However, others have theorized that consumer interpretations of medication instructions may be culturally determined and relatively consistent, regardless of age, gender or educational level.[23]

Demographic Characteristics

The number of elderly people has been increasing since 1900, while the number of individuals aged 19 and under has declined.[8] This is a significant change because the

---

TABLE 5 Factors that influence individual decisions to seek professional health care versus other options

How the symptoms are perceived

Degree to which symptoms are recognizable as being abnormal in some way

Extent to which symptoms are perceived as serious

Perception as to how susceptible the individual is to a particular illness

Anxieties and fears regarding symptom interpretation

Disruptive nature of the symptoms

Extent to which symptoms disrupt family, work, and other functions

Frequency of the appearance or recurrence of symptoms

Persistence of symptoms

Tolerance of the individual and others to symptoms

Other factors

Awareness of decision options (see Table 1)

Available information, knowledge, cultural assumptions, and understanding of the individual

Others who affect the individual's interpretation of symptoms

Perceived benefits of and barriers to taking action regarding symptoms

Availability of treatment resources

Anxiety and suspicion regarding health care professionals and the health care industry

Reprinted from Wolinsky FD. *The Sociology of Health: Principles, Professions and Issues*. 2nd ed. Boston: Little, Brown and Co; 1988.

types of problems addressed by self-care vary with age. For example, younger adults (those under age 55) are more likely to report acute problems (e.g., minor cuts and scratches, colds, sinus problems, acne, lip and dental problems), whereas older individuals are more likely to report chronic problems (e.g., arthritis; rheumatism; problems involving the back, ears, and feet; and sleeping difficulties).[4,6] The use of nonprescription products appears to remain relatively constant with age. However, younger people are less likely to see health care professionals or to self-medicate with prescription drugs already in the home.[4] Young couples, and especially young parents, have been shown in one study to be most influenced by the advice of a pharmacist. Single individuals, on the other hand, seem least influenced by a pharmacist's advice.[22]

The use of prescription medications and professional visits increases with age.[4] Elderly people tend to take some form of action regarding their health problems rather than ignore them.[24] Conversely, the elderly may minimize or disguise their medical problems because they fear that revealing these difficulties may increase their chances for institutionalization.[14,25]

Gender is also an important consideration. Men are more likely to ignore problems, which may reflect a cultural belief that men should be able to tolerate discomfort.[4] Women, on the other hand, have been more likely to make medication purchases, contact health professionals, and use nonprescription drug products.[4,25] Women have tended to have responsibility for family health care matters, especially regarding care for children. Historically, this has been because women were at home. As more women enter the work force, however, this has been changing because women have less time to attend to these responsibilities. Additionally, changes in women's careers and traditional cultural roles are affecting educational and income levels, both of which, in turn, affect health care behaviors.[8]

Men and women report different problems for which self-medication may be used. This may reflect career choices, cultural roles, and cultural imagery, as well as obvious physiological differences. For example, women are more likely to report problems involving anxiety, stomach and indigestion, headaches, fatigue, sleep, arthritis, the lips and skin, and overweight. Men are more likely to report muscle aches and pains, minor cuts and scratches, colds, and dental problems.[4]

Individuals from lower socioeconomic groups appear more likely to seek professional care and use prescription medications already in the home.[4] Self-treatment has been shown to be relatively high among members of large households because these individuals may be more cost-conscious than other consumers.[26]

Accessibility and Availability

The availability of health services affects their use. For example, people are less willing to travel to a health care service facility as the distance to that facility increases. Additionally, people appear to be more willing to travel greater distances when they perceive that the illness involved is more serious.[1,8]

Availability of health personnel is a similar consideration. The American public does not have unlimited access to professional care, especially for minor problems. Consumer demands far exceed the available resources of the health care industry. It has been estimated that if only 2% of self-treating consumers were suddenly to seek professional care, the annual number of physician visits would increase by 300 million—a more than 60% increase.[27] In this way, self-treatment is thought to encourage optimal use of medical resources both by promoting effective and efficient product use and by conserving professional resources for individuals for whom such care is essential. This approach also results in increased professional satisfaction because professionals are freed to address health problems that require greater knowledge and skills and that are more rewarding.

Products

Obviously, the availability of products influences self-medication practices. Consumers are more likely to use products that are promoted and available within their geographic region.

As a result of the Food and Drug Administration (FDA) OTC review program, the switch of some prescription products to nonprescription status, and changes in federal regulations over the years, nonprescription products have become increasingly effective for their self-care indications. Studies indicate that many consumers are satisfied with the products available to them and are able to self-medicate with a high degree of success.[4]

In part, the success of self-treatment may be a result of the nature of the conditions being treated. It has been suggested that more than 75% of all illness episodes are self-limiting or have no specific remedies.[13] Other studies have suggested that more than 87% of illness episodes were addressed without professional intervention.[4,24] Many patients who see physicians have minor ailments or chronic health problems, neither of which are often amenable to energetic or dramatic therapeutic efforts. Thus, it is suggested that many patients who see physicians could benefit from varying degrees of self-treatment.

A significant product consideration is consumer safety. Nonprescription drugs are designed to be safe and effective for self-medication. However, no drug can be considered to be absolutely safe. Any drug can cause significant adverse reactions; mask the existence of potentially serious conditions; interact with foods, other drugs, and laboratory tests; or result in other health hazards. (See Chapter 3, "FDA's Review of OTC Drugs.") Even so, most consumers who use nonprescription products as directed should not experience significant problems. Side effects should be minor and predictable.

Economics

Hospital charges, professional fees, and costs of other health-related products and services have risen significantly and have contributed to consumer demands for low-cost alternatives. The advantage discussed most often as a rationale for self-care is that it is a less expensive form of health care.

Four times as many health problems are treated with nonprescription drugs as are taken to physicians, and 60–

95% of all illness episodes are initially treated with some form of self-care, including self-medication.[4] Total sales of the major groups of nonprescription drugs in 1990 were $11.3 billion, or about $40 per capita. Although 60% of medications purchased by American consumers are nonprescription, these purchases account for only 1.7% of the U.S. health care dollar. This percentage represents an 11% decrease from 1989, while total health expenditures increased by 10.5% during this same 1-year period.[28,29] This suggests that self-medication is a significant and cost-effective component of the U.S. health care system.

The economic advantages proposed for self-care efforts include not only cost-effective purchases but also cost reductions due to reduced health care spending. For example, research suggests that Americans would have spent $10.5 billion more for health care in 1987 if nonprescription products were not available. This figure could rise to $34.1 billion by the year 2000. These estimates include time lost from work, medical fees, prescription costs, insurance services, and travel.[30] Other studies cite prescription-to-nonprescription switches, which have resulted in significant savings to the health care system; for example, it has been estimated that Americans saved $600 million in the first 2 years after the switch of 0.5% hydrocortisone in 1979.[31] And more recently, 12 switches of cough/cold medications have saved the health care system $750 million annually.[32]

Cost concerns are complicated by an aging population because health care costs tend to increase with advancing age. Statistically, more people can expect to reach old age today than in 1900. As the average age of the population increases and health care becomes less affordable, self-medicating may become more attractive.

At any one time, more than 25 million Americans have no health insurance coverage of any kind, and as many as 34 million may be uninsured for some period during the year. Approximately 18 million are without insurance for the entire year, and 16 million are uninsured for some portion of the year. Without health insurance or cash, people may be turned away from hospitals, even in emergency situations. Others may neglect care, allowing some conditions to become life-threatening. Such a lack of insurance creates serious strains in society at all levels.[33] Understandably, many individuals may turn to self-care measures.

In addition to monetary costs, self-treatment is considered cost-effective in terms of time savings. Traditional health care involves time lost from work, time for physician visits, and time required to obtain prescriptions from a pharmacy. Self-treatment can reduce many of these time investments.

Finally, the decision to self-medicate may be largely a matter of convenience. Nonprescription products can be purchased at more than 700,000 locations, including nonpharmacy outlets (e.g., convenience stores, grocery stores, and gas stations). The number of pharmacy outlets is estimated at 70,000 or less.[34,35]

Labels

Labels should provide detailed information so that consumers can properly select and use products without the advice of a health professional.[34,36] And, in fact, label language has been a significant determinant of product eligibility for nonprescription status.[7] FDA regulations require that labeling be "stated in terms that are likely to be read and understood by the average consumer, including those of low comprehension under customary conditions of purchase and use."[37]

Nevertheless, concerns have been raised regarding the potential for problems in reading or understanding labels. One study suggests that consumers may have difficulty reading labels because inappropriate color combinations are used, or print is too small. This study also indicates that many labels are written at a ninth-grade reading level or higher, sometimes even at a college level.[38] Yet the average consumer reads at a sixth- to eighth-grade level, and 20% of American adults are functionally illiterate (reading below a fifth-grade level).

At least one study has indicated that consumers may misinterpret even simple language on labels and that it may be impossible to write labels so as to avoid errors.[23] Studies such as this raise questions regarding the effectiveness of labels alone to enable consumers to self-medicate appropriately.

Recently, the nonprescription drug industry implemented an "improved readability program" in response to consumer and health professional demands for greater readability. The NDMA has adopted guidelines that nonprescription drug manufacturers will follow voluntarily to make drug labels easier to read.[39]

Despite these advances, it is not reasonable to expect the industry to solve all readability problems. The inability of some consumers to read and understand product labels also involves problems with vision (e.g., poor eyesight or ocular diseases), comprehension, and lighting in retail environments.[39]

The Pharmacist's Role in Self-Care

Pharmacists can have an enormously expanded role in providing information, advice, and counseling, and pharmacies can become information and education centers in the community.[34,40] Functioning in the midst of an extraordinary information network, the pharmacist can remain current and disseminate information on all drug products, thereby serving the public well by promoting safe and effective products and self-care practices.

Even though studies indicate that consumers can and do interact with pharmacists, those consumers do not always receive the information they seek.[41,42] Pharmacists are sometimes unavailable because of their dispensing responsibilities, and the advice they give has been criticized as being inadequate and inappropriate in some cases.[41,42] Consumer perceptions of this nature can alienate pharmacist from the consumer, and mar the image of the pharmacist as an essential component of self-care practices.

The irony of these concerns is that the pharmacist is the most available and accessible learned intermediary to assist consumers in nonprescription drug selection and use. They are uniquely qualified and strategically positioned in the community to intervene on the patient's behalf. And studies reveal considerable consumer confidence regarding pharmacists and the professional (e.g., informational and clinical) services they provide.[42]

The Future of Nonprescription Drugs

Current trends may shape the nonprescription drug industry from now until well into the next century. The future will likely reveal increasingly sophisticated products, more prescription-to-nonprescription switches, more self-diagnostics, and a greater variety of products for the aging.

As nonprescription drug companies advance further into their high-tech stage, it is predicted that research and development will result in a wider range of products for both treatment and diagnosis. In addition, new products will likely emerge as a result of biotechnology.

There can be no doubt regarding the role that pharmacists can have in fostering the safe, appropriate, effective, and economical use of nonprescription products by consumers. For pharmacists the issue is not only one of new role responsibilities, but also one of potentials for professional satisfaction.

References

1. Wolinsky FD. *The Sociology of Health: Principles, Professions and Issues.* 2nd ed. Boston: Little, Brown and Co; 1988: 122–60.
2. Lough C, Stewart B. In: Lee PR, Brown N, Red I, eds. *The Nation's Health.* San Francisco: Boyd and Fraser Publishing Co; 1981: 445–53.
3. *Facts and Figures.* Washington, DC: The Nonprescription Drug Manufacturers Association; July 1991.
4. *Health Care Practices and Perceptions—A Consumer Survey of Self-Medication.* Pub No HHR–72792. Washington, DC: Harry Heller Research Corp; Feb 1984.
5. Maiman L, Marshall HB, Katlic AW. How mothers treat their children's physical symptoms. *J Comm Health* 1985 Fall; 10 (3): 136–55.
6. Holt GA, Beck D, Williams MM. *Interview Analysis Regarding Health Status, Health Needs and Health Care Utilization of Ambulatory Elderly.* Unpublished report presented at 40th Annual Conference of the National Council of Aging, Washington, DC; April 1990.
7. Fink JL. *Pharmacy Law Digest.* St. Louis: Facts and Comparisons; 1991.
8. Donabedian A et al. *Medical Care Chartbook.* 8th ed. Ann Arbor, Mich: Health Administration Press; 1986.
9. Stoller EP. Prescribed and over-the-counter medicine use by the ambulatory elderly. *Medical Care* 1988 Dec; 26 (12): 1149–57.
10. Montagne M, Bleidt BA. How to help the elderly self-medicate. *U.S. Pharmacist* 1989 Jun; 14: 53–60.
11. Kleinman A. The Failure of Western Medicine. In: Lee PR, Brown N, Red I, eds. *The Nation's Health.* San Francisco: Boyd and Fraser Publishing Co; 1981: 18–20.
12. *Health, Information and the Use of Questionable Treatments: A Study of the American Public.* Study 833015. A study conducted by Louis Harris & Associates for the U.S. Department of Health and Human Services; 1987.
13. Ingelfinger FJ. Medicine: Meritorious or Meretricious. In: Lee PR, Brown N, Red I, eds. *The Nation's Health.* San Francisco: Boyd and Fraser Publishing Co; 1981: 478–84.
14. Hooyman N, Lustbader W. *Taking Care: Supporting Older People and Their Families.* New York: Free Press; 1986.
15. Dolinsky D. Psychological Aspects of the Illness Experience. In: Wertheimer A, Smith M, eds. *Pharmacy Practice—Social and Behavioral Aspects.* 3rd ed., Baltimore: Williams & Wilkins; 1989: 127–42.
16. Levin LS. *Self-Medication: The Social Perspective. Self-Medication: The New Era—A Symposium.* Washington, DC: The Nonprescription Drug Manufacturers Association; March 1980: 44–57.
17. Nelson MV. Promotion and selling of unnecessary food supplements: quackery of ethical pharmacy practice. *Am Pharm* 1988 Oct; 28 (10): 34–6.
18. *U.S. Consumer Knowledge: The Results of a Nationwide Test.* Consumer Federation of America; September 1990.
19. Gallup poll on self-medication. *Am Health*; March 1989.
20. *A Study of Attitudes, Concerns and Information Needs for Prescription Drugs and Related Illnesses.* New York: The CBS Consumer Model, CBS Television Network; 1984: 8.
21. Thomas L. On magic in medicine. In: Lee PR, Brown N, Red I, eds. *The Nation's Health.* San Francisco: Boyd and Fraser Publishing Co; 1981: 68–71.
22. Laverty R. Price, convenience, variety behind OTC decisions. *Drug Topics* 1984 May 21: 54–60.
23. Holt GA et al. Patient interpretation of label instructions. *Am Pharm* 1992 March; 32 (3): 58–62.
24. *Aging and Health—The Role of Self-Medication: Current Practices, Costs and Benefits, Importance of Information.* Washington, DC: Nonprescription Drug Manufacturers Association; April 1991.
25. Shanas E, Maddox G. Aging, Health, and the Organization of Health Resources. In: Binstock R, Shanas E, eds. *Handbook of Aging and the Social Sciences.* New York: Van Nostrand Reinhold; 1985.
26. Consumers and the OTCs they use. *Drug Topics* 1980 Apr 11: 31–4.
27. Rottenberg S. *Self-Medication: The Economic Perspective. A symposium: Self-Medication: The New Era*; Washington, DC: The Nonprescription Drug Manufacturers Association; March 1990.
28. *Executive Newsletter of the Nonprescription Drug Manufacturers Association.* 1991 Nov 1; No. 41–91: 1.
29. Medicine is 8.2% health costs. *Pharmacy Today* 1991 Nov 22; 30: 15.
30. Kline CH. *The Economic Benefits of Self-Medication. Self-Care, Self-Medication in America's Future: A Symposium.* Washington, DC: The Proprietary Association; 1988.
31. Temin P. Cost and benefits in switching drugs from Rx to OTC. *J Health Econ* 1983; 2: 187–205.
32. Temin P. FDA and Self-Medication: Problems, Priorities, Opportunities. Testimony to the subcommittee on drugs and biologics of the HHS Advisory Committee on FDA. Washington, DC: Nonprescription Drug Manufacturers Association; August 2, 1990.
33. Davis K, Rowland D. Uninsured and Underinsured: Inequalities in Health Care in the United States. In: Lee PR, Estes CL, eds. *The Nation's Health.* 2nd ed. San Francisco: Boyd and Fraser Publishing Co; 1981: 298–308.
34. Palumbo FB. The impact of the Rx to OTC switch on practicing pharmacists. *Am Pharm* 1991 Apr; 31 (4): 41–44.
35. NDMA counters "new" third class push. *Executive Newsletter of the Nonprescription Drug Manufacturers Association* 1991 Sep 6; No. 33–91: 1.
36. *Voluntary Codes and Guidelines of the OTC Medicines Industry.* Washington, DC: Nonprescription Drug Manufacturers Association; December 1990.
37. *Federal Food, Drug and Cosmetic Act,* Section 502(c), 21 USC 352(c).
38. Holt G et al. OTC labels: can consumers read and understand them? *Am Pharm* 1990 Nov; 30 (11): 51–4.

39. Walden JT. NDMA Label Readability Guidelines. Washington, DC: Letter from the Nonprescription Drug Manufacturers Association; June 19, 1991.
40. Martin S. Is a third class of drugs in pharmacy's future? *Am Pharm* 1991 Apr; 31 (4): 36–40.
41. Hall EL, Baker D, Holt GA. Patron choices. *California Pharmacist* 1983; 30 (12): 20.
42. *The Schering Report XIV. Improving Patient Compliance: Is There a Pharmacist in the House?* Kenilworth, NJ: Schering Laboratories; 1992.

CHAPTER 2

Patient Assessment and Consultation

Wendy Klein-Schwartz and J. Michael Hoopes

Self-care, self-diagnosis, and self-medication are important components of the health care system in the United States. Rather than seek the attention of a physician, many people self-diagnose and treat their symptoms with nonprescription drugs and home remedies. Several factors increase the extent of self-treatment, including age (over 75 years), sex (female), socioeconomic status (income under $6,000 per year), and symptomatology (the number of distinct and separate symptoms).[1] Another factor is the trend of reclassifying prescription drugs to nonprescription status.

In 1990, more than $10 billion was spent on nonprescription drugs. Of the total sales, 45.6% of expenditures for these products were made in pharmacies, 3.6% above such sales in 1989.[2] The remaining expenditures were made in food stores and mass merchandising outlets.

The Professional Opportunity

Nonprescription drugs allow individuals to manage many medical problems rapidly, economically, and conveniently without unnecessary visits to a physician. However, appropriate use of nonprescription products, like that of any other drug, requires certain restrictions and limitations. Although warnings are required on the labels of these products, labeling alone may be inadequate; the patient may often need assistance in selecting and properly using nonprescription drugs. Because inappropriate use and misuse of nonprescription drugs can increase the risk of drug misadventures, resulting in increased cost and a more seriously ill patient, the pharmacist's counseling role can be crucial.

Many patients do not appreciate or are not aware of the need for professional assistance in selecting nonprescription drugs. This attitude has recently become more evident by the large number of nonprescription products purchased in nonpharmacy outlets, such as supermarkets and local convenience stores, where such assistance is not available.[2] Figure 1 gives a general indication of the percentage of nonprescription products purchased in nonpharmacy outlets.

The pharmacist is what differentiates the nonprescription drug department in a pharmacy from a similar department in a food store; to serve patients better, pharmacies need to maximize the personal service of the pharmacist. Patient inquiries should always be referred to the pharmacist, who must actively promote the value of his or her guidance in selecting and monitoring treatment with a nonprescription drug. It is essential to increase the patient's awareness of the importance of consulting the pharmacist, not only when considering a drug for the first time but also when making subsequent purchases.

The pharmacist's professional responsibility to participate in the patient's drug therapy has led to the development of the concept of pharmaceutical care. Pharmaceutical care means designing, implementing, and monitoring a therapeutic plan, in cooperation with the patient and other health professionals, that will produce specific therapeutic outcomes.[3] Under this concept, the pharmacist is directly responsible to the patient for the quality of care. The pharmacist works with the patient to select a product, monitors the patient for the desired therapeutic outcome, and prevents drug-related problems. The pharmacist also helps the patient make medication decisions based on an understanding of personal choices (e.g., the patient's own values, lifestyle, environment, and attitudes) and associated risks.[4] This concept of pharmaceutical care, which is provided for the direct benefit of the patient and should enhance the patient's quality of life, should extend to the use of nonprescription drugs.

A number of factors influence the patient's choice of a pharmacist. One study found that patients choose a particular pharmacist because that pharmacist is always available to give advice, recommends nonprescription drugs, and discusses instructions for using those products. Friendliness and courtesy are also important attributes. Nine out of 10 patients said they would follow a pharmacist's advice, particularly if the pharmacist advised seeking medical help for a possibly serious medical disorder.[5]

In a study of 400 community pharmacists, 85% responded that patients usually follow their suggestion, 12% responded that patients always follow their suggestion, and 3% responded that patients sometimes follow their suggestion when a specific brand of nonprescription drug is recommended.[6] But even though a pharmacist's advice is often followed, more than half the patients do not seek the pharmacist's advice regularly.[5] Another analysis of patient use of nondispensing pharmacy services found that, although patients had not used most of the services available, most had obtained advice on nonprescription medications and on minor health problems. The majority of patients considered pharmacists to be competent and to have a professional relationship with their patients.[7]

Pharmacists are increasingly aware of the importance of patient counseling as a professional function. Of 200 community pharmacists surveyed, 72% indicated that their role in counseling has increased over the past 5 years. The reported frequency of counseling patients on nonprescription drugs was more than 10 times daily for 69% of pharmacists.[8] Similarly, the aforementioned 400 community pharmacists reported providing an average of 320 nonprescription drug recommendations a month, resulting in almost 4,000 such recommendations per pharmacist annually.[6] Moreover, of 394 independent and chain pharmacists surveyed, 63% reported that patients often come to them instead of consulting a physician, and 49% indicated that they are often consulted until a medical appointment can be arranged.[9] Patients usually ask pharmacists about usage, dosage, product safety, and side effects, as well as about product efficacy, price, and product ingredients.

Not all evaluations of pharmacists' counseling, however, are positive or encouraging. Patients have indicated that community pharmacists make themselves available to answer drug-related questions but generally do not *voluntarily* provide counseling. Patients rank providing nonprescription drug information as a very important pharmacy service, but indicate that pharmacists do not always provide such information to them.[10]

Advising patients on self-treatment is an important part of pharmacy practice and provides the pharmacist with an opportunity to act in a primary care role. Often the patient's first contact with the health care system, the pharmacist can assess the situation and recommend a course of action, which may include recommending a nonprescription drug, dissuading the patient from buying medication when drug therapy is not indicated, recommending nondrug treatment, or referring the person to another health care practitioner. If the pharmacist deters healthy people from using more costly health care services or products and refers more seriously ill patients to physicians, health care delivery in the United States will be improved.

Communication

To counsel a patient successfully, the pharmacist must have effective communication skills.

Patients' past experiences with and attitudes toward pharmacists as information sources determine whether they continue to use a pharmacist's counseling service.[7] When communication between patients and health care professionals is poor, it produces frustration for both and reduces patient compliance. When an effective relationship is established, however, the patient will probably return for further advice on self-treatment and for prescription medication as well. Thus, effective patient counseling for nonprescription drugs can contribute to an increased demand for other professional services. Communication may be initiated by either the patient or the pharmacist; however, many patients are reluctant to ask questions. In 1991, the American Pharmaceutical Association (APhA) adopted a policy statement affirming the pharmacist's responsibility for "initiating pharmacist–patient dialogue, [and] assessing the patient's ability to comprehend and communicate so as to optimize the patient's understanding of and compliance with drug therapy."[11]

General Principles of Communication

An effective pharmacist–patient relationship will be established if the pharmacist is a capable, empathetic source of information. The pharmacist's underlying attitude toward the patient will influence the quality of communication. The effective pharmacist must eliminate barriers by avoiding biases toward a patient's level of education, socioeconomic or cultural background, interests, or attitude. In addition, the patient must be assured that any information discussed with the pharmacist will be strictly confidential.

Because people may resent being told what they already know, the pharmacist should first determine the patient's level of knowledge. When counseling patients, the pharmacist should use words that a layperson can understand and avoid using complex medical terms.

Effective communication occurs when a receiver of a message hears and understands exactly what the sender wishes to communicate. As information is exchanged, the participants change roles as receivers and senders of information. The message received is influenced by the content and context of the message, as well as by how the message is sent. Pharmacists can improve communication by paying attention to the interaction between sender and receiver.

One way to ensure good communication is known as "active listening." In this process, the receiver repeats the information back to the sender. For example, after a patient describes a symptom, the pharmacist could say, "You have a sharp, stabbing pain in your wrist, is that right?" To be sure that a patient understands dosage instructions, the pharmacist could ask, "So that I know that I haven't forgotten to tell you anything, would you please tell me how you're supposed to take this medicine?"

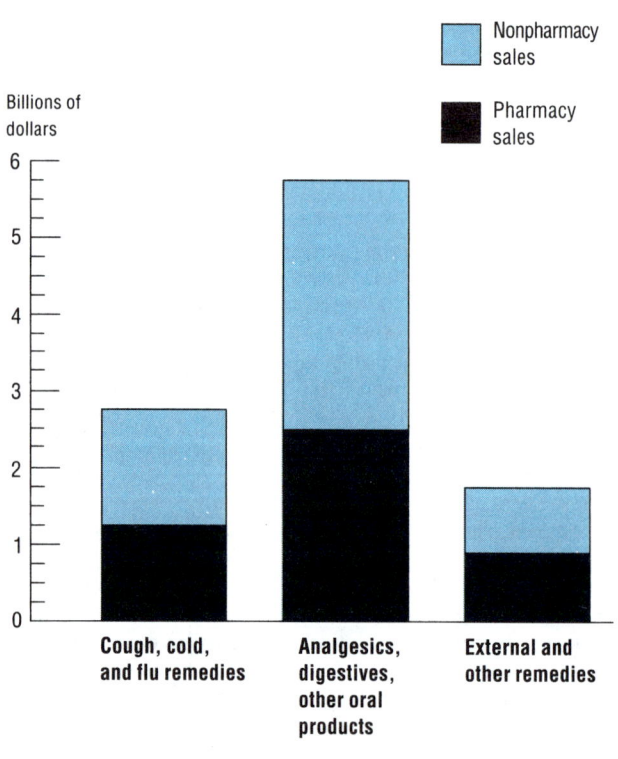

FIGURE 1 Expenditures for nonprescription drugs in 1990 (sales in billions of dollars). Data extracted from *Drug Topics* 1991 Apr; 135: 52–65.

Effective Questioning

Skillful questioning is a mark of a good communicator. The patient should feel that the pharmacist's questions convey a genuine desire to be of help. Because a patient may be uncooperative if the questions suggest only superficial curiosity, the pharmacist should explain the reason for asking personal questions: for example, "For me to select a product for your specific problem, I need some additional information."

Generally, two types of questions are used. Open-ended questions—for example, "Can you tell me more about the symptoms you have?"—are valuable for gathering information regarding a medical problem. Such questions allow more flexibility and provide more information than questions that can be answered with only "yes" or "no." They also enable a good interviewer to collect more information faster and establish better communication. If the patient's response wanders, however, the pharmacist must keep the conversation focused.

Summarizing the important points or redirecting the conversation with a specific, closed-ended question may also be useful. Closed-ended questions—for example, "How long have you had this pain?"—help the pharmacist to gather specific information or to clarify information obtained through open-ended questions. It is important to ask one question at a time. The use of two questions in rapid succession or of multiple-choice questions will only cause confusion and restrict communication.

Effective Listening

Listening is an important component of communication. It means that the patient is free to state the problem completely and receive the pharmacist's undivided attention. The pharmacist must focus on the patient and exclude distracting elements such as the telephone and the computer screen. The pharmacist often must clarify the details of the patient's problem and should be receptive to the patient's response to questions. In addition, the pharmacist should respond with empathy, perhaps by paraphrasing the patient's words or by reflecting on what was said in terms of the pharmacist's own experience. For instance, after listening to a complaint of pain, the pharmacist should describe the pain just related by the patient and end with a statement such as "That must be very uncomfortable." Interrupting or demonstrating disinterest or disapproval may inhibit the patient's discussion of problems and concerns. Alternatively, encouraging the patient to talk, exploring the patient's comments, and expressing understanding will facilitate communication. The pharmacist should reinforce correct decisions the patient has made while reserving judgment, and should communicate warmth, feeling, and interest in the patient's concerns.

Nonverbal Communication

Nonverbal communication skills are also important in counseling patients. Body language, such as posture and facial expression, communicates strong, direct messages. The pharmacist should be very aware both of his or her own nonverbal behavior as well as of the patient's. An open body posture—facing the patient with arms and legs uncrossed—indicates openness, honesty, and a willingness to communicate and listen. It is important to maintain an appropriate distance from the patient; the pharmacist should be close enough for confidential communication to occur without making the patient uncomfortable. If the patient backs away or moves closer, the pharmacist should maintain the new distance that the patient has established. It is also important for the pharmacist to maintain eye contact with the patient and to control his or her facial expressions to avoid showing negative emotions such as disapproval or shock.

The patient's nonverbal communication is equally important. If a patient has a closed body posture—arms crossed, legs crossed, body turned away from the pharmacist—the pharmacist may need to find out why the patient is uncomfortable and allay those concerns. The pharmacist should also watch the patient's facial expressions for signs of anxiety, nervousness, and even physical symptoms such as pain.

Physical Barriers to Communication

For good communication, physical barriers should be removed or minimized. High counters, glass separators, and elevated platforms inhibit communication; the pharmacist should try to be at the same eye level as the patient. Discussions between the patient and the pharmacist should be as private and uninterrupted as possible. If the pharmacist expects or perceives that a patient is uncomfortable discussing the problem, a quiet or private counseling area should be used. Ideally, a specific private area of the pharmacy should be designated for patient consultation.

Communication Techniques for Special Populations

Special techniques may be required with some patients.[12,13] Writing down the information may be necessary if the patient is deaf or hearing impaired. However, pharmacists should also remember that up to 20% of Americans are functionally illiterate.[14] If a hearing-impaired patient reads lips, the pharmacist should be physically close to and directly in front of the patient, and should maintain eye contact while speaking. A quiet, well-lighted environment is essential because background noise and dimness can markedly diminish a hearing-impaired individual's ability to communicate. The pharmacist should also use visual reinforcement such as pointing to the part of the body that hurts or to the directions on the container. In addition, the pharmacist should speak slowly and distinctly in a low-pitched, moderately toned voice. Yelling only serves to distort the sound further.

When counseling a blind patient, a pharmacist should first identify him or herself as a pharmacist. Because a blind patient cannot perceive most nonverbal communication, the pharmacist should depend on tone of voice and verbal feedback to convey empathy and interest in the patient's problem. If touching seems appropriate, the pharmacist should first ask the blind person if it would be acceptable.

The Patient Interview

Counseling patients about self-treatment is a primary care activity that carries with it a great professional responsibility. The initial interaction between the patient and the pharmacist is often initiated by the patient (Figure 2). The patient may approach the pharmacist with a symptom, often in the form of a question such as "What do you recommend for. . . ?" Or the patient may ask a product-related question such as "Which of these two products do you recommend?" The pharmacist should also intervene when a patient selects a product that seems contraindicated or has significant potential for causing problems.

Historical Data

The patient information the community pharmacist has is limited almost exclusively to the patient history. Therefore, the pharmacist must develop good history-taking skills.

Rather than focusing only on drug therapy, the pharmacist should view the patient and the problem as a whole. This entails concentrating on the patient's medical history to assess the problem. This broader approach enables the pharmacist to make the most appropriate recommendation, which may or may not include a drug.

The first step in the decision-making process is to identify the condition that the patient seeks to treat. Patients may initially present incomplete and vague information. By listening carefully and asking questions, the pharmacist can determine the patient's real needs and obtain a problem- and patient-oriented history. The objective is to determine what the specific symptoms are and whether they are amenable to self-treatment.

The pharmacist can determine the specific problem by asking the following questions:

- Can you describe the problem?
- When did the problem start?
- How long does it last? Does it come and go, or is it continuous?
- Does the problem limit your daily activities (sleeping, eating, working, walking, etc.)?
- Is this a new problem or is it the recurrence or worsening of an old one?
- Are there other problems that occur concurrently?
- Does any food, drug, or physical activity make the problem worse?
- Does anything relieve the problem? What has relieved it in the past?
- What has been done so far to treat the problem?

The next step in the process is to gather patient-related data. The pharmacist should selectively elicit the following information:

- Who is the patient? Is the patient the person in the pharmacy or is the patient someone else?
- How old is the patient?
- Is the patient male or female? If the patient is female, is she pregnant or breast-feeding?
- Does the patient have any other medical problems that may alter the expected effects of a given nonprescription drug or be aggravated by the drug's effects? Is the complaint related to a chronic disease?

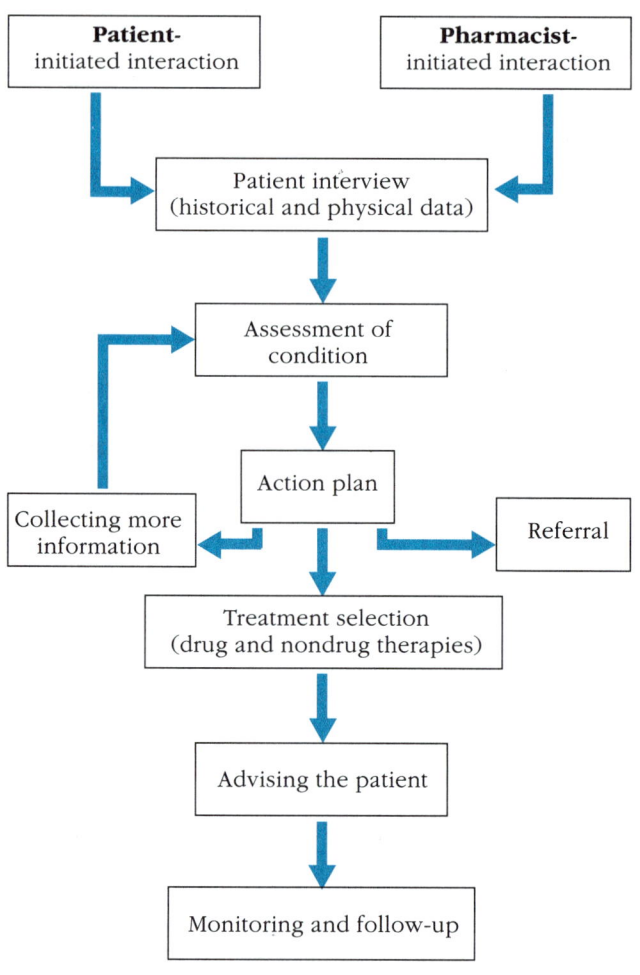

FIGURE 2 Patient–pharmacist consultation process.

- Is the patient on a special diet? Does the patient have any special nutritional requirements?
- Is the patient using any prescription, nonprescription, or social drugs (e.g., vitamins or food supplements, caffeine, nicotine, alcohol, or marijuana)? How long has the patient been taking these drugs?
- Does the patient have any allergies?
- Has the patient experienced adverse drug reactions in the past?

After taking the patient's medical history, the pharmacist should determine if the drug considered for recommendation has any absolute or relative contraindications. In addition, the pharmacist should ascertain if the patient is in a high-risk group because of age, other illnesses, or pregnancy. Similarly, the pharmacist should determine whether the patient has misinterpreted the condition, done any harm by waiting to seek advice, or worsened the condition by previous self-treatment.

Before formulating a plan for self-treatment or physician referral, the pharmacist must obtain enough information to identify and assess the problem and must do it within certain time constraints. This can be done by approaching the problem logically and keeping the questioning direct and to the point. The pharmacist must decide which of the given questions are appropriate to the patient's condition. With experience, the pharmacist will be able to gather the necessary information to assess a particular condition within a few minutes.

Observed Physical Data

Besides the historical data, physical data are extremely helpful in assessing the medical problem. Physical data include pulse rate, heart sounds, respiration rate, age, and weight. Pharmacists have been routinely collecting physical data for years, and some have acquired additional skills that have greatly expanded their ability to assess and monitor patients' medical conditions. Depending on the pharmacist's training and skill, physical data are collected by all or some of the following techniques: observation or inspection, palpation or manipulations, percussion, and auscultation. The importance of each technique in the process of data collection depends on the body system involved. For example, the skin is easily assessed by inspection and palpation, the lung requires percussion and auscultation, and all four skills are essential in examining the abdomen. However, most pharmacists obtain physical data exclusively through observation.

Good observational skills are very valuable. Many clues to a patient's general health and to the seriousness of a condition can come from simple observation. The degree of discomfort caused by pain may be judged from a patient's facial expressions or lack of use of a particular limb. Toxicity from an infection may be manifested by lethargy and pallor. The pharmacist would need to inspect the patient's skin before offering advice about a skin rash, which may result from a simple contact phenomenon or may suggest systemic disease. If a serious disease is suspected, the pharmacist should immediately refer the patient to a physician for diagnosis.

Assessment of Condition

Assessment is the evaluation of all the data (historical and physical) collected from the patient to determine the etiology (cause) and severity of the medical condition.

Assessment of severity will vary depending on the problem. Some conditions may be considered severe only when they reach certain levels, such as diabetes with hyperglycemia or polyuria. Other conditions may be considered severe only when they become symptomatic or when the symptoms begin to impair the activity of the patient; for instance, the pharmacist may elect not to recommend a cough suppressant for a patient with an intermittent cough unless the cough is keeping the patient awake at night. Still other conditions should be considered severe whenever they are present—for example, when ketonuria is noted by a diabetic patient or when an insulin-dependent diabetic is unable to take in calories because of vomiting.

Determining etiology and severity is essential for reaching appropriate conclusions about treatment and the need for referral. Many times, however, the determination cannot be conclusive because certain data may not be accessible. In such situations, referral may be required because the information suggests that a certain etiology is responsible or that the condition is particularly severe. For example, an acutely inflamed joint that is swollen, warm to the touch, tender, and painful may be caused by trauma, bacterial infection, gout, or rheumatoid arthritis. Because a final assessment may require examination of the joint fluid, the patient should be referred immediately to a physician. In general, the more severe the problem is, the greater the potential for referral.

Finally, certain groups of patients are at greater risk of complications and require more careful evaluation. These groups include elderly patients; infants and children; patients with certain chronic diseases, such as diabetes or renal or heart disease; patients with multiple medical conditions and those who are taking multiple medications; recently hospitalized patients; and patients treated by several physicians.

Action Plan

After collecting all the available information and assessing the patient's condition, the pharmacist must quickly formulate an action plan. Often the pharmacist must do this without having all the desired information. Areas of uncertainty will always exist, but a well-considered plan can help ensure proper management of the patient. A sound action plan requires paying careful attention to four specific areas:

- Collecting more information;
- Selecting physician referral;
- Selecting self-treatment;
- Advising the patient on self-treatment.

Collecting More Information

The pharmacist may need more information to assess the patient's condition. This may require specific action, such as talking to a parent or another adult, or calling a physician. Communication between pharmacists and physicians is often desirable to avoid conflict in the management of the patient and to overcome the problem of overlapping responsibilities. In some situations, communication between the pharmacist and the physician may even be necessary. This occurs when the pharmacist must:

- Obtain data on preexisting medical conditions to determine whether self-treatment is appropriate;
- Determine if the physician wants to see the patient, or if the patient should be referred to an urgent care center or a hospital emergency department;
- Determine if the physician wants to deal with the problem over the phone with the patient;
- Provide information on the reason for referral.

Selecting Physician Referral

When enough information is available to assess the condition, the pharmacist must decide whether to refer the patient to a physician or to advise self-treatment. If the plan involves physician referral, the pharmacist must consider both the type of treatment center to which the patient will be referred (physician's office or emergency care facility) and the urgency for treatment. Some conditions do not require the immediate attention or extensive evaluation of emergency care treatment.

When advising a patient to see a physician, the pharmacist should use tact and firmness so that the patient is not frightened unnecessarily but is convinced of the value of the advice. When making a referral, the pharmacist should tell the patient to whom and why the referral is being made. Physician referral is indicated in any of the following situations:

- The symptoms are too severe to be endured by the patient without definitive diagnosis and treatment;
- The symptoms are minor but have persisted and do not appear to be due to some easily identifiable cause;
- The symptoms have returned repeatedly for no readily recognizable cause;
- The pharmacist is in doubt about the patient's medical condition.

Selecting Self-Treatment

Advising self-treatment requires the pharmacist to consider several factors. First, a measurable and achievable therapeutic objective must be identified, based on the condition and the patient. Then, with this determined, a therapeutic modality—either drug or nondrug—may be recommended. For example, the objective in a patient who has a productive cough but is having difficulty producing sputum would be to increase sputum production. Thus, an expectorant would be the agent of choice. However, in a patient with a dry, nonproductive cough, the therapeutic objective would be to suppress the cough, in which case a cough suppressant would be selected. Selecting a specific treatment requires reviewing drug variables (dosage forms, ingredients, side effects, adverse reactions, relative effectiveness, and price) and matching them with patient variables (age, sex, drug history, other physiologic problems, and ability to pay).

Should self-treatment without drugs be indicated, selection of the nondrug modality would similarly be modified based on patient variables. For example, the pharmacist may recommend that a patient with vomiting and diarrhea only drink fluids for a 24-hour period to provide bowel rest. However, if the patient is an insulin-dependent diabetic, the pharmacist must modify this recommendation because diabetic patients must maintain a specific caloric intake. Communicating with the physician is a must in this situation.

To measure the success of treatment, the pharmacist should set indices based on the therapeutic objective, the toxic or adverse effects of the treatment, the nature of the condition, and the ability of the patient to understand the condition and its treatment. The objectives in treating sinusitis with decongestants, for example, are to (1) facilitate drainage and (2) relieve symptoms such as headache. Achievement of the first objective can be determined by observing or asking about the nature of nasal discharge (quantity, color, and viscosity); of the second, by simply asking about the headache. Indices of toxicity are those symptoms indicative of too high a dose or of an untoward reaction. Finally, indices that indicate that the problem may be worsening and may require special attention should be identified.

Advising the Patient on Self-Treatment

The final step in the action plan is to advise the patient on self-treatment. The primary purposes of this step are to educate the patient and to gain the patient's acceptance of the plan. Specifically, the pharmacist should give advice in the following areas:

- Reasons for self-treatment;
- Description of the drug and/or treatment;
- Administration of the drug and/or treatment;
- Side effects and precautions;
- General treatment guidelines.

In advising the patient about the suggested treatment plan, the pharmacist should summarize the patient's condition, explaining the significance of the symptoms and outlining the reasons for treatment. The therapeutic objective(s) should be clearly explained. The pharmacist should also present alternate treatments, with their relative merits. The pharmacist should then discuss the nonprescription drug(s) selected, describing both the therapeutic action of the ingredients (e.g., decongestants, antihistamines, or laxatives) in lay terms and the effect the product(s) will have on the patient's symptoms and condition. Finally, the patient should be told about the available dosage forms and the availability of any generic product.

Administration guidelines should be explained clearly and concisely. Some thought should be given to deciding what is most important for the patient to remember because many patients may remember only part of the information. Covering a few of the most important points is better than overwhelming a patient with a lot of information. Additionally, patients will remember dosage instructions better if administration is linked to specific times of the day rather than just assigned "three times daily." Having patients review their normal daily activities will help them establish the best times to take their medication. It is also important to include information about length of treatment.

The patient should be told about the most common side effects or adverse reactions associated with a drug and instructed on how to manage them. Special warnings about activities, other drugs, foods, or beverages that should be avoided, and about medical conditions that may be complicated by use of the drug, should also be discussed.

Finally, the pharmacist should offer the patient general treatment guidelines that may be helpful in managing the condition. These guidelines might include lifestyle changes, additional products or services, and informational sources, as well as a list of signs and symptoms that indicate whether the drug is working or causing adverse effects and when a physician's advice is needed. In addition, patients should be told of the normal response time to the treatment and time required to resolve the condition, and of what to do if response is delayed.

Follow-up for most problems encountered by the pharmacist is usually not necessary. However, the patient should be encouraged to check back if the condition does not improve within a specific period of time or if problems with the medication develop. To this end, the pharmacist might state: "Please let me know whether you feel better in a couple of days," or "If your cough is not better in a few days, you should see your physician. Be sure to tell your physician that you have been taking this medicine." Follow-up provides feedback that allows pharmacists to assess whether their communication skills require modification and whether they have provided useful information. At the same time, the patient will sense that the pharmacist cares. The pharmacist's concern for the correct use of the nonprescription drugs will also reinforce that these products are drugs and must be used carefully.

High-Risk and Special Groups

Four groups of patients (elderly persons, the very young, pregnant patients, and nursing mothers) often experience a higher incidence of adverse drug effects, which could have dire consequences. Thus, these high-risk patients require special attention. Awareness of their physiologic state, possible pathologic conditions, and special social context is necessary for the proper assessment of their medical conditions and recommendation of treatment.

Geriatric and Pediatric Patients

Social, economic, physiologic, and health factors place elderly patients at high risk of medical problems and prompt them to be large consumers of nonprescription drugs. Indeed, the elderly as a group consume more drugs than any other age segment of our society. A 10-year study of more than 4,509 elderly individuals found that nonprescription drug use in this population increased significantly from 1978 through 1988.[15] Nonprescription drug use must be considered high in elderly persons and should be remembered during the patient interview.

In many respects, geriatric and pediatric patients require surprisingly similar considerations. Both groups share a need for drug dosages different from those for other age groups because of:

- Their altered pharmacokinetic parameters;
- Their decreased ability to cope with illness or drug side effects because of physiologic changes associated with either normal aging or child development;
- Their patterns of impaired judgment because of either altered sensory function or immaturity;
- The different drug effects unique to their age groups;
- The adverse drug effects unique to their age groups;
- A need for special consideration in administering medications.

Yet, because each group is heterogeneous, it is also important to consider these features for each individual patient.

Physiologic State

Normal aging is associated with physiologic changes that alter the pharmacokinetics of certain drugs.[16] These changes include documented significant increases in the proportion of body fat and decreases in renal function, total body water, lean body mass, concentration of plasma albumin, organ perfusion, and hepatic microsomal enzyme activity. Such changes may lead to altered absorption, distribution, metabolism, and elimination of certain drugs. The result is often an unexpected accumulation of the drug to toxic levels. Thus, drug dosing in elderly patients requires constant attention.

The body and organ functions of the pediatric patient are in a continuous state of development. Data on pharmacokinetics in neonates, infants, and children have been more extensively studied for prescription than for nonprescription drugs. In the neonate, factors such as decreased gastric acidity, prolonged gastric emptying, irregular peristalsis, immature biliary function, and altered intestinal enzyme systems are responsible for alterations in the oral absorption of drugs.[17] Changes in body weight, relative body composition (lipid content and body water compartments), and protein binding account for the differences in drug distribution. Drug metabolism is usually slower in neonates and young infants than in older infants and children. Similarly, renal drug elimination is impaired in neonates and young infants but improves rapidly over the first year of life.

Illness in children and elderly people is potentially more serious because their physiologic states are less tolerant of changes. Both groups are very susceptible to fluid loss; therefore, fever, vomiting, or diarrhea represent greater potential risks to them. The common cold can be serious in the first few years of life because children are more susceptible to infections such as otitis media and pneumonia. Decreased pulmonary function in elderly people predisposes them to the complications of respiratory tract infections. Although some physiologic changes are common to all elderly people, the effects of these changes may be quite varied among individuals, making the elderly a very heterogeneous group. These examples show the need not only for treatment plans that vary according to the age of the patient, but also for closer monitoring of the very young and the elderly.

Judgment may be altered in pediatric and elderly patients. In the young, immaturity requires that others provide information and carry out parts of the plan. The same may apply to elderly patients when an organic brain syndrome has developed. Subtle changes in mental status, such as confusion, should be anticipated in elderly patients where an illness has caused anxiety over their state of health. Additionally, central nervous system depressants can have more effect on judgment in the elderly than in the younger adult.

Drugs may have unusual yet predictable effects in elderly patients and in children. For example, antihistamines and central nervous system depressants may cause excitation. Paradoxical reactions of this type are rare, however, in younger adults. Similarly, certain adverse effects are seen more often in the young and the elderly. Elderly patients frequently have altered urinary bladder function and must make a conscious effort to maintain good bladder control. Incontinence may be precipitated in such patients by administration of antihistamines, which have sedative properties that may reduce bladder control.[18] Anticholinergic agents, on the other hand, may cause urinary retention.

Diseases

Children have different diseases than adults, or often have different causes for similar conditions. For example, rashes in children are often the result of common viral illnesses such as measles or chickenpox, which rarely cause rashes in adults. Other conditions such as otitis media and febrile seizures occur more often in children. Certain symptoms have particular significance in children. Fever in any infant under 6 weeks of age is a very serious sign and requires immediate attention because of the increased risk of a serious infection such as bacterial septicemia.

Elderly people also differ from other age groups in that they tend to have serious and multiple diseases such as coronary artery disease, chronic renal failure, or congestive heart failure. These conditions can be aggravated by concurrent therapy for other acute problems. Also, the nutritional status of elderly persons is often marginal, making them more susceptible to illness. Moreover, physiologic changes associated with aging may alter the presentation of certain illnesses and confuse their assessment. For example, elderly patients do not mount fevers to the same degree as younger patients and have altered pain perception, which may cause them to overlook a serious condition. Lastly, elderly patients also lack social supports to supply the aid required by an illness.

Dosage Considerations

Special dosage considerations may be necessary for children and elderly patients. Because of memory lapses, some elderly patients may require unique drug delivery systems to help them adhere to their dosage regimen. Also, elderly patients with cognitive impairment are less likely to read and interpret labels and to differentiate colors correctly,[19] which further emphasizes their need for special dosage considerations.

Because infants and children are unable to swallow tablets and capsules, chewable tablets and liquid preparations are required. This may benefit some elderly patients as well. To assist in the accurate delivery of liquid preparations, devices such as calibrated droppers and spoons are needed. Parents may need instructions on using these devices to measure dosages accurately, as well as advice on giving medications to reluctant or struggling children. Written directions may be needed for other individuals such as day-care providers. Involving the child in the counseling can be effective.[20] Some tips for pediatric counseling include explaining what the medication is; using the word *medicine*, not *drug*; discussing different dosage forms and the importance of medication timing; preparing special vials for school; preparing the child for the medicine's taste; and demonstrating how to take the medicine.

The Pregnant Patient

Drug use during pregnancy is declining. Studies reported in 1978 and 1980 found that the average number of drug products used during pregnancy was 11.0 and during the last trimester was 8.7, with 6.9 (80%) of these drugs taken without the supervision or knowledge of a physician.[21,22] A later study, conducted between 1980 and 1982, among 4,186 women during the first trimester, found that 66% used at least 1 drug, with a mean number of drugs for all subjects and for drug users being 1.3 and 2.9, respectively.[23] Nonprescription drugs accounted for 68% of the drugs used. The most frequently used nonprescription drugs were internal analgesics (acetaminophen and aspirin), antacids, and cold and allergy products. Surveys from other countries also indicate a substantial decline in drug use during pregnancy over the past 2 decades.[24]

Pregnancy introduces a very important variable in drug therapy. Drug therapy during pregnancy may be necessary to treat medical conditions or may be considered to manage common complaints of pregnancy such as vomiting or constipation. However, because most drugs cross the placenta to some extent, a mother who takes a drug might expose her fetus to it. Thus, the desire to ease the mother's discomfort must be balanced with concern for the developing fetus.

Potential Problems

Several factors are important in determining whether a drug taken by a pregnant woman will produce an adverse effect in the fetus. The stage of pregnancy and the ability of the drug to pass from maternal circulation via the placenta to fetal circulation are important factors in determining teratogenic susceptibility. The first trimester, when organogenesis occurs, is the period of greatest teratogenic susceptibility for the embryo and is the critical period for inducting major anatomical malformations. However, exposure at other periods of gestation may be no less important because the exact critical period depends on the specific drug in question.

Unequivocal evidence of teratogenesis is available for some drugs such as thalidomide, androgens, cancer chemotherapeutic agents, tetracyclines, hydantoins, and oral anticoagulants.[25] Many more drugs are suspect, and each year additional drugs are shown to be potentially harmful if used during pregnancy. Still, a major problem faced by the pregnant patient, her physician, and her pharmacist is the lack of readily available information on the teratogenic effects of various drugs. This lack of information has been partly remedied by the Food and Drug Administration's labeling revision program, which places all prescription drugs into one of five categories (A, B, C, D, X) according to the level of risk to the fetus.[26] But although this categorization may increase the amount of information readily available on prescription drugs, a paucity of data on nonprescription drugs still exists. Therefore, knowing the potential danger many nonprescription drugs pose to pregnant women is essential in preventing unnecessary exposure of unborn children to drugs.

Generally, it is prudent to avoid the use of any drug during pregnancy. Evidence of teratogenicity has even implicated drugs such as aspirin, which is available in various prescription and nonprescription products and is often taken during pregnancy. Available data on the teratogenicity of aspirin are in conflict, however;[23,27] several retrospective studies in humans have found a relationship between aspirin and congenital defects, but biases in these studies could account for the results. Similarly, there are conflicting reports on the relationship between the prenatal use of aspirin and the incidence of stillbirths, neonatal deaths, or reduced birthweight. Use of aspirin late in pregnancy has been associated with increases in the length of gestation and in the duration of labor. These effects are related to aspirin's inhibition of prostaglandin synthesis. In addition, because aspirin affects platelet function, perinatal aspirin ingestion has been found to increase the incidence of hemorrhage in both the pregnant woman and the newborn during and following delivery. Therefore, aspirin use during pregnancy should be avoided, especially during the last trimester. Because acetaminophen is generally considered safe for use in pregnancy, it is the nonprescription drug of choice for antipyresis and analgesia when taken in standard therapeutic doses.[23]

Caffeine is also in many nonprescription products such as headache, cold, allergy, and stimulant preparations. There is no evidence of an association between the use of caffeine and congenital malformations.[28,29] Similarly, after controlling for other factors such as smoking and alcohol intake, there is no relationship between caffeine and low birthweights and shorter gestation. However, although pregnant women do not necessarily need to eliminate caffeine from their diets, they might be wise to moderate their caffeine intake.

A possible link between the use of nonprescription vaginal spermicides and congenital disorders in infants has been reported. However, weaknesses in these studies, as well as subsequent negative reports, seem to suggest that these spermicides do not cause teratogenicity.[29] Cigarette smoking and alcohol have also been associated with increased risk to the fetus and with congenital abnormalities.[30–33]

Management of the Pregnant Patient

The pharmacist can aid the self-treating pregnant woman in deciding which drug or nondrug treatments she should consider and when self-treatment may be harmful to her or her unborn child. The decision to suggest a drug must be based on both an up-to-date knowledge of the literature and a very critical risk-to-benefit evaluation of the mother and the fetus. The assessment and management of the pregnant patient require observation of the following principles.

The pharmacist must be alert to the possibility of pregnancy in any woman of childbearing age who has certain key symptoms of early pregnancy, such as nausea, vomiting, and frequent urination. Any woman who fills this description should be warned not to take a drug that might be of questionable safety if she is pregnant.

The pharmacist should similarly advise the pregnant patient to avoid using drugs, in general, at any stage of pregnancy.

The pharmacist should advise the pregnant patient to increase her reliance on nondrug modalities as treatment alternatives. For example, the first approach to nausea and vomiting should be eating small, frequent meals and avoiding foods, smells, or situations that cause vomiting. Next, taking an effervescent glucose or buffered carbohydrate solution may be effective. Only if these measures are ineffective should an antihistamine or antiemetic be considered.

Lastly, the pharmacist should refer the patient to a physician for certain problems that carry increased risk of poor outcomes in pregnancy (e.g., high blood pressure, vaginal bleeding, urinary tract infections, rapid weight gain, or edema).

The Nursing Mother

Drug use while breast-feeding can cause an adverse effect in the infant. The concentration of a drug in the mother's milk depends on a number of factors, including the concentration of the drug in the mother's blood; the drug's molecular weight, lipid solubility, degree of ionization, and degree of binding to plasma and milk proteins; and the active secretion of the drug into the milk. Other important considerations include the relationship between the time of taking a drug and the time of a breast-feeding, as well as the drug's potential for causing toxicity in infants. Additionally, some drugs (e.g., decongestants) may decrease milk supply.

When advising a nursing mother on self-treatment, the pharmacist should decide if the drug is really necessary, recommend the safest drug (e.g., acetaminophen instead of aspirin), and advise the mother to take the medication just after a breast-feeding or just before the infant's lengthy sleep periods.[34]

When taken in therapeutic dosages, most drugs are not present in breast milk in sufficient amounts to cause significant harm to the infant. However, several drugs are contraindicated for use while breast-feeding, and several others should be used cautiously by nursing mothers. The amount of caffeine in caffeine-containing beverages is not harmful, but higher doses could cause irritability and poor sleep patterns in infants. There are also many nonprescription drugs for which data on their transfer into breast milk and their possible clinical effects are not available.

The American Academy of Pediatrics Committee on Drugs recently published a statement on drugs in human milk.[34] Of the nonprescription drugs included in the statement, aspirin and other salicylates are the only ones that were considered to have had significant effects on some nursing infants and that nursing mothers should therefore take with caution. Nonprescription drugs that are usually considered compatible with breast-feeding include:[34,35]

- *Analgesics:* acetaminophen and ibuprofen;
- *Antacids;*
- *Antidiarrheals;* kaolin–pectin and attapulgite;
- *Antihistamines:* brompheniramine, chlorpheniramine, diphenhydramine, and triprolidine;
- *Cough preparations:* dextromethorphan and guaifenesin;
- *Decongestants:* phenylephrine, phenylpropanolamine, and pseudoephedrine;
- *Fluoride;*
- *Laxatives:* bran type, bulk-forming type, docusate, glycerin suppositories, magnesium hydroxide, and senna;
- *Vitamins.*

Summary

The use of nonprescription drugs represents an important component of the health care system. Many people diagnose their own symptoms, select a nonprescription drug product, and monitor their own therapeutic response. Properly used, nonprescription drugs can relieve the minor physical complaints of patients and permit physicians to concentrate on more serious illnesses. If used improperly, however, these products can create a multitude of problems.

To be of greatest service to patients, pharmacists must continually update their therapeutic knowledge and improve their interpersonal communication skills. As pharmacists continue to expand their patient-counseling services, people will learn of these services and will seek their pharmacist's assistance whenever they are in doubt about self-treatment. The result will be better-informed patients, who will not only use the professional services of pharmacists but also recognize the contributions of pharmacists to health care.

References

1. Montagne M, Bleidt B. How to help the elderly self-medicate. *US Pharmacist* 1989 Jun; 14: 53–60.
2. The OTC/HBA battleground. *Drug Topics* 1991 Apr; 135: 52–65.
3. Hepler CD, Strand LM. Opportunities and responsibilities in pharmaceutical care. *Am J Hosp Pharm* 1990 Mar; 47: 533–43.
4. Schulz RM, Brushwood DB. The pharmacist's role in patient care. *Am Pharm* 1991 Dec; NS31: 882–8.
5. The Schering Report VII. What's right with pharmacy! The pharmacist's growing influence in the expanding OTC market. Kenilworth, NJ: Schering Laboratories; 1985.
6. Gannon K. Hot, hot, hot new switches to brighten OTC market. *Drug Topics* 1991 Aug; 135: 32–55.
7. Monsanto HA, Mason HL. Consumer use of nondispensing professional pharmacy services. *Drug Intell Clin Pharm* 1989 Mar; 23: 218–23.
8. Meade V. APhA survey looks at patient counseling. *Am Pharm* 1992 Apr; NS32: 27–9.
9. Gannon K. What do patients want to know about OTCs? *Drug Topics* 1989 Aug; 133: 28–30.
10. Hirsch JD, Gagnon JP, Camp R. Value of pharmacy services: perceptions of consumers, physicians, and third party prescription plan administrators. *Am Pharm* 1990 Mar; NS30: 20–5.
11. New policies adopted by the 1991 APhA House of Delegates. *Am Pharm* 1991 Jun; NS31: 28–30.
12. Chermak G, Jinks M. Counseling the hearing-impaired older adult. *Drug Intell Clin Pharm* 1981 May; 15: 377–82.
13. Smith DL. The patient and his medications. In: *Medication Guide for Patient Counseling*. 2nd ed. Philadelphia: Lea and Febiger; 1981: 3–46.
14. Epstein D. More counseling called for in medicating the illiterate. *Drug Topics* 1988 Nov; 132: 15.
15. Steward RB, Moore MT, May FE, et al. Changing patterns of therapeutic agents in the elderly: a ten-year overview. *Age Ageing* 1991; 20: 182–8.
16. Montamat SC, Cusack BJ, Vestal RE. Management of drug therapy in the elderly. *N Engl J Med* 1989 Aug; 321: 303–9.
17. Morselli PL, Franco-Morselli R, Bossi L. Clinical pharmacokinetics in newborns and infants: age-related differences and therapeutic implications. *Clin Pharmacokinet* 1980; 5: 485–527.
18. Willington FL. Urinary incontinence: a practical approach. *Geriatrics* 1980 Jun; 35: 41–8.
19. Meyer ME, Schuna HH. Assessment of geriatric patients' functional ability to take medication. *Drug Intell Clin Pharm* 1989 Feb; 23: 171–4.
20. Martin S. Catering to pediatric patients. *Am Pharm* 1992 Jan; NS32: 47–50.
21. Doering PL, Stewart RB. The extent and character of drug consumption during pregnancy. *JAMA* 1978 Feb; 239: 843–6.
22. Blyer WA, Au WYW, Lange WA, et al. Studies on the detection of adverse drug reactions in the newborn: I. fetal exposure to maternal medication. *JAMA* 1970 Sep; 213: 2046–8.
23. Buitendijk S, Bracken MB. Medication in early pregnancy: prevalence of use and relationship to maternal characteristics. *Am J Obstet Gynecol* 1991 Jul; 165: 33–40.
24. Rubin PC, Craig GS, Gavin K, et al. Prospective survey of use of therapeutic drugs, alcohol and cigarettes during pregnancy. *Br Med J* 1986 Jan; 292: 81–3.
25. Shepard TH. Teratogenicity of therapeutic agents. *Curr Prob Pediatr* 1979 Dec; 10: 1–43.
26. *Federal Register* 1980; 44:37434–67.
27. Briggs GG, Freeman RK, Yaffe SJ. *Drugs in Pregnancy and Lactation*. 2nd ed. Baltimore: Williams and Wilkins; 1986: 26–31.
28. Briggs GG, Freeman RK, Yaffe SJ. *Drugs in Pregnancy and Lactation*. 2nd ed. Baltimore: Williams and Wilkins; 1986: 53–5.
29. Cordero JF, Oakley GP. Drug exposure during pregnancy: some epidemiologic considerations. *Clin Obstet Gynecol* 1983 Jun; 26: 418–28.
30. American Academy of Pediatrics Committee on Environmental Hazards. Effects of cigarette smoking on the fetus and child. *Pediatrics* 1976 Mar; 57: 411–3.
31. Fielding JE. Smoking and pregnancy. *N Engl J Med* 1978 Feb; 298: 337–9.
32. Clarren SK, Smith DW. The fetal alcohol syndrome. *N Engl J Med* 1978 May; 298: 1063–7.
33. Shaywitz SE, Cohen DJ, Shaywitz BA. Behavior and learning difficulties in children of normal intelligence born to alcoholic mothers. *J Pediatr* 1980 Jun; 96: 978–82.
34. American Academy of Pediatrics Committee on Drugs. Transfer of drugs and other chemicals into human milk. *Pediatrics* 1989 Nov; 84: 924–36.
35. Nice FJ. Breastfeeding and OTC medications. *Pharm Times* 1992 Mar; 58: 114–24.

CHAPTER 3

FDA's Review of OTC Drugs

William E. Gilbertson

Most medications used by American consumers are nonprescription drugs, commonly referred to as over-the-counter (OTC) drugs. Historically, the Food and Drug Administration (FDA) has also recognized the term *OTC drug*, and that term will be used throughout this chapter.

The last 2 decades have seen a trend toward individuals' assuming greater responsibility for personal and family health care. Rising health care costs as well as safer and more effective OTC products have motivated and enabled patients to self-treat conditions previously requiring professional medical intervention. Contributing to this trend is the expanding availability of former prescription drugs that have been reclassified to OTC status; these drugs provide the consumer with even greater choices and opportunities. (See Chapter 1, "The Self-Care Movement.")

The pharmaceutical industry provides a constant flow of new drug products into the marketplace. Approximately 400,000 drug products are currently being marketed in the United States, of which more than 300,000 are OTC drugs. In this country, there are two major channels for drug acquisition: either under a doctor's prescription or by direct OTC purchase by the consumer. Although a number of countries have a class of products with limited availabilities, no widespread pharmacy-only drug distribution system exists in the United States. Several states have been considering such a class, especially as a transition mechanism for products being reclassified from prescription to OTC status. However, at this time only Florida recognizes a select number of drugs that are available only from a pharmacist.

The Approval Process

The first major federal legislation enacted to regulate drugs was the Pure Food and Drugs Act of 1906. "Unsafe" and "nonefficacious" drug products were not actually prohibited by the statute; drugs were only required to meet the standards of strength and purity claimed by manufacturers. Drug safety was not mandated by law until the passage of the 1938 Federal Food, Drug, and Cosmetic Act. Legislation for this new law had been under consideration since 1933, but final passage was compelled by the deaths of more than 100 individuals, many of them children, who used the newly marketed elixir of sulfanilamide incorporating the toxic solvent ethylene glycol (antifreeze) as the vehicle. The 1938 Act required that all new drugs—that is, new drug products introduced after 1938—be proven safe for human use before being marketed and be cleared in advance through a new drug application (NDA). Products marketed prior to 1938 were exempted from the NDA provision under what is commonly referred to as the grandfather clause. Some currently marketed OTC drugs, such as aspirin, still fall under this clause. However, the FDA's OTC drug review has evaluated all OTC drugs for safety, effectiveness, and labeling, regardless of the date of marketing entry.

Even today the 1938 Act, as amended, defines a market divided into "new" drugs, which are defined by law as being recognized as safe and effective (RASE), and those that are generally recognized as safe and effective (GRASE); often these latter drugs are referred to as "old" drugs, but such a legal definition does not exist. New drugs are defined by law as "recognized as safe and effective," commonly referred to as "RASE", whereas other drugs are defined as "generally recognized as safe and effective" or "GRASE". A new chemical entity never before marketed in the United States would be classified as a new drug and, in most cases, initially approved for prescription use only.

Through NDA procedures, a prescription drug may be reclassified to OTC status but remain a new drug. An NDA for an OTC drug product can also be approved directly (without reclassification), such as occurred with ibuprofen 200 mg (a dose that was never available by prescription). When a new drug is used for many years by many patients (referred to in the law as "used for a material time and material extent"), it can be considered GRASE. Another mechanism to gain general recognition status for OTC drugs has been provided by the FDA's OTC drug review. When the review is completed, all OTC drugs that are not approved new drugs will be subject to OTC drug monographs. There is also a group of prescription GRASE drugs (e.g., phenobarbital and atropine sulfate) that continue to be marketed without NDAs; the FDA tentatively plans to address their continued marketing at a later date. Perhaps it will require NDAs or develop monographs.

The legal distinctions between OTC NDAs and OTC drug monographs result in explicit differences in regulatory approaches for product approval (Table 1).

New Drug Application

An NDA is necessary for a drug that is defined by law as being not recognized as safe and effective (NRASE) until it has been precleared and approved by the agency. Under existing public procedures, some data related to the approval and contained in the NDA (e.g., a summary of the safety data and clinical studies) are publicly available. However,

---

This chapter was prepared by a federal employee as part of his official duties and is considered to be in the public domain. Therefore, this chapter is exempt from all copyright protection and may be copied freely.

TABLE 1	Differences in regulatory approach	
Criteria	New drug application	Monograph regulation
Status	New[a]	Old[b]
Reference	RASE[c]	GRASE[d]
Preclearance	Necessary	None
Marketing	Exclusive	Inclusive
Data	Private (some)	Public (all)
Labeling	Restricted	Flexible
Approval	Final formulation	Active ingredient
Reporting	Required	None

[a] OTC drugs approved after the 1938 Federal Food, Drug, and Cosmetic Act.
[b] OTC drugs approved through the OTC drug review.
[c] Recognized as safe and effective.
[d] Generally recognized as safe and effective.

trade information (e.g., final formulation ingredients and quantities) is held confidential.

The approved NDA is manufacturer-specific and allows only the sponsor to market the product. Any other manufacturer interested in marketing a similar product would also first need to seek FDA approval through an appropriate NDA. In some cases, a full NDA is not necessary for the second manufacturer; an abbreviated application may be submitted instead, eliminating the need for duplicative testing.

All NDAs must contain complete (exact) labeling information with final printed labeling usually being the last step prior to approval. Most subsequent revisions in labeling require preapproval through a supplement to the application. Therefore, labeling is highly restricted and often takes considerable time to change. Similarly, except for some minor changes, the final product formulation cannot be changed without an applicable approved supplement to the application. Finally, periodic submissions—for example, a brief summary of significant new information from the previous year that might affect the safety, effectiveness, or labeling, including any actions taken by the sponsor as a result of these findings—are required, to report postmarketing information. Distribution data, minor labeling revisions, chemistry, and manufacturing and control changes must also be reported.

Monographs

In contrast, an OTC monograph is developed for a drug that is defined by law as GRASE. A manufacturer desiring to market a monographed drug need not seek clearance from the FDA prior to marketing. In this case, marketing is not exclusive; any manufacturer may market a similar product without specific approval. Under the monograph approach, all data and information supporting GRASE status are publicly available. The OTC drug review has established the monographs through a complex, public process. Each individual rulemaking (e.g., for antacids, which resulted in an OTC antacid monograph) has resulted in an extensive administrative, public record.

For the final monograph, the manufacturer has considerable flexibility in labeling. All the required monograph labeling must be included; for example, antacids must include terms such as *heartburn, acid indigestion,* and *sour stomach*. In addition, language not included in the monograph may be used in the label without prior approval. For example, *hospital tested* or *pleasant-tasting antacid* are terms considered outside the scope of the monograph but permissible in antacid labeling. However, even though these permissible terms are not precleared, they are subject to the general labeling provision of the 1938 Act and may not be false or misleading.

Monographs primarily address active ingredient(s) in the product, and in most cases, final formulations are not subject to monograph specifications. Manufacturers are free to include any inactive ingredients that serve a pharmaceutical purpose, provided those ingredients are safe and do not interfere with either product effectiveness or any required final product testing. In a few instances, even though the product contains GRASE ingredients, it may need to meet a monograph testing procedure. (For example, antacids must pass an acid-neutralizing test.)

Because the drugs in the monograph system are GRASE, there has been to this point no requirement to report adverse events. Historically, any changes in ingredient status and labeling for these drugs have occurred as a result of adverse drug findings reported in the literature or through similar public mechanisms. With the ever-increasing use of OTC drugs, however, the FDA believes it is important to develop a new and more effective formal mechanism to monitor and screen reports of adverse drug effects and unexpected events associated with their usage.

New Drug Approval

Of the drugs approved since the laws were established to require evidence of safety and efficacy, nearly 90% are considered new in both a medical and legal sense. Most have been approved for prescription use only.

The new drug approval process requires that all new drugs be proven effective as well as safe before they can be marketed. No drug is absolutely safe; there is always some risk of an adverse reaction. When the benefits outweigh the risks, however, the FDA considers a drug safe enough to approve. This risk-to-benefit assessment is critical for drug approval.

Most approved OTC NDAs were approved prior to the OTC drug review. When the program began, most potential applications with ingredients or claims that were also within the purview of the review were deferred. Until the review is completed, interim marketing of products is permissible, but these products are subject to the appropriate final monograph. At that time, products with any marketing factors outside the monograph (e.g., ingredient, dosage, or claim) will require new drug approvals.

TABLE 2 Product categories by which the FDA is reviewing OTC drug ingredients

Acne
Anorectal
Antacid
Anthelmintic
Anticaries
Antidiarrheal
Antiemetic
Antiflatulent
Antifungal
   Diaper rash[a]
Antimicrobials
   Alcohol (topical)
   Antibiotics, first aid
   Antiseptics (topical)
   Diaper rash[a]
   Mercurials
Antiperspirant
Aphrodisiac
Benign prostatic hypertrophy
Boil ointments
Camphorated oil
Cholecystokinetic
Corn/callus removers
Cough/cold/allergy bronchodilator/antiasthmatic combinations
   Anticholinergic
   Antihistamine
   Antitussive
   Bronchodilator
   Expectorant
   Nasal decongestant
Dandruff/seborrhea/psoriasis
Daytime sedative
Deodorants (int.)
Digestive aids
Exocrine pancreatic insuff.
External analgesic
   Astringents (wet dressings)[b]
   Diaper rash[a]
   Fever blister/cold sore (ext.)[b]
   Insect bites and stings
   Male genital densitizers
   Poison (ivy/oak/sumac) treatment/prevention[b]

Fever blister/cold sore (int.)
Hair grower/loss
Hexachlorophene
Hormone (topical)
Hypo/hyperphosphatemia
Ingrown toenail relief
Insect repellents (int.)
Internal analgesic
   Leg muscle cramps
Laxative
Menstrual products
Nailbiting/thumbsucking deterrents
Nighttime sleep-aid
Ophthalmic products
Oral health care
Oral mucosal injury
Overindulgence remedies
   Ingredients intended to minimize or prevent inebriation
Pediculicides
Poison treatment
   Antidotes—toxic ingestion
   Emetic
Relief of oral discomfort
Salicylanilides (TBS)
Skin bleaching
Skin protectant
   Astringents (wet dressings)[b]
   Diaper rash[a]
   Fever blister/cold sore (ext.)[b]
   Insect bites and stings[b]
   Poison (ivy/oak/sumac) treatment/prevention[b]
Smoking deterrent
Stimulant
Stomach acidifier
Sunscreen
Sweet spirits of nitre
Topical otic (earwax)
Topical otic (swimmer's ear)
Vaginal contraceptive
Vaginal drug products
Vitamin/mineral
Wart remover
Weight control

[a]See also antimicrobial, external analgesics, and skin protectants.
[b]See also skin protectants.

NDAs are also necessary for unique delivery systems to ensure bioavailability of the active component. For example, whereas an ingredient in the monograph could be marketed in an immediate-release form, the same ingredient in a sustained-release product would require an NDA.

More recently, NDAs have been the route of approval for many ingredients (not considered in the review) that have been reclassified from prescription to OTC status. These include ibuprofen, loperamide, miconazole, clotrimazole, clemastine, and permethrin. This process is discussed extensively in the section on reclassification of drugs by mechanism 2.

The OTC Drug Review

The 1962 drug amendments to the 1938 Act require that all new drugs be shown to be effective for their intended uses. This legislation thus required the FDA to review the effectiveness of the 4,500 new drug products, including

512 OTC drugs, that had been approved for safety since 1938.

In the mid-1960s, the FDA contracted for a review of these drugs through the National Academy of Sciences/National Research Council (NAS/NRC). The agency took the information from the NAS/NRC and, by a procedure called the Drug Efficacy Study Implementation (DESI), determined the effectiveness of all prescription drugs. As the DESI was nearing completion, it became clear that it was time for an extensive examination of the OTC drug marketplace. In 1972, the FDA initiated a massive scientific review of the active ingredients in OTC drug products to ensure that they were safe and effective and bore fully informative labeling.

Although an estimated 300,000 individual OTC drug products are currently being marketed, these products contain only about 700 active ingredients. The number of individual products may seem high; however, each manufacturer's or distributor's labeled product is considered a separate drug product. Thus, in determining the logistics of the review, the FDA decided that a DESI-type, product-by-product determination would not be feasible because of the sheer volume of OTC pharmaceuticals. Pragmatism dictated a review that focused on the ingredients used in these products, subdivided by therapeutic category (Table 2). For example, instead of examining individual antacid products, of which there are estimated to be more than 8,000, the FDA evaluated only the active ingredients, such as aluminum hydroxide, magnesium carbonate, and sodium bicarbonate. Because the process focuses on active ingredients, the FDA's OTC drug review is vastly different from that applied to a new OTC ingredient as part of an NDA, which evaluates final dosage forms.

The Rulemaking Process

The OTC drug review is a three-phase rulemaking process, with each phase requiring publication in the *Federal Register*. (The *Federal Register* is a daily publication in which federal agencies publicly announce their regulations and legal notices.) The process culminates in the promulgation of regulations establishing standards for both the active ingredients and labeling in each OTC therapeutic drug category (Figure 1).

Phase I: Advisory Panel Review

The first phase of the OTC drug review was accomplished by FDA-appointed advisory review panels. Panel members were scientifically qualified individuals and nonvoting technical liaison members representing consumer and industry interests. These panels were charged with reviewing the ingredients and labeling of marketed OTC drug products to determine whether they could be classifed as GRASE for use in self-treatment.

The panels classified ingredients of OTC drug products into three categories:

- *Category I*: generally recognized as safe and effective (GRASE) for the claimed therapeutic indication;
- *Category II*: not generally recognized as safe and effective (NRASE) or having unacceptable indications;

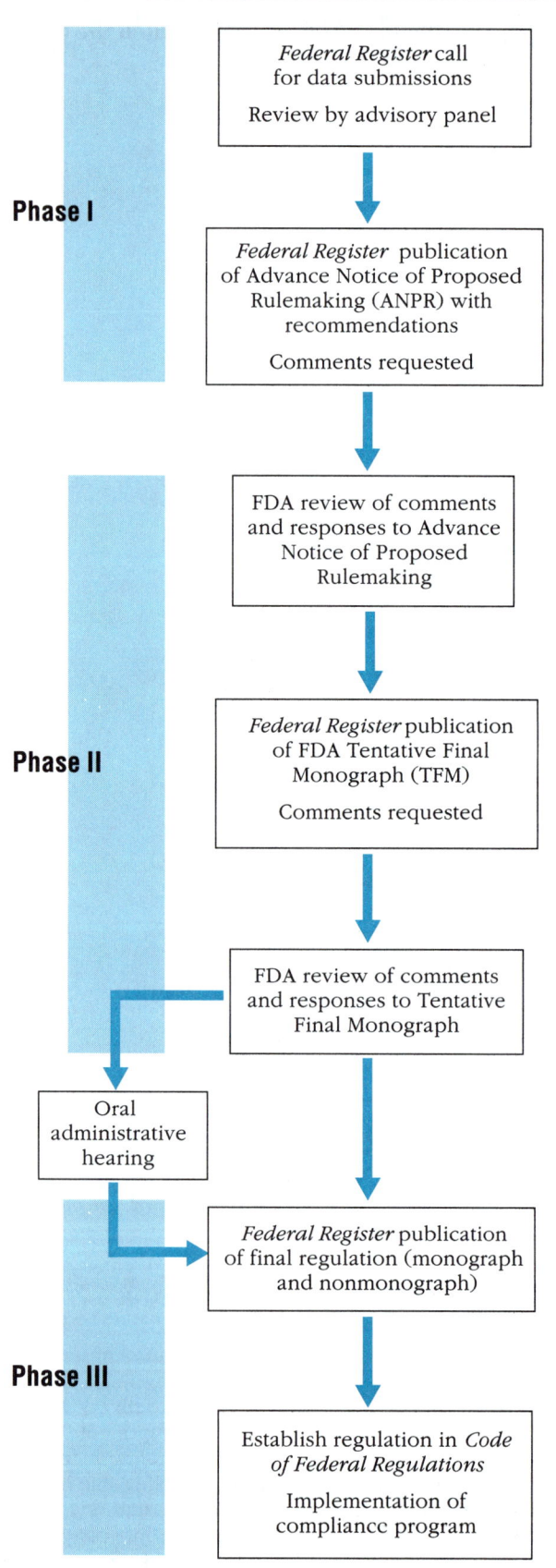

FIGURE 1 FDA's OTC drug review.

- *Category III*: insufficient data available to permit final classification.

The panels also recommended labeling (including therapeutic indications), dosage instructions, and warnings about side effects and potential misuse and abuse.

The panel phase of the review lasted a decade, with more than 300 individuals participating in this unprecedented project. Findings were based on a review of 14,000 volumes of data submitted largely by manufacturers but also by consumers, pharmacists, and other interested parties. The panels also based their judgments on their members' own clinical experience and expertise, on marketing experience of ingredients, and on controlled and uncontrolled clinical trials. The panels heavily relied on the published literature and did not take into account isolated case reports, random experience, testimonials, and reports lacking sufficient details to permit scientific evaluation.

The panels submitted a total of 58 reports to the FDA. These reports and panel-recommended monographs, which summarized the panels' recommendations to the FDA commissioner, were published in the *Federal Register* as advance notices of proposed rulemaking. Each publication invited public comment.

Throughout the OTC drug review, the FDA encouraged manufacturers of drugs under consideration to reformulate and relabel their products to comply with panel recommendations before completion of the rulemaking proceeding, and the pharmaceutical industry's compliance has been outstanding. Consequently, the public has received the benefits of the review before the issuance of final regulations, which often have required years to be completed.

Phase II: Tentative Final Monograph

The second phase of the OTC drug review is the FDA's evaluation of the panels' findings, consideration of public comment, and study of any new data that may have become available. The agency then publishes its tentative conclusions as a proposed rule (tentative final monograph). This document offers the first clear signal of the agency's ultimate intentions. After the tentative final monograph is published, a period of time is allotted for objections or for requests for a public hearing; new data may also be submitted during this period.

Phase III: Final Monograph

After considering objections and new data, and after processing requests for a hearing, the agency issues a final rule, usually in the form of a final monograph. Other final regulations, sometimes referred to as nonmonographs (in which data are insufficient to establish any ingredients or even a monograph) are also developed. These nonmonograph regulations describe ingredients that cannot lawfully be marketed or claims that are unacceptable in labeling.

Preclearance by the FDA (i.e., submission of an NDA for an OTC drug product) is not required if the regulatory standards described in the monographs are met. In essence, the FDA has already precleared the active ingredient(s) and labeling, and the final formulation is consigned to the manufacturer. Each final monograph is included in the *Code of Federal Regulations* (*CFR*), a com-

TABLE 3 Contents of an OTC drug monograph

Subpart A: General Provisions
Manufacturing practices, registration
Suitable inactive ingredients
Product container specifications
General labeling statements

Subpart B: Active Ingredients
Ingredients and concentrations
Combination with other active ingredients

Subpart C: Labeling
Indications for the product
Warnings
Drug interaction precautions
Directions for use
Specialized labeling
Professional labeling

Subpart D: Testing Procedures
Any testing necessary before marketing
Manufacturers have data on file

pilation of the regulations published daily in the *Federal Register*. Usually, monographs become effective 1 year after publication in the *Federal Register*, after which date all affected OTC drug products must meet all regulatory specifications.

After an OTC drug monograph is finalized, new conditions that are not specified in the final regulations (i.e., ingredients, combinations of ingredients, indications, and labeling) will still need to be approved. Manufacturers have two separate approaches to gain marketing clearance: submit supportive data in the form of a petition to amend a final monograph to include the new marketing conditions, or submit an NDA for OTC drug use.

Provisions of OTC Drug Monographs

Monographs contain several components (Table 3). The general provisions section (subpart A) specifies pertinent regulations detailing required conditions (such as those in manufacturing practices and drug registration) common to all OTC drug categories. This section covers inactive ingredients, requiring suitable ingredients that are safe and do not interfere with the effectiveness of the formulation or with tests to be performed on the final product. This section also contains general warning labeling requirements, such as "Keep this and all drugs out of the reach of children" and "As with any drug, if you are pregnant or nursing a baby, seek the advice of a health professional before using this product."

The active ingredients section (subpart B) identifies Category I ingredients that can be used in specific OTC drug products; it also identifies ingredients that may be

PART 338 NIGHTTIME SLEEP-AID DRUG PRODUCTS FOR OVER-THE-COUNTER HUMAN USE

Subpart A   General Provisions

Sec.
338.1   Scope.
338.3   Definition.

Subpart B   Active Ingredients

338.10   Nighttime sleep-aid active ingredients.

Subpart C   Labeling

338.50   Labeling of nighttime sleep-aid drug products.

AUTHORITY: Secs. 201, 501, 502, 503, 505, 510, 701 of the Federal Food, Drug, and Cosmetic Act (21 U.S.C. 321, 351, 352, 353, 355, 360, 371).

SOURCE: 54 FR 6826, Feb. 14, 1989, unless otherwise noted.

Subpart A   General Provisions

§ 338.1   Scope.

(a) An over-the-counter nighttime sleep-aid drug product in a form suitable for oral administration is generally recognized as safe and effective and is not misbranded if it meets each condition in this part and each general condition established in § 330.1 of this chapter.

(b) References in this part to regulatory sections of the Code of Federal Regulations are to Chapter I of Title 21 unless otherwise noted.

§ 338.3   Definition.

As used in this part:

Nighttime sleep-aid. A drug that is useful for the relief of occasional sleeplessness by individuals who have difficulty falling asleep.

Subpart B   Active Ingredients

§ 338.10 *Nighttime sleep-aid* active ingredients.

The active ingredient of the product consists of any of the following when used within the dosage limits established for each ingredient in § 338.50(d):

(a) Diphenhydramine hydrochloride.
(b) Diphenhydramine citrate.

Subpart C   Labeling

§ 338.50 Labeling of nighttime sleep-aid drug products.

(a) *Statement of identity.* The labeling of the product contains the established name of the drug, if any, and identifies the product as a "nighttime sleep-aid."

(b) *Indications.* The labeling of the product states, under the heading "Indications," one or more of the phrases listed in this paragraph. Other truthful and nonmisleading statements, describing only the indications for use that have been established and listed in this paragraph (b), may also be used, as provided in § 330.1(c)(2) of this chapter, subject to the provisions of section 502 of the act relating to misbranding and the prohibition in section 301(d) of the act against the introduction or delivery for introduction into interstate commerce of unapproved new drugs in violation of section 505(a) of the act.

(1) ("Helps you" or "Reduces time to") "fall asleep if you have difficulty falling asleep."
(2) "For relief of occasional sleeplessness."
(3) "Helps to reduce difficulty falling asleep."

(c) *Warnings.* The labeling of the product contains the following warnings under the heading "Warnings":

(1) "Do not give to children under 12 years of age."
(2) "If sleeplessness persists continuously for more than 2 weeks, consult your doctor. Insomnia may be a symptom of serious underlying medical illness."
(3) "Do not take this product if you have asthma, glaucoma, emphysema, chronic pulmonary disease, shortness of breath, difficulty in breathing, or difficulty in urination due to enlargement of the prostate gland unless directed by a doctor."
(4) "Avoid alcoholic beverage while taking this product. Do not take this product if you are taking sedatives or tranquilizers, without first consulting your doctor."

(d) *Directions.* The labeling of the product contains the following information under the heading "Directions":

(1) *For products containing diphenhydramine hydrochloride identified in § 338.10(a).* Adults and children 12 years of age and over: Oral dosage is 50 milligrams at bedtime if needed, or as directed by a doctor.

(2) *For products containing diphenhydramine citrate identified in § 338.10(b).* Adults and children 12 years of age and over: Oral dosage is 76 milligrams at bedtime if needed, or as directed by a doctor.

(e) The word "physician" may be substituted for the word "doctor" in any of the labeling statements in this section.

FIGURE 2 Monograph for OTC nighttime sleep-aid drug products.

combined with other active ingredients, not only from the same monograph but also from other monographs. An example of the latter would be the combination of an antacid with an analgesic; in this case, combinations of specific antacid and analgesic ingredients judged to be safe and effective are identified under the pertinent subsections of each of the two monographs. The regulations also set forth the number (limit) of active ingredients that may be combined in one product.

The labeling section (subpart C) contains the indications for the product; warnings against misuse, including drug interaction precautions; directions for use, including the time interval (frequency); dosage for specific age groups; and any specialized labeling. The label of an OTC drug product is of paramount importance. Unclear or ambiguous directions negate the utility of self-treatment. All instructions must be not only clear, concise, and readable but also written so that a person of low comprehension (i.e., in reading skills or language arts) can fully understand the label. For example, the term *rhinitis* is replaced by *runny nose*, and the writing style is direct and uncomplicated. A monograph may also contain professional labeling—that is, labeling provided only to health professionals but not to the general public. (See the section on labeling for professionals.)

A testing procedures section (subpart D) is included in some monographs for the testing of finished dosage forms. For example, a battery of monograph-specified acid neutralization tests is now required for all antacid products. Each antacid ingredient included in the product must be at a concentration that contributes at least 25% of the total acid-neutralizing capacity of the product, and the finished product must contain at least 5 mEq of acid-neutralizing capacity per dose and must result, at the end of the 10-minute test period, in a pH of 3.5 or greater at prescribed temperatures. Another example is the biologic tests such as enamel solubility reduction, fluoride uptake by enamel, and animal caries reduction conducted to ensure the bioavailability of fluoride ions in fluoride dentifrices. Manufacturers must ensure that their fluoride dentifrice formulations demonstrate the bioavailability of the fluoride ion in two of the three biologic tests.

A good example is the final monograph for nighttime sleep-aid products in Figure 2. A drug manufacturer need only follow the regulation describing the conditions necessary for marketing a product without preclearance by the FDA. The active ingredients are limited to diphenhydramine hydrochloride and diphenhydramine citrate in the amounts specified under directions. Labeling must identify the product as a nighttime sleep-aid and must include one or more of the indications and other truthful or not misleading statements. It is important to emphasize that the indications section is the only part of the monograph that is subject to some interpretation. The reasons for this particular exception for "indications" are discussed in the section on future labeling. All warnings must be included. They may be combined (but not rearranged to eliminate duplicative words or phrases), provided the resulting warning is clear and understandable. Finally, directions may be modified to accommodate the dosage form. For example, a 50-mg capsule product could be labeled "Adults and children 12 years of age and over: Take one capsule at bedtime if needed, or as directed by a doctor." The constraints of the monograph are exemplified in the last paragraph, where the word *physician* may be substituted only for the word *doctor*. Any variations from the monograph other than synonymous indications would result in the product being considered not GRASE.

Establishment of Nonmonographs

Sometimes the publication of the final regulation results in a nonmonograph regulation rather than a monograph regulation. This occurs when an ingredient or an entire class of products fails to demonstrate safety and/or effectiveness or provides insignificant benefits when compared with the risk from use. Thus far, nonmonographs have been established as part of the OTC drug review for the following product categories:

- Anticholinergics;
- Aphrodisiacs;
- Camphorated oil;
- Daytime sedatives;
- Hair grower/hair loss prevention;
- Halogenated salicylanilides;
- Insect repellent—oral;
- Stomach acidifier;
- Sweet spirits of nitre;
- Topical hormones;
- Zirconium aerosols.

More nonmonographs are expected to be established over the next few years. For example, the FDA has not been able to determine the effectiveness of atropine sulfate and all other active ingredients considered for use as anticholinergics in cough and cold products to relieve excessive secretions of the nose and eyes. The tentative final monograph stated that there was a lack of adequate studies available to support the continued use of these ingredients. No substantive data were received in response to the tentative final monograph that would have allowed any anticholinergic ingredient to be upgraded to Category I. Thus, no monograph could be established.

The nonmonograph regulation may also occur when an ingredient or an entire class of products provides insignificant benefits when compared with the risk from use. Zirconium, once widely used in aerosol antiperspirants, was removed from aerosol drug and cosmetic products because of the potential for particulate zirconium to cause granuloma formation in the lungs. Because there was not enough toxicologic data to establish a safe level for use of zirconium and safer products were available, the agency concluded that the poor benefit-to-risk ratio precluded the use of zirconium in aerosol products.

Similarly, the nonmonograph regulation may occur when OTC marketing of a particular ingredient or product is potentially hazardous. For example, camphorated oil, marketed primarily as a topical counterirritant or liniment, was often visually mistaken for castor oil, cod liver oil, mineral oil, olive oil, cough medicine, or other drug products. The OTC marketing of camphorated oil drug products resulted in a large number of accidental ingestions, which often led to toxicity, primarily in infants and young children. Based on the potential hazard of poisoning, the FDA judged the benefits of such products insignificant when compared with the risks.

Daytime sedatives were an interesting and challenging dilemma for the OTC advisory review panel examining them. These products usually contained an antihistamine with labeling claims for tension or anxiety. The central issue debated was whether OTC drugs should be available to sedate people during normal waking hours. While conceding that nighttime sleep-aid drug products (often higher doses of the same drugs) deserve a place in the OTC drug review, the panel concluded that anyone who needed to be sedated during the day had a condition that was not amenable to self-treatment. Subsequently, the entire class of daytime sedatives was removed from the OTC drug marketplace.

Impact of the Review

The review has generated substantial scientific research that has produced impressive amounts of new data on OTC drugs, and additional data have been developed on many of the ingredients to demonstrate their safety and effectiveness. However, ingredients that could not be shown to be both safe and effective for their intended uses have been (and continue to be) dropped from formulations. A few ingredients were found to be so unsafe that they were removed from the market before the full rulemaking process was completed.

Collectively, the review panels examined 722 active ingredients for different uses. Some ingredients have more than one use, resulting in 1,454 ingredients for specific uses with the following results:

- About one-third of the ingredients were judged to be safe and effective for their intended use. Major brand products contain Category I ingredients.
- One-third of the ingredients were found to be largely ineffective, and a few were found to be potentially unsafe. Many of the ingredients in this group had a single or limited use. The very few ingredients whose safety could not be ensured—such as hexachlorophene, methapyrilene, and tribromsalan—have already been removed from the marketplace.
- One-third of the ingredients needed additional data to establish safety and effectiveness. Many have already been upgraded based on new information or additional studies.

The agency also needed to address the marketing of ingredients that the advisory review panels had not found to be effective.

Through a separate rulemaking (commonly referred to as the OTC wrap-up regulation—phase I), the agency proposed to remove 259 ingredients (142 in Category II and 117 in Category III) covering 22 classes of OTC drug products. The FDA gave interested parties 60 days to object but stated that no new scientific data could be submitted. In all instances, it had provided manufacturers with numerous opportunities to prove that the ingredients were effective and had received no significant comments or data. As a result of comments that were received, some minor changes were made, and the final rule, which was published in 1990, removed 223 ingredients.

A second similar rulemaking in 1993 (OTC wrap-up regulation—phase II) removed 415 ingredients (323 in Category II and 92 in Category III) covering seven classes of OTC drug products. In almost every case, the drug manufacturers have already reformulated their products, as illustrated by the significant lack of comment on these proposals.

Drugs Reclassified from Prescription to OTC Status

The OTC drug review is primarily responsible for the reclassification of many drugs from prescription to OTC status. These are often referred to as "switch drugs," and the reclassification process is referred to as "switching from prescription to OTC." Nearly 40 ingredients incorporated into many more drug products have been reclassified since the review began. This reclassification is seen by many as an important health measure, providing consumers with effective medications and curtailing the high cost of health care. Pharmacists should find many new consultative opportunities with this expanding segment of the OTC marketplace. (See Chapter 1, "The Self-Care Movement," and Chapter 2, "Patient Assessment and Consultation.")

Criteria for Reclassification

Until 1951, federal law did not contain criteria for determining whether a drug should be limited to prescription use. This decision was left to the manufacturer, and different manufacturers made different decisions about the same drug formulations, leading to confusion among manufacturers, regulators, health professionals, and the general public. There were serious questions related to the FDA's authority to permit refill authorizations or to limit drug prescribing to physicians. To end the confusion, Congress enacted an amendment to the basic law, specifying three classes of drugs that were limited to prescription use:

- Certain habit-forming drugs listed by name in the Act;
- Drugs not safe for use except under the supervision of a licensed practitioner because of toxicity or other potential for harmful effect, the method of use, or the collateral measures necessary to use;
- Drugs limited to prescription under an NDA.

These statutory definitions, along with the basic statutory language requiring adequate directions for use, are still the principal criteria for determining prescription versus OTC drug classification.

In considering reclassification, the second criterion is probably the most essential and is worthy of close examination. The assessment of the overall margin of safety includes not only those considerations described in the statute (toxicity, potential for harmful effects, method of use, and collateral measures necessary to use), but also the potential for abuse and misuse and the benefit-to-risk ratio.

Many drugs administered to treat serious disease conditions may cause adverse side effects. These drugs must be used carefully to achieve the appropriate level of effectiveness without endangering patient safety. They are therefore too toxic to be used for self-treatment and will continue to be classified as prescription drugs. However, because any

FDA guidelines on soliciting advisors' opinions:

add margin of safety

- What is the product's toxicity?
- Do the methods of use preclude OTC availability?
- Is there other potential for harmful effects (including misuse)?
- Is the product habit forming?
- What is the potential for abuse?
- Do the benefits outweigh the risks?

plus collateral measures necessary to use

- Is the condition self-diagnosable?
- Is the condition self-treatable?

plus adequate labeling

- Can adequate directions for use be written?
- Can warnings against unsafe use be written?
- Can labeling be read and understood by the ordinary individual?

plus additional labeling

equals

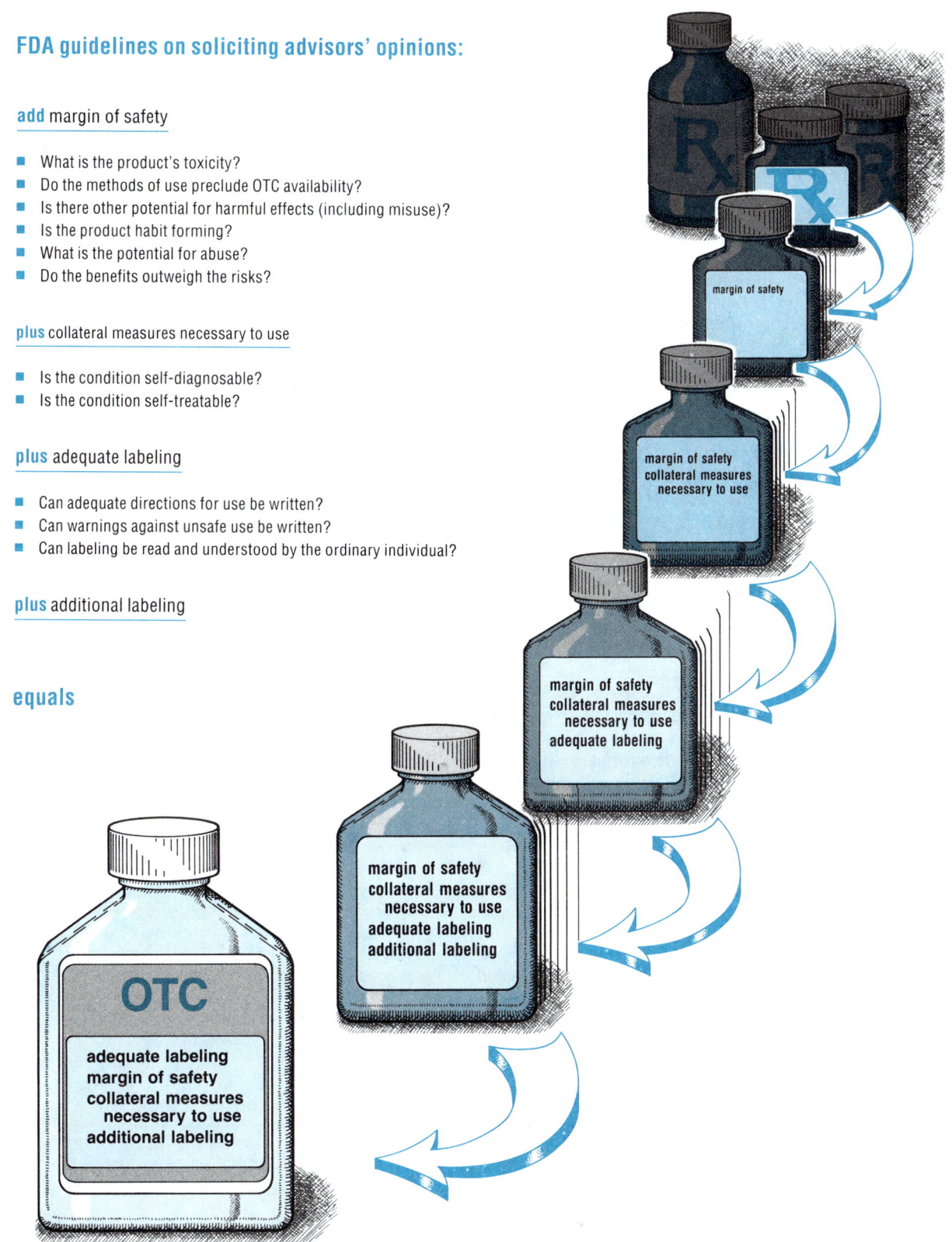

FIGURE 3 Reclassifying prescription drugs as OTC drugs.

drug can be misused with some toxic result, the possibility that a drug can be misused is not the sole basis for prescription classification. Because all drugs have both benefits and risks, some degree of risk must be tolerated for patients to receive the benefits. For example, antihistamine drugs may cause drowsiness. However, consumers can be informed of the risks through adequate directions for use in product labeling.

It is impossible to set exact standards or reclassification criteria because so many factors must be carefully considered as illustrated in Figure 3. The classification is judgmental, based on the various factors related to each drug's use, risks, and benefits. Accordingly, many FDA personnel from diverse agency offices are consulted in an effort to form a consensus on each switch drug candidate. The process is lengthy and extremely thorough. Some drugs have been limited to prescription use, not because the drug is believed to be inherently toxic but because of concerns for adverse effects with intentional abuse; amyl nitrite is an example.

Mechanisms for Reclassification

Four basic mechanisms exist for the reclassification of prescription drugs to OTC status (Figure 4).

Mechanism 1
A new, full NDA may be submitted for a currently marketed prescription drug. The application might contain new clinical studies to support a specific OTC indication using a lower prescription strength. For example, a prescription drug may be available at 25 mg, 50 mg, and 100 mg, and the studies supporting OTC use are conducted using the 25-mg dosage. In this case, because new studies have been conducted, the sponsor of the approved NDA will have marketing exclusivity for several years. Other manufacturers would need to duplicate the studies during that period.

Mechanism 2
The "switch regulation" provides that drugs limited to prescription use under an NDA can be exempted from that limitation if the FDA determines the prescription requirements to be unnecessary for the protection of the public health. The regulation allows a petition for such an exemption to be initiated by the FDA or by any interested person. Before the OTC drug review began in 1972, the FDA used this mechanism to reclassify 25 ingredients to OTC status, the last being the antifungal tolnaftate in 1971.

Mechanism 3
A prescription drug that already has an approved NDA can be reclassified to OTC status through the filing and agency approval of a supplement to the NDA. This alternative has in most respects replaced the switch regulation procedure. The FDA determines whether the drug, which was previously limited under the terms of its NDA, has now been shown to be safe for OTC use. In some cases, the same prescription dosage is considered for OTC status. Heavy reliance is placed on the extent of marketing experience and degree of adverse findings. Under either the switch regulation or the supplement to the NDA, the reclassified drug product remains a "new drug" requiring premarket approval and periodic reports to the FDA.

Mechanism 4
Finally, using a completely different process, nearly 40 ingredients have been switched through the OTC drug review. Asked to make recommendations on any drugs that could be safely converted to OTC status, the advisory panels recommended changing many ingredients—including hydrocortisone, diphenhydramine, nystatin, and oxymetazoline—from prescription use to OTC drug availability. In some cases, the dosage was increased for marketed OTC ingredients (e.g., 2 mg of chlorphemiramine was elevated to 4 mg). Comments and petitions by manufacturers as part of the OTC drug review also have contributed to enlarging the number of available OTC ingredients.

Examples of Reclassification Efforts

Until 1980, most prescription to OTC switches occurred through the OTC review process. As previously mentioned, only the active ingredient was approved for switching and not the entire product. However, most recently, switching has primarily occurred through the new drug approval system, necessitating approval of the entire product. Most future switches will probably occur through this system, which many manufacturers prefer because it ensures some market advantages, given that competitors are required to file NDAs, supplements, or abbreviated NDAs.

Examples of reclassified drugs using the monograph or NDA approach appear in Table 4. Although many drugs have been reclassified, the FDA's experience with reclassification has been varied.

Hydrocortisone
Since 1952, hydrocortisone has been marketed in the United States as a prescription drug. The first effort to change the drug to OTC status occurred in 1956, and public hearings were held to examine a petition request for reclassification. Based on these hearings, the petition was denied. However, in December 1979, an FDA OTC advisory review panel recommended to the agency that hydrocortisone could be considered safe and effective for OTC use at concentrations of 0.25–0.5%. Based on the panel's recommendations, the agency allowed OTC marketing.

After nearly a decade of OTC use of hydrocortisone, some manufacturers stated that reports from consumers and physicians, as well as data from clinical investigators, indicated that these concentrations did not provide the optimal therapy in all individuals for all the conditions for which the drug may be used. They suggested that a 1% concentration of hydrocortisone would provide a more effective treatment for pruritus and inflammation associated with the conditions listed in the OTC labeling. In May 1987, the FDA received a citizen petition requesting OTC marketing status for 1% hydrocortisone. The petition discussed the history of hydrocortisone use, the drug's safety and effectiveness, its approval for OTC use in foreign countries, drug experience reports, and the proposed OTC labeling. The petition also included extensive data and information from published studies on issues related to the safety and

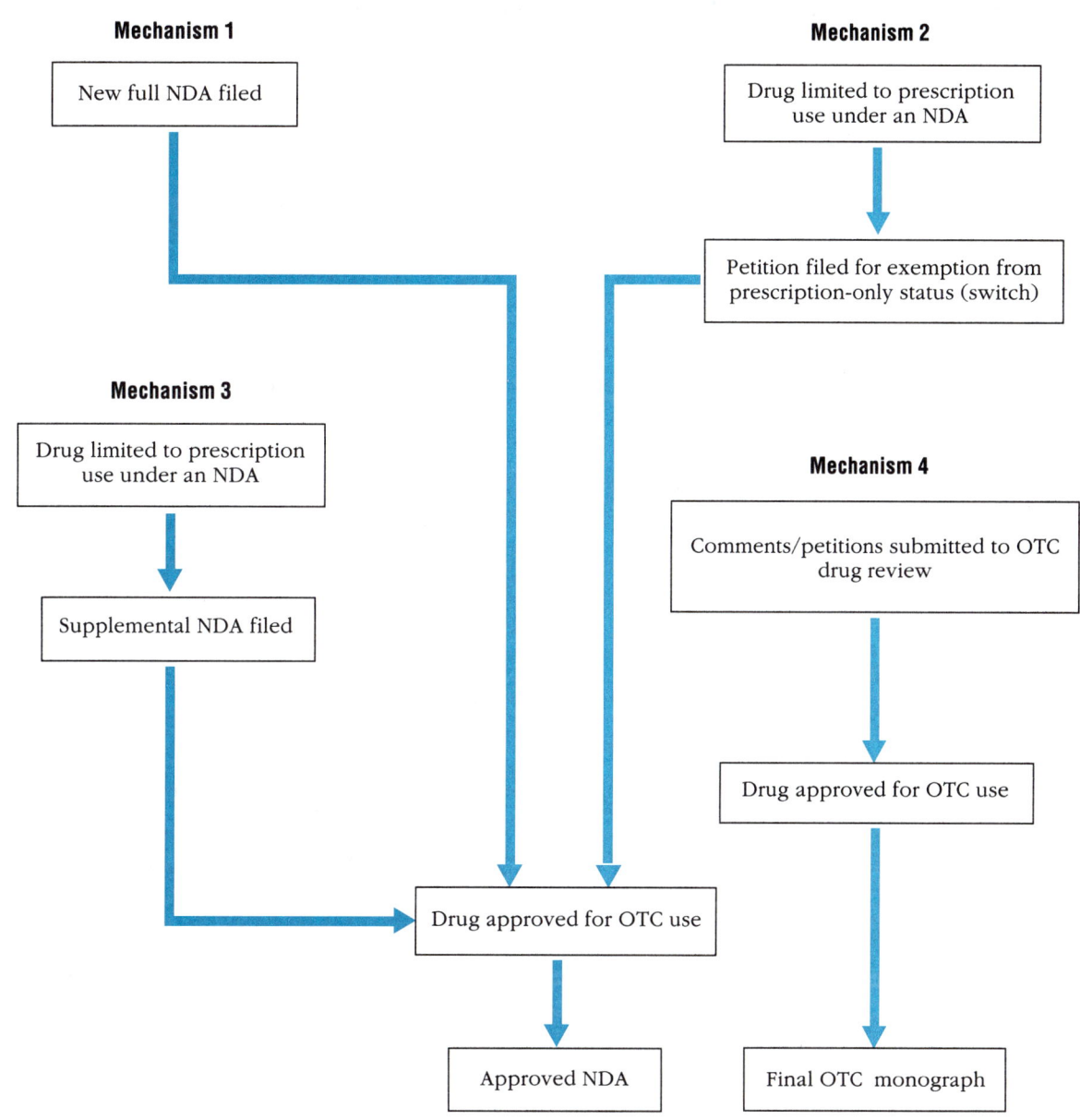

FIGURE 4 Mechanisms for reclassifying prescription drugs to OTC status.

effectiveness of topical hydrocortisone. It noted that more than 130 million OTC units of 0.5% hydrocortisone had been bought in this country to date, and most of the negative reports received by manufacturers of these products involved a lack of effectiveness.

After carefully reviewing the information submitted, the agency postulated that concentrations of hydrocortisone of 0.5–1% could be marketed OTC. Accordingly, in February 1990, the agency published a notice of proposed rulemaking to invite public comment. Numerous comments were received both for and against the proposal; most were of a testimonial nature without substantive data, and no new information was provided. In August 1991, the FDA published a notice allowing 1% hydrocortisone to be available for OTC use. Currently, only the single-ingredient hydrocortisone is marketed for OTC use through the monograph system. However, because of pending submissions to the agency, combinations with other ingredients will probably be available in the future.

Metaproterenol

In October 1982, the FDA proposed a monograph for OTC bronchodilator drug products. In this document was the agency's decision to classify the metaproterenol sulfate in a metered-dose inhalation aerosol as an OTC Category I drug. The agency had carefully reviewed the safety and effectiveness record of the drug, which structurally is a

TABLE 4 Examples of former prescription ingredients now available for OTC use

Status	Ingredient	Purpose
M[a]	Acidulated phosphate fluoride	Dental rinse
M	Brompheniramine maleate	Hay fever, dries runny nose
M	Chlorpheniramine maleate	Hay fever, dries runny nose
N[b]	Clemastine fumarate	Antihistamine
N	Clotrimazole	Antifungal
M	Dexbrompheniramine	Hay fever, dries runny nose
M	Diphenhydramine hydrochloride	Antitussive (cough control)
M	Diphenhydramine hydrochloride	Nighttime sleep aid
M	Diphenhydramine monocitrate	Nighttime sleep aid
N	Doxylamine succinate	Nighttime sleep aid
M	Dyclonine hydrochloride	Oral anesthetic
M	Ephedrine sulfate	Vasoconstrictor (hemorrhoidal)
M	Haloprogin	Antifungal
M	Hydrocortisone	Antipruritic (for itching)
M	Hydrocortisone acetate	Antipruritic (for itching)
N	Ibuprofen	Analgesic
N	Loperamide	Antidiarrheal
N	Miconazole nitrate	Antifungal
M	Oxymetazoline hydrochloride	Nasal decongestant
N	Permethrin	Pediculocide
M	Phenylephrine hydrochloride	Vasoconstrictor (hemorrhoidal)
M	Pseudoephedrine hydrochloride	Nasal decongestant
M	Pseudoephedrine sulfate	Nasal decongestant
M	Pyrantel pamoate	Anthelmintic (pinworm remedy)
M	Sodium fluoride	Dental rinse
M	Stannous fluoride	Dental rinse/gel
M	Triprolidine hydrochloride	Hay fever, dries runny nose
M	Xylometazoline hydrochloride	Nasal decongestant

[a]Reclassification approved under the monograph system.
[b]Reclassification approved under the new drug application system.

member of the same family of drugs as epinephrine. Metaproterenol had a record of safe and effective use under an approved NDA for 9 years. Based on a review of the adverse reaction reports for the drug under clinical studies since the time the drug was approved for marketing, the agency believed the drug could be safely reclassified to OTC use. The agency proposed extensive labeling information for the public.

With the publication of that monograph, immediate marketing was permitted and initiated. This was the first time that the FDA, on its own initiative, had recommended reclassifying the marketing status of a prescription drug as part of the OTC drug review. (Previous reclassifications had been recommended by advisory panels.) Adhering to the OTC rulemaking process, the agency provided an opportunity for public comment that is unavailable when approving an NDA or a supplemental NDA. After OTC marketing began in January 1983, the medical community voiced considerable criticism. By May, the FDA had received approximately 120 letters, many of which expressed concern about the drug's potential for misuse and inappropriate use by young children.

In May 1983 a special meeting of the FDA's standing pulmonary–allergy drugs advisory committee was called to provide a public forum to discuss these concerns. The committee voted 4 to 3 to recommend that the FDA rescind its proposal to make metaproterenol an OTC drug. The committee also believed that this issue merited further discussion. In the interim, products containing metaproterenol were limited to prescription status.

Ibuprofen

Ibuprofen is available for OTC use via NDAs, not monograph. The agency does not consider ibuprofen to be a reclassifed drug because the 200-mg strength currently available OTC was never marketed as a prescription-only drug in the United States. Although experience with ibuprofen marketed at prescription strengths (300, 400, 600, and 800 mg) is pertinent, it is not considered to be support for the proposal that the lower dosage product could be used safely and effectively as an OTC drug.

Some have argued that public data are sufficient to include ibuprofen in the monograph system. However, although the availability of data is clearly necessary for the OTC review, such data do not automatically lead to the general recognition among experts that a prescription drug is safe for OTC use. Published data relating primarily to the prescription strengths of ibuprofen were not regarded as sufficient to support a general recognition of OTC acceptability. Prior to recommending OTC status, the FDA's arthritis advisory committee also reviewed confidential ibuprofen NDA material.

Even if the investigations reported in the medical literature had been sufficient for the 200-mg strength of ibuprofen to be considered GRASE, the FDA concluded that ibuprofen in that strength should be regarded as a new drug because it had not been used to a material extent and for a material time. Such a drug has historically not been considered appropriate for inclusion in a monograph. However, this does not mean that, at some future date and following longer and more extensive marketing experience, ibuprofen could not be incorporated into the OTC internal analgesic drug monograph.

Promethazine

The cough and cold advisory review panel classified promethazine hydrochloride in Category I as an OTC antihistamine, but the FDA dissented. The dissent was based on both the degree of drowsiness produced by the ingredient and the possible adverse effects (e.g., extrapyramidal disturbances) that might occur, especially in children. However, after the 1985 tentative final monograph stated that additional data had adequately addressed concerns regarding extrapyramidal effects and the concern that children seem particularly susceptible to developing adverse central nervous system reactions to promethazine, the FDA did not believe that these possible adverse effects should preclude the use of this ingredient at proposed OTC oral dosages.

Still, the agency noted that promethazine had not been used extensively on a long-term basis as a single ingredient for antihistamine, allergic rhinitis, or antiallergy use, and that consumers who use OTC antihistamines to treat such symptoms often use these products for a prolonged period. Accordingly, it placed single-ingredient products in Category III because of concerns that tardive dyskinesia, a rare but serious central nervous system reaction, might occur with prolonged use. Promethazine as a prescription drug is primarily found in combination products for short-term relief of acute cough and cold symptoms.

In a 1988 tentative final monograph (for OTC combination drug products), the FDA proposed that cough–cold combination products containing promethazine hydrochloride be classified as Category I and used only for short-term (7 days) relief of symptoms of the common cold. That action permitted OTC marketing for this limited use. Claims for the use of these drug products in treating the symptoms of allergic rhinitis were specifically excluded from the labeling. However, the agency later received a citizen petition and letters from a number of physicians objecting to promethazine's OTC drug status based on new information. The major concern was that the drug's use in children under 2 years of age may be associated with sudden infant death syndrome, and that OTC availability could dramatically increase overuse in children of this age. The FDA's pulmonary–allergy drugs advisory committee then met to discuss these issues and evaluate the new information. By a vote of 7 to 1, the committee recommended to the FDA that these drug products not be marketed as OTC products at this time. It should be noted that, during this deliberation period, the major drug manufacturer participated in the proceedings and did not market the product.

Subsequent *Federal Register* notices announced that promethazine-containing combination drug products could not be marketed OTC, but the FDA did reopen the record to allow additional information to be filed. The 1992 OTC antihistamine final monograph did not include promethazine as a single ingredient. The switchability of the drug in cough–cold combination drug products will be discussed in that final rule, yet to be issued.

Future Reclassifications

The reclassification explosion that occurred during the OTC drug review is over. Reclassification will now be less frequent but is expected to continue at a consistent pace. More than 20 switch applications are now under active consideration within the FDA. Some are breakthrough categories in which no comparable OTC drug products are currently available. Interest has been heightened not only by the OTC drug review, but also by the fact that many drugs are available for OTC use worldwide that are currently only marketed by prescription in this country.

Even though switch NDAs are confidential, industry news releases and the trade press have revealed active interest in products in several categories: cough–cold–allergy, analgesics, antacids, smoking cessation, baldness treatment, and cardiovascular conditions.

The FDA has not provided switch guidelines because each product or drug must be considered uniquely and individually. Nevertheless, switch principles have been discussed by agency personnel. The following informal principles are worth noting because they reflect the scientific scrutiny applied by the agency:

- Does the switch candidate have special toxicity in its class?
- Does the candidate have a large margin of safety?

- Does the candidate's frequency of dosing affect its safe use?
- Has the candidate's safety profile been defined at high dose?
- Has the candidate been used for a sufficiently long time (3–5 years) on the prescription market to enable a full characterization of its safety profile?
- What is the worldwide marketing experience of the switch candidate?
- What foreign countries market the candidate for OTC use? What is its experience in those countries?
- What do the "Use Data" (from the National Prescription Audit, the National Drug/Disease Audit, and/or other sources) show?
- Has a vigorous risk analysis been performed?
- Has the efficacy literature been reviewed in a way to support the expected usage and labeling of the switch candidate?
- Is there a full understanding of the pharmacodynamics of the switch candidate?
- Is the minimally effective dose for the proposed OTC indication known? (In some cases, it could be necessary.)
- Have possible drug interactions for the switch candidate been characterized?

Drug Information: Labeling and Advertising

Labeling

For Consumers

The OTC drug regulations require that labeling be in terms that are likely to be read and understood by consumers of low comprehension and under customary conditions of purchase and use. In addition to evaluating the content of the labeling recommended by the panels, the FDA also evaluates the language to ensure that it is likely to be understood by the consumer. A typical OTC drug product and the required labeling information are illustrated for a cough mixture in Figure 5. As a result of the OTC drug review, the labeling of every OTC drug product will be revised.

For Professionals

Some monographs contain professional labeling that provides specific information not included in OTC drug labeling, such as an ulcer therapy indication for antacids. As part of the professional labeling for the internal analgesic tentative final monograph, the FDA has proposed including the ingredient aspirin for "reducing the risk of recurrent transient ischemic attacks (TIAs) or stroke in men" and "to reduce the risk of death and/or nonfatal myocardial infarction in patients with a previous myocardial infarction or unstable angina pectoris." Proposed changes (pending public response) will be implemented upon publication of the final monograph. Obviously, consumers are aware of these uses from the news media, their physicians, and other sources.

Future Labeling

An early policy of the OTC drug review maintained the FDA's long-standing position strictly limiting the labeling terminology to the exact language developed and approved in the applicable monograph. This policy did not allow for synonymous terms or any variation in the labeling.

The agency received many comments on this "exclusivity policy," particularly regarding indications for use. Manufacturers and trade associations contended that the policy was unconstitutional because it unlawfully restrained free speech, was arbitrary and capricious, and was not authorized. Consumer groups urged the FDA to retain the policy to avoid confusion and deception and to ease comparisons among products.

Recognizing that, within limits, there are numerous ways of accurately stating the same concept, the agency concluded that it could still meet its responsibilities of ensuring accurate and truthful labeling while providing greater flexibility. These new regulations, which are now finalized, establish three ways of stating the indications for use in OTC drug labeling.

Style 1 The first style follows the monograph. It requires that the labeling be contained in a prominent and conspicuous location, that it be easily read at the time of purchase, and that it use terminology describing the indications for use that have been established in the applicable final monograph. The terminology should appear within a boxed area designated "Approved Uses" each time it appears in the labeling (e.g., on the outer carton, on the inner bottle label, and in any package insert). The manufacturer could also include other OTC drug labeling requirements within the boxed area. In such cases, the boxed area would be designated "Approved Information" rather than "Approved Uses." A statement that the information in the box was approved by the FDA would appear within or close to the boxed area. In lieu of such a statement, manufacturers could modify the designation of the boxed area to read "FDA Approved Uses" or "FDA Approved Information," as appropriate, or could employ "Uses (or Information) Approved by the Food and Drug Administration" or other similar wording.

The agency anticipates that consumers will look for the approved labeling when purchasing OTC drug products, thereby providing an incentive for manufacturers to use this alternative.

Style 2 The second style follows the monograph but allows interpretations. In addition to the wording required in the boxed area (first style), the label and labeling could contain, outside the boxed area, alternative wording to describe indications for use that have been established in an applicable monograph. This additional wording may not be false or misleading.

Style 3 The third style interprets the monograph and permits manufacturers to state the indications for use in a prominent and conspicuous place in the labeling, using synonymous, truthful, and nonmisleading language. The language describes those indications for use that have been developed in a relevant monograph, subject to the prohibition against false or misleading labeling. However, such alternative terminology cannot be boxed and cannot contain either the "Approved Uses" or "Approved Information" designation or any statement asserting or implying that the

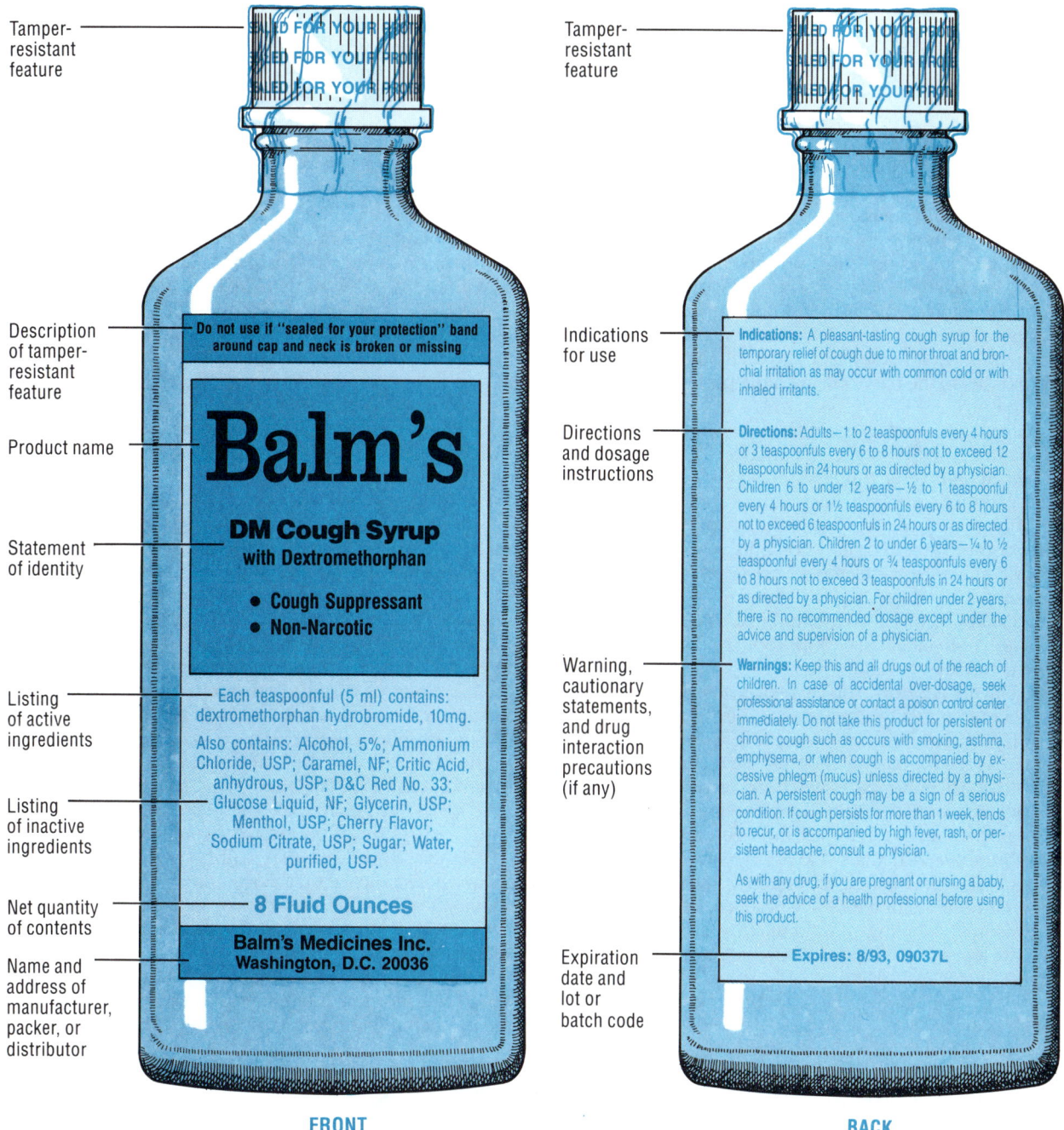

FIGURE 5 Required labeling information on OTC drug products.

indications statement was approved by the FDA. The language must be consistent with that indication for use and must not imply or indicate a use that is not established under a relevant monograph. Alternative language representing or suggesting that use of the drug is safe and effective for indications other than those in an appropriate final monograph would make the drug product a new drug, for which an approved NDA would be required.

Readability

Many individuals have argued that OTC labels are still too difficult to understand and that the print size is often not legible, especially to vision-impaired persons. The monographs establish required labeling but do not address print size. Currently, there are also no specific statutory or regulatory requirements that address the print size and style of the OTC drug product labels. However, regulations do address the prominence of required label statements and describe a number of situations in which information on a drug product's label may lack prominence and conspicuousness. For example, the statement of identity of an OTC drug product must appear in boldface type on the principal display panel, in a size reasonably related to the most prominent printed matter on that panel, and in lines generally parallel to the base on which the package rests when displayed.

Future labels will contain more information and may be difficult to include on small containers. In the past, the FDA has encouraged manufacturers to include a statement on the product container label, carton, or package insert suggesting that the patient retain the carton or insert when all the required labeling does not appear on the container label. Manufacturers are free to design ways of incorporating such labeling (e.g., by using flap, wraparound, or fold-over labels, or by redesigning cartons or containers to provide more label space with room for larger and more legible print).

A citizen petition from a pharmacist has requested that a federal regulation be issued setting optimum standards for print size and style in labels. This petition cites several reasons for these standards: (1) medication misuse and abuse; (2) continued switching of drugs with their attendant side effects and cautions on use; (3) the multitude of packaging of all shapes and sizes; and (4) inability of most people, particularly elderly persons, to read small print and vital information required by FDA. Several congressional subcommittees have also expressed concern that consumer labeling is difficult to read. In 1990, the California legislature enacted a bill that required manufacturers to evaluate labeling of OTC drugs and to provide for labeling to maximize the readability and clarity of label information.

The Nonprescription Drug Manufacturers Association (NDMA), which represents most OTC drug manufacturers, has issued voluntary industry guidelines that identify specific factors to improve the readability of OTC labels. These factors fall into two general categories: layout and design, and typography and printing.

In 1991, the FDA published a notice in the *Federal Register* summarizing the citizen petition for public comment. The agency stated that it was seeking information and views on the feasibility of establishing federal regulations on the print size and style of OTC labeling. Comments were asked for the following questions:

- Are current print sizes, types, colors, contrasts, backgrounds, etc., of OTC drug labeling adequate in providing readable information both for individuals with normal eyesight and for those with poor or deteriorating eyesight?
- Should there be a mandatory minimum print size or other readability standard. If so, what should it be, and should it be established via a regulation or a guideline?
- What relevant data are available and what studies have been performed to determine optimum print size, background, contrast, etc., for package products?
- What adverse effects have been documented that are associated with the inability or failure to read labels on OTC drug products?
- Should a package insert or larger carton be mandatory if a minimum print size standard is implemented that the manufacturer is unable to meet because of package size?
- What impact would a federal legibility/readability regulation have on state laws that relate to "slack-fill"?
- Will the NDMA guidelines be effective and have a positive impact on labeling, and, if so, are these guidelines adequate so that a federal regulation or guideline is not needed?

Many comments have been received from consumers, manufacturers, health professionals, and others. Most favor some form of regulation or guideline to improve label readability. As of the writing of this chapter, the agency had made no decision.

In the meantime, most major OTC drug manufacturers have begun a review of the labeling of currently marketed products using the NDMA guidelines. In addition, the FDA and the Federal Trade Commission (FTC) have begun a two-phase study of OTC drug labels. The first phase will seek to establish legibility criteria for OTC drug labels. Labeling for existing products will be examined, and examples of easy-to-read and hard-to-read labels will be chosen. These labels will then be shown to a sample of consumers, and measurements of the degree to which the consumers can read the material (i.e., discern the words or sentences) will be taken. This study will serve as a basis for FDA standards of legibility. The second phase of the FDA/FTC study will test consumer understanding of OTC labels. Several studies will be performed to test (1) comprehensibility of OTC terminology and alternative terminology, and (2) current formats with revised formats that more clearly communicate important directions, warnings, and precautions.

It would appear reasonable to await the implementation of the industry guidelines and complete the labeling surveys before acting on the citizen petition.

Advertising

The FDA does not regulate or have authority over OTC drug advertising. Such authority rests with the FTC, which, at one time, proposed to allow in OTC drug advertising only those indications established in the final monograph. The FTC, however, has since rejected this approach. It will instead decide such matters on a case-by-case basis, considering the FDA's findings on the safety and effectiveness of OTC drugs in weighing advertising claims.

New Challenges

Office of OTC Drugs

Until the OTC drug review began in 1972, no FDA office existed for the specific purpose of handling currently marketed OTC drugs. Initially, a staff in the Bureau of Drugs assisted the advisory review panels in reviewing ingredients, labeling, and warnings for marketed OTC drugs and promulgated the resulting *Federal Register* documents. In 1977, a larger, more formal organization was created with the Division of OTC Drug Evaluation in the Center for Drug Evaluation and Research (CDER). However, during this time, most issues concerning new drugs (including reclassification applications) were handled in the appropriate new drug divisions of CDER, not by the OTC division.

In 1991, the Division of OTC Drug Evaluation was restructured as the Office of OTC Drug Evaluation. This office now complements the new drug evaluation divisions dealing with NDAs and prescription switches. The new office includes a monograph review staff, a medical review staff, and a drug policy staff, which is designed to address contemporary OTC drug issues such as prescription-to-OTC switching, new OTC drugs, international harmonization, and the need to control health care costs.

Nonprescription Drug Advisory Committee

Since the termination of the last OTC drug advisory panel in 1981, no specific advisory body has routinely examined OTC issues. At times, standing prescription drug advisory panels have considered OTC ingredients.

In 1991, the FDA announced the establishment of the Nonprescription Drug Advisory Committee to review and evaluate the safety and effectiveness of OTC drug products and serve as a forum for the exchange of views regarding the prescription and nonprescription status of various drugs. A core committee of 10 members with broad experience and expertise was established. Members include knowledgeable experts in the fields of internal medicine, obstetrics and gynecology, dermatology, epidemiology, pharmacy, clinical pharmacology, pediatrics, and related specialties. The first chairperson is a pharmacist. The core committee may draw on members of other FDA committees for specific expertise on individual issues. For example, if a topical preparation were being considered, several dermatologists could be included. The new committee also includes a voting consumer representative and a nonvoting industry liaison. The first meeting was held in December 1992 to consider the pharmaceutical role of alcohol in OTC products. New lower limits were recommended for products intended for oral ingestion.

Chapter 4

In-Home Testing and Monitoring Products

Susan M. Meyer

Questions to ask in patient assessment and counseling

Blood Pressure Monitoring

- *Do you or any family members have a history of high blood pressure?*
- *Are you taking any medications to control high blood pressure?*
- *Has your physician told you what blood pressure values are normal for you? Do you know what your blood pressure values have been?*
- *Do you monitor your blood pressure? If so, when do you normally take your blood pressure readings (i.e., time of day, before or after certain activities)? Do you take your blood pressure readings by yourself or does someone assist you?*

Fecal Occult Blood Test Kits

- *How old are you?*
- *Have you ever suffered from any bowel disorder? Have you or anyone in your family had colorectal cancer? Have any family members suffered from stomach or colon problems (e.g., ulcers or hemorrhoids)?*
- *What nonprescription or prescription medications are you currently taking?*

Ovulation Prediction Test Kits

- *Are you currently taking any nonprescription or prescription medications?*
- *Do you have any chronic medical conditions?*
- *Are you consulting or have you consulted a doctor who specializes in fertility problems?*
- *Have you ever used a product like this? If so, how did you use it?*
- *Tell me about how "regular" your periods are.*

Pregnancy Test Kits

- *How late is your period?*
- *Are you currently taking any nonprescription or prescription medications on a routine basis? Do you have any chronic medical conditions?*
- *Have you ever used a pregnancy test before? If so, which one?*

In-home test kits are becoming more important in health care because of increased emphasis on preventive medicine, increased public health awareness, and the strong trend toward self-care. Sales of in-home tests are expected to exceed $1 billion by the early 1990s.[1,2] Contributing to the success of these tests are the increased acceptance of technology by the public and improvements in biotechnology, resulting in more tests that are easy to use. These advances in biotechnology have made it possible for an increased variety of tests to be done at home.[3] A major technological development has been the use of an enzyme-linked immunoassay (ELISA) with monoclonal antibodies. These organic molecules bind uniquely to a target antigen. Because of this specificity and ability to detect small amounts of the target antigen (i.e., sensitivity), the use of monoclonal antibodies has led to the development of highly accurate and reliable tests for in-home use.

In-home kits contribute to the overall health care of a patient by encouraging early detection and treatment and, if necessary, careful monitoring of various conditions.[4] Some test kits are designed to detect the signs of a condition (e.g., fecal occult blood in colorectal cancer), whereas others monitor a chronic condition and its treatment (e.g., blood glucose testing in diabetes).

The in-home test kit market creates an important role for pharmacists in patient education because these test kits can provide useful information and be cost-effective only if they are used and interpreted correctly.[5] Most manufacturers of in-home test kits claim better than 95% accuracy if the user *strictly* adheres to the instructions and recommended procedure. For example, patients need to know when to use a particular in-home test, how to use it properly, and how to interpret test results. Thus, it is increasingly important for the pharmacist to remain current and knowledgeable as products are simplified and moved out of the physician's office into the pharmacy and as new products are introduced.

Home Blood Pressure Monitoring

Hypertension affects approximately 60 million Americans; several million more individuals suffer from the disease but remain undiagnosed. Left untreated, high blood pressure can result in stroke, heart disease, or kidney disease, all of which may be fatal. Through early diagnosis, compliance with a treatment regimen, and appropriate monitoring of blood pressure over time, hypertension can be controlled and the long-term complications avoided.[6,7]

Blood pressure has two components: systolic and diastolic. Systolic pressure refers to the pressure exerted by the blood against the arterial wall during cardiac contraction.[8] Diastolic pressure is resting pressure, or the pressure exerted by the blood against the arterial wall between cardiac contractions. Factors known to affect an individual's blood pressure include recent exercise, time of day, body position at the time of pressure measurement, stress, emotional excitement, illness, current drug therapy, and diet.[9]

There are two types of indirect measurement of blood pressure: auscultatory (i.e., measurement of sound) and oscillometric (i.e., measurement of force). Mercury and aneroid meters involve auscultation with the use of a stethoscope to detect Korotkoff's sounds, which are produced by the motion of the arterial wall in response to changes in arterial pressure. As cuff pressure increases during the measurement procedure, the brachial artery is compressed and blood flow is obstructed. As cuff pressure is gradually released, blood flow is reestablished and Korotkoff's sounds can be heard in different phases. Phase I, which corresponds to systolic pressure, can be identified when at least two consecutive "taps" are heard as cuff pressure is decreased. The nature of the sounds changes over the next three phases. Diastolic pressure is identified as Phase V, the disappearance of sound.[8]

Oscillometric cuffs measure blood pressure by detecting blood surges underneath the cuff as it is deflated. Blood pressure measurements are calculated from changes in the force of the surges.

Types of Blood Pressure Meters

Mercury

There are different types of blood pressure meters. The first is the mercury sphygmomanometer, which consists of a cuff attached to a column of mercury encased in a glass gauge (Figure 1); the mercury rises and falls in relation to cuff pressure. Use of this type of meter requires a stethoscope. The mercury sphygmomanometer is the most accurate and reliable type of blood pressure meter available.[10] It is factory calibrated and requires recalibration only if the mercury gauge does not read "0" when the cuff is deflated. However, the mercury sphygmomanometer is bulky and inconvenient to transport. It contains breakable glass parts and carries with it the potential for toxic leaks of mercury. Proper use of the mercury meter and stethoscope requires that an individual with good eyesight and hearing take the readings; it is also necessary that the gauge be properly positioned (i.e., the mercury column must be vertical).[11]

Anerold

The aneroid blood pressure meter consists of a cuff with an attached circular dial that displays pressure readings (Figure 2). The needle on the dial moves clockwise as cuff pressure increases and counterclockwise as cuff pressure decreases. Like the mercury sphygmomanometer, the aneroid meter requires the use of a stethoscope. This type of meter is relatively compact and portable and the gauge works in any orientation. Aneroid meters are relatively inexpensive, but they require calibration by an expert at least once a year. Good eyesight and hearing are essential for accurate blood pressure measurements with an aneroid meter.[11]

Automated

Auscultatory and oscillometric battery-operated electronic or digital blood pressure meters can also be purchased for in-home use (Figure 3). Because a microphone is included in the design of electronic auscultatory cuffs to detect blood sounds automatically, a stethoscope and good hearing are not required. However, it is important that the cuff be placed so that the microphone is directly over the artery so that blood sounds can be detected.

Electronic oscillometric monitors do not monitor blood sounds; therefore, placement of the cuff is not a significant factor in obtaining an accurate measurement. Cuffless oscillometric meters require the patient only to place a finger in the appropriate area of the monitor to obtain a blood pressure reading.

Automated blood pressure meters are convenient for patients to use and require less skill than meters that require auscultation of Korotkoff's sounds. However, automated meters are relatively expensive, require calibration at least yearly, and may be less accurate than mercury and aneroid devices.[12,13]

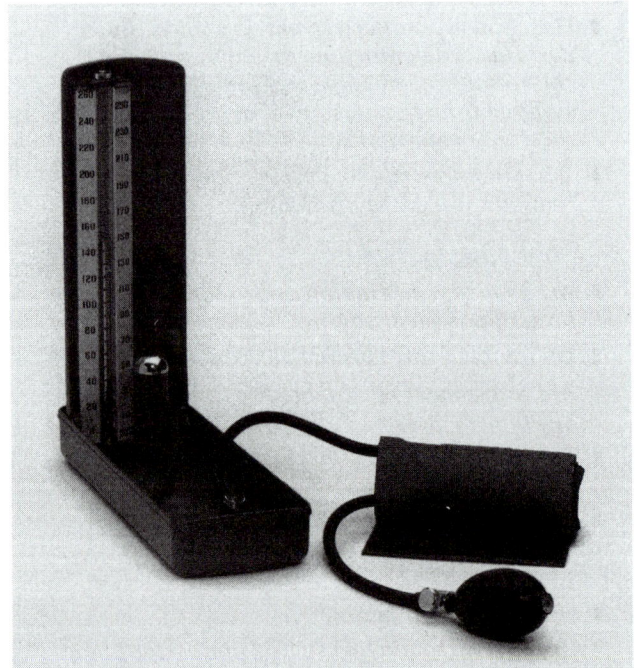

FIGURE 1 Mercury sphygmomanometer. Reprinted from *Am Pharm* 1989; NS29: 578.

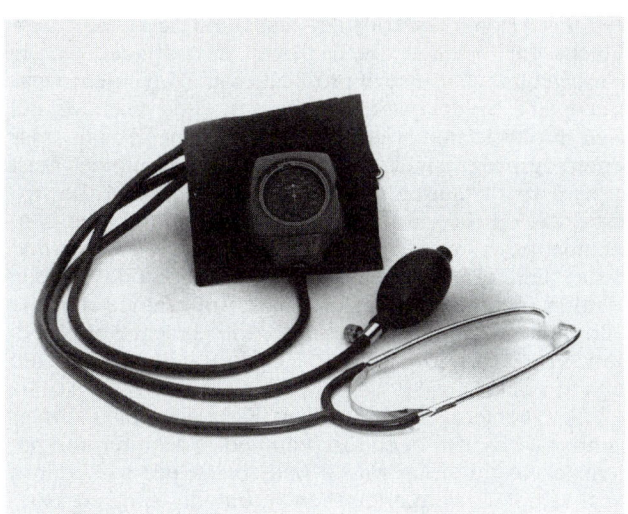

FIGURE 2 Aneroid sphygmomanometer. Reprinted from *Am Pharm* 1989; NS29: 579.

Advantages of Ambulatory Blood Pressure Monitoring

Ambulatory blood pressure monitors facilitate multiple blood pressure measurements over a 24-hour period. These battery-operated, programmable monitors are designed to be worn by the patient for 24 hours. Up to three blood pressure and heart rate readings per hour can be stored in the device's memory for evaluation and follow-up in the physician's office.[14]

Measurements of blood pressure taken in a clinic or physician's office may result in a diagnosis of mild to moderate hypertension because the patient's blood pressure may be artificially elevated. The artificial elevation of blood pressure in response to the stress associated with a visit to a physician is referred to as the white coat phenomenon. Blood pressure measurements taken at home over a 24-hour period provide more valuable data for use in evaluating blood pressure status. Such ambulatory measurements are also more predictive of end organ damage and cardiovascular complications associated with hypertension.[15–18]

General blood pressure monitoring in the community (e.g., with stationary patient service monitors in pharmacies or through health fair screenings) increases the chances of detecting elevated blood pressure in persons who have not been evaluated recently.[13] There are also advantages to ambulatory blood pressure monitoring for persons diagnosed with hypertension. Self-monitoring affords the hypertensive patient the opportunity to actively participate in his or her health care. Close observation and measurement of the effects of medications and lifestyle on blood pressure may make the patient more motivated and compliant with therapy. Compliance and tight control of blood pressure can help avoid the long-term health complications of hypertension. Better monitoring and reporting of blood pressures measured between visits to the physician can help the physician evaluate the effectiveness of therapy and determine appropriate changes in therapy.

Patient Counseling

The pharmacist can provide many services for the hypertensive patient. Compliance with drug and nondrug therapies is often a problem for hypertensive patients, and it is important to monitor a patient's drug therapy regimen for timely refills. In addition, the pharmacist can offer encouragement and stress the importance of lifestyle changes (e.g., sodium restriction, weight loss, and exercise) that are often an integral part of the overall control of hypertension.[19]

The pharmacist can also provide important information to users of in-home blood pressure monitors. Accuracy and consistency in blood pressure readings are crucial to the overall effectiveness of in-home blood pressure monitoring and care of the hypertensive patient. The importance of proper monitoring technique, a properly fitted and positioned cuff, and adherence to the manufacturer's instructions should be emphasized. A first-time user of a blood pressure monitor should be encouraged to compare initial readings with readings taken by a health care professional to ensure that the monitor is calibrated and working properly.

The pharmacist should educate the patient about activities and factors that may affect blood pressure readings. The patient should recognize that blood pressure may fluctuate by 20 to 30 mm Hg if multiple readings are taken each day.[18,20] To increase the accuracy of a blood pressure reading, the patient should be calm and should be seated comfortably, legs uncrossed, with feet flat against the floor. Also, the patient should refrain from eating or smoking for at least 30 minutes before measuring blood pressure. Measurements should be taken at the same time every day.[21]

The pharmacist should caution the patient against adjusting his or her own medication dosage on the basis

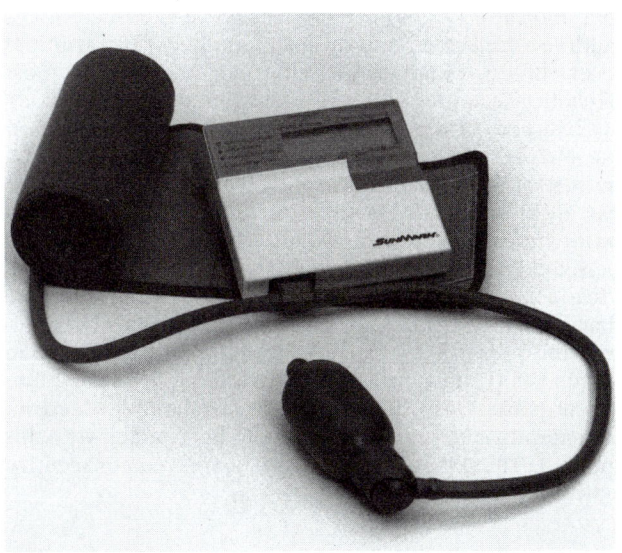

FIGURE 3 Electronic blood pressure meter. Reprinted from *Am Pharm* 1989; NS29: 579.

of in-home blood pressure readings. The patient should be encouraged to consult a physician if a problem occurs or pressure remains uncontrolled. All hypertensive patients should be encouraged to continue to visit a physician regularly for evaluation.

Fecal Occult Blood Test Kits

Patients at Risk

Colorectal cancer is the second most common fatal cancer in the United States after lung cancer for both males and females.[22,23] Colorectal cancer most often begins as a superficial lesion, which, as it progresses, tends to invade the intestinal wall and metastasize to other organs. However, if detected early, colorectal cancer may be successfully treated through surgery and other therapies. Therefore, detection of the cancerous lesion while it is still localized can improve the prognosis and significantly increase survival rates.[24] Certain subgroups of the population are at higher risk for the development of cancers of the anus, colon, or rectum: individuals with a history of inflammatory bowel disease, previous colorectal cancer, female genital cancer, or breast cancer; persons with a positive family history for polyposis, colorectal polyps, or colorectal cancer;[25] and persons aged 40 and older (this risk doubles with each decade after age 50 and appears to peak at age 70).[22] The American Cancer Society has recommended that routine screening for colorectal cancer begin at age 40 with an annual digital rectal exam. In addition, persons aged 50 and older should have a fecal occult blood test performed each year and a sigmoidoscopy every 3–5 years after two initial negative sigmoidoscopies 1 year apart.[26]

Biochemical Basis for Fecal Occult Blood Tests

One indicator of colorectal cancer is the presence of occult (i.e., concealed and in small quantities) blood in the feces. Blood found on the surface of the stool is most likely from a source in the lower gastrointestinal (GI) tract. Matrixed blood (i.e., blood found within the stool, not on the surface) is most likely from a source in the upper GI tract, such as a bleeding peptic ulcer. Tests for in-home use are designed to detect fecal occult blood with a colorimetric assay for hemoglobin. Hemoglobin possesses peroxidase activity and oxidizes the test reagent to produce a noticeable color change. It is important to note that a positive result with this type of test does not indicate the presence of cancer, only the presence of blood within the GI tract, which may be indicative of any number of conditions. Also, cancerous lesions may bleed intermittently and therefore may fail to be detected with this method. Thus, it is recommended that three consecutive bowel movements be tested.

Product Information

The original in-home fecal occult blood tests required the patient to obtain a stool specimen from the toilet bowl and place a smear onto a slide. Marketing of these tests—Hemoccult Home Test® (Menley James) and Fleet DeteCAtest® (Fleet)—for in-home use has been discontinued by the manufacturers because of problems with convenience and acceptance by the patient. However, slide tests are still used in physicians' offices and clinics, as well as in mass screening programs. For the slide tests, the patient must apply a small sample of fecal matter to each of the two test areas on the cardboard slide for each of three consecutive bowel movements. The slides are then returned to the clinic or laboratory for application of a developing solution and interpretation of results. Appearance of a blue color indicates a positive result for the presence of blood. Both matrixed and stool surface blood can be detected with this method.

Another fecal occult blood test, Early Detector® (Warner-Lambert), has also been discontinued. It required the patient to pat the anus with a pad (provided) to obtain a fecal sample. The patient then repeatedly sprayed a developer solution to wet the entire test area and the two control spots on the bottom of the pad. The pad was made of biodegradable material and could be flushed down the toilet after the results were recorded.[27]

The currently available fecal occult blood tests are known as bowl tests. They do not require the patient to handle the stool. Each of these test kits—ColoScreen Self-Test® (Helena Labs), EZ Detect® (NMS Pharmaceuticals), and ColoCare® (Helena Laboratories)—contains materials with which to test three consecutive bowel movements.

In the bowl tests, a test pad is dropped into the toilet bowl after a bowel movement and observed for color change. The premise is that if there is a clinically significant amount of blood on the surface of the stool, it disperses and floats on the surface of the toilet bowl water. The hemoglobin oxidizes the reagent contained within the layers of the test pad and causes a visible color change. Because blood from lesions in the lower GI tract is usually within the outer mucous surface of the stool, it is more likely to be detected with these tests than is blood from lesions in the upper GI tract.

The reagents used in these third-generation tests are susceptible to interference by toilet bowl cleaners, deodorants, and disinfectants. Therefore, the test user should remove any cleaner from the tank, flush three times before testing, and refrain from throwing toilet paper into the bowl before the test is complete.

The ColoScreen Self-Test® pad is floated in the toilet bowl, printed side up, immediately after a bowel movement. The pad is observed for 15–30 seconds for the appearance of a red–orange color in any of the four stool test areas on the pad. This color change, which results from the oxidation of guaiacol derivatives, should be considered a positive sign of the presence of hemoglobin. There are two pad check areas in the middle of the pad; one should turn red–orange and the other should not. If one pad check area does not react appropriately, the test results are considered invalid. The patient should not touch the pad at any time. The pad is composed of biodegradable materials and should be flushed after the results are recorded.[28]

The ColoCare® pad contains tetramethylbenzidine and cumene hydroperoxide as the test reagents. The test procedure is the same as described for the ColoScreen Self-Test®. However, the appearance of a blue or green color in the test area within 15–30 seconds is a positive result. ColoCare® has two check areas at the bottom of the pad; the area on the left should always turn blue or green and the area on the right should not change color.[29]

The EZ Detect® kit contains five test pads and a positive control chemical package. Before using EZ Detect®, the patient should use one test pad to perform a water quality check. If any trace of blue appears in the cross-shaped area when the pad is floated in the toilet water, another toilet bowl should be used for the tests. The same testing procedure is used with the EZ Detect® test pad as with ColoScreen Self-Test®. Three consecutive bowel movements are tested. The reagent in the EZ Detect® test pad is a reduced chromogen, tetramethylbenzidine, which produces a blue cross on the test pad when oxidized in the presence of hemoglobin. The reaction may take up to 2 minutes to occur. If no positive results are obtained in the three tests, a test pad quality check may be performed with the remaining pad. The patient should flush the toilet and empty the contents of the positive control chemical package into the bowl as it refills. The remaining test pad should be floated in the water, printed side up. A blue cross should appear within 2 minutes, indicating that the test pads were working properly. If the blue cross does not appear, the test results are invalid and the patient should call the assistance line provided with the product.[30]

Patient Counseling

The pharmacist can play an important role in community health care by encouraging persons over the age of 50 years to perform a fecal occult blood test annually, to participate in public screening programs, or to see their physician for such a test. Colorectal lesions and polyps grow slowly and may remain asymptomatic for an extended period of time.

When providing a test kit for home use, there are several instructions and warnings the pharmacist should provide to the patient. To ensure accurate results, it is important for the patient to read the manufacturer's instructions thoroughly before testing and to follow the recommended testing procedure exactly. For at least 2 to 3 days before performing the first test and during the testing period, the patient should avoid ingesting medications such as aspirin, potassium products, and iron-containing products. These agents may cause GI irritation and bleeding and positive results may occur with any fecal occult blood test. Use of rectal ointments and medications should also be avoided for 2 days before and during testing. The reagents in ColoScreen Self-Test®, guaiacol derivatives, are prone to interference from dietary sources of peroxidase or hemoglobin, such as red meats, broccoli, horseradish, turnips, cucumbers, grapefruit, and cauliflower. Therefore, the pharmacist should instruct users of ColoScreen Self-Test® to avoid these foods for at least 2 days before and during testing for fecal occult blood. Also, ingestion of ascorbic acid may give false-negative results with this product. Literature accompanying the ColoCare® product also instructs the user to avoid red meats and ascorbic acid before and during testing.

The patient should be encouraged to increase the amount of roughage in his or her diet before and while using any fecal occult blood test kit. Roughage aids in the passage of the stool and facilitates detection of lesions that may bleed only intermittently. Examples of foods that can be used to achieve this goal are popcorn, peanuts, bran cereal, whole grains, and vegetables (other than those that are high in peroxidase).

The pharmacist should also stress precautions associated with concurrent medical conditions that may cause positive results, such as peptic ulcers and colitis. However, a positive outcome of the use of an in-home fecal occult blood test kit is that it may detect blood produced by these conditions and lead to their subsequent diagnosis and treatment. A test for fecal occult blood should not be performed if the patient is experiencing menstrual bleeding, bleeding hemorrhoids, or constipation.

Because interpretation of the results of these tests involves evaluation of a color change, color-blind or visually impaired persons will require assistance in "reading" the test area on the pad.

It is important for the pharmacist to stress to users of in-home fecal occult blood test kits that a positive result does not indicate that colorectal cancer is present. These tests are designed only to detect hidden blood in the stool, a sign of many different GI disorders associated with bleeding. Any person obtaining a positive result with a fecal occult blood test should immediately be referred to a physician for a complete evaluation. Only after further testing by medical personnel can colorectal cancer be diagnosed or ruled out.

Ovulation Prediction and Pregnancy Test Kits

The Female Reproductive Cycle

The female reproductive cycle, which is approximately 28 days in length, is under hormonal control. At the beginning of the cycle (day 1 through approximately day 13), low levels of circulating estrogen and progesterone cause the hypothalamus to secrete gonadotropin-releasing hormone (GnRH), which in turn stimulates the release of follicle-stimulating hormone (FSH) and low levels of luteinizing hormone (LH) from the anterior pituitary. This combination of hormones is responsible for promoting the development of several follicles within an ovary during each cycle. At one point in the development, one follicle is singled out and continues to mature while the others regress. At midcycle (approximately day 14 or 15), circulating LH levels significantly increase and cause final maturation of the follicle. Ovulation (rupturing of the follicle and release of the ovum) occurs approximately 20–48 hours after this LH surge. Cells in the ruptured follicle then luteinize and form the corpus luteum, which begins to secrete progesterone and estrogen. For approximately 7 to 8 days after ovulation, the corpus luteum continues to develop and to secrete estrogen and progesterone, which inhibit further secretion of FSH and LH.

If fertilization occurs, the hormone human chorionic gonadotropin (HCG) is produced by trophoblastic cells. HCG causes the corpus luteum to continue to produce progesterone and estrogen, which forestall the onset of menses while the placenta develops and becomes functional. As early as day 7 after conception, the placenta produces HCG, the concentration of which continues to increase during early pregnancy. Some HCG is excreted in the urine and maximum levels of HCG are reached 6 weeks after conception. HCG levels decline over the following 4–6 weeks and then stabilize for the remainder of the pregnancy.

If fertilization does not occur during a cycle, the corpus luteum degenerates, circulating levels of progesterone and estrogen diminish, and menstruation occurs (days 1–5). Resulting low levels of progesterone and estrogen cause release of GnRH from the hypothalamus and the hormonal cycle begins again.[31,32]

Basal Thermometry

Before the introduction of in-home ovulation prediction test kits, basal body temperature readings were used to help determine when ovulation occurred. The basal resting temperature is usually below normal during the first part of the female reproductive cycle. After ovulation, this temperature rises to a level closer to 98.6°F (37°C). However, because the temperature increase is not detected until after ovulation has occurred, only a few hours (less than 24) of the woman's fertile period (the time during which conception is most likely to occur) remain.

The only equipment necessary for basal body temperature monitoring is a basal thermometer; thus, this method is much less expensive than the use of in-home ovulation prediction test kits. Basal temperatures can be measured orally, rectally, or vaginally each morning before a woman arises. However, it is important that the woman be consistent in her method and time of measurement. Basal body thermometry may be a useful initial approach for a couple attempting to conceive. It is inexpensive, and if after a few months fertilization has not occurred, the woman has accurate data about her cycle length, which will facilitate the selection of an in-home ovulation prediction test kit.

Ovulation Prediction Test Kits

In-home ovulation prediction test kits help to determine a woman's fertile period. These monoclonal antibody tests detect increasing concentrations of LH in the urine. The LH surge precedes ovulation by approximately 20–48 hours and can usually be detected in the urine 8–12 hours after it occurs in the serum. Therefore, depending on the in-home test kit used, ovulation should be expected to occur within 1 to 2 days after the surge is detected in the urine. The ovum remains viable for 12–24 hours after ovulation. Because sperm can survive for up to 72 hours after intercourse, the optimal days for fertilization include the 2 days before ovulation, the day ovulation occurs, and the day after ovulation. Therefore, detection of the LH surge indicates the beginning of the fertile period. However, it is important for the patient to understand that the ovulation prediction tests are not indicated for contraceptive use because intercourse before ovulation may still result in pregnancy.

Product Information

In-home ovulation prediction tests kits were first marketed in the United States in 1985. These tests contain monoclonal antibodies specific for LH and use an ELISA to elicit a color change proportional to the level of LH in the urine. A significant increase in the intensity of the color over baseline is indicative of the LH surge. Different ovulation prediction test kits contain supplies for five to nine tests. Theoretically, the earlier testing begins in a cycle and the more consecutive days tested, the greater the likelihood of predicting ovulation.

Before using an ovulation prediction test kit, the woman must determine the period of time when ovulation is most likely to occur. To do so, she should calculate the average length of her most recent three menstrual cycles. Each product kit contains a chart to assist the patient in determining, on the basis of her calculated average cycle length, on which day of her cycle she should begin testing. Calculation of the time period in which ovulation is most likely to occur should be done carefully so that a baseline can be established and the LH surge detected. If the patient's cycle is irregular, varying by more than 3 to 4 days each month, she should use the length of the shortest cycle to determine when to start testing. If the time is calculated correctly, 6 days of testing is adequate to detect the LH surge and predict ovulation in approximately 66% of ovulating women. Increasing the testing period to 10 consecutive days increases the probability of detecting the LH surge to 95%.[33]

Because in-home ovulation prediction test kits use monoclonal antibodies, the possibility of interference from other substances is minimal. Commonly used nonprescription drug products, such as analgesics, decongestants, antihistamines, antitussives, and expectorants, should not interfere with the results.[34] However, medications used to promote ovulation (e.g., menotropins) may interfere and give false-positive results because LH levels are artificially elevated. The true LH surge can be detected in patients receiving clomiphene if testing does not begin until the second day after drug therapy ends. Medical conditions associated with high levels of LH, such as menopause and polycystic ovary syndrome, may cause false-positive results. A false-positive result may also be obtained if the user is already pregnant.[34] If the patient has recently discontinued using oral contraceptives, the start of ovulation may be delayed for one to two cycles. Use of an in-home ovulation prediction test kit by such an individual would not be appropriate until fertilization has been attempted unsuccessfully for several months following discontinuation of the oral contraceptives.

Patient Counseling

The pharmacist can provide the user of an in-home ovulation prediction test kit with some very important information to ensure proper use of the test and to increase the probability of accurate results. Because these tests involve multiple steps, there is a potential for procedural errors. The pharmacist should review the proper procedure with the patient and should emphasize the importance of strict adherence to the manufacturer's instructions. Timing of the component steps in the procedure is crucial, so the patient should have a clock or timer readily available. If the patient is unable to conduct the test immediately after the sample is collected, the urine may be stored in a refrigerator for up to 12 hours. Before conducting the test on a refrigerated sample, the patient should allow the sample to reach room temperature by letting it stand for approximately 20–30 minutes. Some sediment may accumulate on the bottom of the sample container while it is refrigerated. It is important that the patient not shake the sample or redisperse the sediment.

Some of the test kits require first morning urine, in which LH is most highly concentrated. Other tests will provide accurate results with a sample taken at any time during the day and still others state specifically that first morning urine is not to be used. Whatever the test, it is important for the user to obtain the urine sample at the same time each day and to restrict her fluid intake for 1 to 2 hours before obtaining the sample so that the urine will not be too dilute.[35] Once the LH surge is detected, the patient can discontinue testing. If a woman obtains an intense color on the first day of testing, she has started too late in the cycle and ovulation may have already occurred. She should stop testing for that cycle and, if pregnancy does not occur, begin testing a few days earlier in the next cycle.

It is important for the pharmacist to realize that the desire to conceive can be an emotional issue for the couple using an ovulation prediction test kit and that empathy is important in communicating with these patients. It is advisable for couples who have not conceived after several cycles, even though ovulation was detected, to consult a gynecologist or fertility specialist.

Pregnancy Test Kits

In-home testing makes it possible to detect pregnancy early in the first trimester, when the mother can make crucial behavioral and lifestyle changes to avoid causing harm to the fetus.[35] In-home pregnancy tests have undergone two major stages of development. The first generation of in-home pregnancy test kits used the hemagglutination inhibition reaction method to detect HCG in the urine. The limitations of this method for detecting pregnancy led to the discontinuance of hemagglutination inhibition reaction pregnancy tests in November 1992. Early in the 1980s, a second type of in-home pregnancy test became available as a result of developments in biotechnology, particularly monoclonal antibody technology.

Hemagglutination Inhibition Reaction Tests

Hemagglutination inhibition reaction tests included a test tube containing red blood cells coated with HCG–antibody and an antiserum to the antibody. If HCG was present in the urine sample, it complexed with the antibody and uncoated the red blood cells. The uncoated red blood cells fell to the bottom of the test tube and formed a donut-shaped ring, which was considered a positive indicator of pregnancy. Because the rather high levels of HCG required to produce a positive result with this test are usually not achieved until approximately 9 days after the missed onset of menses, a false-negative result could be obtained if the test was used too early after conception, or too late into the pregnancy when circulating HCG levels have decreased. Other disadvantages of the hemagglutination inhibition reaction tests include the length of time required to perform the test (30–60 minutes) and their sensitivity to vibration.

Monoclonal Antibody Tests

These second-generation pregnancy tests use an immunoassay to produce a color change to indicate a positive result. If HCG is present in the sample, it is trapped by the HCG–antibody. A second antibody attached to an enzyme complexes with the trapped HCG and the enzyme produces a color change on a plastic test stick. The in-home pregnancy tests using monoclonal antibodies and color changes are very sensitive and can detect low levels of HCG. Monoclonal antibody pregnancy tests require less time to complete (1–30 minutes, depending on the specific product) than did the hemagglutination inhibition tests. Also, many of the newer kits are simpler to use, often involving just one step. If correctly used, monoclonal antibody pregnancy tests for in-home use are reported to be more than 95% accurate.[36-38]

Sources of Interference

The monoclonal antibody pregnancy tests are less susceptible to interference from other substances than were the original hemagglutination inhibition tests. However, false-negative results may occur with monoclonal antibody pregnancy tests if the test is performed too soon after conception or if the urine sample was refrigerated and not allowed to return to room temperature.

Patient Counseling

The pharmacist should review the proper test procedure with the patient and should emphasize the importance of strict adherence to the manufacturer's instructions. With most of the in-home pregnancy tests, timing of the component steps is crucial. If the patient is unable to conduct the test immediately after the sample is collected, the urine may be stored in a refrigerator for up to 12 hours. Before conducting the test on a refrigerated sample, the patient should allow the sample to return to room temperature by letting it stand for approximately 20–30 minutes. Some sediment may accumulate on the bottom of the sample container while it is refrigerated. It is important that the patient not shake the sample or redisperse the sediment before testing. If the urine sample is cloudy or pink or has a strong odor, it should not be used for an in-home pregnancy test because the results are likely to be inaccurate.

If the result of an in-home pregnancy test is negative, the patient should review the procedure to make sure that she performed the test properly. Then she should wait the number of days suggested by the manufacturer and repeat the test if menstruation has not yet begun. If the second test is negative and menstruation still has not begun, the patient should contact her physician. There may be underlying medical reasons for the lack of menstruation that would require diagnosis and treatment.

If the result of an in-home pregnancy test is positive, the patient should assume that she is pregnant and arrange for an appointment with a physician. Behaviors known to be harmful to the fetus, such as alcohol ingestion, smoking, and drug use (including oral contraceptives), should be immediately discontinued. Pregnant diabetics should monitor their blood glucose levels very carefully, because normoglycemia decreases fetal morbidity and mortality.

When assisting a patient with product selection, the pharmacist should consider specific product features and patient characteristics. For example, if a woman is testing soon after possible conception, it may be appropriate for her to purchase a kit that contains materials for two tests in case she tests too early to detect the presence of HCG. Other factors to be considered in product selection include the number of component steps (i.e., the complexity of the testing procedure), time to achieve results, and overall ease of use.

Tests for Urinary Tract Infections

Basis for the Test

Test strips to detect the presence of urinary nitrites are available to screen patients at risk for asymptomatic bacteriuria, such as children, patients with a history of urinary tract infections, and pregnant women. These tests can also be used to monitor the effectiveness of antibiotic therapy for urinary tract infections. Nitrites, not normally present in the urine, result from the reduction of dietary nitrates by most Gram-negative bacteria. Therefore, detection of nitrites is an indirect measure for the presence of these bacteria.

A test strip is dipped into a sample of urine for 1 second and observed for the appearance of a pink–red color within 30–60 seconds. The intensity of the color corresponds to the concentration of nitrites in the urine and therefore to the number of organisms per milliliter of urine.[39]

Patient Counseling

Because there is a potential for interference with the chemical basis of the test, the patient should be aware of several things when using a test for urinary nitrites. Ingestion of ascorbic acid, an antioxidant, should be avoided for at least 10 hours before obtaining the urine sample. Foods that cause alkalinization of the urine, such as citrus fruits and juices and dairy products, should be avoided because the test requires acidic urine. Because the test is colorimetric, medications that cause discoloration of the urine (e.g., phenazopyridine) should also be avoided before testing. Patients who are color blind or visually impaired will need assistance in evaluating test results.

False-negative results will be obtained in cases of urinary tract infections caused by Gram-positive bacteria or yeast. There is also a potential for false-negative results if the urine tested was voided without having been held in the bladder for at least 4 hours, the time required for adequate reduction of nitrates to occur.

The Future

As the products of biotechnology become more sophisticated, easier to use, and less costly, more tests will become available on a nonprescription basis for in-home use. Manufacturers will continue to strive to make their products more accurate and reliable. Some tests that are expected to become available on a nonprescription basis in the near future include tests to determine and monitor blood cholesterol levels; tests to detect the presence of sexually transmitted diseases, yeast infections, and streptococcal throat infections; self-administered Pap smears; and tests for use in therapeutic drug monitoring.[1,40,41] Self-monitoring of drug levels may play an important role in the overall health care and maintenance of patients with hypertension, arrhythmias, seizure disorders, asthma, and other chronic conditions. However, pharmacists and other health care professionals must inform patients on the use, interpretation, and limitations of these tests. The interpretation of test results related to an individual patient and the diagnosis of medical conditions remain in the domain of the physician. The role of the pharmacist as patient educator on the use of in-home test and monitoring products should continue to grow as more tests become available. Because of the concern that patients may not interpret test results correctly or act appropriately after they obtain the test results, some manufacturers of diagnostics may allow these products to be disseminated only through health professionals, such as pharmacists. Such a policy would help to ensure that the intended outcome of the test will be achieved.

References

1. Home diagnostics on the rise as more consumers self-diagnose. *Med Advertising News* 1988 Dec 16: 6–7.
2. Smith MC, Garner DD. Tackling the $1 billion home diagnostic market. *U.S. Pharmacist* 1987 Jun; 12 (6): 24–28.
3. Wilson M. New technology boosts home test kit sales. *Am Druggist* 1986 Feb; 193 (2): 107–13, 147.
4. Ratafia M. The diagnostics revolution. *Med Marketing Media* 1985 Aug: 15–25.
5. Feierman R, Shea PV. Diagnostic products that RPHs recommend. *Am Druggist* 1989 May; 199 (5): 62–68.
6. Moser M. *High Blood Pressure and What You Can Do About It*. Elmsford, NY: The Benjamin Co; Dec 1987: 3.
7. *Questions about Weight, Salt, and High Blood Pressure*. Pub. No. 87-1459NIH. Bethesda, Md: U.S. Department of Health and Human Services; May 1987.
8. Hill MN. What can go wrong when you measure blood pressure. *Am J Nurs* 1980; 80 (5): 942–46.
9. Moser M. *High Blood Pressure and What You Can Do About It*. Elmsford, NY: The Benjamin Co; Dec 1987: 7.
10. Schmidt GR, Wenig JH. An evaluation of home blood pressure monitoring devices. *Am Pharm* 1989; NS29 (9): 25–30.
11. Miller RY. What you should know about blood pressure monitors. *U.S. Pharmacist* 1986 Aug; 11 (8): 60–64.
12. Bagley J. Assessing blood pressure monitors. *Am Druggist* 1986 Nov: 102–7.
13. Grim CM. Providing blood pressure screening devices for your patients. *California Pharmacist* 1989; 37 (3): 31–35.
14. McCormick, EM. A new monitoring technique for blood pressure? *Pharm Times* 1991 Oct; 57 (10): 116, 119.
15. Weber MA. Evaluating the diagnosis and prognosis of hypertension by automated blood pressure monitoring: outline of a symposium. *Am Heart J* 1988; 116 (4): 1118–23.
16. Pickering TG. Blood pressure monitoring outside the office for the evaluation of patients with resistant hypertension. *Hypertension* 1988; 11 (3 pt. 2): II96–100.
17. Mancia G, Parati G. Experience with 24-hour ambulatory blood pressure monitoring in hypertension. *Am Heart J* 1988; 116 (4): 1134–40.

18. Lavie CJ, Schmeider RE, Messerli FH. Ambulatory blood pressure monitoring: practical considerations. *Am Heart J* 1988; 116 (4): 1146–51.
19. Fedder DO. How involved should you be in monitoring high blood pressure? *U.S. Pharmacist* 1986 Jul; 11 (7): 66–72.
20. Pickering TG. The influence of daily activity on ambulatory blood pressure. *Am Heart J* 1988; 116 (4): 1141–45.
21. Oed, ML. Measuring blood pressure and blood cholesterol: the need for accuracy and precision. *U.S. Pharmacist's Cardiovascular Disease Supplement* 1990 Jun; 15 (6): 52–56.
22. Stajich GV, Roskos J Jr. Gastrointestinal cancer. In: Herfindal ET, Gourley DR, Hart LL, eds. *Clinical Pharmacy and Therapeutics*. 4th ed., Baltimore: Willliams & Wilkins; 1988: 920.
23. Winawer SJ, Fleischer M, Baldwin M, et al. Current status of fecal occult blood testing in screening for colorectal cancer. *CA* 1982; 32 (2): 100–112.
24. Nostrant TT, Wilson JAP. How good is screening for colorectal cancer? *Postgrad Med* 1986 Jun; 73 (6): 131–39.
25. Stajich GV, Roskos J Jr. Gastrointestinal cancer. In: Herfindal ET, *Therapeutics*. 4th ed., Baltimore: Williams & Wilkins; 1988: 921.
26. American Cancer Society. Guidelines for the cancer-related checkup: cancer of the colon and rectum. *CA* 1980; 30 (4): 208–15.
27. Early Detector® product information. Morris Plains, NJ: Warner-Lambert Company, Inc; 1987.
28. ColoScreen Self-Test® product information. Beaumont, Tex: Helena Laboratories; Mar 1987.
29. ColoCare® product information. Beaumont, Tex: Helena Laboratories; Dec 1988.
30. EZ-Detect® product information. Newport Beach, Calif: NMS Pharmaceuticals, Inc; Oct 1987.
31. Reiders TP, Ruggiero RJ, Steadman S. *Methods of Birth Control: Assessment Skills for Pharmacists*. Palo Alto, Calif: Syntex Laboratories; 1985: 2–5.
32. Inglis JK. *A Textbook of Human Biology*. 3rd ed., New York: Pergamon Press; 1986: 252–53.
33. QTest for Ovulation Prediction® product information. Franklin Lakes, NJ: Becton-Dickinson and Co; 1986.
34. *USP DI, Drug Information for the Health Care Professional*. vol. IB. 12th ed., Rockville, Md: The United States Pharmacopeial Convention, Inc; 1992: 2115.
35. Planning a pregnancy via home testing kits. *Pharm Times* 1989; 55 (3): 107–8.
36. Clearblue Easy® product information. New York: Whitehall Laboratories.
37. Answer Quick and Simple® product information. Cranbury, NJ: Carter Products; Jan 1989.
38. e.p.t. Stick® product information. Morris Plains, NJ: Parke-Davis Consumer Products.
39. Miyahara RK, Nykamp D. On the shelf and in the future. *U.S. Pharmacist* 1990 Dec; 15: 50–62.
40. Chi J. What's new in home test kits. *Drug Topics* 1986 Aug 4; 130 (15): 28–34.
41. Robinson B. Next: home kits for checking drug therapies. *Drug Topics* 1988 Mar 7; 132 (5): 42.

CHAPTER 5

Internal Analgesic Products

W. Kent Van Tyle

Questions to ask in patient assessment and counseling

- *Where is the pain? Is it in one place, such as a particular muscle or area of skin, or does it spread to other parts of the body? Is any part of your body red and swollen? Have you recently sustained a physical injury?*
- *What type of pain do you have? Is it sharp, dull, aching, knifelike, etc.? Is it constant or does it come and go? Did it develop suddenly?*
- *Does the pain occur at any particular time of the day? Does anything make it worse or better? Is it relieved by changing your body position?*
- *Do you have any other symptoms that you feel might be associated with the pain (e.g., visual disturbances, numbness, weakness, a tingling sensation, dizziness, unusual drowsiness, nausea, vomiting, fever, mental confusion, or unusual sensitivity to light or sounds)?*
- *Have you had this pain before? If so, what medications did you take to relieve or manage the pain?*
- *What have you already taken? How much and for how long?*
- *Do aspirin or other pain relievers upset your stomach?*
- *Have you ever had an allergic reaction to aspirin?*
- *Do you now have or have you ever had asthma, allergies, ulcers, gout, high blood pressure, heart failure, kidney disease, or a blood-clotting disorder?*
- *Are you now taking medication for gout, arthritis, asthma, high blood pressure, or diabetes?*
- *Are you currently taking any drug that may thin your blood? Have you taken any such drug within the last week?*
- *What other prescription or nonprescription drugs are you now taking?*
- *Does the intended child or young adult consumer of an aspirin-containing product have a viral influenza or chickenpox?*
- *Are you pregnant? Are you breast-feeding? If you are pregnant, do you plan to breast-feed?*
- *(If appropriate) How high is your fever, and how long have you had it?*

Origin and Perception of Pain

Depending on its origin, pain is categorized as either somatic or visceral. Somatic pain arises from the musculoskeletal system or skin; visceral pain arises from the organs or viscera of the thorax and abdomen.

Stimuli that elicit the perception of acute pain do so most often by injuring tissue and causing the release of intracellular chemical mediators such as histamine, bradykinin, and prostaglandins from the damaged tissue. These chemical mediators stimulate free nerve endings that are diffusely distributed in various tissues, including skin, muscle, tendon, joint surfaces, and the membrane that covers bone. This results in the production of a pain impulse, which enters the spinal cord and travels through two ascending pathways to the brain. One pathway ends in areas of the brain that make the patient aware of the intensity and location of pain. Stimulation of the second pathway contributes to the emotional reaction or suffering component of the pain experience.[1]

Visceral pain results from ischemia, chemical damage (e.g., acid and proteolytic erosion in peptic ulcer disease), spasm, or distention of the visceral structure. Visceral pain differs in one important aspect from pain of musculoskeletal or skin origin. Damage to a visceral structure rarely causes localized intense pain, and intense pain of visceral origin means that nerve endings have been diffusely stimulated. Thus, visceral pain cannot generally be recognized as coming from a specific organ. Instead, the brain may interpret it as coming from various areas of the skin. Such pain is called "referred pain" because it is referred to various body surface areas.[2] Figure 1 provides a reasonable correlation of the location of referred pain with its site of visceral origin.

Neuropathic pain results from injury to or chronic changes in somatic sensory pathways, and it may develop and persist without obvious tissue injury. Neuropathic pain may be accompanied by sensory loss, muscle weakness, a burning or aching sensation, paroxysmal jabs of sharp pain, or an exaggerated response to touch.

Patient Assessment

When evaluating a patient's pain, the pharmacist should ask several well-chosen questions to make the best recommendations for treatment. For example, what is the location, quality, frequency, severity, and duration of the pain? Does the pain recur at the same time daily, or is it associated with a specific activity such as movement or eating? Is the patient taking any medication that could interact adversely with the use of certain nonprescription

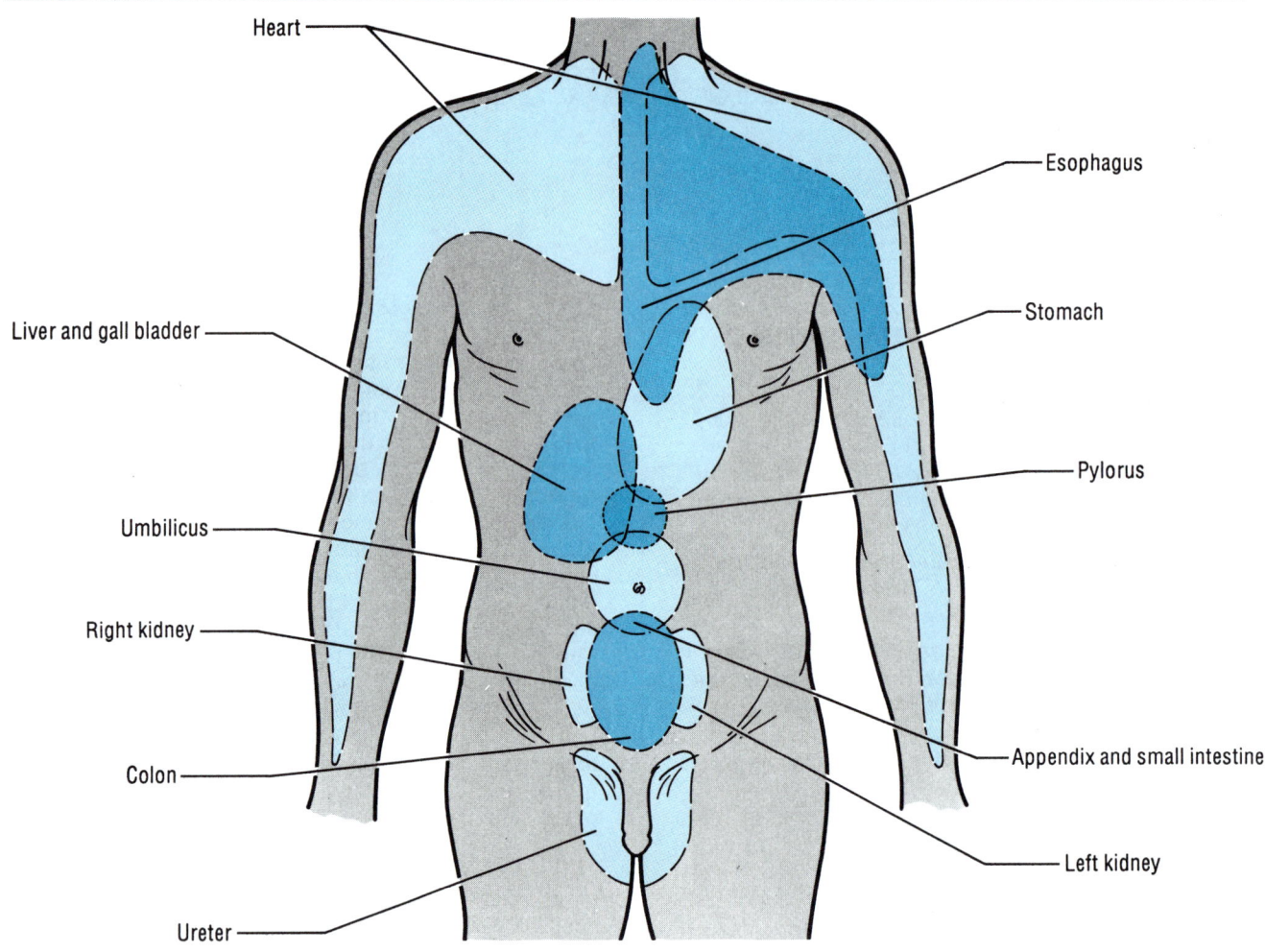

FIGURE 1 Surface areas of referred pain originating from different visceral organs. Adapted with permission from *Guyton's Textbook of Medical Physiology*. Philadelphia: W. B. Saunders Co; 1986: 599.

analgesics? Has the patient ever experienced an adverse reaction (e.g., gastrointestinal [GI] upset or allergic reaction) to nonprescription analgesics? It is important that the pharmacist develop, at a very minimum, this patient database to differentiate those types of pain appropriate for nonprescription analgesic management and those requiring referral and further medical attention.

Selected Conditions Responsive to Nonprescription Analgesics

Headache

Headache is a common experience of diverse etiology. Headache pain may be due to causes such as:

- Distention or dilation of intracranial arteries;
- Traction or displacement of large intracranial veins or their meningeal covering;
- Compression or disease of cranial or spinal nerves;
- Spasm, inflammation, or trauma of cranial or cervical muscles;
- Meningeal inflammation;
- Cerebral hypoxia;
- Diseases of the eye, nose, throat, teeth, and ear;
- Fatigue;
- Fever or "hangover."

Pain arising from intracranial structures is often referred to surface areas of the head and may be associated with tenderness of the scalp.

Although the incidence of headache pain being a symptom of serious pathology is relatively low, the pharmacist must always be alert to that possibility. For example, the headache associated with cerebral aneurysm has a sudden onset with very acute pain reaching a peak within minutes. Neurologic disturbances such as visual defects, unilateral numbness, weakness, or aphasia may precede or occur after onset. Headache and dizziness of fluctuating severity, followed by drowsiness, stupor, coma, and hemiparesis, are the usual manifestations of chronic subdural hematoma. Headache is also a prominent feature of brain tumor. The character of the pain associated with a brain tumor is highly variable; the pain may recur at different times during the day, and its duration may be from a few minutes to an hour or more. The headache may first be localized in the area of the tumor and may be relieved a bit by a change in posture, but it tends to become generalized when intracranial pressure increases.[3] Severe headache with constant, intense pain that is often at the base of the skull and is associated with stiffness of the neck on bending the head forward is suggestive of meningeal infection or hemorrhage. If a headache recurs frequently; is of prolonged duration; is of severe intensity; or is associated with nausea, vomiting, fever, dizziness, seizures, mental confusion, neck stiffness, vision disturbances, or neurologic symptoms, the pharmacist should refer the patient immediately for medical evaluation.

Migraine headache is a recurring, hemicranial, throbbing headache and is subdivided into either classic or common types. Classic migraine usually begins with neurologic symptoms, including shimmering or flashing areas or blind spots in the visual field, difficulty speaking, and one-sided muscle weakness. These symptoms may last for up to half an hour, and the throbbing headache pain that follows may last from several hours to 1 to 2 days. Common migraine does not have the antecedent neurologic symptoms of the classic type, but begins immediately with the headache pain. Both forms of migraine are often associated with nausea, vomiting, photophobia, and phonophobia. Women have a higher incidence of migraine headache than men, and for some women, migraine headache tends to recur at specific times during the menstrual cycle.[3] Aspirin, ibuprofen, or acetaminophen can effectively control the headache pain of migraine if dosed properly and may actually abort a migraine headache if taken very soon after headache onset.

Cluster headache is characterized by intense, nonthrobbing, unilateral pain around the eye and is often associated with tearing, nasal congestion, rhinorrhea, and facial flushing. The pain can last up to 1 to 2 hours, and it usually occurs nightly for days to weeks within 2 to 3 hours of falling asleep. Cluster headache does not respond well to self-medication with nonprescription analgesics and should be referred for medical evaluation and treatment.

Sinus headache occurs when infection or blockage of the paranasal sinuses results in inflammation or distention of the sensitive sinus walls. Sinus headache is usually localized to the periorbital area or forehead. Sinus pain tends to occur upon awakening and may subside gradually after the patient has been upright for a while. Stooping and blowing the nose often intensifies the pain. In addition to nonprescription analgesics, decongestants are often useful in facilitating drainage of the sinuses and thus in relieving pain.[3] (See Chapter 8, "Cold, Cough, and Allergy Products.") Persistent sinus pain and/or discharge suggests possible bacterial infection and requires referral for medical evaluation.

Headache of ocular origin is usually located in the orbit, forehead, or temple and tends to produce a steady, aching type of pain. It usually follows prolonged, close work with the eyes and is believed to result from ocular muscle imbalance. Correction of any refractive error prevents its recurrence and makes the subsequent use of nonprescription analgesics unnecessary. The pharmacist should be aware that intense ocular pain can be symptomatic of acute, angle-closure glaucoma, in which case it may coexist with a fixed and dilated pupil in the affected eye. Such an attack may also be associated with decreased visual acuity, throbbing pain, upper lid edema, lacrimation, nausea, and possible vomiting and is considered a medical emergency. Immediate medical intervention is required to prevent visual loss.

Tension headache is characterized by bilateral, diffuse pain, often over the top of the head and extending to the rear and base of the skull. Patients often describe the pain as "tight" or "pressing," as if the head were constricted by a band. The pain is usually more gradual in onset than it is in migraine, and it has more of an aching than throbbing quality. Tension headache may be associated with emotional stress or anxiety and may continue for several days.[3] Chronic or continuous tension headaches do not respond well to nonprescription analgesics and may require psychiatric or psychologic evaluation and intervention to accomplish effective treatment.

Neuralgia

Facial pain arising from inflammation of the trigeminal nerve (trigeminal neuralgia, or tic douloureux) is characterized by brief episodes of severe pain in the lips, gums, cheek, or chin. These episodes rarely last for more than 1 to 2 minutes, but they can recur many times during the day or night. The pain is not associated with either motor or sensory loss. The intense facial pain of trigeminal neuralgia does not respond well to nonprescription analgesics and requires medical evaluation to distinguish it from facial pain arising from unrelated pathology of the jaw, teeth, or sinus structures. Inflammation of the trigeminal nerve producing facial pain may also result from herpes-zoster infection. This pain, which can be described as burning or stabbing, tends to be unilateral and may be associated with paresthesia or slight sensory loss. Posttherapeutic neuralgia requires medical management beyond that available with nonprescription analgesics.[3]

Myalgia

Diffuse muscle pain is common and can result from various systemic infections (e.g., influenza, Coxsackie virus, measles, or other viral illness) and from strenuous exertion of the unconditioned body. Prolonged tonic contraction produced by exercise, tension, or maintenance of a certain body position for extended periods may also produce muscle pain. Additionally, diffuse muscle soreness and aching may be the initial symptom of rheumatoid arthritis, preceding the signs of joint involvement by weeks or months.[4] Myalgia usually responds well to nonprescription analgesics and adjunctive treatment with heat or massage.

Periarticular Pain

Joints consist of cartilage covering the articulating surfaces of bone; a surrounding synovial membrane; and periarticular supporting structures, including ligaments and tendons. Bursae resemble synovial membranes and provide the surface and lubrication on which these supporting structures move. Pain can arise secondary to injury or inflammation of the tissues surrounding a joint (i.e., the joint capsule, tendons, ligaments, and bursae). Localized tenderness is usually present upon examination, and the pain can be elicited by maneuvers that stress the structure but not the associated joint. Periarticular pain tends to be nocturnal and often involves the shoulder, elbow, or knee. It responds well to nonprescription analgesics and limitation of motion in the affected joint.[5]

Arthralgia

Joint pain frequently involves inflammation of the synovial membrane (synovitis). Cartilage loss with associated synovitis can be the result of mechanical stress and wear, such as in degenerative joint disease (DJD) (osteoarthritis), or of erosive processes, such as in rheumatoid arthritis.

DJD affects 85% of persons over the age of 70, and symptoms usually begin in the fifth or sixth decade of life. The primary complaint is joint stiffness and an aching type of pain in motion and weight-bearing joints. Joint stiffness lasts only a few minutes following the initiation of joint motion. Degenerative changes of the upper extremities usually affect the joints of the fingers but rarely involve wrists, elbows, or shoulders. However, DJD of the hip, knee, and spine does occur and can be particularly disabling. Earlier stages of DJD respond well to nonprescription analgesics such as aspirin or ibuprofen, and local heat is often beneficial. Progressive disease, especially of weight-bearing joints, requires orthopedic management beyond the scope of nonprescription analgesics.[6]

Rheumatoid arthritis symptoms usually appear between the third and seventh decade, and the disease occurs more often in women than in men. It may begin with a prodrome of fatigue, weakness, joint stiffness, arthralgia, and myalgia appearing several weeks before joint swelling. Multiple joints of the hands, wrists, and feet show symmetrical involvement. Involved joints become warm, red, and swollen and develop limited range of motion. Rheumatoid arthritis persists in affected joints and is a progressive disease that leads to joint deformity. Duration of morning stiffness can be used to assess the disease's severity and progression.

Because the onset and progression of rheumatoid arthritis is slow and often subtle, many patients may attempt self-medication in its initial stages. However, the therapeutic goal of managing rheumatoid arthritis—to control inflammation and induce remission—is beyond the scope of self-medication with nonprescription analgesics, although aspirin is a mainstay of therapy. Thus, because rheumatoid arthritis is a progressive, disabling disease, the pharmacist must encourage the patient to seek medical attention to maintain maximum joint mobility.[7]

Nonprescription Analgesic Options

Aspirin and Other Salicylates

Although ineffective in treating pain of visceral origin, salicylates are effective in treating mild to moderate pain arising from musculoskeletal structures. While prostaglandins sensitize peripheral pain receptors to the chemical or mechanical initiation of pain impulses, salicylates inhibit prostaglandin synthesis from arachidonic acid by inhibiting cyclo-oxygenase, an enzyme essential for their synthesis. The resulting decrease in prostaglandins reduces the sensitivity of pain receptors to the initiation of pain impulses at sites of inflammation and trauma.[8] Although some evidence suggests that aspirin might also produce analgesia through a central mechanism, more recent work supports the conclusion that its site of action is totally peripheral and that its analgesia does not result from effects on the brain or spinal cord.[9]

Inflammation is characterized by erythema or redness, edema, and tenderness or hyperalgesia at the site. Multiple mediators, including histamine, bradykinin, 5-hydroxytryptamine, leukotrienes, and prostaglandins of the E-series, participate in the inflammatory response. Salicylates are thought to exert their anti-inflammatory effect, at least in part, through the inhibition of prostaglandin synthesis; however, additional mechanisms are probably involved.[8]

The adult oral aspirin dosage considered to be safe and effective for self-medication in the management of mild to moderate pain is 325–650 mg every 4 hours, or 325–500 mg every 3 hours, or 650–1,000 mg every 6 hours while symptoms persist, not to exceed 4 g in 24 hours.[10] The recommended pediatric analgesic dose is provided in Table 1. It must be noted, however, that

TABLE 1	Pediatric analgesic oral dosing recommendations for aspirin and acetaminophen	
Age (yr)	Number of 80-mg or 81-mg[a] dosage units	Number of 325-mg[a] dosage units
<2	Consult physician	Consult physician
2 to <4	2	1/2
4 to <6	3	3/4
6 to <9	4	1
9 to <11	4–5	1–1 1/4
11 to <12	4–6	1–1 1/2

[a]Doses may be repeated every 4 hours, up to four times daily, while symptoms persist, or as directed by a physician.

the nonprescription use of aspirin in children with viral influenza or chickenpox is not recommended because of the increased risk of Reye's syndrome.

Aspirin doses in the range of 4–6 g per day are often required to produce anti-inflammatory effects. Because the maximum analgesic dose for self-medication with aspirin is 4 g per day in divided doses, it is unlikely that anti-inflammatory efficacy can be optimal in all cases with aspirin doses appropriate for self-medication.

Therapeutic Considerations for Use

Impaired Platelet Aggregation and Hematologic Effects Platelet aggregation is an important hemostatic mechanism for controlling the oozing type of capillary bleeding. Aspirin (but not other salicylates) may compromise hemostasis by irreversibly inhibiting platelet aggregation. Aspirin can potentiate bleeding from capillary sites such as those found in the GI tract, posttonsillectomy tonsillar beds, and tooth sockets following dental extractions. In fact, a single 650-mg dose of aspirin doubles the bleeding time to 4–7 days. Consequently, aspirin therapy should be discontinued at least 1 week prior to surgery and should not be used to relieve the pain of tonsillectomy, dental extraction, or other surgical procedure except under the close supervision of a physician or dentist.[8]

Because of its effect on hemostasis, aspirin is also contraindicated in patients with hypoprothrombinemia, vitamin K deficiency, hemophilia, a history of any bleeding disorder, or a history of peptic ulcer disease. By contrast, acetaminophen does not affect platelet aggregation or bleeding time. A daily dose of 1,950 mg of acetaminophen for 6 weeks was found to have no effect on bleeding time in hemophiliacs.[11] Consequently, acetaminophen is an appropriate analgesic to recommend for self-medication in patients when aspirin's effect on hemostasis is a concern. Salicylates do not normally affect the leukocyte, platelet, or erythrocyte count; the hematocrit; or the hemoglobin content. However, chronic blood loss from the GI tract resulting from continued use of aspirin-containing products can cause iron deficiency anemia and alter hematologic indices.

Impaired Uric Acid Elimination Salicylates can affect uric acid secretion and reabsorption by the renal tubules. The resulting effect on plasma uric acid depends on the dose of salicylate administered. Low doses (1 to 2 g per day) inhibit tubular uric acid secretion without affecting reabsorption, may increase plasma uric acid levels, and may precipitate or worsen an attack of gout. Moderate doses (2 to 3 g per day) have no effect on uric acid secretion, and high doses (>5 g per day) may decrease plasma uric acid by increasing its renal excretion. Because of the dose-dependent nature of salicylate on uric acid excretion, all salicylates should be avoided in patients with a history of gout or hyperuricemia.

Gastrointestinal Irritation and Bleeding Aspirin produces local GI damage by penetrating the protective mucous and bicarbonate layers covering the gastric mucosa and permitting the "back diffusion" of acid, causing cellular and vascular erosion. Contributing mechanisms include inhibition of mucosal prostaglandin synthesis, reduction and alteration of mucous secretion, and reduction of bicarbonate secretion.[12] Endoscopic evaluation of healthy volunteers showed that 650 mg of aspirin produced multiple gastric petechiae and erythema within 1 hour in all subjects. A second group taking 650 mg aspirin every 6 hours for 24 hours showed multiple antral erosions in all subjects and duodenal erosions and petechiae in half the volunteers.[12] In a prospective endoscopic analysis of patients taking aspirin (2.5 g per day) for at least 3 months, 20% had gastric ulcers, 40% had gastric erosions, 75% had gastric erythema, and 4% had duodenal ulceration.[12]

GI blood loss with aspirin is dose-dependent. Normal subjects with no aspirin exposure lose approximately 0.5 mL of blood per day in the stool. Moderate aspirin intake increases this amount to 2–6 mL per day, and up to 15% of patients will lose in excess of 10 mL per day. Chronic GI bleeding of this magnitude can deplete total body iron and thus produce iron deficiency anemia. Patients experiencing aspirin-induced blood loss may or may not be positive for fecal occult blood, depending on the dose and duration of aspirin therapy. Aspirin use should be discontinued for at least 3 days prior to a test for fecal occult blood.

In a small percentage of patients, aspirin use can produce massive GI bleeding (acute hemorrhagic gastritis), resulting in the vomiting of blood (hematemesis) or the presence of large amounts of digested blood in the stools (melena). Recent aspirin ingestion has been associated with about half of all cases of acute hemorrhage gastritis, and the incidence of hospital admissions for major upper GI bleeding attributable to regular aspirin use is estimated to be about 15 cases per 100,000 admissions per year.[13] Elderly patients, patients with a history of gastric ulceration or bleeding, and those with alcoholic liver disease are at increased risk for acute hemorrhagic gastritis with aspirin use and therefore should avoid taking aspirin. In addition, patients who take aspirin should be advised that ingesting aspirin with alcohol appears to increase the incidence of GI bleeding.[14]

Aspirin Intolerance Manifestations of aspirin intolerance include hives (urticaria), edema, difficulty breathing, bronchospasm, rhinitis, or shock, and they usually occur within 3 hours of aspirin ingestion. Aspirin intolerance occurs most commonly in patients with chronic urticaria (up to 28%), in asthmatic patients (up to 19%), and in patients with nasal polyps (up to 23%). Patients with chronic urticaria usually develop an urticarial reaction to aspirin, and those with asthma or nasal polyps normally develop bronchospasm and/or rhinorrhea. The incidence of aspirin intolerance in adults and children without one of the above predisposing factors is about 0.3%.

Patients intolerant to aspirin may also cross-react with other chemicals or drugs. Up to 15% percent of aspirin-intolerant patients may cross-react when exposed to tartrazine dyes, which can be found in many drugs, in foods such as soft drinks and colored candy, and in colored desserts such as puddings and frostings. The cross-reaction rate for acetaminophen and ibuprofen in documented aspirin-intolerant patients is 6% and 97%, respectively. High cross-reaction rates in aspirin-intolerant patients are also reported with prescription nonsteroidal anti-inflammatory drugs (NSAIDs). Thus, patients with a history of aspirin intolerance should be advised to avoid all aspirin- and ibuprofen-containing products and to use acetaminophen for analgesic self-medication. However, even though the cross-reaction rate for acetaminophen is low, aspirin-intolerant patients may exhibit urticarial or bronchospastic symptoms with this drug.[15] Other nonprescription analgesics that have a low risk of cross-reactivity include sodium salicylate and choline salicylate.[16] In 182 documented aspirin-intolerant patients given either sodium or choline salicylate, no symptoms of intolerance were observed.[17]

Pregnancy and Breast-Feeding   Aspirin consumption during pregnancy may produce adverse maternal effects including anemia, antepartum or postpartum hemorrhage, and prolonged gestation and labor. The increased duration of gestation and labor results from the inhibition of prostaglandin synthesis. Regular aspirin ingestion during pregnancy may increase the risk for complicated deliveries, including cesarean sections and breech and forceps deliveries; however, data supporting this concern are lacking.

Aspirin readily crosses the placenta and can be found in higher concentrations in the neonate than in the mother. Salicylate elimination is slow in the neonate because of the immature and underdeveloped capacity to form glycine and glucuronic acid conjugates in the liver and reduced urinary excretion resulting from low glomerular filtration rates.[18,19]

Fetal effects of in-utero aspirin exposure include intrauterine growth retardation, congenital salicylate intoxication, decreased albumin-binding capacity, and increased perinatal mortality. In-utero mortality results, in part, from antepartum hemorrhage or premature closure of the ductus arteriosus. In-utero aspirin exposure within 1 week of delivery can produce hemorrhagic episodes and/or pruritic rash in the neonate. Reported neonatal bleeding complications include petechiae, hematuria, cephalhematoma, subconjunctival hemorrhage, and bleeding from circumcision. An increased incidence of intracranial hemorrhage in premature or low-birthweight infants has also been reported after maternal aspirin use near birth.[20]

The relationship between maternal aspirin ingestion and congenital malformation is unresolved. An association between maternal aspirin ingestion, oral clefts, and congenital heart disease has been reported. However, other studies have failed to demonstrate any increased risk for fetal malformation resulting from maternal aspirin exposure.[20]

Aspirin and other salicylates are excreted into breast milk in low concentrations. Following single-dose oral salicylate ingestion, peak milk levels occur at about 3 hours, producing a milk to maternal plasma ratio of 0.03:0.08. Adverse effects on platelet function in the nursing infant exposed to aspirin via the mother's milk have not been reported but still must be considered a potential risk.[20]

In summary, both increased maternal morbidity and fetal morbidity and mortality have been reported with perinatal aspirin exposure. The role of salicylates in producing fetal malformation during first-trimester exposure is unresolved. Women should be advised to avoid aspirin during pregnancy, especially during the last trimester, and when breast-feeding. At these times, acetaminophen is the preferred analgesic for self-medication.

Reye's Syndrome   Reye's syndrome is an acute, potentially fatal illness occurring primarily in children and young adults. It is characterized by vomiting, progressive central nervous system (CNS) damage, signs of hepatic injury, and hypoglycemia. The onset usually follows a viral infection with influenza (type A or B) or varicella-zoster. Within 1–7 days, persistent vomiting generally occurs along with stupor, possibly progressing to generalized convulsions and coma. Other neurologic symptoms include listlessness, lethargy, disorientation, hostility, combativeness, inability to recognize family members, incessant moaning or screaming, twitching, and jerking. The mortality rate may be as high as 50%.[21]

Three case-controlled retrospective studies reported in the early 1980s by the state health departments of Arizona, Michigan, and Ohio suggested an association between the development of Reye's syndrome and the ingestion of aspirin during the antecedent viral illness. After reviewing the available data, the Centers for Disease Control, the American Academy of Pediatrics (AAP), the Food and Drug Administration (FDA), and the U.S. Surgeon General issued a warning that aspirin and other salicylates should be avoided in children and young adults who have influenza or chickenpox. In 1986, the FDA issued a final regulation requiring that a uniform Reye's syndrome warning be added to the labels of nonprescription aspirin and aspirin-containing products. The required labeling states:

> **WARNING**   Children and teenagers should not use this medicine for chicken pox or flu symptoms before a doctor is consulted about Reye's syndrome, a rare but serious illness.

The Public Health Service (PHS) Reye's Syndrome Task Force conducted its study in the peak influenza season between January 1985 and May 1986 in 70 pediatric tertiary care centers throughout the United States and reported its findings in 1987.[22] Greater than 90% of the subjects who developed Reye's syndrome had taken salicylates. The independent risk of nonaspirin-salicylate use could not be assessed. The study also found that risk of developing Reye's syndrome correlated with the salicylate dose, with those subjects who received higher doses being at greater risk.

The dose dependency of Reye's syndrome risk was further evaluated using data from the PHS's Main Study of Reye's Syndrome and Medications.[23] Aspirin doses as low as 15 mg/kg per day were associated with a sevenfold increase in the risk for developing Reye's syndrome. Based on these data, it was concluded that there is no safe minimum dose of aspirin in children and teenagers with influenza or chickenpox and that the drug should be completely avoided.

Because of concerns of potential bias in the above-cited PHS study, an epidemiologic investigation was conducted to assess whether the findings of that study were flawed.[24] After controlling for five potential sources of bias in the study, a strong association was confirmed between the use of salicylate during an antecedent viral infection and the subsequent development of Reye's syndrome. Thus, it is imperative that pharmacists warn against giving products containing aspirin or nonaspirin salicylate to children and teenagers who have influenza or chickenpox. In such cases, acetaminophen is the preferred nonprescription analgesic/antipyretic. A simple viral upper respiratory infection (the "common cold") is not a contraindication to aspirin use, but symptoms may mimic some of those seen in influenza and chickenpox; therefore, many consumers and clinicians recommend a conservative approach of aspirin avoidance when symptoms resembling influenza occur.

Drug Interactions

Analgesic doses of aspirin can increase the free fraction of valproic acid in plasma up to 43%, possibly causing enhanced neurologic toxicity such as drowsiness and behavioral disturbances. The mechanism is thought to be a combination of protein-binding displacement and decreased clearance of valproic acid. Thus, patients taking valproic acid should avoid salicylates; acetaminophen appears to be a safe nonprescription analgesic alternative.[25]

The hypoglycemic effect of sulfonylureas (e.g., glipizide, glyburide, and tolazamide) may be enhanced by the concurrent administration of any salicylate. The mechanism appears to be a salicylate-induced increase in insulin secretion, which occurs with salicylate doses greater than 2 g per day. The decreased protein binding of the sulfonylurea may also play a role. Thus, patients taking sulfonylurea oral hypoglycemic drugs to control diabetes should avoid all salicylate-containing products and consider acetaminophen as an appropriate alternative.[26]

The uricosuric effect of both probenecid and sulfinpyrazone may be antagonized by the concurrent administration of salicylate, resulting in the worsening of hyperuricemia and the possible exacerbation of gout. The effect and magnitude of this interaction is salicylate dose-dependent. Although an occasional dose of aspirin or other salicylate is unlikely to cause serious problems in patients taking uricosuric drugs, all salicylates are best avoided in such patients. Again, acetaminophen is an acceptable nonprescription analgesic alternative.[26]

Ethanol increases fecal blood loss resulting from aspirin ingestion, possibly doubling daily GI blood loss when compared with that induced by aspirin in the absence of ethanol. This effect results both from the GI erosive effects of ethanol and aspirin and from an enhanced prolongation of bleeding time due to ethanol's potentiation of the antiplatelet effect of aspirin. Additionally, it has been reported that the ingestion of ethanol plus 1 g of aspirin 1 hour after a standard breakfast significantly elevated the blood alcohol concentration compared with that of subjects who did not receive aspirin. In such patients, ethanol bioavailability is increased because gastric alcohol dehydrogenase is inhibited, thus allowing greater GI absorption of ethanol.[26,27] Pharmacists should advise patients not to consume ethanol and aspirin together because of the potential for enhanced irritation or GI bleeding, or enhanced neurologic impairment from the ethanol. If ethanol is to be consumed during analgesic use, acetaminophen should be recommended for self-medication as an alternative to aspirin.

Salicylates may increase the toxicity of methotrexate (MTX) by displacing MTX from protein-binding sites and decreasing its renal excretion. Serious sequelae including pancytopenia have been reported with this drug combination. Patients receiving MTX must be warned against self-medication with any nonprescription analgesic containing any form of salicylate. Acetaminophen has been used concurrently with MTX without producing an increase in MTX toxicity.[26]

Aspirin in doses greater than 3 g per day can have a hypoprothrombinemic effect that can be additive to that produced by oral anticoagulants such as warfarin. In addition, the GI erosion and the inhibition of platelet aggregation produced by aspirin may further increase the bleeding risk if aspirin is used concurrently with an oral anticoagulant. An increased incidence of GI bleeding has been reported in patients receiving warfarin and as little as 500 mg per day of aspirin. Thus, patients receiving oral anticoagulants should be cautioned to avoid all nonprescription analgesic products containing aspirin or other salicylates and to consider acetaminophen as an appropriate nonprescription analgesic alternative.[26]

A large number of additional drug–drug interactions have been documented, many of which are not as potentially significant as those mentioned above. Nevertheless, standard drug interaction reference books and databases should be consulted, especially when patients are chronically taking large salicylate doses.

Overdose

Mild salicylate intoxication (salicylism) occurs with chronic therapy that produces toxic salicylate plasma concentrations. Chronic intoxication in adults generally requires taking salicylate doses of approximately 90–100 mg/kg within 24 hours for at least 2 days. Symptoms include headache, dizziness, ringing in the ears, difficulty in hearing, dimness of vision, mental confusion, lassitude, drowsiness, sweating, thirst, hyperventilation, nausea, vomiting, and occasional diarrhea.[8] These symptoms are all reversible upon lowering the plasma concentration to a therapeutic range.

Acute salicylate intoxication is categorized as mild (<150 mg/kg), moderate (150–300 mg/kg), or severe (>300 mg/kg). Symptoms depend on serum salicylate levels and include lethargy, tinnitus, tachypnea and pulmonary edema, convulsions, coma, nausea, vomiting, hemorrhage, and dehydration. Acid–base disturbances are prominent and range from respiratory alkalosis to metabolic acidosis. Initially, salicylate affects the respiratory center in the medulla, producing hyperventilation and respiratory alkalosis. In severely intoxicated adults and in most salicylate-poisoned children under 5 years of age, respiratory alkalosis rapidly progresses to metabolic acidosis.[28] Children are more prone to develop high fever in salicylate poisoning. Hypoglycemia resulting from increased tissue glucose use may be especially serious in children.[8] Bleeding may occur from the GI tract or mucosal surfaces, and petechiae are a prominent feature at autopsy.

Emergency management of acute salicylate intoxication is directed toward preventing the absorption of salicylate from the GI tract. Because such absorption occurs rapidly, emptying the stomach at home or en route to an emergency medical facility is desirable. Vomiting should be induced even if the patient has vomited spontaneously. Adults and children over the age of 12 should be given 30 mL of syrup of ipecac followed by 8 oz of water, clear liquids, or carbonated beverages, and should be ambulated to stimulate emesis. If emesis does not occur in 20–30 minutes, the process should be repeated with the same ipecac dose.

For children 1–12 years of age, the recommended dose of ipecac syrup is 15 mL (1 tbsp or 3 tsp) followed by 8 oz of water, clear liquids, or carbonated beverages. The same 15-mL dose of ipecac syrup should be repeated if vomiting does not occur within 20–30 minutes. In children under 1 year of age, vomiting should be induced only under medical supervision.

Administering ipecac syrup or other oral liquids to a person who is convulsing or not completely conscious is absolutely contraindicated because of the potential for aspiration.[29,30] Further guidelines on the use of ipecac syrup or activated charcoal in preventing absorption of salicylate are included in Chapter 12, "Emetic and Antiemetic Products."

Biopharmaceutics of Salicylate-Containing Products

Salicylates are absorbed by passive diffusion of the nonionized drug in the stomach and small intestine. Factors affecting absorption include dosage form, gastric pH, gastric emptying time, dissolution rate, and the presence of antacids or food. Because enteric-coated aspirin is absorbed only from the small intestine, its absorption is markedly slowed by food, which increases the gastric residence time. Buffered aspirin products are absorbed more rapidly than nonbuffered products, but this has little therapeutic significance in terms of onset of drug effect.[8,31] Rectal absorption of salicylate is slow and unreliable. By the rectal route, the drug is only 60–75% bioavailable and produces peak salicylate levels of about half those achieved with an equivalent oral dose.[32]

Endoscopic evaluation comparing the gastric damage produced by buffered and nonbuffered aspirin products suggests that there is no difference in the amount of gastric damage produced by either product.[33] However, enteric coating eliminates the gastric injury produced by aspirin.[34,35] Equivalent doses of plain, buffered, or enteric-coated aspirin produce essentially the same plasma levels of salicylate; however, the time to peak is delayed with the enteric-coated product.[36] Thus, for patients requiring rapid pain relief, enteric-coated aspirin is inappropriate because of the delay in absorption and time to analgesic effect. However, for patients requiring prolonged aspirin therapy, such as that required for the management of osteoarthritis, enteric-coated aspirin is often preferred because it produces less gastric mucosal injury than either plain or buffered aspirin.

Timed-release aspirin is formulated to prolong the product's duration of action by slowing dissolution and absorption. Because of this delayed absorption, such products are not useful for rapid pain relief but may be useful as bedtime medication. Bioavailability comparison of a single 1.3-g dose of plain aspirin versus 1.3 g of a timed-release formulation (Measurin®) revealed plasma salicylate concentrations to be higher for the first 4 hours following administration with the plain aspirin product and higher during the 4- to 8-hour interval with the timed-release product.[37] But although comparisons of three timed-release aspirin products (Measurin®, Verin®, and Zorprin®) demonstrated all three to be equally bioavailable, they were not bioequivalent. Fifty percent of the administered dose was recovered in the urine approximately 9 hours following administration of Measurin® compared with 18 to 19 hours for both Verin® and Zorprin®.[38] These data suggest that the release profiles are not identical for the various sustained-release aspirin products and that the duration of therapeutic efficacy is, therefore, product-dependent.

It has been suggested that sustained-release aspirin products produce less GI irritation than regular aspirin.[39] However, aspirin-induced reversible deafness has been reported to occur to a much greater extent with high-dose sustained-release aspirin than with equivalent daily doses of plain aspirin.[40]

Effervescent aspirin solutions (e.g., Alka-Seltzer®) are rapidly absorbed because disintegration does not have to occur; however, there is no evidence that such products produce more rapid or effective analgesia than solid-dose forms containing salicylates. Moreover, effervescent aspirin solutions contain large amounts of sodium and must be avoided by patients requiring restricted sodium intake (e.g., those with hypertension, heart failure, or renal failure).

Aspirin and Myocardial Infarct Prophylaxis

As noted previously, aspirin is known to inhibit prostaglandin synthesis within the platelet irreversibly and to retard platelet aggregation for the life span of the aspirin-exposed platelet. Because platelet aggregation participates in thrombin clot formation, aspirin's antithrombotic activity has been used clinically under medical supervision to prevent transient ischemic attack (TIA), thrombotic stroke, myocardial infarct (MI) in unstable angina patients, postmyocardial reinfarct, and vascular reocclusion following both percutaneous transluminal coronary angioplasty and coronary artery bypass grafts.

Recent evidence as described below suggests a potential primary preventive role for aspirin in MI in adult patients with no history or symptomatology of coronary artery disease. Pharmacists and other health professionals should be cognizant of these study results to counsel patients effectively on the potential benefits and risks of self-medication with aspirin to prevent heart attack.

The final report of the aspirin component of the U.S. Physicians' Health Study was published in 1989.[41] This study was a randomized, double-blind, placebo-controlled trial designed to determine whether low-dose aspirin (325 mg every other day) would decrease overall cardiovascular mortality. Following a rigid selection process, 11,037 physicians were randomly assigned to receive aspirin and 11,034 to receive aspirin placebo. Average follow-up time for the 22,071 participants was 60.2 months.

There was a 44% reduction in the risk of MI, both fatal and nonfatal, in the aspirin group as compared with the placebo group; however, analysis showed that the reduction was apparent only among those who were 50 years of age and older. The benefit was also present at all levels of cholesterol but appeared greatest at low levels. Analysis also showed that aspirin did not reduce all-cause cardiovascular mortality. An approximate 15% increase was observed in the incidence of hemorrhagic stroke in the aspirin group, but this increase was not statistically significant. The relative risk of ulcer development in the aspirin group was 1.22 and was also not significantly different from that of the placebo group. GI discomfort was reported in approximately 26% of both the aspirin and placebo groups.

Platelets are postulated to play a role in atherogenesis and myocardial ischemia, and data from the Physicians' Health Study were analyzed to determine whether low-dose aspirin therapy could prevent the development of angina. Analysis revealed no significant difference between the aspirin and placebo groups with regard to the development of angina pectoris or the need for coronary revascularization.[42]

A subset analysis was reported for 333 physicians with baseline chronic stable angina but with no history of MI, stroke, or TIA.[43] The purpose of this analysis was to evaluate the efficacy of low-dose aspirin (325 mg every other day) in the primary prevention of MI among patients with chronic stable angina. Among these subjects, those treated with aspirin showed an 87% risk reduction for MI; however, they also showed a statistically significant increase in nonhemorrhagic stroke. This finding contrasts with an apparent beneficial effect of aspirin on stroke risk reported in the Second International Study of Infarct Survival (ISIS-2), in which low-dose aspirin therapy given for suspected evolving MI produced a 46% reduction in overall stroke risk.[44]

Contrary to the Physicians' Health Study, a similar 6-year British study conducted among 5,139 healthy male physicians found no beneficial effect of aspirin in the primary prevention of MI.[45] Two-thirds of the subjects were randomly assigned to take aspirin (500 mg per day); the remaining third were randomly assigned to avoid aspirin and aspirin-containing products.

No significant difference in the rate of fatal or nonfatal MI was found between the aspirin-treated and control groups. The aspirin-treated group experienced an approximate 50% reduction in TIA and an increase in stroke that was not statistically significant. However, peptic ulcer disease did increase significantly in the aspirin-treated group.

The primary findings of these two studies are nonconfirmatory, but differences between them may be accounted for by major differences in subject numbers, mean subject age, study design, and statistical analysis. An overview analysis of the two studies found a statistically significant 32% reduction in the incidence of nonfatal MI in the aspirin-treated groups and no significant difference in the incidence of nonfatal stroke or total cardiovascular death.[46]

To determine whether aspirin is also beneficial in reducing MI in women, a prospective cohort study of 87,678 U.S. registered nurses, aged 34–65, was conducted with 6 years of follow-up to evaluate the association between regular aspirin use and the risk of a first MI.[47] Among women under 50 years of age, there was no reduction in risk of MI for any amount of aspirin use. Among those aged 50 years and older who took one to six aspirin per week, there was a 39% risk reduction in MI; however, there was no reduction for those taking seven or more aspirin per week. The risk of stroke or cardiovascular death was unaltered by any degree of aspirin intake.

Based on the above studies, it appears that low-dose aspirin does reduce the risk of a first MI in both men and women over the age of 50. It may be more effective in patients who have other associated atherosclerotic risks such as hypercholesterolemia. However, patients under the age of 50 receive no apparent benefit from aspirin prophylaxis for MI. The dose of aspirin appears important, and based on the Physicians' Health Study, 325 mg of aspirin every other day is sufficient and carries a very low risk of GI erosion and bleeding. The potential for increased risk of stroke during low-dose aspirin prophylaxis remains unresolved.

Nonacetylated Salicylates

Choline Salicylate Choline salicylate (Arthropan®) is a liquid salicylate preparation. It is absorbed from the stomach more rapidly than aspirin tablets, but this property has little clinical significance.[10] A 5-mL dose of choline salicylate (174 mg/mL, or 870 mg) is equivalent to 650 mg of aspirin in terms of salicylate content. The recommended adult dosage is 435–870 mg every 4 hours, or 435–670 mg every 3 hours, or 870–1,340 mg every 6 hours, not to exceed 5,325 mg in 24 hours.[10] Because some patients find the fishy odor of the liquid product unacceptable, choline salicylate oral solution may be mixed with fruit juice, a carbonated beverage, or water just before administration; however, it should not be mixed with any alkaline solution (e.g., antacid) because the liberation of choline exaggerates the fishy odor of the product. Comparative analgesic/anti-inflammatory efficacy studies are not available for choline salicylate. However, the product was found to be less effective than either aspirin or acetaminophen as an antipyretic in children.[48]

Magnesium Salicylate A study comparing the analgesic efficacy of 500 mg of aspirin taken four times daily with 500 mg of magnesium salicylate taken four times daily in patients with chronic degenerative arthritis found similar reductions in objective pain scores for the two drugs at the end of 12 weeks.[49] Magnesium salicylate is available as the tetrahydrate; as a consequence, the salicylate content of 377 mg of magnesium salicylate tetrahydrate is equivalent to that of 325 mg of sodium salicylate. The recommended adult dosage for nonprescription use is 377–754 mg every 4 hours, or 377–580 mg every 3 hours, or 754–1,160 mg every 6 hours, not to exceed 4,640 mg in 24 hours.[10] The maximum 24-hour dose of magnesium salicylate contains 264 mg (11 mEq) of magnesium. Thus, patients with compromised renal function must avoid using magnesium salicylate because of the potential for decreased renal excretion of magnesium with its subsequent accumulation and the production of systemic magnesium toxicity.

Sodium Salicylate Divided oral doses of enteric-coated aspirin and enteric-coated sodium salicylate, 4.8 g per day, have been shown to be equally effective in the treatment of rheumatoid arthritis. Both drugs have produced similar degrees of pain relief, increased grip strength, reduced joint tenderness, and decreased digital joint circumference.[50] Patients hypersensitive to aspirin may be able to tolerate sodium salicylate. However, sodium salicylate is less effective than an equal dose of aspirin in reducing pain or fever. The recommended adult nonprescription anti-inflammatory dosage of sodium salicylate is 325–650 mg every 4 hours, or 325–500 mg every 3 hours, or 650–1,000 mg every 6 hours, not to exceed 4 g in 24 hours.[10] The maximum 4-g dose of sodium salicylate contains 560 mg (25 mEq) of sodium; consequently, patients on sodium restriction should avoid using sodium salicylate.

Comparison of Aspirin and Nonacetylated Salicylates When doses containing equivalent amounts of salicylate are given, it appears that aspirin and the nonacetylated salicylates are equally well absorbed and produce similar plasma salicylate levels. However, choline salicylate oral solution produces peak plasma salicylate levels sooner than the oral solid-dosage forms.[51]

Because aspirin's effect on platelet aggregation with a prolongation of bleeding time requires the participation of the acetyl moiety, nonacetylated salicylates do not affect platelet aggregation or bleeding time significantly.[52–55] But except for this difference, all nonacetylated salicylates can be expected to have all the same contraindications and interactions as aspirin because all other salicylate effects result from the production of salicylic acid by both aspirin and the nonacetylated salicylates. However, nonacetylated salicylates are much weaker prostaglandin synthesis inhibitors than aspirin and, as such, appear to cause less GI erosion and bleeding, fewer renal complications, and a low level of cross-reactivity in aspirin-intolerant patients.[16,56]

Acetaminophen

Acetaminophen is an effective analgesic and antipyretic; however, it has only weak anti-inflammatory activity, as has been demonstrated in animals in doses much greater than those required for analgesia.[8] Nonprescription analgesic doses of acetaminophen do not produce any therapeutically significant anti-inflammatory effect, apparently because acetaminophen is a weak inhibitor of prostaglandin synthesis. Unlike salicylates, acetaminophen produces analgesia through a central rather than a peripheral effect on the nervous system.[9]

Acetaminophen is effective in relieving mild to moderate pain of nonvisceral origin. The recommended adult dosage of acetaminophen is 325–650 mg every 4 hours, or 325–500 mg every 3 hours, or 650–1,000 mg every 6 hours, not to exceed a total of 4 g in 24 hours.[10] Table 1 gives the recommended pediatric analgesic oral dosage. Rectal bioavailability of acetaminophen is approximately 50–60% that of oral administration. Comparative efficacy studies suggest that equivalent doses of acetaminophen and aspirin by the same route produce equivalent degrees of analgesia.[57]

Therapeutic Considerations for Use

Acetaminophen crosses the placenta but is considered safe for use during pregnancy. It appears in breast milk, producing a milk to maternal plasma ratio of 0.50:1.0. Based on a 1,000-mg maternal dose, the estimated maximum infant dose is 1.85% of the maternal dose. The only adverse effect reported in nursing infants exposed to acetaminophen through breast milk is a rarely occurring maculopapular rash, which subsides when drug exposure is discontinued. The AAP considers acetaminophen use to be compatible with breast-feeding.[20]

Acetaminophen has no effect on the urinary excretion of uric acid, on prothrombin synthesis, or on platelet aggregation and bleeding time.[58] In addition, it produces less GI irritation, erosion, and bleeding than aspirin or salicylates. Acetaminophen also has a very low incidence of cross-reactivity in aspirin-intolerant patients. Thus, for patients who cannot take aspirin or a salicylate because of contraindications due to adverse effects on bleeding time, uric acid excretion, GI bleeding, aspirin intolerance, or concurrent drug therapy, acetaminophen is an appropriate nonprescription analgesic alternative.

Drug Interactions

Acetaminophen produces no therapeutically significant drug interactions with the possible exception of zidovudine (azidothymidine, or AZT). It has been reported that patients with acquired immunodeficiency syndrome (AIDS) and AIDS-related complex who were taking zidovudine experienced an increased incidence of bone marrow suppression if they concurrently received acetaminophen.[59] Both acetaminophen and zidovudine are metabolized by hepatic glucuronidation; competition for the same metabolizing system may produce increased levels of zidovudine, resulting in increased bone marrow suppression. In a subsequent attempt to clarify this interaction, four patients receiving 200 mg of zidovudine were administered 650 mg of acetaminophen every 6 hours for 48 hours. Acetaminophen had no significant effect on peak times of zidovudine plasma levels or on the plasma half-life of zidovudine. However, the total availability of zidovudine to plasma with concurrent acetaminophen decreased by 19%.[60] In a study to ascertain whether concurrent treatment with acetaminophen impairs the clearance of zidovudine, 27 patients with AIDS or AIDS-related complex receiving 200 mg of zidovudine were concurrently treated with one of three acetaminophen regimens: 325 mg for 3 days, 650 mg for 3 days, or 650 mg for 7 days. Neither zidovudine clearance nor the production of the zidovudine glucuronide conjugate was impaired by the concurrent acetaminophen treatment. In fact, zidovudine clearance was actually increased by 5%, 11%, and 33%, respectively, with the three acetaminophen regimens. The increased total clearance of zidovudine probably resulted from increased nonhepatic or renal clearance of zidovudine. From baseline until 2 weeks after the last dose of acetaminophen was administered, there were no statistically significant changes in hemoglobin concentration, leukocyte count, absolute neutrophil count, or platelet count in the three acetaminophen treatment groups.[61]

In summary, it appears that acetaminophen does not decrease the hepatic clearance of zidovudine and, in fact, may increase the rate of nonhepatic clearance. These studies suggest that concurrent administration of acetaminophen with zidovudine does not produce increased plasma levels of zidovudine and that the short-term use of acetaminophen (less than 7 days) does not increase the risk of myelosuppression and neutropenia in AIDS patients receiving zidovudine. Aspirin should probably be avoided by AIDS patients receiving zidovudine because the prolonged antiplatelet effect of aspirin could increase their bleeding risk. For these patients, the short-term or intermittent use of acetaminophen is the recommended nonprescription analgesic for self-medication.

Overdose

Data from the American Association of Poison Control Centers reveal that acetaminophen accounted for the most overdoses with nonprescription analgesics (48%), followed by aspirin (37%) and ibuprofen (15%). Forty-seven percent of analgesic overdoses were in children under 12 years of age, and 95–99% of these overdoses were accidental. Fifty-three percent of the nonprescription analgesic poisonings were in adults, with three-fourths of these poisonings being intentional—presumably suicide gestures. Approximately three-fourths of adult nonprescription analgesic overdoses occurred in women.

Of 4,801 nonprescription analgesic overdoses in children, only 0.3 to 0.4% resulted in severe or life-threatening effects, and there were no deaths in this group. In 5,333 adult exposures, severe or life-threatening results occurred in 5.4% taking aspirin, 5.2% taking acetaminophen, and 1.6% taking ibuprofen; 11 deaths occurred with aspirin, 10 with acetaminophen, and none with ibuprofen.[62]

Symptoms during the first 2 days after an acute overdose may not reflect the potential seriousness of the exposure. Early symptoms of acetaminophen intoxication include nausea, vomiting, drowsiness, confusion, low blood pressure, and abdominal pain. In severe poisoning, CNS stimulation, excitement, cardiac arrhythmias, low blood pressure, and delirium may occur initially, followed by CNS depression with stupor, hypothermia, shock, and coma.[63] Clinical manifestations of hepatotoxicity begin 2–4 days after the acute ingestion of acetaminophen and include increased plasma transaminases (both aspartate and alanine aminotransferase), increased plasma bilirubin with jaundice, and prolonged prothrombin time. In nonfatal cases, the hepatic damage is reversible over a period of weeks or months.[8] The most serious adverse effect of acute overdose with acetaminophen is a dose-dependent, potentially fatal hepatic necrosis. Renal tubular necrosis and hypoglycemic coma may also occur.[8] In adults, hepatotoxicity may occur after ingestion of a single dose of 10–15 g (150–250 mg/kg) of acetaminophen; doses of 20–25 g or more are potentially fatal.

Because of the potential seriousness of acetaminophen overdose, all cases should be referred to a poison control center or other medical personnel experienced in managing such cases. Approximately 65% of acetaminophen intoxication in children is effectively managed in the home, compared with only about 18% for adult acetaminophen overdose.[62] Immediate first aid management of acute acetaminophen poisoning includes the induction of vomiting with ipecac syrup. Activated charcoal may also be effective in reducing the absorption of acetaminophen; however, it can also adsorb the specific antidote for acetaminophen hepatotoxicity, N-acetylcysteine, and presumably reduce its efficacy. If activated charcoal is administered on an in-home, first-aid basis for acetaminophen overdose, this information must be made known to emergency medical personnel administering N-acetylcysteine so that appropriate dose adjustments can be made.[63,64] Dosing recommendations for both ipecac syrup and activated charcoal are included in Chapter 12, "Emetic and Antiemetic Products." Pharmacists and other caregivers are strongly encouraged to coordinate with a poison center any nonhospital-based management of poisoning or drug overdose.

Ibuprofen

Ibuprofen has analgesic, antipyretic, and anti-inflammatory activity; it is also useful in managing mild to moderate pain of nonvisceral origin and dysmenorrhea. Its analgesia apparently results from the peripheral inhibition of cyclo-oxygenase and the subsequent inhibition of prostaglandin synthesis.

The nonprescription analgesic dose of ibuprofen is 200–400 mg every 4–6 hours, not to exceed 1,200 mg in 24 hours. A dose–effect relationship has been demonstrated for ibuprofen analgesia in the range of 100–400 mg. On a milligram-to-milligram basis, ibuprofen is approximately 3.5 times more potent than aspirin as an analgesic, and the analgesic effect may last up to 6 hours.[65–67] The anti-inflammatory dose of ibuprofen is 300–600 mg every 4–6 hours, exceeding the maximum daily dose of ibuprofen recommended for nonprescription use. However, anti-inflammatory efficacy can be achieved within that recommended maximum daily dose range.

Primary dysmenorrhea is estimated to occur in up to 50% of women during their reproductive years. It is characterized by uterine cramps, backache, vomiting, diarrhea, headache, mild fever, and malaise. The symptoms occur shortly before and during the onset of menses and result from increased endometrial production of prostaglandins during this period.[68] In numerous clinical trials, ibuprofen has been shown to be superior to aspirin, nonacetylated salicylates, and acetaminophen for the symptomatic relief of primary dysmenorrhea.[68] Symptomatic relief appears to result from the inhibition of prostaglandin production in the uterus. The recommended dose of ibuprofen for primary dysmenorrhea is 400 mg every 4–6 hours as needed for the 2 to 3 days that symptoms persist.[8]

Therapeutic Considerations for Use

The most frequent adverse effects of ibuprofen involve the GI tract and include dyspepsia, heartburn, nausea, anorexia, and epigastric pain. Ibuprofen produces less GI bleeding than aspirin. In patients receiving one of those two medications for at least 1 year, aspirin produced a 15-mL blood loss over 4 days in contrast to only a 3-mL loss with ibuprofen.[69] A gastroscopic evaluation of patients on either ibuprofen or aspirin for 3–12 months revealed that 50% of those receiving aspirin evidenced gastric lesions compared with only 18% of those receiving ibuprofen.[70]

In dosages of 600–1,800 mg per day, ibuprofen increased bleeding time by inhibiting platelet aggregation. However, ibuprofen's effect on platelet aggregation, unlike that of aspirin, is reversible within 24 hours after medication is discontinued.[71] Ibuprofen does not significantly affect whole blood clotting time or prothrombin time. Because alcohol ingestion has been shown to increase by 3.5-fold the prolongation of bleeding time produced by ibuprofen, patients self-medicating with ibuprofen should be cautioned against the concurrent use of alcohol.[72] In dosages of 1,200–2,400 mg per day, ibuprofen does not appear to affect the hypoprothrombinemia produced by warfarin.[73] However, because plasma protein-binding displacement of warfarin by ibuprofen can occur and because of the drug's antiplatelet activity and its potential for increased GI bleeding, ibuprofen should not be recommended for self-medication to patients who are concurrently taking anticoagulants.

Ibuprofen may decrease renal blood flow and glomerular filtration rate as a result of inhibition of renal prostaglandin synthesis. The result may be increased blood urea nitrogen or serum creatinine values, often with concomitant sodium and water retention. This effect is of greatest clinical importance in patients with preexisting renal impairment or congestive heart failure. Advanced age, hypertension, use of diuretics, diabetes, or atherosclerotic cardiovascular disease appear to increase the risk of renal toxicity with ibuprofen.[74-76] As a result, patients with a history of impaired renal function, congestive heart failure, or diseases that compromise renal hemodynamics should not self-medicate with ibuprofen.

Ibuprofen is contraindicated in patients with a history of intolerance to aspirin or to any other NSAID. Cross-reactivity with ibuprofen is reported to be 97% in documented aspirin-intolerant patients. Patients with a history of asthma may experience a worsening of their bronchospastic symptoms with ibuprofen.

There is no evidence that ibuprofen is teratogenic in either humans or animals. However, because all potent prostaglandin synthesis inhibitors can cause delayed parturition, increased postpartum bleeding, prolonged labor, and adverse fetal cardiovascular effects (closure of the ductus arteriosus), ibuprofen use is contraindicated during the third trimester of pregnancy. In lactating women taking up to 2.4 g of ibuprofen per day, there is no measurable excretion of ibuprofen into breast milk. The AAP considers ibuprofen compatible with breast-feeding.[20]

Drug Interactions

Ibuprofen has been reported to increase plasma digoxin concentrations when coadministered to patients receiving digoxin. However, the clinical significance of this interaction is uncertain. Worsening heart failure with fluid overload and blunting of furosemide responsiveness may occur with the administration of ibuprofen to patients with congestive heart failure. Because of the uncertainty of a possible ibuprofen–digoxin interaction and the potential for ibuprofen-induced furosemide refractoriness with symptomatic deterioration, pharmacists should advise patients with a history of congestive heart failure to avoid self-medicating with any ibuprofen-containing products.[26]

Ibuprofen has been shown to antagonize the blood pressure–lowering effects of certain antihypertensive drugs, including diuretics, beta blockers, and centrally acting antihypertensives. Forty-five patients with essential hypertension controlled with at least two antihypertensive drugs were given ibuprofen (400 mg every 8 hours), acetaminophen (1 g every 8 hours), or placebo (2 capsules every 8 hours) for 3 weeks. At the end of 3 weeks, the ibuprofen-treated group experienced a 5.8 mm Hg increase in sitting mean arterial pressure and a 6.6 mm Hg increase in supine mean arterial pressure, both of which were statistically significant when compared with placebo treatment. By contrast, the acetaminophen-treated group showed no change in blood pressure during the 3-week test interval.[77] Thus, pharmacists should advise hypertensive patients selecting a nonprescription analgesic that ibuprofen may antagonize their blood pressure medication and that acetaminophen is a better choice.

The concurrent use of ibuprofen in lithium-stabilized patients is reported to produce increased plasma lithium levels and enhanced lithium toxicity. In a study of nine psychiatric patients on chronic lithium therapy (600–900 mg per day), the administration of ibuprofen, 1,800 mg per day for 6 days, decreased lithium clearance by 34% and increased serum lithium by 34% (range 12–66%). Three patients showed increased tremor, a dose-dependent adverse reaction to lithium.[78] Similar results have been obtained in healthy subjects concurrently given lithium (900 mg per day) and ibuprofen (1,200 mg per day) for 7 days.[79] Based on limited controlled studies, it appears that aspirin does not adversely affect lithium clearance.[80] Consequently, it is imperative that pharmacists advise patients taking lithium to avoid all ibuprofen-containing nonprescription analgesics. For such patients, acetaminophen is considered the best alternative analgesic because it has little, if any, effect on renal prostaglandin synthesis. Based on limited studies, lithium-treated patients may also safely self-medicate with aspirin.

Limited information is available regarding a potentially serious interaction between MTX and ibuprofen. Of four patients who experienced severe MTX toxicity resulting from concurrent ketoprofen administration, three ultimately died from MTX toxicity.[81] A recent anecdotal report of an 18-year-old male undergoing intravenous MTX therapy for osteogenic sarcoma supports the potential severity of the MTX–ibuprofen interaction. Unknown to the oncology team, this patient was self-medicating with ibuprofen (400 mg every 4 hours) for his leg pain. Twenty hours into his MTX infusion, his serum creatinine, which was 0.9 mg/dL before he began infusion, was now found to be 2.3 mg/dL, and folinic acid rescue was begun immediately. It is postulated that ibuprofen competes with MTX for renal proximal tubular secretion, causing decreased renal clearance of MTX and resulting in nephrotoxicity.[82] Based on limited reports, it is imperative that patients receiving MTX as outpatient therapy be warned not to self-medicate with nonprescription analgesic products containing either ibuprofen or aspirin. For such patients, acetaminophen is the only nonprescription analgesic considered safe.

Overdose

Overdose of ibuprofen usually produces minimal symptoms of toxicity and is rarely fatal. In an analysis of more than 1,500 reports of overdose with ibuprofen, only 0.4% of children and 1.6% of adults exhibited major or life-threatening effects; there were no fatalities. Eighty-six percent of children and 41% of adults evidenced no symptoms from the drug exposure.[62] In a prospective study of 329 cases of ibuprofen overdose, it was found that GI and CNS symptoms (in 42% and 30% of patients, respectively) were most common and included nausea, vomiting, abdominal pain, lethargy, stupor, coma, nystagmus, dizziness, and lightheadedness. Hypotension, bradycardia, tachycardia, dyspnea, and painful breathing were also reported. In this study, 43% of ibuprofen-overdose patients were asymptomatic.[83] Unless contraindicated by convulsions or unconsciousness, appropriate first-aid treatment of ibuprofen overdose includes the induction of vomiting with ipecac syrup or the administration of activated charcoal. (See Chapter 12, "Emetic and Antiemetic Products.")

Comparative Efficacy of Aspirin, Acetaminophen, and Ibuprofen

Numerous controlled studies have demonstrated the equivalent analgesic efficacy of aspirin and acetaminophen on a milligram-for-milligram basis in various pain models, including postoperative pain, cancer pain, episiotomy pain, and oral surgery pain. Aspirin and acetaminophen have similar dose–response and time–effect curves and are equipotent and equianalgesic for the relief of most pain.[57,84] In a controlled study involving 269 patients, acetaminophen (1 g) and aspirin (650 mg) produced similar efficacy in the treatment of moderate to severe headache. The apparent superiority of aspirin on a milligram-for-milligram basis may be the result of an inflammatory component to the headache pain that would be unresponsive to acetaminophen.[85] However, acetaminophen (1 g) has been shown to be superior to aspirin (650 mg) in the control of pain secondary to dental surgery or episiotomy.[86,87] This apparent superiority of acetaminophen is thought to result from the dose-responsive nature of pain control with aspirin and acetaminophen.

Ibuprofen has been shown to be at least as effective as aspirin in treating various types of pain, including dental extraction pain, dysmenorrhea, and episiotomy pain. In fact, a double-blind, single-dose study of postepisiotomy pain found ibuprofen (400 mg) to be more effective than aspirin (600 mg).[88] And another double-blind, single-dose study that compared the efficacy of oral ibuprofen (100, 200, or 400 mg) with that of aspirin (650 mg) in treating moderate to severe pain after the extraction of impacted teeth estimated 100 mg of ibuprofen to be as effective as 650 mg of aspirin.[89]

Controlled clinical trials have shown that ibuprofen is as effective as but not superior to aspirin in the treatment of rheumatoid arthritis. A double-blind, crossover, randomized study with 18 rheumatoid arthritic patients compared aspirin (3.6 g per day), ibuprofen (1.2 g per day), and placebo. Both aspirin and ibuprofen were superior to placebo for symptomatic control but were not different from each other. Both drugs reduced morning stiffness and improved grip strength to an equivalent degree. However, aspirin appeared superior to ibuprofen in the reduction of joint size.[90]

Efficacy comparisons between ibuprofen and acetaminophen support the greater potency of ibuprofen over acetaminophen on a milligram-for-milligram basis. In postpartum patients with moderate to severe episiotomy pain, a single ibuprofen dose (400 mg) was found to be superior to acetaminophen (1,000 mg) in producing analgesia. This superior analgesic effect was manifested by a more rapid onset and prolonged effect and by a greater area under the analgesic time–effect curve.[91] In reducing the severity and duration of migraine headache, ibuprofen at 400 mg every 4 hours was found to be significantly superior to acetaminophen at 900 mg every 4 hours.[92] And in a multicenter study involving 706 patients, a single oral dose of ibuprofen (400 mg) provided superior analgesia following oral surgery compared with acetaminophen (1,000 mg).[93] Numerous comparisons of oral ibuprofen and acetaminophen in various pain models suggest that 100–200 mg of ibuprofen is approximately equianalgesic to 650 mg of acetaminophen. Ibuprofen has a clear superiority, however, in pain conditions associated with inflammation.

Analgesic Adjuvants

Many nonprescription analgesics are combination products containing aspirin, ibuprofen, or acetaminophen as primary ingredients plus caffeine or an antihistamine. The adjuvant ingredients are claimed to enhance the analgesic efficacy of the product. Although the FDA has not yet published a final ruling on this claim, there is some evidence, as reported below, to support the enhanced efficacy of combination products containing adjuvant ingredients.

Thirty clinical studies involving more than 10,000 patients have been analyzed to assess the value of caffeine as an analgesic adjuvant. These studies were based on various pain models, including postpartum uterine cramping, episiotomy pain, oral surgery pain, and headache. Caffeine was combined with aspirin or acetaminophen alone and with aspirin–acetaminophen combinations. In 21 of 26 studies reviewed, the relative potency of the analgesic with caffeine was greater than that of the analgesic in the absence of caffeine. The pooled relative potency estimate for caffeine-containing analgesics is 1.41 (95% CI 1.23–1.63), as compared with an analgesic potency of 1.0 for the analgesic in the absence of caffeine. This analysis suggests that to obtain the same amount of response from an analgesic without caffeine would require a dose approximately 40% greater than that required in the presence of caffeine.[94]

The same adjuvant effect of caffeine has been reported for ibuprofen analgesia. In a double-blind study, a single oral dose of ibuprofen (100 or 200 mg) with and without caffeine (100 mg) was evaluated for pain relief in 298 patients with postoperative pain after the surgical removal of impacted third molars (wisdom teeth). Subjects self-rated their pain relief hourly for 8 hours. Relative potency estimates indicated that the caffeine–ibuprofen combination was 2.4–2.8 times as potent as ibuprofen alone. The combination also had a more rapid onset and a longer duration of analgesic action than ibuprofen alone.[95]

Enhanced analgesia has been reported for various antihistamine–analgesia combinations, including orphenadrine–acetaminophen and phenyltoloxamine–acetaminophen. The adjuvant effect of phenyltoloxamine citrate (60 mg) in combination with acetaminophen (650 mg) was evaluated in 200 female inpatients experiencing episiotomy pain using a self-rating pain relief scale. Compared with acetaminophen alone, the phenyltoloxamine–acetaminophen combination produced significantly greater pain relief at all points from one-half hour through 6 hours postadministration, and it produced a longer duration of analgesia with a peak effect at 3 hours compared with 2 hours for acetaminophen alone.[96] A growing body of clinical literature supports the enhancement of analgesia by the inclusion of either caffeine or an antihistamine in a nonprescription analgesic combination.

Nonprescription Analgesic Selection Guidelines

In determining the medication to recommend, the pharmacist must consider the condition being treated; the nature and origin of the pain; the accompanying symptoms; any history of asthma, urticaria, aspirin or NSAID intolerance, peptic ulcer, gout or hyperuricemia, clotting disorders, hypertension, or diabetes; and the concurrent use of both prescription and nonprescription medications. In addition, product selection must include evaluation of the product's proven efficacy for the condition being treated, formulation factors that may give the patient more prompt relief or fewer side effects, and the potential for adverse effects and drug interactions from the product ingredients.

Aspirin has proven efficacy for nonvisceral pain and is especially useful if the pain has an inflammatory component. However, it may be contraindicated because of its effects on hemostasis, uric acid excretion, and GI mucosal surfaces. Aspirin should not be recommended for use during the third trimester of pregnancy. It should also be avoided in teenagers or children with viral influenza or chickenpox because of the increased risk of Reye's syndrome. Aspirin is contraindicated in patients receiving MTX. Buffered aspirin, enteric-coated aspirin, choline salicylate, and effervescent aspirin solutions are associated with a lower incidence of GI intolerance. However, the onset of analgesia is delayed with enteric-coated aspirin, so that product should not be recommended when prompt pain relief is desired. Additionally, effervescent aspirin solutions have a high sodium content and should be avoided in sodium-restricted patients such as those experiencing congestive heart failure or moderate to severe renal failure.

In many patients, acetaminophen is the nonprescription analgesic of choice. It is unlikely to trigger bronchoconstriction in patients with asthma, and it has a very low cross-reactivity rate in persons who are intolerant to aspirin or NSAIDs. Because it does not affect platelet aggregation or bleeding time and produces minimal gastric erosion, acetaminophen is the preferred analgesic for patients with a history of a bleeding disorder, GI bleeding, or ulceration and in patients taking oral anticoagulant drugs. It is also an appropriate recommendation for patients with a history of gout or hyperuricemia because it does not affect the renal excretion of uric acid. Used on a short-term (less than 7 days) or intermittent basis, acetaminophen is preferred over aspirin for self-medication in AIDS patients receiving zidovudine (AZT). Because of its minimal anti-inflammatory activity, however, acetaminophen is not as effective as either aspirin or ibuprofen for conditions having an inflammatory component. Acetaminophen is the analgesic drug of choice in children because of its relative absence of adverse effects and its availability in both oral pediatric solutions and pediatric suppositories. However, its decreased rectal bioavailability may necessitate larger acetaminophen doses if the medication is administered rectally.

Ibuprofen is more potent as an analgesic than either aspirin or acetaminophen and also possesses anti-inflammatory efficacy within the approved nonprescription dose range. Ibuprofen produces a reversible, transient effect on platelet aggregation and bleeding time, and it does not affect prothrombin synthesis. However, even though ibuprofen's effects on the GI mucosa are less than those produced by aspirin, acetaminophen is still the preferred drug for patients with a history of a bleeding disorder, GI bleeding, or anticoagulant therapy. Ibuprofen appears more effective than either aspirin or acetaminophen for the relief of dysmenorrhea and should be recommended as the nonprescription drug of choice for this purpose. Ibuprofen should be avoided by patients with congestive heart failure, hypertension, or moderate to severe renal failure because it may cause sodium and water retention, decrease furosemide-induced diuresis, and antagonize the blood pressure–lowering effect of antihypertensive drugs.

Ibuprofen should not be taken by patients concurrently taking lithium because of the potential for producing lithium toxicity due to decreased renal clearance of lithium. Like aspirin, ibuprofen is absolutely contraindicated in patients taking MTX because of the potential for ibuprofen to induce decreased renal clearance of MTX, which can result in increased MTX toxicity and even death. Ibuprofen must also be avoided by patients with a history of aspirin or NSAID intolerance because of a high degree of cross-reactivity. And it should be avoided by patients with asthma because of the increased potential for producing bronchospasm. Ibuprofen does not affect blood glucose in diabetic patients; thus, it can be used by patients whose conditions are controlled with insulin or oral hypoglycemic drugs. Ibuprofen also does not affect uric acid excretion and so can be safely used by patients with a history of gout or hyperuricemia. Finally, ibuprofen should be avoided during the third trimester of pregnancy but appears safe for use by women who are breast-feeding.

Combination analgesic products may produce enhanced analgesia resulting from the inclusion of caffeine or an antihistamine. However, the same degree of analgesia can be produced by increasing the dose of a single ingredient product. Further, combination analgesic products are often more expensive than single-ingredient, generic products containing either aspirin, acetaminophen, or ibuprofen. This cost consideration should be factored into the pharmacist's recommendation of a nonprescription analgesic product.

References

1. Maciewicz R, Martin JB. Pain: pathophysiology and management. In: Wilson JD, Braunwald E, Isselbacher KJ, et al., eds. *Harrison's Principles of Internal Medicine.* 12th ed. New York: McGraw-Hill, Inc; 1991: 93–8.
2. Guyton AC. *Textbook of Medical Physiology.* 8th ed. Philadelphia: W. B. Saunders; 1991: 520–9.
3. Martin JB. Headache. In: Wilson JD, Braunwald E, Isselbacher KJ, et al., eds. *Harrison's Principles of Internal Medicine.* 12th ed. New York: McGraw-Hill, Inc; 1991: 108–15.
4. Griggs RC. Pain, spasm, and cramps of muscle. In: Wilson JD, Braunwald E, Isselbacher KJ, et al., eds. *Harrison's Principles of Internal Medicine.* 12th ed. New York: McGraw-Hill, Inc; 1991: 173–6.
5. Gilliland BC. Relapsing polychondritis and miscellaneous arthritides. In: Wilson JD, Braunwald E, Isselbacher KJ, et al., eds. *Harrison's Principles of Internal Medicine.* 12th ed. New York: McGraw-Hill, Inc; 1991: 1484–90.
6. Brandt KD, Kovalov-St. John K. Osteoarthritis. In: Wilson JD, Braunwald E, Isselbacher KJ, et al., eds. *Harrison's Principles of Internal Medicine.* 12th ed. New York: McGraw-Hill, Inc; 1991: 1475–9.
7. Lipsky PE. Rheumatoid arthritis. In: Wilson JD, Braunwald E, Isselbacher KJ, et al., eds. *Harrison's Principles of Internal Medicine.* 12th ed. New York: McGraw-Hill, Inc; 1991: 1437–43.
8. Insel PA. Analgesic-antipyretics and antiinflammatory agents; drugs employed in the treatment of rheumatoid arthritis and gout. In: Goodman AD, Rall RW, Nies AS, Taylor P, eds. *Goodman and Gilman's The Pharmacological Basis of Therapeutics.* 8th ed. New York: Pergamon; 1990: 638–81.
9. Piletta P, Porchet HC, Dayer P. Central analgesic effect of acetaminophen but not of aspirin. *Clin Pharmacol Ther* 1991 Apr; 49 (4): 350–4.
10. Internal analgesic, antipyretic, and antirheumatic drug products for over-the-counter human use: tentative final

monograph. *Federal Register* 1988 Nov 16; 53 (221): 46255–7.
11. Mielke CH, Heiden D, Britten AF, et al. Hemostasis, antipyretics, and mild analgesics: acetaminophen vs. aspirin. *JAMA* 1976 Feb 9; 235 (6): 613–6.
12. Ivey KJ. Mechanisms of nonsteroidal anti-inflammatory drug-induced gastric damage. *Am J Med* 1988 Feb; 84 (suppl 2A): 41–8.
13. Levy M. Aspirin use in patients with major upper gastrointestinal bleeding and peptic ulcer disease: a report from the Boston Collaborative Drug Surveillance Program, Boston University Medical Center. *N Engl J Med* 1974 May 23; 290 (21): 1158–62.
14. Needham CD, Kyle J, Jones PF, et al. Aspirin and alcohol in gastrointestinal haemorrhage. *Gut* 1971 Oct; 12 (10): 819–21.
15. Settipane GA. Aspirin and allergic diseases: a review. *Am J Med* 1983 Jun 14; 74 (6A): 102–9.
16. Savitsky ME, Wiens JA. Cross-reactivity in aspirin-sensitive patients. *Drug Intell Clin Pharm* 1987 Apr; 21 (4): 338–9.
17. Samter M, Beers RF Jr. Intolerance to aspirin: clinical studies and consideration of its pathogenesis. *Ann Intern Med* 1968 May; 68 (5): 975–83.
18. Levy G, Procknal JA, Garrettson LK. Distribution of salicylate between neonatal and maternal serum at diffusion equilibrium. *Clin Pharmacol Ther* 1975 Aug; 18 (2): 210–4.
19. Levy G, Garrettson LK. Kinetics of salicylate elimination by newborn infants of mothers who ingested aspirin before delivery. *Pediatrics* 1974 Feb; 53 (2): 201–10.
20. Briggs GG, Freeman RK, Yaffe SJ. *Drugs in Pregnancy and Lactation*. 3rd ed. Baltimore: Williams and Wilkins; 1990.
21. Isselbacher KJ, Podolsky DK. Infiltrative and metabolic diseases affecting the liver. In: Wilson JD, Braunwald E, Isselbacher KJ, et al., eds. *Harrison's Principles of Internal Medicine*. 12th ed. New York: McGraw-Hill, Inc; 1991: 1352–5.
22. Hurwitz ES, Barrett MJ, Bregman D, et al. Public Health Service study of Reye's syndrome and medications: report of the main study. *JAMA* 1987 Apr 10; 257 (14): 1905–11.
23. Pinsky PF, Hurwitz ES, Schonberger LB, et al. Reye's syndrome and aspirin: evidence for a dose-response effect. *JAMA* 1988 Aug 5; 260 (5): 657–61.
24. Forsyth BW, Horwitz RI, Acampora D, et al. New epidemiologic evidence confirming that bias does not explain the aspirin/Reye's syndrome association. *JAMA* 1989 May; 261 (17): 2517–24.
25. Goulden KJ, Dooley JM, Camfield PR, et al. Clinical valproate toxicity induced by acetylsalicylic acid. *Neurology* 1987 Aug; 37 (8): 1392–4.
26. Tatro DS, ed. *Drug Interaction Facts*. St. Louis, Mo: Facts and Comparisons Inc; 1992.
27. Roine R, Gentry RT, Hernandez-Munoz R, et al. Aspirin increases blood alcohol concentrations in humans after ingestion of ethanol. *JAMA* 1990 Nov 14; 264 (18): 2406–8.
28. Temple AR. Pathophysiology of aspirin overdosage toxicity, with implications for management. *Pediatrics* 1978 Nov; 62 (5 pt, suppl 2): 873–6.
29. Danel V, Henry JA, Glucksman E. Activated charcoal, emesis, and gastric lavage in aspirin overdose. *Br Med J* 1988 May 28; 1: 1507.
30. Curtis RA, Barone J, Giacona N. Efficacy of ipecac and activated charcoal/cathartic: prevention of salicylate absorption in simulated overdose. *Arch Intern Med* 1984 Jan; 144 (1): 48–52.
31. Mason WD. Kinetics of aspirin absorption following oral administration of six aqueous solutions with different buffer capacities. *J Pharm Sci* 1984 Sep; 73 (9): 1258–61.
32. Kanto J, Klossner J, Mantyla R, et al. Bioavailability of rectal aspirin in neurosurgical patients. *Acta Anaesthesiol Scand* 1981 Feb; 25 (1): 25–6.
33. Lanza FL. Endoscopic studies of gastric and duodenal injury after the use of ibuprofen, aspirin, and other nonsteroidal anti-inflammatory agents. *Am J Med* 1984 Jul 13; 77 (suppl 1A): 19–24.
34. Hoftiezer JW, Silvoso GR, Burks M, et al. Comparison of the effects of regular and enteric-coated aspirin on the gastroduodenal mucosa of man. *Lancet* 1980 Sep; 2 (8195, pt 1): 609–12.
35. Hawthorne AB, Mahida YR, Cole AT, et al. Aspirin-induced gastric mucosal damage: prevention by enteric-coating and relation to prostaglandin synthesis. *Br J Clin Pharmacol* 1991 Jul; 32 (1): 77–83.
36. Lanza FL, Royer GL, Nelson RS. Endoscopic evaluation of the effects of aspirin and enteric-coated aspirin on gastric and duodenal mucosa. *N Engl J Med* 1980 Jul 17; 303 (3): 136–8.
37. Hollister LE. Measuring Measurin®: problems of oral prolonged-action medications. *Clin Pharmacol Ther* 1972 Jan–Feb; 13 (1): 1–5.
38. Lobeck F, Spigiel RW. Bioavailability of sustained-release aspirin preparations. *Clin Pharm* 1986 Mar; 5 (3): 236–8.
39. Brandslund I, Rask H, Klitgaard NA. Gastrointestinal blood loss caused by controlled-release and conventional acetylsalicylic acid tablets. *Scand J Rheumatol* 1979; 8 (4): 209–13.
40. Miller RR. Deafness due to plain and long-acting aspirin tablets. *J Clin Pharmacol* 1978 Oct; 18 (10): 468–71.
41. Steering Committee of the Physicians' Health Study Research Group. Final report of the aspirin component of the ongoing physicians' health study. *N Engl J Med* 1989 Jul 20; 321 (3): 129–35.
42. Manson JE, Grobbee DE, Stampfer MJ, et al. Aspirin in the primary prevention of angina pectoris in a randomized trial of United States physicians. *Am J Med* 1989 Dec; 89 (6): 772–6.
43. Ridker PM, Manson JE, Gaziano JM, et al. Low-dose aspirin therapy for chronic stable angina: a randomized, placebo-controlled clinical trial. *Ann Intern Med* 1991 May 15; 114 (10): 835–9.
44. Second International Study of Infarct Survival Collaborative Group. Randomized trial of intravenous streptokinase, oral aspirin, both or neither among 17,187 cases of suspected acute myocardial infarction: ISIS-2. *Lancet* 1988 Aug 13; 2: 349–60.
45. Peto R, Gray R, Collins R, et al. Randomized trial of prophylactic daily aspirin in British male doctors. *Br Med J* 1988 Jan 30; 1: 313–6.
46. Hennekens CH, Buring JE, Sandercock P, et al. Aspirin and other antiplatelet agents in the secondary and primary prevention of cardiovascular disease. *Circulation* 1989 Oct; 80 (4): 749–56.
47. Manson JE, Stampfer MJ, Colditz GA, et al. A prospective study of aspirin use and primary prevention of cardiovascular disease in women. *JAMA* 1991 Jul 24-31; 266 (4): 521–7.
48. Wilson JT, Brown RD, Bocchini JA, et al. Efficacy, disposition and pharmacodynamics of aspirin, acetaminophen and choline salicylate in young febrile children. *Ther Drug Monit* 1982; 4 (2): 147–80.
49. Stern SB. Clinical evaluation of the analgesic effect of magnesium salicylate. *Med Times* 1967 Oct; 95 (10): 1072–6.
50. Preston SJ, Arnold MH, Beller EM, et al. Comparative analgesic and anti-inflammatory properties of sodium salicylate and acetylsalicylic acid (aspirin) in rheumatoid arthritis. *Br J Clin Pharmacol* 1989 May; 27 (5): 607–11.
51. McEvoy GK, ed. *AHFS Drug Information*. 1992 ed. Bethesda, Md: American Society of Hospital Pharmacists, Inc; 1992: 1062–4.
52. Sutor A, Bowie EJ, Owen CA. Effect of aspirin, sodium salicylate, and acetaminophen on bleeding. *Mayo Clin Proc* 1971 Mar; 46 (3): 178–81.
53. Binder R, Durocher J, Mielke H. Treatment of pain in hemophilia: effect of drugs on bleeding time. *Am J Dis Child* 1974 Mar; 127 (3): 371–3.
54. Stuart JJ, Pisko EJ. Choline magnesium trisalicylate does not impair platelet aggregation. *Pharmatherapeutica* 1981; 2 (8): 547–51.
55. Estes D, Kaplan K. Lack of platelet effect with aspirin analog, salsalate. *Arthritis Rheum* 1980 Nov; 23 (11): 1303–7.

56. Roth SH. Salicylates revisited: are they still the hallmark of anti-inflammatory therapy? *Drugs* 1988 Jul; 36 (1): 1–6.
57. Mehlisch DR. Review of the comparative analgesic efficacy of salicylates, acetaminophen, and pyrazolones. *Am J Med* 1983 Nov 14; 75 (suppl 5A): 47–52.
58. Clissold SP. Paracetamol and phenacetin. *Drugs* 1986; 32 (suppl 4): 46–59.
59. Richman DD, Fischl MA, Grieco MH, et al. The toxicity of azidothymidine (AZT) in the treatment of patients with AIDS and AIDS-related complex: a double-blind, placebo-controlled trial. *N Engl J Med* 1987 Jul 23; 317 (4): 192–7.
60. Steffe EM, King JH, Inciardi JF, et al. The effect of acetaminophen on zidovudine metabolism in HIV-infected patients. *J Acq Immune Defic Syn* 1990; 3 (7): 691–4.
61. Sattler FR, Ko R, Antoniskis D, et al. Acetaminophen does not impair clearance of zidovudine. *Ann Intern Med* 1991 Jun 1; 114 (11): 937–40.
62. Veltri JC, Rollins DE. A comparison of the frequency and severity of poisoning cases for ingestion of acetaminophen, aspirin, and ibuprofen. *Am J Emerg Med* 1988 Mar; 6 (2): 104–7.
63. McEvoy GK, ed. *AHFS Drug Information*. 1992 ed. Bethesda, MD: American Society of Hospital Pharmacists, Inc; 1992: 1172.
64. Ekins BR, Ford DC, Thompson MI, et al. The effect of activated charcoal on N-acetylcysteine absorption in normal subjects. *Am J Emerg Med* 1987 Nov; 5 (6): 483–7.
65. Ibuprofen without a prescription. *Med Lett Drugs Ther* 1984 Jul 6; 26 (665): 63–5.
66. Cooper SA. New peripherally acting oral analgesic agents. *Ann Rev Pharmacol Toxicol* 1983; 23: 617–47.
67. Miller RR. Evaluation of the analgesic efficacy of ibuprofen. *Pharmacotherapy* 1981 Jul–Aug; 1 (1): 21–7.
68. Chan WY. Prostaglandins and nonsteroidal antiinflammatory drugs in dysmenorrhea. *Ann Rev Pharmacol Toxicol* 1983; 23: 131–49.
69. Schmid FR, Culic DD. Antiinflammatory drugs and gastrointestinal bleeding: a comparison of aspirin and ibuprofen. *J Clin Pharmacol* 1976 Aug–Sep; 16 (8–9): 418–25.
70. Caruso I, Bianchi, Porro G. Gastroscopic evaluation of anti-inflammatory agents. *Br Med J* 1980 Jan 12; 280 (6207): 75–8.
71. Royer GL, Seckman CE, Welshman IR. Safety profile: fifteen years of clinical experience with ibuprofen. *Am J Med* 1984 Jul 13; 77 (1A): 25–34.
72. Deykin D, Janson P, McMahon L. Ethanol potentation of aspirin-induced prolongation of the bleeding time. *N Engl J Med* 1982 Apr 8; 306 (14): 852–4.
73. Penner JA, Albrecht PH. Lack of interaction between ibuprofen and warfarin. *Curr Ther Res Clin Exp* 1975 Dec; 18 (6): 862–71.
74. Schooley RT, Wagley PF, Lietman PS. Edema associated with ibuprofen therapy. *JAMA* 1977 Apr 18; 237 (16): 1716–7.
75. Ciabattoni G, Cinotti GA, Pierucci A, et al. Effects of sulindac and ibuprofen in patients with chronic glomerular disease. *N Engl J Med* 1984 Feb 2; 310 (5): 279–83.
76. Blackshear JL, Davidman M, Stillman MT. Identification of risk for renal insufficiency from nonsteroidal anti-inflammatory drugs. *Arch Intern Med* 1983 Jun; 143 (6): 1130–4.
77. Radack KL, Deck CC, Bloomfield SS. Ibuprofen interferes with the efficacy of antihypertensive drugs: a randomized, double-blind, placebo-controlled trial of ibuprofen compared with acetaminophen. *Ann Intern Med* 1987 Nov; 107 (5): 628–35.
78. Ragheb M. Ibuprofen can increase serum lithium level in lithium-treated patients. *J Clin Psychiatry* 1987 Apr; 48 (4): 161–3.
79. Kristoff CA, Hayes PE, Barr WH, et al. Effect of ibuprofen on lithium plasma and red blood cell concentrations. *Clin Pharm* 1986 Jan; 5 (1): 51–5.
80. Ragheb M. The clinical significance of lithium-nonsteroidal anti-inflammatory drug interactions. *J Clin Psychopharmacol* 1990 Oct; 10 (5): 350–4.
81. Thyss A, Milano G, Kubar J, et al. Clinical and pharmacokinetic evidence of a life-threatening interaction between methotrexate and ketoprofen. *Lancet* 1986 Feb 1; 1 (8475): 256–8.
82. Cassano WF. Serious methotrexate toxicity caused by interaction with ibuprofen. *Am J Pediatr Hematol Oncol* 1989 Winter; 11 (4): 481–2.
83. McElwee NE, Veltri JD, Bradford DC, et al. A prospective, population-based study of acute ibuprofen overdose: complications are rare and routine serum levels not warranted. *Ann Emerg Med* 1990 Jun; 19 (6): 657–62.
84. Cooper SA. Comparative analgesic efficacies of aspirin and acetaminophen. *Arch Intern Med* 1981 Feb 23; 141 (3): 282–5.
85. Peters BH, Fraim CJ, Masel BE. Comparison of 650 mg aspirin and 1,000 mg acetaminophen with each other, and with placebo in moderately severe headache. *Am J Med* 1983 Jun 14; 74 (6A): 36–42.
86. Mehlisch DR, Frakes LA. A controlled comparative evaluation of acetaminophen and aspirin in the treatment of postoperative pain. *Clin Ther* 1984; 7 (1): 89–97.
87. Hopkinson JH III, Smith MT, Bare WW, et al. Acetaminophen (500 mg) versus acetaminophen (325 mg) for the relief of pain in episiotomy patients. *Curr Ther Res* 1974 Mar; 16: 194–200.
88. Sunshine A, Olson NZ, Laska EM, et al. Ibuprofen, zomepirac, aspirin, and placebo in the relief of postepisiotomy pain. *Clin Pharmacol Ther* 1983 Aug; 34 (2): 254–8.
89. Jain AK, Ryan JR, McMahon FG, et al. Analgesic efficacy of low-dose ibuprofen in dental extraction pain. *Pharmacotherapy* 1986 Nov–Dec; 6 (6): 318–22.
90. Huskisson EC, Shenfield GM, Taylor RT, et al. A new look at ibuprofen. *Rheumatol Phys Med* 1970; 10 (suppl 10): 88–98.
91. Schachtel BP, Thoden WR, Baybutt RI. Ibuprofen and acetaminophen in the relief of postpartum episiotomy pain. *J Clin Pharmacol* 1989 Jun; 29 (6): 550–3.
92. Pearce I, Frank GJ, Pearce JM. Ibuprofen compared with paracetamol in migraine. *Practitioner* 1983 Mar; 227 (1377): 465–7.
93. Mehlisch DR, Sollecito WA, Helfrick JE, et al. Multicenter clinical trial of ibuprofen and acetaminophen in the treatment of postoperative dental pain. *J Am Dent Assoc* 1990 Aug; 121 (2): 257–63.
94. Laska EM, Sunshine A, Mueller F, et al. Caffeine as an analgesic adjuvant. *JAMA* 1984 Apr 6; 251 (13): 1711–8.
95. Forbes JA, Beaver WT, Jones KF, et al. Effect of caffeine on ibuprofen analgesia in postoperative oral surgery pain. *Clin Pharmacol Ther* 1991 Jun; 49 (6): 674–84.
96. Sunshine A, Zighelboim I, DeCastro A, et al. Augmentation of acetaminophen analgesia by the antihistamine phenyltoloxamine. *J Clin Pharmacol* 1989 Jul; 29 (7): 660–4.

CHAPTER 6

Antipyretic Drug Products
Thomas E. Lackner

Questions to ask in patient assessment and counseling

- *How long have you been ill?*
- *What is your temperature? How did you measure it (i.e., by the oral, axillary, or rectal method)?*
- *How long have you had this fever?*
- *What activities preceded this fever?*
- *Do you have any other symptoms?*
- *What medication or other treatment have you used to treat the fever?*
- *What other prescription or nonprescription medications are you taking?*
- *Do you take any anticoagulants or medications that interfere with blood clotting?*
- *Do you have any type of bleeding problem or blood-clotting disorder?*
- *Do you have gout?*
- *Have you ever had a convulsion, seizure, or brain disorder?*
- *Have you ever had an ulcer or stomach problem?*
- *Have you ever had asthma, nasal polyps, or a breathing problem?*
- *Have you ever had hives or a recurrent skin rash?*
- *Have you ever had chickenpox?*
- *What allergies or reactions have you ever had to drugs, foods, dyes, or food additives?*
- *How old are you?*
- *Are you pregnant? If so, for how long?*
- *Are you breast-feeding?*

Fever is one of the most common symptoms of a medical disorder. Yet fever continues to be misunderstood and poorly treated. One study revealed that 20% of the population apparently does not know how to measure body temperature properly; many more persons do not know how to interpret the results.[1] Pharmacists and other health professionals must educate patients about fever and teach them how to measure and manage it appropriately.

Fever, a sign of an upward displacement of the body's thermoregulatory "set-point," is manifested as an abnormally elevated body temperature.[2] Fever can occur with or without serious underlying pathophysiology. A fever is generally recognized as a rectal temperature above 101°F (38.3°C), an oral temperature above 99.5°F (37.5°C), or an axillary (armpit) temperature above 98.6°F (37.0°C).[3] The average rectal temperature at 18 months of age is 100°F (37.8°C) although 50% of infants may have normal rectal temperatures exceeding 100°F. Rectal temperatures in healthy children may approach 101°F (38.3°C) in the late afternoon or after physical activity.

Fever may result from a variety of factors, ranging from a relatively harmless, transient viral infection to a condition associated with malignancy. Attention to related signs and symptoms helps distinguish between such disorders. The symptoms associated with fever may include headache, sweating, generalized malaise, tachycardia, arthralgia, myalgia, back pain, irritability, and anorexia.[4] High body temperatures may cause dulled intellectual functioning, disorientation, and delirium, especially in individuals with preexisting dementia, cerebral arteriosclerosis, or alcoholism. Reducing a high temperature may alleviate central nervous system (CNS) symptoms in some individuals, depending on the underlying cause and coexisting pathology.

The foremost reason for treating fever is to alleviate patient discomfort. When possible, such treatment should be directed against the underlying cause. Serious complications of fever are uncommon and are usually the result of inappropriate treatment rather than of the fever itself.

The perception of fever among individuals is highly variable. Although some individuals quite accurately perceive an elevation in their body temperature, others (e.g., those with tuberculosis) may be unaware of temperatures as high as 103°F (39.4°C).[5] Furthermore, fever may be ignored because of more unpleasant concomitant symptoms.

Mechanisms of Normal Thermoregulation and Fever

Body temperature is determined by the body's ability to produce and maintain heat relative to the rate at which heat is lost. Body heat is primarily the product of basal metabolic processes and muscle activity. When the body is at rest, the liver is the principal source of body heat. During exercise, muscles elicit a substantial amount of heat. Metabolic activity is largely influenced by adrenal medullary catecholamines and thyroxine. Heat loss is associated with conduction, evaporation, and radiation from the skin. The rate of heat loss is directly proportional to the rate of cutaneous blood flow.

Body temperature is regulated by a thermoregulatory center located in the anterior hypothalamus.[2] Temperature-sensitive neurons in both the hypothalamus and the skin continuously transmit information about body temperature to the hypothalamic "thermostat." Physiologic and behavioral homeostatic mechanisms can then be invoked to maintain body temperature within the normal range. Examples of behavioral adaptations to temperature changes or extremes include putting on additional clothing, adjusting air conditioning, rubbing the hands together, or seeking out shade for relief from the hot sun. Compensatory physiologic mechanisms involve heat dissipation (e.g., sweating, vasodilation, and hyperventilation) in response to heat, or heat production or conservation (e.g., shivering and vasoconstriction) in response to cold. Compensatory effects are mediated by alterations in the secretory rates of thyroid-stimulating hormone and catecholamines. Normal thermoregulation prevents wide fluctuations in body temperature so that the average body temperature is usually maintained at 97.7°–99.5°F (36.5°–37.5°C).

An individual's normal body temperature varies consistently throughout the day, peaking daily between 5 and 7 PM, and reaching its lowest point between 3 and 5 AM.[2,6] Except in neonates and infants under 2 years of age, this predictable circadian rhythm occurs regardless of age (although it is more pronounced in children than in adults), sleep state, or work pattern. The body temperature during a 24-hour period can vary by as much as 1.8°F (1°C) in adults and as much as 2.5°F (1.4°C) in children. Because circadian variation is even manifest during febrile illness, many individuals with a febrile illness can have a relatively normal temperature in the early morning. Furthermore, a moderately high evening temperature associated with circadian variation should not be misinterpreted as a fever.

Numerous fever-producing substances called pyrogens can increase the thermoregulatory set-point.[2] Pyrogens can be categorized as exogenous (originating outside the body) or endogenous (growing from within). Most febrile episodes can be attributed to infection by various microorganisms (exogenous pyrogens), including viruses, bacteria, fungi, yeasts, and protozoa. Despite some evidence that elevated temperatures associated with bacterial infection are generally higher than those associated with viral infection, there is no absolute temperature at which these infections can be differentiated. Nor is there any basis for differentiating viral from bacterial infections according to the magnitude of temperature reduction with antipyretic drug therapy.[7] In addition, clinical data suggest that the febrile response to exogenous pyrogens, such as infection, is often diminished somewhat in elderly patients (Table 1).[8] Consequently, the presence of infection may not be easily recognized in elderly persons if fever response is the primary assessment criterion.

Other causes of fever include malignancies, certain drugs, tissue damage (e.g., myocardial infarct and surgery), metabolic disorders (e.g., thyroid and gout), antigen–antibody reactions, and dehydration. Each of these factors can cause the production and release of low molecular weight proteins (endogenous pyrogens). These chemicals are released primarily from liver and spleen cells, monocytes, eosinophils, and neutrophils. Fever caused by the release of endogenous pyrogens from the malignant cells of acute leukemia, histiocytic lymphoma, and Hodgkin's disease is difficult to distinguish from an infectious etiology in such patients.

Experimental evidence suggests that prostaglandins of the E series are produced in response to circulating endogenous pyrogens and act on the anterior hypothalamus to elevate the thermoregulatory set-point.[2] In response to E prostaglandins and to changes in monoamine concentration, the hypothalamus appears to direct the reestablishment of body temperature to correspond to the new, elevated set-point.[2] Within hours the body temperature reaches this new set-point, and fever results. During the period of upward temperature readjustment, the patient experiences symptoms of chills as homeostatic peripheral heat mechanisms, such as peripheral vasoconstriction and increased skeletal muscle tone, are activated. The new set-point is regulated by a negative feedback system so that body temperatures rarely exceed 106°F (41.1°C).[2] Drugs that inhibit the synthesis of E prostaglandins in response to endogenous pyrogens possess antipyretic activity.

Hyperthermia

Temperature elevation may occur in a condition referred to as hyperthermia. In contrast to fever, in hyperthermia a normal thermoregulatory set-point is maintained. Body temperature rises when the compensatory homeostatic thermoregulatory response to heat production or retention is inadequate and heat production and retention exceed the rate of heat dissipation. For example, strenuous and excessive physical activity on a hot, humid day can greatly increase body temperature and overcome compensatory vasodilation and sweating, resulting in heat stroke. The loss of large amounts of fluid by sweating may further increase the morbidity and mortality of hyperthermia by causing dehydration. Heat dissipation by evaporation of perspiration may be suppressed by high humidity while heat production is accelerated during exercise. Body temperatures associated with heat stroke generally exceed 107.6°F (42°C) and can result in delirium, coma, anhidrosis (suppression of perspiration with hot, dry skin), and death.[9,10] Without early detection and aggressive management, the mortality rate of hyperthermia may approach 80%, and those who survive may be afflicted with permanent neurologic deficits such as ataxia (muscular incoordination) and severe dysarthria (difficulty in speaking clearly and fluently). Early symptoms may include unsteadiness, stumbling or clumsiness, dizziness, headache, nausea, profuse sweating, and mental status changes. Thus, suspected heat stroke and a temperature of 102°F (38.9°C) or higher should be considered a medical emergency, and the patient should be treated by a physician.

Elderly persons are at particularly high risk of heat stroke when overexposed to heat because of the physiologic changes that generally occur with the normal aging process (Table 1). Their risk is then compounded by the higher prevalence of conditions such as cardiovascular disease and consumption of certain medications (e.g., diuretics, anticholinergics, phenothiazines, tricyclic antidepressants, beta blockers, and monoamine oxidase inhibitors), which may further compromise their thermoregulatory function.[11–13] In addition, psychotropic drugs, physical restraints, and disabilities such as severe arthritis may

TABLE 1	Thermoregulatory alterations in the elderly

Impaired central thermoregulation with decreased capacity to sense heat

Diminished ability to accelerate heat dissipation with decreased ability to increase cardiac output, dilate cutaneous blood vessels, and perspire

Increased propensity to dehydration (more labile extracellular fluid volume and decreased thirst reflex)

Diminished heat evasion behavior

prevent an individual from moving from a hot environment. Some drugs (e.g., psychotropics) may suppress the thirst reflex, thus increasing risk.

Children are also at high risk of heat stroke because of their slower physiologic response to temperature change, high physical activity level, fewer sweat glands, and inability or failure to recognize and/or react to warning signs of heat stroke.

Management of heat stroke calls for removing most clothing and placing the patient in a cool and ventilated location. Ice-water sponging and vigorous manual skin massage to prevent reflex vasoconstriction should be initiated as a first-aid measure pending further medical treatment to facilitate heat loss. The cornerstone of hospital medical treatment of heat stroke is immersion of the patient in an ice-water bath to ensure heat dissipation. However, ice-water immersion should not be used at home to lower a high fever unless it is recommended by a physician. Intravenous rehydration is often needed owing to hypovolemia and hypernatremia; this also provides venous access for other treatments in the event of additional complications. However, antipyretic agents such as aspirin and acetaminophen are of no benefit in treating hyperthermia because the thermoregulatory set-point is not elevated in this condition.

Hyperthermia may also accompany endocrine disorders such as thyrotoxicosis and pheochromocytoma, both of which increase the basal metabolic rate.[14]

Drug-Induced Fever

Many drugs are reported to induce fever as an adverse effect. Table 2 lists the drugs most often implicated in this iatrogenic condition. The actual incidence of drug-induced fever is unknown, but this condition likely accounts for more than 3% of all adverse drug reactions. Recognition of drug-induced fever is important because failure to discontinue use of the offending agent can result in substantial morbidity and even mortality. However, drug-induced fever often goes unrecognized because consistent signs and symptoms are lacking.[15]

Drug-induced fever is probably not related to atopy, gender, age, or systemic lupus erythematosus, as was previously believed. It mostly occurs as a hypersensitivity reaction or is idiosyncratic in nature.[16] However, drugs may also elicit fever by interfering with peripheral heat dissipation, increasing the basal metabolic rate, invoking a cellular immune response, structurally mimicking endogenous pyrogens, and inflicting direct tissue damage.

TABLE 2	Selected agents responsible for episodes of drug-induced fever		
Cardiovascular Methyldopa Quinidine Procainamide Hydralazine Nifedipine **Antimicrobial** Penicillin G Ampicillin Methicillin Cloxacillin Cephalothin Cephapirin Cefamandole Tetracycline Lincomycin Sulfonamide	Sulfamethoxazole–trimethoprim Streptomycin[a] Vancomycin Colistin Isoniazid Para-aminosalicylic acid Nitrofurantoin Mebendazole **Antineoplastic** Bleomycin Daunorubicin Procarbazine Cytarabine Streptozocin	6-Mercaptopurine L-Asparaginase Chlorambucil Hydroxyurea **Central nervous system** Phenytoin Carbamazepine Chlorpromazine Nomifensine Haloperidol Triamterene Benztropine[a] Thioridazine Trifluoperazine[a] Amphetamine	**Anti-Inflammatory** Ibuprofen Tolmetin Aspirin **Other** Iodide Cimetidine Levamisole Metroclopramide Clofibrate Allopurinol Folate Prostaglandin E_2 Ritodrine Interferon Prophylthiouracil

[a]Fever seen during drug overdose.
Adapted with permission from Mackowiak PA, LeMaistre CF. *Ann Intern Med* 1987; 106: 729.

Sometimes it is the method of administration, rather than the drug itself, that induces fever. Such reactionary fevers may be due to thrombophlebitis and septicemia from intravenous catheterization, phlebitis from careless administration of potentially caustic agents (e.g., the excessively rapid infusion of vancomycin), or the release of endogenous pyrogens from sterile abscesses formed after multiple intramuscular injections.

Some drugs can elevate body temperature by altering normal thermoregulatory mechanisms. Large doses of phenothiazines or anticholinergic agents can decrease sweating and thus reduce heat dissipation. Thyroid hormones may increase the metabolic rate and thus increase heat generation. Other drugs may modify the behavioral response to the climatic temperature. For example, obtundation (a decreased level of consciousness) from sedatives may impair the usual behavioral withdrawal response from high environmental temperature and result in hyperthermia.

Occasionally, fever may be a direct result of the pharmacologic effect of a drug. For example, the release of endotoxin from bacteria following the initiation of antibiotic therapy (e.g., penicillin for syphilis) can result in high fever, chills, hypotension, myalgia, and leukocytosis.[16] This phenomenon (the Jarisch–Herxheimer reaction) may occur within hours after parenteral antibiotic therapy is begun. Fever may also result from the release of endogenous pyrogens associated with cellular injury or death following cancer chemotherapy. Similarly, the administration of drugs that possess oxidizing activity to individuals who have a glucose-6-phosphate dehydrogenase deficiency may cause fever secondary to the release of endogenous pyrogens from damaged erythrocytes.[16]

Drugs, or drug metabolites, and certain biologic preparations can behave as antigens and produce a hypersensitivity reaction. Although drug fever usually develops after 7–10 days of treatment, fever and other symptoms may occur shortly after initiation of drug therapy when previous exposure and sensitization has occurred.[16] The onset of drug fever caused by antineoplastic agents often comes within 7 days after therapy begins. Fever caused by cardiac drugs may not occur until more than 10 days have passed.[15]

Drug fever is distinguished by (1) fever occurring during or shortly after treatment with a drug previously reported to cause fever or other allergic symptoms, (2) fever accompanied by other manifestations of allergy, and (3) temperature elevation despite patient improvement.[17] One study of drug-induced fevers identified skin rash in only 18% of patients, and fewer than half of these individuals experienced urticaria.[15] Furthermore, a generally mild eosinophilia was present in only 22% of the patients. The presence of high fever and shaking chills may make it hard to differentiate a drug fever from an infection. Bradycardia is uncommon with drug fever.[15] Drug fever should not be excluded on the basis of a left shift of the white blood cell differential count because this occasionally accompanies drug-induced fever.[18] And because diurnal (circadian) temperature variation accompanying a drug fever is often minimal, this fever pattern is not a reliable diagnostic sign of a drug fever, either.

The management of drug-induced fever involves the discontinuation of the suspected drug whenever possible. If feasible, all medications should be temporarily discontinued. If the fever is drug induced, the patient's temperature will generally decrease within 24–48 hours after the offending drug is withdrawn. After patient safety and the need to definitively identify the offending drug have been considered, each medication may then be restarted, one at a time, with observation for fever recurrence. If an implicated drug cannot be discontinued, systemic corticosteroids may be given to suppress fever and minimize other allergic symptoms. A fever associated with parenteral drug administration may be prevented if (1) proper catheter placement and care are provided, (2) frequent intramuscular injections are avoided, and (3) recommended infusion rates are followed. Dosage reduction of phenothiazines, anticholinergic agents, and thyroid hormone may decrease an elevated temperature and should be considered if these drugs are suspected of causing fever, particularly in elderly individuals.

The onset of fever in persons taking neuroleptic medication (e.g., phenothiazines, butyrophenones, or thioxanthenes) suggests the possibility of neuroleptic malignant syndrome, a potentially life-threatening condition.[19] The high fever of neuroleptic malignant syndrome is often accompanied by muscle rigidity, abnormal body movements, sweating, tachycardia, hypo- or hypertension, incontinence, and altered consciousness including delirium, stupor, or coma. Although neuroleptic malignant syndrome may occur in anyone taking these medications, it is most common in young males and possibly individuals who are dehydrated. When this syndrome is suspected, the neuroleptic medication should be discontinued and a physician contacted immediately.

Complications of Fever

Serious complications of fever are rare. Harmful effects (e.g., dehydration, delirium, seizures, coma, and irreversible neurologic or muscular damage) are most likely to occur at temperatures in excess of 106°F (41.1°C). However, even lower body temperature elevations may be life-threatening in patients with heart disease because of an increased demand for oxygen in conjunction with increased cardiac output and heart rate.[2] A greater risk and poorer tolerance of elevated body temperature also exist in infants and in patients with brain tumors or hemorrhage, CNS infections, preexisting neurologic damage, and/or decreased ability to dissipate heat.[20,21]

Febrile seizures—that is, seizures associated with fever and occurring in the absence of another cause (e.g., acute metabolic disorder or CNS inflammation)—occur in about 2–4% of all children between 6 months and 6 years of age.[22,23] Simple febrile seizures generally last no longer than 15 minutes, have no features characteristic of a focal origin, and do not recur during a single febrile episode.[24] Significant neurologic sequelae (e.g., impaired intellectual development) are believed to be unlikely following a single pediatric febrile seizure that is not complicated by status epilepticus.[25] However, the prevalence of epilepsy may be somewhat higher following a febrile seizure, particularly after a complex seizure or when severe electroencephalogram abnormalities exist.[25]

Unlike simple febrile seizures, complex febrile seizures in children are repetitive during the course of a single febrile episode, generally last longer than 15 minutes, and exhibit signs characteristic of a focal origin. Complex seizures are believed to be precipitated by fever in children with preexisting epilepsy or a predilection for that disorder.[22]

Although both the magnitude and rate of temperature increase appear to be critical determinants in precipitating febrile seizures, the temperature at which a particular child will experience a seizure is unpredictable. Most initial febrile seizures occur in children under 3 years of age.[23] Seizures occurring after that age are usually unrelated to fever. The risk of a febrile seizure is increased in children who have experienced a previous febrile seizure (especially if it occurred before 1 year of age or was a complex febrile seizure) or have a documented seizure or other CNS disorder, or whose family history includes febrile seizures.[23,25]

It is generally recommended that chronic prophylaxis against febrile seizures with antiepileptic drugs be reserved for individuals at high risk of subsequent epilepsy. For such chronic therapy, phenobarbital or sodium valproate have been the prophylactic drugs of choice. However, new evidence raises doubt about the benefit of continuous prophylaxis with phenobarbital: two reports failed to find a decrease in the seizure recurrence rate with this therapy, and cognitive performance may be impaired even after the drug is discontinued.[26,27]

Status epilepticus, which is characterized by recurrent or repetitive seizures without intervening periods of normal consciousness, occurs in only about 1 to 2% of children who experience a febrile seizure. Unlike simple febrile seizures, status epilepticus can result in permanent brain damage, renal failure, cardiorespiratory arrest, and death if not controlled. Any person experiencing such seizures requires immediate medical attention.

Temperature Measurement

Normal body temperature varies according to the individual's age and level of physical and emotional stress, the environmental temperature, the time of day, and the anatomical site at which the temperature is measured.[2,3,6] Body temperature may be measured at rectal, axillary, oral, or tympanic (ear canal) sites. The rectal method is generally regarded as yielding the most accurate measure; however, most individuals, particularly children, prefer the axillary or oral methods of temperature measurement.

Body temperature may also be measured using various types of thermometers. During the course of an illness, however, the same thermometer should be used because the accuracy of different brands of thermometers may vary. And regardless of the site or method used, thorough hand washing should precede and follow all temperature measurements.

Types of Thermometers

Mercury-in-glass and electronic thermometers are commonly used for temperature measurement. Both are accurate when used appropriately. The advantages of mercury-in-glass thermometers over electronic thermometers are (1) patient familiarity, (2) low cost, (3) light weight, and (4) compact size. However, mercury-in-glass thermometers can break, rendering them useless and potentially dangerous. Although the elemental mercury contained in modern-day thermometers is nonabsorbable through the gastrointestinal (GI) tract and is nontoxic, many patients still fear mercury poisoning from a broken thermometer. In fact, the real danger is from glass fragments. Patients should be instructed to discard chipped thermometers. In addition, mercury-in-glass thermometers register slowly and must be disinfected before each subsequent use. Finally, these thermometers should be stored in a cool location and out of direct sunlight because they may be damaged by excessive heat.[28]

Electronic thermometers register quickly (about 30 seconds for equilibration) and are not subject to glass breakage and the risk of cuts. The use of disposable covers with these thermometers eliminates the need for disinfection following their use. In addition, the electronic digital temperature display makes this thermometer much easier to read than the traditional glass thermometer.

Glass thermometers intended for oral use have a long, thin bulb designed to reach well under the tongue. In contrast, the bulb of the rectal thermometer is short and thick, permitting insertion in the rectum with little risk of breakage. Although a rectal thermometer can be used for oral temperature measurement, an oral thermometer should never be inserted into the rectum because oral thermometers are more fragile and likely to break and injure rectal tissue. The same thermometer should never be used both rectally and orally because effective disinfection is difficult and cross-infection is a risk. To ensure a reliable measurement, the patient should not engage in vigorous physical activity or heat or cool the oral cavity artificially by smoking or by drinking hot or cold beverages for at least 5 minutes (preferably 20 minutes) before the temperature is measured.

Experience with skin thermometers—adhesive temperature strips that are applied to the skin and change color over a particular temperature range—indicates that they are not sufficiently accurate or reliable.[29] In one study, temperature strips failed to detect 66% of fevers of 100°F (37.8°C) or higher.[30] Thus, this method of temperature measurement is not recommended.

Subjective assessment of fever typically involves palpating a part of the body, such as the forehead. However, it has been found that fever was unrecognized by this method in up to 26% of children with documented fever, whereas 6% of children who were thought to have a fever did not.[31]

Oral Measurement

Before a patient's oral temperature is measured using a mercury-in-glass thermometer, the thermometer should be inspected for cracks or imperfections. It should then be disinfected by drawing it through a swab moistened with an antiseptic (e.g., alcohol or Betadine®), and then rinsed with cool water. (Hot water should never be used because this may break the thermometer.) After disinfection, the thermometer should be calibrated by rotating it at or slightly below eye level to confirm that the displayed temperature is below 96°F (35.6°C). If the reading exceeds this value, the thermometer should be shaken in a rapid, downward snapping motion until the height of the mercury column falls below the 96°F level. When counseling patients about mercury-in-glass thermometers, the pharmacist should demonstrate the correct shaking motion. The user should also be advised to shake the thermometer over a bed, carpet, or other soft surface to reduce the likelihood of breakage if the thermometer should slip from the hand.

The thermometer should then be placed under the tongue, positioned slightly to one side of the mouth, and left in place for 3 to 4 minutes. Although the literature recommends insertion for 6–10 minutes, there is evidence that 3 to 4 minutes is sufficient. Further research is necessary, however, to resolve this controversy.[32] The patient's lips should be sealed to hold the thermometer in place and to prevent air from flowing over the thermometer. Saliva should be removed from the thermometer by wiping from the stem toward the bulb. After the recorded temperature is noted, the mercury should be shaken down to less than the 96°F (35.6°C) level and disinfected as described previously.

To measure an oral temperature with an electronic thermometer, the probe should be removed from the thermometer base in which it is stored. The temperature set-point should be verified as specified by the manufacturer. The thermometer probe should then be inserted into a probe sheath following the same instructions for placement in the mouth as those for the glass thermometer. After the electronic thermometer indicates that the temperature has been measured, the probe should be removed from the mouth, the contaminated sheath discarded, and the temperature display read. Finally, the probe should be returned to the base to reset the thermometer. Electronic thermometers can be used with a child as young as 3 years of age because they are not breakable if bitten and pose no risk of accidental cuts.

An oral temperature should not be taken when an individual is mouth breathing or hyperventilating; has recently had oral surgery; is not fully alert; is uncooperative, lethargic, or confused; or is under 3 years of age.[28,33] (Maintaining a tight seal around the oral thermometer is difficult for young children.)

Rectal Measurement

To measure a rectal temperature using a mercury-in-glass thermometer, a rectal (security bulb) thermometer should be disinfected and calibrated in the same manner as an oral thermometer. The thermometer bulb should then be lubricated with a water-soluble lubricant such as K-Y Lubricating Jelly® to allow easy passage through the anal sphincter and reduce the risk of trauma.

Adults should lie on their side with their legs flexed to about a 45° angle from their abdomen, and the bulb should be inserted about 1.5–2 in. into the rectum. The thermometer can be held about 1.5–2 in. from the bulb and inserted until the finger touches the anus. To facilitate passage of the thermometer through the anal sphincter, the patient should be told to take a deep breath; this helps to divert the patient's attention to another activity. If the patient has hemorrhoidal tissue, insertion of a thermometer into the rectum should be particularly gentle so as not to cause pain and injury.

Rectal body temperature measurement in infants and young children is best accomplished by placing the child face down over the parent's lap, separating the buttocks with the thumb and forefinger of one hand, and inserting a rectal thermometer gently and calmly in a direction pointing toward the child's umbilicus with the other hand.[3] In infants, the thermometer should be inserted to the length of the bulb; in young children, it should be inserted about 1 in. into the rectum.[3] The thermometer should be held in place for at least 3 minutes, in a straight line along its angle of insertion, and cleaned of feces by wiping from the stem toward the bulb. The temperature should be read at or slightly below eye level. Finally, the thermometer should be disinfected as previously described for the oral method, and any remaining lubricant should be wiped away from the anus.

Risks associated with taking a rectal temperature include (1) injuries resulting from broken glass, (2) retention of the thermometer, (3) rectal or intestinal perforation, and (4) peritonitis.[34] The patient should never be left unattended while the rectal thermometer remains in place because a positional change may cause the thermometer to be expelled or broken. Rectal temperature measurement is relatively contraindicated in patients who (1) are neutropenic, (2) have had recent rectal surgery or injury, or (3) have rectal pathology (e.g., obstructive hemorrhoids), as well as in newborns (who are more susceptible to mucosal perforation).[34] Many parents cannot use a rectal thermometer correctly or read it accurately.[1] In addition, confusion often results from the difference between the Celsius and Fahrenheit scales and from normal variations in temperature among rectal, oral, and axillary sites of measurement. These differences should be emphasized when instructing individuals on the proper use of fever thermometers.

Axillary Measurement

An axillary temperature measurement is recommended for adults who are not candidates for oral or rectal temperature measurement (e.g., somnolent individuals recovering from rectal surgery or severe diarrhea). Axillary temperature measurement may also be preferred in children 3 months to 5 years of age because intrusive rectal procedures can be very frightening to preschool children, children with diarrhea, or infants with severe diaper rash. However, because axillary temperature measurement is generally considered to be unreliable for detecting fever in infants and young children, rectal temperature measurement is preferred for infants under 3 months of age.[35–37]

Axillary temperatures range from 0.72°F (0.4°C) higher to 3.6°F (2°C) lower than rectal temperature measurement. This discrepancy cannot be ascribed to improper measurement technique. Axillary-measured temperatures are considered meaningful when they exceed 100.4°F (38°C), whereas the rectal temperature will usually exceed 100.4°F.

Axillary temperature measurement is accomplished by placing a thermometer under the arm (in the armpit) and holding the arm pressed against the body for at least 10 minutes.

Treatment

The decision to treat fever is based on several considerations. Although patient discomfort associated with fever warrants treatment with antipyretic analgesics, arguments against treatment include (1) the generally benign and self-limited course of fever, (2) the possible elimination of a diagnostic or prognostic sign, (3) the attenuation of enhanced host defenses, (4) the possible therapeutic effect of fever, and (5) the untoward effects of antipyretic drugs.

The diagnostic or prognostic value of fever alone does not generally warrant withholding antipyretic therapy. Additionally, there is no correlation between the magnitude or pattern (i.e., persistent, intermittent, recurrent, or prolonged) of temperature elevation and the underlying etiology or severity of the disease.[38] Furthermore, when associated with an infectious disease, effective antibiotic therapy is generally guided by microbiologic cultures, sensitivity data, and laboratory and radiographic parameters. In the febrile neutropenic patient with negative cultures, antipyretic therapy should be periodically interrupted to determine the need for continued antibiotic therapy.[39] An agent lacking anti-inflammatory activity, such as acetaminophen, should be used when anti-inflammatory effects may mask the clinical signs of a particular disease (e.g., septic joint or rheumatic fever).[40]

The issue of the physiologic benefit of fever with respect to disease is quite controversial. If fever is considered to be an adaptive response, one can argue that some therapeutic benefit might result from the presence of elevated body temperature. Although the growth of some pathogenic microorganisms is impaired by higher than normal temperatures, the benefits of fever appear to be restricted to regional infections (e.g., cutaneous infection).[41] Despite the possibility that a low-grade fever might enhance certain host defense mechanisms (e.g., antigen recognition, T helper lymphocyte function, and leukocyte motility), there is no conclusive evidence that fever favorably alters the course of infectious diseases.[42] Moreover, data from animal studies suggest that the abolition of fever may actually enhance and prolong viral shedding;[43] aspirin, for example, has been associated with increased shedding or rhinovirus in adults.[44]

Treatment of fever with oral antipyretic agents is recommended if the oral temperature exceeds 102°F (38.9°C).[2] When a lower temperature and its associated discomfort is present, nonpharmacologic or pharmacologic intervention may be used. All nonprescription antipyretic agents are also analgesics, and the discomfort associated with a fever of less than 102°F may be the primary indication of antipyretic analgesics (e.g., acetaminophen, aspirin, and ibuprofen), with the antipyretic effect being a value-added secondary benefit.

A physician should be contacted at the first sign of fever in a child predisposed to seizures. In such individuals, antipyretic medication should be given regularly every 4 hours with one dose given during the night, and therapy should be continued for at least 24 hours. The need for additional therapy, such as anticonvulsant medication, should be determined by the physician.

If a fever-induced seizure occurs, sponging with tepid (lukewarm) water should be initiated and the physician notified immediately. Nonpharmacologic treatment should consist of parental reassurance in the case of the febrile child, an adequate fluid intake to replenish imperceptible fluid losses, light clothing, removal of blankets, and maintenance of the room temperature at 78°F (25.6°C).

When the body temperature exceeds 104°F (40°C), body sponging with tepid water can be started to facilitate heat dissipation. However, body sponging is not routinely recommended for children with a temperature under 104°F because this procedure is usually uncomfortable and often causes the child to shiver, which could raise the temperature even higher. Ideally, sponging should follow oral antipyretic therapy by 1 hour to permit the therapeutic reduction of the hypothalamic set-point and thereby permit a more sustained temperature-lowering response. Unlike acetaminophen, ibuprofen, and salicylates, topical sponging does not reduce the hypothalamic set-point; it is sufficient, however, because only a small temperature gradient between the body and the sponging medium is necessary to achieve an effective antipyretic response.[45] Ice-water baths or spongings with hydroalcoholic solutions (e.g., isopropyl or ethyl alcohol) are uncomfortable, unnecessary, and not generally recommended. In addition, serious alcohol poisoning can result from the cutaneous absorption or inhalation of topically applied alcohol solutions.[45] In the case of extreme hyperthermia, in which the temperature exceeds 106°F (41.1°C), medically supervised sponging or immersion in ice water may be appropriate.[10]

In addition to the above-mentioned measures to lower body temperature, fluid intake should be increased with water, soft drinks, juices, soups, or popsicles (at least 1 oz an hour for children).

Any rectal temperature above 101°F in an infant is considered a potential medical emergency. Should it occur, the physician should be contacted immediately and antipyretic medication withheld pending the physician's directive.

Pharmacologic Agents

The selection of an antipyretic agent should be based on the agent's clinical effectiveness, the incidence and severity of adverse effects associated with its use, its absolute and relative contraindications, the convenience of its administration, and the cost of therapy. Acetaminophen, aspirin, and ibuprofen are the most popular and effective antipyretic agents available today. Under most circumstances, all three of these nonprescription agents are equally effective and have similar times to onset of effect, similar times to peak antipyretic activity, and similar duration of action. These agents exert antipyretic activity by lowering the elevated set-point, which they do largely by inhibiting prostaglandin synthesis and release at the thermoregulatory center. When concurrent anti-inflammatory effects are desired, salicylates and ibuprofen should be used because acetaminophen lacks significant anti-inflammatory activity. All three agents are also effective analgesics and contribute to the relief of numerous discomforting symptoms (e.g., myalgia, arthralgia, and headache), which are often associated with fever.

The onset of antipyretic activity after an oral dose of one of these agents occurs within about 30 minutes to 1 hour. Maximum temperature reduction is evident between 2 and 3 hours after the dose, and antipyretic effects are generally sustained for 4–6 hours. Because the average maximum reduction in temperature is usually only 2 to 3°F (1.1 to 1.7°C), "normalization" of temperature may not occur and should not necessarily be a goal of therapy. The most important objective of fever management is to relieve patient discomfort.

Because acetaminophen, aspirin, and ibuprofen have similar antipyretic activity, product selection should be based primarily on patient acceptance, the side effects of each agent, concurrent diseases that may preclude the use of one or more of the drugs, convenience of administration, and cost of therapy.

Ibuprofen, one of several nonsteroidal anti-inflammatory drugs with documented antipyretic activity, is approved for the treatment of fever in adults and in children as young as 6 months of age. Oral ibuprofen suspension in doses of 5–10 mg/kg of body weight is as safe and effective as acetaminophen (12.5 mg/kg) and aspirin (10 mg/kg) for the short-term treatment of fever in children.[46] Ibuprofen may, in fact, be a better tolerated alternative to acetaminophen than aspirin. It is as effective as acetaminophen in reducing elevated body temperature, and it is also effective in relieving discomfort, the symptom for which antipyretic therapy is usually recommended.[46] Moreover, it has a somewhat longer duration of antipyretic effect than acetaminophen and aspirin, which permits dosing every 6–8 hours in children.[46]

The adverse-effect profile of ibuprofen in adults has been established by long-term clinical experience. Adverse effects associated with ibuprofen given over a short period of time (a few days) are uncommon and rarely serious. However, widespread use in children is relatively new, so all untoward effects in this age group may not yet be documented. In addition, the safety and efficacy of ibuprofen suspension in children below the age of 6 months have not been established. Finally, the suspension of ibuprofen that is approved for use in children in the United States is only available by prescription.

Adverse Reactions/Drug Interactions

For a detailed discussion of adverse reactions and drug interactions associated with antipyretics, see Chapter 5, "Internal Analgesic Products."

Dosage Considerations

Acetaminophen is often underdosed, especially in young patients. This occurs when parents reuse the 0.8 mL dropper provided with infant drops (80 mg/0.8 mL) to measure a dose of an equivalent volume of acetaminophen elixir in a concentration of 160 mg/5 mL, incorrectly assuming the same strength. In addition, rapidly growing infants quickly outgrow previous dose requirements. Therefore, recalculation of the pediatric dose according to present age and body weight is recommended at the time of each treatment course.[47]

The recommended oral antipyretic dose of aspirin and acetaminophen for children 2–11 years of age is 10–15 mg/kg of total body weight every 4–6 hours as needed, up to a maximum daily dose of 65 mg/kg for up to 5 days. Although a dose that is calculated according to body weight is most accurate, age-related dose instructions are a more practical guide for the lay public (Table 3). The dosing of either aspirin or acetaminophen in children under 2 years of age should be directed by a physician. In adults, the recommended dose of either agent is 650 mg every 4–6 hours, or 1 g three to four times daily for acetaminophen as needed for up to 10 days;[47] the daily adult dose of acetaminophen should not exceed 4 g.

Excessive aspirin dosage should be avoided because the manifestations of early salicylate toxicity (e.g., nausea, vomiting, restlessness, irritability, tinnitus [ringing in the ears], hyperthermia, and hyperpnea [rapid breathing]) may mimic the signs and symptoms of the disease being treated.

Rectal suppositories of aspirin and acetaminophen should be avoided because rectal absorption is slower, incomplete, and less reliable than oral administration. However, when aspirin or acetaminophen cannot be given orally (e.g., when the patient is vomiting), rectal suppositories at a dosage of 25–50% greater than the usual oral dosage have been recommended.[48]

Repeated dosing (i.e., for more than 5 days) of acetaminophen or salicylates should be avoided whenever possible in infants and children under 12 years of age. This recommendation is based on a lack of pharmacokinetic and pharmacodynamic data in this patient population. Moreover, drug clearance in neonates may be significantly lower than expected with liver and renal immaturity, so the appropriate frequency of dosing in neonates is uncertain.

Neither the dose nor the frequency of administration of salicylates or acetaminophen requires alteration in elderly patients.

TABLE 3	Recommended antipyretic doses: acetaminophen and acetylsalicylic acid	
Body weight	**Age (yr)**	**Single dose (mg)[a]**
Acetaminophen		
(10–15 mg/kg)	< 2	Physician directed
	2–3	160
	4–5	240
	6–8	320
	9–10	400
	11–12	480
	Adult	650
Acetylsalicylic acid		
(10–15 mg/kg)	< 2	Physician directed
	2–3	162
	4–5	243
	6–8	324
	9–10	405
	11–12	486
	Adult	650

[a]Individual doses may be repeated every 4–6 hours as needed, up to four to five daily doses. Do not exceed five doses in 24 hours.

The dosage guidelines for ibuprofen in fever reduction in adults and in children 12 months to 12 years of age are presented in Table 4.

Product Selection Guidelines

Acetaminophen is often considered the preferred antipyretic agent, particularly for children. It is recommended as a fever-lowering agent in individuals with blood coagulation defects, a predisposition to bleeding (e.g., platelet defects or ongoing treatment with anticoagulant drugs), active bleeding, steroid-dependent asthma, chronic urticaria, nasal polyps, peptic ulcer disease, alcoholism, or gout, as well as for patients who have cancer or are undergoing cancer chemotherapy (especially with methotrexate) and patients in the last 3 months of pregnancy.

Acetaminophen is available as a taste-free powder (Feverall®) in a sprinkle capsule, which is emptied onto a teaspoon containing a small amount of cold water or a favorite drink. The powder may also be sprinkled onto a teaspoon of nonheated soft food. Mixing the powder in a glass of liquid is not advised, however, because a larger number of drug particles may adhere to the side of the glass. Mixing with a hot beverage should also be avoided as this can result in a bitter taste.

Adults may be given aspirin or ibuprofen in the absence of a specific contraindication (e.g., a previous episode of intolerance to a nonsteroidal anti-inflammatory agent or an allergy to tartrazine dye) and when concomitant anti-inflammatory activity is desired. However, salicylates are not recommended for individuals, especially children and teenagers, who have a viral illness (e.g., influenza or chickenpox). Aspirin and ibuprofen may be taken with food or milk to minimize GI upset, even though this does not prevent GI bleeding. Oral administration of aspirin, ibuprofen, or acetaminophen is preferred over rectal administration because of the inferior and unreliable bioavailability of the latter route of administration.

The combined use of salicylates, ibuprofen, and acetaminophen or the use of any two of the three drugs in an alternating schedule is not currently recommended. It is true the concurrent administration of acetaminophen and aspirin or ibuprofen has resulted in a greater temperature reduction than that achieved with either agent alone, and that the antipyretic effect after combined therapy is sustained beyond that of either agent when used alone. However, further study is needed to evaluate the possible clinical benefits of such administration. There is also concern that the hepatotoxic potential of acetaminophen and the untoward effects of salicylate may be increased with combined treatment.[39] Alternating the administration of salicylates and acetaminophen has not been proven to be significantly clinically superior to the use of either agent alone in managing fever. In addition, an alternating schedule is likely to be confusing and more likely to result in medication error.

All oral antipyretic agents are ineffective in the treatment of hyperthermia and drug fever; for fevers exceeding 104°F (40°C), nonpharmacologic therapy should be instituted under the direction of a physician.

Patient Information

Pharmacists and other health professionals should counsel patients about the proper assessment and treatment of fever so as to reduce medication errors and optimize therapeutic outcomes. Patients should also be instructed on the proper use of the various types of fever thermometers. Furthermore, parents should be reminded that rectal temperatures are generally about 1°F (0.6°C) higher than oral temperatures.

Patients and parents should be assured that fever is usually a benign, self-limited disorder and that the primary purpose of treatment is to alleviate the patient's discomfort. Acetaminophen is the preferred antipyretic agent for infants, children, and young adults; salicylates and ibuprofen should not be used to treat fever associated with chickenpox, viral upper respiratory infections, or influenza-like illness in these individuals. Oral antipyretic agents can be withheld until the temperature exceeds 102°F (38.9°C) or the patient's fever-associated discomfort

TABLE 4 Recommended antipyretic doses: ibuprofen

Age (yr)	Single dose	Maximum daily dose	Guidelines	Comments
1–12	5 mg/kg	40 mg/kg	Fever ≤ 102.5°F (39.2°C)	Fever should be reduced for 6–8 hr
1–12	10 mg/kg	40 mg/kg	Fever > 102.5°F (39.2°C)	Fever should be reduced for 6–8 hr or slightly longer
Adult	200 mg/4–6 hr	1.2 g/24 hr	Preferred dose	Physician should evaluate and treat fever of > 3 days
Adult	400 mg/4–6 hr	1.2 g/24 hr	If unresponsive to lower dose	Physician should evaluate and treat fever of > 3 days

TABLE 5	Equations to convert temperatures °Celsius ↔ °Fahrenheit and selected temperature conversions

Celsius = 5/9 (°F−32)

Fahrenheit = (9/5 × °C) + 32

Sample conversions

Celsius	Fahrenheit
36°	96.8°
37°	98.6°
38°	100.4°
39°	102.2°
40°	104.0°
41°	105.8°
42°	107.6°

warrants treatment. Fevers of more than 3 days' duration should be evaluated by a physician.

Temperatures may be lowered by nonpharmacologic as well as pharmacologic measures. Sponging with tepid water should be reserved for temperatures exceeding 104°F (40°C) that follow a seizure or that have not responded to treatment with oral antipyretic agents at recommended doses. Except in the case of an individual predisposed to seizures, sleep should not be interrupted to administer an antipyretic agent or to measure the temperature because a restful sleep is also presumed to be important.

Unnecessary antipyretic medication in adults can be avoided by measuring body temperature before administering each dose. Body temperature should be remeasured 1 hour after the initial dose of an antipyretic drug to establish its effectiveness. If the presence of fever is uncertain or if discomfort persists despite treatment, body temperature should be remeasured. Because frequent temperature measurements may not be acceptable to a child or adhered to by parents, the child's behavior, complaints, and discomfort level should serve as useful guides to the need for repeated, scheduled doses in children. Patients should also be alerted to the fact that aspirin and acetaminophen may be components in many other nonprescription products, and that the use of more than one agent may result in inadvertent overdosage of acetaminophen or aspirin.

In the case of a febrile child who has experienced a previous febrile seizure, who has a documented history of seizures or another CNS disorder, or whose family history includes seizures, a physician should be notified and antipyretic therapy instituted routinely. If a seizure occurs, topical sponging should be initiated and a physician notified immediately.

Other conditions that warrant physician consultation are fever relapse or delayed fever associated with an otherwise mild cold, persistent vomiting, diarrhea, back or abdominal pain, painful urination, headache or stiff neck, earache, productive cough, sore throat, swollen glands, and mental status changes such as increasing lethargy, irritability, whimpering, and delirium. The appearance of tinnitus, difficulty in breathing (or rapid breathing), nausea, vomiting, restlessness, spontaneous or uncontrolled bleeding, small subcutaneous hemorrhages (petechiae), or dysuria during salicylate therapy warrants immediate referral to a physician. A physician should also be contacted in the case of a temperature exceeding 104°F (40°C) despite the administration of antipyretic agents or of fever relapse and fever associated with any illness or more than 72 hours' duration. The possibility of subtle manifestations of life-threatening infections in infants and children under 6 months of age mandates physician consultation when a fever of more than 100°F (37.8°C) occurs.

Antiplatelet effects of salicylates in the nursing infant are unlikely to be clinically significant, but acetaminophen can be substituted if this is a concern.

Parents should be instructed to keep antipyretic agents, as well as all other medications, in a cool, dry location out of the reach of children. A poison control center or physician should be contacted immediately if an overdose occurs or an unknown amount of acetaminophen, ibuprofen, or a salicylate is ingested. (See the appendix in Chapter 12, "Emetic and Antiemetic Products," for a listing of major poison control centers.) Table 5 contains Celsius-to-Fahrenheit and Fahrenheit-to-Celsius conversion formulas and selected equivalent temperatures.

Summary

Fever is generally a benign, self-limited disorder. The primary purpose of treatment is to alleviate discomfort. Selection of an antipyretic drug should be based on the pharmacotherapeutics of the drug and the medical history of the patient.

References

1. Eskerud JR, Hoftvedt BO, Laerum E. Fever: management and self-medication. Results from a Norwegian population study. *Fam Pract* 1991; 8: 148–53.
2. Mackowiak PA, ed. *Fever: Basic Mechanisms and Management.* New York: Raven Press; 1991.
3. Hoekelman RA. The physical examination of infants and children. In: Bates B, ed. *A Guide to Physical Examination and History Taking.* 5th ed. Philadelphia: Lippincott; 1991: 136–7, 577.
4. Dale DC. The febrile patient. In: Wyngaarden JB, Smith LH, Bennett JC, eds. *Cecil Textbook of Medicine.* 19th ed. Philadelphia: W. B. Saunders; 1992: 1567–8.
5. MacGregor RR. A year's experience with tuberculosis in a private urban teaching hospital in the postsanatorium era. *Am J Med* 1975 Feb; 58: 221–8.
6. Stephenson LA, Kolka MA. Effect of gender, circadian period, and sleep loss on thermal responses during exercise. In: Pandolf KB, Sawka MN, Gonzalez RR, eds. *Human Performance Physiology and Environmental Medicine at Terrestrial Extremes.* Indianapolis: Benchmark Press; 1988: 267–304.
7. Wasserman M, Levinstein M, Lee S, et al. Utility of fever, white blood cells, and differential count in predicting bacterial infections in the elderly. *J Am Geriatr Soc* 1989 Jun; 37(6): 537–43.
8. Jones PC, Kauffman CA, Bergman AG, et al. Fever in the elderly: production of leukocyte pyrogen by monocytes from elderly persons. *Gerontology* 1984 May/Jun; 30(3): 182–7.

9. Ferris EB Jr, Blankenhorn MA, Robinson HW, et al. Heat stroke: clinical and chemical observations on 44 cases. *J Clin Invest* 1938 May; 17(3): 249–62.
10. Knochel JP. Environmental heat illness: an eclectic review. *Arch Intern Med* 1974 May; 133(5): 841–64.
11. Wongsawat N, David BB, Morley JE. Thermoregulatory failure in the elderly. *J Am Geriatr Soc* 1990 Aug; 38: 899–906.
12. Rousseau PC. Hyperthermia in the elderly. *Geriatr Consult* 1988; 7(1): 13–4.
13. Birrer RB. Heat stroke: don't wait for the classic signs. *Emerg Med* 1988 Jun 30; 20: 9–16.
14. Stitt JT. Fever versus hyperthermia. *Fed Proc* 1979 Jan; 38(1): 39–43.
15. Mackowiak PA, LeMaistre CF. Drug fever: a critical appraisal of conventional concepts. *Ann Intern Med* 1987 May; 106: 728–33.
16. Patterson R, Anderson J. Allergic reactions to drugs and biologic agents. *JAMA* 1982 Nov; 248(20): 2637–45.
17. Murray HW, Mann JJ. *Ann Intern Med* 1975 Jul; 83(1): 84–5.
18. Lysy J, Oren R. Drug fever with a shift to the left. *DICP Ann Pharmacother* 1990 Jul/Aug; 24(7/8): 782.
19. Guze BM, Baxter LR Jr. Neuroleptic malignant syndrome. *N Engl J Med* 1985 Jul 18; 313(3): 163–6.
20. McCarthy PL, Dolan TF. Hyperpyrexia in children. *Am J Dis Child* 1976 Aug; 130: 849–51.
21. Akerren Y. On hyperpyretic conditions during infancy and children: a clinical study of fever. *Acta Pediatr* 1943; 31: 1–72.
22. Fishman MA. Febrile seizures: the treatment controversy. *J Pediatr* 1979 Feb; 94(2): 177–84.
23. Verity CM, Butler NR, Golding J. Febrile convulsions in a national cohort followed up from birth: I. prevalence and recurrence in the first five years of life. *Br Med J* 1985 May 4; 290: 1307–10.
24. Ellenberg JH, Nelson KB. Febrile seizures and later intellectual performance. *Arch Neurol* 1978 Jan; 35(1): 71–21.
25. Verity CM, Butler NR, Golding J. Febrile convulsions in a national cohort followed up from birth: II. medical history and intellectual ability at 5 years of age. *Br Med J* 1985 May 4; 290: 1311–5.
26. Newton RW. Randomized controlled trial of phenobarbital and valproate in febrile convulsions. *Arch Dis Child* 1988 Oct; 63(10): 1189–91.
27. Farwell JR, Lee YJ, Hirtz DG, et al. Phenobarbital for febrile seizures—effects on intelligence and on seizure recurrence. *N Engl J Med* 1990 Feb 8; 322(6): 364–9.
28. Erickson R. Oral temperature differences in relation to thermometer and technique. *Nurs Res* 1980 May/Jun; 29: 157–64.
29. Reisinger KS, Kao J, Grant DM. Inaccuracy of the Clinitemp skin thermometer. *Pediatrics* 1979 Jul; 64: 4–6.
30. Lewit EM, Marshall CL, Salzer JE. An evaluation of a plastic strip thermometer. *JAMA* 1982 Jan 15; 247(3): 321–5.
31. Siebenaler ME. Taking a baby's temperature: is it common knowledge? *Am J Maternal Child Nurs* 1985 Jan/Feb; 10: 71.
32. Baker NC, Cerone SB, Gaze N, et al. The effect of type of thermometer and length of time inserted on oral temperature measurements of afebrile subjects. *Nurs Res* 1984 Mar/Apr; 33(2): 109–11.
33. Tandberg D, Sklar D. Effect of tachypnea on the estimation of body temperature by an oral thermometer. *N Engl J Med* 1983 Apr 21; 308(16): 945–6.
34. Greenbaum EI, Carson M, Kincannon WN, et al. Rectal thermometer-induced pneumoperitoneum in the newborn. *Pediatrics* 1969 Oct; 44(4): 539–42.
35. Eoff MJ, Joyce B. Temperature measurements in children. *Am J Nurs* 1981 May; 81: 1010–1.
36. Weisse ME, Reagen MS, Boule L, et al. Axillary vs. rectal temperatures in ambulatory and hospitalized children. *Pediatr Infect Dis J* 1991 Jul; 10: 541–2.
37. Ogren JM. The inaccuracy of axillary temperatures measured with an electronic thermometer. *Am J Dis Child* 1990 Jan; 144(1): 109–11.
38. Musher DM, Fainstein V, Young EJ, et al. Fever patterns: their lack of clinical significance. *Arch Intern Med* 1979 Nov; 139: 1225–8.
39. Done AK. Treatment of fever in 1982: a review. *Am J Med* 1983 Jun 14; 74(6A): 27–35.
40. Done AK. Uses and abuses of antipyretic therapy. *Pediatrics* 1959 Apr; 23: 774–80.
41. Rodbard D. The role of regional body temperature in the pathogenesis of disease. *N Engl J Med* 1981 Oct 1; 305(14): 808–14.
42. Roberts NJ Jr. Impact of temperature elevation on immunologic defenses. *Rev Infect Dis* 1991 May/Jun; 13(3): 462–71.
43. Brunell PA. Contagion and varicella-zoster virus. *Pediatr Infect Dis* 1982 Sep/Oct; 1(5): 304–7.
44. Stanley ED, Jackson GG, Panusarn C, et al. Increased virus shedding with aspirin treatment of rhinovirus infection. *JAMA* 1975 Mar 24; 231(12): 1248–51.
45. Steele RW, Tanaka PT, Lara RP, et al. Evaluation of sponging and of oral antipyretic therapy to reduce fever. *J Pediatr* 1970 Nov; 77(5): 824–9.
46. Wilson JT, Brown D, Kearns GL, et al. Single-dose, placebo-controlled comparative study of ibuprofen and acetaminophen antipyresis in children. *J Pediatr* 1991 Nov; 119: 803–11.
47. Gribetz B, Cronley SA. Underdosing of acetaminophen by parents. *Pediatrics* 1987 Nov; 80: 630–3.
48. Lorin MI. In: *The Febrile Child: Clinical Management of Fever and Other Types of Pyrexia*. New York: John Wiley & Sons, 1982: 227–8.

Chapter 7

Menstrual Products

Leslie A. Shimp

Questions to ask in patient assessment and counseling

- *What symptoms are you currently experiencing?*
- *Describe the severity of your symptoms.*
- *At what time in the menstrual cycle do your symptoms occur?*
- *Are these symptoms the same as or different from symptoms you have experienced in other menstrual cycles?*
- *Are your menses heavier or lighter than usual?*
- *Have you experienced unusual menstrual bleeding? Has this occurred at midcycle or at the usual time of menses?*
- *Is your menstrual cycle shorter or longer than usual?*
- *Have you missed a period?*
- *Have you experienced an abnormal vaginal discharge? Has it been accompanied by itching and burning?*
- *Have you experienced vaginal dryness and/or difficult or painful sexual intercourse? Do you experience hot flashes?*
- *Have you experienced any abdominal pain, lower abdominal pain, or lower back pain? Would you classify your abdominal pain as cramps?*
- *Have you experienced one or more of the following symptoms as you near your period: mood swings, low self-esteem, depression, anger, hostility, anxiety, tension, jumpiness, lack of energy, difficulty concentrating, food craving, overeating, insomnia, weight gain, fluid retention, breast tenderness and/or bloating?*
- *Are you now experiencing a high fever, dizziness, nausea, vomiting, diarrhea, sunburn-like rash, muscle aches and/or mental confusion?*
- *Do you use menstrual pads or tampons?*
- *What medication(s) are you currently taking?*
- *What medication(s) have you taken previously to control your symptoms?*
- *Are you allergic or hypersensitive to any drugs? If yes, which one(s)?*

This chapter is based in part on the chapter with the same title that appeared in the 9th edition but was written by Catherine Angell Sohn and Barbara H. Korberly.

The menstrual cycle is a regular physiologic event for women beginning during adolescence and continuing through late middle age. During the menstrual cycle, some women experience unpleasant symptoms such as abdominal pain and cramping, headache, and fluid retention. Many women use nonprescription products and seek advice from a pharmacist on how best to manage their symptoms.

The pharmacist should be familiar with common menstrual symptoms and disorders, as well as the risks associated with the misuse of menstrual products (e.g., toxic shock syndrome). The pharmacist should be able to interview a woman, assess her symptoms, determine their severity, recommend a product or activity to produce symptomatic relief, or refer the patient to a physician when appropriate. The pharmacist should be particularly expert in evaluating available nonprescription preparations and recommending safe and effective therapy, including nondrug adjunctive measures, for symptom relief.

Menstrual Cycle

Menstruation results from the monthly cycling of female reproductive hormones. In contrast to male fertility, which is relatively constant, female fertility is cyclic, occurring once monthly around the midpoint of the menstrual cycle. A single menstrual cycle is the time between the onset of one menstrual flow (menstruation or menses) and the beginning of the next. Two principal reproductive events, each hormonally controlled, occur during each menstrual cycle. The first is the maturation and release of an ovum (egg) from the ovaries; the second is the preparation of the endometrial lining of the uterus for the implantation of a fertilized ovum.[1,2] However, the first 12–18 months of the menstrual cycle may be irregular and anovulatory (not associated with ovum release) as the complex endocrine system involved in the reproductive cycle achieves synchronization and maturation.[2,3]

The average age at which menarche (the initial menstrual cycle) occurs in U.S. women is 12.5 years. However, menarche may occur as early as age 9 or 10 or as late as age 16 or 17. The onset of menstruation may be influenced by race, genetic factors, nutritional status, exercise intensity, and psychologic factors. The variability in the onset of menstruation parallels the variation in onset of puberty, which can begin as early as age 9 and as late as age 14. Two of the earliest signs of puberty are a growth spurt and the beginning of breast development. On average, there is a 2-year lag period between the beginning of breast development and the onset of menarche.[4]

The average menstrual cycle lasts 28 days; the normal range for cycle length is 21–35 days.[5] The first day of the menstrual flow is called day 1 of the cycle. Menses usually last 4–6 days (± 2 days). Most of the blood loss occurs during days 1 and 2.[1,6] The major components of menstrual fluid are endometrial cellular debris and blood. Average blood loss is 30–35 mL (range 20–80 mL) per cycle. A loss of more than 80 mL per cycle is considered abnormal.

Menopause is defined as the cessation of menstrual flow, or the last menstrual cycle. However, this term is also commonly used to refer to the perimenopausal or climacteric period, the years just before and after menopause. Menopause is associated with a depletion of ovarian follicles. The average age for onset of menopause in women is 51 years; however, menopause may occur as early as age 45 and as late as age 55. The age at which it occurs is not related to race, body size, age of menarche, number of pregnancies, lactation, or prior oral contraceptive use.[7] Alterations and irregularities in the menstrual cycle, which are often one of the earliest signs of the climacteric, typically begin when a woman is 40–45 years of age. These changes are related to changing hormone levels. The usual overt change is for the menses to become lighter and irregular; ovulation may occur less often. The anovulatory cycles are related to a decline in progesterone levels.[7] The decline in estrogen levels affects many tissues because estrogen receptors are located throughout the body. Some degree of estrogen-deprivation symptoms are experienced by almost all peri- and postmenopausal women. The most common of these symptoms are hot flashes, sleep disturbances, psychologic symptoms, and vaginal dryness.[8]

Menstrual Physiology

The menstrual cycle results from the hormonal activity of the hypothalamus, pituitary gland, and ovaries (hypothalamic–pituitary–ovarian axis). The hypothalamus is a cluster of nerve cell bodies located in the center of the brain. The arcate nuclei of the hypothalamus play an important role in regulating the menstrual cycle via production of gonadotropin-releasing hormone (GnRH). Low levels of estradiol and progesterone, occurring at the end of the previous menstrual cycle, stimulate the hypothalamus to release GnRH, which is then immediately transported to the anterior pituitary. The pituitary gland is located adjacent to the hypothalamus in a bony depression called the sella turcica. GnRH stimulates pituitary gonadotrope cells to synthesize and secrete luteinizing hormone (LH) and follicle-stimulating hormone (FSH) into the general circulation. FSH released from the anterior pituitary gland stimulates a group of ovarian graafian follicles to mature. These maturing follicles then begin to secrete the estrogen estradiol, which influences follicular development and promotes the growth of the uterine endometrium. In addition, the increasing estradiol levels promote the midcycle surge in LH from the pituitary gland. This LH surge then stimulates the cells of the graafian follicles to secrete progesterone, which helps to maintain the endometrial lining and to inhibit hormonal secretions of the hypothalamus and pituitary gland.

The events of the menstrual cycle can be described in phases and by changes in the uterine endometrium (menstrual, proliferative, and secretory phases) or in the ovary (follicular, ovulatory, and luteal phases). Cycle day 1 (the first day of menstrual blood flow) is the beginning of the follicular phase in the ovary and of the menstrual phase in the uterus. The follicular phase, during which the final maturation of a graafian follicle occurs, is quite variable in length; it lasts an average of 14 days but can range in length between 7 and 22 days.

By about cycle day 7, a single ovarian follicle becomes dominant. This follicle continues to develop and secrete increasing amounts of estradiol while the other follicles regress and degenerate. Once it is mature and capable of ovulation, this follicle is known as the graafian follicle. The ovulatory phase of the cycle is approximately 3 days in length. During this phase, the LH surge occurs. This is a 36- to 48-hour period when several large waves or pulses of LH are released, thus increasing serum LH levels as much as 10-fold. The LH surge catalyzes the final steps in the maturation of the ovum and also stimulates the production of prostaglandins and proteolytic enzymes, which are necessary for the rupture of the follicle wall and ovulation (release of a mature ovum). Increasing levels of progesterone also play a role in stimulating the production of proteolytic enzymes. During the LH surge, levels of estradiol decrease, sometimes accompanied by midcycle endometrial bleeding. Ovulation typically occurs within 24 hours after the LH surge; however, this time has been reported to be as little as 16 hours and as many as 48 hours after the surge. Ovulation releases 5–10 mL of follicular fluid, which contains the oocyte mass; this event may cause abdominal pain (mittelschmerz) for some women.[1–5]

The luteal phase is the time between ovulation and the beginning of menstrual blood flow. In contrast to the follicular phase, the luteal phase is more constant in length, averaging 13 to 14 days (± 2 days). After the graafian follicle ruptures, its walls collapse and its cells take up lipid and lutein pigment, which gives it a yellow appearance. This transformed graafian follicle is now referred to as the corpus luteum. The duration of the luteal phase is consistent with the functional period (about 10–12 days) of the corpus luteum, during which time the corpus luteum secretes progesterone, estradiol, and androgens. The increased levels of estrogen and progesterone alter the character of the two outer layers of the uterine endometrial lining. The glands of the endometrium mature, proliferate, and become secretory in nature (secretory phase) as the uterus prepares for the implantation of a fertilized egg. Progesterone and estrogen levels reach their peaks in the middle of the luteal phase, and levels of LH and FSH decline in response to the increase in these two hormones. If pregnancy occurs, human chorionic gonadotropin (HCG) released by the developing embryo supports the function of the corpus luteum until the placenta develops enough to begin secreting estrogen and progesterone. If pregnancy does not occur (no production of HCG), the corpus luteum ceases to function and estrogen and progesterone levels decline, causing the endometrial lining of the uterus to become edematous and necrotic. The decrease in progesterone also allows prostaglandin synthesis. Prostaglandins initiate vasoconstriction and uterine contractions, and the sloughing of the outer two endometrial layers occurs. The decline in estrogen and progesterone also results in an increase in GnRH and the renewed production of LH and FSH, which begins a new menstrual cycle.[1–5]

Figure 1 presents a graphic display of the events of the normal menstrual cycle.

Menstrual Dysfunction

Dysmenorrhea

Dysmenorrhea is a term meaning difficult or painful menstruation.[9] One of the most common gynecologic problems in the United States, dysmenorrhea is estimated to occur in approximately 50% of postpubescent women. Approximately 40% of adult women experience some degree of painful menstrual cramps and up to 10% may be functionally impaired for 1–3 days per month. This dysfunction translates into an estimated 650 million work hours lost per year at a cost in excess of $3 billion in lost productivity. Similarly, 10–18% of adolescent girls report missing school regularly due to dysmenorrhea.[4,9–11]

Dysmenorrhea is divided into primary and secondary disease. Primary dysmenorrhea is idiopathic and associated with pain at the time of menstruation with no identifiable organic pelvic disease. It occurs most often in young women, usually developing within 6–12 months of menarche and generally affecting women during their teenage years and early twenties. Primary dysmenorrhea occurs only during ovulatory cycles; therefore, its prevalence rises between early adolescence, when about 39% of 12-year-olds ovulate, and older adolescence, when approximately 72% of 17-year-olds ovulate.[4] Its prevalence decreases after 30–35 years of age.[9,10]

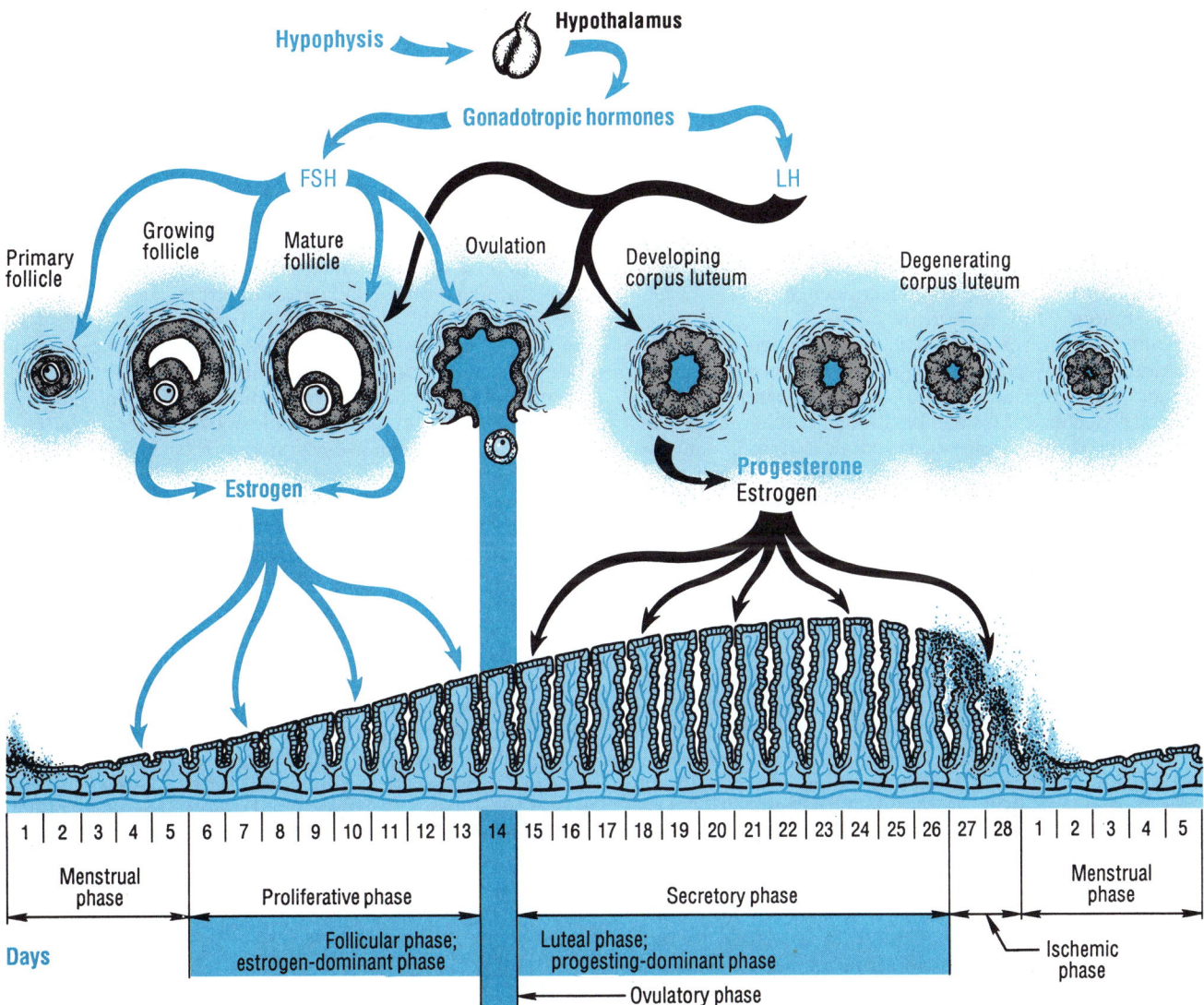

FIGURE 1 Schematic drawing illustrating the interrelations of the hypothalamus, hypophysis (pituitary gland), ovaries, and endometrium. One complete menstrual cycle and the beginning of another are shown. Changes in the ovaries, called the ovarian cycle, are promoted by the gonadotropic hormones, (FSH and LH). Hormones from the ovaries (estrogens and progesterone) then promote changes in the structure and function of the endometrium. Thus, the cyclical activity of the ovary is intimately linked with changes in the uterus. From Moore KL. *The Developing Human.* 2nd ed. Philadelphia: W. B. Saunders; 1977.

Secondary dysmenorrhea is usually associated with pelvic pathology. Possible causes include endometriosis, congenital abnormalities, pelvic inflammatory disease, ovarian cysts, benign uterine tumors, endometrial cancer, adhesions, and cervical stenosis. Secondary dysmenorrhea may also be caused by the presence of intrauterine devices.[4,9]

Symptoms of dysmenorrhea are similar to those of ectopic pregnancy and pelvic inflammatory disease; therefore, physician evaluation is necessary to rule out the presence of secondary causes of dysmenorrhea. Primary dysmenorrhea pain usually begins with the onset of menses and lasts from a few hours up to 48–72 hours.[9,10] Although it is experienced as lower midabdominal or suprapubic pain, which is cramping in nature, the pain may radiate to the lower back and upper thighs, and may be accompanied by symptoms such as nausea, vomiting, fatigue, nervousness, dizziness, diarrhea, and headache.[4]

Evidence suggests that dysmenorrhea is related to prostaglandin levels. Both the endometrium and the myometrium of the uterus have the capacity to synthesize prostaglandins. Prostaglandin levels in the endometrium and menstrual fluid of women with dysmenorrhea have been found to be elevated. Researchers have reported prostaglandin serum levels to be 5–13 times greater in women with dysmenorrhea compared with women without dysmenorrhea. The symptoms of primary dysmenorrhea are very similar to those produced by the administration of a prostaglandin to induce labor. Finally, administration of prostaglandin synthesis inhibitors such as nonsteroidal anti-inflammatory drugs (NSAIDs) has been shown to reduce the symptoms of dysmenorrhea.[9,10,12]

Prostaglandin serum levels rise as progesterone levels decrease during the luteal phase of the menstrual cycle. Concurrently, the levels of prostacyclin (a smooth-muscle relaxant) decrease. This combination of biochemical events can lead to strong uterine contractions and significant vasoconstriction, resulting in uterine hypoxia and pain in some women.[10] Four physiologic changes have been identified that contribute to development of this pain: (1) an elevation of myometrial resting tone to above 10 mm Hg, (2) an elevation of contractile myometrial pressure to above 120 mm Hg, (3) increased frequency of uterine contractions, and (4) dysrhythmia of contractions. Both the intrauterine pressure and the number of uterine contractions have been shown to be directly related to the pain of dysmenorrhea because both of these conditions produce a decrease in blood flow and tissue hypoxia.[4,9,10]

In a subset of women with primary dysmenorrhea, prostaglandin levels were not found to be elevated and administration of prostaglandin synthesis inhibitors did not alleviate their pain. One hypothesis suggests that leukotrienes may cause the pain. The prostaglandin precursor, arachidonic acid, can also be converted to leukotrienes. Leukotrienes induce uterine contractions and vasoconstriction similar to the action of the prostaglandins. In addition, there is some evidence that vasopressin (a substance that can produce dysrhythmic uterine contractions) may also be involved in the etiology of primary dysmenorrhea.[10]

A number of factors have been associated with the occurrence or severity of dysmenorrhea. As mentioned previously, dysmenorrhea is most common in young women and less so in women beyond the late twenties. This decrease in incidence and severity may be related to pregnancy, given that during late pregnancy, uterine adrenergic nerves virtually disappear and only a portion regenerate after childbirth.[13] Lifestyle alterations may also alleviate symptoms to varying degrees. Smoking tobacco or consuming excessive amounts of ethanol has been associated with more severe dysmenorrhea; the severity reportedly increases with the number of cigarettes smoked per day. The basis for this effect is unknown although it has been hypothesized that nicotine-induced vasoconstriction is involved in the adverse effect noted from tobacco smoking.[13,14] Evidence regarding the benefit of exercise is conflicting.[4,10,13]

Amenorrhea

Amenorrhea is defined as the absence or cessation of menses. This disorder has many etiologies. *Primary amenorrhea* is the term used for the disorder when a female adolescent does not begin menstruation. Amenorrhea is diagnosed if menses has not occurred by age 14 if the female has not had any secondary sexual development, or by age 16 if secondary sexual development has occurred. *Secondary amenorrhea* refers to a cessation of menses for 3 months or longer in a woman who was previously having menses. Possible causes of amenorrhea include gonadal failure, reproductive tract anomalies, emotional stress, weight loss or gain, poor nutrition, anorexia nervosa, excessive exercise, hyperthyroidism, and hypothyroidism.[15]

Exercise-induced amenorrhea can be manifested as either primary or secondary amenorrhea, depending on the age at which intense athletic training occurs. If such training is begun before the onset of menarche, it can delay onset and increase the likelihood of menstrual cycle irregularity. More than 80% of competitive swimmers and runners who begin athletic training before menarche experience irregular menses or amenorrhea; this incidence is lower (approximately 40%) among athletes who experienced menarche before beginning strenuous training.[16] Although the exact cause of exercise-induced amenorrhea has not been established, this condition has been shown to correlate with exercise intensity, nutrition, emotional stress, and anxiety associated with competition. Changes in levels of hormones involved in the normal menstrual cycle have also been noted; estradiol, progesterone, and LH levels have all been found to be decreased during strenuous athletic training.[16,17] Fortunately, exercise-induced amenorrhea is readily reversed with a decrease in the intensity of training and/or a 2 to 3% increase in body weight.[17] The major risk associated with this type of amenorrhea is loss of bone density and associated stress fractures of bones. It is unclear whether the decrease in bone density (peak bone mass) from exercise-induced amenorrhea will contribute to a greater risk for osteoporosis and bone fractures postmenopausally.[16,17]

Menorrhagia

Menorrhagia is excessive menstrual blood loss with either menses lasting for more than 7 days or a total blood loss of more than 60–80 mL of blood. Women who repeatedly experience a cyclic menstrual blood loss of more than 80 mL may develop low hemoglobin, low hematocrit, and low serum iron levels. About 15–20% of healthy women have experienced menorrhagia,[18] which is one of the most common causes of iron deficiency in reproductive-age women.[6] A number of systemic illnesses and endocrine disorders (e.g., renal and hepatic disease, uterine tumors or polyps, thyroid dysfunction, and diabetes mellitus) may cause menorrhagia. In addition, a number of medications, including anticoagulants, oral contraceptives, postmenopausal hormone replacement therapy, oral or intramuscular progestins, neuroleptics, and chemotherapy, can cause abnormal vaginal bleeding. Intrauterine devices may also cause excessive menses.[18]

Estrogen–progestin combination oral contraceptives, which suppress ovulation, are effective in decreasing the thickness of the endometrial lining and thus reducing menstrual blood loss. NSAIDs are also effective in decreasing menorrhagia. These agents may achieve their effect by altering the balance between the vasoconstrictor thromboxane A_2 and the vasodilator prostacyclin. An increased production of leukotrienes, which are powerful vasoconstrictors, has also been suggested as a mechanism by which NSAIDs benefit the patient.[6] NSAIDs are most effective when given for several days premenstrually and then every 6 hours during the menses.[18]

Dysfunctional Uterine Bleeding

Dysfunctional uterine bleeding (DUB) is a syndrome of irregular menses with periods of prolonged, heavy menstrual flow alternating with amenorrhea for which there is no identifiable etiology.[6,19] DUB most commonly occurs during the first 2 years following menarche and during the perimenopausal period. It is usually the result of anovulatory cycles. In the first year following menarche, about 50% of menstrual cycles are anovulatory.[6]

The amount of bleeding during menses is a function of the number of days the endometrium has been exposed to estrogen stimulation. Normally, menses occurs about 13 to 14 days following ovulation. In anovulatory cycles, there is no midcycle surge in LH, so the endometrium remains in the proliferative phase rather than switching to a secretory phase. Bleeding will then eventually occur when the endometrium has grown to such a thickness that it can no longer be supported. Excessive fibrinolytic activity and changes in uterine prostaglandin production also appear to contribute to DUB.[6,19]

The management of DUB is directed toward regulating the menstrual cycle to avoid excessive bleeding and anemia. In mild cases, therapy is usually initiated with just iron supplementation. If the DUB is more severe, an estrogen–progestin combination oral contraceptive may be prescribed to regulate the menstrual cycle. Hormone therapy is usually continued until the hemoglobin level and iron store are normalized. Iron therapy is continued for at least 3 months after hemoglobin is normalized in order to restore body iron stores.[19]

Midcycle Pain and Bleeding

Midcycle bleeding (spotting) is a relatively common phenomenon; microscopic bleeding is demonstrated in 60–94% of women at midcycle. This type of intermenstrual bleeding, which may be accompanied by short-lived abdominal pain, is typically due to the decrease in ovarian estrogen production, which occurs at midcycle. At the time of ovulation, estrogen levels may decrease by 25–33%. Bleeding of this type is self-limited and does not require therapy.[6]

Premenstrual Syndrome

Premenstrual syndrome (PMS) is a condition surrounded by controversy owing to the lack of agreement regarding its etiology, definition, and treatment. It can be defined as a cyclic disorder composed of a combination of physical and emotional (mood) changes that occur during the luteal phase of the menstrual cycle and improve significantly or disappear within the first several days of menstrual flow. Attempts have been made to standardize the diagnosis and study of PMS, also known as late luteal phase dysphoric disorder, by specifying a strict set of criteria for diagnosis (Table 1).

TABLE 1 Criteria for diagnosing premenstrual syndrome

1. Symptoms must occur in most menstrual cycles, beginning after ovulation and decreasing within several days after the onset of menses.

2. Symptoms must include at least five of the following (and at least one of the first four):

    Marked mood swings;

    Persistent and marked anger or irritability;

    Marked anxiety, tension, or feeling of being "keyed up" or "on edge";

    Markedly depressed mood, feeling of hopelessness, low self-esteem;

    Decreased interest in usual activities;

    Lack of energy; feeling of being easily fatigued;

    Difficulty concentrating;

    Marked change in appetite, overeating, food cravings;

    Hypersomnia or insomnia;

    Other physical symptoms, such as breast tenderness or swelling, headaches, joint or muscle pain, bloating, or weight gain.

3. The condition seriously interferes with work or usual activities, or with social relationships with others.

4. The condition is not merely a worsening of the symptoms of another disorder (e.g., depression, panic disorder, or personality disorder).

5. The criteria specified above are confirmed by prospective daily self-ratings during at least two symptomatic menstrual cycles.

Information extracted from Robinson GE, Garfinkel PE. *Can J Psychiatry* 1990; 35 (3): 199–206.

Almost all women experience some physical or mood changes prior to the onset of menses. These changes are regarded as part of the normal menstrual cycle and are referred to medically as molimina. Common symptoms include minor weight gain, abdominal bloating, mild fatigue, and irritability; some women report positive change such as increased energy and increased work productivity. Very few women who experience premenstrual symptoms experience a decline in their ability to function normally. Less than 1% reported regularly missing work as a result of their symptoms.[20,21] Only a small percentage of women, probably less than 10%, experience symptoms severe enough to meet the criteria in Table 1.[20,22,23]

Many theories have been developed to explain the etiology of PMS, but it remains unknown. Nonetheless a variety of therapies paralleling these theories have been advocated. One of the more publicized theories has been the progesterone-deficiency theory. However, inadequate progesterone levels have not been clearly demonstrated as an etiologic factor in studies, and well-controlled clinical trials have not shown a benefit from progesterone therapy.[21-24] Similarly, neither aldosterone, endorphin, nor prolactin levels have been found to be different in control versus symptomatic patients.[21,24,25]

Another relatively popular theory suggests that vitamin B_6 might be an effective treatment for PMS. The theory hypothesizes that a deficiency of vitamin B_6 might occur secondary to depletion by estrogen. However, controlled trials have not found vitamin B_6 to be any more efficacious than placebo, and no evidence exists for altered vitamin B_6 absorption or metabolism.[21-24] Still, one study reported a high percentage of physicians (60%) who prescribed vitamins for women with premenstrual symptoms, and a significant number of patients (40%) had taken vitamin B_6.[26] Vitamin B_6 supplementation is not without risk; high doses (2–6 g per day) have been associated with the development of peripheral neuropathy,[22,24] and one report suggests that doses of about 50 mg per day might also be associated with neuropathy.[23]

Evening primrose oil has also been advocated for the treatment of PMS based on the theory that PMS is caused by a prostaglandin E_1 deficiency. Evening primrose oil contains gamma linoleic acid (efamol), which is a prostaglandin E_1 precursor. Several placebo-controlled trials have shown an improvement in breast tenderness and depression, but response to placebo was also high and more studies are needed.[24,25] The dose of efamol used for the treatment of breast tenderness is 4 g daily throughout the cycle for at least three to four cycles.[24] The NSAIDs have also shown some evidence of efficacy in managing symptoms. These agents may be most useful for women who experience both dysmenorrhea and PMS; reducing symptoms associated with dysmenorrhea may help improve a woman's ability to tolerate PMS-related symptoms.[21,22,24,25] Both psychologic and nutritional theories for the etiology of PMS have been suggested. There is some evidence that PMS severity may be affected by disturbed family relationships and negative attitudes toward menstruation.[25] In addition, women's expectations may affect their rating of symptoms such as fluid retention; in one study, women who were told they were premenstrual reported a greater degree of fluid retention than those who were told they were intermenstrual.[25] In two well-controlled double-blind studies, the benzodiazepine alprazolam was rated by both patients and physicians as more effective than placebo in alleviating symptoms.[24] The benefit of nutritional therapy for PMS is unproven; nonetheless, many clinicians recommend a balanced diet and the avoidance of salty foods (which aggravate fluid retention) and caffeine (which increases irritability).[21,22,24]

Patient Assessment

Most women who purchase nonprescription drugs for menstrual cycle–related symptoms are healthy. Before recommending any product for a patient, the pharmacist should gather pertinent information, such as current drug medication therapy; treatment previously tried; outcome of prior therapy (efficacy, dose, duration, side effects); drug allergies, hypersensitivities, or intolerances; and whether symptoms were evaluated by a physician. The pharmacist also needs to obtain a clear and complete description of the patient's current symptoms including their severity, recentness of onset, similarity to symptoms experienced during other menstrual cycles, and the patient's explanation for their occurrence. The pharmacist should instruct the patient to see a physician for any of the following problems:

- Abnormal vaginal bleeding or discharge;
- Atrophic vaginitis;
- Dyspareunia (difficult or painful sexual intercourse);
- Irregular menstrual cycles or amenorrhea or dysmenorrhea;
- Significant alterations in mood;
- Breast tenderness.

Recommendations for any nonprescription drug should be accompanied by adequate patient counseling regarding the appropriate use of the product and other adjunctive measures.

Vaginal Dryness

Among the common complaints associated with menopause are atrophic vaginitis and associated dyspareunia.[27,28] Atrophic vaginitis is inflammation of the vagina related to atrophy of the vaginal mucosa secondary to decreased estrogen levels. Symptoms include vaginal irritation, burning, itching, and dyspareunia.[29] At menopause, vaginal lubrication declines secondary to the decrease in estrogen levels. The most common cause of secondary superficial dyspareunia is a lack of adequate vaginal lubrication.[27,28] This condition is most common in postmenopausal women and breast-feeding women. The pharmacist should inquire about the onset of these symptoms; self-treatment is most appropriate for those women who have previously been able to maintain adequate vaginal lubrication. Severe vaginal dryness or dyspareunia should be evaluated by a physician, however.

Dysmenorrhea

Before recommending any product for a patient experiencing symptoms of dysmenorrhea, the pharmacist should establish the onset of pain in relation to the onset of menses.

Primary dysmenorrhea produces abdominal and lower back pain that begins within 1 to 2 days prior to the onset of menses and ceases during the first several days of menstrual blood flow. Pain that does not follow this pattern and that is severe or different in character from pain occurring during previous menstrual cycles should be evaluated promptly by a physician. It is important that adolescents who experience symptoms be educated about dysmenorrhea and that they realize this condition can be treated with products that can provide symptomatic relief. They should also be reassured about the "normality" of dysmenorrhea.

Menstrual Dysfunction

All conditions of menstrual dysfunction, (i.e., amenorrhea, menorrhagia, DUB, and midcycle pain and bleeding) with the exception of minor midcycle pain and bleeding, should be evaluated by a physician. There are many possible etiologies for these conditions, and appropriate therapy depends on an accurate diagnosis and a determination of the severity and prognosis for the disorder. Although symptoms may not be bothersome, pharmacists should encourage patients to seek medical evaluation to avoid potential long-term adverse consequences (e.g., osteoporosis associated with long-term amenorrhea) or the delayed diagnosis and treatment of a potentially serious medical condition.

Premenstrual Syndrome

Pharmacists discussing premenstrual symptoms with patients should emphasize that minor symptoms such as bloating and weight gain, fatigue, irritability, mood swings, changes in appetite, and breast tenderness are not uncommon. If these symptoms are more severe, evaluation by a physician is encouraged. In addition, pharmacists should inquire about prior self-treatment and discuss any potential dangers inherent in prior therapy (e.g., neuropathy associated with vitamin B_6 therapy). Pharmacists should also dispel some common myths about the adverse effect of the menstrual cycle on the ability of women to function normally.

Drug Therapy Management

Vaginal Dryness

Treatment of vaginal dryness can often be accomplished with application of topical lubricants. One study found that about half the women who experienced vaginal dryness had tried "something," including substances such as butter, baby oil, and Vaseline®, before seeking medical attention.[28] The pharmacist should question patients about the use of any vaginal or feminine hygiene products because such products may cause or worsen vaginal irritation and dyspareunia.[30]

Water-soluble lubricants (e.g., Gyne-moistrin®, KY Jelly®, and Replens®) and moisturizing skin lotions (e.g., Lubriderm® and Keri-lotion®) are acceptable vaginal lubricants.[28] Vaseline® should not be used because it is difficult to remove from the vagina. If the patient is using a condom or diaphragm, only water-soluble lubricants should be used. Water-soluble lubricant gels can be applied both externally and internally. Initially, the patient should be instructed to use a liberal quantity of lubricant (up to 2 tbsp) and then to tailor the quantity and frequency of use to her specific needs. If the patient is treating dyspareunia, the lubricant should be applied to both the vaginal opening and the penis. If the use of nonprescription lubricants does not produce adequate benefit or if the patient finds the use of lubricants aesthetically unappealing, oral or topical estrogen replacement therapy may be prescribed.[28]

Dysmenorrhea

The treatment of dysmenorrhea varies with the severity of symptoms. For mild symptoms, an analgesic agent such as aspirin, ibuprofen, or acetaminophen and the application of local heat to the abdomen or lower back may be adequate.[1] Many nonprescription menstrual products contain aspirin, ibuprofen, or acetaminophen as the analgesic agent. However, aspirin has only a limited effect on prostaglandin synthesis and is therefore only moderately effective in treating women with more than minimal symptoms.[9] When used for menstrual discomfort, the dosing of aspirin or acetaminophen is 325–650 mg every 4 hours, 325–500 mg every 3 hours, or 650–1,000 mg every 6 hours as needed, not to exceed 4,000 mg per day. Aspirin is best taken with food or a full glass of water. Ibuprofen is typically taken at doses of 400 mg every 4–6 hours as needed.

Before recommending aspirin therapy, the pharmacist should question the patient about allergy or intolerance to aspirin, disease states that are relative contraindications to aspirin therapy (e.g., peptic ulcer disease, gastritis, bleeding disorders, asthma, or renal insufficiency), and current medication usage. Clinically significant aspirin–drug interactions occur with anticoagulants, probenecid, phenytoin, oral hypoglycemics, and high doses of antacids (e.g., 60–120 mL of an aluminum–magnesium hydroxide suspension).

The principal nonprescription agent for the treatment of moderate dysmenorrhea is ibuprofen, an NSAID that inhibits the production and action of prostaglandins. In clinical trials, ibuprofen was found to be effective in 66–100% of patients.[10] Therapy should begin at the onset of pain after menstrual flow begins. Optimal pain relief is achieved when ibuprofen is taken on a scheduled rather than an as-needed basis; therefore, ibuprofen should be taken every 4–6 hours for the first 48–72 hours of menstrual flow because this is when prostaglandin release is maximal.[10] It should be explained to patients that ibuprofen is used as much to prevent cramps as to relieve pain.[1] The recommended ibuprofen dose is 400 mg taken initially and every 6 hours thereafter as needed. However, the nonprescription dose of 200 mg taken every 4–6 hours may be used at first; if it is not effective, 400 mg taken every 6 hours should be recommended. For nonprescription use, the maximum daily ibuprofen dose should not exceed 1,200 mg.

Ibuprofen (or any other NSAID) should be taken for three to four menstrual cycles before a judgment is made as to its effectiveness.[9] Side effects from a few days of use are limited. Those most commonly associated with short-term ibuprofen therapy include gastrointestinal (GI) symptoms (e.g., upset stomach, vomiting, heartburn, abdominal pain, diarrhea, constipation, and anorexia) and central nervous system side effects (e.g., headache and dizziness). The GI side effects of this agent may be decreased by taking ibuprofen with food. Relative contraindications to the use of ibuprofen include a history of allergy to aspirin (bronchospastic reaction) or to any other NSAID, active GI disease (e.g., peptic ulcer disease, gastroesophageal reflux disease, or ulcerative colitis), and bleeding disorders.[1,10] The patient with more severe dysmenorrhea or with dysmenorrhea that does not respond to nonprescription therapy should be referred to a physician. A trial with a prescription NSAID from another class or therapy with an oral contraceptive may be prescribed.

Premenstrual Syndrome

The initial treatment of the symptoms of PMS is generally conservative and consists of education and nondrug measures. Women with symptoms of PMS should be educated about the syndrome and encouraged to elicit family support and understanding. Other management recommendations include avoiding stress, developing coping mechanisms for effectively managing stress, learning relaxation techniques, incorporating regular exercise into the lifestyle, and making appropriate dietary alterations (e.g., lowering sodium intake and avoiding caffeine).[24] A woman who believes she has symptoms of PMS should be evaluated by a physician. For symptoms that are not responsive to nondrug therapy, medications previously shown to be effective in controlled trials may be useful. These include evening primrose oil and alprazolam.[21,22,24] A woman who has symptoms of dysmenorrhea in conjunction with PMS may benefit from nonprescription ibuprofen.

One of the most common premenstrual complaints is fluid accumulation. The Food and Drug Administration (FDA) has examined the usefulness and safety of nonprescription diuretics to relieve water retention, weight gain, bloating, swelling, and a full feeling. Three nonprescription diuretics—ammonium chloride, caffeine, and pamabrom—are contained in commercially available menstrual products. Ammonium chloride is an acid-forming salt with a short duration of effect. It is taken in oral doses of up to 3 g per day (divided into three doses) for no more than 6 consecutive days. Larger doses of ammonium chloride (4–12 g per day) can produce significant GI and central nervous system adverse effects. Ammonium chloride is contraindicated in patients with renal or liver impairment because metabolic acidosis may result.[31]

Caffeine, a xanthine, promotes diuresis by inhibiting the renal tubular reabsorption of sodium and water. It is safe and effective as a diuretic in doses of 100–200 mg every 3 to 4 hours. Tolerance to the diuretic effect may occur. Patients should be reminded that caffeine may cause anxiety, restlessness, or insomnia (if taken within several hours of bedtime), and that additive side effects (nervousness, irritability, nausea, or tachycardia) might occur if other caffeine-containing beverages, foods, or medications are consumed concurrently. Patients taking monoamine oxidase inhibitors or other xanthine medications (e.g., theophylline, aminophylline, oxtriphylline, or dyphylline) should avoid caffeine-containing diuretics. Caffeine may cause GI irritation; patients with a history of peptic ulcer disease should avoid caffeine.[31,32]

Pamabrom, a derivative of theophylline, is contained in combination products (along with analgesics and antihistamines) and is marketed for the treatment of PMS. It is taken in doses up to 200 mg per day (50 mg four times daily).[31]

Several smooth-muscle relaxants, antihistamines, sympathomimetic amines, and herbal preparations have been evaluated for the treatment of dysmenorrhea and PMS. None of these agents is classified as Category I (safe and effective).[31]

Related Menstrual Products

Feminine Cleansing Products

The pharmacist should be familiar with feminine hygiene products and should know how to advise a patient regarding their appropriate use and which symptoms related to their use require referral to a physician. (See Chapter 27, "Personal Care Products.")

Feminine Pads and Tampons

Feminine pads are used to absorb menstrual or other vaginal discharges. They are made of absorbent cotton, synthetic, or cellulose (derived from wood pulp) material that is covered with a lightweight paper gauze to reduce irritation. A layer of cellulose or thin plastic is incorporated into the side of the pad worn away from the perineum to minimize leakage and the soiling of undergarments. Most styles are held in place with adhesive strips on the underside of the pad, which affix to the undergarment.

Feminine pads are available in a wide variety of sizes and absorbencies. Because most women experience their heaviest menstrual flow on day 2 of the menstrual cycle, "super" or "maxi" pads may be used at this time. During the days of heaviest flow, pads may need to be changed every 2–4 hours; changing them every 4–6 hours may be adequate for days of lesser menstrual flow. Frequent changing of sanitary pads minimizes the development of unpleasant odors arising from the breakdown of blood products and vaginal secretions; it also helps to minimize irritation and chafing of the perineum and upper inner thighs. Applying powder to the inner thighs may also alleviate chafing.

"Mini" or "light" pads and "junior" or "teen" pads are designed to accommodate the smaller anatomy and lighter flow of the adolescent female. The narrower width of these pads may reduce chafing and irritation. Many women prefer the new, less cumbersome light pads for the first and last days of their cycles. These light pads or the thin shields may also be used to protect undergarments from being stained by vaginal creams, vaginal tablets, suppository leakage, or normal vaginal secretions.

Tampons are intravaginal inserts made of cellulose, cotton, or synthetic materials (viscose rayon or polyacrylate rayon) and designed to absorb menstrual or other vaginal discharge. They have the advantage over feminine pads

TABLE 2	CDC[a] case definition of toxic shock syndrome

Fever: temperature ≥ 102°F (38.9°C)

Rash: diffuse macular erythroderma

Desquamation: 1 to 2 weeks after onset of illness, particularly on palms and soles

Hypotension: systolic blood pressure ≤ 90 mm Hg, orthostatic drop in diastolic ≥ 15 mm Hg; orthostatic syncope or dizziness

Involvement of three or more of the following organ systems:

    Gastrointestinal: vomiting or diarrhea at onset of illness

    Muscular: severe myalgia or twice-normal creatine phosphokinase

    Mucous membranes: vaginal, oropharyngeal, or conjunctival hyperemia

    Renal: twice-normal blood urea nitrogen or creatinine or pyuria (more than five white blood cells in a high-power field)

    Hepatic: twice-normal bilirubin or transaminases

    Hematologic: platelets <1,000,000/mm^3

Central nervous system: disorientation or alterations in consciousness without focal neurologic signs when fever and hypotension are absent

Negative results on the following tests, if obtained: blood, throat, or cerebrospinal fluid cultures (blood culture may be positive for *S. aureus*)

Serologic tests for Rocky Mountain spotted fever, leptospirosis, or measles

[a]Centers for Disease Control.

of being worn internally, which lessens chafing, odor, bulkiness, and irritation. Some tampons are "scented," and some fragrances may cause local irritation and allergic reactions, such as allergic contact dermatitis. The FDA evaluated feminine pads and tampons and classified unscented menstrual pads into performance Class I, which indicates that the device meets only the general controls applicable to all devices. The FDA has classified scented menstrual pads and both unscented and scented menstrual tampons into performance Class II, which requires the future development of standards to ensure the safety and efficacy of the products.[33]

Both high absorbency and the composition of tampons have been associated with toxic shock syndrome (TSS).[34] In response to this association, and in an effort to decrease the likelihood of TSS, tampon manufacturers have altered the composition and lowered the absorbency of tampons.[34] In addition, the FDA changed the requirement for the labeling of tampons so that terms such as *regular* and *super*, which are used to indicate the absorbency of tampons, have a uniform meaning and indicate a specific range of absorbency.[35] Four descriptive terms are now used: *junior* (6 g or less of fluid absorbed per tampon), *regular* (6–9 g), *super* (9–12 g), and *super-plus* (12–15 g). Higher absorbency products (15–18 g or more) are not prohibited, but no products are currently marketed with these higher absorbencies.[35]

Toxic Shock Syndrome

Toxic shock syndrome was a term coined by Todd and coworkers in 1978 to describe a severe multisystem illness characterized by high fever, profound hypotension, severe diarrhea, mental confusion, renal failure, erythroderma, and skin desquamation.[36] In 1980 it was recognized that these symptoms were affecting a relatively large number of young, previously healthy, menstruating women, and the term *toxic shock syndrome* was applied to their illness. The Centers for Disease Control case definition of TSS is shown in Table 2.[37]

Obviously, TSS is a severe, life-threatening disease. Known to result from infections (at any site) caused by toxin-producing strains of *Staphylococcus aureus*, TSS is essentially a consequence of the systemic effects of the toxin. The major cause of TSS is an exotoxin, produced by *S. aureus*, called toxic shock syndrome toxin 1 (TSST-1). This exotoxin is produced by 90–100% of the strains of *S. aureus* associated with menstrual TSS and by 60–75% of the strains associated with nonmenstrual TSS.[37,38] The effects of TSST-1 are due to both the direct effects of the toxin and the toxin's ability to induce production of two other cytokines. The biologic properties of TSST-1, either directly or via the other cytokines, include induction of fever, enhanced susceptibility to endotoxin shock, blockade of the reticuloendothelial system, lymphocyte mitogenicity, enhancement of delayed-type hypersensitivity skin reactions, inhibition of neutrophil chemotaxis, and suppression of immunoglobulins. Further study of *S. aureus* has shown that the presence of *Escherichia coli* can facilitate its growth and the production of TSST-1. Other toxins are also associated with the production of TSS; some isolates of *S. aureus* associated with nonmenstrual TSS do not produce TSST-1.[37]

The clinical manifestations of TSS characteristically evolve quite rapidly. Within 8–12 hours an individual can move from a state of good health to full-blown TSS, which includes high fever, myalgias, vomiting and diarrhea, erythroderma, decreased urine output, severe hypotension, and shock.[36,37] The hypotension is characteristically profound; even individuals with mild cases often experience syncope.[37] This hypotension is due to several factors, including a decrease in vasomotor tone, which allows for the pooling of blood in the periphery; a leaking of fluid from the intravascular space to the interstitial space ("second-spacing"); depressed heart function; and volume depletion caused by vomiting, diarrhea, and fever. Multisystem organ involvement typically occurs in TSS. Myalgias, muscle weakness, arthralgias, and the GI symptoms (vomiting, diarrhea, and abdominal pain) typically occur early in the illness and affect almost all patients. Neurologic manifestations also occur in almost all cases. Encephalopathy, from cerebral edema, can be manifested as headache, confusion, agitation, lethargy, and seizures. Finally, both acute renal failure and adult respiratory distress syndrome are common in TSS.

Dermatologic manifestations are also characteristic of TSS, and both the early rash and subsequent skin desquamation are required for a definite diagnosis. The early rash is often described as a sunburn-like, diffuse, macular erythroderma that is not pruritic. It usually appears on the lower abdomen and thighs, or it may involve the perineum, torso, or extremities. This rash is often most intense in the area of infection, perhaps reflecting a high local concentration of toxin or mediators. It usually disappears after 3 days, and about 1–3 weeks later, desquamation of the skin on the patient's soles and palms begins to occur. A second rash (very erythematous, pruritic, and maculopapular) occurs in more than 50% of patients. Telogen effluvium, a late dermatologic manifestation that is a common, nonspecific reaction to severe sepsis and stress, may also be seen. Telogen effluvium describes the loss of hair and/or nails, which can occur after 4–16 weeks; growth is restored in 5 to 6 months.[37,39]

TSS is commonly divided into menstrual and nonmenstrual cases. Nonmenstrual TSS is much less common; only about one-third of TSS cases are of the nonmenstrual type. TSS can occur in both men and women; currently, about one-third of the nonmenstrual cases occur in males. The current incidence of TSS in the United States is unknown, but it has declined dramatically since 1980, when 812 cases of menstrual TSS were reported to the Centers for Disease Control; in 1988, only 53 cases were reported.[37]

Menstrual TSS has been found to affect primarily young women between the ages of 15–19 years. One reason for the greater incidence in young women is the absence of preexisting antibodies to the TSS toxin. By the age of 20–25, more than 90% of both men and women have detectable antibodies to this toxin.[36] However, in almost all cases of TSS, an absent or low titer of antibody to TSST-1 has been found.[39] TSS is also more common in Caucasian women than in women of other racial groups. This is primarily owing to a difference in the usage of menstrual products (i.e., tampons versus menstrual pads). Other explanations include a difference both in the susceptibility to TSS and in the ability to recognize the characteristic early rash in dark-skinned individuals.[37] The early data also indicated a possible difference in the geographic distribution of menstrual TSS; in 1981 and 1982, there were more cases occurring in the Mountain and North Central states than on either coast.[40] However, current data do not reveal any geographic variation in incidence.[36]

Risk factors for menstrual TSS have been identified. The strongest predictor of risk is use of tampons. One study found that women who used tampons had a 33 times greater risk than those who did not.[37,40] A case-control study from 1986 to 1987 found that the use of all major tampon brands was associated with the increased risk, although the risk varied by the brand of tampon.[34] The risk also varied with the absorbency of the tampon. Two studies found that for every increase in absorbency of 1 g, the risk of TSS increases 34–37%.[34,40] Additionally, the occurrence of TSS has been related to tampon composition, which can alter the presence of several factors (e.g., oxygen, magnesium, and glucose) that can influence the production of toxin by *S. aureus*.[36] Since the early 1980s, when the association between tampon usage and TSS was first noted, the absorbency and composition of tampons have changed dramatically. Nonetheless, the risk for TSS continues to be greater in tampon users, and the greatest risk is associated with the use of higher absorbency tampons. Finally, patterns of tampon use may affect risk of TSS. Continuous use of tampons for at least 1 day of menses has been shown to correlate with an increased risk of menstrual TSS.[34] This association persisted after the investigators controlled for the absorbency of the tampon product.

The question of whether tampons induce changes in vaginal microflora has received considerable attention. Both qualitative and quantitative changes in vaginal microflora (aerobic and anaerobic) occur during the menstrual cycle. Neither the type of menstrual product used nor the composition of tampons affected either of these parameters for women who had previously used tampons.[41] However, one study found a change in the number of staphylococci present when women who had previously used menstrual pads switched to tampons.[34] Tampons do not appear to act as a focus for microbial growth. Bacterial counts from vaginal swabs were consistently higher than those obtained from tampons; lower levels of bacterial counts were obtained from tampons after both 2 and 6 hours of use.

In addition to tampons, the risk for TSS has been associated with the use of all barrier contraceptives including diaphragms, cervical caps, and cervical sponges. This risk has been calculated to be about 10–12 times greater for women who use these forms of contraception than for women who do not. Neither oral contraceptive use nor use of an intrauterine device has been related to the development of TSS.[42]

A pharmacist should be able to counsel a patient about the prevention of TSS. It is important to emphasize that the risk for TSS is quite small; recent data suggest an incidence of 1–2.5 per 100,000 menstruating women.[34] Avoidance or reduction of risk can be accomplished if patients follow the guidelines listed below:

- To reduce the risk for TSS to almost zero, women should use sanitary pads instead of tampons.
- To lower the risk for TSS while using tampons, women should use the lowest absorbency tampons compatible with their needs and should alternate the use of menstrual pads (e.g., at night) with the use of tampons. Although frequent changing of tampons has not been found to reduce the risk for TSS, changing them at least 4–6 times per day is often suggested.
- Women should wash their hands with soap before inserting anything into their vagina (e.g., a tampon, a diaphragm, a contraceptive sponge, or a vaginal medication).
- Women should follow instructions for vaginal contraceptive products carefully. A sponge or diaphragm or cervical cap should not be left in place in the vagina longer than recommended and should not be used during a menstrual period.
- During the first 12 weeks after childbirth, women should not use tampons, contraceptive sponges, or a cervical cap, and it may be best to avoid using a diaphragm as well.
- Every woman should be encouraged to read the package insert on TSS enclosed in the tampon package and familiarize herself with the early symptoms of TSS.

- Early symptoms of TSS include a high fever, muscle aches, a sunburn-like rash appearing after a day or two, weakness, fatigue, nausea, vomiting, and diarrhea. If these symptoms occur, the tampon should be removed immediately and emergency medical treatment should be sought.[36] In severe cases, TSS can cause dizziness, faintness, shock, and even death.

Women who have had TSS are at higher risk for recurrent episodes, especially during the first year after the illness, because it takes at least that long for protective antibodies to reappear. Prevention of TSS for these patients includes avoidance of tampons; administration of oral antistaphylococcal antibiotics during menses until there is a rise in the TSST-1 titer;[37,39] and the use of nonbarrier forms of contraception, at least until the TSST-1 titers rise.[42]

Summary

Most women function normally and require minimal or no pharmacologic intervention for menstrual cycle–related symptoms. If necessary, relief of many minor menstrual symptoms may be accomplished with nonprescription products. However, more severe symptoms and specific menstrual disorders, such as amenorrhea, dysmenorrhea, menstrual dysfunction, and significant PMS symptoms, may require referral to a physician for evaluation.

References

1. Hatcher RA, Stewart FH, Trussel J, et al. The Menstrual Cycle. In: *Contraceptive Technology 1990–1992*. 15th ed. New York: Irvington Publishers Inc; 1990: 39–46.
2. Espey LL, Halim IA. Characteristics and control of the normal menstrual cycle. *Obstet Gynecol Clin North Am* 1990; 17 (2): 275–98.
3. Kustin J, Rebar RW. Menstrual disorders in the adolescent age group. *Prim Care* 1987; 14 (1): 139–66.
4. Neinstein LS. Menstrual problems in adolescents. *Med Clin North Am* 1990; 74 (5): 1181–203.
5. Franz WB. Basic review: endocrinology of the normal menstrual cycle. *Prim Care* 1988; 15 (3): 607–16.
6. Field CS. Dysfunctional uterine bleeding. *Prim Care* 1988; 15 (3): 561–74.
7. Willis J. Demystifying menopause. *FDA Consumer* 1988; 22 (Jul–Aug): 24–9.
8. Shimp LA. Hormone replacement therapy. *J Mich Pharm Assoc* 1991; 29 (6): 218–21.
9. Avant RF. Dysmenorrhea. *Prim Care* 1988; 15 (3): 549–59.
10. Dawood MY. Dysmenorrhea. *Clin Obstet Gynecol* 1990; 33 (1): 168–78.
11. Johnson J. Level of knowledge among adolescent girls regarding effective treatment for dysmenorrhea. *J Adolesc Health Care* 1988; 9: 398–402.
12. Jensen DV, Andersen KB, Wagner G. Prostaglandins in the menstrual cycle of women. *Dan Med Bull* 1987; 34 (3): 178–81.
13. Sundell G, Milsom I, Andersch B. Factors influencing the prevalence and severity of dysmenorrhea in young women. *Br J Obstet and Gynaecol* 1990; 97: 588–94.
14. Barry JA. Dysmenorrhoea: periods can be a pain. *Aust Fam Physician* 1988 17 (3): 174–5
15. Doody KM, Carr BR. Amenorrhea. *Obstet Gynecol Clin North Am* 1990; 17 (2): 361–87.
16. Henley K, Vaitukaitis JL. Exercise-induced menstrual dysfunction. *Ann Rev Med* 1988; 39: 443–51.
17. Olson BR. Exercise induced amenorrhea. *Am Fam Physician* 1989; 39 (2): 213–21.
18. Long CA, Gast MJ. Menorrhagia. *Obstet Gynecol Clin North Am* 1990; 17 (2): 343–59.
19. Coupey SM, Ahlstrom P. Common menstrual disorders. *Ped Clin North Am* 1989; 36 (3): 551–71.
20. Johnson SR. The epidemiology and social impact of premenstrual symptoms. *Clin Obstet and Gynecol* 1987; 30 (2): 367–76.
21. Chihal HJ. Premenstrual syndrome: an update for the clinician. *Obstet Gynecol Clin North Am* 1990; 17 (2): 457–79.
22. Robinson GE. Premenstrual syndrome: current knowledge and management. *Can Med Assoc J* 1989; 140: 605–10.
23. Wickes SL. Premenstrual syndrome. *Prim Care* 1988; 15 (3): 473–87.
24. Robinson GE, Garfinkel PE. Problems in the treatment of premenstrual syndrome. *Can J Psychiatry* 1990; 35 (3): 199–206.
25. Lurie S, Borenstein R. The premenstrual syndrome. *Obstet Gynecolog Surv* 1990; 45 (4): 220–8.
26. Kendall KE, Schnurr PP. The effects of vitamin B_6 supplementation on premenstrual symptoms. *Obstet Gynecol* 1987; 70 (2): 145–9.
27. Gass ML, Rebar RW. Management of problems during menopause. *Compr Ther* 1990; 16 (2): 3–10.
28. Sarazin SK, Seymour SF. Causes and treatment options for women with dyspareunia. *Nurse Pract* 1991; 16 (10): 30–41.
29. Chantigian PDM. Vaginitis: a common malady. *Prim Care* 1988; 15 (3): 517–45.
30. Sandberg G, Quevillon RP. Dyspareunia: an integrated approach to assement and diagnosis. *J Fam Pract* 1987; 24 (1): 66–9.
31. *Federal Register* 1988; 53: 46194–202.
32. Leonard TK, Watson RR, Mohs ME. The effects of caffeine on various body systems: a review. *J Am Diet Assoc* 1987; 87: 1048–53.
33. *Federal Register* 1980; 45: 12713.
34. Reingold AL, Broome CV, Gaventa S, et al. Risk factors for menstrual toxic shock syndrome: results of a multistate case-control study. *Rev Infect Dis* 1989; 2 (suppl 1): S35–41.
35. Nightingale SL. New requirements for tampon labeling. *Am Fam Physician* 1990; 41 (3): 999–1000.
36. Reingold AL. Toxic shock syndrome: an update. *Am J Obstet Gynecol* 1991; 165: 1236–9.
37. Freedman JD, Beer DJ. Expanding perspectives on the toxic shock syndrome. *Adv Intern Med* 1991; 36: 363–97.
38. Chow A. Microbiology of toxic shock syndrome: overview. *Rev Infect Dis* 1989; 2 (suppl 1): S55–60.
39. Chesney PJ. Clinical aspects and spectrum of illness of toxic shock syndrome: overview. *Rev Infect Dis* 1989; 2 (suppl 1): S1–7.
40. Broome CV. Epidemiology of toxic shock syndrome in the United States: overview. *Rev Infect Dis* 1989; 2 (suppl 1): S4–21.
41. Onderdonk AB, Delaney ML, Zamarchi GR, et al. Normal vaginal microflora during use of various forms of catamenial protection. *Rev Infect Dis* 1989; 2 (suppl 1): S61–7.
42. Schwartz B, Gaventa S, Broome CV, et al. Nonmenstrual toxic shock syndrome associated with barrier contraceptives: report of a case control study. *Rev Infect Dis* 1989; 2 (suppl 1): S43–9.

CHAPTER 8

Cold, Cough, and Allergy Products

Bobby G. Bryant and Thomas P. Lombardi

> **Questions to ask in patient assessment and counseling**
>
> - *What symptoms do you have? Do you have a runny or stuffy nose, sore throat, cough (productive or nonproductive), fever, muscle aches, joint pain, or earache? Do you have red eyes, itchy eyes, an itchy nose, sneezing, or postnasal drip? Do you have chest congestion? Do you have chills, fever, or a feverish feeling?*
> - *How long have you had these symptoms?*
> - *Do you or members of your family have a history of allergies, asthma, or atopic dermatitis (chronic skin problems)?*
> - *Do you have any respiratory disease (breathing problems) such as asthma, bronchitis, or emphysema?*
> - *Do you have diabetes, glaucoma, heart disease, thyroid problems, or high blood pressure? Are you under a physician's care for any of these conditions? Are they controlled? If so, how?*
> - *What prescription and nonprescription medications are you taking? How long have you been taking them?*
> - *Which products have you used for your cold and allergy symptoms? Have they been effective? Have they caused any adverse effects?*
> - *Does your job require mental alertness, coordination, or physical dexterity?*

Although the common cold and allergic rhinitis present with similar symptoms they are etiologically different and require different management. This chapter provides the pharmacist with information necessary to identify and distinguish between the common cold and allergic rhinitis, as well as other disorders that may mimic them, and to advise the patient on the proper use of cold and allergy products.

Types of Disorders

The common cold is a symptom complex affecting the upper respiratory tract (Figure 1). It is also called a cold, acute rhinitis, infectious rhinitis, coryza, or catarrh. The symptoms, which are usually acute and self-limiting, may be caused by one of many viruses. The main anatomical sites of infection may vary; therefore, a cold may present symptoms, individually or in combination, of the nose (rhinitis), throat (pharyngitis), larynx (laryngitis), or bronchi (bronchitis). The intensity of symptoms may vary from hour to hour. A reasonable approach is to treat the patient symptomatically and as specifically as possible with single-entity agents.[1]

Allergic rhinitis is the antibody-mediated reaction of the nasal mucosa to one or more inhaled antigens. It may be perennial because of the year-round presence of antigenic substances, or it may be seasonal and correspond with the periodic appearance of offending antigens. The most common type of allergic rhinitis, hay fever (pollenosis), is seasonal.

Upper Respiratory Tract

The nose is a respiratory organ. As a passageway for airflow into and out of the lungs, it humidifies and warms inspired air and filters inhaled particles. Several anatomical features aid the performance of these functions. The nasal cavity is divided by a central septum and finger-like projections (turbinates) that extend into the cavity, increasing the nasal surface area (Figure 2).

The surface of the nasal passageway is coated with a thin layer of mucus, a moderately viscous mucoproteinaceous liquid that is secreted continuously by the mucous glands. Foreign bodies such as dust, pollen, bacteria, powder, and other airborne pollutants are trapped in the film and carried out of the nose posteriorly into the nasopharynx, where they may be expectorated or swallowed. The turbinates facilitate this action by causing many eddies in the flowing air, forcing particulates to rebound in different directions. This rapid change in the direction of airflow causes air-suspended particles to land on nasal mucosal surfaces. High vascularity and resultant high-blood flow within the nasal mucosa help warm and humidify the inspired air, thus decreasing trauma to the respiratory passages and helping to prevent opportunistic infections in the lungs.

The nasopharyngeal vascular bed is controlled by both sympathetic and parasympathetic divisions of the autonomic nervous system. Stimulation of the sympathetic fibers causes decreased activity of the mucous glands and vasoconstriction that widens the nasal passageway. Parasympathetic (cholinergic) stimulation increases mucus production and narrows the airways by vasodilation and vascular engorgement of the mucosal tissue. Treatment may be directed toward eliciting a sympathetic response, blocking a parasympathetic response, or both.

The epithelium of the nasal passageways is ciliated. The constant beating of the cilia continually moves the mucus film, together with trapped particles to be expectorated

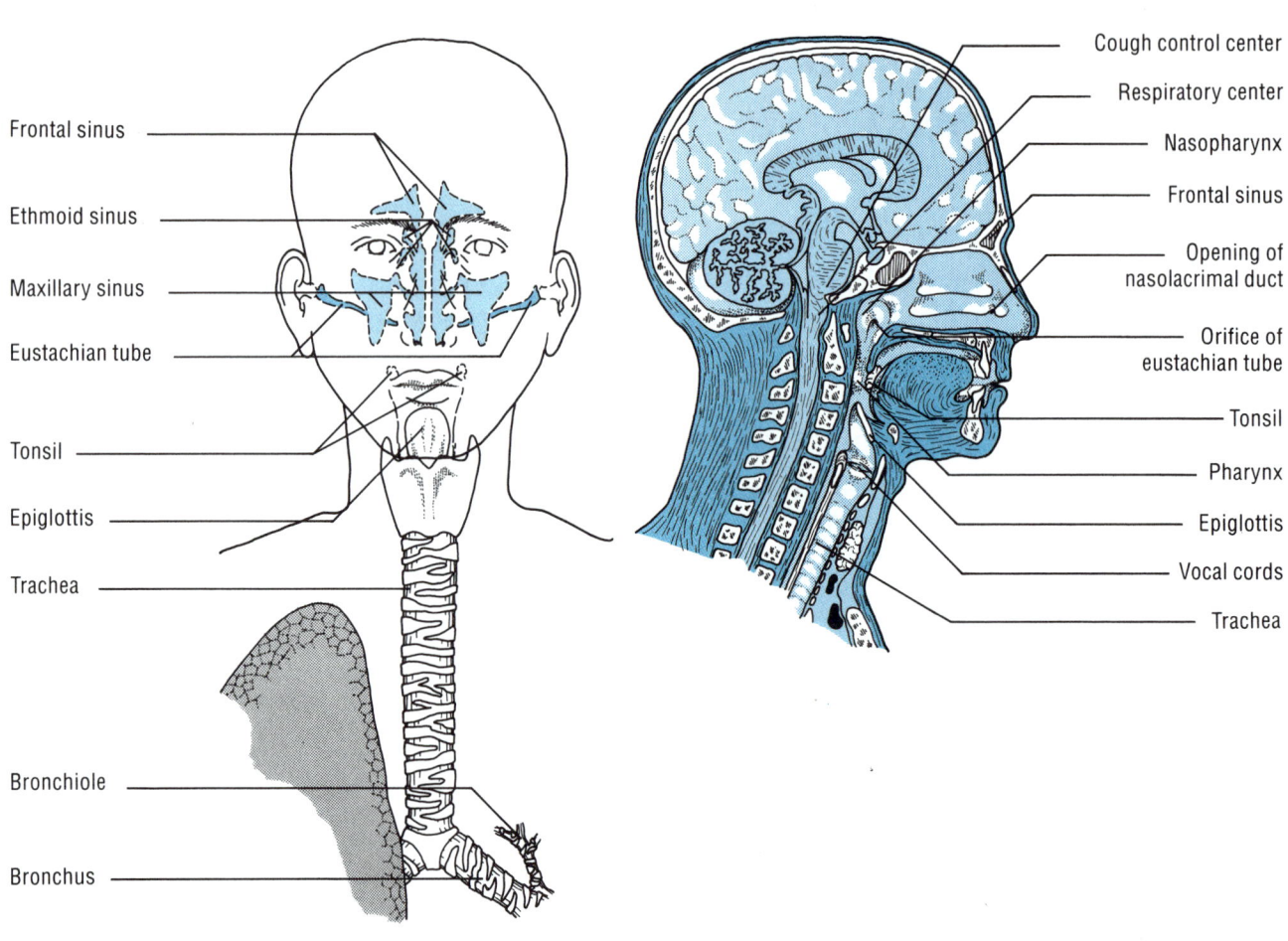

FIGURE 1 Anatomy of the respiratory passages.

or swallowed, toward the nasopharynx. Because this ciliary movement is a major defense mechanism, agents that impair it should be avoided. Such agents include oils, especially mineral oil, in addition to dust, fumes, and smoke. A lack of humidity or the overuse of topically applied decongestants may also interfere with normal ciliary movement.

The mucus is rich in lysozymes and contains glycoproteins and immunoglobulins.[2] Lysozymes are an important defense against bacteria because they readily attack and destroy lipids and carbohydrates of the cell walls of some bacteria and pollens, as well as antigenic substances that are subsequently released. Mucus glycoproteins may temporarily inhibit some viruses by combining with the virus protein coat. The union of inhibitor and virus is reversible; therefore, mucus glycoproteins probably do no more than delay host cell invasion by the virus particles. Immunoglobulins, mainly IgA and IgG, also are contained in the mucus secretion. Although present in low concentrations, they may decrease the infectivity of certain viruses.

Viruses that attach to and invade respiratory tract host cells stimulate the infected cell to produce interferon. Interferon protects neighboring, noninfected cells by inducing them to produce an antiviral protein that inhibits viral replication, thus preventing subsequent viral infection. Interferon is active not only against the virus that caused its production but also against other unrelated viruses.[3] Although endogenous interferon appears to play a positive role in attenuating symptoms of the cold, administration of recombinant interferon nasal drops or spray does not appear to be markedly effective.[4]

The cough reflex is an essential body defense mechanism by which the respiratory airways leading to the lungs are kept free of foreign debris. All areas of the respiratory tract (e.g., trachea, larynx, bronchi, and terminal bronchioles) are sensitive to foreign matter and other causes of irritation such as irritant gases and infection. A cough may be produced by stimulation of the receptors (mechanoreceptors and chemoreceptors) located in the mucosa of the airways and lungs. Afferent impulses pass along nerve pathways to the cough center in the medulla, which coordinates efferent impulses to the diaphragm and intercostal and abdominal muscles. An automatic sequence of events leads to the cough response—the rapid expulsion of air from the lungs—which helps remove the foreign bodies that initiated the reflex. Localized bronchoconstriction may

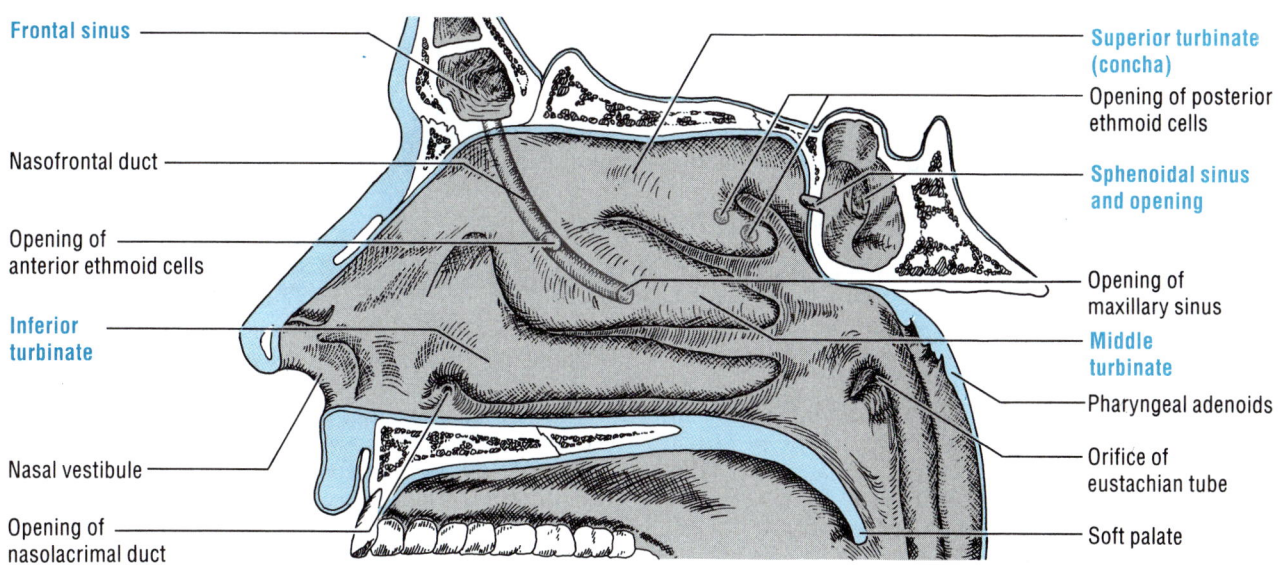

FIGURE 2 The nose and paranasal sinus. Reprinted with permission from *Medical Notes on the Common Cold*. Pub. No. PI99–2. Research Triangle Park, NC: Burroughs Wellcome Co; 1972.

also play an important role in stimulating the cough reflex.

The sneeze reflex is similar to the cough reflex, except that it clears the nasal passages instead of the lower respiratory tract. Irritation in the nasal passages initiates the sneeze reflex. The afferent impulses from the nose travel to the medulla, where the reflex is triggered. A series of reactions similar to those for the cough reflex occur. In addition, the uvula is depressed so that large amounts of air pass rapidly through the nose as well as through the mouth, helping to clear the nasal passages of foreign matter.

The passageways of the trachea and lungs are lined with a ciliated, mucus-coated epithelium that aids in removing foreign matter. As in the nasal passageways, the cilia in the trachea and lungs sweep toward the pharynx, carrying mucus and trapped particles out of the respiratory tract to be expectorated or swallowed.

The Common Cold

The common cold has been described as the single most expensive illness in the United States. In fact, the common cold causes more time lost from work and school than all other diseases combined. It accounts for more than 160 million days of restricted activity, more than 26 million days of school absence, and approximately 23 million days of work absence each year, according to the National Health Interview Survey of 1985.[5,6]

The common cold leads to approximately 27 million physician visits per year. Surveys report that drugs were prescribed or recommended in 94% of visits for upper respiratory tract infections. An average of two drugs are prescribed per patient.[7]

Most colds do not require or result in medical attention but can instead be self-treated. With approximately 50% of cough and cold preparations purchased in pharmacies, pharmacists should interact with and assist the self-treating patient in selecting and using such products properly.

The common cold can be spread directly from person to person with no intermediate vector such as food, water, or animals. The only way to prevent its spread is by isolating the infected individual. However, by the time a cold has been detected, the virus undoubtedly has been transmitted to others through respiratory droplets or hand-to-hand contact.[3]

There is an apparent relationship between the season of the year and the common cold. The exact etiologic relationship is not known, but there are typically three peak seasons of common colds per year: one occurs in the autumn, a few weeks after schools open; another in midwinter; and a third in the spring. These separate epidemics are generally associated with different viruses, each of which may have its own seasonal epidemiology. The U.S. Public Health Service studies show that, during the winter quarter, approximately 50% of the population experience a common cold; during the summer quarter, only about 20% are so stricken.

The patient's age is related to both the incidence of the common cold and its complications. Children 1–5 years of age are most susceptible, averaging 6–12 respiratory illnesses per year, most of which are common colds. Some practitioners believe that infants under 6 months of age are somewhat resistant to the various cold viruses, but this finding may be attributed to the infants' relatively infrequent exposure to different environments. Individuals 25–30 years of age average about six respiratory illnesses per year; older adults average two or three. Women, primarily those 20–30 years of age, appear to be afflicted by colds more often than men of the same age or older patients. This could be attributed to exposure to children with colds.[5] Young children are more prone to complications of the common cold, such as otitis media (middle ear inflammation and infection) and pneumonia. Adults also suffer from these complications but with a much lower frequency.[2]

Poor nutritional state, fatigue, emotional disturbances, and compromised host defenses are associated with greater susceptibility as well as with increased severity of infection and greater likelihood of complications.[8] Body chills or wet feet do not induce the common cold.

Allergic disorders involving the nasopharynx, such as hay fever, may facilitate viral infection. The probable mechanism is the inflammatory changes that occur in the mucosa as a result of the antigen–antibody reaction, which may pave the way for subsequent viral invasion.

Etiology

Viruses cause the common cold. More than 120 different viral strains that produce common cold symptoms in humans have been isolated. Known causative organisms include rhinoviruses (of which there are approximately 60 serologic types), coronaviruses, adenoviruses, coxsackieviruses, influenza viruses, parainfluenza viruses, and respiratory syncytial viruses. Of these, the rhinoviruses comprise the largest etiologic group, probably accounting for more than half of all common colds in adults. A significant percentage, 5–10%, of common colds is associated with more than one virus, and evidence of simultaneous infection with two viruses is common.[2]

Viruses differ from bacteria by their existence within the host cell, their chemical composition, their mode of replication, and their relative lack of responsiveness to traditional anti-infective drug therapy.[2] The process of a viral infection is divided into three states: entry into the host cell and nucleic acid release, genome replication and viral protein synthesis, and assembly of new virus particles and their release from the cell to infect additional host cells. There are probably several mechanisms by which the virus penetrates a host cell, but none are well defined. Once inside the host cell, the virus is attacked by host cell enzymes and possibly other substances, releasing the viral nucleic acid. In the second state of infection, the virus uses the metabolic pathways of the host cell itself to duplicate the viral genome and synthesize viral proteins. Finally, these components are assembled into new, mature virus particles and are released by the host cell. The release may be rapid and may be accompanied by lysis and death of the host cell although cell death may not always result. The new virus particles then infect other cells by the same cycle.

When host cell injury or death occurs, the body's inflammatory defense mechanism is activated, causing pathologic changes and subsequent symptoms. These clinical manifestations of infection are not evident, however, until after extensive viral replication and inflammation have occurred.

Specific immunity against illness from reinfection with the same strain of virus was demonstrated in volunteers; this clinical immunity is apparent for about 2 years after infection. Reinfection, however, is not entirely prevented and usually results in a modified illness. The specificity of the antibody and its concentration at the infection site appear to be critical in the likelihood and extent of reinfection.[2] These characteristics also underscore the difficulty in developing comprehensive vaccines to prevent the common cold.

Pathophysiology and Symptoms

Symptoms associated with the common cold are a manifestation of the pathologic changes (inflammation) that occur in the respiratory epithelium secondary to viral invasion. The inflammatory responses to one or more viruses are hyperemia (excess blood flow in the area), edema (abnormal fluid accumulation in the intercellular spaces), and rhinorrhea (profuse watery discharge from the nasal mucous membrane).

The severity of cellular damage (i.e., the degree of inflammation and symptoms) is related to the type of infecting virus and extent of the infection. Various strains of influenza virus may cause more damage to the respiratory epithelium than other viruses that cause the common cold. Therefore, flu symptoms are usually more severe than cold symptoms, and the predisposition to secondary bacterial complications is greater with influenza.

Although colds commonly involve the nasal structure, other sites along the respiratory tract may be affected. This is because of both the predilection of certain viruses for pharyngeal, laryngeal, or bronchial cells and the extension of the infectious process from the original invasion site.[3]

Because the incubation period for viral infections is relatively short (1–4 days), patients often report a rapid onset and progression of symptoms. Viral shedding usually begins 1 to 2 days before the onset of symptoms and is associated with epithelial sloughing and regeneration. A few days later, during the symptomatic phase, peak viral replication and host cell injury occur. With the intervention of host defenses, such as the production and release of interferon, symptoms decrease after several days.[2]

The clear, watery fluid that initially flows from the irritated nasal epithelium is the cardinal symptom of the common cold. Although it is initially clear, this fluid is followed by a more viscous, tenacious secretion that is composed largely of dead epithelial cells and white blood cells. The quantity of shed epithelial cells may be so high at times as to make the secretion appear purulent. It is commonly assumed that these mucopurulent secretions are the result of secondary bacterial infection; however, this is not always the case. Viruses cause inflammatory reactions, and secretions occur even when there has been no change in the nasal bacterial flora.

Nasal congestion (engorgement of the nasal vasculature and swelling of the nasal turbinates) encroaches on the nasal lumen, which is also burdened with increased secretions. Nasal discharge and congestion are the most commonly described discomforts associated with the common cold.

The combination of nasal irritation, discharge, and congestion gives rise to sneezing. Sneezing is not as discomforting as the discharge and congestion, and it subsides when the infection and secretions clear.

Pharyngitis may also occur during a cold.[2] This throat symptom is usually described as a dryness or soreness rather than as actual pain, such as that associated with bacterial pharyngitis or acute tonsillitis. Nonbacterial pharyngitis is attributed to edema of the pharyngeal mucosa, which activates sensory nerve fibers as the viral infection spreads to deeper tissue.

Diseases in which pharyngitis may be a symptom include not only the common cold but also streptococcal infection of the throat (strep throat), scarlet fever, tonsillitis, influenza (the flu), and measles. Environmental factors, such as overuse of tobacco, ingestion of alcohol, or exposure to other irritating substances, may produce or worsen preexisting pharyngitis. It is important that the etiology be determined so that appropriate treatment measures may be taken. An acute sore throat of nonbacterial origin usually has a much slower onset than bacterial pharyngitis. Nonbacterial pharyngitis is characterized by milder constitutional symptoms; normal or slightly elevated temperature; and a dry, raspy, or tickling sensation in the throat.

This irritation of the pharynx may also cause a cough. The cough may also be due to irritation of tracheal or bronchial mucous membranes caused by the direct extension of the inflammation or by infectious material dripping from the nasopharynx (postnasal drip). At its onset, the cough is usually dry and nonproductive. At later stages of the common cold, however, heavy bronchial congestion may result as the cellular debris of local phagocytic activity adds to the respiratory tract fluids in the bronchial and nasal passage secretions and drains into the lower respiratory tract. Because normal physiologic ciliary activity of respiratory passages may not be sufficient to remove these fluids, coughing is necessary to clear the lower respiratory tract of accumulated secretions.

Another possible manifestation of the common cold is laryngitis, which is associated with hoarseness or loss of voice. It may be caused by the spread of infection to the larynx or by irritation secondary to drainage from the nasopharynx.

A hot or warm sensation (feverishness) is another fairly common complaint. In general, however, little or no fever is actually present. Finally, headache, which usually occurs in the early stages of the cold, may be caused by the infection and inflammation of the nasal passages and paranasal sinuses.

Complications

In an otherwise healthy individual, the common cold is self-limiting; the course of symptoms is 5–7 days. It is not uncommon, however, for complications to develop during or immediately following a common cold. The pharmacist should be familiar with possible complications, their causes, and their treatment. Viral infection induces swelling and some exudation, but it causes no significant change in the bacterial flora of the nasopharynx. If the inflammatory changes are of sufficient magnitude, passages connecting the paranasal sinuses and middle ear become obstructed; under these conditions, infection may occur from secondary bacterial growth. In addition, it has been reported that viral infections trigger a substantial proportion of wheezing attacks in young asthmatic children, chronic bronchitics, and patients with emphysema.[9,10]

The most common bacterial complications of colds are purulent sinusitis, otitis media, bacterial pneumonia, and tonsillitis.[9,11] Young children are especially prone to pneumonia and otitis media. Approximately 5% of children develop otitis media following a cold.[11] This occurs largely because a child's eustachian tubes are short, relatively horizontal, and rather narrow. This configuration facilitates fluid accumulation in the middle ear as well as rapid narrowing of the eustachian tube in response to only a slight degree of inflammation. A young child's bronchial passages are also smaller in diameter than those of older children and adults. Narrower passages and a child's lack of conscious effort to cough up accumulated fluids and cellular debris in the lower respiratory tract may lead to stasis of the fluid and accumulated debris, inflammation, and secondary bacterial infection.

These complications usually manifest themselves by a worsening of local symptoms (e.g., earache, headache, and cough), the development of a fever, and the failure of the cold to improve over a 5- to 7-day period. Such manifestations in a person with a recent cold are probably caused by secondary bacterial invaders, for which culture and sensitivity tests and appropriately prescribed antibiotic therapy are indicated.

Conditions Mimicking the Common Cold

Other infectious diseases present initial symptoms similar to those of the common cold.[12] The pharmacist should be aware of these disorders so that minor self-limited conditions can be differentiated from potentially serious ones for which a physician should be consulted. Using strictly palliative therapy to provide symptomatic relief in situations that may not be self-limiting has little or no effect on the underlying problem and may delay necessary and more appropriate treatment.

A patient's sore throat, for example, alone or in conjunction with other symptoms, may be caused by bacteria, a virus, or another irritative process.[13] Care should be taken to note additional symptoms that may help differentiate bacterial from viral infection (Table 1). A sore throat that may be bacterial in origin (i.e., bacterial pharyngitis) should be evaluated by a physician as soon as possible. In a child, a sore throat may be a bacterial pharyngitis caused by Group A beta-hemolytic species of *Streptococcus*, or strep throat. In such a case, symptomatic therapy should be used to provide relief until a physician can be seen. If only symptomatic therapy is recommended, rheumatic fever or glomerulonephritis may develop. Appropriate antibiotic therapy may help prevent these dangerous sequelae. Sore throat in adults may be due to various causes, some of which may be amenable to self-treatment. Again, if bacterial pharyngitis is suspected, the patient should be referred to a physician immediately for appropriate evaluation and follow-up.

The influenza A viral respiratory tract infection that may mimic a cold is called influenza, or the flu (Table 2). Flu is usually distinguishable from the common cold by its epidemic or pandemic occurrence, especially during the winter months, and by its symptoms of fever, dry cough, generalized joint and muscle ache, and more significant

TABLE 1	Distinguishing bacterial from nonbacterial sore throats	
	Bacterial sore throat	**Nonbacterial sore throat**
Onset	Rapid	Slower
Soreness	Marked	Seldom marked
Constitutional symptoms	Marked	Mild
Upper and lower respiratory symptoms	Present in 50% of cases	Usual
Lymph nodes	Large, tender	Slight enlargement, not tender

Adapted from Bulteau V. *Med J Aust* 1966; 2: 1053.

malaise. Complications, especially secondary bacterial infections, are more likely to develop, especially in elderly and debilitated patients, who should be referred to a physician when influenza is suspected. Influenza vaccines are readily available and generally recommended for annual prophylaxis in high-risk patient populations. Amantadine hydrochloride, a prescription medication, may be useful for the prophylaxis and treatment of influenza A viral disease.

Measles

Measles (rubeola), also known as red measles, is a highly contagious disease caused by a virus. Although the incidence of measles has been drastically reduced by active immunization practices, it appears to be increasing and occurs in localized outbreaks. One possible explanation for the increase in measles cases may be the failure of a primary vaccine. A recent study has shown that infants demonstrating cold symptoms at the time of their initial measles vaccination have a lower rate of seroconversion.[13]

When measles does occur, it is associated with a prodrome that includes fever, rhinitis, dry cough, and conjunctivitis. Initially, it is difficult to distinguish measles from the common cold. However, in about 3 days, a red rash develops over the face, trunk, and extremities. Koplik's spots, which are characteristic of measles, usually appear 1 to 2 days before the rash. They are white or gray marks often described as "table salt crystals," and they appear most often on the mucous membranes of the oral cavity and throat. The patient should be isolated, and although treatment is symptomatic, a physician should be notified because secondary bacterial infection and postmeasles encephalitis or subacute sclerosing panencephalitis may develop. These complications rarely occur in the United States. Infection with rubeola provides long-lasting immunity to the disease.[14]

Pharmacists should be aware of both local public health regulations that require the reporting of measles and local or state vaccination requirements.

German Measles

Another viral disease in which arthralgia, fever, malaise, lymphadenopathy, and rhinitis coincide with the eruption of a fine red rash is German measles (rubella). It is recommended that this disorder be brought to a physician's attention because of possible complications. An important concern is the devastating effect rubella infection may have on a developing fetus. Maternal infection has been associated with miscarriage, spontaneous abortion, and numerous

TABLE 2	Symptoms that differentiate influenza from the common cold	
Symptom	**Common cold**	**Influenza**
Fever	Rare	Sudden onset; lasts 3–4 days; temperature above 102–104°F
Headache	Rare	Prominent
General muscle and joint aches and pains	Slight	Prominent
Fatigue, weakness, and exhaustion	Mild	Extreme; early; may last up to 2–3 weeks
Runny, stuffy nose	Common	Uncommon
Sneezing	Common	Uncommon
Sore throat	Common	Uncommon
Cough	Mild to moderate; hacking; usually nonproductive	Common; may become severe
Complications	Sinus congestion; earache	Bronchitis; pneumonia

Adapted from *U.S. Pharm* 1987; 12 (8): 77.

fetal abnormalities. If a pregnant woman is exposed to a case of rubella (proven or suspected), she must be referred to a physician to determine her degree of immunity to the virus via a rubella titer. Vaccination against rubella has significantly decreased the incidence in the United States. Immunization is encouraged for all children by the age of 18 months.[14]

Chronic Fatigue Syndrome

Chronic fatigue syndrome is an ill-defined, debilitating disease of varying severity, with fatigue as the primary symptom. The disease is often reported to occur with a sudden onset following an initial flulike illness. Other common features are low-grade fever, myalgias, sleep disorder, impaired cognition, depression, headaches, and pharyngitis. The symptoms are present virtually all the time and may be severe enough to impair normal functioning or produce occupational disability. Patients who are experiencing prolonged debilitating fatigue with other symptoms listed above should be referred to their physician.[15]

Allergy

A history of allergy and a review of symptoms help differentiate seasonal or perennial allergic rhinitis from the common cold. Hay fever may be suspected in young children who suffer from repeated coldlike symptoms in a seasonal pattern. Persistent symptoms of a cold are often the first clue to allergic rhinitis. Because a cold usually lasts only several days, a patient who has a stuffy nose for weeks to months may have allergic rhinitis or some other form of noninfectious rhinitis.

Treatment of the Common Cold

Self-treatment of the common cold is intended to relieve symptoms. There are no curative remedies; there are only drugs that bring temporary relief while the cold runs its course and normal body defenses attempt to remove the viral invaders and repair the damage. In general, additional bed rest and prevention of chilling add to the patient's comfort. Adequate fluid intake is necessary to prevent dehydration and enhance expectoration. Humidification of room air may contribute to a loosening of respiratory secretions. A well-balanced diet should be maintained.

Single-agent therapy offers the ability to design a specific regimen directed at each symptom; however, many products contain multiple medications. These combination products may be effective and provide a convenient dosage form when the patient has multiple symptoms. However, combination products are usually more expensive, are limited by fixed doses in the preparation, and may have additive adverse effects.[16]

Nasal Congestion and Discharge

Treatment of nasal congestion not only relieves the discomfort but also prevents excessive nose blowing, which may further irritate mucous membranes and the nostrils. Excessive nose blowing also may force infected fluids into nasal sinuses and the eustachian tubes, extending the infection and the discomfort. Decongestants (sympathomimetic amines) applied as drops or spray to the nasal mucosa or administered systemically are effective vasoconstrictors that help decrease edema and swelling of the nasal mucosa, thereby enlarging the nasal airways.

Cough

The first step in attempting to control a cough is to provide the respiratory tract with adequate fluids. This is done by increasing oral fluid intake, humidifying the inspired air, or both. If the cough is productive and its frequency is tolerable, ensuring adequate fluid intake may be all that is needed. If the cough is dry, nonproductive, hyperactive, annoying, and related to asthma, a cough suppressant (antitussive) may be indicated, especially if the cough interferes with sleep. Expectorants have been used if the cough is productive or if respiratory congestion is marked; however, their use is somewhat controversial.[17] Any increase in cough by persons with a chronic obstructive lung disease (e.g., asthma, chronic bronchitis, or emphysema) should be referred to a physician. (See Chapter 9, "Asthma Products.") The tickling sensation in the pharynx that may cause a cough may be treated initially with a demulcent such as hard candy or cough drops, but if the cough becomes more intense, a cough suppressant may be recommended.

Dry or Sore Throat

A sore throat in a child is difficult to evaluate and should not be self-treated. Accordingly, the child should be seen by a physician.

Lozenges and gargles containing antiseptics and topical anesthetics are heavily promoted for treating sore throat. Aside from a demulcent effect, however, the use of such products is irrational in treating sore throats caused by a viral infection because the antibacterial ingredients are not effective against viruses.

If the throat is dry or raspy, hard candy may be used to stimulate saliva flow, which acts as a soothing demulcent. An often overlooked measure in soothing an inflamed throat is the regular use of a warm, saline gargle (1–3 tsp of salt per 8–12 oz of warm water). If these measures do not provide adequate relief, lozenges or sprays containing a local anesthetic (e.g., benzocaine) may be used every 3 to 4 hours for temporary symptomatic relief. Systemic analgesics such as acetaminophen, aspirin, or ibuprofen have also been promoted to provide symptomatic relief of sore throat as well as to relieve other discomforting symptoms associated with a cold.

Laryngitis

Acute laryngitis presents a therapeutic problem: the only direct way to reach the inflamed laryngeal tissue is via inspired air. Lozenges and gargles do nothing to relieve hoarseness; their ingredients or the saliva they stimulate does not reach this area. Water vapor inhalation (e.g., cool mist) several times a day may be beneficial in acute laryngitis. The value of adding any medications to steam has not been established. Active or passive inhalation of irritants such as cigarette smoke should be avoided. The voice should be rested as much as possible.

Feverishness and Headache

Vague complaints of feverishness and headache, although not necessarily occurring together, may be treated with the same remedies. Proper analgesic dosages of aspirin, acetaminophen, or ibuprofen are usually effective in relieving discomforting symptoms because of their analgesic/antipyretic properties. Fever (oral temperature higher than 98.9–99.6°F [37.2–37.6°C] or rectal temperature higher than 99.9–100.6°F [37.7–38.1°C]) is seldom associated with the common cold. When a fever persists for more than 24 hours, a physician should be consulted. In the interim, an analgesic/antipyretic will provide temporary relief of fever symptoms. (See Chapter 6, "Antipyretic Drug Products.")

Evidence suggests a relationship between aspirin use for fever associated with viral infection such as influenza and chickenpox, and the increased incidence of Reye's syndrome. Therefore, aspirin should be used with extreme caution in children and adolescents with fever associated with known or suspected viral infection. (See Chapter 6, "Antipyretic Drug Products" for further discussion of Reye's syndrome.)

Physician-directed treatment is usually unnecessary unless there is concern that the patient has a disease other than a cold, the symptoms are severe, or secondary complications are present or suspected. Severely debilitated patients, however, should consult their physician, as should patients with other chronic disorders (e.g., emphysema, chronic bronchitis, asthma, diabetes, or cystic fibrosis) for whom respiratory infection may pose serious problems or the usual nonprescription remedies are contraindicated.

Allergic Rhinitis

Etiology

Allergic rhinitis may occur at almost any age; however, the incidence of first onset is greatest in children and young adults and decreases with advancing age. Heredity seems to play a role. Although, allergic rhinitis itself is not genetically transmitted, the heightened predisposition to become sensitized after exposure to adequate concentrations of an allergen is genetically transferred.[18] Studies suggest that the condition is transferred as an autosomal dominant characteristic with variable expression.[19]

Pollens and mold spores are the main agents responsible for seasonal allergic rhinitis. Ragweed pollen accounts for about 75% of seasonal allergic rhinitis in the United States; grass pollens, 40%; and tree pollens, about 9%. Approximately 25% of individuals with this condition suffer from both grass and ragweed allergic rhinitis, and about 5% suffer from all three allergies.[20]

The seasonal appearance of symptoms reflects the presence of pollen or spores in the air and is influenced by the geographic location and specific hypersensitivities. Of the airborne mold spores, species of *Alternaria* and *Hormodendrum* are the most common.[21] These spores are most prevalent from mid-March to late November. Tree pollination begins in late March and extends to early June. Grasses generally pollinate from mid-May to mid-July. Ragweed pollen has a long season, extending from early August to early October or to the first killing frost. The pollinating season for a particular plant in a given locale is relatively constant from year to year. Weather conditions such as temperature and rainfall influence the amount of pollen produced but not the actual onset or termination of a specific season.

Perennial allergic rhinitis is usually caused by environmental proteins, such as house dust mite, animal dander, and feathers. Occupational causes include exposure to certain proteins of wheat flour, various grains, cotton and flax seeds, enzymes used in detergents, paint fumes, topical sprays, and industrial solvents. Foods and medications may also contain allergens such as sulfites. Nonspecific irritants such as tobacco smoke, chalk dust, road dust, and heavily polluted air may also contribute to symptoms in an allergic patient. The continued presence of the allergens results in symptoms that persist more or less year-round. Some patients may exhibit perennial allergic rhinitis symptoms with seasonal exacerbations.

Vasomotor rhinitis is a nonallergic, noninfectious rhinitis characterized by watery, profuse nasal discharge and nasal congestion. Often the symptoms are provoked by changes in environmental temperature or posture and by exposure to volatile irritants. This form of rhinitis can be differentiated by the lack of eosinophils in the nasal secretions; no evidence of sensitization to specific antigens can be demonstrated.

Pathophysiology

Symptoms of allergic rhinitis may be due to many different allergens. These allergens, which are primarily protein in nature, may, when deposited on the nasal mucosa, initiate an inflammatory response by the body and produce symptoms characteristic of allergic rhinitis.

The pathologic inflammatory process of seasonal allergic rhinitis develops within minutes after an allergen is deposited on the nasal mucous membrane of an allergy-prone individual. Pollen itself is not believed to be directly antigenic. However, the body reacts to the pollen, as it does to any foreign substance, and the lysozyme component of nasal mucus degrades the pollen cell wall to allow for the release of the proteinaceous contents. This released protein may be an antigen. The antigen stimulates plasma cells in the respiratory tract to produce a specific type of immunoglobulin, IgE (reagin). These reaginic antibodies have a special affinity for circulating basophils and tissue mast cells. The cells pick up many IgE molecules on their surfaces and thus become sensitized. Subsequent exposure to the same antigen, by its deposition on nasal mucosa, causes an antigen–antibody reaction, which in turn causes the sensitized mast cells to release vasoactive chemical mediators. These mediators of inflammation include histamine, eosinophilic and neutrophilic chemotactic factors, and mast cell proteases. Prostaglandin D_2, leukotrienes, and platelet-activating factor are also released.[22]

The nasal mucosa is particularly vulnerable to this immediate type of allergic reaction because the allergen is deposited directly where it may act locally and because the mediators are very active vasodilators that are released in a highly vascularized area. The immediate effects are vasodilation, increased vascular permeability, and increased mucus secretion, all of which are responsible for the symptoms.

The clinical picture seen with seasonal allergic rhinitis has been divided into early and late phases. The early phase, described above, is due to the immediate effect of the antigen–antibody reaction. The late phase is characterized by engorgement of the nasal passageways, congestion,

TABLE 3 Characteristics of the various types of rhinitis

Rhinitis	Allergic		Infectious	Nonallergic (vasomotor)
	Seasonal	Perennial		
Etiology	IgE-mediated immunologic reaction	IgE-mediated immunologic reaction	Respiratory infection	Autonomic nervous system disorder
Seasonal pattern	Yes	Present year-round	Often worse in winter	Worse in changing seasons
Recurrences	Mild symptoms between attacks	Mild symptoms between attacks	Clears completely	Frequently continuous
Family history of allergy	Common	Common	Occasional	Occasional
Systemic symptoms	Rare	Rare	Common	Rare
Other allergic symptoms (asthma, eczema)	Common	Common	Occasional	Occasional
Pruritus	Yes	Yes	No	Mild or absent
Fever	No	No	Occasional	No
Conjunctivitis	Yes	Yes	No	No
Discharge	Water-like	Water-like	Mucopurulent	Water-like
Paroxysmal sneezing	Yes	Yes	No	Yes

and less watery rhinorrhea, reflecting the accumulation of products from cellular inflammation. To the self-treating person, this distinction may be lost during the appearance of disturbing symptoms. In addition, the late phase is often more effectively treated with topical intranasal corticosteriods, which are not available as nonprescription drugs. However, prevention of the early phase of the disorder, often with nonprescription drugs, will prevent the later phase.

The longer the symptoms persist, from whatever cause, the more likely the patient is to develop chronic and irreversible changes such as thickening of the mucosal epithelium, proliferation of connective tissue, loss of epithelial cilia, and development of polyps of the nose or sinuses.

Symptoms

Major symptoms of allergic rhinitis are mucosal edema and those resulting from the engorgement of the nasal mucosa, such as sneezing, rhinorrhea, nasal pruritus, and nasal congestion (Table 3). Sudden sneezing attacks may consist of 10–20 sneezes in rapid succession. Rhinorrhea is typically a clear, watery discharge that may be profuse and continuous. Purulent discharge does not usually occur in uncomplicated allergic rhinitis; its presence may indicate a secondary infection. The nasal congestion of allergic rhinitis is due to swollen turbinates. If the nasal obstruction is severe, it may cause headaches or earaches. With continuous, severe nasal congestion, loss of smell and taste may occur. Itching of the nose, particularly in children, may cause frequent nose rubbing.

Conjunctival symptoms commonly associated with allergic rhinitis include itching and lacrimation. These symptoms are caused by pollen grains becoming trapped in the conjunctival sac and the subsequent antigen–antibody reaction, as well as by possible lacrimal duct congestion caused indirectly by the nasal congestion. Patients may complain of photophobia and sore, tired eyes. Dark circles or greater than normal discolorations beneath the eyes are called allergic shiners. These discolorations are more common in perennial rhinitis than in the seasonal variant.

A characteristic of seasonal allergic rhinitis is the periodicity of its appearance. A careful patient history indicates when the symptoms began and at what intervals they are exacerbated. With seasonal rhinitis, the allergic reaction often begins with sneezing and progresses to rhinorrhea, and then possibly to severe nasal obstruction, at which time sneezing may be absent and rhinorrhea minimal. Perennial rhinitis is more likely to begin with nasal obstruction and postnasal discharge than with sneezing and rhinorrhea.

The symptoms of allergic rhinitis may exhibit periodicity, even within the season. Most patients tend to exhibit more intense symptoms in the morning and on windy days because of increased pollen in the air. Symptoms may diminish when it rains and the pollen is cleared from the air.

It is more difficult to associate perennial rhinitis than seasonal rhinitis with the environment; the patient history may be helpful in these cases. The most common perennial allergens are house dust mite and household pet dander. Many patients with perennial allergic rhinitis have continuous symptoms because of the presence of such irritants in their environment. However, other patients who have overlapping allergies can be symptomatic each season for different reasons. The patient with allergies to mold, grass, ragweed, and house dust may be symptomatic year-round.

Allergic rhinitis tends to show increasingly severe symptoms for 2 or 3 years until a somewhat stable condition is reached. With the seasonal variant, symptoms tend to be exacerbated annually. There is no effective means of predicting whether symptoms will increase or decrease in severity. In fact, for reasons not well understood, hypersensitivity may disappear after several years.

The pharmacist may differentiate seasonal allergic rhinitis from perennial allergic rhinitis by questioning the patient about the appearance and disappearance of symptoms. The presence of acute exacerbations is important in making this differentiation. Patients with seasonal allergic rhinitis generally have a marked increase in symptoms corresponding to an increase in the amount of allergen in the air. The treatment of both is similar.

Complications

Patients with allergic rhinitis may develop complications of chronic nasal inflammation, including recurrent otitis media with hearing loss, sinusitis, and loss of epithelial cilia. Hyposmia (decreased sense of smell acuity), nasal polyps, and vocal changes may be caused by chronic mucosal inflammation, which is more often seen in patients with the perennial form.

Complications of allergic rhinitis seem to be more prominent in children. Often a child develops a characteristic manner of rubbing the nose upward with the palm of the hand to relieve itching and spread the nasal wall, producing better nasal ventilation. This persistent rubbing is called the allergic salute and may lead to the development of a fold on the bridge of the nose called an allergic crease. Nasal allergy in children may also lead to bony structural changes in the palate and to a depression of cheekbone prominence. The resultant crowding of the incisor teeth is called the Gothic arch. Other related facial growth patterns have been identified in children with allergic rhinitis as well. In addition, children with chronic, recurrent rhinitis may develop a hearing impairment because of the involvement of the eustachian tube and middle ear. Approximately 20% of patients with allergic rhinitis have middle ear abnormalities.[23]

Allergic rhinitis and asthmatic attacks may be precipitated by the same agents. If symptoms of allergic rhinitis are prolonged, a persistent cough and asthmatic wheezing or a feeling of constriction in the chest may follow. These are dangerous signals—a warning of possible asthma onset. Because one-third or more of all patients with allergic rhinitis may develop asthma, these signs warrant directing the patient to a physician for diagnosis and treatment. (See Chapter 9, "Asthma Products.")

Perennial allergic rhinitis may be associated with chronic symptoms that may lead to anatomical changes within the nasal and sinus cavities. The resulting complications include loss of epithelial cilia and development of nasal polyps.

Conditions Mimicking Allergic Rhinitis

It is important for pharmacists to recognize common disease entities that may mimic signs and symptoms of allergic rhinitis. The main clinical entity in differential diagnosis of seasonal allergic rhinitis is infectious rhinitis. A mucopurulent discharge, fever and other systemic symptoms, and the lack of pruritus often distinguish infectious rhinitis (Table 3). Chronic sinusitis; recurrent infectious rhinitis; abnormalities of nasal structures such as septal deviations; and nonseasonal, nonallergic, noninfectious rhinitis of unknown etiology (vasomotor rhinitis) may be confused with perennial allergic rhinitis.[12] A physician should be consulted to differentiate among these conditions.

Other conditions that may mimic allergic rhinitis symptoms are rhinitis medicamentosa, reserpine rhinitis, foreign bodies in the nose, and cerebrospinal rhinorrhea. Rhinitis medicamentosa results from the overuse of topically applied vasoconstrictors. The pharmacist may identify this condition by questioning the patient about past use of nose drops or sprays for nasal congestion. Preparations containing reserpine or other antiadrenergic antihypertensives may cause marked nasal congestion. This side effect is generally transient and subsides with continued antihypertensive administration. However, if it persists and is bothersome, topical decongestant treatment may be tried for a few days. In rare instances, the presence of a foreign body in the nose may be mistaken for chronic allergic rhinitis; examination by a physician is necessary. Lastly, cerebrospinal rhinorrhea, which may follow a head injury, is characterized by the discharge of a clear, watery fluid, usually from one nostril, and the presence of glucose within the nasal discharge.

Treatment

Allergic rhinitis treatment may involve:

- Avoidance of allergens, when possible, to prevent the immunologic response;
- Pharmacologic treatment to minimize or counteract the consequences of the immunologic response once it has occurred;
- Injection of allergen extracts to alter the immunologic response to the allergens (immunotherapy).

In most cases of allergic rhinitis, total avoidance of the allergen is difficult because airborne allergens are so widely distributed and most patients are sensitive to more than one allergen. However, avoidance of certain situations (e.g., burning leaves, sleeping with the bedroom windows open, or driving in the countryside when pollen counts are especially high) decreases exposure to potential allergens. The mechanical filters in most air conditioners help reduce the number of allergens if the filters are changed regularly, if doors and windows are kept closed, and if the air is recirculated. An electrostatic precipitator or other high-efficiency mechanical filter used in conjunction with a central heating and air-conditioning unit is even more effective in reducing house dust and other potential allergens. An effective environmental control for allergy to house dust mite is covering the bed mattress (where the dust mite lives) with a plastic cover and sealing the pillow in a plastic casing.

When brief exposure to an allergen is unavoidable, such as when mowing the lawn, a proper face mask may effectively filter the inhaled air. Such masks are sold by industrial or scientific supply firms as well as by pharmacies for protection against noxious dust. The commonly used gauze masks are ineffective.

Immunotherapy (hypersensitization) is regarded as less effective than avoidance or pharmacologic management; however, it may be used in combination with other approaches in more severe allergic disease. Immunotherapy attempts to raise a person's threshold for developing symptoms following exposure to an allergen. Although the mechanisms of immunotherapy are not understood completely, it is believed that blocking antibodies are produced when the patient is given a continuing series of allergen injections in specified incremental doses. A successful treatment regimen enables the patient to develop increased allergen tolerance. The indications for immunotherapy, which is generally a long-term treatment, are relative rather than absolute. For example, if a patient's symptoms are mild and last only a few weeks, the patient may be managed by symptomatic therapy alone. For the patient whose reaction to the allergens is much more severe or who cannot tolerate symptomatic treatment, however, immunotherapy may be considered.

Immunotherapy begins with the proper identification of the offending allergen, most commonly by skin tests measuring the patient's response to test allergens introduced intradermally. After the offending allergen is identified, an extract is injected subcutaneously in small amounts at frequent intervals. Studies indicate that, in pollen allergy, 70–80% of the patients treated with immunotherapy experience beneficial results.[18] However, most of the studies on the efficacy of immunotherapy relate to successes with ragweed and grass.

Immunotherapy does not cure the condition, but it may reduce the frequency and severity of symptoms, making it easier to control the allergy with symptomatic therapy. Patients who experience symptoms of allergic rhinitis throughout the year, whose allergic reactions tend to be severe, and who do not demonstrate a beneficial response from pharmacologic management may be candidates for immunotherapy and should be advised by the pharmacist to seek the advice of a physician.

Pharmacologic Agents

The primary pharmacologic agents used in treating these disorders are antihistamines and decongestants. Antihistamines are valuable because they competitively inhibit the effects of any histamine released as a result of the antigen–antibody reaction. The alpha-adrenergic agonist decongestants constrict dilated blood vessels, thereby diminishing nasal congestion.

Antihistamines

Histamine is a potent biogenic amine found in every body tissue; most histamine, however, is stored in granules in the mast cells and basophils. Mast cells are located primarily in the skin, respiratory, and gastrointestinal (GI) tract. Histamine generally becomes active only when these cells are activated; it may be released as a result of an antigen–antibody reaction (allergy) or physical damage (trauma or infection). Histamine has its most significant effects on the cardiovascular system, exocrine glands, and smooth muscles. Its major effects in allergic rhinitis are profound vasodilation, increased capillary permeability, and edema. These effects are more pronounced in highly vascularized areas such as the nose.

Research into the immunology and biochemistry of the allergic reaction continues to illustrate additional substances that are released as a result of cellular lysis. These substances may not be affected by commonly used drugs and continue to contribute to a patient's symptoms.[24]

As noted, histamine is released in allergic reactions. It may also be released in colds, but this remains controversial. The symptomatology varies according to the amount of histamine released. In allergy, the antigen–antibody reaction leads to the activation of specific sensitized cells (mast cells) and the consequent release of histamine, which initiates the local inflammatory response. In colds, the local inflammatory response results from widespread cellular injury caused by the invasion of virus particles. Therefore, the vasodilation and resultant edema associated with a cold may be attributed predominantly to the body's inflammatory defense and the release of other inflammatory chemical mediators.

Antihistamines are chemical agents that exert their effect in the body primarily by competitively blocking the actions of histamine at H_1-receptor sites. They are classified as "pharmacologic antagonists" of histamine, with a mechanism of action analogous to that of other pharmacologic antagonists such as antiadrenergics and anticholinergics. They do not prevent histamine release but act by competitive inhibition; therefore, if the histamine concentration at the receptor site exceeds the drug concentration, histamine effects predominate.

Antihistamines are typically classified as H_1-receptor blockers. H_2-receptor blockers, whose primary effect is blocking histaminic stimulation of gastric acid secretion, are used primarily in treating peptic ulcer disease and other related GI problems. Those antihistamines that block the H_1-receptor are potentially useful in treating allergic rhinitis.

Although antihistaminic activity is the dominant effect of these agents, antihistamines are structurally similar to other pharmacologic classes of drugs (e.g., anticholinergic, local anesthetic, and ganglionic- and adrenergic-blocking agents), and exert various combinations and degrees of side effects. In some cases, the side effects have been used to achieve a therapeutic goal, such as central nervous system (CNS) depression for insomnia and local anesthetic effects for pruritus. However, the side effects, especially drowsiness, may be bothersome and potentially dangerous.

The most commonly used nonprescription antihistamines and their usual dosages are listed in Table 4. Brompheniramine maleate, chlorpheniramine maleate, diphenhydramine hydrochloride and nitrate, doxylamine succinate, phenindamine tartrate, pheniramine maleate, pyrilamine maleate, thonzylamine hydrochloride, and triprolidine hydrochloride are recognized by the Food and Drug Administration (FDA) Advisory Review Panel on Over-the-Counter Cold, Cough, Allergy, Bronchodilator, and Antiasthmatic Drug Products as being safe for

TABLE 4 Dosage guidelines for selected nonprescription antihistamines

Drug (by chemical class)	Dosage (maximum/24 hr)		
	Adults	Children 6 to <12 yr	Children 2 to <6 yr
Ethanolamines			
Clemastine fumarate	1.34 mg every 12 hr (2.68 mg)	—	—
Diphenhydramine hydrochloride	25–50 mg every 4–6 hr (300 mg)	12.5–25 mg every 4–6 hr (150 mg)	6.25 mg every 4–6 hr (37.5 mg)
Ethylenediamines			
Pyrilamine maleate	25–50 mg every 6–8 hr (200 mg)	12.5–25 mg every 6–8 hr (100 mg)	6.25–12.5 mg every 6–8 hr (50 mg)
Thonzylamine hydrochloride	50–100 mg every 4–6 hr (600 mg)	25–50 mg every 4–6 hr (300 mg)	12.5–25 mg every 4–6 hr (150 mg)
Alkylamines			
Pheniramine maleate	12.5–25 mg every 4–6 hr (150 mg)	6.25–12.5 mg every 4–6 hr (75 mg)	3.125–6.25 mg every 4–6 hr (37.5 mg)
Brompheniramine maleate	4 mg every 4–6 hr (24 mg)	2 mg every 4–6 hr (12 mg)	1 mg every 4–6 hr (6 mg)
Chlorpheniramine maleate	4 mg every 4–6 hr (24 mg)	2 mg every 4–6 hr (12 mg)	1 mg every 4–6 hr (6 mg)
Triprolidine hydrochloride	2.5 mg every 4–6 hr (15 mg)	1.25 mg every 4–6 hr (7.5 mg)	Consult physician
Miscellaneous			
Phenindamine tartrate	25 mg every 4–6 hr (150 mg)	12.5 mg every 4–6 hr (75 mg)	6.25 mg every 4–6 hr (37.5 mg)

nonprescription use and effective in suppressing the symptoms of allergic rhinitis when taken in the dosage specified. Conclusive evidence is still lacking as to the safety and effectiveness of phenyltoloxamine citrate. Antihistamines are most effective in controlling allergic rhinitis and are rarely effective in treating vasomotor rhinitis.

Some regular antihistamine users may find that they do not obtain the same degree of relief after several consecutive weeks or months of using a particular antihistamine. One reason for this decreased effectiveness is that some antihistamines are capable of hepatic enzyme induction, resulting in increased metabolism in the liver. Enzyme induction by antihistamines can also diminish the effectiveness of other drugs; however, the clinical significance of such interactions is undetermined. The various antihistamine classes differ in their capacity to induce hepatic enzymes. Some practitioners have found that if tolerance develops, some patients may benefit by switching to an alternative antihistamine from a different chemical class. Further studies are needed to evaluate the effectiveness of this technique objectively.

Although antihistamines have no ability to prevent or abort the common cold, they are found in many cold remedies, probably because their anticholinergic action decreases the amount of mucus secretion, thus relieving the rhinorrhea. Although some people experience a drying effect, the anticholinergic activity of the antihistamines is actually very weak and may even be insignificant at the recommended dosage levels of the various nonprescription preparations.[25]

In general, antihistamines possess a high therapeutic index (toxic dose/therapeutic dose), and serious toxicities are seldom noted in adults. At recommended labeled doses, most nonprescription antihistamines are also safe for use in children. As with most drugs, however, accidental overdosage in children may lead to profound symptoms such as excitement, ataxia, incoordination, muscular twitching, generalized convulsions with pupillary dilation, and flushing. Treatment is symptomatic and supportive.

The major precaution associated with antihistamine use relates to its sedative property. Degrees of drowsiness associated with antihistamine use vary. The ethanolamines (e.g., diphenhydramine hydrochloride) have a pronounced tendency to induce sedation; the alkylamines (e.g., chlorpheniramine maleate) possess weak sedative properties; and the ethylenediamines (e.g., pyrilamine maleate) have intermediate sedative properties. Although most individuals acquire a tolerance to this effect, the alkylamines probably are the most suitable nonprescription agents currently available for daytime use. Persistent drowsiness is relatively uncommon when therapy is initiated with a low dose of the drug at bedtime and the dose is increased gradually and progressively over a 10-day period as tolerated. If a person's job or other activities require a high degree of mental alertness, physical coordination, or physical dexterity, any antihistamine must be used cautiously until its effect is determined. Antihistamines may also enhance the sedative effects of alcohol and other CNS depressants, including hypnotics, sedatives, analgesics, antidepressants, antipsychotics, and antianxiety agents. If concurrent administration is necessary, caution must be exercised because of the increased possibility of drowsiness, impaired coordination, and delayed reaction time. Patients should be warned of "hidden" sources of alcohol contained in some nonprescription liquid medications (e.g., elixirs and syrups).

Recently, a number of prescription antihistamines have been introduced that offer the advantage of low sedation. These newer agents are characterized by weak anticholinergic effects, longer duration, and less ability to "cross over" the blood brain barrier into the CNS. It is believed that this latter effect in what makes these agents less sedating. Although these newer agents (e.g., terfenadine and astemizole) are restricted to prescription use in the United States at this time, manufacturers are attempting to have them reclassified to nonprescription status, as they are in several foreign countries.

Many commercial products contain both an antihistamine and a decongestant. These combination products may have a lower tendency to cause sedation because of the CNS stimulant properties of the decongestant.

A paradoxical effect from antihistamines often seen in children and elderly persons is CNS stimulation rather than depression, which may cause insomnia, nervousness, and irritability. For this reason, antihistamines must be used cautiously in individuals with seizure disorders or children with hyperkinesis.[1]

The anticholinergic properties of an antihistamine may predominate in some individuals, producing side effects of dry mouth, blurred vision, urinary retention (in older men suffering from an enlarged prostate), and constipation. These effects, however, are usually associated with high doses. In the past, some health practitioners believed that antihistamines should not be given to asthmatics because of the potential drying effect on the respiratory tract. However, these products have proven useful in patients whose asthma has an allergic component.

The anticholinergic effect of antihistamines also has a quantitatively unpredictable additive effect with anticholinergic drugs. Although excessive blocking effects are usually of minor clinical significance, effects such as urinary retention, constipation, and dry mouth may be bothersome in certain individuals. Moreover, these cholinergic-blocking properties may pose a problem for patients taking an anticholinesterase agent to control angle-closure glaucoma. Because of the potential consequences, such patients probably should take antihistamines only under a physician's supervision. Approximately 95% of all patients with glaucoma have the wide-angle type, and antihistamines are not contraindicated in these patients.

Hypersensitivity reactions may develop with the antihistamines, but this effect is more common with topical application than with systemic use. Antihistamine overdose may cause dermatitis, psychosis, convulsions, and various dyskinesias.

Topical Decongestants

Various sympathomimetic amines have been used to provide relief from the nasal stuffiness of colds and allergic rhinitis (Table 5). These drugs, which differ primarily in their duration of action, are contained in many nonprescription products promoted for treating symptoms of allergic rhinitis and colds. Nasal decongestants stimulate the alpha-adrenergic receptors of the vascular smooth muscle, constrict the dilated arteriolar network within the nasal mucosa, and reduce blood flow in the engorged edematous nasal area. This constriction results in shrinkage of the engorged mucous membranes, which promotes drainage, improves nasal ventilation, and relieves the feeling of stuffiness.

The ideal topical decongestant agent should have a prompt and prolonged effect. It should not produce systemic side effects, irritation to the mucosa with resultant harmful interference with the action of the respiratory tract cilia, or rebound congestion. Such a product, however, has not yet been found.

It is very important that the patient strictly follow the decongestant's label directions regarding the frequency and duration of use. When these agents are misused or overused, a rebound phenomenon (rhinitis medicamentosa) may occur in which the nasal mucous membranes become even more congested and edematous as the drug's vasoconstrictor effect subsides. This secondary congestion is believed to result from ischemia caused by the drug's intensive local vasoconstriction and from local irritation of the topically applied agent itself. If the use of a topical nasal decongestant is restricted to 3 or 4 days or less, rebound congestion is minimal. With chronic use or overuse of the agent, however, rebound nasal stuffiness may become quite pronounced. This phenomenon may then produce a dependency and begin a vicious cycle because it leads to more frequent use of the agent to get the pharmacologic effect initially received. To determine the possible existence of this condition, the pharmacist should question a patient about prior use of nasal sprays or drops. If the pharmacist suspects that the patient is experiencing this rebound phenomenon, the patient should be referred to a physician. Attempts to treat the iatrogenic symptoms with additional topical sympathomimetic drugs create a cycle that is extremely difficult to break. Topical decongestant therapy should be discontinued, and systemic decongestants or isotonic saline drops or spray or intranasal steroids may be used instead.

The patient should be instructed on the proper use of topical decongestants to obtain maximum relief without systemic side effects. Nasal decongestant sprays are packaged in flexible plastic containers that produce a fine mist when squeezed. The nasal passages should first be cleared by gently blowing the nose. The patient should administer nasal sprays in the upright position, squeezing once into each nostril. The nose should be blown to remove mucus 3–5 minutes after spraying. If the nose is still congested, the patient should administer another dose, which should reach farther into the nasal passages and to the surfaces of the turbinates.

TABLE 5 Topical nasal decongestant dosages

Drug	Concentration (%)	Adults (drops or sprays)	Children 6 to <12 yr (drops or sprays)	Children 2 to <6 yr[a]
Ephedrine	0.5	2–3 (≥4 hr)	1–2 (≥4 hr)	—
Naphazoline hydrochloride	0.05	2 (≥4–6 hr)	Not recommended (refer to 0.025%)	—
	0.025	—	1–2 (≥6 hr)	—
Oxymetazoline hydrochloride	0.05	2–3 (morning and evening)	Same as for adults	Not recommended (refer to 0.025%)
	0.025	—	—	2–3 (morning and evening)
Phenylephrine hydrochloride	1	1–2 (≥4 hr)	Not recommended (refer to 0.25%)	Not recommended (refer to 0.125%)
	0.5	1–2 (≥4 hr)	Not recommended (refer to 0.25%)	Not recommended (refer to 0.125%)
	0.25	1–2 (≥4 hr)	1–2 (≥4 hr)	Not recommended (refer to 0.125%)
	0.2	1–2 (≥4 hr)	1–2 (≥4 hr)	Not recommended (refer to 0.125%)
	0.125	—	—	1 drop (≥4 hr)
Xylometazoline hydrochloride	0.1	2–3 (8–10 hr)	Not recommended (refer to 0.05%)	Not recommended (refer to 0.05%)
	0.05	—	2–3 (8–10 hr)	2–3 (8–10 hr)

Note: The FDA Advisory Review Panel on OTC Cold, Cough, Allergy, Bronchodilator, and Antiasthmatic Drug Products has recommended these ingredients as safe and effective (Category I) at the dosages specified. Only drops should be used in children 2 to under 6 years of age because the spray is difficult to use in small nostrils. These products should not be used in patients with chronic rhinitis because of the risk of rhinitis medicamentosa.

[a]For children under 6 years of age, there is no recommended dosage of ephedrine, naphazoline, or oxymetazoline except under the advice and supervision of a physician.

Some persons prefer to administer the decongestant solution with a nasal atomizer. Most commercial spray containers are designed to deliver the approximate dose with one squeeze; the atomizer, however, is not so calibrated. Also, using an atomizer may increase the possibility of contaminating the solution. If the patient prefers to use a nasal atomizer, instructions should be provided on the proper use of the particular atomizer, including the liquid level, proper placement within the nostril, and hazards of misuse. The patient should be instructed to remove the solution and rinse the atomizer after use to guard against solution contamination. Naphazoline solutions should not be used in atomizers containing aluminum parts because drug degradation will result.

Nasal drops usually do not cover the entire nasal mucosa and may pass to the pharynx, where they may be swallowed. Although systemic absorption through the nasal mucosa is minimal because of the local vasoconstriction induced by the drug, absorption and systemic effects are possible if an excess amount drains through the nasal passage and is swallowed. Proper use minimizes the amount of medication swallowed.

To administer nasal drops, the patient should clear the nasal passages and recline on a bed either with the head tilted back over the edge or on the side with the head held lower than the shoulders. The drops should be placed in the lower nostril; the dropper should not touch the nasal surface. After the drops have been instilled into each nostril, the patient should breathe through the mouth and remain in the reclining position for about 5 minutes. To ensure more uniform absorption of the medication, the head should be turned from side to side while the patient is reclining.

A topical decongestant in spray form is probably more convenient for adults and older children. Sprays also may afford better decongestion by reaching greater areas of the mucous membranes. Drops are the most effective means of administering a topical decongestant to children under 6 years of age. Dosage guidelines for topical decongestants are included in Table 5.

Ephedrine Ephedrine, though not the preferred therapeutic agent today, is the prototype of the topical sympathomimetic decongestant. Various ephedrine salts provide rapid nasal decongestion when applied topically in 0.5–1.0% concentrations. Ephedrine's peak effects are achieved 1 hour after administration. Aqueous solutions of topical ephedrine as drops or sprays are preferred over oily solutions, which may lead to lipoid pneumonia. Products containing ephedrine should be shielded from direct light, which will hasten its decomposition. Discolored ephedrine solutions should not be used. Ephedrine in a concentration of 0.5% should be administered as two or three drops or sprays for adults and as 1 or 2 drops or sprays for children 6–12 years of age no more frequently than every 4 hours. Ephedrine is not recommended for children under 6 years of age except under the advice and supervision of a physician.

Phenylephrine Phenylephrine hydrochloride is an effective topical (and systemic) nonprescription nasal decongestant. A 0.25–1.0% solution is commonly applied topically as one or two drops or sprays every 4 hours in adults. Children over 6 years of age should use the 0.25% spray or drops. The 0.125%, 0.16%, and 0.2% solutions are available for use in children under 6 years of age; however, a physician should be consulted first. The use of stronger solutions is hazardous except under a physician's direction. This agent may produce a marked irritation of the nasal mucosa in some individuals; if this occurs, phenylephrine use should be stopped immediately.

Phenylephrine hydrochloride is also available as an aqueous jelly. A small amount of jelly is placed in each nostril and snuffed well back into the nasal passage. This dosage form is neither convenient nor widely used, and its effectiveness has not been established. Theoretically, a more prolonged decongestant effect may be achieved with nasal jellies alone exerting an emollient and protective action on the nasal mucosa, but these effects also have not been objectively demonstrated. Nasal decongestant jellies are used most commonly by otorhinolaryngologists for office examination or treatment.

Naphazoline Naphazoline hydrochloride is a more potent vasoconstrictor than phenylephrine hydrochloride. When absorbed systemically, it produces CNS depression rather than stimulation. Because of its systemic effects, this agent is not recommended for use in children under 6 years of age except under the advice and supervision of a physician. Naphazoline hydrochloride is commonly administered as two drops or sprays of a 0.05% solution every 4–6 hours. It may irritate the mucosa and sting when administered; its use should be discontinued if these effects persist or worsen.

Oxymetazoline and Xylometazoline Longer acting topical nasal decongestants, such as oxymetazoline hydrochloride and xylometazoline hydrochloride, have a decongestant effect that may last 5 to 6 hours or longer, with a gradual decline thereafter. Because of their long duration of action, these agents are used only twice a day; therefore, they are more convenient to use. Overuse or chronic use of these topical agents is associated with chronic rhinitis, nasal congestion, and nasal irritability. Oxymetazoline (0.05%) may be administered as two or three drops or sprays in the morning and evening in adults and in children over 6 years of age. Xylometazoline (0.1%) may be administered in the same amount every 8–10 hours in adults and in children over 12 years of age. The less concentrated solutions of both products can be used in children as young as 2 years of age if they are under a physician's supervision.

Levodesoxyephedrine and Propylhexedrine Levodesoxyephedrine and propylhexedrine are volatile sympathomimetic amines commonly used in inhalants. Both of these aromatic amines are classified as Category I (safe and effective) when used as two inhalations in each nostril no more often than every 2 hours. Although children 6 years of age and over may use the adult dose of propylhexedrine, the dose of levodesoxyephedrine should be halved to one inhalation no more often than every 2 hours for such patients. Neither product is promoted for use in children under 6 years of age.

The use of nasal inhalers is associated with potential problems, such as the loss of the active agent when the cap is not properly replaced. Also, there may not be sufficient nasal airflow to distribute the agent throughout the nasal cavity. Like all effective topical nasal decongestants, these agents have been implicated as being irritating to the nasal mucosa and as interfering with ciliary action. And like other topical amines, overuse produces side effects of local irritation and rebound congestion.

Oral Decongestants

Oral administration of sympathomimetic amines distributes the drug throughout the systemic circulation and to the vascular beds of the nasal mucosa. The oral decongestant agents have a longer duration of action than certain topically applied decongestants. However, they cause less intense vasoconstriction than the topically applied sprays or drops and have a slower onset of action. Oral agents have not been associated with rebound congestion because of their lesser degree of vasoconstriction and the lack of local drug irritation.

These agents do not exert their action exclusively on the vasculature of the nasal mucosa; in doses large enough to bring about nasal decongestion, they also affect other vascular beds of the body. Although the vasoconstriction they produce does not usually increase blood pressure, individuals predisposed to hypertension may experience an elevation in blood pressure when using them. These decongestants may also produce cardiac stimulation and the development of arrhythmias in predisposed individuals. Sympathomimetic agents may also be a problem in patients with glucose intolerance or insulin-dependent diabetes mellitus because these drugs may increase blood glucose levels (hyperglycemia). However, hyperglycemia is a beta$_2$-adrenergic effect and most oral decongestants (except ephedrine) contain primarily alpha-adrenergic stimulating properties. Instruction labels on products containing

TABLE 6 Oral nasal decongestant dosages

	Dosage (maximum/24 hr)		
Drug	Adults	Children 6 to <12 yr	Children 2 to <6 yr[a]
Phenylephrine	10 mg every 4 hr (60 mg)	5 mg every 4 hr (30 mg)	2.5 mg every 4 hr (15 mg)
Phenylpropanolamine	25 mg every 4 hr (150 mg)	12.5 mg every 4 hr (75 mg)	6.25 mg every 4 hr (37.5 mg)
Pseudoephedrine	60 mg every 6 hr (240 mg)	30 mg every 6 hr (120 mg)	15 mg every 6 hr (60 mg)

Note: The FDA Advisory Review Panel on OTC Cold, Cough, Allergy, Bronchodilator, and Antiasthmatic Drug Products has recommended these ingredients as safe and effective (Category I) at the dosages specified.
[a]There is no recommended dosage for children under 2 years of age except under the advice and supervision of a physician.

---

sympathomimetics should indicate that patients with hypertension, hyperthyroidism, diabetes mellitus, or ischemic heart disease should use these products only on the advice of a physician. (See Chapter 16, "Diabetes Care Products and Monitoring Devices.")

Sympathomimetic amines are contraindicated in patients receiving monoamine oxidase inhibitor therapy for depression or selegiline therapy for Parkinson's disease because a hypertensive crisis may result. These products should be used cautiously in hypertensive patients stabilized with guanethidine. These warnings apply largely to the oral agents and are not likely to be necessary with topically applied drugs.

Apart from hypertension, adverse effects that may occur with oral decongestant therapy include CNS stimulation and headache. Because the agents may also cause sleep disturbance, patients may benefit most from using them at times other than bedtime.

Phenylpropanolamine hydrochloride, phenylephrine hydrochloride, and pseudoephedrine are oral sympathomimetic amines commonly incorporated into cold and allergy products. Dosage guidelines are included in Table 6. According to the FDA, only these three products have been shown to be effective as oral decongestants.

Ephedrine According to the FDA, ephedrine is effective as a bronchodilator for asthma but has not been proven effective as a nasal decongestant. Ephedrine has CNS stimulatory effects.

Phenylpropanolamine Phenylpropanolamine hydrochloride resembles ephedrine in its action, but it is somewhat more active as a vasoconstrictor and less active as a bronchodilator. The peak effect occurs approximately 3 hours after administration. Adverse effects include hypertension, headache, jitteriness, irritability, insomnia, and cardiac rhythm irregularities. Although these effects are more common following administration of higher doses, as is seen when the agent is used as a diet aid, patients with underlying hypertension or a cardiac rhythm disturbance should use these agents with caution.[26]

Phenylephrine Phenylephrine hydrochloride is rapidly metabolized in the GI tract, and the amount delivered to the bloodstream through oral administration is difficult to predict even though its effectiveness as an oral decongestant has been demonstrated. Phenylephrine is a common ingredient of nonprescription cold preparations. Because of the unique properties of this agent, it is important to select products that contain the full and appropriate FDA recommended dosage.

Pseudoephedrine Pseudoephedrine is an effective systemic vasoconstrictor. It has less vasopressor and cardiac stimulant action than other systemic decongestants and causes little CNS stimulation. The dosages in Table 6 reflect a relabeling requirement following an FDA decision that data on safety and effectiveness do not support the advisory review panel's original recommendation for a 360-mg maximum adult daily dosage of pseudoephedrine. The FDA's latest labeling requirement sets the total adult daily dosage at 240 mg. The daily dosage for children 6–12 years of age has been changed from 180 mg to 120 mg and for children 2–6 years of age, from 90 mg to 60 mg. The peak effect of a single 60-mg adult dose occurs approximately 4 hours after administration. Because pseudoephedrine has a short duration of effect, several companies have marketed slow-release formulations to maintain more constant relief from nasal airway obstruction. Patients whose nasal stuffiness interferes with nighttime sleep may benefit from such a formulation.

Expectorants and Antitussives

The cough associated with the common cold may be either productive or nonproductive. The productive cough is useful if it helps to remove accumulated secretions and debris (phlegm) from the respiratory passages of the lung. Although a patient with chest congestion is expected to expectorate phlegm during coughing, this does not always occur. Differentiation of the cough as productive or nonproductive is very important in the drug selection and use process. For the sake of developing a rationale for product selection, a cough will be classified in one of the following categories:

- *Congested/productive:* cough associated with chest congestion and the expectoration of phlegm;

- *Congested/nonproductive:* cough associated with chest congestion and scant expectoration of phlegm;
- *Dry/nonproductive:* cough not associated with chest congestion or the expectoration of phlegm.

By referring to these categories, the pharmacist will be able to determine when and which type of an agent should be used.

Coughs in the first two categories could be undiagnosed symptoms of asthma because intermittent asthmatics may only develop symptoms during a viral respiratory infection. Cough may also indicate other disorders such as pneumonia, bronchitis, or congestive heart failure.

Excessive coughing, particularly if it is dry and nonproductive, not only is discomforting but also tends to be self-perpetuating; this is because the rapid air expulsion further irritates the tracheal and pharyngeal mucosa. The general classes of pharmacologic agents available for self-treatment are expectorants and cough suppressants. Table 7 indicates both the mechanism of these agents and the sites at which the cough reflex may be blocked.

Expectorants

Use of expectorants in clinical practice is controversial because of doubts regarding their therapeutic efficacy. The controversy stems from a lack of strong, supportive, objective data showing that an expectorant truly decreases sputum viscosity or eases expectoration. One study evaluating guaifenesin concludes that "from a scientific point of view this drug probably has no rational use in clinical medicine as an expectorant."[27] Clinicians appropriately question the efficacy of expectorants and suggest that their use is based primarily on tradition and on the widespread subjective clinical impression that they are effective. The apparent difficulty in accumulating objective evidence of efficacy stems from three factors: (1) insufficient evidence as to which physiochemical property of respiratory secretions correlates best with ease of expectoration, (2) a lack of appropriate techniques and instrumentation to measure the effect of expectorants on respiratory secretions, and (3) a lack of an adequate animal or in-vitro model.

The FDA advisory panel has classified guaifenesin as the only expectorant in Category I (generally recognized as safe and effective). All other expectorants remain classified as Category III (available data are insufficient to classify as safe and effective, and further testing is required). Moreover, the FDA issued a warning effective July 30, 1992, regarding the use of nonprescription expectorants in children under age 12. This warning states that, unless directed by a physician, expectorants should not be given if there is a persistent or chronic cough such as occurs with asthma or if the cough is accompanied by excessive phlegm (mucus).

Increasing fluid intake and maintaining adequate humidity of the inspired air are important for the production and expectoration of respiratory tract fluid mucus. These measures may be accomplished by increasing fluid intake to 6–8 glasses (8 oz per glass) a day in patients who do not have fluid restrictions and by using a cool mist or hot steam vaporizer. Maintaining a well-hydrated body may be a primary way to enhance expectoration.

TABLE 7 Blockage of cough reflex

Site	Mechanism	Blocking agents
Sensory nerves	Reduction of primary irritation; inhibition of bronchoconstriction; inhibition of afferent impulses	Demulcents/expectorants; bronchodilators; local anesthetics
Cough center (medulla)	Depression	Opiate and nonopiate suppressants
Motor nerves	Inhibition of efferent impulses	Local anesthetics

Adapted from Salem H, Aviado DM. *Drug Inform J* 1974; 8: 111.

Subjective findings constitute the basis for continued expectorant use. Table 8 lists the usual doses and dosage ranges of the most commonly used expectorants.

The toxicity associated with expectorant drugs varies among agents. Although they lack objective evidence of effectiveness, most expectorants are considered to be safe. In general, the adverse effect most likely to occur is gastric upset.

Ammonium Chloride Ammonium chloride is a Category III agent; it allegedly increases the removal of respiratory tract fluid by reflex stimulation of bronchial mucous glands that results from irritation of the gastric mucosa, but it is of questionable efficacy. Moreover, in the presence of renal, hepatic, or chronic heart disease, ammonium chloride doses of 5 g have caused severe poisoning. Symptoms of toxicity include nausea, vomiting, thirst, rash, headache, bradycardia, mental confusion, hyperventilation, hyperreflexia, and electroencephalogram abnormalities. A relative contraindication exists when ammonium chloride is used in patients with hepatic, renal, or pulmonary insufficiency; doses larger than those recommended may predispose to hyperammonemia and metabolic acidosis. Because ammonium chloride acidifies the urine, it may also affect the excretion of other drugs. This effect is probably not significant, however, because the usual daily dosage range as a systemic acidifier is 4–12 g, which exceeds the safe range for nonprescription use.

Guaifenesin Guaifenesin, in the doses recommended in Table 8 for nonprescription use, is thought to act as an expectorant by reflex gastric stimulation. Despite its mechanism of action, its use at these doses is seldom associated with gastric upset and nausea. There are no apparent absolute contraindications to the use of guaifenesin.

Iodides Iodides, iodinated glycerol, and hydriotic acid are all prescription-only expectorants. The American

TABLE 8 Expectorant dosages, where specified, considered safe

Drug	Dosage (maximum/24 hr)		
	Adults	Children 6 to <12 yr	Children 2 to <6 yr[a]
Ammonium chloride	300 mg every 2–4 hr	150 mg every 2–4 hr	75 mg every 2–4 hr
Beechwood creosote	250 mg every 4–6 hr (1,500 mg)	125 mg every 4–6 hr (750 mg)	62.5 mg every 4–6 hr (375 mg)
Guaifenesin	200–400 mg every 4 hr (2,400 mg)	100–200 mg every 4 hr (1,200 mg)	50–100 mg every 4 hr (600 mg)
Potassium guaiacolsulfonate	Not established	Not established	Not established
Ipecac syrup	0.5–1.0 mL (of syrup containing not less than 123 mg and not more than 157 mg of total ether-soluble alkaloids of ipecac per 100 mL) 3 or 4 times a day	0.25–0.5 mL (of syrup containing not less than 123 mg and not more than 157 mg of total ether-soluble alkaloids of ipecac per 100 mL) 3 or 4 times a day	Not recommended
Terpin hydrate	200 mg every 4 hr (1,200 mg)	100 mg (of terpin hydrate alone or in a nonalcoholic mixture, not the elixir for children under 12) every 4 hr (600 mg)	50 mg (of terpin hydrate alone or in a nonalcoholic mixture, not the elixir for children under 12) every 4 hr (300 mg)

Note: The FDA Advisory Review Panel on OTC Cold, Cough, Allergy, Bronchodilator, and Antiasthmatic Drug Products has concluded that available data are sufficient to classify guaifenesin as Category I. All other expectorants lack data to permit reclassification in Category I and remain in Category III.

[a]There is no recommended dosage for children under 2 years of age except under the advice and supervision of a physician. The FDA issued a warning, effective July 30, 1992, which states that, unless directed by a physician, expectorants should not be given to children under 12 years of age if they have a persistent or chronic cough such as occurs with asthma, or if the cough is accompanied by excessive phlegm (mucus).

Academy of Pediatrics recommends that iodides not be used as expectorants in children. If used chronically, they may produce iodism, hypothyroidism, and goiter. Hypersensitivity reactions to iodine may occur. These drugs are contraindicated in pregnancy, nursing mothers, children, and patients in hyperkalemic and hyperthyroid states.

Ipecac Syrup Administration of 0.5–1.0 mL of ipecac syrup (see Table 8 for concentration) three or four times a day has been alleged to increase respiratory secretion flow by gastric irritation and is of questionable efficacy and safety. Although the fluidextract of ipecac is no longer commercially available as an expectorant, special care should be taken not to use it. Little is known regarding the toxicity associated with ipecac at dosages used for expectoration; however, the chief alkaloids, emetine and cephaeline, are very cardiotoxic. Cardiac and neuromuscular toxicity have caused deaths. Fatalities have also occurred from the administration both of ipecac in emesis-producing dosages over prolonged periods of time and of the more potent fluidextract of ipecac. Ipecac is not recommended for use in children under 6 years of age except as an emetic in a confirmed or suspected poisoning.

Terpin Hydrate Terpin hydrate, a Category III agent and a volatile oil derivative, is claimed to act as an expectorant in the dosage recommended for nonprescription use by direct stimulation of lower respiratory tract secretory glands. Evidence of its efficacy, however, is lacking. Because of the elixir's high alcohol content, the potential for alcohol abuse should be recognized. Misuse has been associated with terpin hydrate and codeine elixir, but this product is no longer commercially available. Terpin hydrate elixir is not recommended for use in children under 12 years of age. Some GI distress, such as nausea and vomiting, has been noted with the recommended dosage.

Other ingredients of unproven effectiveness that may be added to cold products for their claimed but unproven expectorant properties include:

- Beechwood creosote/potassium guaiacolsulfonate;
- Benzoin preparations;
- Camphor;
- Eucalyptus oil;
- Menthol;
- Peppermint oil;

TABLE 9 Antitussive dosages			
	Dosage (maximum/24 hr)		
Drug	Adults	Children 6 to <12 yr	Children 2 to <6 yr[a]
Codeine[b]	10–20 mg every 4–6 hr (120 mg)	5–10 mg every 4–6 hr (60 mg)	2.5–5 mg every 4–6 hr (30 mg)
Dextromethorphan	10–20 mg every 4 hr or 30 mg every 6–8 hr (120 mg)	5–10 mg every 4 hr or 15 mg every 6–8 hr (60 mg)	2.5–5 mg every 4 hr or 7.5 mg every 6–8 hr (30 mg)
Diphenhydramine hydrochloride	25 mg every 4 hr (150 mg)	1.25 mg every 4 hr (75 mg)	6.25 mg every 4 hr (37.5 mg)
Noscapine hydrochloride[c]	15–30 mg every 4–6 hr (180 mg)	7.5–15 mg every 4–6 hr (90 mg)	3.75–7.5 mg every 4–6 hr (45 mg)

Note: The FDA Advisory Review Panel on OTC Cold, Cough, Allergy, Bronchodilator, and Antiasthmatic Drug Products has recommended all of these ingredients as safe and effective (Category I) except noscapine hydrochloride, for which there is insufficient evidence (Category III).
[a]There is no recommended dosage for children under 2 years of age except under the advice and supervision of a physician.
[b]The FDA recommends that the labels on nonprescription agents containing codeine not give dosage information for children under 6 years of age.
[c]Category III, additional evidence of safety and effectiveness required.

- Pine tar;
- Sodium citrate;
- Tolu balsam;
- Turpentine oil.

Antitussives

Antitussives (cough suppressants) are indicated when there is a need to reduce the frequency of a cough, especially one that is dry and nonproductive. Antitussives may be counterproductive when used in a productive cough because cough suppression may impair expectoration; however, judicious use of these agents may be warranted if the productive cough is particularly bothersome or sleep disrupting. Otherwise, antitussives should not be used in patients with productive or congested coughs.

The mechanism by which the narcotic and non-narcotic antitussives affect a cough's intensity and frequency depends on the principal site of drug action.

Codeine Codeine is the standard antitussive against which all other antitussives are compared.[23] An FDA advisory panel has concluded that, under usual conditions of therapeutic use as a cough suppressant, codeine has low-dependency liability.

Nonprescription availability of codeine-containing products varies between states. There is no significant danger of psychologic or physical dependence when codeine is used in recommended amounts for short periods; however, dependence may develop after prolonged use.[28] The average adult antitussive dose is 15 mg (with a range of 10–20 mg). At this dosage, codeine generally provides effective cough relief in adults (see Table 9 for adult and child dosages). Stringent controls have been placed on codeine-containing nonprescription products because of their abuse and misuse potential.

The respiratory depressant effect of codeine is about one-fourth that of morphine. Even when the codeine dose is increased, a commensurate increase in respiratory depression does not necessarily occur. In otherwise healthy persons, codeine does not have any apparent adverse effect on respiration when taken in dosages commonly used in nonprescription cough products. Some investigators believe codeine has a slight drying effect on the respiratory mucosa. This property is not well documented but would be detrimental in asthma, emphysema, and bronchitis sufferers because of the drug-induced increased viscosity of respiratory fluids and decreased cough reflex, which lead to a decreased ability to expectorate respiratory tract debris.

An FDA advisory panel has suggested limiting label dosage recommendations for products containing codeine to patients over 6 years of age and dispensing a measuring device when the product is to be used in children between the ages of 2 and 6 years.[29] Physician consultation is suggested for children under 6 years of age because codeine causes a slightly greater chance of respiratory depression.[29]

In clinical practice, the adverse effects most commonly encountered with codeine include nausea, drowsiness, lightheadedness, and constipation. Allergic reactions and pruritus may also occur but are not as common. Hypersensitivity reactions may be more common in patients who are atopic or are prone to allergic reactions; however, nonprescription antitussive codeine doses are generally well tolerated. Codeine's CNS effects are additive to those of other CNS depressants; therefore, such agents should be used cautiously when given concurrently.

Codeine use is contraindicated in individuals with chronic pulmonary disease, in whom mucosal drying and slight respiratory depression, in addition to impairment of expectoration, may be detrimental. Codeine should be avoided by patients who have experienced codeine-induced allergic manifestations (pruritus or rash). It is, however, generally considered safe and effective when used as directed for cough.

Dextromethorphan Dextromethorphan is the methylated dextro-isomer of levorphanol, but, unlike its narcotic analgesic relative, it has no significant analgesic properties and does not depress respiration or predispose to addiction. Some investigators believe that dextromethorphan and codeine are equipotent, others give a slight edge to codeine, and still others support dextromethorphan as the superior antitussive.[30] Therefore, because of the probable equal effectiveness and a favorable side effect profile, dextromethorphan may be indicated in patients for whom the adverse effects of codeine may be particularly bothersome. Increasing the dose of dextromethorphan to 30 mg does not increase its antitussive effects but may extend its duration of action by a few hours. This may be particularly useful in treating a nonproductive, sleep-disrupting cough because a 30-mg bedtime dose in an adult may provide an antitussive effect throughout the normal sleeping period.

Adverse effects produced by dextromethorphan hydrobromide at recommended nonprescription dosages are mild and infrequent. Drowsiness and GI upset are the most common complaints. Accidental poisonings in children have resulted in symptoms of stupor and gait disturbances, with rapid recovery after emesis and activated charcoal. Larger dosages in the abuse range have produced intoxication with bizarre behavior but no drug dependence.

Dextromethorphan hydrobromide at nonprescription dosages (Table 9) is a safe and effective antitussive for which there are no apparent contraindications except hypersensitivity to this agent.

Diphenhydramine Diphenhydramine hydrochloride is both an antihistamine and an antitussive. Objective results indicate that diphenhydramine, in 25- and 50-mg doses, significantly reduces coughing in patients with a chronic cough. Diphenhydramine's antitussive effect is due to a central mechanism involving the medullary cough center. A peripheral action may also contribute to its effectiveness, but further studies are required to establish this point. (See Table 9 for dosage recommendations.)

The adverse effects associated with diphenhydramine hydrochloride are similar to those of other antihistamines but are of varying intensity. The most commonly encountered adverse effects are sedation and anticholinergic (atropine-like) effects. Because of these properties, diphenhydramine hydrochloride should not be taken by individuals in whom anticholinergics are contraindicated (e.g., those with narrow-angle glaucoma or prostatic hypertrophy) or in situations in which mental alertness or physical coordination and dexterity are required, (e.g., driving a car or operating motor equipment).

Because of its additive CNS depressant effects, diphenhydramine should be used cautiously by individuals taking antianxiety agents, sedatives, hypnotics, antidepressants, or narcotics. Similarly, ingesting alcohol will have additive depressant effects. Because of its additive anticholinergic effects, diphenhydramine hydrochloride should also be used cautiously by patients taking other anticholinergic drugs as well as by patients combining this agent with other antitussives such as codeine. Diphenhydramine hydrochloride, like codeine and dextromethorphan hydrobromide, is a safe and effective antitussive; however, when recommending it, pharmacists must keep in mind its high likelihood of producing side effects.

Camphor-Containing Ointments The FDA has reclassified camphor-containing ointments as Category I agents. The antitussive action of these products is believed to occur because inhalation of the aromatic vapors causes a local anesthetic action. Camphor has been shown to be safe and effective for reducing cough when externally applied to the chest and throat of young children. Products used for the antitussive effect contain approximately 5% camphor. However, an FDA advisory panel has concluded that topical agents containing as much as 11% of camphor are safe for external use.

Toxicity may occur if the camphor is ingested. The primary toxic effect reported is seizures. Patients should be counseled to avoid use near the mouth and nose to prevent accidental internal ingestion.

Noscapine Noscapine, an opium alkaloid related to papaverine, is used in only a few nonprescription preparations. Noscapine is apparently safe at currently available nonprescription dosages; however, its effectiveness is unproven, and the FDA advisory review panel has suggested additional testing to establish its effectiveness. Noscapine's antitussive efficacy appears to be dose related, and although some investigators believe that it is equipotent on a weight basis to codeine, safe nonprescription adult dosages range from 15 to 30 mg every 4–6 hours, not to exceed 180 mg a day (Table 9).

In therapeutic doses, noscapine shows little or no effect on the CNS or respiratory system, and has neither analgesic properties nor addictive liability. Constipation and other GI reactions have not been encountered to a significant degree.

The following additional ingredients may have antitussive properties but need to be tested objectively for effectiveness and safety:

- Beechwood creosote;
- Benzonatate;
- Camphor (lozenges);
- Caramiphen edisylate (ethanedisulfonate);
- Carbetapentane citrate;
- Cod liver oil;
- Elm bark;
- Ethylmorphine hydrochloride;
- Eucalyptol/eucalyptus oil (topical/inhalant);
- Horehound (horehound fluidextract);
- Menthol/peppermint oil (topical/inhalant);
- Thymol (topical/inhalant);
- Turpentine oil (spirits of turpentine or rectified turpentine oil) (topical/inhalant).

Oral Antibacterials and Anesthetics

A sore throat may indicate a more serious disease that demands medical attention (e.g., streptococcal pharyngitis), and self-treatment may mask the symptoms. When the sore throat symptom is not related to environmental factors, allergic rhinitis, or a cold, a physician should be consulted. Failure to do so may result in a worsening of the condition and development of complications.

For self-treatment of sore throat symptoms, many products promote relief, but only those containing local anesthetics have any basis for effectiveness. Because most of these products are lozenges, sprays, mouthwashes, gargles, and throatwashes, effectiveness is limited to the mucous membranes of the oral tract that can be reached by the dosage form. Local anesthetics have no beneficial effect in the treatment of laryngitis because the drug cannot be delivered to the site of inflammation.

Antibacterial Agents

The primary purpose of a mouthwash is to cleanse and soothe. Most mouthwashes are promoted for bad breath, with the suggestion that these products kill germs. However, much of the controversy surrounding the use of these products stems from problems associated with substantiating germicidal or germistatic claims. There is no method that effectively compares the germicidal activity in the test tube (in vitro) with that in the oral cavity (in vivo). There is also no adequate evidence that individuals benefit substantially from a nonspecific change in the flora of the oral cavity. It is possible that alteration of the normal oral cavity flora may actually allow invasion by pathogenic organisms. In addition, most infectious sore throats are viral in origin, and using a lozenge or gargle promoted as an antibacterial does not influence the viral pharyngitis. Thus, the American Dental Association Council on Dental Therapeutics does not recognize substantial contributions to oral health from medicated mouthwashes.[31]

The antimicrobial substances in most commercial mouthwashes are phenols, alcohol, quaternary ammonium compounds, volatile oils, oxygenating agents, and iodine-containing preparations. These agents are believed to be of little value in treating sore throat symptoms.

Anesthetic Agents

A possible benefit of oral mouthwashes, gargles, and lozenges is derived from the local anesthetics (e.g., benzocaine) they contain. These agents temporarily desensitize the sensory nerves in the pharyngeal mucosa, affording transient relief. The danger remains, however, of masking a symptom or condition that may be harmful.

Much controversy surrounds the effectiveness of the different local anesthetic ingredients in lozenges and mouthwashes promoted for relief of sore throats. The value and effectiveness of such an agent is usually established by testing on human skin, oral mucosa, or tongue, but not by pharyngeal tests. Consequently, patient satisfaction is probably the best current indicator of product effectiveness.

The pharmacist should recommend a product that contains an effective and well-tolerated dose or strength of a local anesthetic and a minimum of extraneous compounds. Not only is the effectiveness or value of extraneous compounds doubtful, but such agents may also increase the risk of a hypersensitivity reaction. The pharmacist should also try to follow up on patient responses to recommended agents to suggest alternative nonprescription therapy for pharyngeal soreness.

Benzocaine Benzocaine, the most commonly utilized local anesthetic in commercially available medicated lozenges, will produce local anesthesia in concentrations of 5–20%. Concentrations of less than 5% are not considered beneficial.

Phenol and Phenol-Containing Salts Phenol and phenol-containing compounds are included in several nonprescription liquids and lozenges as local anesthetics. These compounds are also effective antibacterial agents in concentrations of 0.5–1.5% if contact time with susceptible bacteria is adequate.[32]

Benzyl Alcohol Benzyl alcohol is a nonprescription oral anesthetic agent used in concentrations up to 10%.

Anticholinergics Although anticholinergics, such as atropine, have been shown to have no effect on sneezing or congestion caused by the common cold, they can theoretically dry excessive nasal secretions associated with a cold. High dosages are necessary, however, to achieve a therapeutic drying effect. Because the dosages of anticholinergics commonly found in nonprescription cold medications (0.06–0.2 mg of total alkaloids) are generally ineffective if given alone, these agents are often found in products that also contain an antihistamine. The additive anticholinergic effect obtained from such a combination could, in theory, help reduce secretions resulting from the common cold, but this claim remains to be objectively proven. Such a combination does, however, expose the patient to unwanted sedative effects of the antihistamine. Thus, it seems irrational to combine the therapeutic effect of one drug (in subtherapeutic amounts) with an unpredictable side effect of another in an attempt to achieve the effects obtainable with a larger (therapeutic) dose of a single agent.

Drug interactions involving anticholinergics are unlikely at doses used in nonprescription cold or allergy remedies that do not contain other ingredients with anticholinergic effects. However, hypersensitivity to these relatively small amounts does occur. If a hypersensitive individual also suffers from angle-closure glaucoma or an enlarged prostate, a physician should be contacted before a preparation containing an anticholinergic is taken. These products should also be used with caution in nonhypersensitive patients with cardiovascular disease.

The anticholinergics currently available in nonprescription products should not be considered primary contributors to the relief of cold or allergy symptoms. The FDA has determined that no anticholinergic agent is appropriate on efficacy or safety grounds for the treatment of the common cold. Any nonprescription product containing any anticholinergic intended for such a purpose is considered misbranded.

Antipyretics/Analgesics

Patients experiencing a common cold seldom have an actual clinical fever. More often they have a feeling of warmth or feverishness but little or no temperature elevation. The usefulness of aspirin, acetaminophen, or ibuprofen lies in relieving the discomforts of generalized aches and pains or malaise associated with the viral infection. (See Chapter 5, "Internal Analgesic Products.")

Ascorbic Acid (Vitamin C)

The claim that ascorbic acid is effective in preventing and treating the common cold is controversial. Linus Pauling, who popularized the use of ascorbic acid for this purpose, recommends 1–5 g per day as a prophylactic measure and as much as 15 g per day to treat a cold.[33] Many clinical studies have been conducted, however, and although some have shown trends in favor of ascorbic acid's effectiveness, they have not shown the vitamin to be unequivocally effective in any dosage in either preventing colds or reducing their severity or duration.

The potential for adverse effects associated with these large dosages of ascorbic acid is real. The most frequently noted adverse effect is diarrhea. Precipitation of urate, oxalate, or cystine stones in the urinary tract has been seen, and the potential for this problem increases with daily dosages of 1 g or above. The effects on the urinary excretion of other drugs also must be investigated because of ascorbic acid's ability to acidify the urine, thus increasing the elimination of basic drugs or the potential to reabsorb acidic drugs and their metabolites.

Urinary acidification increases the possibility of aminosalicylic acid crystalluria in patients receiving aminosalicylic acid in the free acid form. It also increases the excretion of drugs that are weak bases (e.g., amphetamines), reducing their effect, and it increases renal tubular salicylate reabsorption, increasing serum salicylate concentrations. Ascorbic acid in dosages large enough to acidify the urine (2–10 g per day) should not be given with aminosalicylic acid and should be used cautiously when salicylates are taken in large dosages (3–5 g per day).

Diabetic patients who are taking ascorbic acid and monitoring their condition by testing their urine using glucose oxidase test kits may encounter false-negative results; the copper reduction method may produce false-positive results.

Adjunctive Therapy

Inhaling water vapor as humidified air is an adjunctive therapeutic measure that provides a soothing effect to the respiratory mucosa. Humidifying inspired ambient air may aid in the relief of the cough and hoarseness that accompanies laryngitis and associated colds. Inhalation of humidified warm air has been shown to reduce symptoms of allergic rhinitis and the common cold and to increase nasal patency without adverse effects.[34] Another study, however, showed the use of heated vapor to have limited effectiveness in treating the cold.

Humidification may be a prophylactic measure against upper respiratory infections when people are exposed to low relative humidities. This is usually the case during the winter months when doors and windows are closed and heat-generating systems dry the air. The mucus viscosity increases with inspiration of dry air, and irritation of the respiratory mucosa may develop, creating a favorable environment for viral or bacterial invasion. The relative humidity may be as low as 10% in the home on a cold day; 40–50% is necessary for comfort, and 60–80% is better for persons with respiratory problems. However, at the higher level, condensation on windows and walls is a limiting factor.

The oldest method of humidifying air involves generating steam from a pot of boiling water or, more commonly, from an electric steam vaporizer. Newer methods involve formation of a cool mist by pumping water through a fine screen or by ultrasonically dispersing the water. Both methods disperse fine droplets of water. Therapeutically, the steam vaporizer does not seem to offer any readily apparent advantage over the cool mist vaporizer. Cool mist vaporizers are safe in that they do not generate heat or hot water. However, they are noisier and humidify somewhat more slowly than steam vaporizers. Moreover, unlike steam vaporizers, cool mist vaporizers become contaminated quickly, and may lower room temperature as the water particles absorb heat from the surrounding air, thereby chilling the air and causing air saturation at a lower temperature. In one study, 24 hospitalized patients contracted systemic infections with *Acinetobacter calcoaceticus* during a 4-month period; cold-air humidifiers at patients' bedsides were implicated as the source of infection in six patients. The outbreak ended with the removal of the humidifiers.[35] It is important to follow the manufacturer's directions for cleaning the cool mist unit to avoid bacterial overgrowth.

If humidification is supplemented with a volatile substance (menthol or compound benzoin tincture), a steam vaporizer must be used. It has not been established as to whether these volatile substances are of therapeutic value. They do not appear to have any advantage over unmedicated water vapor; in some cases, they may even cause irritation of the respiratory tract and could be potentially dangerous if they reached high concentrations in a small, enclosed room.

As an adjunctive measure, humidifying inspired air is important. Either a steam-generated unit or a cool mist vaporizer may be used as prophylaxis and should be used at the onset of a cold. It is also important to increase oral fluid intake (6–8 glasses of fluid a day) to prevent dehydration and encourage expectoration during a cold.

Devices have been introduced that force dry, hot air into the nose and mouth in an unproven attempt to "destroy" the virus and therefore treat and "cure" the common cold.[36] A solution of 0.05% hexylresorcinol has also been marketed for use in the "viralizer" device. However, there is no objective evidence to support any claims that these forced-air devices relieve symptoms or cure the common cold, and the FDA has disallowed product marketing of 0.05% hexylresorcinol for inhalation.

Controlled studies have shown that regular sauna bathing for longer than 3 months appears to decrease the incidence of the common cold.[37] Patients who take insulin, suffer from infection or anhidrosis, have consumed alcohol, or are pregnant should abstain from using a sauna.

Product Selection Guidelines

The effectiveness of many products available for self-treatment of cold symptoms may be questionable, but most such products are safe when used as directed. Experience may influence drug selection. The pharmacist must be prepared to distinguish between the common cold and allergic rhinitis on the basis of symptoms, recognize complications that may arise or have arisen, and recommend the proper approaches to control the symptoms (self-treatment or consultation with a physician), including drug therapy and adjunctive measures.

Patient Considerations

When symptoms typically associated with the common cold are present, recognizing the underlying disorder is not difficult. However, recognizing allergic rhinitis is often more difficult. In both conditions, the pharmacist should conduct a brief but careful history of the present illness. This history should provide information that is useful in distinguishing one disorder from another and in identifying those disorders or symptoms that should or should not be self-treated. The following specific points should be investigated:

- Abruptness of onset;
- Symptomatology;
- Intensity;
- Duration;
- Recurrence;
- Other medications being used;
- Concurrent medical problems;
- Family history of atopy.

Common cold onset is generally associated with a prodrome ("running nose" or dry throat); in fact, it is very common for people to predict that they are "coming down with a cold." Early in a cold's development, the symptoms are not very intense. As the infection runs its course, however, the symptoms may get worse, subject to patient variability and the infecting organism.

The intensity of symptoms in allergic rhinitis is based on the amount of allergen encountered and the degree of individual hypersensitivity. Generally, the symptoms are most intense following allergen exposure, and they subside over time unless additional exposures occur.

Duration of symptoms is a very important factor in differentiating a cold from allergic rhinitis. Typically, the common cold lasts 4–7 days. If symptoms persist beyond 7–10 days with no apparent improvement or if they tend to recur, a physician should be consulted for an evaluation. Duration of the symptoms of allergic rhinitis is extremely variable, partially because of individual sensitivity to the allergen. If the patient has received no relief in 10 days of self-treatment, physician evaluation and proper management are indicated.

The recurrent nature of seasonal allergic rhinitis is a hallmark in differentiating this condition from other nonallergic respiratory conditions. Symptoms often recur following high pollen counts or patient activities that result in increased allergen exposure. If the symptomatology is present throughout the year or persists after the first killing frost, the condition may be perennial allergic rhinitis. In this case, referral to a physician is desirable because of the prolonged duration of symptoms and the potential for developing complications.

Information regarding medications that have already been tried will aid the pharmacist not only in assessing the patient's current status but also in selecting a product. If, in the pharmacist's judgment, the measures were appropriate but were not effective, the patient should be encouraged to see a physician. If no medication was tried or if inadequate or inappropriate measures were taken, the pharmacist should recommend a more appropriate course of therapy. When a patient seeks the pharmacist's assistance in selecting a cold or allergy remedy, the pharmacist should question the individual about the presence of other acute or chronic illnesses. This process may identify patients for whom certain preparations should be used cautiously, if at all.

Orally administered preparations containing sympathomimetics should be given only on the advice of a physician to patients with hyperthyroidism (who are already predisposed to tachycardia and arrhythmias), hypertension (especially moderate to severe, in whom additional peripheral vasoconstriction may cause significant blood pressure elevation), diabetes mellitus (especially insulin-dependent diabetics and those in whom glycogenolysis may complicate glycemia control), or ischemic heart disease or angina (for whom an increase in heart rate may precipitate an acute angina attack and possibly a subsequent myocardial infarct). These concerns center primarily on the oral administration of sympathomimetic decongestants, in which systemic effects are predictable. Judiciously administered decongestant drops, sprays, or inhalations provide a local intranasal action without significant concern of systemic absorption.

Theoretically, all these effects may occur when a sympathomimetic reaches the systemic circulation. In practice, however, the effect on diabetic patients has not been a particular problem except in those who are extremely unstable (e.g., labile or brittle). The question often arises: "Should a diabetic patient take a liquid cough or cold preparation containing sugar?" The syrup vehicle may contain as much as 85% (weight per volume) sucrose, and each gram of sucrose has about 4 cal (17 kcal/tsp). If 4 tsp (about 70 kcal) are taken in 1 day, the additional (nondietary) calories may be clinically significant in a labile, brittle diabetic patient. Consequently, a sugar-free preparation is preferable. In a stable diabetic patient, however, these additional calories probably would be of little concern. (See Chapter 16, "Diabetes Care Products and Monitoring Devices.")

Another factor that pharmacists should consider when counseling a diabetic patient is the alcohol content of the product to be used. Alcohol, like sucrose, will provide calories—more calories, in fact, than an equal weight of sucrose. Because most liquid cough remedies contain alcohol (1–25%, each gram providing about 7 kcal), it is clear that a brittle diabetic patient taking a recommended dose might experience some difficulty with diabetes control. Persons taking disulfiram must be particularly mindful of alcohol in cough syrups. The minimum amount of alcohol necessary to trigger an adverse reaction or interaction in a disulfiram user has not been established. Products containing alcohol should also be used with caution in children.

The anticholinergic properties of antihistamines are usually not prominent in nonprescription preparations. In cases of glaucoma or urinary retention secondary to prostatic hypertrophy, preparations containing anticholinergic agents and antihistamines, especially in combination, should be used only on a physician's advice.

The pharmacist should obtain a medication history to avoid possible drug interactions and to identify and avoid drug allergies or idiosyncrasies. A history of chronic use of topical nasal decongestants may help identify rhinitis medicamentosa.

Product Considerations

Because of the large number of cold and allergy products (single entity and combinations), it is important that the pharmacist become familiar with a few preparations, especially those Category I products found to be safe and effective by the FDA. These products should be recommended preferentially. The pharmacist who recommends a nonprescription product must know what effect is sought, which drug entity will produce this effect, how much of the drug is necessary to produce this effect, and which nonprescription product satisfactorily meets these needs. The dosage of each ingredient should follow the FDA recommended dosage for the appropriate age of the user.

When only one effect is sought (e.g., nasal decongestion), a preparation with a single agent in a full therapeutic dose should be used. When more than one effect is desired, selection becomes more complex. Several single-entity products may be used, but a combination product will usually be preferable to the patient because of cost and convenience. The pharmacist should be selective in recommending combination products because many of these multidrug preparations are extreme examples of shotgun therapy.

Combinations recommended by the FDA advisory review panel provide a reasonable basis for selection when directions for use are followed carefully. The panel initially proposed that nonprescription products contain no more than three products from different pharmacologic groups. The FDA has subsequently adopted a policy of no fixed limit on the number of ingredients as long as the product can be shown to be rational, safe, and effective.

The pharmacist should select a combination product that deals as specifically as possible with the symptoms and that contains the desired agents in full therapeutic doses, with as few additional ingredients as possible. The pharmacist must decide which pharmacologic effects are most important and select the combination on the basis of the agents that will produce those desired effects.

There is no evidence that incorporating secondary agents or other ingredients of the same pharmacologic class in a subtherapeutic dose provides more relief or even as much relief as one agent at its full therapeutic dose. There is also no evidence that supports increased efficacy when two or more antihistamines are combined within a product. Adding a sufficient dosage of decongestant to an antihistamine in a product designed to treat allergic rhinitis is rational, and the decongestant may provide additional relief of symptoms and counteract some drowsiness produced by the antihistamine.

Combination products containing analgesic and antipyretic agents should generally not be recommended. Their routine use carries the risk of masking a fever that might indicate a bacterial infection. Also, if an adverse effect should occur, confusion would exist as to which agent was the cause. Such agents should be administered separately and only when needed.

Similarly, preparations that do not disclose the amounts of ingredients on the package should not be recommended. It would be difficult for a pharmacist to justify recommending a product to ameliorate a symptom when there is no indication as to how much of the active ingredients the product contains.

In general, the use of timed-release preparations allows better patient compliance and increased patient convenience. The recommendation of a timed-release preparation should be based on the presence of one or more pharmacologic agents in therapeutic doses and on the product's record of efficacy and safety.

Much controversy surrounds the use of oral nasal decongestants over the topical agents. Proponents of oral decongestants state that these agents can affect all respiratory membranes, are unaffected by the character of mucus, do not induce pathologic changes in the nasal mucosa, and relieve nasal obstruction without the additional irritation of locally applied medication.

There is also evidence to support the value of using short-term, topically applied vasoconstrictors. Although nasal sprays and drops do not represent the ideal dosage form, they do provide rapid relief. Because the relief is so dramatic, however, the patient may tend to overuse topical agents, risking drug-induced irritation of the nasal mucosa, alteration of the mucosal ciliary movement, and rhinitis medicamentosa.

Patient Consultation

In almost all cases of self-treatment, the pharmacist is the first health professional contacted. If the pharmacist takes the time to identify the patient's problem and ensure proper product selection, advice regarding proper use of the product must also be considered essential to fulfilling professional responsibility.

Patients cannot always be depended on to read, understand, and follow the package instructions. There is a tendency to believe in the philosophy that "if one is good, two are better." Because of the movement toward formulating nonprescription drug products in accordance with FDA recommended dosages, however, this is not the case. Pharmacists should caution patients against increasing the dosage or frequency of administration of any medication.

Even when antihistamines are taken in recommended amounts, they may cause transient drowsiness. Patients should be advised of this effect, especially if they are taking a prescription medication that also depresses the CNS. Patients should also be advised of possible additive effects, and they should determine what sedative effect the antihistamine has on them before engaging in activities requiring mental alertness, such as driving an automobile or operating heavy machinery. The patient should also be specifically warned of the additive sedation that will occur if the antihistamine is combined with alcohol.

Nasal solutions may become contaminated. The pharmacist should recommend that the tip of the dropper or the spray applicator be rinsed in hot water after use, that only one person use the spray or drop applicator, and that the bottle or spray be discarded when the medication is no longer needed. Contamination of the nasal dropper also may be minimized by keeping it out of direct contact with the nose or nasal surface.

In patients with allergic rhinitis, the presence of coughing; wheezing; tightness in chest (asthma); earache; and pain above the teeth, on the sides of the nose, or around the eyes (sinusitis) are all indications for medical referral. The patient should also consult a physician if nonprescription drugs are not markedly effective or if side effects persist even at reduced dosages.

Nondrug measures (humidification, increased fluid intake, and local heat) may be recommended, and although these suggestions may not seem acceptable to the patient who desires a medication, they may be quite beneficial. Saline gargles several times a day may help relieve an inflamed throat. However, patients using saline gargles should be warned against swallowing the solution. These solutions should also be used with caution by patients with cardiac disease, hypertension, or renal failure and by patients who are on salt-restricted diets.

A cold usually lasts approximately 7 days. The duration of therapy depends on which day in the course of the cold the medication is begun. If symptoms persist beyond the arbitrary, yet fairly reliable, 7-day limit despite adequate therapy, a physician should be consulted. If, after 2 or 3 days of therapy, the symptoms either do not improve or become more intense, or if a fever, a very painful sore throat, or a cough associated with mucopurulent sputum develops, the patient should seek a physician's diagnosis of the condition.

It is important for the patient to realize that a cold will usually resolve itself despite the medication and other measures recommended, that the medication is intended only to relieve discomfort, and that relief should occur in a week or less. The concern for duration of self-treatment stems not only from the potential adverse effects of some medications but also from the minority of cold sufferers who may develop complications, such as secondary bacterial infections. If the pharmacist does not stipulate a time limit for therapy, patients may unknowingly continue self-treating with little effect, prolonging their discomfort and delaying a physician's diagnosis and appropriate treatment.

Product selection must be based not only on the presence of an effective agent in a therapeutic amount but also on underlying disorders that may be influenced adversely by the recommended therapy. Having chosen the product, the pharmacist must then ensure that the patient knows how to take the medication, how long to take it, and what to expect from it with regard to both symptomatic relief and adverse effects. Lastly, the pharmacist should always encourage the patient to return or call back if there are any questions.

Summary

By evaluating the presenting symptoms, the pharmacist can usually distinguish the common cold from disorders such as influenza or allergic rhinitis. The pharmacist can then offer both proper suggestions for treatment and medications to provide the allergic rhinitis sufferer with symptomatic relief. By conducting a careful history and recognizing the pertinent symptoms, the pharmacist may achieve a partial diminution of the symptoms through advice and medication.

Recommendations for the common cold should be directed at relieving symptoms; those for allergic rhinitis should be directed first at preventing symptoms and then at relieving them. The pharmacist's endorsement of a shotgun remedy is generally irrational, as is recommending a particular product if it contains the needed drug in less than therapeutic amounts.

Common cold treatment objectives include reducing nasal secretions, opening congested nasal passages, reducing the frequency of a cough, soothing a sore throat, overcoming the hoarseness of laryngitis, and relieving feverishness and headache. For allergic rhinitis, the treatment is directed at blocking or competing with the effect of released histamine, relieving nasal congestion, and diminishing secondary symptoms such as pharyngitis and headache.

The very few oral nasal decongestants available as single-entity products should be recommended for managing symptoms of the common cold. Topically applied products should contain only the decongestant. Oral antihistamines in combination with nasal decongestants may be indicated in allergic rhinitis; they should be avoided in treating the common cold, however, because of the lack of evidence to support the beneficial effect of antihistamine use in this regard.

The frequency of cough resulting from a cold may be controlled by humidification of the inspired air (with a steam or cool mist vaporizer) or the use of cough-suppressing medication. A demulcent to the oral and pharyngeal mucosa (hard candy or cough drop), an expectorant (guaifenesin), a cough suppressant (codeine or dextromethorphan), and the antihistamine diphenhydramine used as an antitussive are included in the armamentarium for the treatment of a cough associated with a cold. Products that contain a cough suppressant in combination with an expectorant should not be recommended. In the case of a dry cough, the dosage of the cough suppressant is the criterion by which a product is selected. Productive coughs should not generally be treated with cough suppressants. Administration of 15 mg of codeine or dextromethorphan usually decreases the cough's frequency and intensity adequately.

The dry, sore throat present in colds and, to a lesser extent, in allergic rhinitis may be relieved by dissolving a piece of hard candy in the mouth to stimulate saliva flow. Frequent warm, normal saline gargles may also relieve symptoms. Significant relief may be obtained from a lozenge or throat spray containing an anesthetic such as benzocaine in sufficient concentration. Topical antibacterials for a viral infection or allergic rhinitis are of no value. A throat that is markedly sore and accompanied by swollen lymph nodes, fever, and constitutional symptoms may be caused by bacterial rather than viral infection. The patient should be directed to seek medical care for appropriate diagnostic tests and antimicrobial therapy. For nonbacterial pharyngitis, a sore throat product may be used for as long as the symptom persists.

Laryngitis may be managed by water vapor inhalation, voice rest, and avoidance of inhaled irritants such as tobacco smoke. Dissolving lozenges in the mouth, gargling, or using a throat spray does little to soothe the inflamed laryngeal tissues.

Relief from feverishness and headache may be provided by using an analgesic/antipyretic, such as aspirin, acetaminophen, or ibuprofen. Products containing these agents in combination with other ingredients are not recommended. Taking an antipyretic agent regularly during a common cold or acute allergic rhinitis masks the possible development of fever, which could indicate a secondary bacterial infection. An antipyretic agent should be used to bring acute relief only as needed. Products containing aspirin or other salicylates should be avoided in children and adolescents when influenza, chickenpox, or another viral infection is suspected because of the associated risk of Reye's syndrome.

Antihistamines are effective in relieving symptoms of allergic rhinitis; however, their role in the treatment of symptoms associated with the common cold is controversial and, at best, only adjunctive because of mild anticholinergic drying effects. There is marked individual variability among the different antihistamines in both pharmacologic effect and sedation. The pharmacist should be aware of this variability and should be prepared to suggest an alternative if relief is not obtained with the original agent or if side effects are poorly tolerated. Most antihistamines in commercial products are found in combination with other ingredients. A combination of these agents may be best used to treat allergic rhinitis, for which the only rational combination is an oral antihistamine with an oral nasal decongestant. Other ingredients found in nonprescription products are of dubious efficacy.

The duration of therapy in managing symptoms of a cold depends on when during the course of a cold the patient decides to start treatment. In any case, the patient should be able to stop treatment on the sixth or seventh day of the cold. However, slight symptoms, such as cough, may persist for another day or so and may be treated, if necessary.

The duration of treatment of allergic rhinitis should be limited to 3 days when topical nasal decongestants are used in order to minimize the chances of rhinitis medicamentosa. Generally, oral decongestant therapy should be limited to 10 consecutive days; the patient's need for such therapy beyond 10 days may indicate the development of complications, and the patient should be referred to a physician. An antihistamine product may be used prophylactically for acute allergic rhinitis during periods when exposure to allergens is increased.

Patients who have a common cold or allergic rhinitis offer the pharmacist many opportunities to be involved. Although pharmacists cannot counsel every cold or hay fever sufferer, they should be available as a health and drug information resource as other professional responsibilities permit.

References

1. Establishment of a monograph for OTC cold, cough, allergy, bronchodilator and antiasthmatic products. *Federal Register* 1976 Sept 9; 41: 38312.
2. Wyngarden JB, Smith LH. *Cecil Textbook of Medicine*. 18th ed. Philadelphia: W. B. Saunders; 1988: 1750–7.
3. Christie AG. *Infectious Disease—Epidemiology and Clinical Practice*. 4th ed. New York: Churchill Livingston; 1987: 416–7, 442, 444–5, 459.
4. Sperber SJ, Levine PA, Sorrentino JV, et al. Ineffectiveness of recombinant interferon—beta serine nasal drops for prophylaxis of natural colds. *J Infect Dis* 1989 Oct; 160: 700–5.
5. Sperber SJ, Hayden FG. Chemotherapy of rhinovirus colds. *Antimicrob Agent Chemother* 1988 Apr; 32: 409–19.
6. Current estimates from the National Health Interview Survey. *Vital and Health Statistics,* Series 10, No. 160. Washington, DC: Public Health Service; 1986.
7. Cypress BK. Medication therapy in office visits for selected diagnosis. National Ambulatory Medical Care Survey. *Vital and Health Statistics,* Series 13, No. 71. Washington, DC: Public Health Service; 1983: 1–47.
8. Cohen S, Tyrell DAJ, Smith AP. Psychological stress and susceptibility to the common cold. *N Engl J Med* 1991 Aug 29; 325: 606–12.
9. Price J. Asthma in children: diagnosis. *Br Med J* 1984; 288: 1666–8.
10. Gregg I, Gotoh T, Ueda S, et al. Protein components of bronchoalveolar lavage fluids from non-smokers. *Eur J Respir Dis* 1983; 64: 369–77.
11. Marchant CD, Shurin PA. Therapy of otitis media. *Pediatr Clin North Am* 1983; 30: 281–96.
12. Jackler RK, Kaplan MJ. In: Schroeder SA, Krupp MA, Tierney LM, et al., eds. *Current Medical Diagnosis and Treatment 1989*. Norwalk, Conn: Appleton and Lange; 1989: 116.
13. Krober MS, Stracener CE, Bass JW. Decreased measles antibody response after measles–mumps–rubella vaccine in infants with colds. *JAMA* 1991 Apr 24; 265: 2095–6.
14. Bolinger AM, Serrano Murphy VA, Bubica G. General pediatric therapy. In: Young LY, Koda-Kimble MA, eds. *Applied Therapeutics: The Clinical Use of Drugs*. 4th ed. Vancouver, Wash: Applied Therapeutics, Inc; 1988: 1817–60.
15. Komaroff AL, Buchwald D. Symptoms and signs of chronic fatigue syndrome. *Rev Infect Dis* 1991; 13 (suppl 1): S8–S11.
16. Refinetti P, Novahistine in the treatment of congestive processes of the respiratory tract. *Curr Ther Res Clin Exp* 1981 Jul; 30: 33–37.
17. Cold, cough, allergy, bronchodilator, and antiasthmatic drug products for over-the-counter human use; Expectorant drug products for over-the-counter human use; Final monograph; Final rule. *Federal Register* 1989 Feb 28; 54: 8495.
18. Ricketti AJ. *Allergic Diseases—Diagnosis and Management*. Philadelphia: Lippincott; 1985: 207–31.
19. Cookson W, Sharp PA, Faux JA, et al. Linkage between immunoglobulin E responses underlying asthma and rhinitis and chromosome 11q. *Lancet* 1989 Jun 10; 1: 1292–5.
20. Sherman WB. *Hypersensitivity Mechanisms and Management*. Philadelphia: W. B. Saunders; 1968.
21. O'Loughlin JM. Non-allergics' guide to allergic rhinitis. *Drug Ther* 1974 Aug; 4: 47–48, 52–55.
22. Trigg CJ, Davis RJ. Allergic rhinitis. *Arch Dis Child* 1991 May; 66: 565–7.
23. Bernstein JM, Ellis E, Li P. The role of IgE-mediated hypersensitivity in otitis media with effusion. *Otolaryngol Head Neck Surg* 1981 Sept–Oct; 89: 874–8.
24. Naclerio RM. Allergic rhinitis. *N Engl J Med* 1991 Sept; 325: 860–69.
25. Hutton N, Wilson MH, Mellits ED, et al. Effectiveness of an antihistamine-decongestant combination for young children with the common cold: a randomized, controlled clinical trial. *J Pediatr* 1991 Jan; 118: 125–30.
26. Lake CR, Gallant S, Masson E, et al. Adverse drug effects attributed to phenylpropanolamine: a review of 142 case reports. *Am J Med* 1990 Aug; 89: 195.
27. Hirsch SR. What role expectorants. *Drug Ther* 1976; 5 (4): 179–89.
28. Borde M, Nizamie SH. Dependence on the common cough

syrup. *Lancet* 1988 Apr 2; 1: 760.
29. Cold, cough, allergy, bronchodilator, and antiasthmatic drug products for over-the-counter human use; Final monograph for OTC antitussive drug products; Final rule. *Federal Register* 1987 Aug 12; 52: 30049.
30. Matthys H. *J Intern Med* 1983; 11: 92.
31. *Accepted Dental Therapeutics*. 38th ed. Chicago: American Dental Association; 1979.
32. Valle-Jones JC. Chloraseptic liquid in sore throat. *Practitioner* 1983 Jun; 227: 1037–40.
33. Pauling L. *Vitamin C and the Common Cold*. San Francisco: W. H. Freeman; 1970.
34. Ophir D, Elad Y. Effects of steam inhalation on nasal patency and nasal symptoms in patients with the common cold. *Am J Otolaryngol* 1987 May; 8: 149–53.
35. Smith PW, Massanari RM. Room humidifiers as the source of *Acinetobacter* infections. *JAMA* 1977 Feb 21; 237: 795–7.
36. The viralizer for the common cold. *Med Lett Drug Ther* 1989 Jan 27; 31: 8.
37. Ernst E. Sauna—a hobby or for health? *J R Soc Med* 1989 Nov; 82: 639.

CHAPTER 9

Asthma Products

H. William Kelly and Mary Beth O'Connell

Questions to ask in patient assessment and counseling

- *Has a physician diagnosed your condition as asthma?*
- *Are you under the care of a physician?*
- *Do you have any other medical problems, such as heart disease, seizures, high blood pressure, hyperthyroidism, or diabetes?*
- *What prescription or nonprescription medications are you currently taking?*
- *Have you used any asthma products in the past? If so, which ones? Were they effective? Did they cause any problems (side effects)? If so, what were they?*
- *How often during each day and during each week do you use a bronchodilator inhaler?*
- *Would you demonstrate how you use your inhaler?*

An estimated 10 million persons in the United States—including 3 million children—have asthma. From 1980 to 1987, the reported prevalence rate increased 29% to 40.1 per 1,000 population.[1] The estimated cost of treating asthma in the United States in 1990 was approximately $6.2 billion.[2] The largest single direct medical expenditure was inpatient hospital services (emergency care), reaching almost $1.5 billion. Loss of school days was the largest single indirect cost, approaching $1 billion. In total, approximately 43% of the economic impact of asthma was associated with emergency room use, hospitalization, and death.

The increased morbidity and mortality from asthma in the United States and worldwide in the last decade has been a major concern and was the impetus for the National Heart, Lung, and Blood Institute to establish the National Asthma Education Program (NAEP) and an expert panel to provide guidelines for the diagnosis and management of asthma.[1]

Anatomy of the Respiratory Tract

The respiratory system is a series of airways, starting with the nose and mouth and leading ultimately to the terminal air sacs or alveoli. The mouth and nasal passages lead to the pharynx, which branches out into the esophagus and the trachea. The trachea divides into the two large mainstem bronchi that supply air to the lungs. Each bronchus progressively divides into smaller airways (bronchioles), leading through the alveolar ducts to the alveoli.[3] Layers of smooth muscle are wrapped around the airways in diminishing amounts as the airways progress toward the alveoli. As an airway branches, the walls become progressively thinner. At the level of the alveoli, all that remains is a thin layer of cells surrounded by pulmonary capillaries. Respiration, which is the exchange of gases, occurs in the alveoli. Inspired oxygen passes across the alveolar walls into the capillaries, and carbon dioxide diffuses in the opposite direction and is expired.

The lungs are essentially elastic air sacs suspended in the airtight thoracic cavity. The movable walls of this cavity are formed by the sternum, ribs, and diaphragm. The ribs are attached to the spinal vertebrae and join together at the sternum (breastbone). As the thoracic cavity expands, the pressure within it becomes less than the atmospheric pressure, air enters, and the lungs expand. This process is accomplished by means of two simultaneous mechanisms. The diaphragm, a dome-shaped muscle (when relaxed) that extends upward into the thoracic cavity, contracts. As it contracts, the diaphragm becomes flattened and moves downward into the abdomen, increasing the longitudinal size of the thoracic cavity. Simultaneous contraction of the external intercostal muscles raises the ribs, causing an elevation and forward movement of the sternum and an increase in the diameter of the chest cavity. During inspiration, the diaphragm and ribs move simultaneously, expanding the thoracic cavity and thus allowing the lungs to fill with air. Expiration results from relaxation of the ventilatory muscles and the elastic recoil force of the alveoli and airways.

The nasal cavities are lined with highly vascular mucous membranes and ciliated epithelial cells interspersed with mucus-producing goblet cells. During normal inspiration, as air passes over these areas enroute to the alveoli, it is warmed, humidified, and filtered. Dust particles, bacteria, and other foreign matter are trapped in the mucus and propelled upward with it toward the pharynx by the wavelike movement of the nasal cilia; they are then deposited in the oral cavity, where they are either expelled or swallowed. The humidification and filtration processes continue as air passes through the trachea, bronchi, and bronchioles.

Bronchial smooth muscle tone and mucus secretion are under neural and humoral control (Figure 1).[4] Afferent nerves leading from irritant receptors in the mucosal epithelium produce reflex bronchoconstriction, increased mucus production, and cough through cholinergic

---

Editor's Note: This chapter is based in part on the chapter with the same title that appeared in the 9th edition but was written by H. William Kelly and Celeste Lindley.

innervation of bronchial smooth muscle and goblet cells from the vagus nerve. Smooth muscle of the airway is only sparsely innervated by the adrenergic system; however, smooth muscle throughout the entire airway contains beta-adrenergic receptors. Alpha-adrenergic stimulation produces smooth muscle contraction (primarily vascular), and $beta_2$-adrenergic stimulation produces smooth muscle relaxation. The nonadrenergic, noncholinergic (NANC) nervous system is the principal inhibitory system of the airways, counteracting the cholinergic excitatory system.[4] Stimulation of the NANC system through the vagus nerve primarily produces bronchodilation but can also produce bronchoconstriction. Neurotransmission through the NANC system is mediated by neuropeptides, which have not been conclusively identified. It appears that vasoactive intestinal peptide acts as an inhibitory transmitter and that substance P acts as an excitatory transmitter.[4] Under normal circumstances, these systems assist in maintaining normal bronchomotor tone.

Epidemiology and Etiology of Asthma

The NAEP expert panel report defines asthma as a lung disease with the following characteristics:

- Airway obstruction that is reversible (but not completely so in some patients) either spontaneously or with treatment;
- Airways inflammation;
- Increased airway responsiveness to a variety of stimuli.[1]

The death rate from asthma increased 31% from 1980 to 1987, with 4,360 deaths reported in 1987.[1] The cause of the increase in mortality is unknown, but the increase has been greater in elderly and urban populations. Among persons aged 15–44 years, African-Americans have a death rate five times that of Caucasians. Recently, the excessive use of sympathomimetic metered-dose inhalers has been implicated as a risk factor for asthma mortality.[5,6] In addition, retrospective studies of asthma deaths both outside and inside the hospital indicate that underassessment of the severity of illness by both patients and the medical profession has led to inadequate therapy and is a major contributing factor in most asthma-related deaths.[1] And because most deaths occur outside the hospital, impaired access to medical care has also been proposed as a contributing factor.

Symptomatic asthma is more common in children, with the age of onset being under 10 years of age for 50% of all subjects.[7] The prevalence rate is slightly higher in males until puberty, at which time the gender ratio is approximately equal. Often, symptoms significantly decrease in severity as patients age, so the overall prognosis for children who develop asthma is good. Longitudinal studies indicate that 50–70% of asthmatic children have a permanent or temporary symptom-free remission by adulthood. However, 30% of asthmatic children continue to have chronic symptoms into adulthood. Asthma is present in 3.8% of men and 7.1% of women over age 65.[8] Evidence increasingly suggests that chronic asthma can result in irreversible chronic obstruction.[7]

The precise etiology of asthma is not known. However, epidemiologic studies in families and twins suggest a genetic component.[7] Respiratory infections, particularly respiratory syncytial virus bronchiolitis, appear to be a significant environmental factor. Chronic exposure to allergens and respiratory irritants such as passive smoke may also be contributing environmental factors. However, the relationship between atopy and asthma is complex. Atopy in parents and children predicts an increased risk of developing asthma but is not essential, and not all allergic patients develop asthma.[7] Although underlying lung pathology is common to all asthmatics, patients often differ in what incites their asthma, and are therefore often classified according to their predominant trigger. But regardless of whether they are classified as extrinsic (allergic) or intrinsic asthmatics, all patients with asthma have elevated serum levels of immunoglobulin E.

Asthma is generally exacerbated by respiratory tract infections, primarily viral ones; inhaled allergens such as pollen, dust, or mold; inhaled air pollutants; exercise; or occupational and industrial irritants, sulfites, or drugs. An identifiable allergen is the major precipitating factor in 35–55% of the asthmatic population, and respiratory infections are a major factor in about 40%.[1] About 2–10% of asthmatics develop acute asthma following ingestion of aspirin or other nonsteroidal anti-inflammatory drugs.[4]

Pathophysiology of Asthma

Although the cellular defect in asthma is still unknown, it is now recognized that unchecked inflammation of the airways is the principal cause of their excessive reactivity to various triggering events.[1,4,9] This bronchial hyperreactivity (BHR) is characterized by (1) smooth muscle contraction (bronchoconstriction), (2) mucus hypersecretion, (3) mucosal edema, and (4) epithelial desquamation (Figure 2). The inflammatory process in asthma is characterized by submucosal infiltration of eosinophils and lymphocytes, with epithelial shedding and hyperplasia of the basement membrane.[9] Tissue mast cells increase in number and often appear to be activated.[4] Mast cell degranulation, which is produced by exercise, exposure to allergen, hyperosmolar conditions from hyperventilation, or occupational or environmental irritants, may release preformed mediators such as histamine; eosinophil chemotactic factor; platelet activating factor; prostaglandins; and leukotrienes C-4, D-4, and E-4. This is known as the early asthmatic response (EAR). Although the relative importance of each mediator in the pathogenesis of asthma is still unknown, each is capable of producing bronchoconstriction; stimulating mucus secretion; increasing vascular permeability; and attracting and activating eosinophils, neutrophils, and lymphocytes.[4] The activated eosinophils are then capable of releasing toxins such as major basic protein, which can desquamate epithelium. The lymphocytes release cytokines capable of retaining and priming eosinophils in the airways as well as amplifying effects of other mediators.[10]

The bronchial smooth muscle hypertrophy, goblet cell hypertrophy, and excessive mucus production are secondary to the ongoing inflammatory process. Although imbalances in neural control of the airways have been

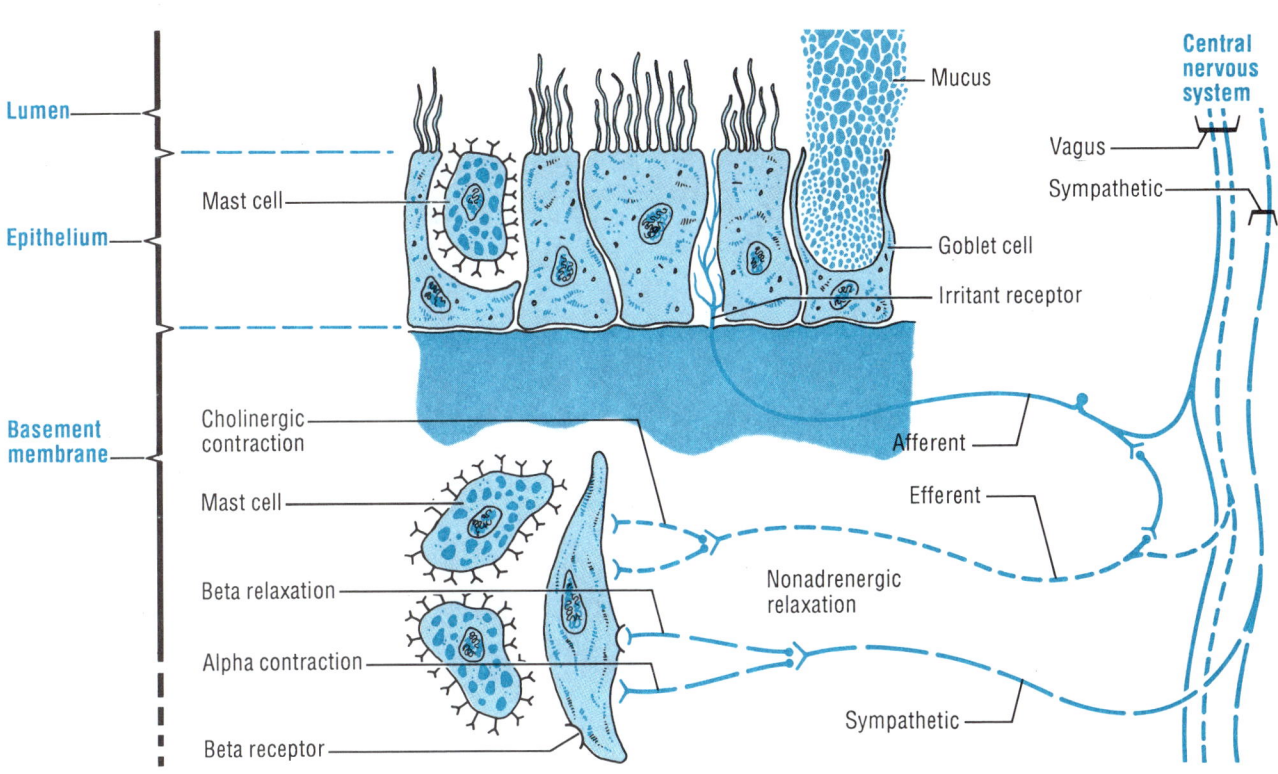

FIGURE 1 Innervation of the airways by the sympathetic, cholinergic, and nonadrenergic inhibitory systems. Mast cell concentration increases from the epithelial lumen to the submucosa. Adapted with permission from *Pharmacotherapy: A Pathophysiologic Approach.* 2nd ed. Dipiro J. et al., eds. New York: Elsevier Science Publishing; 1992: 410.

postulated as a primary cause of BHR, it now appears that, if such imbalances exist, they are more likely to play a role in amplifying the inflammation and bronchoconstriction.[4] Bronchial smooth muscle from asthmatics taken out of the inflammatory milieu of the airways does not react any differently to contracting or relaxing substances than does bronchial smooth muscle from nonasthmatics.

The characteristic feature of the asthmatic is excessive BHR to various stimuli. The clinical severity and need for therapy correlate with the degree of BHR; acute exacerbations are associated with an increase in BHR.[11] The degree of BHR can be measured with a number of pharmacologic (histamine, methacholine, or propranolol), physical (cold air or hypertonic saline), or physiologic (exercise or eucapnic hyperventilation of dry air) stimuli. The standard approach is bronchoprovocation with inhaled histamine or methacholine, which are defined as "nonspecific" bronchoprovocation stimuli to differentiate them from "specific" allergen bronchoprovocation stimuli. Patients inhale increasing concentrations in doubling increments of either histamine or methacholine, and spirometric measurements are made after each increment. The provocative dose or concentration that produces a 20% drop in forced expiratory volume exhaled in 1 second (FEV_1) is calculated, and that value is used as a measure of tissue reactivity.[11] A lower provocative concentration indicates greater BHR.

BHR is increased following allergen exposure, viral respiratory tract infections, and environmental exposure to pollutants. It is decreased as a result of allergen avoidance and therapy with certain anti-inflammatory drugs. A positive bronchoprovocation challenge is consistent with but not diagnostic of asthma.[11] Positive bronchoprovocation challenges can occur in cystic fibrosis, chronic obstructive lung disease, and allergic rhinitis as well, although symptomatic asthmatics have greater BHR. Studies using bronchoalveolar washings and biopsies have now demonstrated a good correlation between the numbers of various inflammatory cells and desquamated epithelial cells and the degree of BHR.[10,11] In the past, asthma could only be diagnosed if reversibility (defined as at least a 15% improvement in FEV_1 following treatment with a bronchodilator) was present with spirometry. Now the diagnosis can be confirmed by bronchoprovocation in patients with normal spirometry on examination but a history consistent with asthma. Spirometry often does not correlate with BHR, so bronchoprovocation is a more sensitive indicator of airway inflammation.

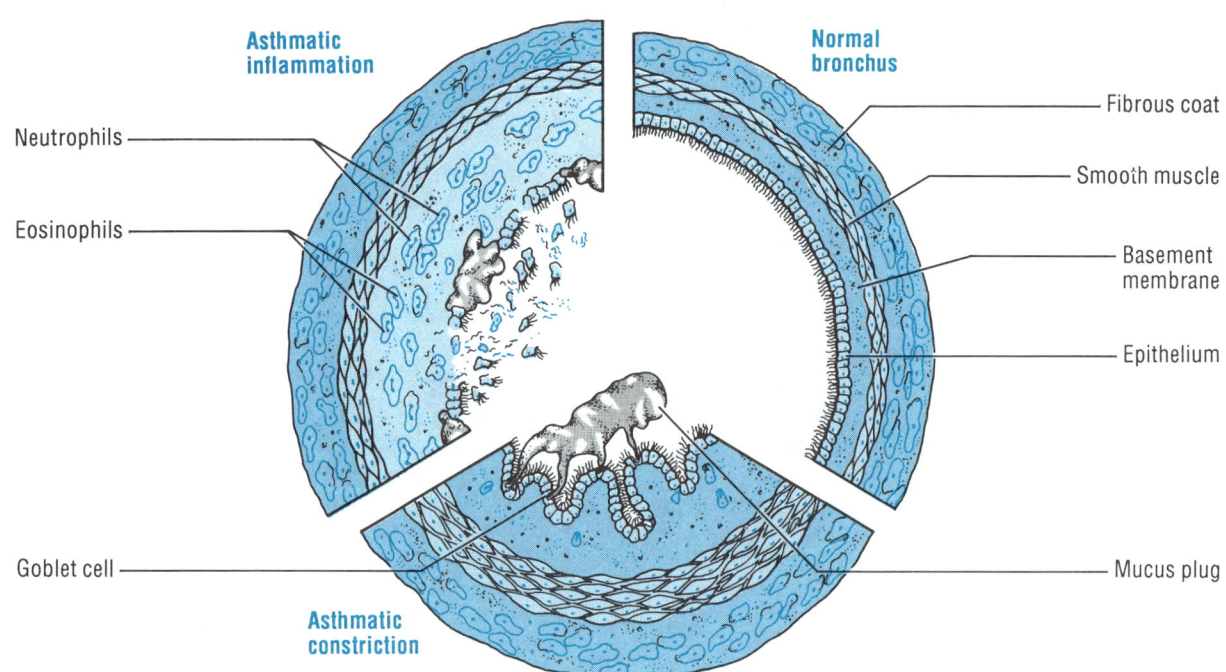

FIGURE 2 Representative illustration of the pathology found in the asthmatic bronchus compared with a normal bronchus (upper right section). Each section demonstrates how the lumen is narrowed. Edema of the basement membrane, mucus plugging, smooth muscle hypertrophy, and construction contribute (lower section). Inflammatory cells producing epithelial desquamation fill the airway lumen with cellular debris and expose the airway smooth muscle to other mediators (upper left section). Adapted with permission from *Pharmacotherapy: A Pathophysiologic Approach*. 2nd ed. Dipiro J. et al., eds. New York: Elsevier Science Publishing; 1992: 409.

Within 5 minutes of inhaling a specific allergen, asthmatics demonstrate a drop in pulmonary functions that bottoms out in 10–20 minutes and then spontaneously improves within 1 hour. Many asthmatics will undergo a second bronchoconstrictive response 4–12 hours later, which may persist for 2–4 hours. This response, known as the late asthmatic response (LAR), is one key factor involved with increasing BHR and maintaining that increase. The LAR occurs after inflammatory cells infiltrate the airways and is associated with an increase in BHR that does not occur with an EAR alone. Drugs that effectively block the LAR prevent the increase in BHR and can lower BHR with chronic use (Table 1). Specific allergen avoidance can also prevent the usual seasonal increases in BHR in asthmatics as well as lower their BHR over time.

Symptoms of Asthma

By definition, asthma is episodic in nature. Periods of airway obstruction may last from a few minutes to several days. The severity of obstruction is highly variable, producing mild symptoms or rapidly progressing to respiratory failure. Patients with more severe disease may have continuous symptoms that require chronic medication for control; others may have normal pulmonary function between episodes and require only periodic medication.

The classic symptom of asthma is wheezing (a fine whistling sound) on expiration; in more severe obstruction, wheezing may occur on inspiration as well. Coughing as a result of stimulation of the irritant receptors is common. Chronic cough may be the only presenting symptom in some patients with asthma. Patients may have normal spirometric pulmonary function tests between episodes, but many asthmatics have an increased bronchomotor tone, which is readily reversed with a bronchodilator drug. During attacks, asthmatics demonstrate a marked decrease in all measures of expiratory flow rate and often complain of a tightness in their chest and of dyspnea (difficult breathing). Because outflow of air is obstructed to a greater degree than inflow, the lungs actually become overinflated and the patient has to breathe at higher lung volumes, which makes breathing more difficult. Patients then become "air hungry" and apprehensive. About 30–50% of asthmatic patients complain of excessive sputum production. The sputum is usually yellowish and, upon microscopic examination, full of eosinophils.

Patient Assessment

As with other diseases, medical diagnosis of asthma is essential to rule out other causes of pulmonary symptoms such as physical obstruction from a tumor, congestive heart failure, and chronic bronchitis. For example, if a patient with new pulmonary symptoms describes a history of hypertension or heart disease, physician referral is critical. A patient who awakens in the middle of the night with dyspnea and cough resulting from pulmonary edema ("cardiac asthma") may have congestive heart failure. As another example, shortness of breath and chest pain in women taking oral contraceptives may be signs of pulmonary emboli rather than asthma, and such patients should also be referred to a physician immediately. Patients with chronic bronchitis and emphysema experience some symptoms similar to those associated with asthma. However, these symptoms are usually continuous, not episodic, and should not be treated with nonprescription drugs except under a physician's direction.

If a diagnosis of asthma has been previously established, it is important to determine how severe the symptoms are and which self-treatment approaches have already been attempted. Patients need immediate medical intervention if shortness of breath makes them unable to complete a full sentence without stopping, if discomfort persists while they are at rest after using a bronchodilator, or if the bronchodilator does not completely relieve their symptoms. If a bronchodilator is being used but the dyspnea becomes worse, a severe attack may be imminent or in progress, and the patient should see a physician immediately. Patients with progressive dyspnea and wheezing and who are dependent on nonprescription products may be in danger of severe pulmonary obstruction, which may require hospitalization.

Nonprescription medications may be appropriate for the treatment of patients with documented mild asthma. More potent medications, available by prescription, are required for the treatment of moderate and severe asthma. The pharmacist should be actively involved in the patient's decision process to use nonprescription medications. If the underlying disease is asthma, self-treating may delay the patient seeking necessary medical care and result in resistant acute severe asthma attacks. Furthermore, the nonprescription asthma medications are predominantly bronchodilators, and the evolving philosophy for treating chronic asthma also involves the use of anti-inflammatory agents.[1]

It is extremely important for the pharmacist to determine the pattern of use for patients using nonprescription bronchodilator inhalers. Patients with symptoms greater than one to two times weekly with nocturnal asthma should be strongly encouraged to seek medical advice and to consider using a home peak flow meter for a more objective physical assessment. If the symptoms are new and the patient has not been diagnosed by a physician as having asthma, physician referral for evaluation is essential.

In most cases, the patients themselves make the diagnosis of asthma after several episodes of intermittent shortness of breath and wheezing.[12] Tightness in the chest and cough are often present and usually come and go with each attack. In some cases, however, chronic cough and shortness of breath may occur. Many patients have mild asthma that does not progress; in others, the condition may worsen and be accompanied by dyspnea and wheezing, cough, tachycardia, retraction of the sternocleidomastoid muscle, apprehension, chest distention, tenacious sputum, and flaring nostrils. Sinus tachycardia with a pulse rate up to 120 beats per minute is a very common finding, as is sternocleidomastoid muscle retraction in patients with severe airway obstruction.[12]

It is extremely important to recognize that delay in seeking medical care is a major contributing factor to asthma mortality.[1] Subjective symptoms of wheezing and dyspnea are notoriously poor measures of lung function and contribute to such delay. Thus, the NAEP expert panel has recommended home monitoring of peak expiratory flow rate (PEFR) with portable peak flow meters in all chronic, moderate to severe asthmatics.[1]

Various brands of peak flow meters are available, but they all work similarly to achieve the same objective: to determine the PEFR, or the maximum rate of air flow following forced expiration. The PEFR correlates well with a patient's FEV and provides an objective at-home measurement of airway obstruction. These devices are to asthmatics what a home blood pressure monitor is to hypertensive patients and what a blood glucose meter is to diabetic patients. Thus, proper use of these devices is important and pharmacists should ensure proper technique.

In using a peak flow meter, the patient should:

- Set the meter indicator on the bottom of the scale before each forced expiration;
- Take all measurements while standing;
- Not cover the hole in the back of the meter;
- Take a deep breath;
- Purse the lips tightly around the mouthpiece;
- Rest the mouthpiece on the tongue but not obstruct the opening of the mouthpiece with the tongue;
- Expire hard and fast (forcefully);
- Record the best of three efforts as the peak flow value.

The NAEP's expert panel recommends that the patient and physician determine the patient's best peak flow. Once an asthma patient's personal best peak flow has been adequately determined, the "three-zone" system may be used to relate peak flow readings to

TABLE 1 Phase activity of asthma medications

Medication	Early asthmatic response	Late asthmatic response
Beta$_2$ agonist	+	−[a]
Theophylline	+	−
Steroids	−	+
Cromolyn	+	+
Nedocromil	+	+
Anticholinergics	+	−
H$_1$ antihistamines	−	−

Key:
+ means medication inhibits this response.
− means medication does not inhibit this response.
[a]Long-acting investigational beta$_2$ agonists may inhibit the LAR.

Information extracted from:
Lipworth BJ, McDevitt DG. *Br J Clin Pharmacol* 1992; 33: 129–38.
Twentyman OP et al. *Lancet* 1990 Dec 1; 336: 1338–42.

TABLE 2	Three-zone system of asthma management	
Zone	Peak flow values	Patient guideline
Green	≥80–100% of the patient's personal best, or the predicted flow value indicated by a standard chart	*Go!* Continue regular activity and regular asthma maintenance therapy
Yellow	50–80% of the patient's personal best, or the predicted flow value indicated by a standard chart	*Caution!* Patient may require additional medication or increase in regular maintenance therapy
Red	<50% of the patient's personal best, or the predicted flow value indicated by a standard chart	*Stop!* Seek medical advice or medication immediately

asthma management (Table 2). However, this color-coded scheme, which uses a traffic light analogy, should serve as a guideline only: the patient and his or her physician should individualize the system by defining the peak flow values for each zone that will provide optimal therapy for the patient.

Treatment of Asthma

The role of the pharmacist in an ambulatory setting should focus on (1) patient education; (2) evaluation of compliance; (3) safe, effective, and appropriate use of medications and devices; and (4) patient monitoring for therapeutic efficacy and drug-induced toxicity. To assist with the appropriate treatment plan for a specific asthmatic patient, the pharmacist must consider the goals of treatment, the severity of the disease, specific patient characteristics, past medical history, and the benefits and risks of the various drug classes for asthma treatment. A stepped-care approach, as outlined by the NAEP expert panel report, may be instituted.[1] The stepped-care approach includes prevention, "as-needed" drug usage, chronic regular drug usage, rescue, and reduction. An integral part of this approach is patient education and evaluation of compliance and response.

The clinical goals of asthma treatment are to:

- Maintain normal activity levels (including exercise);
- Maintain normal or near normal pulmonary function rates;
- Prevent chronic and troublesome symptoms;
- Prevent recurrent exacerbations of asthma;
- Avoid adverse effects from asthma medications.[1]

The primary focus and first step of asthma therapy is prevention of the inflammatory response. Patients should be instructed on the home use of a peak flow meter so that therapy can be initiated as soon as significant obstruction is measured. If "as-needed" or "chronic" medications do not abate the asthma attack, the patient should be instructed to seek medical attention early. Caregivers and significant others of patients with asthma should also be educated on how to assess the severity of and treat asthma attacks as well as on how and when to seek medical assistance. Patients should learn what triggers their asthma attacks so they can either avoid these triggers or appropriately premedicate prior to exposure. All patients with pulmonary diseases (e.g., chronic bronchitis, emphysema, or cystic fibrosis) should receive the Pneumovax® vaccine[13] and yearly flu vaccines.[14]

The NAEP expert panel treatment plan for asthma[1] is as follows: Mild asthma can be treated using a $beta_2$-agonist inhaler when needed. The patient can use the inhaler either to prevent attacks when exposure to known triggers associated with difficulty in breathing are anticipated or to abate dyspnea. The patient should maintain a record of inhaler usage and peak flow measurements so the need for chronic therapy can be evaluated.

For the moderate asthmatic who has at least two asthma attacks a week, chronic therapy with an anti-inflammatory should be initiated. The anti-inflammatory should be combined with an as-needed or a continuously inhaled bronchodilator. Recent studies suggest that continuous, chronic use of inhaled, short-acting bronchodilators may lead to worsening pulmonary functions and asthma, so it may be better to use these agents as needed.[5,15]

Inhaled corticosteroids are the most potent anti-inflammatories, but issues such as long-term sequelae and use in children need to be resolved before inhaled steroids are used as first-line treatment agents in all patients. If a patient's symptoms occur predominantly in the night, drug therapy that will protect the patient for at least 8 hours (e.g., sustained-release theophylline or a sustained-release oral $beta_2$ agonist) should be prescribed.[9] In young children and in adults with predominantly allergen-induced or seasonal asthma, cromolyn or nedocromil may be considered as first-line therapy. Anticholinergics have a minor role in the initial treatment of asthma and should be reserved for resistant patients. Combinations of asthma medications may be needed if single-agent therapy is not effective. Combinations of drugs that work on the different phases of asthma (i.e., inflammation and bronchoconstriction) are preferred.

For patients with severe asthma, chronic multiple drug use is required. Chronic use of both a $beta_2$ agonist and a steroid inhaler, supplemented with an additional inhaled $beta_2$ agonist as needed, may be required. Theophylline, an oral $beta_2$ agonist, and oral steroids may also be needed.[1]

TABLE 3 Selected characteristics of bronchodilator drugs

Drug	Route of administration	Availability	Sympathomimetic Alpha	Sympathomimetic Beta$_1$	Sympathomimetic Beta$_2$	Anticholinergic	Duration of action (hr)
Albuterol[a]	Inhalation	Rx		+	+++		3–6
	Oral: tablets	Rx		+	+++		5–8
Bitolterol[a]	Inhalation	Rx		+	+++		4–6
Epinephrine[a]	Inhalation	OTC	+++	+++	+++		1–3
	Subcutaneous	Rx	+++	+++	+++		1–4
Ephedrine	Oral: syrup, capsules, tablets	OTC	+++	++	++		3–5
	Intramuscular, subcutaneous	Rx	+++	++	++		<1
Isoproterenol[a]	Inhalation	Rx		+++	+++		0.5–2
	Sublingual	Rx		+++	+++		1–2
Isoetharine[a]	Inhalation	Rx		++	+++		1–3
Metaproterenol[a]	Inhalation	Rx		+++	+++		2–4
	Oral: tablets, syrup	Rx		+++	+++		4
Pirbuterol[a]	Inhalation	Rx		+	+++		4–6
Terbutaline[a]	Inhalation	Rx		+	+++		3–6
	Oral: tablet	Rx		+	+++		4–8
	Subcutaneous	Rx		+	+++		1.5–4
Theophylline[b] (various salts)	Oral: liquid, tablets	OTC	+	++	++		4–12
(sustained release)	Oral: liquid, tablets	Rx	+	++	++		8–24
Atropinm	Inhalation	Rx	—	—	—	+++	4
Ipratropium	Inhalation	Rx	—	—	—	+++	4–6

Key: + indicates relative intensity of effect.
[a]Inhalation confers more bronchial activity than systemic administration.
[b]Although theophylline is not a sympathomimetic drug, it causes the release of endogenous catecholamines.

General Pharmacology

Asthma medications can be categorized by their ability to inhibit the EAR and/or LAR. Medications that prevent the EAR are bronchodilators or inhibitors of mast cell mediator release.[4,9] Medications that modify the LAR inhibit the inflammatory response that is characteristic of asthma.[4,9] Table 1 lists the various asthma medications according to which phase they prevent or reverse. Only those drugs that inhibit the LAR can reduce BHR. A comparison of the dosage forms, prescription status, receptor activity, and duration of action of the bronchodilators is presented in Table 3.

Beta agonists

Stimulation of beta$_2$ receptors by sympathomimetic amines in turn stimulates the enzyme adenylate cyclase, producing an increased intracellular cyclic adenosine monophosphate concentration. In the airways, this results in smooth muscle relaxation, prejunctional inhibition of cholinergic neurotransmission, increased mucociliary clearance, reduced mucosal edema, and inhibition of mast cell mediator release.[4] The currently available short-acting beta$_2$ agonists have no significant anti-inflammatory effect and therefore have no significant effect on the LAR. The effect of the long-acting beta$_2$ agonists, salmeterol and formoterol, on the LAR and BHR requires further study.[16,17]

Beta receptors found in other tissues explain the other effects seen with beta-agonist medications. Because 30–50% of cardiac beta receptors are beta$_2$ receptors, beta$_2$ agonists can produce tachycardia by directly stimulating these receptors. Other effects of beta$_2$-receptor stimulation include peripheral vasodilation; skeletal muscle tremor; hypokalemia; uterine relaxation; increased release of glucose, lactate, pyruvate, insulin, and high-density lipoproteins from the liver and pancreas; and increased urinary excretion of magnesium, calcium, and phosphate.[18] Peripheral vasodilation from systemic beta$_2$-adrenergic stimulation decreases blood pressure and produces a compensatory increase in the heart rate to maintain cardiac output.

The nonprescription and some prescription beta$_2$ agonists also influence other adrenergic receptors (Table 3). The alpha-adrenergic stimulation produces bronchoconstriction, vasoconstriction, urinary retention, and mydriasis, which are not beneficial in asthma. Stimulating beta$_1$ receptors results in increased cardiovascular inotropic and chronotropic activity. Isoproterenol and metaproterenol stimulate beta$_1$ and beta$_2$ receptors equally. The newer agents such as albuterol, bitolterol, pirbuterol, and terbutaline selectively stimulate beta$_2$ receptors; however, with higher inhaled doses or oral and intravenous administration, beta$_1$ receptors are also stimulated.

Route of administration has a profound effect on pulmonary selectivity and on the adverse effects of sympathomimetic bronchodilators. Beta$_2$ agonists produce few adverse reactions when administered in standard doses via inhalation; when these drugs are inhaled, much less drug reaches the systemic circulation because the dose is smaller and the portion of the dose that is deposited in the mouth is swallowed and metabolized in the gut and liver.[19] However, high-dose inhalation and oral and intravenous therapy will produce higher serum concentrations and more systemic adverse reactions. For example, at the same degree of bronchodilation, terbutaline taken orally or intravenously produces more tremor, hypotension, and tachycardia than it does when inhaled.[9] Up to 33% of patients receiving oral terbutaline therapy may experience skeletal muscle tremor, which can be severe.[4]

The selective beta$_2$ agonists also have a longer duration of activity (Table 3). The available beta$_2$ agonists will provide 4–6 hours of bronchodilation but only 2 to 3 hours of protection against bronchoprovocation. Investigational, long-acting beta$_2$ agonists, formoterol and salmeterol, provide bronchodilation and protection for up to 12 hours.[9,17]

The long-term use of beta$_2$ agonists may produce tolerance or tachyphylaxis. Down regulation (decreased number) and a decreased affinity at the beta$_2$ receptor may develop.[20] A plateau response is reached within 2–8 weeks with no further deterioration; the duration of action is affected more than the intensity of effect.[20] However, the clinical consequence of beta$_2$-agonist tolerance appears minor in that beta$_2$ receptors in the airways are not as susceptible to tolerance as other beta$_2$ receptors.[21] Moreover, corticosteroid therapy can prevent and reverse the tolerance.[20]

Methylxanthines

Methylxanthines attenuate the bronchospasm component of the LAR, but they do not prevent the increase in BHR. Thus, they do not have any significant anti-inflammatory activity.[4,9]

Theophylline has pharmacologic effects on multiple organs. Theophylline increases cardiac contractility and rate, dilates peripheral arteries, and constricts arteries in the brain. The cardiac output may increase in patients with congestive heart failure secondary to reduced preload and improved contractility. In asthmatic patients with normal cardiovascular function, therapeutic concentrations of theophylline increase the heart rate by approximately 10 beats per minute. Theophylline can produce diarrhea, nausea, vomiting, and anorexia through local irritation and central nervous system (CNS) stimulation. Acutely, it produces a diuresis through an increase in the glomerular filtration rate. Theophylline also produces numerous CNS effects such as irritability, insomnia, altered behavior, and seizures at high concentrations.

Cromolyn and Nedocromil

Cromolyn effectively blocks both the EAR and LAR.[22] Cromolyn inhibits the degranulation of mast cells and stabilizes epithelial cells, but the exact mechanism by which it inhibits the LAR is unknown.[9] Cromolyn can be used to treat intermittent, seasonal, and chronic asthma or allergen-, sulfite-, aspirin-, and exercise-induced asthma. Its use may permit a lowering of the systemic steroid dose. A trial of cromolyn for 8–12 weeks should be conducted before determining cromolyn ineffective.[22] Because the drug is not orally absorbed, minimal adverse reactions exist. Dry mouth and hoarseness may result from inhalation therapy.

Nedocromil is a recently approved drug whose pharmacology is similar to that of cromolyn, but nedocromil is more potent on a weight basis.[9] As a result, it inhibits both the EAR and LAR. Nedocromil is effective for chronic stable asthma and exercise-induced asthma. After the addition of nedocromil, theophylline and beta$_2$-agonist doses can be decreased. Nedocromil is well tolerated, with reported side effects of altered taste (25%), coughing (8%), bronchospasm (8%), and headache (3%).

Corticosteroids

Because asthma is predominantly an inflammatory disease, inhaled corticosteroids are becoming the mainstay of chronic asthma therapy.[1] However, because their long-term sequelae are unknown in children, inhaled corticosteroids have not been universally adopted as a drug of choice in the pediatric patient. Corticosteroids prevent the LAR but not the EAR. Proposed mechanisms include decreased peripheral blood eosinophils, basophils, lymphocytes, and monocytes; altered chemotaxis; impaired mediator synthesis and release; enhanced beta-adrenergic receptor activity; and decreased vascular permeability.[23] Few adverse reactions result from standard doses of inhaled corticosteroids, the most notable being oral candidiasis and hoarseness. These adverse effects may be minimized by using a spacer device or by rinsing the mouth after each usage.

Antihistamines

The classic antihistamines competitively inhibit histamine at type I receptors (H$_1$) in vascular smooth muscle. However, most of the first-generation antihistamines also influence other receptors such as cholinergic, serotonin, and alpha-adrenergic receptors, producing adverse effects. The newer, more selective H$_1$-antagonist antihistamines block the EAR by blocking histamine release from the mast cell. As a result, vascular permeability and prostaglandin generation are decreased, smooth muscle is relaxed, and activation of airway vagal afferent nerves is inhibited.[4] Some of these drugs, such as ketotifen and cetirizine, possess additional anti-inflammatory activity.

Anticholinergics

Although they are not anti-inflammatory medications, anticholinergics can cause bronchodilation. Anticholinergic bronchodilators (atropine, glycopyrrolate, and ipratropium) inhibit the formation of cyclic guanosine monophosphate, which increases the release of mediators causing bronchoconstriction and inflammation. Atropine and glycopyrrolate are used in nebulizers. Atropine, which is well absorbed through the lung parenchyma, causes anticholinergic adverse reactions such as tachycardia, urinary retention, decreased mucociliary clearance, mydriasis, and altered mentation. The quaternary ammonia derivatives, ipratropium bromide and glycopyrrolate, though poorly absorbed, provide greater bronchoselectivity and fewer side effects than atropine. Anticholinergic medications are more effective for chronic obstructive lung diseases but have shown additive bronchodilation to beta$_2$ agonists and theophylline in asthmatic patients.

Specific Ingredients in Nonprescription Products

As understanding of the pathophysiology of asthma increases, the importance of prescribing anti-inflammatory medication as first-line therapy for mild, moderate, and severe asthma is becoming more apparent and the usefulness of currently available nonprescription drugs is becoming less obvious. The recent evidence that regular bronchodilator use may worsen chronic asthma underscores the need for anti-inflammatory drug therapy in managing asthma. Prescription therapy with an as-needed selective beta$_2$-agonist inhaler or chronic use of one of the anti-inflammatory medications (e.g., inhaled corticosteroids or cromolyn) should be instituted if nonprescription drug therapy does not provide adequate symptom relief.

The primary nonprescription medications for treating mild forms of asthma include epinephrine, ephedrine, and theophylline. These agents provide bronchodilation with little anti-inflammatory activity. Nonprescription combination products usually contain theophylline and ephedrine with phenobarbital, antihistamines, expectorants, and/or antitussives. Prescription bronchodilators for inhalation usually have greater potency, a longer duration of effect, and fewer adverse side effects.

Epinephrine

Epinephrine can be used to treat periodic and acute severe bronchospasm. For periodic asthma, epinephrine is administered by inhalation. Although the various epinephrine-containing products differ slightly in the dose delivered, no significant difference between prescription and nonprescription epinephrine for inhalation exists. Acute, severe asthma attacks can be treated by subcutaneous injection or by inhalation. However, inhalation of beta$_2$ agonists is currently considered the therapy of first choice for both indications.[1]

Epinephrine has equipotent alpha-, beta$_1$-, and beta$_2$-agonist effects, all of which are dose-dependent. These effects are terminated as the drug is taken up by sympathetic nerve endings and surrounding tissues. Epinephrine is metabolized in the nerve endings by monoamine oxidase and in the tissues by catechol-o-methyltransferase (COMT). Epinephrine is ineffective when taken by mouth because nearly complete metabolism by COMT and sulfatase occurs in the gastrointestinal tract and the liver. Adverse effects due to epinephrine (e.g., tachycardia, cardiac arrhythmia, hypertension, tremor, and anxiety) are almost always associated with the parenteral route of administration. These effects would not generally be expected by the inhalation route except in an overdose situation.

Some patients may tend to overuse these products, particularly when relief of symptoms does not occur. The peak effect of epinephrine aerosol for inhalation occurs within 5–10 minutes after use.

The Food and Drug Administration (FDA) has classified as Category I epinephrine, epinephrine bitartrate, and epinephrine hydrochloride (racemic) in pressurized, metered-dose aerosol dosage forms and aqueous solutions equivalent to 1% epinephrine for use with hand-held rubber-bulb nebulizers. These drugs are not to be used unless a doctor has made a diagnosis of asthma, the patient has not been hospitalized for asthma, and no other medications are being taken for asthma unless directed by a physician.[24] Patients with preexisting disease or conditions such as heart disease (e.g., coronary artery disease, heart failure, or cardiac rhythm disturbance), high blood pressure, thyroid disease, diabetes, or difficulty urinating due to enlargement of the prostate should avoid self-treatment with these products except under the advice and supervision of a physician.[24] In addition, patients taking a prescription antihypertensive or antidepressant drug should consult their physician or pharmacist before using the asthma products.[24]

Each epinephrine inhalation should contain the equivalent of 0.16–0.25 mg of epinephrine base.[24] For adults and children 4 years of age and older, the dosage recommendation adopted for metered-dose delivery systems is one inhalation followed by a second inhalation if symptoms have not been relieved after at least 1 minute;[24] usage should not then be repeated for at least 3 hours. When an aqueous solution at a concentration equivalent to 1% epinephrine base is used with a hand-held rubber-bulb nebulizer, the inhalation dosage for adults and children 4 years of age or older is one to three inhalations no more often than every 3 hours. For children under 4 years of age, no dosage recommendations exist and the doctor should be consulted. The solution should not be used if it is brown or cloudy. An adult should supervise the use of these products by children to avoid under- or overuse.

These products also require statements warning against exceeding the recommended dosages unless directed by a physician. The following warnings must appear in boldface type in the package labeling:

> Do not continue to use this product, but seek medical assistance immediately if symptoms are not relieved within 20 minutes or become worse. Patients should be warned that excessive use of epinephrine-containing products may cause nervousness, rapid heart beat, and possibly adverse effects on the heart. Epinephrine may increase certain symptoms of Parkinson's disease such as tremor and rigidity.[25]

Ephedrine

Ephedrine is useful for treating only mild forms of seasonal or chronic asthma. Ephedrine is also FDA approved for treating enuresis, hypotension, nasal congestion, penile erection, rhinorrhea, and sinusitis. Although ephedrine sulfate is available on a nonprescription basis for use as a single entity in a 25-mg capsule and a syrup, the most abundantly available preparations are combination tablets, elixirs, and suspensions containing ephedrine with theophylline, phenobarbital, guaifenesin, and/or pyrilamine maleate.

Ephedrine has equivalent alpha-, beta$_1$-, and beta$_2$-activity. These effects are primarily produced indirectly through the release of norepinephrine from sympathetic nerve endings. The peak bronchodilation effect from orally administered ephedrine occurs in 1 hour and lasts about 5 hours. Tachyphylaxis or tolerance may develop with long-term use. Ephedrine is predominantly eliminated unchanged in urine. Although the average elimination half-life is 6 hours, the half-life is decreased by urinary acidification and increased by urinary alkalinization.

Ephedrine is available as a base, as hydrochloride and sulfate salts, and as racemic ephedrine hydrochloride. The FDA considers nonprescription ephedrine to be a safe and effective bronchodilator; however, the drug is not to be used unless the doctor has made a diagnosis of asthma, the patient has not been hospitalized for asthma, and no other medications are being taken for asthma unless directed by a doctor. Patients with heart disease, high blood pressure, thyroid disease, diabetes, or difficulty urinating due to enlargement of the prostate should avoid self-treatment with these products except under the advice and supervision of a physician. In addition, patients taking a prescription antihypertensive or antidepressant drug should consult their physician or pharmacist before using the products.

Severe hypertension could develop in a patient who has been receiving ephedrine while taking a monoamine oxidase inhibitor (MAOI). This is because the MAOI decreases the degradation and increases the storage of norepinephrine. Tricyclic antidepressants may partially block the action of ephedrine.[25] Ephedrine may also increase the effect of ergotamine on the heart and blood vessels[25] and decrease the blood pressure–lowering ability of guanethidine. The effects of ephedrine may be minimized if it is taken with methyldopa or reserpine. Because of alkalinization of the urine, the concentrations of ephedrine may be increased with concomitant administration of acetazolamide, dichlorphenamide, or a large dose of sodium bicarbonate. Blood pressure may be increased if ephedrine is taken with clonidine, procarbazine, furazolidine, and selegiline.

The dosage recommendation for ephedrine in adults and children over 12 years of age is 12.5–25 mg every 4 hours, not to exceed 150 mg in 24 hours.[24] For children 6–12 years of age, the recommended dosage is one-half to one tablet every 3–5 hours, depending on the specific combination product; the American Medical Association suggests 3 mg/kg per day divided into four to six doses. The manufacturers suggest that a doctor be consulted for use of ephedrine in children under 6 years of age. The maximum daily adult ephedrine dosage recommendation (150 mg a day) is approximately one-half the current maximum ephedrine hydrochloride dosage allowable with current Tedral® labeling (288 mg per day). This ephedrine dosage is likely to produce adverse effects in many patients; this is because Tedral® contains both ephedrine and theophylline, and these two agents share similar toxicity profiles and can be dangerous in selected patients.

Labeling requirements for ephedrine-containing products include a warning statement against exceeding the recommended dosage unless directed by a physician. If symptoms are not relieved within 1 hour or become worse, the product should be discontinued and a physician consulted immediately.[24]

TABLE 4 Factors that influence theophylline metabolism

Increase metabolism	Decrease metabolism
Diseases	**Diseases**
Cystic fibrosis	Acute hepatitis
Hyperthyroidism	Acute respiratory failure
	Cholestasis
Social habits	Congestive heart failure
Charcoal-broiled beef diet	Cor pulmonale
High-protein/low-carbohydrate diet	Hepatic cirrhosis
Smoking cigarettes, marijuana	Hypoxia
	Pulmonary edema
	Systemic viral infection
Medications	**Social Habits**
Benzodiazepines	High-carbohydrate/low-protein diet
Carbamazepine	
Felodipine	**Medications**
Isoniazid[b]	Allopurinol
Isoproterenol	B C G vaccine
Moricizine	Caffeine
Phenobarbital	Cimetidine
Phenytoin	Ciprofloxacin
Rifampin	Clarithromycin
Sulfinpyrazone	Diltiazem
Terbutaline	Disulfiram
	Enoxacin
	Erythromycin
	Furosemide[a]
	Interferon
	Methotrexate
	Metoprolol
	Mexiletine
	Norfloxacin
	Oral contraceptives
	Pefloxacin
	Propranolol
	Single ingestion of alcohol
	Thiabendazole
	Ticlopidine
	Trivalent flu vaccine
	Troleandomycin
	Verapamil

[a]This medication has also been reported to decrease theophylline concentration.
[b]This medication has also been reported to decrease theophylline clearance.

The principal adverse effects of ephedrine are CNS stimulation, sleeplessness, nausea, loss of appetite, tremors, tachycardia, and urinary retention. To prevent insomnia, ephedrine should be taken a few hours before bedtime. Reports indicate that chronic ephedrine overdosage may result in either severe cardiac toxicity or psychosis.[26,27] One report indicated that ephedrine may be a potential drug of abuse. Like amphetamines, it produces the release

TABLE 5	Maximum daily doses of theophylline
Age	**Dose**
Infants	(0.3 × age in weeks) + 8 mg/kg daily in divided doses
Children 1–9 yr old	24 mg/kg daily in divided doses
Children 9–12 yr old	20 mg/kg daily in divided doses
Children 12–16 yr old	18 mg/kg daily in divided doses
Adults 16 yr and older	13 mg/kg daily or 900 mg daily, whichever is less, in divided doses

of catecholamines in the CNS. Ephedrine, caffeine, and phenylpropanolamine are frequent ingredients of drugs manufactured to physically resemble amphetamine-containing dosage forms. To prevent drug abuse with ephedrine, some states, including Oregon, Washington, and New Mexico, have changed or are considering changing single-entity ephedrine to prescription-only status.

Theophylline

Theophylline is considered third- or fourth-line therapy for asthma.[1,9] Theophylline has a narrow therapeutic window, interacts with multiple medications, is influenced by various disease states, and requires therapeutic monitoring for safety and efficacy. It is reserved for patients who are unresponsive to inhaled medications (e.g., beta$_2$ agonists or steroids), are unable or unwilling to use inhalers, or have nocturnal asthma. Theophylline is contraindicated in patients allergic to theophylline, caffeine, and theobromine. It should be used cautiously in patients with peptic ulcer disease, hyperthyroidism, glaucoma, diabetes mellitus, severe hypoxemia, hypertension, compromised cardiac or circulatory function, angina pectoris, and acute myocardial infarct.

To determine the correct dose for a patient on theophylline, the health care practitioner should review the patient's medical history and characteristics to assess their potential impact on absorption, distribution, metabolism, and elimination. Theophylline products are generally well absorbed. Different salts are used in nonprescription and prescription theophylline products. Theophylline equivalents need to be calculated to determine dose and for pharmacokinetic analysis. The theophylline equivalent of the various compounds is as follows: anhydrous theophylline, 100%; hydrous theophylline, 91%; hydrous aminophylline, 80%; anhydrous aminophylline, 86%; oxtriphylline, 64%; theophylline calcium salicylate, 48%; theophylline sodium glycinate, 46%; and theophylline monohydrate, 91%. The formulation and release profiles of the various sustained and rapid-release products will produce serum concentration–time curve differences, peak–trough differences, and extent-of-absorption differences. An understanding of the pharmacokinetics of theophylline is required for the optimal use of the drug.

Theophylline's volume of distribution is 0.45 L/kg. Conditions such as prematurity, pulmonary edema, cirrhosis, pregnancy, and obesity can alter this average volume. Theophylline crosses the placental barrier and is secreted in breast milk. Because theophylline is only 40% protein bound, drug interactions due to protein binding and displacement are unlikely.

Theophylline is predominantly metabolized in the liver with less than 15% eliminated unchanged in the urine. The cytochrome P-450 mixed-function oxidase enzyme system produces inactive metabolites via hydroxylation and N-demethylation. For some patients, the enzyme systems may become saturated, resulting in nonlinear kinetics.[28] However, for most patients the assumption of first-order (linear) pharmacokinetics is sufficient for clinical dosage adjustments. Age, coexisting disease, other drugs, and social habits may influence the metabolism of theophylline and must be considered when dosing is initiated or when other diseases or drugs are added, controlled, or eliminated. Theophylline metabolism is slow during the neonatal period, but it increases to its highest levels during the first 9 years, after which it decreases with age. Table 4 lists the influence of various conditions and medications on theophylline metabolism.[28–30]

Dosing guidelines have been published (Table 5). Maximum bronchodilation occurs at a serum concentration between 10 and 20 mcg/mL. Due to the logarithmic nature of the concentration–response curve and the potential for serious toxicity at levels just above 20 mcg/mL, the NAEP expert panel now recommends a therapeutic goal of 5–15 mg/mL.

If theophylline is used to relieve an acute asthmatic attack, the patient should receive a loading dose of theophylline. For a patient with stable asthma, a lower than therapeutic dose should be initiated and increased slowly over 7–10 days to the therapeutic dose needed to reduce the incidence of adverse reactions.[28]

The dosage guidelines for theophylline are based on single-entity treatment. The nonprescription theophylline-containing products often contain other medications, such as ephedrine, that may produce synergistic toxicity with theophylline and do not allow individualization of theophylline dosage. The dosage recommendation for Tedral® (130 mg of theophylline, 24 mg of ephedrine hydrochloride, and 8 mg of phenobarbital) for adults is one or two tablets every 4 hours and for children over 25 kg, one-half or one tablet every 4 hours. At the maximum daily adult dose of 1,560 mg of theophylline, the average steady-state concentration—assuming complete absorption and a clearance of 39 ± 11.4 mL/kg per hour[28] in a 45-year-old, nonsmoking, 70-kg adult who is in generally good health and without any interferences in theophylline absorption or clearance—would be 23.8 mcg/mL (range for ± 2 S.D. 9.9–96.8 mcg/mL). With the same dose, complete absorption, and a clearance of 35.4 ± 4.2 mL/kg per hour,[28] the average steady-state theophylline concentrations in an 85-year-old, 50-kg adult would be 36.7 mcg/mL (range for ± 2 S.D. 29.7–48 mcg/mL). Using a similar projection for a 25-kg child taking one Tedral® tablet every 4 hours and having a theophylline clearance of 96 ± 24 mL/kg per hour,[28] the average steady-state concentration would be 13.5 mcg/mL (range for ± 2 S.D. 9.0–27.1 mcg/mL). Substantial potential for theophylline toxicity exists for a patient who uses the maximally recommended dose of nonprescription theophylline combination products, especially if there are factors that affect theophylline clearance or if the patient is already on a prescription theophylline product.

Many theophylline-induced adverse effects involve the gastrointestinal, cardiovascular, and central nervous systems. The local and centrally mediated gastrointestinal adverse reactions include nausea, vomiting, epigastric pain, abdominal cramps, anorexia, and, rarely, diarrhea and hematemesis. Theophylline can increase gastric acidity and decrease lower esophageal sphincter pressure. Some patients receiving theophylline may experience heartburn, gastroesophageal reflux, gastric or duodenal ulcers, or an exacerbation of these conditions.

Cardiovascular adverse effects include palpitation, sinus tachycardia, extrasystole, flushing, hypotension, circulatory failure, and ventricular arrhythmia. In 100 hospitalized patients, 20% of those with theophylline serum concentrations of less than 10 mcg/mL, 48% of those with theophylline serum concentrations of between 10 and 20 mcg/mL, and 56% of those with theophylline serum concentrations of greater than 20 mcg/mL had arrhythmias on electrocardiograms.[31]

CNS toxicity includes headache; irritability; restlessness; nervousness; insomnia; dizziness; reflex hyperexcitability; seizures; and a potentially impaired learning ability, memory, and attention span in children. Miscellaneous adverse effects include increased urinary frequency, dehydration, finger and hand twitching, tachypnea, increased serum aspartate aminotransferase (AST) concentration, and hypersensitivity. Women with fibrocystic breast disease may experience an increase in symptoms.[25] Patients should be instructed to contact a health care practitioner if adverse reactions occur.

The advent of fingerstick theophylline analytical analyses has enabled pharmacists to monitor theophylline serum levels in their pharmacies or at nursing homes. Some patients have been given these fingerstick tests (e.g., Acculevel® by Syntex Medical Diagnostics, Palo Alto, Calif.) to measure serum concentrations at home and have been asked to call the results in to a health care practitioner for evaluation and adjustment of theophylline dosage.[32]

Antihistamines

Antihistamines, although certainly not primary therapy, should not be considered contraindicated for asthmatics. Antihistamines have proven useful in children and adults who have a strong allergic component to their asthma. Originally, there was concern about the anticholinergic activity of antihistamines and their potential to dry and thicken mucous secretions. However, when anticholinergics have been used to treat acute and chronic asthma, the bronchodilator effect has prevailed and the drying of secretions has been minimal and without clinical significance.

Because histamine produces bronchospasm, inflammation, and edema, antihistamines have an adjunctive role in the treatment of asthma.[33] The second-generation antihistamines (e.g., terfenadine, astemizole, cetirizine, ketotifen, loratidine, and azelastine) have been found to partially prevent the EAR.[33] Some of these more H_1-selective antihistamines, such as ketotifen, cetirizine, and azelastine, also have anti-inflammatory activity unrelated to their antihistamine activity.[33] These newer agents are lipophobic, do not cross the blood brain barrier, act more peripherally, and therefore produce less sedation than the older antihistamines. Further information on available nonprescription antihistamines can be found in Chapter 8, "Cold, Cough, and Allergy Products."

Expectorants

Many asthma products contain expectorants, especially guaifenesin and potassium iodide. Guaifenesin, at proper doses, is considered to be a safe and effective expectorant, but other nonprescription expectorants are probably no more effective than adequate hydration of the patient and are therefore of questionable clinical value. A change in mucus production may be a sign of worsening asthma or infection, both requiring medical evaluation rather than self-assessment and self-treatment. Because of the concern for iodide toxicity, an FDA advisory panel has recommended that iodide-containing products (expectorants) be restricted to prescription status. The FDA also states that, unless ordered by a physician, guaifenesin should not be taken for persistent or chronic cough such as occurs with asthma or is accompanied by excessive sputum.[24] Further information on expectorants can be found in Chapter 8, "Cold, Cough, and Allergy Products."

Antitussives

Coughing is the major physiologic host defense mechanism for removing bronchial secretions and mucus plugs. Antitussives should generally not be used for asthma because a productive cough has a highly useful effect. The reflex cough induced by bronchospasm is often relieved by bronchodilators, not antitussives. However, nonprescription antitussives, such as codeine and dextromethorphan, are occasionally used in asthma products.

According to the FDA, codeine should not be taken by patients with a chronic pulmonary disease or shortness of breath unless directed by a physician.[24] Similarly, dextromethorphan should not be used without a doctor's prescription if cough persists for longer than 1 week; tends to recur; or is accompanied by fever, rash, or persistent headache.[24] Further information on antitussives can be found in Chapter 8, "Cold, Cough, and Allergy Products."

Phenobarbital

Phenobarbital has been used in nonprescription products containing theophylline and ephedrine to decrease the incidence and severity of their adverse reactions. However, phenobarbital does not alleviate all the adverse reactions of these drugs and may add to the toxicities experienced by the patient. Phenobarbital is contraindicated in patients who are hypersensitive to barbiturates or have porphyria or marked liver and pulmonary impairment.

The amount of phenobarbital in a nonprescription tablet is 8 mg; in a nonprescription liquid, it is 0.8 mg/mL. The phenobarbital dose present in the maximum daily adult dose of Tedral® is 96 mg. For comparison, the adult dose of phenobarbital for sedation is 30–120 mg daily; for hypnosis (sleep), 100–200 mg daily; and for seizures, 60–200 mg daily. The sedative dose for children is 6 mg/kg daily and for pediatric seizure control, 3–6 mg/kg daily. Therapeutic doses of phenobarbital may require tapering after regular usage to prevent withdrawal symptoms.

The half-life of phenobarbital is 2–6 days. Most of the drug is metabolized. Metabolism may be enhanced by alkalinization of the urine. About 25–50% of the drug is excreted unchanged in the urine and may require a downward dosage adjustment in patients who have impaired renal function.

Phenobarbital is a potent liver enzyme inducer and may enhance the metabolism of certain other drugs. When it is ingested from nonprescription medications, the drug interaction significance of small, occasional doses of phenobarbital may vary from the effect of therapeutic doses used regularly for seizure control. Drugs whose clearance is enhanced by phenobarbital include anticoagulants, corticosteroids, theophylline, and other steroidal hormones. Women using oral contraceptives should take additional precautions with concomitant phenobarbital usage.[25]

Phenobarbital may cause CNS depression or excitation. Sedation is a very common adverse effect; children are more likely than adults to experience excitation. The CNS effects of phenobarbital are enhanced with concomitant administration of other drugs with CNS depressant activity (e.g., alcohol, narcotics, tranquilizers, antipsychotics, antidepressants, sedative/hypnotics, muscle relaxants, antihistamines, and anesthetic agents). Decreased respiratory function, confusion, hyperkinesia, ataxia, nightmares, nervousness, insomnia, anxiety, dizziness, learning dysfunction, nausea, vomiting, constipation, headache, osteomalacia, bradycardia, and megaloblastic anemia may also occur.

Combination Products

To increase efficacy but reduce toxicity, combination products are designed to include ingredients with different mechanisms of action or lower doses of each agent. The nonprescription asthma products usually combine theophylline and ephedrine. Although these two drugs have different mechanisms of action, they have similar side-effect profiles. A disadvantage of combination products is the inability to titrate one drug dosage to an individual's unique need. Of note, when a patient is dosed with a combination product to achieve therapeutic theophylline concentrations, the ephedrine dose may exceed the recommendation for single-entity ephedrine[24] and produce adverse reactions with chronic administration.

The combination of epinephrine inhalations and combined theophylline–ephedrine in an oral dosage form is an effective bronchodilator, and the oral combination has been shown to be as effective as or, in some cases, less effective than the newer, orally active beta$_2$ agonists.[1,2,4] Ephedrine has been variously shown to produce additive bronchodilation with theophylline, or no added bronchodilation when compared with optimal theophylline doses.[34,35]

Phenobarbital and hydroxyzine have been added to some theophylline–ephedrine combination products to decrease CNS stimulation; however, this effect is not always achieved. These products add additional toxicity potential themselves. A patient who takes the maximum dose of Tedral® might consume 96 mg of phenobarbital per day. Assuming complete absorption and average clearance, the average steady-state phenobarbital concentration would be approximately 15 mcg/mL.[36] The therapeutic range for phenobarbital for seizure control is 10–30 mcg/mL.

The fixed-dose combinations of theophylline and ephedrine may offer no advantage over single-drug therapy and will probably produce more adverse effects. With the availability of newer, longer acting, selective beta$_2$ agonists and the increased usage of anti-inflammatories (e.g., steroids or cromolyn), currently available nonprescription bronchodilators, particularly combination products, may be used to a significantly lesser extent in managing any form of asthma except mild asthma.

Delivery Systems: Traditional Inhalers

Correctly used, an inhaler deposits only about 8.8% of medication into the lungs.[37] Incorrect inhaler technique can reduce drug delivery and efficacy. Incorrect technique can result from incorrect or conflicting instruction, lack of instruction, and patient confusion and forgetfulness. Health care practitioners need to be more aware of correct inhaler technique. Patient and health care practitioner education, as well as evaluation programs on proper inhaler technique and use of spacers, can improve therapeutic response.

Up to 89% of patients using inhalers do not perform all the drug administration steps correctly.[38] Results from two evaluations revealed that 50–79% of nonpulmonary physicians, 35–53% of medical residents, 71% of pharmacists, 43% of nurses, and 8% of respiratory technicians did not perform or identify at least four of the steps required for correct inhaler usage.[39,40] The number and nature of specific steps taught by various health care practitioners may also differ. Currently, both the closed- and open-mouth techniques are taught; however, manufacturers' package instructions are for the closed-mouth technique. Many health practitioners instruct patients on only the basic steps; others include specific complete instructions on every aspect of inhaler use. As a result of this inconsistency in education, patients may be confused on how to use inhalers.

Investigators have found that patients perform inhaler technique better when they receive both written and verbal education.[41] Yet 87% of patients visiting a community pharmacy did not receive any verbal education on inhaler use.[39] Moreover, a patient's inhaler technique may actually worsen over time. Therefore, repeated education and assessment of inhaler technique is strongly encouraged.

The steps for correct inhaler use with the open- and closed-mouth technique for metered-dose inhalers are listed in Table 6. Shaking the canister distributes the drug particles evenly throughout the suspension. The open-mouth technique is advocated to decrease the amount of drug making contact with and adhering to the back of the throat; the risk with this technique, however, is that patients may miss their mouth when they spray. The slower the breath, the greater the likelihood that the drug will reach the smaller

TABLE 6	Correct inhaler technique

1. Remove duster cap.
2. Shake canister.
3. Position mouthpiece to bottom.
4. Tilt head back.
5. Breathe out to functional volume.
6. Close lips on inhaler or hold inhaler 1 to 2 in. from open mouth.
7. Actuate while inhaling slowly and deeply.
8. Hold breath 5–10 seconds or as long as possible.
9. Breathe out slowly.
10. Wait 1–10 minutes before second inhalation.
11. If steroid inhaler is being used, rinse mouth after use.

airways. The longer the breath is held and the slower it is exhaled, the greater the amount of drug that is retained in the airways. Waiting between inhalations allows the bronchodilator to work and may increase delivery of drug to the airways with subsequent inhalations. Because most $beta_2$ agonists begin to work within minutes after inhalation, reaching their peak effect within 5–15 minutes, $beta_2$-agonist inhalers may be used first to open the airways for other inhaled medications. Ipratropium and steroids take longer to reach onset and peak activity, and should follow the $beta_2$ agonists.

The number of sprays remaining in the canister can roughly be determined by submerging the canister in water. When the canister is full, it will sink to the bottom of the water. When the canister is completely empty, it will float on its side on the water line.

Delivery Systems: Nontraditional Inhalers, Spacers, and Other Devices

Because up to 89% of patients use an inadequate inhaler technique, spacer devices or specialized inhalers are advocated. The most commonly used spacer devices are the Aerochamber®, InspirEase®, Inhal-Aid®, and Volumatic®. Brethancer®, Maxair®, and Azmacort® inhalers are manufactured with a collapsible tube device. The Brethancer® will support some other inhalers whereas the Azmacort® and Maxair® device will not. Breath-activated dry powder inhalers are being developed to decrease the usage of chlorofluorocarbon propellant. Ventease® can be attached to an inhaler to facilitate actuation for elderly and arthritic patients.

Spacers or extender devices can improve delivery of the drug to the airways.[42] The distance between the inhaler mouthpiece and the mouth allows the chlorofluorocarbons to evaporate, resulting in smaller droplet sizes and greater lung deposition.[42] Use of a spacer lessens impaction of the drug on the oropharynx and thereby decreases the incidence of oral candidiasis that can occur with regular use of steroid inhalers.[38]

Aerochamber® and InspirEase® are two devices that provide the patient with feedback on the appropriate rate of inhalation. If a whistle is heard on inhalation, it indicates that the patient inhaled too quickly. These devices also have inhalation valves to eliminate drug loss from the device until the patient is ready to inhale, obviating the need for good hand–lung coordination. Patients should be instructed to inhale the drug within 15 seconds after actuating the aerosol into the device.

The inhalation technique for dry powder inhalers such as Rotahaler® is significantly different from that for MDIs. After inserting the device in the mouth the patient should breathe in deeply and rapidly.

Specific Patient or Disease Considerations

Geriatric Implications

Elderly patients may have altered pharmacodynamic and pharmacokinetic responses to asthma medications. Some investigators have reported decreased beta-agonist activity in elderly patients due to decreased receptor number, decreased receptor affinity, or altered biochemical pathways.[43–45] Because most of the receptor studies have been in vitro or in vivo on cardiovascular and endocrine receptors, the effect of aging on beta receptors in the lungs is largely unknown. Bronchodilation from theophylline for a given serum concentration was found to be less in elderly asthmatics than in younger asthmatics.[46] This was due to differences in asthma severity or duration, concomitant bronchitis and emphysema, or aging. Many investigators have reported decreased theophylline elimination in elderly patients.[28] Because of the potential for lower clearances in such patients, lower doses of theophylline should be initiated and therapy monitored with serum theophylline concentrations. Increased age is a risk factor for the development of life-threatening events (e.g., seizures or cardiac arrhythmias) with theophylline overdosage. Because other prescription and nonprescription medications are used significantly, an elderly patient's medication profile should be closely scrutinized for potential drug interactions with theophylline (Table 4).[47]

The percentage of elderly patients unable to perform correctly most of the steps required for proper inhaler use is greater than that of younger adult patients. Reasons for their inappropriate inhaler technique include arthritis, decreased muscle strength, dementia, inability to read or comprehend the instructions, and/or inadequate prior patient education on inhaler technique. One-third of elderly patients may not have sufficient hand strength to actuate the inhaler.[48] Ventease® can facilitate inhaler usage in elderly patients with arthritis. Specialized inhaler instruction should be repeatedly given to the elderly patient. Spacers or nebulizers should be used with elderly patients who are unable to use inhalers correctly.

Pediatric Implications

Generally, children under the age of 5 will not be able to use an inhaler; nebulizers may be required for administration in this age group. For children over the age of 5,

TABLE 7 Classification of fetal risk from asthma medications by FDA pregnancy categories[a]

Medication	Category	Medication	Category
Anti-Inflammatories		**Bronchodilators**	
Beclomethasone dipropionate	C	Albuterol	C
Cromolyn sodium	B	Atropine	C
Flunisolide	C	Bitolterol	C
Prednisone	B	Ephedrine	C
Triamcinolone	D	Epinephrine	C
		Glycopyrrolate	B
Antihistamines		Ipratropium	B
Astemizole	C	Isoproterenol	C
Brompheniramine	C	Metaproterenol	C
Chlorpheniramine	B	Pirbuterol	C
Diphenhydramine	C	Terbutaline	B
Hydroxyzine	C	Theophylline	C
Pyrilamine maleate	C		
Terfenadine	C	**Decongestants**	
Tripelennamine	B	Phenylephrine	C
Triprolidine	C	Phenylpropanolamine	C
		Pseudoephedrine	C
		Miscellaneous	
		Guaifenesin	C
		Iodinated glycerol	X
		Phenobarbital	D

Key to pregnancy categories:

A: Adequate studies in pregnant women have not demonstrated a risk to the fetus in the first trimester of pregnancy, and there is no evidence of risk in later trimesters.

B: Animal studies have not demonstrated a risk to the fetus, but there are no adequate studies in pregnant women...or...Animal studies have shown an adverse effect, but adequate studies in pregnant women have not demonstrated a risk to the fetus during the first trimester of pregnancy, and there is no evidence of risk in later trimesters.

C: Animal studies have shown an adverse effect on the fetus, but there are no adequate studies in humans; the benefits from the use of the drug in pregnant women may be acceptable despite its potential risks...or...There are no animal reproduction studies and no adequate studies in humans.

D: There is evidence of human fetal risk, but the potential benefits from the use of the drug in pregnant women may be acceptable despite its potential risks.

X: Studies in animals or humans demonstrate fetal abnormalities, or adverse reaction reports indicate evidence of fetal risk. The risk of use in a pregnant woman clearly outweighs any possible benefit.

[a]Regardless of the designated pregnancy category or presumed safety, no drug should be administered during pregnancy unless it is clearly needed and potential benefits outweigh potential risks.

---

an inhaler with a large volume spacer may be used. Children over the age of 8 can generally use an inhaler without a spacer. The child's technique should be assessed often and the need for a spacer ascertained. Thirty percent of children who previously showed good administration technique were found to develop an incorrect technique over time.[49] Spacer devices with whistles may help a child learn the appropriate rate for breathing during an inhalation.

Concerns exist about the impact of theophylline on learning, attention, behavior, and cognitive function. Negative theophylline effects have not been found in all studies, and, in fact, improvement has been reported in some studies or in some children. Patients who appear to demonstrate a higher incidence of compromised cognitive function with theophylline may have had prior attention and achievement problems. The FDA has reviewed this issue and concluded that the evidence of theophylline-induced cognitive impairment is inconclusive.[50] However, children on long-term phenobarbital may develop psychologic and cognitive dysfunction as well as hyperactivity.[51]

Implications in Pregnancy and Lactation

The use of asthma medications in a pregnant or lactating asthmatic patient is based on the balance between adverse drug reactions and the sequelae of an asthma attack on the developing fetus or nursing infant. Theophylline can cause tachycardia, jitteriness, irritability, gagging, vomiting, and breathing disorders in newborns. Regular phenobarbital use during the last 3 months of pregnancy can cause fetal dependency and produce withdrawal in the baby at delivery. Further, teratogenicity has been reported with phenobarbital.

Information on drug safety during pregnancy has been compiled by the Collaborative Perinatal Project Study, case reports, and manufacturer's information. Information for newer medications have been obtained from the package insert. The classification of fetal risk from asthma medications can be found in Table 7.

Certain asthma medications can be delivered to a nursing infant via mother's milk. The American Academy of Physicians' Committee on Drugs lists the following medications as potentially problematic: atropine, dexbrompheniramine maleate with d-isoephedrine, iodinated glycerol, pseudoephedrine, prednisone, prednisolone, terbutaline, theophylline, and triprolidine.[52] Examples of drug-related toxicities experienced by breast-fed infants include insomnia (theophylline); altered thyroid function (iodinated glycerol); and irritability, crying, and poor sleep patterns (dexbrompheniramine with isoephedrine).[52] Phenobarbital may be used by mothers who breast-feed; however, adverse reactions have occurred in some babies, and all babies should be monitored for increased sedation or hyperactivity.[52]

Exercise-Induced Asthma

Exercise-induced asthma may be treated by modifying the exercise regimen or using inhaled beta$_2$ agonists or cromolyn sodium.[53] Patients with exercise-induced asthma may minimize the adverse impact of exercise by choosing exercises that are conducted in warm, humid areas (e.g., swimming); extending their warm-up period; increasing their fitness level; refraining from food ingestion 2 hours before exercise; or wearing a face mask.[53] Theophylline's efficacy in preventing exercise-induced asthma is concentration-dependent and is less than that of inhaled beta$_2$ agonists.[1,4,9] Beta$_2$-agonist therapy should generally be administered approximately 15 minutes before the onset of exercise. Ephedrine, epinephrine, barbiturates, isoetharine, isoproterenol, metaproterenol, oral albuterol, oral terbutaline, prednisone, theophylline–ephedrine–phenobarbital combination, and ephedrine–phenobarbital combination are banned by the U.S. Olympic Committee. The committee allows inhalation therapy with albuterol, bitoterol, pirbuterol, procaterol, terbutaline, cromolyn, ipratropium, and corticosteroids; and it allows oral therapy with theophylline, guaifenesin, and pyrilamine maleate.[25] Even though a drug is prescribed by a physician, it may not be approved by the U.S. Olympic Committee. The patient or health care providers may consult with the committee to determine the current status of accepted drug use in amateur competitive athletic competition (1–800–233–0393). The National Collegiate Association of America (NCAA) and other national and international sports rules are generally consistent with guidelines established by the U.S. Olympic Committee.

Nocturnal Asthma

Pharmacologic therapy is often selected to provide treatment throughout the sleeping period. Sustained-release beta agonists and sustained-release theophylline can be used to provide full coverage during the sleeping period.[9] Because increased eosinophils and histamine levels have been measured during nocturnal asthma, most patients' nocturnal asthma will improve by increasing their daytime anti-inflammatory therapy with cromolyn or inhaled steroids.[9]

Product Selection Guidelines

Once the assessment of asthma has been confirmed, the pharmacist should ask the patient a series of questions to gather the necessary information for product choice and determine if there is a need to seek medical attention. If the patient does not have hypertension, diabetes, uncontrolled thyroid disease, heart disease, or difficulty urinating due to an enlarged prostate; has never been hospitalized for asthma; and is not currently receiving prescription antiasthmatic medications, the pharmacist can consider using a nonprescription antiasthmatic drug. The patient's pharmacy profile and use of other nonprescription medications must then be reviewed for drugs, diseases, smoking, and dietary factors known to alter theophylline pharmacokinetics; for drugs that interact with any of the products available in the nonprescription drugs; or for any allergies to the nonprescription products or aspirin. Specific patient factors such as age, pregnancy, lactation, and finances also need to be considered. From the profile, the pharmacist may also determine the patient's compliance with other asthma medications. The dilemma associated with the use of nonprescription drugs to treat bronchospasm from asthma is that the nonprescription bronchodilators are usually effective in mild disease; however, mild disease can progress to more moderate to severe disease if it is not appropriately treated with anti-inflammatories, and bronchodilators may potentially mask a worsening of asthma by treating only overt symptoms. To tread this fine line can be dangerous, and the patient and the patient's family should know when to abandon self-treatment and immediately seek medical care. In most cases of death from asthma, the severity of the obstruction had been underestimated by the physician or patient. Thus, the NAEP expert panel recommends that patients rely more heavily on peak flow measurements in making treatment decisions.

Epinephrine and ephedrine are nonselective with short durations of activity. Ephedrine is less potent and potentially more toxic, particularly in hypertensive patients, than the newer, orally active, selective beta$_2$ agonists. The combination products prevent individualization of drug therapy and their ingredients may produce additive adverse effects. In some patients with bronchospasm and rhinorrhea, decongestant effects may be desirable. However, patients with bronchospasm and rhinorrhea who need a nasal decongestant may be treated more effectively with an alpha-adrenergic nasal spray for the short term and with intranasal cromolyn or steroids for chronic allergic rhinitis. The primary roles of the pharmacist when caring for the asthmatic patient and family include educating the patient, assessing the patient's response, monitoring for toxicity, determining patient compliance, and directing the patient to obtain additional medical care when appropriate.

Patient Education

When counseling asthmatic patients, the pharmacist should provide general information about the use and storage of medications, instructions on the use and care of inhalers (if appropriate), and pertinent pharmacologic information about a patient's particular medication.

Patients should be told the following about the use and storage of medications:[25]

- Because asthma medication can produce significant toxicity with an overdose, patients should not exceed dosages stated on the labeling.
- Asthma medications should be stored away from a child's access, outdated medications should be discarded, discarded medications should not be accessible to a child's reach, and medication in use should not be stored in a damp or hot place or in direct sunlight.
- Patients should contact a health care practitioner if they experience decreased responsiveness to a drug because this may indicate a worsening of the asthma.

To educate patients adequately on inhaler use, pharmacists should provide both written and verbal instructions.[41] Patients should then demonstrate their inhaler technique to the pharmacist.

If a patient's technique is not adequate after repeated inhaler instruction, the pharmacist should suggest the use of a spacer. If epinephrine aerosols are being used, the patient should be advised to wait at least 1 minute between inhalations. Patients should also be told that dryness of the mouth and throat and oral candidal infections may be prevented by rinsing the mouth after inhaler use or using a spacer.

Besides instructing patients on correct inhaler technique, the pharmacist should discuss the following tips on care and disposal of the canister.

- The inhaler mouthpiece should be washed daily with warm water to prevent clogging and should always be kept free of particles.
- The inhaler devices should be cleaned routinely and air dried.
- The patients should not puncture the unit because the contents are under pressure.
- The canisters should not be stored near heat (temperatures greater than 120°F [48.9°C]) or open flames. They also should not be discarded into fires or incinerators.

An important element in educating patients about their asthma therapy is telling them which precautions to take with their medications and what side effects might occur. Key precautions for nonprescription asthma medications include:[25]

- Patients taking theophylline should avoid large amounts of foods and beverages that contain caffeine and should tell their pharmacist if they are on a special diet.
- Theophylline doses should not be increased beyond recommended doses, and a doctor should be contacted if the patient develops a systemic viral infection.
- Phenobarbital should not be taken with alcohol or other medications affecting the CNS.
- Patients taking oral contraceptives should be warned that phenobarbital may lessen the effectiveness of the contraceptives.
- The patient should use caution if driving or using machinery because phenobarbital can cause sedation and decreased alertness.
- Antihistamines may be associated with increased CNS side effects if taken with other CNS medications such as phenobarbital, pain medications, and alcohol.

From 4–28% of asthmatics will have bronchospasm induced by aspirin.[54] A cross-sensitivity may exist with other nonsteroidal anti-inflammatory drugs. Patients should be cautioned that some nonprescription allergy, cough/cold, and pain preparations contain aspirin. To treat pain, aspirin-sensitive patients can usually use acetaminophen as an analgesic or antipyretic.[54]

Asthmatic patients also need to be educated about the potential of sulfites and sulfur dioxide to elicit bronchospasm. Sulfites are used as preservatives in the pharmaceutical, food, and fermentation industries. Foods and beverages that may contain sulfur dioxide or sulfites include dried and packaged fruits and beverages; beer, wines, and other fermented beverages; salads and salad bar ingredients; guacamole and other dips; potatoes (chips or fries); cider and wine vinegars; pickled vegetables; shrimp and other seafood; and processed, preserved, and "ready to eat" foods and beverages.[55] Certain medications also contain sulfites; however, by FDA regulations, such medications must list sulfites as an ingredient in the package insert.

Various pharmaceutical companies, agencies, and foundations offer patient education materials and services. A complete list of educational material can be obtained from the National Asthma Education Program.

Summary

Hyperactivity of the airways to various physical, chemical, or pharmacologic stimuli is the hallmark of asthma. Therapy is directed at preventing severe attacks and normalizing an asthma patient's lifestyle. Treatment involves both drug and nondrug measures. Nonprescription medications that are currently available for managing asthma are best suited for managing mild attacks. Patients whose asthma is not responding to nonprescription products should consult their physician.

References

1. National Heart, Lung, and Blood Institute, National Asthma Education Program, Expert Panel Report. *Guidelines for the Diagnosis and Management of Asthma*. Pub. No. 91–3042. Bethesda, Md: U.S. Department of Health and Human Services; 1991.
2. Weiss KB, Gergen PJ, Hodgson TA. An economic evaluation of asthma in the United States. *N Engl J Med* 1992 Mar 26; 326: 862–6.
3. West JB. *Respiratory Physiology—the Essentials*. 3rd ed. Baltimore: Williams & Wilkins; 1985.
4. Kaliner MA, Barnes PJ, Persson CGA. *Asthma: Its Pathology and Treatment*. New York: Marcel Dekker, Inc; 1991.

5. Sears MR, Taylor DR, Print CG, et al. Regular inhaled beta-agonist treatment in bronchial asthma. *Lancet* 1990 Dec 8; 336: 1391–6.
6. Spitzer WO, Suissa S, Ernst P, et al. The use of beta agonists and the risk of death and near death from asthma. *N Engl J Med* 1992 Feb 20; 326: 501–6.
7. Coultas DB, Samet JM. Epidemiology and natural history of childhood asthma. In: Tinkelman DG, Falliers CJ, Naspitz CK, eds. *Childhood Asthma: Pathophysiology and Treatment*. New York: Marcel Dekker, Inc; 1987: 131–57.
8. Burrows B, Barbee RA, Cline MG, et al. Characteristics of asthma among elderly adults in a sample of the general population. *Chest* 1991; 100: 935–42.
9. Barnes PJ. A new approach to the treatment of asthma. *N Engl J Med* 1989 Nov 30; 321: 1517–27.
10. Djukanovic R, Roche WR, Wilson JW, et al. Mucosal inflammation in asthma. *Am Rev Respir Dis* 1990; 142: 434–57.
11. Hargreave FE, Gibson PG, Ramsdale EH. Airway hyperresponsiveness, airway inflammation, and asthma. *Immunol Allergy Clin North Am* 1990 Aug; 10: 439–48.
12. Kelly HW, Davis RL. Asthma. In: DiPiro JT, Talbert RL, Hayes PE, et al., eds. *Pharmacotherapy: A Pathophysiological Approach*. New York: Elsevier; 1989: 347–67.
13. Immunization Practices Advisory Committee. Update on adult immunizations. *MMWR* 1991; 40 (RR–12): 42–4.
14. Immunization Practices Advisory Committee. Prevention and control of influenza recommendations. *MMWR* 1991; 40 (RR–6): 1–14.
15. Van Schayck CP, Dompeling E, van Herwaarden F, et al. Bronchodilator treatment in moderate asthma or chronic bronchitis: continuous or on demand? A randomized controlled trial. *Br Med J* 1991 Dec 7; 303: 1426–31.
16. Lipworth BJ, McDevitt DG. Inhaled β_2-adrenoceptor agonists in asthma: help or hindrance? *Br J Clin Pharmacol* 1992; 33: 129–38.
17. Twentyman OP, Finnerty JP, Harris A, et al. Protection against allergen-induced asthma by salmeterol. *Lancet* 1990 Dec 1; 336: 1338–42.
18. Lipworth BJ. Risks versus benefits of inhaled β_2-agonists in the management of asthma. *Drug Safety* 1992; 7: 54–70.
19. Jenne JW, Ahren RC. Pharmacokinetics of beta-adrenergic compounds. In: Jenne JW, Murphy S, eds. *Drug Therapy for Asthma: Research and Clinical Practice*. New York: Marcel Dekker, Inc; 1987: 213–58.
20. Kelly HW. New β_2-adrenergic agonist aerosols. *Clin Pharm* 1985; 4: 393–403.
21. Lipworth BJ, Struthers AD, McDevitt DG. Tachyphylaxis to systemic but not to airway response during prolonged therapy with high dose inhaled salbutamol in asthmatics. *Am Rev Respir Dis* 1989; 140: 586–92.
22. Murphy S, Kelly HW. Cromolyn sodium: a review of mechanisms and clinical use in asthma. *Drug Intell Clin Pharm* 1987; 21: 22–35.
23. Szefler SJ. Glucocorticoid therapy for asthma: clinical pharmacology. *J Allergy Clin Immunol* 1991; 88: 147–65.
24. Cold, cough, allergy, bronchodilator, and antiasthmatic drug products for over-the-counter human use. *Federal Register* 1991 Apr 1; 190–7.
25. *USP DI 1992, Vol II, Advice for the Patient*. Rockville, Md: US Pharmacopeial Convention Inc; 1992.
26. Van Mieghem W, Stevens E, Cosemans J. Ephedrine-induced cardiopathy. *Br Med J* 1978; 1: 816.
27. Roxanas MG, Spalding J. Ephedrine abuse psychosis. *Med J Aust* 1977; 2: 639–40.
28. Hendeles L, Massanari M, Weinberger M. Theophylline. In: Evans WE, Schentas JJ, Jusko WJ, eds. *Applied Pharmacokinetics*. 2nd ed. Spokane, Wash: Applied Therapeutics, 1986; 1105–88.
29. Upton RA. Pharmacokinetic interactions between theophylline and other medication (part I). *Clin Pharmacokinet* 1991; 20: 66–80.
30. Upton RA. Pharmacokinetic interaction between theophylline and other medication (part II). *Clin Pharmacokinet* 1991; 20: 135–50.
31. Bittar G, Friedman HS. The arrhythmogenicity of theophylline: a multivariate analysis of clinical determinants. *Chest* 1991; 99: 1415–20.
32. Chandler MHH, Clifton GD, Louis BA, et al. Home monitoring of theophylline levels: a novel therapeutic approach. *Pharmacotherapy* 1990; 10: 294–300.
33. Holgate ST, Finnerty JP. Antihistamines in asthma. *J Allergy Clin Immunol* 1989; 83: 537–47.
34. Pinnas JL, Schachtel BP, Chen TM, et al. Inhaled epinephrine and oral theophylline-ephedrine in the treatment of asthma. *J Clin Pharmacol* 1991; 31: 243–7.
35. Weinberger M, Bronsky E, Bensch GW, et al. Interaction of ephedrine and theophylline. *Clin Pharmocol Ther* 1975; 17: 585–92.
36. Levy RH, Wilensky AJ, Friel PN. Other antiepileptic drugs. In: Evans WE, Schentas JJ, Jusko WJ, eds. *Applied Pharmacokinetics*. 2nd ed. Spokane, Wash: Applied Therapeutics, 1986; 540–69.
37. Newman SP, Pavia D, Moren F, et al. Deposition of pressurized aerosols in the human respiratory tract. *Thorax* 1981; 36: 52–5.
38. Toogood JH, Baskerville J, Jennings B, et al. Use of spacers to facilitate inhaled corticosteroid treatment of asthma. *Am Rev Respir Dis* 1984; 129: 723–9.
39. Mickel TR, Self TH, Farr GE, et al. Evaluation of pharmacists' practice in patient education when dispensing a metered-dose inhaler. *DICP Ann Pharmacother* 1990; 24: 927–30.
40. Guidry GG, Brown WD, Stogner SW, et al. Incorrect use of metered-dose inhalers by medical personnel. *Chest* 1992; 101: 31–3.
41. Self TS, Brooks JB, Lieberman P, et al. The value of demonstration and role of the pharmacist in teaching the correct use of pressurized bronchodilators. *Can Med Assoc J* 1983; 128: 129–31.
42. Konig P. Spacer devices used with metered-dose inhalers: breakthrough or gimmick? *Chest* 1985; 88: 276–84.
43. Schocken DD, Roth GS. Reduced beta-adrenergic receptor concentrations in aging man. *Nature* 1977; 267: 856–8.
44. Stressman J, Eliakim R, Cahan C, et al. Deterioration of beta-receptor–denylate cyclase function in elderly, hospitalized patients. *J Gerontol* 1984; 39: 667–72.
45. Vestal RE, Wood AJJ, Shand DG. Reduced β-adrenoceptor sensitivity in the elderly. *Clin Pharmacol Ther* 1979; 26:181–6.
46. Chandler MHH, Clifton GD, Burki NK, et al. Pulmonary function in the elderly: response to theophylline bronchodilation. *J Clin Pharmacol* 1990; 30: 330–5.
47. Sims JA, doPico GA, Reed CE. Bronchodilating effect of oral theophylline–ephedrine combination. *J Allergy Clin Immunol* 1978; 62: 15–21.
48. Armitage JM, Williams SJ. Inhaler technique in the elderly. *Age Ageing* 1988; 17: 275–8.
49. Lee H, Evans HE. Evaluation of inhalation aids of metered-dose inhalers in asthmatic children. *Chest* 1987; 91: 366–9.
50. Nicklas RA. Theophylline, school performance, and Food and Drug Administration [letter]. *Pediatrics* 1989; 83: 146–7.
51. Camfield CS, Chaplin S, Doyle A-B, et al. Side effects of phenobarbital in toddlers; behavioral and cognitive aspects. *J. Pediatr* 1979; 95:361–5.
52. American Academy of Physicians, Committee on Drugs. Transfer of drugs and other chemicals into human milk. *Pediatrics* 1989; 84: 924–36.
53. Pierson WE. Exercise-induced bronchospasm in children and adolescents. *Pediatr Clin North Am* 1988; 25: 1031–40.
54. Slepian IK, Mathews KP, McLean JA. Aspirin-sensitive asthma. *Chest* 1985; 87: 386–91.
55. Mathison DA, Stevenson DD, Simon RA. Precipitating factors in asthma: aspirin, sulfites, and other drugs and chemicals. *Chest* 1985; 87: 50S–4S.

CHAPTER 10

Sleep Aid and Stimulant Products

M. Lynn Crismon and Donna M. Jermain

Questions to ask in patient assessment and counseling

Sleep Aid and Sedative Products

- *How long have you had trouble sleeping?*
- *How severe is your sleep disturbance?*
- *Do you generally have trouble falling asleep? Do you wake up frequently or too early?*
- *Do you feel rested when you awake in the morning?*
- *Do you have trouble functioning or staying alert during the day?*
- *How often do you take naps?*
- *What do you think is causing your sleep problem?*
- *Has there been increased stress in your life lately?*
- *Do you have any health problems or physical complaints?*
- *What prescription and nonprescription medications do you take?*
- *How often and at what times during the day do you drink coffee or other caffeinated beverages? Alcoholic beverages?*
- *Do you smoke?*
- *Have you ever been treated for psychiatric problems?*
- *Would you describe yourself as a nervous or anxious person?*
- *Have you felt depressed or disinterested in your usual activities?*
- *Have you ever been told you snore loudly or are a restless sleeper?*
- *What methods or medications have you used to treat insomnia thus far? How long did you use them? Were they effective?*

Stimulant Products

- *Why do you want to use this product?*
- *How long do you intend to use this product?*
- *Have you ever used a stimulant product before? Did you experience any adverse effects?*
- *Do you regularly consume coffee, tea, cola, or other caffeinated beverages? Have you experienced adverse effects from drinking them?*
- *What other medications, prescription and nonprescription, do you take?*
- *Are you under a physician's care? What types of medical problems do you have?*
- *Do you have anxiety, irritability, or any other nervous condition?*
- *Do you have problems sleeping? (If patient has problems sleeping, see sleep aid questions.)*
- *Are you pregnant or breast-feeding?*
- *Do you smoke cigarettes or chew tobacco?*
- *Do you drink alcohol? If so, how much and how often?*

Sleep Aids

Insomnia is one of the most common patient complaints, ranking third behind headache and the common cold. Annually, approximately one-third of all Americans report at least occasional difficulty sleeping, and about 15% of the U.S. population experiences insomnia severe enough to warrant seeing a physician. Nearly 2% of adult Americans will receive a prescription for a hypnotic medication annually, and about 1 out of every 100 patients with insomnia will buy a nonprescription sleep product.[1] The frequency of this complaint, and the widespread use of both prescription and nonprescription medications and other remedies make treating insomnia a significant concern for the pharmacist.

Insomnia is not a disease. It is a symptom or patient complaint for which there are no precise criteria or definitions. Patients may complain of difficulty falling asleep (sleep latency insomnia), frequent nocturnal awakening, early morning awakening, or poor quality of sleep. There is no ideal duration of sleep, and patients complaining of a sleep disturbance may actually sleep for the same length of time as other individuals who feel they sleep well. However, these patients usually report that it takes them more than 30 minutes to fall asleep, and their sleep duration is less than 6 to 7 hours nightly.[1] Moreover, their perceived sleep pattern and quality of daytime functioning may be more important than their duration of sleep. Thus, patients with insomnia are those who feel they sleep poorly at night and function poorly during the day.

This chapter is based in part on the chapter with the same title that appeared in the 9th edition but was written by James P. Caro and Susan R. Dombrowski.

Sleep Physiology

Physiologically, sleep can be categorized into different stages by using the sleeping electroencephalogram (EEG) in conjunction with electro-oculography and electromyography. State 1 sleep is a transitional stage, which occurs as the patient falls asleep; the EEG resembles the waking state more than sleep. Stage 2 sleep, in which approximately 50% of sleep time is spent, is light sleep. Stages 3 and 4, collectively known as deep sleep or delta sleep, are characterized by the patterns of delta waves on the EEG. Rapid eye movement (REM) sleep is neither light nor deep. It is characterized by the body being more physiologically active than during other sleep stages while skeletal muscles are actively inhibited. The eyes move rapidly from side to side, and the blood pressure, heart rate, temperature, respirations, and metabolism are increased.[2,3]

Upon falling asleep, one progresses through the four stages of sleep and reaches the first REM period in about 70–90 minutes. This time, from falling asleep to the first REM period, is referred to as the REM latency. The first REM period is of short duration, usually 5–7 minutes. The sleep cycle then repeats about every 90 minutes, with each progressive REM period becoming longer and the time in deep sleep becoming shorter.[2,3] Although the effects of medication on the sleep stages are thought to be important, their relative importance on the different stages of sleep is unclear. However, prolonged suppression of REM may result in psychologic and behavioral changes.

Sleep physiology changes with increasing age. Among elderly persons, less time is spent in stage 4 sleep, the total duration of sleep becomes shorter, sleep becomes more shallow and disrupted, the number of nocturnal awakenings increases, and sleep latency usually remains normal. Elderly individuals may take more daytime naps. Although these changes alone do not indicate insomnia, there is an increased prevalence of sleep complaints in this population. Elderly individuals are frequent consumers of nonprescription sleep products, and 35% of all hypnotic prescriptions are written for older people.[1]

Insomnia: Classification and Assessment

Based on the duration of sleep disturbance, insomnia can be classified as transient, short-term, or chronic.[4] It is extremely important that the pharmacist ask the patient questions to determine the etiology and duration of the insomnia. Although nonprescription sleep products have not been extensively evaluated, it is assumed they work best in transient and short-term insomnia.

Transient insomnia is usually situational and is commonly caused by environmental changes or life stresses such as travel, hospitalization, or anticipation of an important or stressful event. Transient insomnia is often self-limiting, lasting only a few days. However, if more severe stresses are present (e.g., the death of a loved one, the loss of a job, or divorce), transient insomnia may become short-term insomnia, usually lasting no longer than 3 weeks. Unless it is managed appropriately, short-term insomnia may progress to chronic insomnia. Chronic insomnia lasts from months to years and is often the result of medical problems, psychologic dysfunction, or substance abuse.[1,4] Individuals with psychophysiologic insomnia experience chronic insomnia and are thought to develop faulty sleep habits during transient or short-term insomnia that progress to a long-term sleep problem. Thus, it is critical to identify the problem that is responsible for long-term insomnia if the sleep disturbance is to be appropriately managed.[5]

Patients with other sleep disorders may also seek a nonprescription hypnotic from the pharmacist. Among these disorders are sleep apnea, narcolepsy, and nocturnal myoclonus. Sleep apnea is characterized by patient and family complaints of poor sleep quality, gasping, snoring, and

TABLE 1 Drugs that may exacerbate insomnia

Drugs that may cause insomnia	Drugs that may produce withdrawal insomnia
Alcohol	**Alcohol**
Antidepressants Buproprion Fluoxetine Monoamine oxidase Tricyclic antidepressants	**Antihistamines** **Barbiturates** **Benzodiazepines**
Antihypertensives Beta blockers Clonidine Methyldopa Reserpine	**Hypnotics (miscellaneous)** Bromides Chloral hydrate Ethchlorvynol Glutethimide
Hypnotic use (chronic) **Nicotine**	**Monoamine oxidase inhibitors** **Tricyclic antidepressants**
Sympathomimetic amines Amphetamines Appetite suppressants Beta-adrenergic agonists Caffeine Decongestants (e.g., phenylpropanolamine, phenylephrine)	**Miscellaneous** Amphetamines Cocaine Marijuana Opiates Phencyclidine
Miscellaneous Corticosteroids Levodopa Methysergide Oral contraceptives Phenytoin Quinidine Theophylline Thyroid preparations	

TABLE 2	Etiology of chronic (long-term) insomnia
Medical problems	**Psychiatric problems (30–70% of cases)**
Pain	Depression
Angina pectoris	Anxiety disorder
Arthritis	Schizophrenia
Cancer	Bipolar disorder
Peptic ulcer/gastrointestinal reflux	Substance abuse
Respiratory difficulty	**Sleep disorders**
Asthma	Sleep apnea
Bronchitis	Nocturnal myoclonus
Chronic obstructive pulmonary disease	Delayed sleep phase syndrome (night shift workers)
Congestive heart failure	Drug-related insomnia
Other medical problems	Psychophysiological insomnia (idiopathic insomnia)
Hyperthyroidism	
Parkinson's disease	
Renal insufficiency	

daytime fatigue and sedation. This disorder appears to be more common in men, and the stereotype is the middle-aged, overweight, hypertensive male. Although it is usually caused by some form of airway obstruction, sleep apnea may be produced through central nervous system (CNS) mechanisms. Narcolepsy is characterized by daytime sleep attacks, cataplexy (sudden loss of muscle tone), hypnagogic hallucinations, and sleep paralysis. The patient with nocturnal myoclonus experiences jerky leg movements throughout the night. This patient may only perceive poor-quality sleep and daytime fatigue; however, the bed partner can confirm the presence of muscle jerks. Patients with nocturnal myoclonus also often complain of "restless legs syndrome," an uncomfortable feeling in their calves and thighs in the evening hours. Patients who complain of any of these types of symptoms should be referred to a physician for a thorough evaluation. Formal assessment by a sleep laboratory, including sleep studies, can be extremely useful in evaluating patients with chronic sleep dysfunction.[1]

Regardless of the etiology of the disorder, sleep-deprived individuals are highly symptomatic and their quality of life is negatively affected. In a telephone survey of 691 untreated insomniacs, 83% reported being "easily upset, irritated, or annoyed"; 80% reported feeling "blue, down in the dumps, or depressed"; 78% said they were "too tired to do things"; and 59% admitted having "more general trouble remembering things," among other complaints.[6]

The pharmacist should evaluate patients carefully before deciding whether to recommend a nonprescription product. Questions such as those at the beginning of this chapter should be asked regarding medical disorders, psychiatric disorders, medications (Table 1), psychologic or situational stresses, or any exogenous problems that may be responsible for the sleep disturbance. Medical and psychiatric problems (Table 2) are often associated with long-term insomnia, and the underlying problem needs to be addressed; thus, the conditions listed in Table 2 warrant referral to a physician rather than the recommendation of a nonprescription sleep aid. Whenever a sleep product is recommended, the pharmacist should stress measures to improve sleep hygiene (Table 3).

Sleep Aid Products

Antihistamines

Subsequent to a comprehensive review of all ingredients in nonprescription sleep products, the Food and Drug Administration (FDA) found the antihistamine diphenhydramine to be the only agent, based upon clinical trials, to be safe and effective for nonprescription use.[7,8] Although the safety of another antihistamine, doxylamine, has not been fully established, the FDA has allowed the drug to remain on the market, pending further studies.[8] No published studies supporting the efficacy of doxylamine as a hypnotic are currently available. Products containing pyrilamine maleate, potassium or sodium bromide, and scopolamine hydrobromide have been removed from the market.[7] The FDA has not addressed products containing diphenhydramine or doxylamine in combination with other agents, and such products continue to be marketed. Clinical trials are currently under way to assess the efficacy and safety of acetaminophen–diphenhydramine products. The FDA is requiring that the study population be composed of patients who require both an analgesic and a sleep aid.[9]

Both diphenhydramine and doxylamine are members of the ethanolamine group of antihistamines. Although the exact mechanism by which the ethanolamines affect sleep is unclear, it is probably related to their affinity for histamine I and muscarinic receptors.[8]

TABLE 3	Principles of good sleep hygiene

1. Go to bed and arise at about the same time daily.
2. Engage in relaxing activities prior to bedtime.
3. Exercise regularly but not late in the evening.
4. Avoid eating meals or ingesting large snacks immediately prior to bedtime.
5. Eliminate daytime naps.
6. Avoid caffeine use after noon.
7. Avoid alcohol or nicotine use later in the evening.
8. Minimize external disruptions (e.g., light and noise).
9. If unable to fall asleep, do not become anxious; leave the bedroom and participate in relaxing activities (e.g., read or listen to music) until tired.

Pharmacokinetics

Selected clinical and pharmacokinetic properties of diphenhydramine and doxylamine are summarized in Table 4. Both drugs are well absorbed from the gastrointestinal (GI) tract and have short to intermediate half-lives. Diphenhydramine is metabolized in the liver through two successive N-demethylations, and its apparent half-life may be prolonged by a factor of approximately 1.5 in patients with chronic liver disease.[10,11] A positive relationship exists between diphenhydramine plasma concentrations and drowsiness and cognitive impairment. Significant drowsiness has been shown to last from 3 to 6 hours after a single 50-mg dose of diphenhydramine whereas impairment in performance on psychomotor tests lasts from 2 to 4 hours.[12,13] How this may be extrapolated to nightly dosing of diphenhydramine is unclear; however, it may indicate that patients can be assured that their ability to perform tasks requiring mental alertness and cognitive ability will not be impaired for any longer than they feel drowsy.

Patient ethnicity may account for differences in drug effect. One study indicates that Orientals have lower diphenhydramine peak plasma concentrations, more rapid clearance, and less subjective sedation than Caucasians have.[10] Thus, Orientals may require as much as 1.7 times more diphenhydramine than Caucasians to experience the same level of sedation. Oriental patients who do not initially respond to a 50-mg dose of diphenhydramine should be advised to try a 75-mg nightly dose.

Efficacy

Of the published clinical trials with diphenhydramine, most but not all indicate efficacy, particularly in decreasing sleep latency.[1] Fifty milligrams of diphenhydramine appear to be the optimal adult dose, and, except in Orientals, doses greater than 50 mg are not more efficacious as a sleep aid but do increase the potential for adverse effects. Patients who have never been treated with hypnotics tend to respond better to diphenhydramine than previously treated individuals.[14] In a study of elderly nursing home patients, subjects rated both diphenhydramine 50 mg and temazepam 15 mg as more effective than placebo in inducing sleep.[15] Although these patients reportedly tolerated diphenhydramine well, the possibility of anticholinergic side effects should not be overlooked. Because no published efficacy and safety studies are available documenting the value of doxylamine as an hypnotic, only diphenhydramine should be recommended to patients for such use at the present time.

Indications

Although the primary indication for nonprescription hypnotics is the symptomatic management of transient and short-term insomnia, the results of a recent telephone survey of insomniac patients in four major U.S. cities question their usefulness. Hypnotic users who responded to newspaper advertisements announcing a survey of consumer opinions concerning sleep products were questioned about multiple aspects of hypnotic effects. These consumers reported nonprescription hypnotics to be less effective in improving nighttime or daytime symptoms of insomnia than three marketed benzodiazepine hypnotics.[6] Although the results of clinical trials have suggested that nonprescription products are effective in treating sleep latency insomnia, the authors of this study concluded that "OTC [over-the-counter] hypnotics provide some relief from insomnia, but from a benefit–risk perspective, their net benefits are meager."[6] Of nocturnal symptoms, "frequent awakenings" is the symptom reported to respond best, but even then this was so for only 26% of 310 respondents. In addition, 11% of nonprescription hypnotic users reported experiencing more morning grogginess while taking the nonprescription product than before taking it. However, when asked the following question—"Taking into account both the positive effects on your sleep and daytime functioning and any negative effects you may have experienced, would you take this medication again for the same purpose?"— 61% of nonprescription hypnotic users answered affirmatively. Although this is a lower overall satisfaction level than that reported by prescription hypnotic users, it does indicate a reasonable level of consumer satisfaction regarding nonprescription hypnotic use.

Although poorly studied, tolerance to the hypnotic effects of diphenhydramine appears to result with repeated use. With the exception of Orientals, adult patients should be advised not to exceed 50 mg nightly, and all patients should limit their use of diphenhydramine to no more than 7–10 consecutive nights. For patients with transient or short-term insomnia—assuming there are no underlying problems—reestablishing the normal sleep cycle with hypnotics should assist in normalizing sleep patterns. Patients complaining of continuing insomnia after 10 days of nonprescription hypnotic use and good sleep hygiene measures should be referred to a physician for a more thorough evaluation.

Adverse Effects and Toxicity

In addition to sedation, the intended effect when they are used as hypnotics, the primary side effects of diphenhydramine and doxylamine are anticholinergic in nature.[8] Commonly occurring adverse effects include dry

TABLE 4 Selected pharmacokinetic and clinical properties of nonprescription hypnotics

	Diphenhydramine	Doxylamine
Time to maximum plasma concentration	1–4 hr	2–3 hr
Maximum sedation	1–3 hr	N/A
Protein binding	80–85%	N/A
Elimination half-life	2.4–9.3 hr	10 hr
Duration of sedation	3–6 hr	N/A
Bioavailability	26–61%	N/A

Key: N/A = not available.
Data extracted from:
AHFS Drug Information 92: 2–5, 17–20.
Clin Pharmacol Ther 1980; 28: 229–34.
Clin Pharmacol Ther 1989; 45: 15–21.
Clin Pharmacol Ther 1978; 23: 375–82.

mouth and throat, constipation, blurred vision, and tinnitus. Older male patients should be asked about prostatic hypertrophy and difficulty urinating. Narrow- (closed-) angle glaucoma is also a contraindication. Patients with cardiovascular disease (e.g., angina or rhythm disturbance) may be particularly susceptible to the anticholinergic adverse effects of diphenhydramine and doxylamine. If these problems exist, ethanolamine hypnotics should not be recommended. In addition, a patient's concomitant medication regimen should be reviewed before a pharmacist recommends diphenhydramine or doxylamine. A patient who is taking other anticholinergics should be alerted to the potential for additive side effects.

Patients should be cautioned not to drive an automobile or operate machinery until their response to the drug is known. They should also be warned of the additive CNS depressant effects of alcohol and encouraged not to drink alcoholic beverages while taking these drugs. Some patients may develop paradoxical excitation. This occurs more often in children, elderly patients, and patients with organic mental disorders. Symptoms include nervousness, restlessness, agitation, tremors, insomnia, delirium, and, in rare cases, seizures. These symptoms may also be a sign of anticholinergic toxicity.

Antihistamine dosage excess can result in anticholinergic toxicity.[16] This may occur as a result of drug interactions, purposeful ingestion of a large amount, or individual sensitivity. Anticholinergic toxicity is particularly common in children, in whom the symptoms are usually more severe. CNS anticholinergic toxicity is one of the primary presenting features of antihistamine excess. Patients may be anxious, excited, delirious, hallucinating, or stuporous; in more severe cases, coma or seizures may occur. Other physical signs may include dilated pupils, hot and dry mucous membranes, and elevated body temperature. Tachycardia is common, and in severe cases, dysrhythmias, cardiovascular collapse, and death may occur.

The primary treatment of anticholinergic toxicity includes emesis to decrease drug absorption if ingestion is acute. If the patient is stuporous or comatose, gastric lavage and activated charcoal may be used. Patients should receive general supportive care such as hydration, antipyretics, and maintenance of vital signs, including ventilatory support. Seizures should be treated with standard anticonvulsants such as diazepam. Despite the potential pharmacologic rationale, physostigmine is not recommended as first-line therapy in anticholinergic toxicity because of its narrow therapeutic index and short duration of action.

Use During Pregnancy and Lactation

The safety of antihistamines during pregnancy has not been clearly established.[8] Therefore, the benefit-to-risk ratio of using these drugs during pregnancy should be carefully evaluated. Doxylamine was formerly marketed as a prescription combination product for treatment of morning sickness during pregnancy. However, the manufacturer voluntarily removed this combination from the market in 1976 following allegations of teratogenicity. Although it is not possible to prove conclusively that doxylamine is not teratogenic, epidemiologic studies indicate that the possibility of such a relationship is remote.[8] Nevertheless, rather than recommending a nonprescription product, pharmacists should advise pregnant women to consult their physician regarding any sleep disturbance.

There appears to be an increased risk of CNS side effects from antihistamine use in neonates. For this reason, and because such drugs may inhibit lactation, most pharmaceutical manufacturers recommend that nursing mothers generally not use antihistamines.[8]

Miscellaneous Products

L-Tryptophan

The efficacy of L-tryptophan in treating insomnia has not been clearly established. Some studies have demonstrated hypnotic efficacy; others have not.[1,17]

Although touted by health food stores in 1- to 3-g doses as being a safe and natural way to induce sleep, L-tryptophan is not an innocuous product. More than 1,500 cases of eosinophilia–myalgia syndrome (EMS), including at least 27 deaths, have been reported in patients taking contaminated L-tryptophan.[1,18] In March 1990, the FDA recalled all products containing L-tryptophan except protein supplements, infant formulas, and parenteral and enteral nutritional products.

The symptoms of EMS develop over several weeks. Primary symptoms are myalgia, which may be severe and incapacitating, and fatigue. Other symptoms include shortness of breath, cough, skin rash, arthralgia, muscle weakness, and peripheral edema. In a few severe cases, congestive heart failure, dysrhythmias, pneumonia, vasculitis, ascending polyneuropathy (similar to Guillain–Barré syndrome), and scleroderma-like skin changes have been reported. Clinical symptoms are accompanied by eosinophilia, often with more than 1,000 cells per cubic millimeter. The natural course of EMS is unpredictable. Although some patients' symptoms will remit when L-tryptophan is discontinued, others will develop into some of the more severe symptoms described above.[1]

EMS has been thought to be caused by a contaminant in the manufacturing process and its development related to the dose of the contaminated product ingested.[1,19] The Centers for Disease Control has traced all EMS cases to products manufactured by Showa Denko KK in Japan. Batches of the implicated L-tryptophan products were found to contain greater quantities of 1-1'-ethylidenebis[tryptophan], or EBT, than other batches. However, results from a recent animal study indicate that high doses of EBT-free L-tryptophan also produced EMS but that such episodes of EMS did not appear to be as severe as those incurred by the contaminated product. These investigators appropriately question whether any L-tryptophan–containing product should be taken in high doses.[18] Pressure has been placed on the FDA to regulate all amino acid–containing products, and it is not known when L-tryptophan products will be remarketed in the United States.

In addition to EMS, L-tryptophan has been associated with causing "serotonin storm" when used in combination with serotonin reuptake inhibitors (e.g., sertraline and fluoxetine) or monoamine oxidase inhibitors. Symptoms of this drug interaction include agitation, restlessness, aggressiveness, tremor, hyperthermia, diarrhea, and cramping.[1] L-tryptophan should not be initiated in combination with one of these agents in outpatients. Given its questionable efficacy and known adverse effects, pharmacists should be reluctant to recommend L-tryptophan as a sleep aid.

Alcohol

Ethanol is a CNS depressant that has been used for both its sedative and disinhibiting properties for centuries. However, alcohol does not have the positive effects on sleep that many people believe it to have. After occasional evening consumption of one or two drinks, alcohol is effective in decreasing sleep latency. However, with heavy or continuous consumption, alcohol disrupts the sleep cycle. Although sleep latency decreases, the patient usually begins to experience restless sleep and often awakens within 2–4 hours. The total duration of sleep also decreases. Moreover, after alcohol is discontinued, rebound insomnia is likely to occur.[20] Chronic alcoholics usually have marked disorganization of their sleep cycle, with shortened REM periods and delta sleep. Approximately 10–15% of chronic insomniacs have problems with substance abuse, especially alcohol abuse.[4] Patients who abuse alcohol are also frequent abusers of other CNS depressants, including benzodiazepines. Patients should be questioned regarding their alcohol use before a nonprescription hypnotic is recommended; those who drink regularly should instead be referred to a physician.

Alcohol is present in some nonprescription combination cold products, such as Nyquil®, which contains 25% alcohol by volume. Products of this type are marketed and sometimes recommended by physicians and pharmacists to induce sleep. Data are limited, however, regarding their efficacy and safety as hypnotics. They contain multiple ingredients, which increases the risk of side effects and interactions with other drugs. At least four cases of liver injury, possibly due to the alcohol–acetaminophen combination, have been reported with Nyquil®.[21]

Alcohol has negative effects on patients with sleep apnea. As little as 3 oz (two shots) of 80-proof ethanol may increase the frequency and severity of apneic episodes, even in patients with mild apnea.[22] Furthermore, alcohol has even been reported to cause apnea in normal individuals.[23]

The pharmacist must acquire the patient's medication history to examine for the possibilities both of additive CNS depression between alcohol and other medications and of substance abuse. Patients who inquire about using alcohol as a sleep aid should be advised to limit such use to one or two drinks on an occasional basis. Most clinicians advise that alcohol never be used as a hypnotic or an adjunct to a sleep aid program.

Summary: Sleep Aids

Sedating antihistamines such as diphenhydramine are effective in treating occasional transient or short-term insomnia, particularly if the sleep disturbance is primarily related to difficulty falling asleep. Because little information is available regarding the hypnotic effects

TABLE 5 Approximate caffeine content of selected beverages and foods

Beverage or food	Caffeine content (mg)
Coffee (5 oz)	
Brewed, automatic drip	60–180
Brewed, percolator	40–170
Instant	30–120
Decaffeinated, instant	1–5
Decaffeinated, brewed	2–5
Tea (5 oz)	
Brewed, imported brands	25–110
Brewed, U.S. brands	20–90
Instant	25–50
Iced (12 oz)	67–76
Soft drinks (12 oz)	
Mountain Dew®	54
Coca-Cola®	45.6
Diet Coke®	45.6
Dr. Pepper®	39.6
Sugar-Free Dr. Pepper®	39.6
Big Red®	38.4
Sugar-Free Big Red®	38.4
Pepsi-Cola®	38.4
Diet Pepsi®	36
7-Up®	0
Sunkist Orange®	0
Ginger ale	0
Chocolate cake (1/16th of 9-in. cake)	13.8
Chocolate ice cream (2/3 c)	4.5
Chocolate pudding, instant (1/2 c)	5.5
Chocolate milk beverage (8 oz)	2–7
Chocolate-flavored syrup (1 oz)	4
Milk chocolate (1 oz)	1–15
Dark chocolate, semisweet (1 oz)	5–35
Baker's chocolate (1 oz)	26
Cocoa beverage (5 oz)	2–20

Data extracted from:
JAMA 1984 Aug 10; 252: 803–6.
FDA Consumer 1984 Mar; 18: 14–6.
Hosp Pharm 1984 Apr; 19: 257–67.

of doxylamine, only diphenhydramine should be recommended as a hypnotic at the present time. Before recommending a nonprescription agent, the pharmacist should question the patient carefully regarding the characteristics and possible etiologies of the sleep disturbance. A patient who appears to have long-term insomnia or sleep disturbance caused by an underlying disorder should be referred to a physician for further evaluation. The patient should also be questioned regarding medical disorders or concomitant medications that may interact with diphenhydramine, and should be counseled regarding diphenhydramine's side effects and particularly the additive effects of alcohol. The patient should be advised that nonprescription hypnotics are intended for short-term use and that a physician should be consulted if sleep problems persist beyond 7–10 nights. Regardless of whether a nonprescription product is recommended, the pharmacist should emphasize the importance of maintaining healthy sleep habits to ensure a good night's sleep.

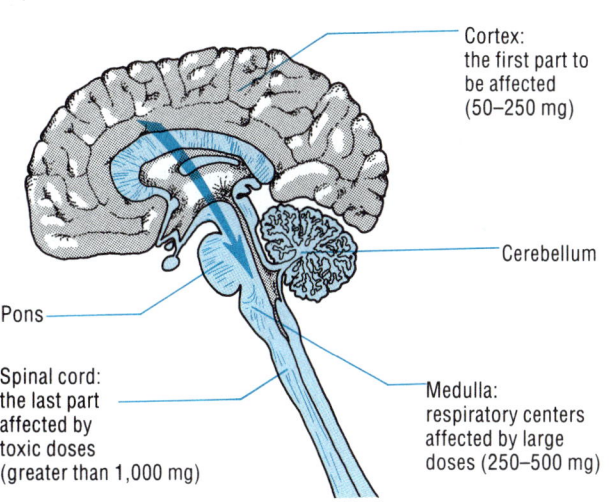

FIGURE 1 Sites of action of caffeine in the central nervous system.

Stimulant Products (Caffeine)

Caffeine is the only FDA-approved stimulant for nonprescription use. Nearly 80% of the U.S. adult population consumes caffeine daily, thus making it one of the most popular drugs.[24] Many children also consume caffeine. For example, mean caffeine intake in children 6–11 months old is 4.2 mg per day; in children 6–17 years old, it increases to 43 mg per day.[25] In adults, mean caffeine intake is 186 mg per day (approximately two cups of coffee daily or the equivalent). Daily caffeine intake correlates with age.

Caffeine is a common ingredient in coffee, tea, soft drinks, and chocolate products[24] (Table 5). It is also present in many prescription and nonprescription drugs, including headache and cold remedies, menstrual pain relief products, diet aids, and stimulant preparations. Caffeine concentrations vary among the products; generally, stimulants contain the highest concentrations, averaging 100–200 mg per tablet.

Physiologic Effects

Central Nervous System Effects

Caffeine is the most potent methylxanthine in terms of CNS stimulation, even at low plasma concentrations. As caffeine plasma concentrations increase, the cortex, then the medulla, and lastly the spinal cord are stimulated (Figure 1). Caffeine doses of 50–200 mg can increase alertness and decrease fatigue and drowsiness. At higher doses (200–500 mg), caffeine may produce tremulousness, nervousness, headache, and irritability. High plasma concentrations may also cause excitement, tinnitus, insomnia, and restlessness.

Caffeine's effect on sleep may be dose-dependent, but it varies greatly among individuals. Caffeine appears to increase stage 2 sleep and decrease delta sleep. Thus, it may increase awakenings and arousability although tolerance may develop to these effects.

Caffeine also has varying effects on mood. Aggressive behavior has been reported to decrease with caffeine reduction. Caffeine may exacerbate anxiety, thus potentially worsening symptoms in patients with anxiety or panic disorder.[26] Depression has been reported in persons consuming large amounts of caffeine (five cups of coffee a day or more).[26] However, it is difficult to know whether depressed patients self-medicate with caffeine or whether caffeine produces depression. Increased caffeine intake has been linked to a worsening in the behavioral symptoms of moderate to severe premenstrual syndrome.[27]

Cardiovascular Effects

Pharmacologic effects of caffeine on the cardiovascular system have long been debated. Caffeine stimulates heart muscle; however, this action is often opposed by simultaneous medullary vagal stimulation. The resultant heart rate changes are variable. As the caffeine dose is increased, the myocardium stimulation overcomes the vagal effect and increased cardiac activity is noted.

Caffeine causes systemic release of norepinephrine, epinephrine, and renin, causing alterations in blood pressure.[24] However, recent studies suggest that caffeine does not produce persistent increases in blood pressure because tolerance develops quickly.[28] Even in individuals who do not regularly consume caffeine, the increased blood pressure resulting from caffeine ingestion rapidly returns to normal. Thus, hypertensive patients can continue to consume moderate amounts of caffeine.

Several reports have suggested that heavy caffeine consumption is associated with coronary heart disease.[24,29] One prospective study involving 1,130 male medical students followed for 19–35 years noted a positive dose–response relationship between caffeine consumption and coronary heart disease.[29] However, another prospective study over 2 years involving 45,589 men with no history of cardiovascular disease found no association between coffee consumption and the risk of coronary heart disease or stroke.[30]

The effect of caffeine on cardiac rate and rhythm, and the possible development of arrhythmias have been studied. In 34 normal adults, high caffeine doses were not associated with any significant change in cardiac rate or rhythm.[31] Moderate caffeine intake, 300–450 mg per day, did not increase the severity or frequency of arrhythmias in normal individuals, in ischemic heart disease patients, or in patients with preexisting serious ventricular ectopy.[32] In contrast, an increased incidence of spontaneous ventricular ectopic beats was noted in persons with preexisting ventricular ectopic beats who received 1 mg of caffeine per kilogram of body weight.[33] Thus, in both healthy individuals and in heart disease patients, the role of moderate amounts of caffeine in cardiac arrhythmias is unclear. In very high concentrations, however, caffeine may cause sinus tachycardia, paroxysmal supraventricular tachycardia, ventricular arrhythmias, or hypotension.[24,34]

Caffeine may also contribute to adverse changes in lipid metabolism.[24] Some epidemiologic studies suggest a link between coffee consumption and increased total and low-density lipoprotein cholesterol concentrations.

Miscellaneous Effects

Caffeine affects the respiratory, endocrine, GI, and renal systems. Caffeine is a bronchodilator, but it is only about 40% as potent as theophylline,[24] and it may increase the respiratory rate. Endocrine effects include increases in renin, cortisol, free fatty acids, blood glucose concentrations, and the metabolic rate. Effects on the GI system include increases in gastric acid and pepsin secretion. Caffeine may either decrease or have no effect upon lower esophageal sphincter pressure, and it relaxes smooth muscle in the biliary and GI tract. Caffeine reduces mesenteric and liver blood flow, the latter by up to 19%. Finally, caffeine has a mild diuretic effect by increasing the glomerular filtration rate and inhibiting sodium tubular reabsorption.

Pharmacokinetics

Caffeine is rapidly and completely absorbed from the GI tract; peak plasma concentrations occur 30–60 minutes after ingestion. Caffeine crosses the blood brain barrier rapidly and has a volume of distribution of 0.5–0.8 L/kg of body weight. It is extensively metabolized in the liver by the microsomal cytochrome P-450 system, primarily through oxidative demethylation and hydroxylation. Furthermore, no significant first-pass effect exists. Paraxanthine, theobromine, and theophylline are active metabolites of caffeine. In adults, the average half-life of caffeine is 4–6 hours. In smokers, the half-life is shorter; in patients with chronic liver disease and in pregnant women, the half-life is extended. In neonates, the half-life may be as long as 100 hours because neonates primarily eliminate caffeine unchanged by the kidneys until they are 3 months old. The half-life of caffeine in elderly patients is not significantly different than that in younger adults.

Indications

Caffeine is commercially available as the sole ingredient in most CNS stimulant products as well as one of the ingredients in many combination products such as headache remedies. Used as a CNS stimulant, caffeine is marketed as a product to help fatigued patients stay awake and to restore mental alertness. Before recommending caffeine for this purpose, however, the pharmacist should ask the patient a number of questions (outlined at the beginning of this chapter) that address the etiology of the patient's fatigue and the patient's medical or psychiatric problems, current medications, dietary caffeine consumption, and intended use of the product. Based on the paucity of data supporting efficacy and the well-known effects of caffeine excess, pharmacists should carefully consider whether caffeine products should be recommended to improve daytime alertness.

Administration and Dosage Guidelines

Oral doses of 100–200 mg are needed to achieve mild CNS stimulation in adults. If a timed-release caffeine preparation is used, the dose should not be taken less than 6 hours before bedtime. The recommended adult dose of timed-release products is 200–250 mg.

Adverse Effects

The primary adverse events associated with caffeine are CNS stimulant effects and GI irritation. Adverse CNS effects include insomnia, nervousness, restlessness, excitement, tinnitus, muscular tremor, headache, lightheadedness, and mild delirium. These effects are more pronounced in children. Adverse GI effects include nausea, vomiting, diarrhea, and stomach pain. Other adverse effects include diuresis, extrasystoles, palpitations, and tachycardia.

Dependence and Withdrawal

Physical dependence may result from prolonged caffeine consumption; withdrawal symptoms can occur following abrupt cessation.[24] The most common withdrawal symptoms are fatigue and headache. Anxiety, nausea, vomiting, impaired psychomotor function, irritability, restlessness, lethargy, and, less commonly, yawning and rhinorrhea are also noted. Withdrawal symptoms generally occur 12–24 hours after cessation of caffeine ingestion, peak in 20–48 hours, and may persist for a week. A throbbing headache, the typical symptom, results from the rebound vasodilatation that occurs following abrupt withdrawal.

Toxicity

Serious symptomatology can occur after caffeine overdose. Caffeinism, the ingestion of high caffeine doses (>250 mg), can produce symptoms mimicking anxiety. The diagnostic criteria for caffeinism include recent caffeine consumption of more than 250 mg and at least five of the following symptoms: nervousness, restlessness, insomnia, excitement, diuresis, facial flushing, muscle twitching, GI disturbance, tachycardia or cardiac arrhythmia, "rambling" flow of thought and speech, psychomotor agitation, or periods of inexhaustibility.[35] Five caffeine overdose deaths have been reported in patients ingesting caffeine-containing nonprescription products.[36] Four of those cases were successful suicide attempts, and the fifth was an accidental death secondary to drug abuse. The lethal dose in adults is 150–200 mg/kg of body weight.[37]

The primary management of caffeine toxicity includes general supportive care. For an acute ingestion, emesis should be initiated with ipecac unless the patient is obtunded, comatose, or convulsing. A cathartic such as magnesium sulfate, magnesium citrate, sodium sulfate, or sorbitol should be given with or without charcoal. If the patient is stuporous or comatose, gastric lavage and activated charcoal should be used. Patients should receive general supportive care such as hydration, antipyretics, and maintenance of vital signs, including ventilatory support and electrocardiogram monitoring. Antacids such as aluminum hydroxide gel can be used for GI irritation. Seizures should be treated with intravenous diazepam and, if they recur, with phenytoin or phenobarbital. For extremely high caffeine serum concentrations, exchange transfusion or hemoperfusion may be considered.

Warnings and Precautions

Caffeine is contraindicated in patients with known hypersensitivity to the drug. It should be used cautiously in patients who have or have had peptic ulcer disease, and in patients with symptomatic cardiac arrhythmias and palpitations. Also, high-dose caffeine intake may result in a hyperglycemic event as it may increase blood glucose concentrations. Lower doses should be used in patients with renal dysfunction. Caffeine has been shown to worsen mental status in some patients with psychiatric disorders, and it should be used cautiously in this population.

Drug Interactions/Laboratory Test Interferences

Drug interactions between caffeine and other agents may be clinically significant. Patients should be informed that caffeine's metabolism is inhibited by disulfiram, mexiletine, cimetidine, oral contraceptives containing estrogen, norfloxacin, enoxacin, ciprofloxacin; and that alcohol acutely inhibits the metabolism of caffeine.[24,38–40] In addition, caffeine may decrease iron absorption, although the clinical significance of this interaction is unclear; patients should be instructed to take iron 1 hour before or 2 hours after caffeine consumption.

GI distress is increased when nonsteroidal anti-inflammatory drugs, aspirin, corticosteroids, or alcohol is administered along with caffeine. Blood pressure may be increased when caffeine and phenylpropanolamine are coadministered. Monoamine oxidase inhibitors in combination with caffeine are of particular concern because patients may develop potentially life-threatening cardiac complications. Caffeine does not typically affect the efficacy of medications used to treat hypertension but may interfere with the therapeutic benefit of antiarrhythmic agents. Furthermore, caffeine and diazepam coadministered have antagonizing effects, depending on the dosage of the two agents and the specific task behavioral tests employed.[41,42] For example, caffeine antagonizes diazepam-induced impairment of psychomotor performance and sedation but does not antagonize diazepam-induced impairment of delayed recognition memory performance or immediate recall.[41] Alternatively, diazepam antagonizes caffeine-induced restlessness, alertness, arousal, and tension.

Caffeine may cause false-positive diagnostic tests for both pheochromocytoma and neuroblastoma because it causes elevations in urine concentrations of vanillylmandelic acid, catecholamines, and 5-hydroxyindoleacetic acid. Also, serum uric acid concentrations may be falsely elevated.

Therapeutic Concerns

Use During Pregnancy and Lactation

The safety of caffeine in pregnancy is a significant issue because caffeine is often consumed by pregnant women and freely crosses the placenta. Based on the teratogenic effects of caffeine in rodents, the FDA issued a warning in 1980 advising pregnant women to limit or avoid caffeine consumption.[43] However, no consistent teratogenic effects have been reported in animal studies that used massive caffeine doses.[44]

Possible teratogenic mechanisms are uncertain, but three hypotheses are proposed. Caffeine may interfere with fetal cell growth by increasing cyclic adenosine monophosphate (cAMP).[45] Because it structurally resembles adenine and guanine, caffeine may directly alter nucleic acids, resulting in chromosome abnormalities. Or caffeine may restrict uteroplacental circulation through vasoconstriction, resulting in fetal hypoxia.

Data on caffeine's teratogenic effect in humans are limited to a few studies, most of which rely on questionnaires or interviews.[46] Based on these limited data, caffeine's teratogenic potential appears to be dose related.[44] One study found an increased risk for late first- and second-trimester spontaneous abortions in women consuming at least 151 mg of caffeine daily.[45] However, the study noted that larger amounts of caffeine were consumed by mothers who were also relatively heavy alcohol users and smokers, both of which practices are known to increase the risk for spontaneous abortion.[47,48]

Caffeine intake of more than 300 mg per day is associated with intrauterine growth retardation and infants of low birthweight.[46,49] These findings are not surprising because caffeine at doses of 200 mg significantly decreases placental blood flow through vasoconstriction within the placental villi,[49] and any decrease in uteroplacental circulation is significantly correlated with decreased fetal growth. Increased fetal breathing activity was noted in mothers consuming two cups of regular or decaffeinated coffee;[50] similar results were found in mothers consuming more than 500 mg of caffeine per day.[51] Consumption of six or more cups of coffee daily during pregnancy has been associated with spontaneous abortion, stillbirth, low birthweight, breech presentation, and decreased activity and muscle tone of neonates.[44] Cleft palate, electrodactyly, and interventricular septal defect have been noted in infants of mothers consuming eight or more cups of coffee per day.[44,52] Furthermore, three cases of arrhythmias have occurred in infants whose mothers ingested large amounts of caffeine.[53]

Although anecdotal case reports suggest adverse fetal effects in mothers ingesting caffeine, case-control studies involving infants with congenital malformations suggest no relationship.[54-56] In a prospective study of 286 mothers, caffeine intake was not associated with an increased incidence of breech birth, miscarriage, premature birth, or caesarian section deliveries.[57] No relationship between caffeine intake and low birthweight was noted in several large prospective and retrospective studies.[58,59] Overall, information is incomplete and the data are conflicting, but no direct correlations can be made between caffeine consumption and birth defects.[46] However, it is prudent to recommend limiting caffeine intake to 300 mg per day or less because decreases in birthweight are reported to occur when intake exceeds this amount.[46,49]

Caffeine has been linked to decreased fertility. One study of 104 women attempting pregnancy noted that women were half as likely to become pregnant if more caffeine than the equivalent of one cup of coffee per day was consumed compared with intake of less than this amount.[60] Another study found similar results in 6,303 women.[61]

Caffeine passes into breast milk; however, the caffeine concentration in breast milk is only 1% of the mother's plasma concentration.[46] Peak caffeine concentrations in breast milk occur within 1 hour of consumption, but infant caffeine plasma concentrations are not correlated with the levels in breast milk. No adverse effects have been reported in infants of nursing mothers consuming 200–336 mg per day of caffeine, although wakefulness and irritability have been noted in infants of nursing mothers consuming 600 mg per day of caffeine. Caffeine, whether from medicinal or food sources, should be ingested immediately after nursing to avoid high maternal plasma and milk concentrations. To avoid the potential for caffeine accumulation in the infant, consumption should be moderate, especially when mothers are nursing infants younger than 4 months of age.

Use in Neonates

Liver metabolic pathways, including the cytochrome P-450 system, are immature in the neonate. Thus, newborns metabolize caffeine very slowly and may accumulate toxic caffeine plasma concentrations. The rate of caffeine elimination increases as liver metabolic function matures. Caffeine clearance and half-life are correlated directly with gestational age.[62] If caffeine is used therapeutically in neonates, dosing intervals should be 24 hours in infants under 1 month old, 12 hours in infants 1 to 2 months old, 8 hours in infants 2–4 months old, and 6 hours for infants over 4 months old.[62]

Malignancy

Clinical studies proposing an association between caffeine intake and increased risk of breast cancer provide conflicting and nonconclusive results.[63-65] The causal relationship between caffeine ingestion and bladder and pancreatic cancers has been evaluated. A case-control study of 75 patients with bladder cancer and 142 control patients found no association between caffeine intake and the risk of bladder cancer.[66] Earlier studies suggest that the relative risk of developing pancreatic cancer is 2.7 in persons consuming three or more cups of coffee per day;[67] however, later studies do not support this conclusion.[68-70] Thus, no conclusive data exist to suggest that caffeine ingestion is associated with any malignancy.

Benign Breast Disease

As results from various studies have been inconsistent, the possibility of a relationship between benign breast disease and caffeine is controversial.[64] Case-control studies suggest no such association.[71,72] Fibrocystic breast disease, however, may be associated with caffeine consumption.[71] Some investigators have noted the complete resolution of benign breast nodules, tenderness, pain, and nipple discharge once women with fibrocystic disease eliminated caffeine from their diet.[73]

Guidelines for Patient Education and Counseling

Pharmacists should be aware of the various prescription and nonprescription products containing caffeine. Dietary caffeine consumption may be substantial; thus, patients should be advised of the additive effects of dietary and medicinal caffeine. This is particularly important for elderly patients, who may be more sensitive to the stimulant effects of caffeine and may present with nervousness, anxiety, insomnia, and irritability. Elderly patients receiving other CNS stimulants should ingest caffeine with caution. Agents such as theophylline, decongestants, amantadine, tricyclic antidepressants, and appetite suppressants added to caffeine may result in disorientation, delirium, and a host of other adverse effects.

Patients need to be advised of the possible drug interactions, as outlined above, that may occur with caffeine. The combination of caffeine and alcohol ingestion needs to be addressed. Caffeine does not antagonize the effect of alcohol, improve a person's driving ability, or lessen any of the detrimental effects of alcohol. Contrary to folklore, caffeine will not "sober up" a person intoxicated on alcohol.

Again, pharmacists should ask themselves whether there is any reason to recommend caffeine-containing products. Although caffeine is commonly used, its use should not be encouraged by health professionals, and it should never be recommended as a substitute for adequate sleep and rest.

Summary: Stimulants

Caffeine is present in many foods, beverages, and drug products. Moderate use is generally considered safe, and no conclusive data exist linking regular caffeine use with various cardiovascular diseases, teratogenic effects, or cancer. However, pregnant or nursing patients and patients with cardiac dysfunction should consume caffeine with moderation, if at all.

Patients should be advised of several issues related to the use of nonprescription stimulants containing caffeine. First, caffeine toxicity may occur if higher than recommended doses are ingested. Second, stimulant products will not reverse alcohol impairment. Third, stimulant use should be discontinued if rapid pulse, dizziness, or heart palpitations occur. Finally, stimulant products are not intended as a substitute for normal sleep. If fatigue persists or recurs, the patient should consult a physician.

References

1. Crismon ML. Insomnia. In: Koda-Kimble MA, Young LY, eds. *Applied Therapeutics: The Clinical Use of Drugs*. 5th ed. Vancouver, Wash: Applied Therapeutics, Inc; 1992: (chp 55) 1–18.
2. Bixler EO, Vela-Bueno A. Normal sleep: patterns and mechanisms. *Semin Neurol* 1987; 7: 227.
3. Hauri P. *The Sleep Disorders, Current Concepts*. Kalamazoo, Mich: Upjohn; 1977.
4. Gillin JC, Byerly WF. The diagnosis and management of insomnia. *N Engl J Med* 1990; 322: 239.
5. Doghramji K. Sleep disorders: a selective update. *Hosp Community Psychiatry* 1989; 40: 29.
6. Balter MB, Uhlenhuth EH. The beneficial and adverse effects of hypnotics. *J Clin Psychiatry* 1991; 52 (7, suppl): 16–23.
7. FDA announces standards for nonprescription sleep-aid products and expectorants. *Clin Pharm* 1989 Jun; 8: 388.
8. Antihistamine drugs. In: McEvoy GK, ed. *AHFS Drug Information 92*. Bethesda, Md: American Society of Hospital Pharmacists; 1992: 2–5, 17–20.
9. NDMA task force to sponsor acetaminophen/diphenhydramine clinicals. *F-D-C Reports* 1992 Jan 27; T&G-12.
10. Spector R, Choudhury AK, Chiang C, et al. Diphenhydramine in Orientals and Caucasians. *Clin Pharmacol Ther* 1980; 28: 229–34.
11. Meridith CG, Christian CD, Johnson RF, et al. Diphenhydramine disposition in chronic liver disease. *Clin Pharmacol Ther* 1984; 35: 474–9.
12. Gengo F, Gabos C, Miller JK. The pharmacodynamics of diphenhydramine-induced drowsiness and changes in metal performance. *Clin Pharmacol Ther* 1989; 45: 15–21.
13. Carruthers SG, Shoeman DW, Hignite CE, et al. Correlation between plasma diphenhydramine level and sedative and antihistamine effects. *Clin Pharmacol Ther* 1978; 23: 375–82.
14. Kudo Y, Kurihara M. Clinical evaluation of diphenhydramine hydrochloride for the treatment of insomnia in psychiatric patients: a double-blind study. *J Clin Pharmacol* 1990; 30: 1041–8.
15. Meuleman JR, et al. Evaluation of temazepam and diphenhydramine as hypnotics in a nursing-home population. *Drug Intell Clin Pharm* 1987; 21: 716.
16. Koppel C, Ibe K, Tenczer J. Clinical symptomatology of diphenhydramine overdose: an evaluation of 136 cases in 1982 to 1985. *Clin Toxicol* 1987; 25: 53–70.
17. Schneider-Helmert D, Spinweber CL. Evaluation of L-tryptophan for treatment of insomnia: a review. *Psychopharmacol* 1986; 89: 1–7.
18. Aldhous P. Yellow light on L-tryptophan. *Nature* 1991; 353: 490.
19. Kamb ML, Murphy JJ, Jones JL, et al. Eosinophilia–myalgia syndrome in L-tryptophan exposed patients. *JAMA* 1992; 267: 77–82.
20. Roth R et al. Pharmacological effects of sedative-hypnotics, narcotic analgesics, and alcohol during sleep. *Med Clin North Am* 1985; 69: 1281.
21. Foust RT, Reddy R, Jeffers LJ, et al. Nyquil-associated liver injury. *Am J Gastroenterol* 1989; 84: 422–5.
22. Scrima L, et al. Increased severity of obstructive sleep apnea after bedtime alcohol ingestion: diagnostic potential and proposed mechanism of action. *Sleep* 1982; 5: 318.
23. Tasan VC, et al. Alcohol increases sleep apnea and oxygen desaturation in asymptomatic men. *Am J Med* 1981; 71: 240.
24. Benowitz NL. Clinical pharmacology of caffeine. *Annu Rev Med* 1990; 41: 277–88.
25. Graham DM. Caffeine—its identity, dietary sources, intake and biological effects. *Nutr Rev* 1978 Apr; 36: 97–102.
26. Clementz GL, Dailey JW. Psychotropic effects of caffeine. *Am Fam Physician* 1988 May; 37: 167–72.
27. Rossignol AM, Bonnlander H. Caffeine-containing beverages, total fluid consumption, and premenstrual syndrome. *Am J Public Health* 1990 Sep; 80: 1106–10.
28. Myers MG. Effects of caffeine on blood pressure. *Arch Intern Med* 1988 May; 148: 1189–93.
29. LaCroix AZ, Mead LA, Liang KY, et al. Coffee consumption and the incidence of coronary heart disease. *N Engl J Med* 1986 Oct 16; 315: 977–82.
30. Grobbee DE, Rimm EB, Giovannucci E, et al. Coffee, caffeine, and cardiovascular disease in men. *N Engl J Med* 1990 Oct 11; 323: 1026–32.
31. Newcombe PF, Renton KW, Rautaharju PM, et al. High-dose caffeine and cardiac rate and rhythm in normal subjects. *Chest* 1988 Jul; 94: 90–4.
32. Myers MG. Caffeine and cardiac arrhythmias. *Ann Intern Med* 1991 Jan 15; 114: 147–50.
33. Sutherland DJ, McPherson DD, Renton KW, et al. The effect of caffeine on cardiac rate, rhythm, and ventricular repolarization. *Chest* 1985 Mar; 87: 319–24.
34. Pentel P. Toxicity of over-the-counter stimulants. *JAMA* 1984 Oct 12; 252: 1898–1903.
35. Organic mental syndromes and disorders. In: Spitzer RL, ed. *Diagnostic and Statistical Manual of Mental Disorders III-R*. Washington, DC: American Psychiatric Association; 1987: 138–9.
36. Garriott JC, Simmons LM, Poklis A, et al. Five cases of fatal overdose from caffeine-containing "look-alike" drugs. *J Anal Toxicol* 1985 May/Jun; 9: 141–3.
37. *Poisindex*. Vol. 72. Englewood, Colo: Micromedex, Inc; 1992.
38. Fazio A. Caffeine, oral contraceptives, and over-the-counter drugs. *Arch Intern Med* 1989 May; 149: 1217–8.
39. Healy DP, Polk RE, Kanawati L, et al. Interaction between oral ciprofloxacin and caffeine in normal volunteers. *Antimicrob Agents Chemother* 1989 Apr; 33: 474–8.
40. Harder S, Fuhr U, Staib AH. Ciprofloxacin–caffeine: a drug interaction established using in vivo and in vitro investigations. *Am J Med* 1989 Nov 30; 87 (5A): 89S–91S.
41. Roache JD, Griffiths RR. Interactions of diazepam and caffeine: behavioral and subjective dose effects in humans. *Pharmacol Biochem Behav* 1987 Apr; 26: 801–12.
42. Ghoneim MM, Hinrichs JV, Chiang CK, et al. Pharmacokinetic and pharmacodynamic interactions between caffeine and diazepam. *J Clin Psychopharmacol* 1986 Apr; 6 (2): 75–80.
43. Caffeine and pregnancy. *FDA Drug Bulletin* 1980 Nov; 10 (3): 19–20.
44. Al-Hachim GM. Teratogenicity of caffeine; a review. *Eur J Obstet Gynecol Reprod Biol* 1989; 31 (3): 237–47.
45. Srisuphan W, Bracken MB. Caffeine consumption during pregnancy and association with late spontaneous abortion. *Am J Obstet Gynecol* 1986 Jan; 154: 14–20.
46. Berger A. Effects of caffeine consumption on pregnancy outcome—a review. *J Reprod Med* 1988 Dec; 33: 945–56.
47. Harlap S, Shiono PH. Alcohol, smoking, and incidence of spontaneous abortions in the first and second trimester. *Lancet* 1980 Jul 26; 2: 173–76.
48. Kline J, Stein Z, Shrout P, et al. Drinking during pregnancy and spontaneous abortion. *Lancet* 1980 Jul 26; 2: 176–80.
49. Fenster L, Eskenazi B, Windham GC, et al. Caffeine consumption during pregnancy and fetal growth. *Am J Public Health* 1991 Apr; 81: 458–61.
50. Salvador HS, Koos BJ. Effects of regular and decaffeinated coffee on fetal breathing and heart rate. *Am J Obstet Gynecol* 1989 May; 160 (5, pt 1): 1043–7.
51. McGowan J, Devoe LD, Searle N, et al. The effects of long- and short-term maternal caffeine ingestion on human fetal breathing and body movements in term gestations. *Am J Obstet Gynecol* 1987 Sep; 157: 726–9.
52. Jacobson MF, Goldman AS, Syme RH. Coffee and birth defects. *Lancet* 1981 Jun 27; 1: 1415–6.

53. Oei SG, Vosters RPL, van der Hagen NLJ. Fetal arrhythmia caused by excessive intake of caffeine by pregnant women. *Br Med J* 1989 Mar 4; 298: 568.
54. Kurppa K, Holmberg PC, Kuosma E, et al. Coffee consumption during pregnancy. *N Engl J Med* 1982 Jun 24; 306: 1548.
55. Rosenberg L, Mitchell AA, Shapiro S, et al. Selected birth defects in relation to caffeine-containing beverages. *JAMA* 1982 Mar 12; 247: 1429–32.
56. Kurppa K, Holmberg PC, Kuosma E, et al. Coffee consumption during pregnancy and selected congenital malformations: a nationwide case-control study. *Am J Public Health* 1983 Dec; 73: 1397–9.
57. Watkinson B, Fried PA. Maternal caffeine use before, during, and after pregnancy and effects upon offspring. *Neurobehav Toxicol Teratol* 1985; 7: 9–17.
58. Brooke OG, Anderson HR, Bland JM, et al. Effects on birth weight of smoking, alcohol, caffeine, socioeconomic factors, and psychosocial stress. *Br Med J* 1989 Mar 25; 298: 795–801.
59. Linn S, Schoebaum SC, Monson RR, et al. No association between coffee consumption and adverse outcomes of pregnancy. *N Engl J Med* 1982 Jan 21; 306: 141–5.
60. Christianson RE, Oechsli FW, van den Berg BJ. Caffeinated beverages and decreased fertility. *Lancet* 1989 Feb 18; 1: 378.
61. Wilcox A, Weinberg C, Baird D. Caffeinated beverages and decreased fertility. *Lancet* 1988 Dec 24/31; 2: 1453–6.
62. Pons G, Carrier O, Richard MO, et al. Developmental changes of caffeine elimination in infancy. *Dev Pharmacol Ther* 1988; 11 (5): 258–64.
63. Wolfrom D, Welsch CW. Caffeine and the development of normal, benign and carcinomatous human breast tissues: a relationship? *J Med* 1990; 21 (5): 225–50.
64. Lubin F, Ron E. Consumption of methylxanthine-containing beverages and the risk of breast cancer. *Cancer Lett* 1990 Sep; 53 (2–3): 81–90.
65. Lubin F, Ron E, Wax Y, et al. Coffee and methylxanthines and breast cancer: a case-control study. *J Natl Cancer Inst* 1984 Mar; 74: 569–73.
66. Najem GR, Louria DB, Seebode JJ, et al. Life time occupation, smoking, caffeine, saccharine, hair dyes and bladder carcinogenesis. *Int J Epidemiol* 1982; 11 (3): 212–7.
67. MacMahon B, Yen S, Trichopoulos D, et al. Coffee and cancer of the pancreas. *N Engl J Med* 1981 Mar 12; 304: 630–3.
68. Hsieh CC, MacMahon B, Yen S. More on coffee and pancreatic cancer. *N Engl J Med* 1987 Feb 19; 316: 484.
69. Hsieh CC, MacMahon B, Yen S, et al. Coffee and pancreatic cancer. *N Engl J Med* 1986 Aug 28; 315: 587–8.
70. Hiatt RA, Klatsky AL, Armstrong MA. Pancreatic cancer, blood glucose and beverage consumption. *Int J Cancer* 1988; 41 (6): 794–7.
71. Boyle CA, Berkowitz GS, LiVolsi VA, et al. Caffeine consumption and fibrocystic breast disease: a case-control epidemiologic study. *J Natl Cancer Inst* 1984 May; 72: 1015–9.
72. Lubin F, Ron E, Wax Y, et al. A case-control study of caffeine and methylxanthines in benign breast disease. *JAMA* 1985 Apr 26; 253: 2388–92.
73. Minton JP, Foecking MK, Webster DJT, et al. Response of fibrocystic disease to caffeine withdrawal and correlation of cyclic nucleotides with breast disease. *Am J Obstet Gynecol* 1979 Sep 1; 135: 157–8.

CHAPTER 11

Antacid Products

Julianne B. Pinson and C. Wayne Weart

Questions to ask in patient assessment and counseling

- Can you describe the pain? How severe is it?
- Are there any other symptoms that accompany this pain?
- How long have you had this pain?
- Is the pain constant or does it come and go?
- Where and when does the pain occur? Do you experience it immediately after meals or several hours later? Does the pain wake you up at night?
- Is the pain worse when you lie down? When you bend over?
- Is the pain relieved by food? Do certain foods, coffee, or carbonated beverages make it worse?
- Do you drink alcohol? How much? Is the pain worse after drinking alcohol?
- Have you lost any weight?
- Have you vomited blood or black material that looks like coffee grounds?
- Have you noticed blood in the stool or have the stools been black or tarry?
- Have you seen a physician about these symptoms? If so, what did your physician tell you to do?
- Have you previously used any antacid to treat this pain? Which ones? How were you taking the antacids? Did they relieve the pain?
- What prescription and nonprescription drugs do you regularly take? Have you recently taken aspirin or ibuprofen-containing products?
- Do you smoke? How much?
- Have you or has anyone in your family ever had an ulcer?
- Do you have any medical problems such as diabetes or kidney or heart disease? Are you currently under a physician's care for any medical conditions?
- Are you on any special diets such as a low-salt diet?

Forty percent of adults in America report having some type of digestive problem in an average 2-week period.[1] Americans currently spend more than $1 billion per year on antacids.[2] Antacids are useful for the short-term relief of indigestion, heartburn, and excessive eating and drinking, as well as for the long-term management of gastroesophageal reflux and peptic ulcer disease. The pharmacist should first be able to distinguish between those patients who are appropriate for self-treatment and those who need medical attention, and then to select appropriate antacid products for patients with mild gastrointestinal (GI) complaints.

Physiology of the Gastrointestinal Tract

A basic understanding of the physiology of the stomach and the duodenum (Figure 1), and of gastric acid secretion and the forces that protect the stomach from acid, is essential to understanding the pathophysiology of GI disorders and the drugs used to treat them.

Gastric Acid Secretion

The stomach is divided into four anatomic regions: the cardia, fundus, body, and antrum. Little is known about the function of the cardia, which is the smallest region of the stomach. The body and fundus make up the largest part of the stomach and contain the cells responsible for acid and pepsin secretion. The two principal cell types of the body and fundus are (1) the parietal cell, which secretes hydrochloric acid (about 2 L is secreted daily[3]) and intrinsic factor (required for vitamin B_{12} absorption); and (2) the chief cell, which secretes pepsinogen (precursor of pepsin). The antrum contains gastrin cells, or G-cells, which secrete the hormone gastrin into the circulation.

Gastric acid serves several important functions. Acid and pepsin are powerful proteolytic substances that hydrolyze protein and other foods so they can be absorbed by the intestine; thus, gastric acid aids in the digestion and absorption of food. In addition, gastric acid kills most bacteria in the stomach and helps to maintain a stable stomach environment.

The primary cell involved in acid secretion is the parietal cell. The outer membrane of the parietal cell has receptors for (1) histamine released from mast cells in the stomach; (2) acetylcholine released from nerve endings in the stomach; and (3) gastrin, which reaches the parietal

---

This chapter is based in part on the chapter with the same title that appeared in the 9th edition but was written by William R. Garnett.

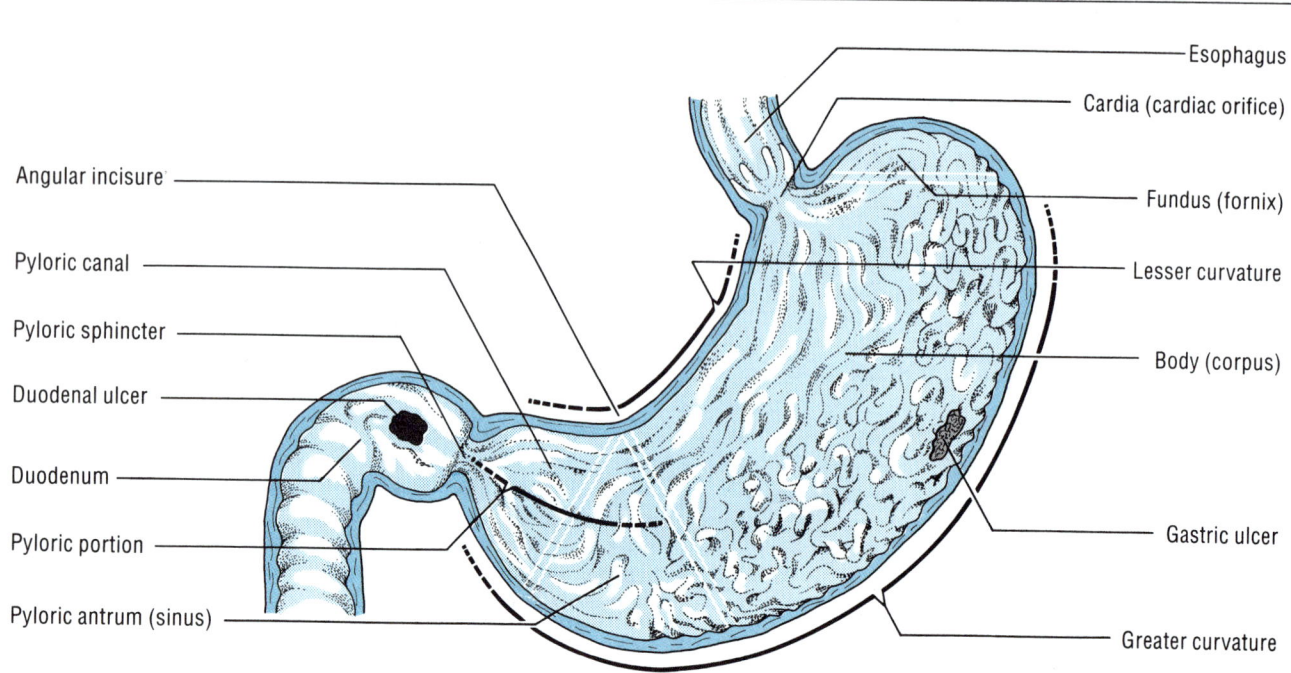

FIGURE 1 Sites of duodenal and gastric ulcers. Adapted from Netter FH. *The Ciba Collection of Medical Illustrations*. Vol. 3, part II. New York: Ciba Pharmaceutical Company; 1962: 49, 52.

cell from distant locations in the blood. When any of these substances come into contact with their receptors on the parietal cell, calcium and cyclic adenosine monophosphate (cAMP) concentrations within the cell increase.[3] The increased levels of calcium and cAMP activate the hydrogen/potassium (H^+/K^+) adenosine triphosphatase (ATPase) enzyme, which is located on the parietal cell and referred to as the proton pump. When stimulated, the proton pump secretes hydrogen ions in the stomach lumen in exchange for potassium. The proton pump can respond directly to calcium and cAMP, as well as indirectly to histamine, acetylcholine, and gastrin. Thus, the proton pump is the final common pathway for acid secretion from any stimuli.

The parietal cell serves as the target for pharmacologic inhibition of acid secretion. Anticholinergic agents inhibit acid secretion by occupying the acetylcholine receptor on the parietal cell. H_2-antagonists reduce acid secretion by blocking the histamine receptor on the parietal cell. However, H_2-antagonists also block acid secretion from other stimuli, including acetylcholine, gastrin, food, and calcium. The recognition that H_2-antagonists inhibit acid secretion from more than one stimulus highlights the interdependency of the pathways involved in controlling acid secretion. Ultimate suppression of acid can be achieved by inhibiting the proton pump with omeprazole. Because the proton pump is the final step in acid secretion, omeprazole abolishes acid secretion regardless of the stimulus.

Another important factor in the control of acid secretion is gastrin, which is released from the G-cells of the antrum. Gastrin stimulates the parietal cell directly by binding to its receptor and indirectly by triggering mast cells to release histamine. The most potent stimulant of gastrin release is the protein in food, but vagal stimulation (acetylcholine), calcium, other cations such as magnesium and aluminum, and mechanical distention by food also contribute to gastrin secretion.[1] In addition, any factor that increases gastric pH stimulates gastrin release. This is important because most drugs used to treat acid-peptic disorders (e.g., antacids, H_2-antagonists, and omeprazole) increase gastric pH and thus increase gastrin concentrations. Gastrin secretion is inhibited by acid within the lumen of the antrum.[1]

Pepsinogen is released by the chief cells of the body and fundus in response to much the same stimuli as acid from the parietal cell—i.e., vagal stimulation, histamine, and acetylcholine. In the presence of acid, pepsinogen is hydrolyzed to the active proteolytic enzyme pepsin. Maximum activity of pepsin occurs at a pH of 2 whereas complete inhibition occurs at a pH of 4.[3]

The rate and amount of acid that the parietal cell secretes depend on whether the stomach has been stimulated or is in the basal state. Both basal and stimulated acid outputs vary considerably among individuals and are generally higher in men than in women. Basal acid secretion also varies within individuals, as it appears to follow a circadian rhythm. The peak time for basal acid secretion is around midnight to the early morning hours, and its lowest point is between 5 and 11 AM.[4] This cyclical variation explains why patients with peptic ulcer disease are often awakened in the middle of the night with pain and also provides the rationale for nighttime dosing of H_2-antagonists. Dosing these agents after dinner or at bedtime ensures that their onset and maximal acid suppression coincide with the peak acid secretion.

Gastric Mucosal Barrier

The concentration of hydrochloric acid in the stomach lumen is 3 million times that in the tissues and blood.[3] Exposure to such enormous concentrations of acid would destroy any other tissues in the body. However, the gastric mucosa is equipped to withstand the acidic environment of the stomach through a combination of defense and repair mechanisms collectively called the gastric mucosal barrier. A major component of this barrier is the epithelial cells that line the entire surface of the stomach as well as the duodenum. These cells secrete both mucus and bicarbonate to form a protective mucus gel layer between the gastric lumen and the mucosa. The high-viscosity mucus limits the penetration of hydrogen ions across the mucosa, while the bicarbonate allows a pH gradient to develop between the acidic stomach lumen and the more alkaline surface of the mucosa. The mucus–bicarbonate layer thus acts as a physical and chemical barrier to prevent diffusion of hydrogen ions across the mucosa. When this mucosal barrier is disrupted, rapid mucosal blood flow removes any hydrogen ion that has diffused across the barrier. When damage does occur, the epithelial cells have a unique ability to repair themselves quickly through rapid cell turnover. This process, known as restitution or reconstitution, is aided by the delivery of oxygen and other nutrients to the cells by the mucosal blood supply.

Prostaglandins are also a vital component of the gastric mucosal barrier. Prostaglandin E_2 is synthesized by the gastric mucosa and works to enhance its protective mechanisms. Prostaglandins inhibit gastric acid secretion from the parietal cells, as well as increase mucus and bicarbonate secretion from the epithelial cells. Prostaglandins also help maintain mucosal blood flow and thus help remove back-diffused hydrogen ions.

Pathogenesis of Gastrointestinal Disease

The maintenance of normal, healthy gastric mucosa is often described as a balance between the aggressive forces of acid and pepsin and the defensive forces of the gastric mucosal barrier. As long as the gastric mucosal barrier is healthy and intact, the stomach is protected from acid and pepsin. When this barrier is disrupted, however, the destructive forces of acid and pepsin predominate and mucosal injury or ulceration occurs. Although acid and pepsin play a critical role in the pathogenesis of acid-peptic diseases, a breakdown in mucosal defense is equally important in determining whether disease will occur. All acid-peptic diseases can be viewed as an imbalance between these aggressive factors and protective mucosal defenses. Similarly, virtually all factors implicated in the etiology of these diseases affect this critical balance by increasing aggressive factors, impairing mucosal defenses, or altering both sides of the balance.

Factors Increasing Gastric Acid Secretion

Acid is necessary for the development of peptic ulcers and most other acid-peptic disorders. However, very few factors disrupt the balance between health and acid-peptic disorders by increasing gastric acid secretion. The most striking cause of increased acid secretion is Zollinger–Ellison syndrome, a disorder caused by a gastrin-secreting tumor (gastrinoma) in the pancreas. Patients with this syndrome have massive hypersecretion of gastric acid and usually develop intractable peptic ulcer disease. Many patients with duodenal ulcers (DUs) appear to be hypersecretors of acid, although not to the same degree as those with Zollinger–Ellison syndrome. Many beverages such as milk, beer, coffee, tea, and colas (both caffeinated and decaffeinated) also increase acid secretion.[5] However, although these substances may exacerbate some peptic disorders, they do not, by themselves, increase the risk of developing peptic ulcer disease. Lastly, there are many environmental factors that impair mucosal defenses, but such factors do not appear to increase acid secretion significantly.

Factors Disrupting the Gastric Mucosal Barrier

Most factors predisposing patients to acid-peptic diseases do so by impairing mucosal defenses. Two factors that appear to play a major role are *Helicobacter pylori* and drugs. Although nonsteroidal anti-inflammatory drugs (NSAIDs) most often weaken mucosal defenses, other drugs, including alcohol, tobacco smoke, caffeine, and corticosteroids, may affect the gastric mucosal barrier.

Helicobacter pylori

Spiral-shaped organisms were observed in ulcerated gastric mucosa of the human stomach as early as 1938.[4] It was not until 1983, however, that this Gram-negative aerobic bacillus was isolated in gastric biopsy specimens from patients with gastritis. The organism was named *Campylobacter pylori*, a name later changed to *Helicobacter pylori* because of its unique structural and biochemical characteristics. Since its discovery, the study of *H. pylori* has progressed rapidly because the organism may be a major factor in the pathogenesis of certain acid-peptic disorders.

H. pylori colonizes the epithelial cells that line the surface of the stomach, where it causes inflammation and potential ulceration.[4] The organism may also adhere to islands of gastric epithelium, or gastric metaplasia, in the duodenum. Other microorganisms would not survive the bactericidal effects of gastric acid, but *H. pylori* has a unique ability to survive in the normal gastric mucosa: *H. pylori* is protected from acid because it works its way under the mucus–bicarbonate layer and adheres to the gastric epithelial cells. The bacterium produces large amounts of urease, an enzyme that generates bicarbonate and ammonium from urea and thus alkalinizes the environment. Its structural features also enable it to move easily through its environment beneath the mucus layer.[4] Although the exact mechanism of damage is not certain, it is thought that *H. pylori* produces an enzyme that degrades gastric mucus. As the organism digests mucus, the mucus layer thins or completely erodes, making it an easy target for back-diffused hydrogen ions. This acid contact with the mucosa is thought to be responsible for the gastric inflammation observed in patients with *H. pylori* infection.

H. pylori is the most common GI infection in humans. Its prevalence in healthy, asymptomatic individuals increases substantially with age, with 10% of persons younger than 30 years and up to 60% of those older than 60 years infected.[6] Virtually all patients (more than 97%) with DUs and 80% of patients with gastric ulcers (GUs) harbor the organism.[6] Up to 70–100% of patients with chronic (Type B) gastritis and 30–50% of patients with nonulcer dyspepsia are also infected with *H. pylori*.[4,6] Despite these strong associations, however, whether *H. pylori* causes these diseases has not been conclusively established. Many persons who harbor the organism do not have symptoms or develop an acid-peptic disorder.

NSAIDs

The mechanisms by which NSAIDs produce gastroduodenal damage and ulceration are twofold. As a primary insult, NSAIDs cause direct acid damage to the gastric mucosa. Aspirin and most other NSAIDs are weak organic acids that remain un-ionized in the acidic stomach lumen. In this form, they easily penetrate the lipophilic surface of the gastric mucosa. Once in contact with the surface epithelial cells, where the pH is much higher, these agents dissociate into their ionized forms and become "trapped" within the cells. As a result, cell membrane permeability is altered, allowing hydrogen ions to back-diffuse across the mucosal surface and cause damage.

In addition to their local damaging effect, NSAIDs inhibit prostaglandin synthesis. As a result, the adaptation measures that protect and restore the gastric mucosa fail. Gastric mucus secretion is inhibited and the thickness and viscosity of gastric mucus are reduced. Chronic administration of NSAIDs also inhibits bicarbonate secretion from epithelial cells, reduces mucosal blood flow, and impairs cell regeneration. Although of lesser clinical significance, the aggressive side of the balance is affected because gastric acid secretion is increased.

Smoking

Smoking has a number of adverse effects on the gastric mucosal barrier that may contribute to the development of peptic disorders, particularly peptic ulcer disease. One of the most damaging effects of smoking is the reduction of mucosal prostaglandins, perhaps by as much as 70%.[7] Smoking also reduces mucosal blood flow, increases reflux of duodenal contents into the stomach, and weakens the ability of H_2-antagonists to heal peptic ulcers.[5]

Considering these effects, it is not surprising that, compared with nonsmokers, smokers (1) are at higher risk for developing peptic ulcers, (2) have ulcers that are larger and more difficult to heal, and (3) suffer ulcer relapses sooner and more often. The risk of these consequences appears to be related to the number and frequency of cigarettes smoked. Therefore, limiting cigarette consumption should substantially lower the risk of peptic ulcer disease. When patients stop smoking entirely, functions adversely affected by smoking recover rapidly.

Alcohol

Though alcohol is often considered a risk factor for acid-peptic disorders, it appears to play a significant role in the development of acute mucosal injury rather than of chronic peptic diseases.[5] Because pure ethanol is lipid soluble, it penetrates the gastric mucosal barrier and may cause acute mucosal erosions and hemorrhages.[5] The extent of damage appears to correlate with the ethanol concentration consumed. Acute mucosal injury does not appear to occur at ethanol concentrations of less than 10% (20 proof) but does occur when concentrations exceed 20% (40 proof).[5] Thus, acute ingestion of alcohol produces predictable, concentration-dependent mucosal damage that may manifest clinically as acute gastritis. However, because the mucosal cells can repair themselves quickly, it is unlikely that acute alcohol ingestion results in chronic mucosal damage—that is, chronic (Type B) gastritis or peptic ulcer disease. In fact, there is evidence that chronic gastritis in alcoholics is due to infection with *H. pylori* rather than to alcohol.[8] Similarly, with the exception of cirrhosis, alcohol consumption has not been found to be positively related to the prevalence of peptic ulcer.

Other Drugs

Apart from NSAIDs, corticosteroids have received the most attention as drugs that may alter the gastric mucosal barrier and predispose patients to the development of acid-peptic disorders. Many studies in arthritic patients receiving corticosteroids have found an increased risk of peptic ulcer disease, but most of these studies have failed to mention whether these patients were also receiving aspirin or other NSAIDs. The risk of peptic ulcer disease in patients receiving corticosteroids appears to be increased in those also receiving NSAIDs.[9] Thus, the effects of corticosteroids alone on both the gastric mucosal barrier and the risk of peptic ulcer disease remain controversial.

Immunosuppressive agents such as cyclophosphamide, methotrexate, and azathioprine may predispose to the development of acid-peptic disorders by preventing epithelial cell turnover and impairing cellular defenses.[10] Colchicine may also be ulcerogenic by a similar mechanism.

Treatment of Acid-Peptic Disorders

The primary aim of pharmacologic therapy for peptic disorders has been either to neutralize existing acid (using antacids) or to reduce the secretion of acid (using anticholinergic agents, H_2-antagonists, or omeprazole). Sucralfate is used to prevent access of acid and pepsin to the ulcer crater. The therapeutic value of enhancing mucosal defenses (cytoprotection) has only recently been explored. The development of prostaglandin analogues (misoprostol) and the attention focused on the cytoprotective properties of antacids, bismuth compounds, and sucralfate highlight this recent interest in enhancing mucosal defenses as a means of treating peptic disorders.

Antacids

Antacids act to neutralize gastric acid secreted by the parietal cells. Antacids only neutralize existing acid; they do not affect the amount or rate of gastric acid secreted. Antacids increase pH in both the stomach and the duodenal bulb, with a greater effect on duodenal pH than on gastric pH. Antacids do not neutralize all stomach acid; with usual therapeutic doses, they do not raise and cannot maintain gastric pH over 4 to 5. However, when the pH is increased from 1.3 to 2.3, 90% of acid is neutralized, and at a pH of 3.3, 99% is neutralized. As a result, both the amount of acid that back-diffuses across the gastric mucosal barrier and the amount that reaches the duodenum are significantly reduced.

Antacids also inhibit the conversion of pepsinogen to pepsin, which depends on the degree of acid neutralization. Pepsin is most active at a pH of 1.5 to 2.5, and progressive inhibition occurs as gastric pH increases. At a pH of 4 or greater, pepsin activity is completely inhibited. Thus, by raising gastric pH, antacids disrupt the two major aggressive factors responsible for damaging the gastric mucosa in acid-peptic diseases.

Apart from the ability to neutralize acid, some antacids have adsorbent properties that reduce aggressive factors and may contribute to their beneficial therapeutic effects. Aluminum-containing antacids may bind pepsin. This effect is controversial, however, because several studies suggest that aluminum may precipitate pepsin rather than bind it.[11] Antacids that contain aluminum hydroxide have a strong binding capacity for bile salts with an affinity comparable to that of cholestyramine.[12] Magnesium hydroxide and aluminum phosphate antacids also appear to bind bile salts, but not as strongly as aluminum hydroxide. Whether this effect can be used clinically to lower cholesterol has recently been considered and is undergoing investigation. The bile salt–binding capacities of aluminum antacids might also help patients with GUs or gastritis, in whom reflux of bile into the stomach is implicated. However, the benefit of this property in such patients has not been adequately studied.

Various pharmacologic actions of antacids have been reported. One study found that the magnesium–aluminum antacid combination increased the volume of acid secretion, particularly in the 2–4 hours after meals.[13] However, most of this acid was neutralized by the antacid, resulting in an increased alkaline load to the duodenum. Aluminum antacids appear to delay gastric emptying, presumably because the aluminum ion relaxes the smooth muscle of the stomach. Alkalinization of gastric contents by antacids generally increases lower esophageal sphincter tone, which may partially account for its benefit in gastroesophageal reflux disease (GERD). Additionally, antacids have been shown in one study to suppress *H. pylori* infection, but this finding has not been reproduced in other trials.[14]

Contrary to popular advertising claims that some products "coat, soothe, and relieve," antacids do not coat the mucosal lining. However, they may protect the gastric mucosa by other mechanisms. Several recent studies suggest that low-dose antacids heal peptic ulcers as effectively as traditional, high-dose (1,000 mEq per day) regimens.[15,16] The buffering capacity of these low-dose regimens (120–200 mEq per day) is modest at best. Thus, it seems that antacids have healing and protective actions beyond and independent of their acid-neutralizing capacities. Antacids may stimulate several components of the gastric mucosal barrier, including bicarbonate and mucus secretion, mucosal cell regeneration, and mucosal blood flow. Because antacids act locally and do not penetrate the mucosa, they may enhance these mechanisms by increasing the release of prostaglandins. One of the few studies in human gastric mucosa demonstrated an increase in mucosal prostaglandins after low-dose antacid therapy.[17] Although much remains to be learned about these effects, a proven cytoprotective benefit of antacids might lead to new therapeutic indications, such as the prevention of NSAID- or alcohol-induced mucosal damage. Additionally, cytoprotection would allow lower doses of antacids to become standard in the treatment of peptic ulcer disease. A dosage reduction of this magnitude would improve the side effect profile of antacids, increase patient acceptance, reduce cost, and possibly restore antacids as a mainstay of therapy for acid-peptic disorders.

Primary Ingredients

All antacids are basic compounds that react with gastric acid to form a salt and water. Four primary neutralizing compounds are found in antacid products: sodium bicarbonate, calcium carbonate, aluminum salts (hydroxide, phosphate), and magnesium salts (hydroxide, chloride). All antacid products contain at least one of these ingredients, which differ significantly in potency, GI side effects, systemic complications, and drug interactions. Most of these properties are determined by the metal cation of the antacid and the degree of its systemic absorption. All of these considerations are important when choosing an appropriate antacid for any given patient.

Sodium Bicarbonate Sodium bicarbonate is a potent, highly soluble compound that reacts almost instantaneously with acid in the stomach to produce sodium chloride, carbon dioxide, and water. The chemical reaction is $NaHCO_3 + HCl \rightarrow NaCl + H_2O + CO_2$. The loss of carbon dioxide as a gas makes the reaction irreversible. Sodium bicarbonate differs from other antacids in that it is a systemic antacid, meaning that it is completely absorbed into the systemic circulation and can alter systemic pH. To understand this concept, one must recall that in the absence of exogenous antacid, gastric acid is neutralized in the small intestine by bicarbonate generated by the pancreas. When sodium bicarbonate is taken orally, gastric acid is neutralized by exogenous antacid instead of by endogenous bicarbonate in the intestinal lumen. Because sodium chloride does not react with bicarbonate in the small intestine, this endogenous bicarbonate is "left over" in the small intestine, where it is absorbed into the systemic circulation. Thus, the amount of sodium bicarbonate taken orally equals the amount that is absorbed into the blood. In patients with normal renal function, this excess bicarbonate is rapidly excreted by the kidneys. However, in patients with poor renal function, sodium bicarbonate can accumulate and cause a clinically significant metabolic alkalosis, or it can offset the metabolic acidosis of renal failure.

A particular form of the systemic alkalosis caused by high doses of sodium bicarbonate is the milk–alkali syndrome. This syndrome can occur whenever there is high intake of calcium combined with any factor producing alkalosis. Many reports involve calcium carbonate as the sole source of both calcium and alkali. Conversely, sodium bicarbonate can result in the development of alkalosis (and the milk–alkali syndrome) when ingested with calcium but not when ingested alone.

The risk of milk–alkali syndrome was greater in the past, when antacid regimens were routinely prescribed with hourly administration of milk for patients with peptic ulcers. Although such regimens are considered antiquated and are no longer recommended, the milk–alkali syndrome may be important in pregnant women, for whom milk or calcium intake is emphasized, as well as in postmenopausal women taking large doses of supplemental calcium carbonate. Other risk factors for the development of the syndrome include factors that may worsen or prolong alkalosis, such as vomiting, gastric aspiration, hypokalemia, and dehydration. Because thiazide diuretics inhibit calcium excretion and increase calcium absorption, they may be involved in the production of hypercalcemia in the milk–alkali syndrome.

Presenting symptoms of the milk–alkali syndrome include hypercalcemia, alkalosis, irritability, headache, vertigo, nausea, vomiting, weakness, and myalgia. If calcium and alkali ingestion continues, neurologic symptoms (e.g., memory loss, personality changes, lethargy, stupor, and coma) may develop. Renal dysfunction occurs early in the course of the disorder and is present in all stages of the syndrome. Most of the symptoms and biochemical abnormalities are reversed rapidly after calcium and alkali ingestion is discontinued; however, renal damage may be irreversible.

Another problem occurring as a result of systemic absorption of sodium bicarbonate is sodium overload. Because each gram of sodium bicarbonate contains 12 mEq of sodium, normal doses deliver large quantities of sodium into the systemic circulation. This sodium load can be dangerous for many patients. Accordingly, sodium bicarbonate is contraindicated in patients with edema, congestive heart failure, renal failure, and cirrhosis and in those on low-salt diets. Hypertensive patients should also avoid the therapeutic use of sodium bicarbonate, even on a short-term basis. For other patients, the sodium load may cause less dangerous, yet troublesome, side effects of fluid retention and weight gain.

Sodium bicarbonate is the active ingredient in baking soda. Some commercial combination products contain effervescent sodium bicarbonate and aspirin. These effervescent preparations may cause gastric distention and flatulence as a result of carbon dioxide being lost during the chemical reaction of sodium bicarbonate and gastric acid. Ingestion of large doses of combination sodium bicarbonate–aspirin products after heavy alcohol ingestion may lead to hematemesis and melena in some fragile and highly susceptible patients.

Because of the risks of systemic alkalosis and sodium overload, sodium bicarbonate should be used only for short-term relief of symptoms of overeating or indigestion. It is not recommended for the treatment of peptic ulcer disease, and it is contraindicated for prolonged or chronic therapy.

Calcium Carbonate Calcium carbonate dissolves more slowly in the stomach than sodium bicarbonate does, but it produces a potent and more prolonged neutralization of gastric acid. It reacts with gastric acid to produce calcium chloride, carbon dioxide, and water. The reaction is $CaCO_3 + 2HCl \rightarrow CaCl_2 + H_2O + CO_2$. Unlike sodium chloride, which is formed from the reaction of sodium bicarbonate and gastric acid, calcium chloride is highly soluble, and about 90% of it reacts with bicarbonate in the small intestine to form insoluble calcium salts. Because these calcium salts are excreted in the feces and not absorbed, calcium carbonate is considered a nonsystemic antacid. However, about 10% of the calcium chloride does not react with intestinal bicarbonate; this small percentage of leftover endogenous bicarbonate is reabsorbed into the systemic circulation.

Clinically significant alkalosis from calcium carbonate ingestion does not usually develop. However, as previously discussed, calcium carbonate may cause or contribute to the development of the milk–alkali syndrome. When calcium carbonate serves as the source of both calcium and alkali, the risk of the syndrome is increased by prolonged administration of calcium carbonate, the concomitant ingestion of milk fortified with vitamin D (which increases intestinal absorption of calcium), renal impairment, and dehydration with electrolyte imbalance.

To the same extent that calcium carbonate and calcium chloride do not react with intestinal bicarbonate (10%), calcium is absorbed into the systemic circulation. Although the amount of calcium absorbed into the blood is minimal, enough may be absorbed after several days of high-dose antacid ingestion to cause hypercalcemia. Hypercalcemia is characterized by neurologic symptoms, renal calculi, and reduced renal function. These side effects are rare in healthy patients, and they do not appear to occur in patients with normal renal function if daily consumption of calcium carbonate is less than 20 g. However, patients with impaired renal function may develop hypercalcemia from as little as 4 g per day. This adverse effect becomes a concern when calcium carbonate is used to bind phosphate in patients with renal failure.

Perhaps the major limiting factor to the chronic use of calcium carbonate is its tendency to cause acid rebound. Acid rebound is described as sustained hypersecretion of gastric acid after antacid has been emptied from the stomach. This phenomenon may be related to increased gastrin concentration, which in turn stimulates acid secretion. Any agent that increases gastric pH causes an increase in gastrin secretion by sending negative feedback signals to the stomach that gastrin (and subsequent acid) is needed. Indeed, all antacids, H_2-antagonists, and omeprazole cause hypergastrinemia and may transiently increase acid secretion. However, only calcium-containing antacids cause intense and prolonged hypersecretion of acid after leaving the stomach. Increased gastric acid secretion begins within 2 hours after administration of calcium carbonate and may last for 3–5 hours. This effect has been reported after large doses (4–8 g) as well as single small doses (500 mg). Acid rebound caused by calcium carbonate is particularly pronounced after meals.

The mechanism of acid rebound caused by calcium is not well defined. Because many agents increase gastrin but only calcium antacids cause acid rebound, the mechanism may be related to a local effect of calcium ions on gastric mucosa in addition to hypergastrinemia.[18]

Despite evidence that acid rebound occurs, there is no evidence that it is clinically significant. Acid rebound has not been shown to delay ulcer healing, and no studies suggest that calcium carbonate is inferior to other antacids in the treatment of peptic ulcer disease. Nevertheless, although acid rebound is primarily a theoretical concern, calcium-containing antacids are not currently recommended for chronic treatment of acid-peptic diseases.

It is a widely held belief that calcium carbonate causes constipation. However, an extensive literature search found that this belief is not substantiated by case reports, controlled studies, or uncontrolled studies.[19] To the contrary, published reports of patients with peptic ulcer disease indicate that calcium carbonate may act as a laxative, increasing fecal bulk in some patients and causing diarrhea in others. Because peptic ulcer disease itself may be constipating, it may be that the constipation noted in patients taking calcium carbonate for peptic ulcer disease may be a consequence of the ulcer rather than of the calcium.

Aluminum Aluminum hydroxide is slowly dissolved in the stomach, where it reacts with gastric acid to form aluminum chloride and water. The reaction is $Al(OH)_3 + 3HCl \rightarrow AlCl_3 + 3H_2O$. In the small intestine, aluminum chloride reacts with bicarbonate to form a series of poorly absorbed basic aluminum salts. Because most of the aluminum chloride reacts with intestinal bicarbonate, very little endogenous bicarbonate is left over, and systemic alkalosis is a minimal risk.

Although the formation of insoluble salts limits aluminum absorption, about 17–30% of the aluminum chloride formed is absorbed.[10] In patients with normal renal function, this aluminum chloride is rapidly excreted by the kidneys. However, patients with impaired renal function who take aluminum antacids chronically may fail to clear aluminum, resulting in hyperaluminemia and accumulation of aluminum in other tissues.

Aluminum absorbed from antacids has adverse effects on phosphate metabolism. All aluminum-containing antacids, except for aluminum phosphate, bind phosphate in the gut, forming insoluble phosphate salts that are excreted in the feces. The result is reduced intestinal phosphate absorption. This effect is beneficial in patients with chronic renal failure who have increased serum levels of phosphorous. However, use of aluminum-containing antacids as phosphate binders in renal failure patients is associated with serious risks. Elevated aluminum concentrations have been reported in the bone, muscle, and brain tissue of such patients taking aluminum antacids.[20] Aluminum is neurotoxic and has been associated with the development of encephalopathy in uremic patients on hemodialysis taking aluminum antacids.[21] However, the relationship between aluminum and this "dialysis dementia" is not well supported. The primary concern with use of aluminum antacids in patients with renal failure is that too much phosphate will be bound by the antacid. The resulting phosphorous depletion can cause calcium to be resorbed from bone, leading to osteomalacia.

In patients with normal renal function, the reduction in phosphate absorption caused by aluminum antacids may lead to clinically significant phosphate depletion. Phosphorous depletion is characterized by anorexia, malaise, and muscle weakness; if severe and prolonged, it may lead to osteomalacia, osteoporosis, and fractures. Although not common, phosphorous depletion may occur as early as the second week of therapy and has been reported with doses of aluminum hydroxide as low as 30 mL three times daily.[22] Although hypophosphatemia is not a concern with most patients taking antacids, it is more likely to occur in those taking large doses of aluminum hydroxide for prolonged periods and those with inadequate dietary intake of phosphorous.[10] Other patients at risk for hypophosphatemia include elderly persons, alcoholics, and those with diarrhea or malabsorption syndromes. Hypophosphatemia can be reversed by administering aluminum phosphate supplements or increasing phosphate in the diet.

The most frequent side effect of aluminum-containing antacids is constipation. This effect may be due to inhibition of intestinal smooth muscle contraction by the aluminum ion. Antacids containing aluminum hydroxide have been reported to cause intestinal obstruction, hemorrhoids, fissures, and fecal impaction.[10] Patients predisposed to obstruction include those with reduced bowel motility, dehydration, and fluid restriction. Constipation from aluminum is thought to be dose related and may be managed with stool softeners or laxatives, or by combining aluminum with magnesium-containing antacids.

Although aluminum may be administered in several different salt forms (carbonate, phosphate, or aminoacetate), the hydroxide salt is the most potent buffer and is used most often. In comparison with magnesium hydroxide, calcium carbonate, and sodium bicarbonate, however, aluminum hydroxide has a relatively low neutralizing capacity.

Magnesium Like sodium bicarbonate, magnesium hydroxide reacts with gastric acid to produce a potent, short-acting neutralizing action. The reaction is $Mg(OH)_2 + 2HCl \rightarrow MgCl_2 + 2H_2O$. Most of the magnesium chloride formed reacts with bicarbonate in the small intestine, thus minimizing the risk of systemic alkalosis. However, about 5–10% of the magnesium chloride is absorbed and rapidly excreted by the kidneys in patients with normal renal function. As with other antacids, the risk of cation absorption and toxicity is significant only in patients with impaired renal function.

Although magnesium toxicity from antacids is rare and occurs primarily in patients with significant renal failure, it can produce life-threatening complications. Magnesium is a strong central nervous system depressant and may cause depressed reflexes, muscle paralysis, nausea, vomiting, hypotension, respiratory depression, coma, and death. Magnesium toxicity can also cause severe cardiac depression, seen clinically as hypotension, electrocardiographic changes, and bradyarrhythmias. Cardiotoxicity does not usually occur until there is severe hypermagnesemia (10–15 mEq/L; normal is 1.8 to 2.4 mEq/L) in patients with renal dysfunction.[23] Considering these risks, magnesium antacids should not be used in patients with marked renal failure; if they are, doses exceeding 50 mEq per day of magnesium should be used cautiously and only under the supervision of a physician who should monitor electrolytes regularly.[10]

The most frequent and limiting side effect of magnesium-containing antacids is diarrhea, which may be severe enough to cause fluid and electrolyte imbalances. Any magnesium hydroxide that does not react with gastric acid is converted in the small intestine to soluble but poorly absorbed magnesium salts. It is likely that these nonabsorbable salts cause an osmotic gradient that is at least partially responsible for the diarrhea associated with magnesium. One study suggests that the laxative effect of magnesium hydroxide is associated with increased output of prostaglandin E_2 in the stool.[24] However, whether these prostaglandins actually cause the diarrhea associated with magnesium therapy requires further study.

Diarrhea associated with magnesium-containing antacids is dose related. The incidence of diarrhea from magnesium ranges from 4% in patients taking low-dose antacid (144 mEq per day) to 76% in patients taking higher doses (1,064 mEq per day). Diarrhea caused by magnesium may differ from diarrhea from other causes in that it does not cause abdominal cramps or nocturnal bowel movements.[24] Efforts to minimize this diarrhea include the use of combination aluminum–magnesium antacid products or alternating aluminum–magnesium therapy with an aluminum antacid only.

Although the hydroxide salt is used most often, other magnesium salts with antacid properties are the oxide (which is converted to hydroxide in water), carbonate, and trisilicate. The neutralizing capacity of magnesium salts is greater than that of aluminum hydroxide but less than that of sodium bicarbonate and calcium carbonate.

Aluminum–Magnesium Combinations Many commercially available antacid products contain a mixture of aluminum and magnesium. Because constipation from aluminum and diarrhea from magnesium are dose related, combining these two agents allows for a potent neutralizing capacity with lower doses of each agent. In theory, the constipating effect of aluminum should balance the diarrheal effect of magnesium, and vice versa. However, the optimal ratio between magnesium and aluminum to achieve this balance has not been found in any commercially available product. Diarrhea appears to be the predominant effect, regardless of the ratio, if doses of magnesium hydroxide exceed 8.5 g per day. Indeed, up to three-fourths of patients taking these combination products experience diarrhea; constipation is rarely reported.

Regardless of whether the GI effects of aluminum and magnesium are reduced with combination products, it is important to realize that the risks of other adverse effects are not reduced. To the contrary, the presence of both salts introduces the possibility of side effects from absorption of two cations. Thus, patients taking combination products may experience hypermagnesemia, aluminum toxicity, hypophosphatemia, or metabolic alkalosis. As with either agent alone, these risks appear to be of concern primarily in patients with reduced renal function.

Magaldrate is a chemical mixture of aluminum and magnesium hydroxides that is converted to aluminum and magnesium ions in hydrochloric acid. Magaldrate has a lower neutralizing capacity than a physical mixture of aluminum and magnesium hydroxides. Because the presence of aluminum is not readily recognized from the term *magaldrate,* the pharmacist should take care not to recommend magaldrate as a non–aluminum-containing product.

Additional Ingredients

Most antacid products contain excipient ingredients that may be clinically important in certain patients. In addition, many products contain ingredients that do not have antacid properties but are used by manufacturers to meet unique advertising claims.

Sugars Some antacids contain considerable amounts of sugars or saccharin. When taken only occasionally or in small doses, the sugar content is not high enough to cause clinical problems. However, when taken in large amounts over long periods of time, enough sugar is ingested to alter glucose control in patients with labile diabetes. When recommending an antacid for diabetic patients, the pharmacist should consider the sugar content. Unfortunately, this information is not required to be listed on the product labeling. An additional concern with the sugar content of antacids is the possibility of tooth decay with extended use.

Sodium Most antacids contain sodium as an impurity, but the amount differs considerably among products. Because of the risks of sodium to certain patients, the sodium content in antacids has been reduced significantly over the past several years. Many antacid products have been developed that contain less than 0.04 mEq (1 mg) sodium per 5 mL, or no sodium at all. These products should be used in patients with hypertension, congestive heart failure, renal failure, edema, or cirrhosis, and in those on salt-restricted diets. The usual amount of sodium allowed in sodium-restricted diets is 3 g or less per day. Antacids containing more than 5 mEq (115 mg) sodium in the total daily dose should not be recommended without first consulting with the patient's physician. Obviously, antacids containing sodium bicarbonate have the largest quantities of sodium and should not be used in these patients.

Simethicone Simethicone is a mixture of inert silicon polymers used as a defoaming agent to relieve gas. Simethicone acts in the stomach and intestine to reduce the surface tension of gas bubbles embedded in mucus in the GI tract. As surface tension changes, the gas bubbles are broken or coalesced so they can be eliminated more easily by belching or passing flatus.[10] The Food and Drug Administration (FDA) considers simethicone safe and effective as an antiflatulent agent, but simethicone has no activity as an antacid.

Many antacid products contain a combination of simethicone and antacids, but use of both agents is often unnecessary. The efficacy of such combination products has not been well studied. However, use of a combination product may be rational for patients with acid-peptic disorders who have symptoms related to gas (e.g., upper GI bloating, pressure, fullness, or flatulence). Conversely, the addition of simethicone to antacids does not benefit patients with peptic disorders if they do not have symptoms suggestive of gas. To the contrary, one study has reported that the addition of simethicone to an aluminum-containing antacid adsorbed the antacid, reducing the bioavailability of both agents.[25]

Alginic Acid Alginic acid is combined with sodium bicarbonate and other antacids in several commercial products. Alginic acid has foaming, floating, and viscous properties that render it beneficial in GERD.[10] However, use of these products is not indicated for other acid-peptic diseases because the amount of antacid ingredients included does not provide sufficient neutralizing capacity to be useful. The FDA considers alginic acid to be safe.

Formulation

The formulation of an antacid is important for both neutralizing capacity and patient acceptance and compliance. The two most popular and often used antacid formulations are liquids (suspensions) and tablets. These formulations differ significantly with regard to both neutralizing capacity and patient acceptance.

TABLE 1 Symptoms and characteristics of selected gastrointestinal disorders

Gastroesophageal reflux disease

Heartburn/pain in lower chest
Pain is worse after meals & when lying down
Pain may wake patient at night
Pain is often relieved by antacids
Pain may be worse after certain foods, smoking, alcohol, caffeine, and medications that reduce lower esophageal sphincter tone

Duodenal ulcer

Gnawing, aching, epigastric pain
Well-localized
Predictable pattern
Begins 1–2 hours after eating & worse before next meal
Relieved by food or antacids
Weight gain common
May wake patient at night
History of smoking

Gastric ulcer

Variable epigastric pain
Unpredictable pattern
Food may worsen pain
Weight loss is common
May be relieved by antacids
History of chronic NSAID use

Acute gastritis

Burning epigastric pain
Possible association with anorexia, nausea, and vomiting
History of alcohol binge or NSAID use

Because only dissolved antacid can react with hydrogen ions, the dissolution rate or ease of solubility is an important determinant of ultimate neutralizing capacity. These factors depend largely on the formulation of the antacid. Antacid suspensions are formulated with smaller particles than tablets; therefore, they provide a larger surface area and are more rapidly and effectively dissolved in gastric acid. Moreover, antacid suspensions are already in a form to dissolve and react with acid, whereas tablets must be chewed so they will disintegrate and dissolve in stomach fluids. Because of these differences, suspensions are more potent than tablets of the same antacid on a milligram-for-milligram basis.

Despite higher potency, many patients find liquid antacids unpalatable or cumbersome and prefer to take tablets. Use of antacid tablets may be appropriate for such patients, particularly those who are noncompliant with liquid antacids. Some patients may prefer to alternate tablets during the day at work with liquids at night at home. Patients should be instructed to chew antacid tablets thoroughly and follow with a full glass of water to ensure maximum therapeutic benefit. Tablets that do not disintegrate may lodge in the intestine and cause obstruction.

The feasibility of using antacid tablets for chronic disorders such as peptic ulcer disease depends on the total neutralizing capacity desired. Studies supporting the efficacy of low-dose antacids have demonstrated DU healing with one or two antacid tablets (20–30 mEq) four times daily.[15,16] On the other hand, high-dose antacid regimens for DU could require the ingestion of 5–40 tablets seven times a day, depending on the neutralizing capacity of the tablet. Patient compliance is likely to be compromised at such a regimen. Cost to the patient may also be prohibitive when large numbers of tablets must be taken. Patients seeking short-term relief from mild GI symptoms may be better suited for therapy with antacid tablets. However, patients with peptic ulcer disease may best be managed with high-potency liquid antacids.

Other formulations of antacids include lozenges, chewing gums with antacid coating, and effervescent tablets and powders to be dissolved in water. These formulations do not appear to offer any advantages over liquids and tablets in either neutralizing capacity or patient acceptance.

Palatability

Because antacids often must be taken frequently and in large amounts, their taste, or palatability, is a critical factor in determining patient compliance. Taste may be especially important to patients with peptic ulcers who no longer have pain or dyspeptic symptoms. A taste test performed with 19 liquid antacids failed to find any overwhelming favorites.[26] Mylanta II® has been well accepted in several taste tests, but there is much individual variation. Unfortunately, it is unlikely than any scientific study can resolve the issue of taste for all patients because taste preference is an individual matter. General recommendations for improving taste tolerability of antacids include refrigerating the product and using high-potency liquid antacids, which can be taken in smaller quantities. However, patients should be advised not to freeze antacid suspensions because this may result in coarse particles that are less reactive to acid. Patients taking antacids on a long-term basis should be questioned about taste preference as a guide to compliance. When they complain or tire of the taste of an antacid, the pharmacist should be prepared to offer alternatives. Some patients may prefer flavored tablets, if an equivalent neutralizing capacity can be provided with a reasonable number of tablets.

Potency

The potency of antacids should be expressed in terms of mEq of acid-neutralizing capacity—that is, the amount of acid buffered per dose over a specified period. The FDA requires that an antacid product neutralize at least 5 mEq per dose and must maintain the pH over 3.5 for 10 minutes in an in-vitro test.[2] Any ingredient in a product must contribute at least 25% of the total acid-neutralizing capacity of the product to be called an antacid.

There are large differences in neutralizing capacities of antacid products depending on ingredient(s), formulation, and manufacturer (Tables 1 and 2). The neutralizing capacity of 15 mL of liquid antacid may vary from 6 mEq in a low-potency formulation to 60 mEq in a concentrated or high-potency formulation. Thus, equal volumes of antacids are not equipotent. Consequently, antacids should be dosed according to the mEq acid-neutralizing capacity

TABLE 2 Antacid–drug interactions

Drug	Al	Mg	Al–Mg	CaCO₃	NaHCO₃	Effect	Mechanism	Clinical implication
Allopurinol	✓					↓ absorption in 3 patients on chronic hemodialysis with failure to reduce uric acid	Unknown	Monitor patient for ↓ allopurinol response. Separate doses by ≥ 2 hr
Amphetamine					✓	↓ urinary excretion, allowing potential for retention & intoxication	↓ renal clearance due to ↑ urine pH	Avoid concurrent use
Antibiotics Nitrofurantoin	✓					↓ rate & extent of absorption		Separate doses by ≥ 2 hr
Tetracycline and Quinolones	✓	✓		✓		↓ absorption (up to 90%), resulting in ↓ serum and urine concentrations	Chelation	May result in treatment failures. Separate dosing ≥ 3 hr
Anticoagulants		✓				↑ absorption of dicumarol by 50%; no effect on warfarin absorption	Chelation	Patients needing antacids & anticoagulants should receive warfarin
Anticonvulsants Phenytoin		✓	✓			↓ rate & extent of absorption with large doses of antacid; no effect with small doses	Unknown	Monitor phenytoin effects/levels
Valproic acid	✓	✓	✓			↑ absorption by 12%	Unknown	Potential for valproic acid toxicity
Beta blockers Propranolol	✓					↓ bioavailability by 50% in 4 of 5 subjects; no effect in another study	Delay in gastric emptying	Clinical significance of long-term therapy not assessed
Metoprolol			✓			↑ bioavailability by 25% after single dose in 6 healthy volunteers	Interference with first-pass metabolism	Probably not significant
Atenolol	✓		✓	✓		↓ bioavailability from 37–51%		May be clinically significant; separate doses by at least 1 hour
Benzodiazepines Diazepam	✓		✓			↑ absorption & ↑ sedative effects; ↓ rate, but not extent, of absorption	Unknown	May result in delay in sedative effect. Important only in acute anxiety with single doses, not in chronic dosing
Chlordiazepoxide Clorazepate			✓			↓ rate, but not extent, of absorption ↓ rate & extent of absorption		
Captopril			✓			↓ absorption by 42% in 10 healthy volunteers	Unknown	No evidence of compromised efficacy
Chlorpromazine			✓			↓ absorption & serum concentration; ↓ therapeutic response reported	Adsorption	Monitor for ↓ therapeutic response. Separate doses by ≥ 2 hr
Corticosteroids Dexamethasone		✓				↓ absorption	Adsorption	Evidence conflicting & clinical significance questionable
Prednisone	✓		✓			↓ absorption in one study, but not confirmed		

Chapter 11 — Antacids

Drug	Antacids Al	Mg	Al–Mg	CaCO₃	NaHCO₃	Effect	Mechanism	Clinical implication
Digoxin	✓	✓	✓			↓ absorption of digoxin up to 30% in some reports, but no effect in others. May be more likely to occur with tablets than capsules	Adsorption	Clinical significance uncertain. Monitor patients for ↓ digoxin effect when antacids given concurrently. Space doses to avoid possible interaction
H₂-antagonists Cimetidine Ranitidine Famotidine	✓✓		✓✓			↓ absorption & peak concentration by 30–40%; clinical failures not reported	Adsorption	Separate doses by at least 2 hr
Iron	✓			✓	✓	↓ absorption by 50–60%	↓ iron solubility due to chelation or ↑ gastric pH	May interfere with patient's response to iron replacement therapy. Separate doses by ≥ 2 hr
Isoniazid	✓	✓				↓ absorption, particularly with aluminum antacids	Delayed gastric emptying due to aluminum	Separate doses by ≥ 1 hr
Ketoconazole	✓		✓		✓	↓ ketoconazole absorption	↑ gastric pH	Separate doses by ≥ 2 hr
Levodopa			✓			↑ absorption in some patients, but effect is variable	↑ gastric emptying due to antacids, thus more levodopa delivered to small intestine for absorption	May be clinically useful in certain patients with delayed gastric emptying. Monitor patient response when adding or stopping antacid
NSAIDs Aspirin			✓	✓		↓ serum concentrations by 30–70%	↑ renal clearance due to ↑ urine pH	Monitor serum salicylate levels & observe symptoms when sustained levels important (e.g., RA, SLE)
Enteric-coated aspirin						Premature rupture of enteric coating & dissolution in the stomach	↑ gastric ph	Separate doses in patients at risk for NSAID gastropathy
Indomethacin Naproxen Diflunisal	✓✓	✓	✓✓			Delayed absorption & possible ↓ peak concentrations	Adsorption	Not clinically important
Pseudoephedrine						↑ rate, but not extent, of absorption in 6 healthy volunteers		Clinical significance unknown
Quinidine		✓		✓		↑ serum concentrations; toxicity has been reported	↓ renal clearance due to ↑ urine pH	Use with caution. Monitor levels & patient response
Sodium polystyrene sulfonate		✓	✓	✓		Metabolic alkalosis	Antacid binds resin instead of intestinal HCO₃, resulting in ↑ reabsorption of HCO₃	Concurrent use may be dangerous. Separate doses by ≥ 2 hr
Sucralfate						↓ dissolution & possible loss of efficacy	↑ gastric pH	Separate doses by ≥ 30 min
Theophylline						↑ & ↓ in rate, but not extent, of absorption observed, depending on the theophylline preparation	Unknown	Not important in chronic dosing

Key:
✓ indicates interactions reported in humans. However, interactions may be likely with other antacids in which interactions are not yet reported.
↑ = increased; ↓ = decreased; ASA = aspirin; RA = rheumatoid arthritis; SLE = systemic lupus erythematosus.

Information extracted from:
Gugler R, Allgayer H. *Clin Pharmacokin* 1990; 18 (3): 210–9.
Gibaldi M et al. *Clin Pharmacol Ther* 1974; 16: 520–5.
Tatro DS, ed., *Drug Interaction Facts*. St. Louis: Facts and Comparisons Division: J. B. Lippincott Co; 1990.
Hansten PD, Horn JR. *Drug Interactions*. 6th ed. Philadelphia: Lea & Febiger; 1989.

rather than by volume or number of tablets. Higher potency antacids can be dosed in smaller volumes or fewer tablets, which is an advantage reflected in lower costs and higher patient acceptance. Antacids containing calcium carbonate or sodium bicarbonate are the most effective neutralizers but are not suitable for long-term, large-dose administration. Aluminum–magnesium combination products offer adequate neutralizing capacity with the least potential for side effects.

Onset and Duration of Action

The onset of the neutralizing action of an antacid depends on the product's solubility (how fast the antacid dissolves in gastric acid). The solubility of an antacid depends on both chemical and physical properties. Sodium bicarbonate and magnesium hydroxide dissolve quickly at gastric pH and provide a rapid buffering effect. Aluminum hydroxide and calcium carbonate dissolve slowly in stomach acid, and it may take 10–30 minutes for any significant neutralization to take place. Antacid suspensions generally dissolve more easily in gastric acid than do tablets or powders. Although a fast antacid effect is advertised by antacid manufacturers as an advantage, its clinical significance is questionable.

The duration of action of antacids is determined by how long the antacid remains in the stomach and is dependent on gastric emptying time. If taken on an empty stomach, antacids are rapidly emptied from the stomach and have a duration of action of only 20–40 minutes.[10] However, gastric emptying is greatly slowed by the presence of food; thus, antacids taken after meals leave the stomach more slowly. When taken 1 hour after meals, antacids may neutralize acid for up to 3 hours. Sodium bicarbonate and magnesium hydroxide have the shortest duration of neutralizing action; aluminum hydroxide and calcium carbonate have the longest. Combination aluminum–magnesium antacids have an intermediate duration of neutralizing action.

Antacid–Drug Interactions

Antacid–drug interactions have been reported with more than 30 classes of drugs. Such interactions are so common that drug regulatory agencies in many countries request interaction studies with antacids as part of the new drug approval process.[27] Despite the large number of drugs that interact with antacids, however, clinical experience with these agents has demonstrated that most such interactions are not clinically significant. Nevertheless, some interactions with antacids may be significant enough to result in clinical treatment failures with one or both drugs (Table 2).

In general, antacids alter the absorption of other drugs by three mechanisms: (1) chelating or binding drugs, (2) increasing gastric pH, and (3) increasing urine pH. Although all antacids may interact in these ways, some are more likely to cause these changes than others. Factors that influence whether an antacid interacts with another drug include the valence of the cation in the antacid, the dose used, the chronicity of dosing, and, most important, the timing of the administration or consumption of the antacid in relation to the other drug.

Drugs That Chelate with Antacids   The most significant drug interactions with antacids are those in which antacids containing divalent (Ca^{2+}, Mg^{2+}) or trivalent (Al^{3+}) cations chelate or bind certain other drugs and reduce their absorption. Antacids containing magnesium hydroxide or magnesium trisilicate appear to have the greatest potential for drug binding, whereas aluminum hydroxide and calcium carbonate have an intermediate ability.[10]

Probably the most well known drug interaction with antacids is that of tetracycline. Polyvalent metallic cations have a strong affinity for tetracycline, resulting in the formation of a chelate. This insoluble compound cannot penetrate the intestinal mucosa for absorption. When antacids are coadministered with tetracycline, response to the antibiotic may vary depending on the extent of chelation. Antacids containing aluminum, magnesium, or calcium are strong inhibitors of tetracycline absorption and have been reported to reduce bioavailability by 50% to more than 90%.[27] Chelation with antacids has also been reported with other tetracyclines, including doxycycline, demeclocycline, and oxytetracycline.[28] Although not reported, this interaction is likely to occur with minocycline as well. Patients taking any form of tetracycline who need an antacid should be advised not to take antacids until at least 3 hours after tetracycline administration.

The metal cations of antacids also have a strong ability to chelate quinolone antibiotics, which may result in impaired GI absorption. Significant reductions (up to 90%) in bioavailability and peak plasma concentrations of ciprofloxacin have been reported with magnesium- and aluminum-containing antacids, as well as with calcium carbonate.[28] Significant reductions in peak serum concentrations have also occurred with ofloxacin, norfloxacin, temafloxacin, lomefloxacin, and enoxacin.[28] Given that these antibiotics may be used to treat serious Gram-negative infections (e.g., osteomyelitis or prostatitis) on an outpatient basis, the importance of this interaction cannot be overstated. Patients taking quinolones who have an indication for an antacid should be instructed to separate doses of these agents by at least 2 hours.

Reduced absorption of H_2-antagonists has been documented with concurrent administration of antacids, but conflicting results exist. Although the antacid is suspected of binding the H_2-antagonists, the precise mechanism is unknown. Single doses of magnesium–aluminum combination antacids have reportedly decreased the absorption of cimetidine, ranitidine, famotidine, and nizatidine.[28] Reductions in serum concentrations of these H_2-antagonists have ranged from 30 to 40% and can be avoided or diminished when the dosing of the antacid and H_2-antagonists is separated by 1 to 2 hours. Other data suggest that antacids do not significantly affect the absorption of H_2-antagonists in long-term therapy.[27] However, until more data substantiate a lack of significant interaction, administration of antacids and H_2-antagonists should be separated by at least 2 hours.[29]

Drugs That Are Affected by Gastric pH   Because antacids increase gastric pH, they can interfere with the absorption of drugs requiring an acidic environment for dissolution or absorption. Theoretically, antacids could interfere with the action of sucralfate, which is thought to need an acidic environment to dissociate and form the viscous gel that binds to gastric and duodenal mucosa. Although antacids have diminished the binding of sucralfate to GUs in animals, it is not known whether they interfere significantly with the binding of sucralfate in humans.[30] Until more is known about this interaction, it is wise to give antacids at least 30 minutes apart from sucralfate. Similarly, drugs such as ketoconazole, which need acid for absorption should be separated by at least 2 hours from antacid dosing.[28]

Drugs That Are Affected by Increased Urine pH By increasing urine pH, antacids may affect the elimination of certain acidic or basic drugs whose renal clearance depends on urine pH. This interaction is particularly pronounced with sodium bicarbonate, the strongest urinary alkalinizer of all antacids. Other antacids have been shown to increase urinary pH significantly in the following order: aluminum–magnesium combination > magnesium hydroxide > calcium carbonate.[31] Antacids that contain only aluminum hydroxide do not appear to increase urine pH.

Aspirin and salicylates are weakly acidic drugs that become ionized in alkaline urine, thus accelerating their renal clearance. Antacid-induced urine pH changes can decrease steady-state plasma salicylate levels by almost one-half.[27] In contrast, the renal excretion of basic drugs such as quinidine and amphetamines may be significantly reduced by antacids.[28] Increased drug concentrations and effects may result from such interactions. In fact, quinidine toxicity has been documented to occur as a result of an increase in urine pH.[27] Concurrent use of these drugs with antacids should be avoided or closely monitored.

Other Drugs

H_2-antagonists

The introduction of the first H_2-antagonist, cimetidine, in 1977 revolutionized the treatment of acid-peptic disorders. Since that time, new and more potent H_2-antagonists have been developed. Four H_2-antagonists are currently available for prescription use in the United States: cimetidine, ranitidine, famotidine, and nizatidine. Nonprescription status for the H_2-antagonists is a possibility in the future.

H_2-antagonists act in the treatment of acid-peptic diseases primarily by reducing aggressive forces rather than by enhancing mucosal defenses. H_2-antagonists inhibit gastric acid secretion by competitively blocking H_2-receptors on the parietal cell. They suppress nocturnal and basal gastric acid secretion by 90–95% and meal-stimulated acid secretion by 70–80%. H_2-antagonists also inhibit up to 90% of acid secretion stimulated by acetylcholine and gastrin receptors on the parietal cell, calcium, and other stimuli.[3] By inhibiting gastric acid secretion, H_2-antagonists increase gastric pH and subsequently inhibit pepsin activity. As a result of increased gastric pH, all H_2-antagonists increase gastrin concentrations, but there is no significant acid rebound such as may occur with calcium carbonate.

The four available H_2-antagonists are not equipotent on a milligram-for-milligram basis. The ability of these agents to inhibit gastric acid secretion varies from 20- to 50-fold, with cimetidine being the least potent and famotidine being the most potent. Equipotent oral doses of the H_2-antagonists are cimetidine 1,200–1,600 mg, nizatidine 300 mg, ranitidine 300 mg, and famotidine 40 mg.[32]

As a class, the H_2-antagonists are well studied and relatively safe. These drugs have been given to more than 24 million people and have rarely caused serious side effects; the overall incidence of side effects is less than 3%.[5] Cimetidine has antiandrogenic effects and reduces the metabolism of estrogen. These effects may result in impotence, loss of libido, and gynecomastia. However, these side effects rarely occur except in men receiving large doses (more than 3 g per day) for Zollinger–Ellison syndrome for prolonged periods, and they are readily reversed by stopping cimetidine or substituting another H_2-antagonist. Use of cimetidine has been associated with mental confusion, primarily in patients with renal or hepatic impairment who consume large doses. Mental confusion has also been reported with ranitidine and famotidine. Adverse hematologic effects (e.g., leukopenia, thrombocytopenia, and anemia) are rare but have been reported with cimetidine, ranitidine, and famotidine.[29]

In general, all four H_2-antagonists are equally effective when taken in equipotent doses. An impending change that may expand the role of H_2-antagonists in GI disorders—and possibly diminish the role of antacids—is the proposed move of cimetidine and ranitidine from prescription to nonprescription status for the treatment of "episodic heartburn."[33] However, it is not clear when this reclassification will be made, or whether a lower dose will be approved so that there is a clear separation between prescription and nonprescription doses.

Omeprazole

Omeprazole is the first of a class of agents known as proton pump inhibitors. Whereas H_2-antagonists inhibit acid secretion by inhibiting the receptors on the parietal cell, which stimulate the proton pump, omeprazole inhibits the pump itself.[32] Because activation of the proton pump is the final step in acid secretion, inhibition by omeprazole abolishes gastric acid secretion in response to any type of acid stimulation. Accordingly, omeprazole is the most potent and effective antisecretory agent currently available. Whereas H_2-antagonists suppress most of the acid secretion, omeprazole provides total acid suppression. Because omeprazole binds irreversibly to the H^+/K^+-ATPase enzyme of the proton pump, new ATPase protein must be made before acid secretion returns. This process takes 3–5 days, which means that omeprazole has a prolonged duration of acid suppression.[34] By reducing gastric acid secretion, omeprazole causes serum gastrin levels to increase significantly; however, acid rebound does not occur.[5] Omeprazole also causes a dose-related reduction in gastric acid volume and pepsin activity. Omeprazole does not alter lower esophageal sphincter tone or GI motility.

Omeprazole appears to be as well tolerated as the H_2-antagonists, with mild GI complaints reported occasionally. The most common side effects of omeprazole are abdominal pain, nausea, vomiting, headache, and diarrhea.[10] The major concern with this drug is the observation that rats treated chronically with high doses of it developed carcinoid tumors of the stomach, some of which were malignant.[32] The tumors may be related to high levels of gastrin induced by omeprazole. Hypergastrinemia appears to stimulate the growth of certain cells in the stomach that may cause tumors.[32] Although there is currently no evidence that carcinoid tumors develop in humans with chronic use of the drug, the carcinogenic potential of omeprazole remains a concern. The drug is not approved or recommended for long-term use, except for the treatment of Zollinger–Ellison syndrome.

Because of its potency and long-lasting reduction of gastric acidity, omeprazole may be regarded as the ultimate medical therapy for acid-peptic diseases.[32] It is the drug of choice for patients with Zollinger–Ellison syndrome, although doses as high as 360 mg per day may be necessary to control this disorder. For treatment of peptic ulcers, omeprazole works faster and more effectively than currently recommended doses of H_2-antagonists.[32] However, omeprazole is also the most expensive of the antisecretory drugs. Cost and concern regarding its carcinogenic potential preclude its use as first-line therapy for uncomplicated acid-peptic disorders.

Anticholinergic Agents

Before the introduction of H_2-antagonists, the only drugs that could reduce gastric acid secretion were anticholinergic agents. These drugs reduce acid secretion by blocking the action of acetylcholine on the cholinergic receptor of the parietal cell. At the optimal effective dose, which differs among patients, anticholinergic drugs reduce basal gastric acid secretion by 40–50% and stimulate acid secretion by 30–40%.[35] However, the doses necessary to achieve this reduction in gastric acid also inhibit other cholinergic receptors in the body. Familiar anticholinergic side effects occur frequently and include dry mouth, blurred vision, tachycardia, urinary retention, constipation, and mental confusion.

Despite three decades of use, the value of such agents in relieving symptoms, healing peptic ulcers, or preventing ulcer recurrence has not been established. Furthermore, these agents delay gastric emptying, resulting in gastric distention and gastric acid retention. This effect was once considered a therapeutic benefit in that it prolonged the time antacids remained in the stomach.[35] However, antacids adsorb anticholinergics and reduce their absorption, further reducing the potency of the anticholinergic agent. A final undesirable effect of anticholinergic agents is a reduction in lower esophageal sphincter tone, which can aggravate GERD.[36]

Although several anticholinergic agents are approved for treating peptic ulcer disease, their use has been superseded by the development of the H_2-antagonists and omeprazole.[5] Considering the higher potency of these newer agents, their efficacy in healing peptic ulcers, and their superior side effect profiles, it is difficult to justify use of an anticholinergic agent for peptic ulcer disease.

Sucralfate

Sucralfate is the only agent approved for the treatment of peptic ulcer disease that does not reduce or neutralize gastric acid. The recognition that sucralfate can heal ulcers by protecting the gastric mucosa supports the idea that cytoprotection is important in the treatment of peptic ulcer disease. Sucralfate is a complex salt of sucrose sulfate and aluminum hydroxide that dissolves in stomach acid, releases aluminum, and forms a viscous gel. This viscous substance has a strong negative charge and binds electrostatically to any positively charged chemical groups, such as proteins at the base of an ulcer. In its active form, sucralfate binds to defective mucosa and forms a barrier that protects the ulcer from the destructive forces of acid and pepsin. Sucralfate also binds to normal GI mucosa, but not as strongly.[30] Numerous other cytoprotective mechanisms have been demonstrated in vitro, but whether these effects occur in human GI mucosa and are clinically significant is not known.

Compliance with sucralfate is rarely compromised because of side effects; however, the large tablet size and multidose regimen may be inconvenient for some patients. Patients who find the large tablets difficult to swallow may find it easier to suspend the tablets in a glass of water. A suspension is currently under development, but it is not known when it will be available. Patients should be advised to take sucralfate on an empty stomach, about 30 minutes before meals. This is when the stomach is most acidic and the potential for sucralfate dissolution is greatest.

Misoprostol

Misoprostol, a prostaglandin E_1 analogue, is the only drug available that has both antisecretory effects and established cytoprotective properties. Its primary action is enhancement or restoration of the gastric mucosal barrier. Misoprostol protects the gastric mucosa by stimulating mucus and bicarbonate secretion, increasing epithelial cell regeneration, and enhancing gastric mucosal blood flow.[37] Misoprostol also causes reduction in acid secretion, which occurs 30 minutes after a dose and persists for at least 3 hours. However, misoprostol at doses of 50–200 mcg is a less potent inhibitor of acid secretion than H_2-antagonists and omeprazole.[37]

Like natural prostaglandins, misoprostol increases smooth muscle contractions in many parts of the body, most notably in the GI tract and uterus. The primary side effect limiting its use is diarrhea. At the approved dose of 200 mcg four times daily for the prevention of NSAID-induced gastropathy, misoprostol has been noted to cause diarrhea in up to 40% of patients.[38] Diarrhea usually occurs within the first 2 weeks of therapy and subsides after 7–10 days. It is generally described as mild, but it may be severe and cause fluid or electrolyte disturbances. Most patients develop tolerance to this side effect, but some will discontinue the drug as a result of it. Because this effect is dose related, initiating therapy with a lower dose (e.g., 100 mcg four times daily) and slowly increasing the dose may help avoid the problem. Patients should be warned that diarrhea may occur and should be advised to take the drug after meals to minimize this side effect. Other common side effects of misoprostol include abdominal cramping, flatulence, nausea, and vomiting.[10] Because misoprostol significantly increases uterine contractions and may cause abortions in pregnant women, it is contraindicated in pregnancy, and special precautions must be taken if it is prescribed to a woman of childbearing age. Such patients should receive adequate contraception, understand the risks involved if pregnancy occurs while taking the drug, and have a negative serum pregnancy test within 2 weeks prior to initiating misoprostol therapy.[37] Overall, misoprostol is not as well tolerated as H_2-antagonists, sucralfate, or omeprazole.

Coadministration of aluminum-only antacids with misoprostol may be beneficial for several reasons. First, absorption of misoprostol is delayed, and peaks are slightly reduced by administration with aluminum-only antacids.[37] Because diarrhea caused by misoprostol is dose related, this interaction may help to reduce the diarrhea. Furthermore, constipation caused by aluminum-containing antacids may offset diarrhea from the misoprostol and help patients tolerate the drug. Because of this diarrhea, antacids containing magnesium only or aluminum–magnesium combinations should be avoided in patients receiving misoprostol.

Bismuth

Bismuth compounds have been used to treat various GI disorders for more than 200 years. These compounds have recently attracted attention because of their ability to suppress *H. pylori* infection and their potential for cytoprotection. The two bismuth compounds used most commonly are colloidal bismuth subcitrate (CBS) and bismuth subsalicylate (BSS). Both compounds have antibacterial activity and have been used alone and in combination with antibiotics to eradicate *H. pylori*.[39]

BBS (Pepto Bismol®) is the only bismuth compound available in the United States. BSS was once called an antacid but has no measurable acid-neutralizing capacity. Currently, it is indicated only for common diarrhea, traveler's diarrhea, and occasional relief of upset stomach or upper GI symptoms. Although BSS has been shown to coat the mucosal lining in animals, it does not appear to form a protective coating in human mucosa and is not recognized as a gastric mucosal protectant. It is generally believed that the benefit of BSS in treating peptic ulcers is derived almost entirely from its ability to suppress *H. pylori*.

The major concern with the use of the bismuth salts is the potential for systemic bismuth absorption and toxicity. The primary manifestation of bismuth toxicity is neurotoxicity. Most reports of bismuth neurotoxicity have been related to other bismuth salts, such as the subnitrate and the subgallate. In the many years in which BSS has been used as an occasional nonprescription medication, only two cases of neurotoxicity have been reported.[40] To date, only one case of neurotoxicity has been linked to CBS.[40] Both compounds are converted by colonic bacteria into bismuth sulfide and thus can cause blackening of the tongue and stools.[39,40] This side effect should not be confused with melena, in which the stools become black and tarry because of blood loss.

GI Disorders and Role of Antacids

Peptic Ulcer Disease

Peptic ulcer disease is a group of chronic disorders characterized by ulcerating mucosal lesions in the upper GI tract. A peptic ulcer is a well-defined erosion or lesion in the GI mucosa whose formation depends on acid and pepsin. The most common sites of peptic ulcer are the duodenum and the stomach. However, peptic ulcer disease can occur anywhere in the GI tract exposed to acid and pepsin. Today, DUs are about four times more common than GUs,[41] and both types of ulcers are two to three times more common in men than in women.

Peptic ulcer disease poses enormous health and economic problems to society. Approximately 500,000 new cases and 4 million recurrences are reported each year in the United States.[5] Considering the number of persons affected with this disease, the mortality rate of 9,000 deaths per year is relatively low. However, more than 400,000 patients are hospitalized annually due to peptic ulcer disease, resulting in more than 4 million inpatient days and more than 130,000 surgical procedures.[42] The annual estimated cost of this disease in the United States, which includes both direct costs for treatment of patients and indirect costs related to time lost from work, is in excess of $5 billion.[5]

Duodenal Ulcer

Estimates for the United States suggest that more than 200,000 new cases of DU occur each year. The DU patient generally responds well to therapy, and rapid pain relief and ulcer healing can be expected. One can also expect the ulcer to recur. The old saying "once an ulcer, always an ulcer" is illustrated by the fact that 65–90% of DU patients will relapse within 1 year of initial healing.[43] Although this rate may be lowered by chronic maintenance therapy or eradication of *H. pylori*, DUs are a chronic, recurrent, and expensive illness for the majority of patients and society as a whole.

Pathogenesis DUs characteristically occur in the first portion of the duodenum, or the duodenal bulb, and are usually from 1 mm to 1 cm in diameter.[44] Because the duodenal bulb is the juncture through which gastric contents enter the duodenum, it makes sense that gastric acid and pepsin are involved in the development of DUs. Indeed, it is generally felt that patients with DUs produce too much gastric acid, giving rise to the phrase "no acid—no ulcer."

Approximately 30–50% of patients with DUs have an increased capacity to secrete acid as well as an increased rate of basal acid secretion.[5] Consequently, the excess acid and pepsin are delivered from the stomach to the duodenal bulb. However, excess acid is not an adequate explanation for DUs as a whole. These ulcers develop in many patients whose gastric acid output is normal, and many patients with high acid output do not develop them. Although effective antisecretory agents such as H_2-antagonists heal most DUs, 20–30% of patients do not heal within 4 weeks, and at least the same percentage have recurrences despite maintenance treatment.[45] Among patients with active DUs, 40–50% heal during placebo therapy within 4 weeks, presumably in the absence of changes in acid/pepsin secretion.[5] Furthermore, pharmacologic agents that do not reduce gastric acid secretion, such as colloidal bismuth and sucralfate, heal DUs as effectively as H_2-antagonists. Clearly, elements other than excess acid are involved in the pathogenesis of DUs.

These other factors are probably related to duodenal mucosal defenses, but they have not been fully evaluated. Indeed, the gastric mucous layer in DU patients has been reported to be significantly thinner than in patients without ulcer.[46] If mucosal defenses are impaired in these patients, the factor most likely responsible is *H. pylori*. The role of *H. pylori* in the pathogenesis of DUs is not yet clear; however, essentially every patient with chronic DUs harbors the organism.[4] Although available evidence does not yet support the conclusion that *H. pylori* alone causes DUs, recent observations do support at least a contributory role for the organism.

Genetic and environmental factors may also be involved in the pathogenesis of DUs. DUs tend to cluster in families, with a threefold increase in the incidence of the disease in first-degree relatives of DU patients.[41] Genetic influence is also demonstrated by a higher concordance in identical than in fraternal twins and by an increased incidence in those who have inherited blood group O.[41] Probably the most important single environmental factor in the development of DUs is smoking. Cigarette smokers are about twice as likely to develop the disease as nonsmokers, and the risk increases with both the number of cigarettes smoked and the number of years of smoking.[5] Alcohol is not a proven risk factor for DUs except in patients with cirrhosis.[41] Additionally, epidemiologic data suggest that DUs occur more commonly in patients with other chronic diseases, including pulmonary disease, pancreatitis, cirrhosis, and rheumatoid arthritis. However, these associations may be explained by cigarette smoking, alcohol abuse, and aspirin and other NSAID use, respectively. Although stress and psychologic factors are widely believed to contribute to DUs, ulcer patients as a group tend to exhibit the same psychologic makeup as the general population.[5]

Clinical Presentation The classic and most frequent symptom of DUs is epigastric pain (in the upper abdomen). This pain is often described as burning, annoying, or gnawing, or a dull ache resembling hunger pain. It is usually so well localized that patients have tenderness to palpation at a small localized point in the epigastrium. The pain of DUs generally occurs when the stomach is empty and when unbuffered gastric acid is in contact with the ulcer. It usually begins 2 to 3 hours after meals and may continue, reaching maximum intensity just before the next meal. The pain is usually relieved within 5–10 minutes of eating or taking antacids. About 50–80% of patients report being awakened with pain at night, usually around 1:00 to 2:00 AM,[42] when gastric acid secretion is maximal and food that could buffer the acid is absent. The pain is usually not present in the morning on awakening. Other symptoms that may accompany ulcer pain include belching, bloating, and abdominal distention. Although not common, nausea, vomiting, and mild diarrhea may occur. Most patients have a good appetite and may even gain weight as they eat more in an effort to relieve pain.

Because DUs typically have periods of exacerbation and remission, the pain is intermittent as well. However, symptoms do not always correlate with the presence or absence of an ulcer. In fact, a substantial percentage (5–25%) of patients with DUs have no symptoms at all. The only physical sign in these patients may be point tenderness in the epigastrium.

Complications The most common complication of DUs is bleeding, which occurs in about 20% of all patients with peptic ulcer disease.[5] Bleeding may occur at all ages but is more common in patients over age 60. If there is bleeding, stools may become black and tarry (melena), and patients may vomit blood (hematemesis). Iron deficiency anemia can be a sign of chronic bleeding and may be recognized by weakness, fatigue, tachycardia, and dyspnea on exertion.

Other major complications of DUs are perforation, penetration, and obstruction. Perforation, which develops in about 7% of patients with peptic ulcer disease and is considered the most serious complication,[5] occurs when the ulcer erodes through the stomach or duodenum and allows gastric contents to spill into the abdominal cavity. It is characterized by a sudden, severe, and generalized abdominal pain; abdominal rigidity; and pneumoperitoneum (air or gas in the abdominal cavity). Penetration occurs when the ulcer crater erodes through the entire wall of the intestine and penetrates a surrounding organ; in the case of DUs, the surrounding organ is usually the pancreas. Patients with penetrating DUs may complain of pain that is constant and unchanging rather than the intermittent pain typical of uncomplicated DUs. Pain that radiates to the back may also indicate that a DU has penetrated another organ. Gastric outlet obstruction occurs in about 2–5% of patients with peptic ulcer disease.[5] Obstruction occurs when the pylorus of the stomach or the duodenum is blocked, preventing the passage of food. Unlike perforation and penetration, obstruction develops slowly over an extended period of time. It may be recognized by the insidious onset of gastroesophageal reflux, early satiety, weight loss, abdominal pain, and, most commonly, vomiting. Patients with any of these complications need immediate medical attention because acute surgical intervention may be required.

Diagnosis A complete patient history and physical examination are the first steps in diagnosing a DU. Epigastric pain is certainly suggestive of a DU, but it is not diagnostic. Patient symptoms may help localize the pain, but they cannot confirm that an ulcer is present, discriminate whether the ulcer is in the stomach or in the duodenum, or rule out other disorders such as gastric carcinoma or nonulcer dyspepsia. Abdominal X-rays (i.e., an upper GI series with barium swallow) ordinarily detect between 30 and 60% of DUs, depending on the technique used.[42] However, the diagnosis of DUs can only be confirmed by visualizing an actual ulcer crater through upper GI endoscopy.

Nonpharmacologic Treatment Special diets have been recommended for the management of peptic ulcer disease since the 1940s. These diets have typically consisted of bland foods given in multiple small feedings throughout the day. However, many studies since 1942 have found no benefit with such diets.[35] Although food relieves ulcer pain and buffers gastric acid for approximately 30–60 minutes, each meal results in an increased acid load for several hours.[32] Therefore, patients should be encouraged to eat three meals a day of their own choosing and should avoid eating snacks at night, which will increase nocturnal acid secretion. The restriction of spicy foods does not speed ulcer healing, but patients should avoid foods that cause dyspeptic symptoms. Coffee (both caffeinated and decaffeinated), caffeine-containing beverages, and alcohol are the only items that ulcer patients should eliminate from their diets. Additionally, ulcer patients should be encouraged to stop smoking because smoking delays ulcer healing and increases the rate of recurrence.

The frequent ingestion of milk has traditionally been recommended to buffer acid in patients with peptic ulcer disease. However, milk is a very poor buffering agent, and the calcium and protein in milk actually stimulate acid secretion.[47] Despite its historical popularity, the use of milk for ulcer disease is without scientific basis and should not be encouraged.

Pharmacologic Treatment The goals of therapy for DUs are to promote ulcer healing, relieve pain, prevent complications, and prevent recurrences. Since the introduction of cimetidine in 1977, H_2-antagonists have been the preferred pharmacologic agents to achieve these goals because of their efficacy, patient acceptance, and favorable side effects profile. All four currently available H_2-antagonists are more effective than placebo in healing DUs.[48] At equipotent doses administered twice daily or once at bedtime, H_2-antagonists can be expected to heal about 70–80% of DUs in 4 weeks and about 85–90% in 8 weeks.[5]

Because nocturnal acid secretion is unbuffered by food, much attention has been focused on single bedtime doses of the H_2-antagonists. When administered in this way, the maximum antisecretory activity of H_2-antagonists occurs in the early morning hours when nocturnal acid secretion is greatest. Many clinical trials have demonstrated equivalent, if not superior, healing rates for single bedtime regiments as compared to twice-daily regimens. Bedtime dosing is generally preferred over twice-daily regimens because of its ease of administration, improved patient compliance, and lower cost.

Other agents approved for the acute treatment of DUs include sucralfate and omeprazole, both of which heal DUs as effectively as H_2-antagonists.[48] It is quite common for DU patients to be treated with a combination of sucralfate and an H_2-antagonist. However, no controlled trial has shown a significant benefit in healing ulcers or for any indication with this combination over either agent alone.[30] Use of such combination therapy should be discouraged because it serves only to increase patient inconvenience and add to the already substantial cost of treating ulcer disease.

The benefit of eradicating *H. pylori* in healing DUs is unclear. Agents with bactericidal effects on the organism have generally shown good results in healing DUs. Triple antibiotic therapy with bismuth, metronidazole, and amoxicillin or tetracycline for 4 weeks appears to be as effective in healing DUs as H_2-antagonists.[49] However, the large doses used (five to eight tablets per day of BSS, 2 g per day of tetracycline, 750 mg per day of metronidazole) are inconvenient for patients and add their own assortment of side effects. The risks of such therapy include diarrhea, pseudomembranous colitis, and the development of antibiotic resistance. Additionally, none of these anti-infective regimens has been approved by the FDA. For these reasons, triple therapy with antibiotics and bismuth should not routinely be added to accelerate DU healing.[50]

Antacids were the mainstay of treatment for peptic ulcer disease until the late 1970s, when H_2-antagonists became available. It was not until 1977, however, that antacids were actually proven effective in healing DUs.[51] A liquid aluminum–magnesium antacid was given to patients seven times a day (1 and 3 hours after each meal and at bedtime). The rationale for this intensive dosing regimen was the assumption that it was necessary to keep the gastric pH continuously elevated throughout the day. Several studies have found such high-dose antacid regimens (560–1,008 mEq neutralizing capacity per day) to be comparable to H_2-antagonists in healing DUs.[16]

Recent interest in the mucosal protective effects of antacids has prompted studies to determine whether lower doses of antacids could heal DUs. Several studies have found that doses as low as 120–200 mEq per day of buffering capacity produce healing rates equivalent to those found in studies using the higher traditional doses.[52] Other studies have demonstrated medium (414 mEq per day) or lower doses of antacids to be comparable to H_2-antagonists.[15,53] Frequency of dosing in these studies, however, has remained six to seven times a day—still an inconvenient schedule for patients. Several studies have shown that neither this frequency of administration nor high doses of antacid are necessary to promote healing.[54,55] In most of these studies, antacid tablets (120 mEq per day) given four times daily (1 hour after meals and at bedtime) healed DUs more effectively than placebo and as effectively as cimetidine.

Whether antacids or any antiulcer agents relieve ulcer pain better than placebo is difficult to determine from clinical trials. A significant problem in interpreting results of these trials is the large placebo response (up to 50%) observed in patients.[5] Accordingly, some DU patients report significant pain relief from antacids while others do not. However, the results of these trials should not discourage the use of antacids for relief of ulcer pain. Even if the pain relief is a placebo response, it is one of the treatment goals, and any regimen that achieves that goal should be encouraged.

An important consideration is the poor correlation between pain relief and ulcer healing. Most DU patients will have significant pain relief within 7–14 days of starting treatment, but ulcer healing cannot be expected for 4–6 weeks.[56] Patients should be encouraged to continue their antiulcer regimens for the full treatment duration even when their symptoms have resolved. Conversely, lack of pain relief with an agent does not mean that a DU is not healing properly. Patients taking antacids or other medications whose pain has not yet resolved should not discontinue their medication because they feel their ulcer is not healing.

Despite an equal ability to heal DUs, antacids are not generally favored as first-line therapy over the H_2-antagonists and sucralfate. Because more data are needed to support using low doses of antacids, the standard dose for healing DUs remains 80–160 mEq of neutralizing capacity taken 1 and 3 hours after meals and at bedtime. Antacids are not given until 1 hour after meals because food buffers gastric acid for about an hour. When given 1 and 3 hours after meals, antacids will neutralize acid for approximately 2 hours. In this way, the gastric pH is continuously elevated throughout the day. However, achieving this goal requires taking 1 to 2 tbsp of a liquid that is often unpalatable seven times a day. Taking a single tablet (e.g., H_2-antagonist) at bedtime is a more acceptable and convenient regimen. Although high-potency liquid antacids can be taken in smaller volumes than low-potency liquids or antacid tablets, they should also be taken seven times a day. The cost to the patient for these intensive antacid regimens is often comparable to that of H_2-antagonists or sucralfate. Additionally, high doses of antacids often cause changes in bowel habits (e.g., diarrhea). If additional studies substantiate the effectiveness of low-dose antacids, these regimens may prove more acceptable to patients. Low-dose antacids would also offer the most cost-effective alternative for healing DUs. If low doses become the new standard for antacid use in treating DUs, antacids may be reconsidered as primary therapy for ulcer disease.

However, the current role of antacids in treating DUs is to provide additional pain relief for patients already taking H_2-antagonists or other antiulcer agents. When antacids are used for supplemental pain relief, patients should be advised to take doses providing 40–80 mEq neutralizing capacity. These doses may be taken on an as-needed basis and may be titrated upward if needed. Because antacids can reduce the bioavailability of H_2-antagonists, doses should be separated by at least 2 hours.[29] Most patients will need supplemental antacids for pain relief only for the first 7–14 days of treatment.

Maintenance Treatment Currently, only H_2-antagonists and sucralfate are approved for maintenance therapy of DUs to prevent recurrences. The maintenance dose of H_2-antagonists is one-half the approved treatment dose, usually given at bedtime. At these doses, all H_2-antagonists reduce DU recurrence rates to 20–50%, as compared with 50–90% for patients on placebo.[5] Sucralfate in doses of 1 g twice daily is as effective as H_2-antagonists in reducing recurrence.[30]

Although these doses have been approved and recommended for use for 12 months, the duration of maintenance therapy of DUs is not certain. A high relapse rate is usually observed after drug therapy is withdrawn. It may be reasonable to discontinue maintenance therapy and reassess ulcer recurrence after 1 to 2 years in most patients.[5] Some data suggest that ulcer disease may "burn out" over 10–15 years in many patients, but other patients at high risk of recurrence and complications may need prophylactic treatment indefinitely. There are no definite criteria for who should receive maintenance therapy. In general, however, consideration should be given to patients who experience frequent ulcer recurrence (two to three attacks in 1 year), those who have had previous complications, and those who are poor surgical risks.[56]

Several studies have demonstrated that eradication of *H. pylori* by bismuth or antibiotic therapy results in dramatically lower rates of DU recurrence than is observed in patients who remain *H. pylori*-positive.[50,57] Although eradication of *H. pylori* to reduce DU recurrence is still considered an active research issue, a reasonable argument can be made for using antibiotics to eradicate this organism in patients with chronic ulcer disease severe enough to warrant continuous maintenance treatment or surgery.[58]

Antacid doses given twice daily (160 mEq per day) have been proven as effective as cimetidine 400 mg at bedtime in preventing DU recurrence.[59] In this study, three aluminum–magnesium antacid tablets were given in the morning and at bedtime. Low-dose antacid (three tablets, or 81 mEq at bedtime) in this trial was less effective than the higher dose (160 mEq per day). Another study found low-dose aluminum–magnesium antacid tablets (80 mEq) given 1 hour after meals to be as effective as cimetidine and sucralfate in preventing DU relapse.[60] However, antacids caused the highest incidence of side effects. Despite its lower cost, antacid therapy for DU maintenance requires that antacids be taken three to four times daily as compared with a single dose of an H_2-antagonist or two doses of sucralfate. Thus, antacids are not typically first-line agents for maintenance therapy because of patient acceptance, compliance problems, and side effects.

Gastric Ulcer

Like DUs, GUs are considered a chronic disease that has serious health and economic consequences for society. Although less common than DUs, GUs affect approximately 3 million Americans and account for more than 100,000 hospitalizations each year.[42] They are associated with higher morbidity and mortality rates than DUs, probably because GUs tend to occur in older persons, typically those between the ages of 55 and 65.[47] Patients with GUs also appear to have more concomitant diseases than patients with DUs, again likely because of the difference in age distribution. Another particular concern is the risk of gastric cancer in patients with an apparently benign GU. The recurrence rate for GUs is lower than that observed for DUs but is still substantial; 40–60% of patients will relapse in the first 1 to 2 years after initial healing.[5]

Pathogenesis Like DUs, GUs represent a heterogeneous disease whose pathology is not well understood. The acid-secretory response in patients with a GU varies with the location of the ulcer.[45,47] In contrast to most DU patients who are hypersecretors of acid, patients with GUs in the body of the stomach secrete normal or less than normal amounts of gastric acid. The mechanism by which ulcers develop in the presence of minimal acid is not clear, but the ulcers are probably due to an impairment of the gastric mucosal barrier.[5] GUs located in the antral or prepyloric areas of the stomach resemble DUs and are associated with excess acid production. GUs and DUs are often found together. GUs found in conjunction with DUs are usually associated with excess acid secretion.[45]

Most GUs occur in the antrum of the stomach and are surrounded by a widespread area of chronic gastritis.[47] The gastritis occurs before the ulcer develops and usually persists after the ulcer has healed. Because *H. pylori* can produce chronic gastritis, the organism may play a role in the development of GUs. Indeed, 70–90% of patients with GUs have *H. pylori* gastritis.[4,6] However, because not all patients with GUs have *H. pylori*-associated gastritis, factors unrelated to the organism must be involved in the development of some cases of GUs.

These other factors are most likely agents that disrupt the gastric mucosal barrier. In the case of GUs, NSAIDs are the most likely offenders. Chronic ulcers due to NSAIDs occur most commonly in the stomach, causing at least a 4:1 predominance of GUs over DUs.[61] NSAID-induced GUs are not surrounded by areas of antral gastritis and are not consistently linked to *H. pylori* infection.[62] Accordingly, it has been suggested that NSAIDs account for the 10–30% of GU patients who do not have associated *H. pylori* gastritis.[62] Other environmental factors such as smoking increase the risk of GUs. A genetic influence is supported by the two- to threefold risk of first-degree relatives of patients with GUs to develop the disease.[44]

Clinical Presentation Epigastric pain is the most common symptom in patients with GUs. However, GU pain may differ from DU pain in that GU pain is much less typical and does not occur in a predictable or rhythmic pattern. As with DUs, the pain is described as a vague, nagging, cramping, or dull ache. However, it is not well localized but rather covers a wide area of the midepigastrium. Some patients with GUs will experience pain relief from food, but pain recurs only a short time after eating.[42] In other patients, food may precipitate or accentuate the pain, and antacids appear to provide less consistent relief.[42] Such patients will associate pain with eating and may even stop eating. Nausea and vomiting, a sense of fullness, and abdominal distention are fairly common with GUs. For these reasons, weight loss is common in patients with GUs (benign and malignant) and may be profound (up to 30–50 pounds).

Complications The complications of GUs are generally the same as with DUs. One important distinction, however, is that patients with GUs who suffer a complication have a higher mortality rate than DU patients. This may be because GUs affect primarily elderly patients who are not as able to survive ulcer complications. The most common complication of GUs is bleeding, but perforation, penetration, and obstruction can also occur. GUs most commonly penetrate into the left lobe of the liver and rarely into the colon.[5] Obstruction due to GUs is uncommon.

Diagnosis Because 5–10% of patients with seemingly benign GUs actually have gastric cancer, an accurate and timely diagnosis is essential.[32] Whether a GU is benign or malignant cannot be distinguished on the basis of patient symptoms. Diagnosis also may be confused by the fact that a malignant GU tends to respond symptomatically to H_2-antagonists. Thus, all patients with suspected GUs should undergo endoscopy, not only to diagnose GUs but also to rule out gastric cancer.[45]

Nonpharmacologic Treatment Dietary restrictions do not accelerate the healing of GUs, nor do they prevent recurrences.[47] Special ulcer diets have no role in GU therapy. Recommendations for GU patients are to eat three nutritious meals a day; avoid coffee, caffeinated beverages, and alcohol; and stop smoking.

Pharmacologic Treatment Despite pathophysiologic differences, treatment strategies for GUs and DUs are very similar. The primary difference is that GUs, regardless of the treatment used, heal more slowly than DUs and need more sustained treatment (about 2–4 weeks longer). Larger GUs (diameter greater than 2.5 cm) may take up to 15 weeks to heal.[47] GUs that do not heal after 12 weeks of treatment should raise the suspicion of a malignancy.

The H_2-antagonists (cimetidine, ranitidine, famotidine and nizatidine) are approved for the treatment of GUs. These agents produce healing rates of 80–90% after 8–12 weeks of therapy.[63] Single bedtime dosing of H_2-antagonists for GU has not been approved for all four agents because healing rates with GUs seem to be more dependent on 24-hour acid suppression than on nocturnal acid suppression.[5]

Although many GUs are associated with abnormal gastric mucosa rather than with excess acid secretion, the value of strengthening mucosal defenses with cytoprotective agents (e.g., CBS, sucralfate, or misoprostol) in GUs has not been well studied. Consequently, the use of sucralfate or the eradication of *H. pylori* with bismuth or antibiotic therapy to heal GUs cannot currently be routinely recommended.

The ability of antacids to heal GUs is less substantiated than their ability to heal DUs. Moderately large doses of liquid antacids (320–560 mEq per day, dosed seven times daily) appear to be as effective as cimetidine in healing GUs, with healing rates approaching 90% after 12 weeks of therapy.[64] Doses as low as 120 mEq per day (taken as tablets four times daily) have healed GUs better than placebo.[65] All of these doses provided pain relief for patients with GUs. However, lower doses of antacids have not been directly compared with high-dose antacids or H_2-antagonists. In the absence of such comparisons, the current standard for dosing antacids in GUs remains 40–80 mEq of neutralizing capacity given 1 and 3 hours after meals and at bedtime. This dose is lower than the recommended dose for DUs because GUs are less dependent on acid secretion. Even at these doses, however, frequency of dosing and side effects may significantly interfere with a patient's lifestyle.

As long as higher antacid doses are recommended for GUs, the role of antacids will most likely remain confined to use on an as-needed basis for pain relief in patients receiving other agents for ulcer healing. As with DUs, antacid doses in this setting should provide 40–80 mEq neutralizing capacity and can be titrated upward if needed.

Maintenance Therapy No pharmacologic agent currently has approval for maintenance therapy of GUs. H_2-antagonists reduce 1-year GU recurrence rates to 6–36%.[5] Both bedtime and twice-daily doses appear to be effective. Sucralfate has not consistently reduced GU recurrence more than placebo.[30] Eradication of *H. pylori* with triple antibiotic therapy plus ranitidine has been shown to reduce the probability of GU recurrence significantly compared with recurrence in patients receiving ranitidine alone.[57]

The ability of antacids to reduce GU recurrence has not been adequately studied. Therefore, antacids currently have no role in maintenance or prophylactic therapy of GUs. Furthermore, it is unlikely that they will have a role in preventing GU recurrence for reasons already discussed: poor patient acceptance, frequent side effects, and lack of proven safety in long-term use.

Gastroesophageal Reflux

The reflux of gastric contents into the esophagus, or gastroesophageal reflux, is generally a benign physiologic process that occurs in normal individuals. In fact, virtually everyone experiences multiple episodes of gastroesophageal reflux throughout the day, particularly after meals. Most of these episodes are unnoticed and do not cause symptoms or mucosal damage to the esophagus. However, gastroesophageal reflux does produce symptoms in some individuals and may cause tissue damage to the esophagus, oropharynx, larynx, and respiratory system.[66] Patients who suffer symptoms or tissue damage as a result of gastroesophageal reflux are said to suffer from GERD. What distinguishes patients with GERD from those with normal physiologic reflux is the frequency and duration of reflux episodes.[67]

The most common form of GERD is reflux esophagitis, which develops when there is prolonged contact of the acidic contents of the stomach with esophageal tissue. This contact may produce a broad range of damage, such as inflammation, hyperplasia, esophageal erosions, or ulcerations.[68] The typical complaint of patients with reflux esophagitis is heartburn, which is probably one of the most common symptoms a pharmacist is asked to treat. The incidence of heartburn is high in the American population; 7% of adult Americans experience it daily and 45% experience it at least once a month.[68] Pregnant women are affected most commonly, with about 25% complaining of heartburn daily. However, patients with heartburn do not necessarily have reflux esophagitis, given that 60–70% of patients complaining of heartburn do not have mucosal injury to the esophagus.[68]

Most individuals with GERD have only mild and sporadic symptoms. Accordingly, most patients do not seek medical attention from a physician but rather seek symptomatic relief from antacid products.[36] In fact, approximately 18 million Americans who have heartburn take antacids on a regular basis. The primary reason for antacid use is relief of heartburn. Thus, it appears that the health care professional most involved with the majority of reflux sufferers is the community pharmacist, who routinely provides antacids. Considering the impact pharmacists may have on this disease, an understanding of the pathogenesis, clinical presentation, and treatment of GERD is essential if pharmacists are to manage and triage such patients effectively.

Pathogenesis

Like that of peptic ulcer disease, the pathogenesis of GERD can be described as an imbalance between aggressive and protective factors. The aggressive side of this balance is determined by the noxious quality of the gastric contents that reflux into the esophagus. Most patients with GERD secrete normal or greater than normal amounts of gastric acid; therefore, most patients have acidic refluxates. The degree of damage to the esophagus appears to be both concentration- and time-dependent—that is, the lower the pH of the refluxate and the longer the refluxate is in contact with the mucosa, the greater the degree of mucosal damage.

Despite the potential for gastric contents to injure the esophageal mucosa, most individuals who have physiologic reflux do not develop GERD. This is because several defense mechanisms normally protect the esophagus from noxious gastric contents. For the refluxed material from the stomach to injure the esophagus, it must enter the esophagus, stay in prolonged contact with the epithelium, and then damage the mucosa. Thus, there are three lines of defense that must be impaired for GERD to develop: (1) antireflux barriers that limit the rate of reflux, (2) clearance mechanisms that limit the duration of contact of refluxate with the epithelium, and (3) esophageal mucosal resistance that minimizes epithelial damage from noxious gastric contents.[66]

The presence of competent antireflux barriers is critical in preventing GERD. Because resting pressure is higher in the stomach than it is in the esophagus, gastric contents would follow the path of least resistance and continually reflux into the esophagus if there were no barriers to prevent it. Although a number of such barriers have been identified, the major barrier to reflux is the lower esophageal sphincter (LES). The LES is an area of specialized smooth muscle located at the lower end of the esophagus, about 2–5 cm above the junction where the stomach meets the esophagus. When at rest, the LES is contracted, creating a high-pressure zone that prevents the passage of stomach contents into the esophagus. When swallowing occurs, the LES relaxes and allows food to pass freely into the stomach from the esophagus.

Because everyone experiences reflux, the LES is an imperfect barrier. Normal individuals experience transient relaxations of the LES multiple times throughout the day. Patients with GERD, however, tend to have more transient relaxations of the LES, and thus reflux more often than healthy individuals. Many patients with GERD also have a weak, or hypotonic, LES.[69] In such patients, the high pressure in the stomach creates enough force to overcome the weak squeeze of the LES and allows reflux to occur. A common misconception is that hiatal hernia causes the decrease in LES tone that is responsible for GERD. Although hiatal hernia may contribute to lowering LES pressure by loss of diaphragmatic and other external support, not all patients with GERD have a hiatal hernia, or vice versa.[68]

After reflux occurs because of an incompetent LES, the resultant symptoms and degree of damage depend on the duration of contact between the gastric contents and the esophageal mucosa. The esophagus normally clears the refluxate by one to two peristaltic contractions induced by swallowing. Gravity speeds up this process when the patient is upright, but it does not operate when the patient is lying down.[66] The residual acid refluxate in the esophagus is then neutralized by bicarbonate-rich saliva that has been swallowed. A defect in one or both of these processes may lead to increased contact time with refluxed material and the development of esophagitis. All these mechanisms are impaired during sleep, when there is neither swallowing nor salivation and when clearance by gravity is not operative. Thus, prolonged acid exposure may occur during sleep and predispose patients to esophagitis.[66,70]

A third protective mechanism is provided by the cells of the esophagus. Although the esophagus does not have a well-defined mucosal barrier like the stomach and duodenum, its cells are structurally designed to limit penetration of hydrogen ions into the epithelium.[66] Currently, the contribution of cellular defense mechanisms to GERD is uncertain, but a further understanding of this line of defense may have significant impact on prevention and treatment of this disease.

A number of factors disrupt the balance between aggressive factors and esophageal defense mechanisms and may potentiate GERD. Most of these factors promote reflux by impairing defensive mechanisms, particularly by reducing LES tone. Foods that decrease LES tone include chocolate, mints (spearmint or peppermint), and foods rich in fat.[36] Other foods may precipitate symptomatic reflux either by directly irritating the esophageal mucosa (citrus juices, tomato products, and coffee) or by increasing gastric acid secretion (colas, beer, and milk).[36] Caffeine, alcohol, and smoking reduce LES tone and increase frequency of reflux episodes.[36] Numerous medications decrease LES pressure, including alpha-adrenergic agonists, prostaglandins E_1 and E_2, anticholinergic agents, dopamine, meperidine, morphine, diazepam, nitrates, and calcium channel blockers. Of the calcium channel blockers, nifedipine causes the most marked reduction in LES tone.[36] Theophylline and $beta_2$ agonists also reduce LES tone, but use of inhaled $beta_2$-agonist preparations may minimize this effect.[36] Estrogens and progesterone lower LES tone, which explains the higher incidence of reflux in pregnant women and in women using oral contraceptives. Reflux also tends to worsen throughout pregnancy as intragastric pressure increases as a result of an enlarging uterus. Other factors that promote reflux by disturbing the gastroesophageal pressure gradient include supine body position, obesity, and tight-fitting clothing around the abdomen.[36]

Clinical Presentation

The classic symptom of GERD is heartburn, or pyrosis, occurring in more than half of patients with this disorder.[71] Heartburn is usually described by the patient as a burning sensation or pain located in the lower chest (substernal area). The pain may radiate up into the chest, to the back, and, less often, into the throat.[67,71] Most patients complain of heartburn soon after meals and upon lying down at bedtime, and they may be awakened from sleep because of the pain. Heartburn may also occur when the patient bends or stoops over and after some forms of exercise. Some patients have brief episodes of heartburn that are readily relieved by antacids or simple dietary measures; others have persistent and severe symptoms that disrupt their daily lives. Regardless of how the pain presents, the severity of the symptoms of GERD does not correlate well with the severity of esophageal mucosal damage.

Some patients with GERD may complain of chest pain that is not typical of heartburn. Atypical chest pain due to reflux is difficult to distinguish from anginal chest pain due to coronary artery disease.[67] This atypical chest pain may be sharp or dull and may radiate widely, extending into the neck or arms. The relationship of the pain to exercise may aid in differentiating GERD from anginal pain. Although the presence of other typical reflux symptoms (e.g., dysphagia or regurgitation) may suggest esophageal chest pain, failure to identify patients with significant myocardial ischemia could result in a fatal outcome. Therefore, patients with angina-like chest pain should be referred for immediate medical attention and appropriate testing.

Other symptoms of reflux disease may occur with or without heartburn. Regurgitation is an extension of the reflux process, with gastric contents entering the mouth. Patients will complain of an acid, burning, or bitter taste and may refer to this problem as "sour stomach." Although some patients may confuse this symptom with vomiting, regurgitation does not cause nausea, retching, or abdominal contractions.[71] Additionally, GERD patients with delayed gastric emptying often complain of bloating, early satiety, belching, and nausea.

Another symptom of GERD is dysphagia, which is a sensation of slow or blocked passage of food from the mouth to the esophagus. Patients may describe dysphagic symptoms as food "hanging up," "slowing down," or "getting stuck." If the complaint is for only solid food, the suspicion of an esophageal stricture or cancer should be raised. If the problem is with both solid food and liquids, the patient most likely has a motor disorder of the esophagus. Although not common in GERD, odynophagia (pain on swallowing) may occur and usually suggests severe mucosal damage in the esophagus.[71] More commonly, odynophagia is associated with esophagitis due to infectious agents (e.g., *Candida*, herpes, or cytomegalovirus) or medication (e.g., tetracycline, quinine, or potassium chloride) rather than to GERD. Symptoms of GERD that affect the throat include water brash (hypersalivation), globus (sensation of a lump in the throat), and hoarseness.[71] Any patient complaining of dysphagic symptoms should be referred to a physician for evaluation.

Complications

Complications of GERD most often affect the esophagus but may affect other sites both inside and outside of the GI tract. Approximately 8–20% of patients with long-standing GERD develop a complication known as Barrett's esophagus.[72] Barrett's esophagus is associated with midesophageal strictures, esophageal ulcers, and histologic changes in the lower esophageal mucosa that may become cancerous in up to 10% of patients.[72] Acute and chronic bleeding has occurred in association with GERD as a result of an esophageal ulcer. Acute bleeding from esophageal ulcers is uncommon but has been reported to account for 6 to 7% of massive upper GI bleeding episodes.[72] Acute bleeding from esophageal ulcers is more common in patients with Barrett's esophagus, in those using NSAIDs, and in neurologically impaired patients. Patients with GERD may suffer chronic GI bleeding from esophageal ulceration and may exhibit signs of iron deficiency anemia or blood in the stools. Approximately 10% of patients who seek medical attention for GERD develop an esophageal stricture (narrowing of the esophageal lumen), which impedes passage of food from the mouth to the stomach.[72]

Pulmonary complications are being noted with increasing frequency in patients with GERD.[72] Patients with severe GERD may aspirate refluxed material into the upper airways and lungs. Such patients may develop chronic nighttime cough, chronic bronchitis, pulmonary fibrosis, or recurrent pneumonia.[72] Typical asthma symptoms of wheezing and bronchoconstriction may also be induced by pulmonary aspiration of refluxed contents. Characteristics that may help distinguish GERD-induced asthma from typical asthma include nocturnal symptoms, adult onset, negative history of allergies, and heartburn experienced immediately before wheezing. Additionally, patients with GERD-induced asthma may have worsening symptoms when treated with theophylline and beta$_2$ agonists, which reduce LES pressure.[72]

Diagnosis

The diagnosis of GERD can often be made on the basis of patient history alone.[68] Patients who describe typical symptoms of heartburn or regurgitation may not require any diagnostic studies if they improve with empiric antireflux therapy (e.g., antacids or simple dietary and other measures).[36,37,68] Patients whose symptoms do not improve with these measures, however, need diagnostic tests to determine whether esophagitis is present and whether complications have developed. Patients who complain of dysphagic symptoms or weight loss or who have signs of anemia should also be referred for further evaluation. As stated previously, patients who present with atypical chest pain should be referred immediately for diagnostic tests to rule out cardiac disease. This is especially important in patients who are older than 40 years and have risk factors for ischemic heart disease (e.g., obesity, family history of heart disease, smoking, or hyperlipidemia). The diagnostic procedures most commonly used for reflux disease are barium esophagography, which provides X-ray visualization of the esophagus; endoscopy, which allows direct visualization of the esophagus; and 24-hour pH monitoring, which provides the most sensitive indication of reflux.[68]

Nonpharmacologic Treatment

Whereas dietary and lifestyle modifications have little proven benefit in treating peptic ulcer disease, conservative nondrug

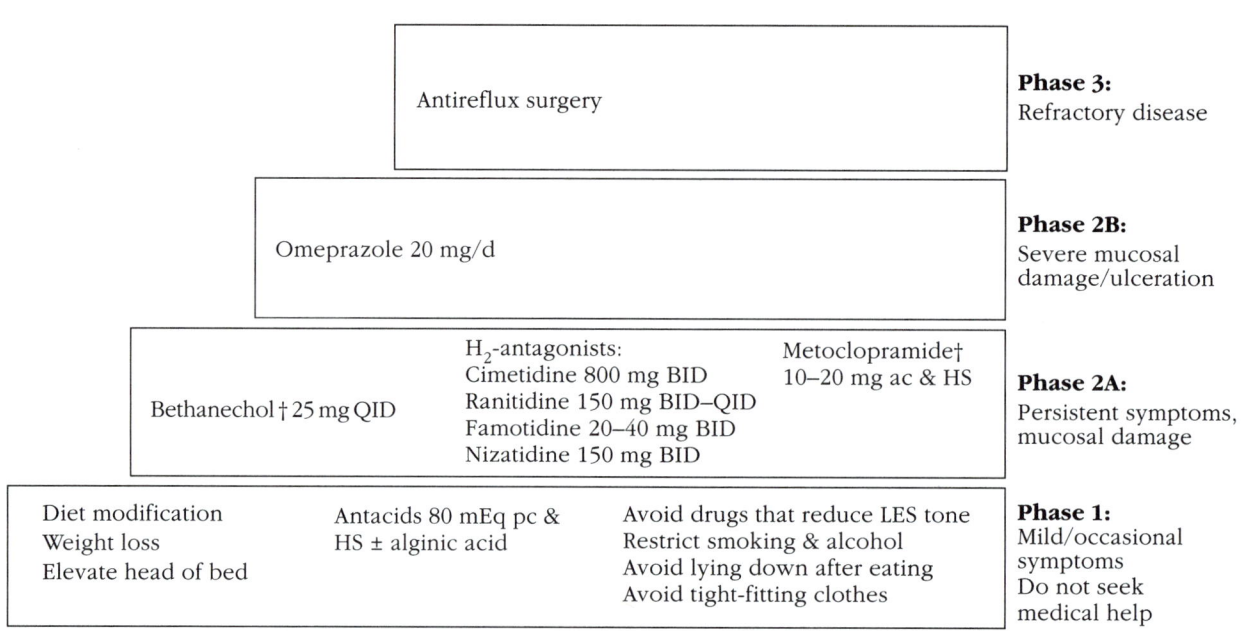

FIGURE 2 Stepped-care approach to managing gastroesophageal reflux disease.

measures are considered a cornerstone of therapy for GERD. Many patients with mild GERD can be managed with such measures alone and without pharmacologic intervention.[36] These measures attempt to reduce or eliminate factors that promote reflux. Because esophageal defenses are impaired during sleep, special effort should be made to reduce nocturnal reflux. Patients should be instructed to elevate the head of the bed 6 in. to improve esophageal clearance and reduce the duration of reflux. This should be done by raising the head of the bed with blocks or by placing a foam wedge under the patient's head. Patients should not try to do this by sleeping on pillows because this will cause them to bend at the waist and will actually increase intragastric pressure. Eating the evening meal at least 3 hours before going to bed to allow adequate time for gastric emptying also reduces reflux during sleep. Dietary suggestions for GERD are to (1) avoid foods that reduce LES tone (e.g., chocolate, mints, and fats); (2) avoid foods that are direct irritants (e.g., citrus juice, tomato products, and coffee); (3) reduce the size of meals; and (4) avoid lying down after meals. Patients with GERD should be encouraged to stop smoking and limit their alcohol intake. Obese patients with GERD may have symptomatic improvement if they lose weight and avoid wearing tight-fitting clothing. It may be helpful to advise patients to avoid aerophagic habits, such as chewing gum, sucking on hard candy, or drinking carbonated beverages. Finally, patients with GERD should be questioned about the use of drugs that decrease LES pressure. When a drug is implicated in causing reflux, switching to a drug with similar therapeutic benefit but without an effect on the LES should be considered.

Pharmacologic Treatment

Role of Antacids   The management of GERD may be viewed as a stepped-care approach, with antacids and nondrug measures forming the basis for the first step (Figure 2). Antacids have long been the pharmacologic mainstay of therapy for GERD. They work to reduce the aggressive factors in GERD by neutralizing gastric acid and increasing the pH of refluxed gastric contents. As a result, the refluxed contents are not as damaging to the esophageal mucosa. Antacids also strengthen defensive forces because gastric alkalinization increases LES pressure.

Conflicting results have been reported regarding the benefit of antacids in GERD. Controlled studies have found antacids to be better than placebo at relieving symptoms of GERD, but other studies suggest that antacids do not offer significant symptomatic relief. Their ability to heal esophageal mucosal damage is even less substantiated, given that healing rates may be as low as 13–36%.[36] Similarly, studies comparing antacids to H_2-antagonists in patients with GERD have provided inconsistent results. Cimetidine (300 mg four times daily) provided superior symptom relief when compared with antacids, while antacids have been reported to be as effective as ranitidine (150 mg twice daily) in reducing symptoms. Despite these conflicting results, many patients subjectively report relief of reflux symptoms with antacids and continue to use these products regularly for GERD.

Doses of antacids used typically range from 80 to 160 mEq of liquid aluminum–magnesium antacids given immediately after meals, 3 hours after meals, and at bedtime. Lower doses of antacid tablets (14 mEq per tablet) given on an as-needed basis (two to six times daily) have been reported to provide symptomatic relief for patients with GERD. The ability of low-dose antacids to heal damaged esophageal mucosa has not been assessed.

The addition of alginic acid to antacids appears to be effective in relieving GERD symptoms. Studies suggest that this combination is superior to antacid alone.[73,74] Alginic acid works by reacting with sodium bicarbonate and saliva to form a viscous solution of sodium alginate. This viscous solution floats on the surface of gastric contents so that, when reflux occurs, sodium alginate rather than acid is refluxed and irritation is minimized. When using antacid–alginic acid combination tablets, patients should understand that the tablets must be chewed to be effective and should be instructed to drink a glass of water after taking the tablets so that the viscous foam (sodium alginate) can float on it in the stomach. In addition, patients should be aware that the formulation only works when they are in the upright position and therefore must not be taken at bedtime or just before they lie down.[75]

Because antacids, whether alone or in combination with alginic acid, do not convincingly heal esophagitis, their use is best suited for patients with mild or occasional symptoms of GERD.[68] Given that most patients with GERD have only mild symptoms and do not seek medical care, antacids continue to be first-line treatment for this disease. As with other drug therapies, use of antacids should be combined with dietary and lifestyle modifications that limit reflux. In the absence of data that support lower doses, patients seeking symptomatic relief from antacids should be instructed to take doses of 80 mEq immediately and 3 hours after meals and at bedtime. Because reflux symptoms are worse after meals, GERD patients should be instructed to take antacids soon after eating rather than waiting 1 hour like ulcer patients.

Other Therapies Patients who fail to respond to conservative treatment with antacids and lifestyle modifications warrant further evaluation and treatment with other pharmacologic agents. H_2-antagonists form the basis for the second phase of therapy for GERD. By decreasing gastric acid secretion, H_2-antagonists reduce the damaging potential of the refluxed gastric contents. Overall, H_2-antagonists produce symptomatic relief in 50–75% of GERD patients within 2 to 3 weeks, as compared with 20–30% of patients treated with placebo.[76] The ability of H_2-antagonists to heal esophageal mucosa is variable, with about 60% of patients showing endoscopic improvement after 8–12 weeks.[76] Damaged mucosa in the esophagus is generally more difficult to heal than that in the duodenum; therefore, higher doses of H_2-antagonists for longer durations are necessary. All currently available H_2-antagonists are approved for symptomatic treatment of GERD. Unlike in peptic ulcer disease, bedtime dosing of these agents does not appear to be effective, and at least twice-daily dosing of these agents is necessary because reflux occurs throughout the day and night.[76]

Although most patients with mild to moderate GERD have an excellent clinical response from H_2-antagonists, patients with severe erosive and ulcerative esophagitis, including Barrett's esophagus, are unlikely to heal in 6–12 weeks with standard doses of H_2-antagonists.[67] Such patients usually require either higher doses of H_2-antagonists for longer periods of time or treatment with omeprazole. More than 90% of patients with severe GERD are healed after 8–12 weeks of omeprazole therapy;[76] the remaining 10% who do not respond to omeprazole are potential candidates for antireflux surgery to restore LES competence. Although antireflux surgery has 85–90% short-term success, it does not always result in a permanent cure. Symptoms recur in about 10% of the cases, and 2–8% of patients have complications from surgery such as dysphagia and an inability to belch or vomit.[66] Thus, antireflux surgery should be considered a last resort.

Because of their ability to increase esophageal motility, bethanechol and metoclopramide have been used as single-agent therapy or in combination with antacids or H_2-antagonists for GERD. However, neither drug has been shown to be consistently beneficial, and both cause significant adverse effects.[76] Studies using sucralfate for GERD have produced mixed results, and use of this agent for GERD remains investigational.

Maintenance Therapy

Despite the success of treatment with H_2-antagonists or omeprazole in most patients with GERD, recurrences occur in about 30% of patients within 6 months after stopping either drug.[77] Long-term, full-dose H_2-antagonists (e.g., cimetidine 800 mg twice daily) are generally required to reduce recurrence; maintenance doses used for peptic ulcer disease (e.g., ranitidine 150 mg per day or cimetidine 400 mg per day) have not been shown to be effective for reflux maintenance.[76] Although omeprazole is probably effective in GERD prophylaxis, lack of established long-term safety and the potential for causing gastric carcinoid tumors limit its use to short-term treatment.

Gastritis

The term *gastritis* is often used too loosely to describe virtually any condition in the stomach. Of the various conditions usually described as gastritis, the one common feature is inflammation of the gastric mucosa. This inflammation can be acute or chronic; it can be focal or diffuse; it may or may not be accompanied by superficial erosions, ulcers, or hemorrhages; and it may or may not be associated with symptoms. Although many classification schemes exist, gastritis may be viewed most simply as either acute erosive gastritis or chronic nonerosive gastritis.[5,78] In both types, the mechanism for injury appears to be a break in the normal gastric mucosal barrier allowing back-diffusion of acid rather than an increase in aggressive factors.

Acute Erosive Gastritis

Acute erosive gastritis is a short-lived inflammatory process characterized by superficial erosions or ulcerations of the stomach. The erosions, which may vary in size and number and may affect any part of the stomach, are associated with varying degrees of inflammation and hemorrhage, and in severe cases may penetrate deep enough to become an acute GU.[78] In acute erosive gastritis, the erosions can be linked to a specific cause; however, there are no distinctive features of these lesions that clearly point to the cause.[78] The agents most often responsible for causing such erosions are alcohol, aspirin, and other NSAIDs. Gastric erosions develop within 24 hours of high-dose (2.5 g) aspirin therapy and have been reported within 6 hours of excessive alcohol ingestion.[78] The pathogenesis of damage caused by these "barrier breakers" was reviewed previously. Other conditions or agents that may cause acute erosive gastritis include uremia, infections (bacterial, viral, and parasitic), direct local trauma, X-ray irradiation, caustic substances, reflux of bile into the stomach, pronounced physiologic stress (i.e., stress ulcers), and a number of other drugs (e.g., colchicine, antineoplastics, and immunosuppressives).

Clinical Presentation/Complications Most patients with acute erosive gastritis are asymptomatic. A few patients complain of epigastric pain or discomfort, typically of a burning nature. Unlike DU pain, pain from acute erosive gastritis is only partially relieved by food. Patients may also experience anorexia, nausea, and vomiting. When present, these symptoms are often intermittent and do not correlate with the number and severity of erosions at any given time. Because most patients do not have symptoms, most cases of acute erosive gastritis remain undiagnosed unless there is bleeding or the patient undergoes endoscopy for some reason.[5]

The most common complication of acute erosive gastritis is upper GI bleeding, in which case the disease is called acute hemorrhagic gastritis. Patients may present with vague, ulcer-like abdominal pain, but more often they have no pain or symptoms to warn of an impending bleed. Most patients who bleed will have signs and symptoms of acute blood loss (hematemesis, melena, hypotension, or tachycardia). Less commonly, patients may have chronic bleeding, which may be detected by more subtle signs (black tarry stools, guaiac-positive stools, and symptoms of iron deficiency anemia). Acute erosive gastritis has been reported to account for up to 30% of all acute GI bleeding episodes.[79] Fortunately, the mortality rate is well below 5% in otherwise healthy persons when the cause of bleeding is aspirin or alcohol.

Treatment The most important step in managing acute erosive gastritis is to remove the offending agent or condition, after which the erosions usually heal within a few days. Patients suspected of having this disorder should be questioned about their use of NSAIDs, alcohol, and other likely causative agents. Hemorrhagic gastritis is the only form of acute gastritis that requires a particular therapeutic effort. When evidence of either acute or chronic bleeding is present, patients should be referred for medical evaluation and management. Bleeding from acute erosive gastritis is usually mild and self-limited, stopping spontaneously in 2–5 days after the cause is removed.[78,79]

Because acute erosive gastritis usually heals spontaneously, pharmacologic agents are rarely needed. Although controlled studies supporting the benefit of antacids or H_2-antagonists in relieving symptoms are not generally available, these agents are often offered to patients to provide symptomatic relief. Patients subjectively appear to obtain relief from antacids after a bout of heavy alcohol drinking or other conditions in which acute erosive gastritis is suspected. Thus, provided there is no evidence of bleeding, it is reasonable to recommend an antacid for such patients. In the absence of controlled trial data, it is logical to recommend standard doses for GUs (i.e., 40–80 mEq 1 and 3 hours after meals and at bedtime), given that neither condition is caused by excess acid.

Chronic Nonerosive Gastritis

Chronic nonerosive gastritis refers to the presence of gastric mucosal inflammation over an extended period of time without associated mucosal erosion or ulceration. Chronic nonerosive gastritis is classified into two types based on the anatomical location in the stomach. Type A gastritis is an autoimmune disease characterized by chronic inflammation of the acid-secreting mucosa of the fundus and body of the stomach.[80] Patients with Type A gastritis develop antibodies directed against parietal cells, leading to reduced acid secretion and eventually to achlorhydria. Because acid secretion is reduced in these patients, dyspeptic symptoms and benign peptic ulcers are uncommon.[4] Therefore, antacids and other antiulcer medications do not play a role in the management of this disorder.

Type B gastritis affects the mucus-secreting epithelial cells that line the antrum of the stomach.[78,80] The epithelial cells are usually abnormal, and there are fewer mucus-secreting glands. Acid secretion is either reduced or normal, whereas mucosal defenses are impaired.[81] Type B gastritis is the more common variety of chronic nonerosive gastritis. As with Type A gastritis, the incidence increases with age. In fact, so many elderly persons have Type B gastritis that many consider it to be a normal process of aging. Type B gastritis occurs in 20% of young adults and 60% of elderly people.[4]

Clinical Presentation/Complications Type B gastritis may be due to reflux of duodenal contents into the stomach (alkaline reflux gastritis), chronic infection with *H. pylori*, or other undefined causes.[80] The strong evidence supporting an association with this organism cannot be disputed: (1) 70–100% of patients with Type B gastritis are infected with *H. pylori*; (2) chronic gastritis has developed in healthy volunteers after ingestion of *H. pylori*; and (3) eradication of *H. pylori* with antibiotic or bismuth therapy often causes resolution of gastritis.[6,82] Accordingly, most experts now believe that *H. pylori* is the cause of Type B gastritis.[6]

Type B gastritis is more important because of the company it keeps (i.e., DUs and GUs) rather than because of the symptoms it produces. With the exception of NSAID-induced GUs, chronic benign GUs almost always occur within an area of chronic gastritis rather than in normal mucosa. *H. pylori*-associated gastritis is also present in more than 95% of patients with DUs.[6,82] Studies have concluded that *H. pylori* gastritis is associated with an increased risk of gastric cancer.[83,84] Despite these strong associations, whether *H. pylori* gastritis actually causes these diseases is not known.

Most patients with Type B gastritis do not have symptoms, but some patients may experience chronic dyspeptic symptoms. When symptoms do occur, they are likely to be epigastric pain, heartburn, anorexia, and vomiting.[85] The pain is not as periodic and predictable as it is with DUs, and it tends to occur after eating, especially after a large meal. Gastritis is slow in progression, may last for years or decades, and rarely heals spontaneously.

Treatment The discovery of *H. pylori* infection in most patients with Type B gastritis has renewed interest in the treatment of this disorder. Currently, there is no clear reason to treat asymptomatic patients with Type B gastritis, whether or not *H. pylori* infection is present.[58] In most settings, this is not a consideration because asymptomatic *H. pylori* gastritis is unnoticed unless the patient has a gastric biopsy for some reason. However, if *H. pylori* gastritis is proven to be the cause of peptic ulcer disease or gastric cancer, routine detection and elimination of the infection may become standard practice.[5]

No treatment has been found that consistently alleviates symptoms of Type B gastritis. Clearance and eradication of *H. pylori* with antibiotic therapy or bismuth compounds usually resolves the gastritis (if it is not associated with a GU).[86] However, eradication of *H. pylori* has not consistently alleviated dyspeptic symptoms in these patients. Although acid secretion is normal in patients with *H. pylori* gastritis, H_2-antagonists are widely used in medical practice for symptomatic relief of chronic gastritis.[87] In one study, sucralfate provided symptomatic relief equivalent to that provided by ranitidine but was better at improving gastritis.[87]

Currently, there is not enough information to support the use of antacids for treatment of chronic gastritis. One study has shown that aluminum–magnesium antacid tablets given four times daily (120 mEq per day) suppressed *H. pylori* infection.[14] However, the antacid did not heal the gastritis or provide symptomatic relief. Still, a recent survey indicated that antacids are the most frequently prescribed drugs for dyspeptic symptoms thought to be related to gastritis.[88] Considering the high placebo response in patients with GI illnesses (20–80%) and the fact that many patients subjectively report relief with antacids, it may be worthwhile to try antacids in patients with symptomatic gastritis. However, because low doses are not effective, higher and more frequent doses (80 mEq seven times daily) should be recommended if the patient can tolerate such a regimen.

NSAID-Induced Ulcer

NSAID-induced ulceration is by far the most common and significant form of drug-induced mucosal injury. *NSAID gastropathy* is a term proposed to represent the broad range of mucosal lesions caused by NSAIDs. These lesions may be as minimal as superficial petechiae or as serious as chronic ulcers that perforate or bleed.[89] NSAID gastropathy is becoming a more prevalent problem because use of NSAIDs has increased dramatically over the last several decades. It is estimated that 15 million Americans use NSAIDs chronically and that 20% of these chronic users will develop an ulcer.[89]

Unlike classic peptic ulcer disease, most NSAID-induced ulcers occur in the stomach, with only 10-25% occurring in the duodenum.[61] Elderly patients, particularly females, are most often affected by NSAID ulceration.[89] The risk of developing an NSAID-induced ulcer increases with the dose and duration of NSAID use or the use of more than one NSAID. Patients taking other ulcerogenic medications (e.g., corticosteroids, methotrexate, colchicine) or medications predisposing to bleeding (e.g., warfarin) with an NSAID are more likely to develop an ulcer.[89] Other risk factors for NSAID gastropathy include previous history of peptic ulcer or GI bleeding, multiple medical problems, smoking, and heavy alcohol intake.[89] Whether patients with NSAID-induced ulcers are more likely to harbor *H. pylori* is controversial, as studies have failed to find a consistent relationship between NSAID users and the presence of the organism.[62]

Pathogenesis

NSAIDs produce a dual insult to the gastric mucosa by (1) causing direct, topical damage and (2) inhibiting prostaglandin synthesis. Acid hypersecretion is not a significant factor in the development of NSAID-induced ulcers. The mechanisms of NSAID-induced damage have been described in detail previously.

Clinical Presentation

NSAIDs may cause a wide variety of complaints that are typical of other acid-peptic disorders, including epigastric pain, dyspepsia, nausea, vomiting, diarrhea, and constipation. However, there is very poor correlation between these symptoms and actual ulceration. More than half of the patients who develop an NSAID-induced ulcer are asymptomatic. In fact, 60–80% of such patients have a major hemorrhage or perforation as the first clinical sign that an ulcer is present.[90,91] Thus, the presence of dyspeptic symptoms is not a reliable indicator for patients at risk for developing an NSAID-induced ulcer or complications.

Complications

Fortunately, most patients with NSAID-induced gastropathy do not develop major complications. The risk of complications appears to correlate with the duration of NSAID exposure. Acute mucosal injury may develop within 1 to 2 weeks of NSAID therapy, but clinically significant ulcers usually do not develop until after 3–6 months of therapy.[5] It is estimated that 1% of patients taking NSAIDs regularly for 3–6 months develop a symptomatic ulcer, gross bleeding, or perforation.[92] This incidence increases to 2–4% when NSAIDs are taken for 1 year. The incidence of complications from an NSAID-induced ulcer, as well as the mortality, is highest in elderly patients.[89]

Prevention

Replacing the protective mechanisms lost owing to NSAID inhibition of prostaglandin appears to be the only effective pharmacologic strategy to prevent both gastric and duodenal NSAID-induced ulcers. Accordingly, the prostaglandin analogue misoprostol is the only agent currently approved for preventing NSAID-induced gastropathy. At the approved dose of 200 mcg four times daily, misoprostol significantly reduces the risk of GUs from NSAID use.[38] Although H_2-antagonists and sucralfate may prevent NSAID-induced duodenal injury, neither has been shown to prevent NSAID-induced gastric injury.[93]

A common misconception is that coadministering antacids with NSAIDs will prevent the development of NSAID-induced ulcers. However, antacids have not been found to prevent NSAID gastropathy. In fact, one study found that low-dose aluminum–magnesium tablets (104 mEq per day) actually increased the number of gastric erosions in patients receiving NSAIDs compared with those receiving placebo.[94] Although antacids may offer symptomatic benefit to patients experiencing side effects from NSAIDs, patients should not be led to believe that taking antacids with NSAIDs will prevent adverse reactions.

Treatment and the Role of Antacids

After an NSAID-induced ulcer has developed, use of the NSAID should be discontinued, if possible, and another agent (acetaminophen or nonacetylated salicylate) substituted for it. If NSAIDs are withdrawn, ulcers usually respond to standard therapies for classic peptic ulcers and heal rapidly.[93] However, optimum management of ulcers during continued NSAID therapy is less clear because no drugs have been approved specifically for this indication. H_2-antagonists heal most NSAID-induced gastric and duodenal ulcers within 8–12 weeks.[93] However, larger GUs often require either longer therapy with standard doses of H_2-antagonists or the more potent acid suppression of omeprazole.[93]

Antacids appear to be effective at healing both gastric and duodenal NSAID-induced ulcers within 12 weeks of therapy, whether or not NSAIDs are continued.[95] In one study, antacids healed 100% of NSAID-induced ulcers when NSAIDs were discontinued;[96] when NSAIDs were continued, the overall healing rate was 85%. Another study compared placebo plus antacids used as needed with H_2-antagonists and found similar healing rates between the two regimens.[97] Overall, antacids heal most small gastric and duodenal ulcers despite continued NSAID therapy, but healing larger GUs may require long periods of time or potent acid suppression (i.e., large doses of H_2-antagonists or omeprazole) to heal.[95] To date, only full doses of antacids have been shown to heal NSAID-induced ulcers effectively. As with ordinary peptic ulcers, use of H_2-antagonists or omeprazole offers a more acceptable regimen for patients than frequent use of large doses of antacids.

Because low-dose antacids have not been studied in healing NSAID-induced ulcers, the role of antacids is more practically aimed at alleviating GI symptoms from NSAID use. Up to 50% of NSAID users experience GI side effects from NSAIDs,[95] and antacids may provide relief for these side effects. Even though their role in this regard has not been well studied, antacids may best be suited to as-needed use in addition to H_2-antagonists for healing. Although only a small percentage of these patients actually have ulcers, relief of ulcer-like symptoms due to NSAIDs may be necessary for patients to tolerate therapy. However, considering the poor correlation between symptoms and NSAID damage, it is unclear whether suppressing these symptoms will benefit patients or mask signs of serious mucosal injury.[95] A reasonable approach is to recommend antacids for NSAID symptoms only to patients who are not at risk for developing an ulcer. Such patients include younger patients without underlying illnesses, nonsmokers, those not taking concurrent ulcerogenic medications, and those intending to use NSAIDs on a short-term basis. The dose for such patients may be initiated at 40–80 mEq and taken as needed. Patients who are at risk for an NSAID-induced ulcer and complain of ulcer-like symptoms, especially elderly patients, should be referred for medical evaluation rather than treated symptomatically with antacids.

Nonulcer Dyspepsia

Dyspepsia is a vague, misunderstood term that literally means "bad digestion." Clinicians and patients use this term to describe any abdominal discomfort, including epigastric pain, heartburn, nausea, bloating, belching, and indigestion. Patients are said to have nonulcer dyspepsia when they present with symptoms that prompt a clinician to believe an ulcer is present, but no ulcer is found on evaluation. Despite the lack of specific defining characteristics, it is believed that one-third of the population suffers from nonulcer dyspepsia. It is at least twice as common as peptic ulcer disease.[98] Nonulcer dyspepsia also produces a substantial economic impact on society in that it often accounts for the nonprescription use of antacids, the empiric treatment of peptic ulcer disease with H_2-antagonists, expensive diagnostic tests, and time lost from work.

Pathogenesis

Although it might be expected that acid plays a role in producing ulcer-like symptoms, most studies indicate that acid secretion is normal in patients with nonulcer dyspepsia.[98] Studies report that 8–82% of patients with nonulcer dyspepsia are colonized with *H. pylori*.[99] However, when the age of these patients is considered, it appears that most of those (50–70%) with nonulcer dyspepsia and *H. pylori* infection are older than 60 years. Because a similar percentage of healthy persons older than 60 years also are colonized with *H. pylori*, the presence of that organism in these studies may be a normal aging phenomenon rather than a major cause of nonulcer dyspepsia. Studies have not found a clear relationship between nonulcer dyspepsia and stress, emotions, personality, food, environmental factors (e.g., smoking, alcohol, or caffeine), genetic factors, or other diseases.[98] Until any of these factors is proven to be a pathogenetic feature, nonulcer dyspepsia remains a disease in search of a cause.

Clinical Presentation and Complications

The typical patient with nonulcer dyspepsia presents with a chronic history (longer than 3 months) of widespread abdominal symptoms, usually in relation to meals.[100] These symptoms are most often epigastric pain and nausea without vomiting, but they may include belching, indigestion, heartburn, bloating, and abdominal distention. Among patients who seek medical care, the condition is more common in women, and the onset of symptoms is usually before 40 years of age.[98] The pain of nonulcer dyspepsia differs from that of DUs in that it (1) is less cyclical, (2) is not as localized, (3) does not usually waken patients from sleep, (4) occurs during or immediately after meals, and (5) is less likely to be relieved by antacids.[100] Although they may complain of heartburn, patients with nonulcer dyspepsia do not experience regurgitation, dysphagia, or other typical symptoms of GERD. These patients do not typically lose weight, and they may look surprisingly healthy given the magnitude and duration of symptoms they describe. Symptoms from the lower GI tract (e.g., diarrhea or constipation) are not part of the syndrome of nonulcer dyspepsia because bowel habits generally remain unchanged.[100] Nonulcer dyspepsia is a chronic condition that may persist over many years and become very troublesome for patients. However, it is generally a benign disease that is not associated with complications. There is no evidence that it leads to peptic ulcer disease or any other disorder.

Treatment and the Role of Antacids

No treatment has been proven to be of benefit in relieving symptoms of nonulcer dyspepsia. Even though patients with this disease do not secrete excess acid, the pharmacologic agents most often used to treat it are antacids and H_2-antagonists. Several studies have found H_2-antagonists superior to placebo in relieving symptoms, while other studies have concluded that these agents are not beneficial.[101] Studies using bismuth or antibiotics to treat *H. pylori* in patients with nonulcer dyspepsia have failed to show consistent symptomatic relief despite clearance of the organism.[102,103]

Antacids have been used to treat dyspepsia since the first century AD, when crushed coral (calcium carbonate) was given to patients complaining of such symptoms. Despite the widespread use of antacids for dyspeptic symptoms, there is little objective proof of their benefit. Neither high doses of liquid aluminum–magnesium antacid (400 mEq per day, given 1 and 3 hours after meals and at bedtime) or low doses of aluminum–magnesium tablets (120 mEq per day, given 1 hour after meals and at bedtime) have proven superior to placebo in controlled trials.[14,104] Nevertheless, antacids subjectively appear to provide relief for some patients with nonulcer dyspepsia, even if they act as a placebo.[105] In patients with mild, intermittent symptoms of nonulcer dyspepsia, it is reasonable to recommend a trial of antacids before incurring the expense of medical care and prescription with H_2-antagonists. When antacids are recommended for nonulcer dyspepsia, the dose may be initiated at 40–80 mEq, given 1 hour after meals and at bedtime, and titrated upwards as needed. However, the patient's response to antacids should be evaluated after 1 to 2 weeks because lack of response or significant improvement may indicate the need for further diagnostic evaluation or therapy with H_2-antagonists.

Miscellaneous Uses of Antacids

Overindulgence/Hangover

The FDA has long recognized antacids as being safe and effective for the symptomatic relief of heartburn, sour stomach, or acid indigestion. However, patients often take antacids for a wide variety of GI complaints, many of which do not fit these indications. One of the most common reasons people take antacids is for relief of symptoms associated with overeating or excessive indulgence in alcohol. A previous review by the FDA concluded that antacids were safe for the relief of immediate postprandial upper abdominal discomfort, but no data supported their efficacy for this indication. More recently, the FDA has reviewed nonprescription oral products for the relief of symptoms associated with overindulgence in food and drink and has endorsed the use of antacids for such purposes.[106] Antacid products can now add to their indications of heartburn, sour stomach, and acid indigestion the statement "and upset stomach associated with these symptoms" or "associated with overindulgence in food and drink." Although the cause of GI discomfort associated with hangover is more likely to be acute erosive gastritis than excess gastric acid, the FDA panel believes that antacids protect the mucosa from gastric acid. The FDA has also approved antacid and acetaminophen combination products for the relief of symptoms associated with hangover or overindulgence in food and drink. Finally, it has reversed a previous recommendation and placed in Category II (not generally recognized as safe and effective) all combination products for hangover that contain both an antacid and caffeine.[106]

Phosphate-Binding Effects

The phosphate-binding effects of antacids are often used clinically to lower serum phosphate in patients with chronic renal failure. Aluminum hydroxide has been the standard phosphate binder for many years. When added to dietary phosphate restriction, aluminum hydroxide in doses of 1.9–4.8 g given three to four times daily significantly reduces serum phosphate concentrations in these patients. However, significant amounts of aluminum may be absorbed in patients with chronic renal failure, resulting in the serious complication of osteomalacia. Recognition of the risks of aluminum accumulation has prompted the use of other antacids, particularly calcium salts, for this indication. Many studies have shown calcium carbonate in doses of 8–12 g per day to be a safe and effective phosphate binder in 70–80% of patients receiving chronic dialysis.[107] Long-term use of calcium carbonate in this setting is limited by the development of hypercalcemia and GI intolerance (diarrhea and constipation). Calcium citrate has been used successfully on a short-term basis as a phosphate binder.[108] However, its long-term safety and efficacy for this indication have not been established.

Cholesterol-Lowering Effects

Recognition of the bile salt–binding properties of aluminum antacids has prompted investigation into the potential lipid-lowering potential of antacids. Because aluminum antacids bind bile acids as strongly as cholestyramine, it is possible that aluminum hydroxide acts like cholestyramine to lower cholesterol. Because bile salts are bound and enterohepatic circulation is interrupted, more cholesterol is converted in the liver to bile acid, and hepatic cholesterol is depleted. This prompts the liver to make more low-density lipoprotein (LDL) cholesterol receptors, thus clearing cholesterol faster and reducing serum cholesterol. A recent study showed that 4 months of treatment with an aluminum–magnesium antacid significantly reduced serum LDL cholesterol and, to a lesser extent, high-density lipoprotein (HDL) cholesterol in hypercholesterolemic patients. However, far more data are needed to establish antacids as a therapeutic modality in treating hyperlipidemia.[109]

Reconstitution of Didanosine

Another use for antacids has been realized with the recent FDA approval of the antiviral agent didanosine (Videx®). Didanosine, which is indicated for the treatment of adult and pediatric human immunodeficiency virus infection, is rapidly degraded at acidic pH. Therefore, all oral forms of the drug contain antacid to increase gastric pH and allow for maximal absorption.[10] The pediatric powder for oral solution does not contain an antacid and must be reconstituted by the pharmacist with a high-potency liquid antacid. The product labeling specifies that either Mylanta Double Strength Liquid® or Maalox TC Suspension® be mixed with the didanosine powder to reach the final dispensing concentration.[10]

Antacid Use in Special Populations

The Elderly

An appreciation for the special concerns of elderly patients with GI complaints is essential to the pharmacist for several reasons. First, antacid use is heaviest in this age group. The frequent purchase of antacids appears to begin around age 45 and increases with age so that 20–25% of people older than 65 years take antacids.[110,111] Frequent use of antacids by elderly patients is to be expected because many GI disorders occur more often in this age group. The elderly have an increased incidence of GUs, NSAID-induced ulcers, and Type B (*H. pylori*) gastritis. Although their incidence of GERD is not greater, elderly patients often take drugs that reduce lower esophageal sphincter tone and predispose them to this disorder. In addition, constipation is an extremely common complaint in the elderly. Magnesium-containing antacids are often used as a laxative in this population rather than as therapy for peptic disorders.

Not only are acid-peptic disorders more common in the elderly, but complications such as perforations and bleeding from peptic ulcers are more likely to occur in these patients. Furthermore, mortality rates are high in this population when complications occur: more than one-third of elderly patients with peptic ulcer complications die.[112] Mortality rates increase with multiple medical illnesses, delay in diagnosis and treatment, and use of NSAIDs. In fact, elderly NSAID users are four times more likely to die from peptic ulcers or GI bleeding than nonusers.[113]

Because of these risks, the pharmacist's ability to assess the need for medical intervention in an elderly patient with GI complaints is often important. However, this task can be difficult because symptoms of peptic ulcer disease in elderly patients are very different from those seen in younger patients and can even be quite misleading. Many elderly patients with GUs, and most patients with NSAID-induced ulcers, have no symptoms at all. The pharmacist should not expect the elderly patient with an ulcer to complain of classic burning epigastric pain; if symptoms are present, they are more likely to be vague abdominal discomfort, anorexia, and severe weight loss.[113] It is very common for a perforation or bleeding to be the first sign that an ulcer is present, especially in those taking NSAIDs.[90,91] Therefore, regardless of whether pain or other symptoms are present, the elderly patient should be questioned about signs or symptoms of these complications. An adequate drug history, especially with regard to NSAID use, should be obtained as well. Because delayed diagnosis and treatment may result in significant morbidity or even mortality in elderly patients, the pharmacist should have an increased awareness of the risk factors for GI diseases in this population and should evaluate even vague or minor complaints. If the pharmacist cannot determine that the symptoms are related to overeating, eating spicy foods, or occasional reflux, it is wise to refer the elderly patient to a physician for further evaluation.

When it is determined that antacid use is appropriate for an elderly patient, selection of an antacid product should be guided by the same principles used in choosing antacids for any patient population. However, the pharmacist should realize that elderly patients are more likely to experience side effects from antacids, less likely to tolerate a large sodium load, and more likely to be taking a drug that can interact with antacids. Because constipation is a troublesome and frequent occurrence in elderly patients, magnesium-containing antacids should be recommended provided the patient does not have severe renal impairment. Antacids containing only aluminum hydroxide are not good choices for elderly patients with constipation and have been reported to cause hypophosphatemia and resultant bone changes in this population.[112] On the other hand, these patients may be more likely to have diarrhea from magnesium or calcium carbonate antacids, and fluid-electrolyte disturbances are more dangerous in elderly patients than in younger persons. Patients should be aware that diarrhea and constipation are possibilities from antacid use and should be encouraged to switch antacids if these side effects occur. Because many elderly patients are on low-salt diets because of hypertension or congestive heart failure, they should avoid sodium bicarbonate, even for short-term use.

Finally, the aging process causes changes that affect the pharmacokinetics of drugs, particularly their metabolism and elimination. Doses of antacids do not generally need to be altered in elderly patients because of these changes but may need to be reduced because of side effects. However, dosage adjustments of H_2-antagonists are often necessary in the elderly, primarily because of reduced renal function. This is especially true for cimetidine, whose clearance is reduced in older patients. Failure to reduce the dose of cimetidine could result in mental confusion that may be misinterpreted as dementia.

Pregnant Women

Because 30–50% of pregnant women have symptomatic gastroesophageal reflux, they often seek advice from the pharmacist about the safe use of antacids.[114] Heartburn in pregnancy occurs most commonly in the third trimester, and is a recurrent problem for more than 75% of women who experienced reflux symptoms in preceding pregnancies.[114] Antacids are generally considered safe in pregnancy as long as chronic high doses are avoided. However, there have been reports of magnesium-, calcium-, or aluminum-containing antacids causing hypermagnesemia, hypomagnesemia, hypercalcemia, and increased tendon reflexes in fetuses and neonates whose mothers were using these antacids chronically in high doses. In addition, it is best not to recommend sodium bicarbonate to pregnant women because of the risks of systemic alkalosis and the sodium load leading to edema and weight gain.

Patient Assessment

The most valuable service the pharmacist can provide to patients with GI complaints is to determine whether their symptoms are amenable to self-treatment with antacids or if they need medical attention. Three types of situations are considered medical emergencies and deserve immediate medical attention: (1) pain that is indistinguishable from angina or a myocardial infarct; (2) signs and symptoms of complicated peptic ulcer disease; and (3) pain that mimics acute pancreatitis.

Heartburn associated with GERD may mimic the pain associated with angina or a myocardial infarct, which is usually described as a crushing pain in the chest that may radiate down the left arm or to the back, may be related to exercise, and is often relieved by sublingual nitroglycerin tablets. However, pain related to gastroesophageal reflux most often occurs immediately after meals, may be worsened by bending over or lying down, and is more likely to be relieved by antacids.[68] The pharmacist should ask appropriate questions to determine which type of pain the patient is experiencing. If there is any suspicion that the pain may be of cardiac origin, the patient should be referred immediately to a physician. This is especially important for patients with a history of cardiac disease.

A peptic ulcer that bleeds, perforates, penetrates another organ, or obstructs a gastric outlet can be a life-threatening event. Vomiting blood or material that looks like coffee grounds (hematemesis), or black tarry stools with a distinctive foul odor (melena) are serious signs. Both of these signal acute blood loss and indicate that bleeding is occurring or has recently occurred. By the time melena develops, the patient has already lost at least 200 mL of blood.[115] A perforated ulcer may be described by a patient as a sudden onset of epigastric pain that radiates to the right shoulder and down into the right lower quadrant. It may be accompanied by nausea and vomiting. Penetration often presents as constant epigastric pain rather than the intermittent pain that is associated with a DU. Gastric obstruction is characterized by a slow onset of vomiting, abdominal pain, and weight loss.[5] The prompt attention and evaluation a pharmacist provides to patients complaining of these symptoms can make a difference in survival, especially for elderly patients.

The pain of acute pancreatitis is like that of peptic ulcer disease in that it generally occurs in the epigastrium. However, unlike typical DU pain, acute pancreatitis is a steady, boring pain that may be severe enough to incapacitate the patient.[44] The pain often radiates to the back, chest, flanks, and lower abdomen; is not relieved by antacids; and is worse when the patient lies down. Nausea, vomiting, and abdominal distention often accompany the pain. Acute pancreatitis is most likely to occur in patients with a history of alcohol abuse, thiazide use, or gallstones. Because a significant percentage of patients with acute pancreatitis die, it is essential to refer patients who present with these symptoms to a physician immediately.

Many patients who seek antacid relief for dyspeptic symptoms or pain will have a disorder that warrants medical evaluation but is not an immediate, life-threatening situation. Important clues to determining what type of problem is present are (1) when the symptoms occur, especially in relation to meals and nighttime; (2) whether the pain is well localized; (3) whether the symptoms are acute or chronic; (4) whether the symptoms are relieved by food or antacids; and (5) whether the symptoms are made worse by certain types of foods (Table 1). It is always important to question the patient about the use of both prescription and nonprescription drugs, paying special attention to the pattern of NSAID use. If the patient is taking a nonprescription drug, the brand name should be specified because patients may not be aware that certain combination products contain aspirin or ibuprofen. The patient's personal and family history of peptic ulcer disease may also provide helpful hints for the pharmacist. On the basis of this information, patients who are suspected of having peptic ulcer disease, severe and/or chronic GERD, or chronic gastritis should be referred for a diagnostic evaluation. Even though some of these disorders can be treated successfully with antacids, medical attention is needed to establish a diagnosis, initiate treatment, and monitor success of therapy. Furthermore, even the most typical ulcer pain may be misleading because the patient could have pancreatitis, pancreatic cancer, gastric or duodenal cancer, gallbladder disease, hiatal hernia, or coronary artery disease or angina.

The disorders that may be treated without medical intervention are acute gastritis without bleeding and occasional gastroesophageal reflux. Patients who complain of acute symptoms that can be related to overeating, eating spicy or certain types of foods, or consuming alcohol probably have one of these disorders and can be treated with antacids. If the symptoms can be related to NSAID ingestion, antacids may be recommended if the patient is not at risk for NSAID-induced ulcers (i.e., if the patient is young, has no concomitant illnesses or drug use, and has made short-term use of NSAID).[5] If antacids are recommended in any of these situations and the patient does not experience prompt relief, the pharmacist should refer the patient to a physician for further evaluation. Similarly, symptoms that are relieved by antacids but return often probably warrant medical attention.

As noted above, assessment of elderly patients with GI complaints is difficult because the elderly often do not have symptoms.

Product Selection Guidelines

Selection of an antacid product should be guided by consideration of the chemical properties of the ingredients, the GI and systemic side effects of the ingredients, potency, formulation, taste, drug interactions, and cost. The choice of product should always be tailored to the specific needs of the patient seeking therapy based on the patient's symptoms, age, lifestyle, concurrent diseases, medication profile, and financial status. After carefully interviewing the patient, the pharmacist should try to select an antacid that is:

- *Potent:* Small amounts of the product should neutralize large amounts of gastric acid. Patients prefer to take smaller amounts of medication.
- *Long-acting:* The antacid should neutralize gastric acid for a prolonged period without causing rebound acid secretion.
- *Safe:* The antacid should not cause troublesome side

effects, disturb electrolyte balance, or alter the systemic acid–base balance. The product should neither interfere with other drugs the patient is taking nor contain large amounts of other ingredients that might exacerbate concomitant diseases.
- *Inexpensive:* The product should be inexpensive so that the patient can afford it, especially if it is intended for long-term use.
- *Palatable:* The taste and formulation should be acceptable to the patient because a product that tastes good is almost a prerequisite for successful antacid therapy.

There is no antacid that meets all these criteria. Thus, an antacid should be chosen that fits as many of these qualities as possible while being suitable for the patient and the disorder to be treated. The label of an antacid is useful in evaluating the content of excipient ingredients, but the amounts of these ingredients should be compared in equipotent volumes to be administered. Contents to consider before selecting an antacid for a patient include sodium, lactose, potassium, magnesium, and sugar. The pharmacist should evaluate the amount of these substances before recommending a product for patients with renal disease, congestive heart failure, edema, or lactose intolerance or those on low-salt diets. In general, all antacids pose a risk of systemic side effects or electrolyte imbalances in patients with chronic renal failure. Specifically, products containing large amounts of sodium or more than 50 mEq per day of magnesium are to be avoided in such patients.

Patients complaining of constipation (common in elderly patients) or hemorrhoids should be given antacids containing magnesium or magnesium–aluminum combinations. Conversely, patients with a history of diarrhea (e.g., ulcerative colitis) should avoid magnesium-containing antacids and may best be treated with aluminum-only antacids.

Apart from listing amounts of certain excipient ingredients, the antacid product labeling contains little information that is helpful to the pharmacist in choosing an antacid for a patient.[116] A listing of the quantity of active ingredients is voluntary, and the milliequivalent neutralizing capacity provided per dose is not specified.

A final consideration in antacid product selection is cost. Although most antacids are relatively inexpensive, the cost may vary considerably when acid-neutralizing capacity is compared. As with all antacid ingredients, the cost should be calculated for equipotent, not equivolume quantities.

Patient Counseling

The patient who purchases an antacid should be given the following specific advice:

- Antacids used for relief of indigestion, upset stomach, or heartburn should not be taken for longer than 2 weeks. If antacids do not relieve symptoms promptly or if symptoms return often, a physician should be contacted.
- If the antacid is being taken for peptic ulcer disease, it should be taken 1 and 3 hours after meals and at bedtime to provide the best benefit.
- If the antacid is being taken for heartburn (reflux), it should be taken immediately after meals and at bedtime, and the patients should (1) not eat within 3 hours of going to bed; (2) elevate the head of the bed with blocks; (3) avoid smoking, caffeine, and alcohol; (4) avoid tight-fitting clothing; and (5) avoid lying down after eating.
- If a product with alginic acid is recommended, the patient should drink a glass of water after taking it and should not lie down or go to bed immediately after taking the product.
- Because the antacid may cause constipation or diarrhea, the patient should seek advice on switching antacids if one of these side effects develops.
- Patients on low-salt diets should know the amount of sodium in the antacid and take only those products with a low sodium content. Patients with renal or cardiac disease should be similarly wary of potassium and magnesium content.
- Tablets are not as potent as liquids. Patients who find liquids bulky and difficult to carry may take antacid tablets during the day at work and more potent liquids at night.
- Chewable tablets should be chewed thoroughly and followed with a full glass of water. Effervescent tablets should be dissolved completely in water, and the bubbles subsided, before drinking.
- Patients should space doses of antacids at least 2 hours apart from interacting drugs.

Summary

The safe and effective use of antacids starts with the pharmacist's ability to distinguish between patients who are appropriate for self-treatment and those who need to be referred to a physician. The pharmacist should take care in selecting a safe antacid product for a particular patient by evaluating a patient's symptoms, history, concomitant disease states, and concomitant medications. To ensure that antacids are used effectively, they should be dosed to provide maximum duration of acid neutralization while minimizing the potential for drug interactions. The success of antacid therapy depends largely on patient compliance. Therefore, high-potency products should be used when possible, the taste should be acceptable to the patient, and the antacid should not cause intolerable side effects.

Although there is little objective evidence of antacid effectiveness for many acid-peptic disorders, their widespread and long-term use by patients can be viewed as a statement of their efficacy. Patients with symptoms of mild heartburn, indigestion, upset stomach, or acute gastritis without bleeding may be relieved by any antacid. Therapy can be initiated with 40–80 mEq of a liquid antacid or 2–4 g of sodium bicarbonate or calcium carbonate. Patients with symptoms of gas may benefit from a product containing simethicone; those with heartburn may benefit from a product containing alginic acid. The pharmacist should instruct the patient not to take the product for more than 2 weeks, at which time the patient should be referred to a physician if symptoms persist. For treatment of peptic ulcer disease, high-potency aluminum–magnesium liquid antacids should be initially recommended provided the patient has no contraindications.

Knowledge of GI diseases is advancing rapidly, and changing with it is the role of antacids. If antacids can protect the gastric mucosa independent of their ability to neutralize acid, dosing recommendations may be lowered to 120–200 mEq per day. Such a reduction would make antacids more attractive to patients in terms of side effects, convenience, and cost. However, as the association of *H. pylori* with acid-peptic disorders grows stronger, the roles of acid neutralization and suppression may change. Antacids continue to be used widely for short-term relief of mild GI complaints; however, the introduction of nonprescription forms of cimetidine and ranitidine could affect the popularity of antacids for such indications. To continue the safe and effective use of antacids, pharmacists should understand the value of these agents in relation to other therapies for acid-peptic disorders and be informed of advances that affect the use of these products.

References

1. Szeinbach SL, Smith MC. Gastroesophageal reflux disease. Pharmacist's role in patient referrals. *Drug Top* 1991 Jan; 4–16.
2. Cramer T. When do you need an antacid? *FDC Consumer* 1992 Jan–Feb; 19–22.
3. Gray GM. Peptic ulcer diseases. *Sci Am* 1988; 4 (2): 1–15.
4. Marshall BJ. Peptic ulcer: an infectious disease? *Hosp Pract* 1987 Aug; 87–96.
5. Isenberg JI et al. Acid-peptic disorders. In: Yamada T, Alpers DH, Owyang C, eds. *Textbook of Gastroenterology*. Philadelphia: J. B. Lippincott Co; 1991; 1: 1231–349.
6. Peterson WL. *Helicobacter pylori* and peptic ulcer disease. *N Engl J Med* 1991; 324 (15): 1043–7.
7. Cryer B, Lee E, Feldman M. Factors influencing gastroduodenal mucosal prostaglandin concentrations: roles of smoking and aging. *Ann Intern Med* 1992 Apr; 116: 636–40.
8. Uppal R, Lateef SK, Korsten MA, et al. Chronic alcoholic gastritis: Roles of alcohol and *Helicobacter pylori*. *Arch Intern Med* 1991 Apr; 151: 760–4.
9. Piper JM, Ray WA, Daugherty JR, et al. Corticosteroid use and peptic ulcer disease: role of nonsteroidal anti-inflammatory drugs. *Ann Intern Med* 1991 May; 114: 735–40.
10. Olin B, ed. *Drug Facts & Comparisons*. St. Louis: J. B. Lippincott Co; 1992: 306, 406k, 653d.
11. Berstad A. Antacids and pepsin. *Scand J Gastroenterol* 1982; 17 (suppl 75): 13–5.
12. Kivilaakso E. Antacids and bile salts. *Scand J Gastroenterol* 1982; 17 (suppl 75): 16–9.
13. Deering TB, Carlson GL, Malagelada JR, et al. Fate of oral neutralizing antacid and its effect on postprandial gastric secretion and emptying. *Gastroenterology* 1979; 77: 986–90.
14. Berstad A, Alexander B, Weberg R, et al. Antacids reduce *Campylobacter pylori* colonization without healing the gastritis in patients with nonulcer dyspepsia and erosive prepyloric changes. *Gastroenterology* 1988 Sep; 95: 619–24.
15. Weberg R, Aubert E, Dahlberg O, et al. Low-dose antacids or cimetidine for duodenal ulcer? *Gastroenterology* 1988 Jun; 95: 1465–9.
16. Walt R, Langman MJS. Antacids and ulcer healing: a review of the evidence. *Drugs* 1991; 42 (2): 205–12.
17. Preclik G, Stange EF, Gerber K, et al. Stimulation of mucosal prostaglandin synthesis in human stomach and duodenum by antacid treatment. *Gut* 1989; 30 (2): 148–51.
18. Hade JE, Spiro HM. Calcium and acid rebound: a reappraisal. *J Clin Gastroenterol* 1992; 15 (1): 37–44.
19. Clemens JD, Feinstein AR. Calcium carbonate and constipation: a historical review of medical mythopoeia. *Gastroenterology* 1977 May; 72: 957–61.
20. Ulmer DD. Toxicity from aluminum antacids. *N Engl J Med* 1976 Jan; 294 (4): 218–9.
21. Alfrey AC, Legendre GR, Kaehny WD. The dialysis encephalopathy syndrome: possible aluminum intoxication. *N Engl J Med* 1976; 294 (4): 184–8.
22. National Institutes of Health. Over-the-counter antacid preparations can have adverse effects on bone. *JAMA* 1977; 238 (10): 1018.
23. Herzog P, Holtermuller KH. Antacid therapy—changes in mineral metabolism. *Scand J Gastroenterol* 1982; 17 (suppl 75): 56–62.
24. Donowitz M, Rood RP. Magnesium hydroxide: new insights into the mechanism of its laxative effect and the potential involvement of prostaglandin E_2. *J Clin Gastroenterol* 1992 Jan; 14 (1): 20–6.
25. Stead JA, Wilkins RA, Ashford JJ. In vitro and in vivo defoaming action of three antacid preparations. *J Pharm Pharmacol* 1978; 30: 350–2.
26. Schneider RP, Roach AC. An antacid testing: the relative palatability of 19 liquid antacids. *South Med J* 1976 Oct; 69 (10): 1312–3.
27. Gugler R, Allgayer H. Effects of antacids on the clinical pharmacokinetics of drugs: an update. *Clin Pharmacokin* 1990; 18 (3): 210–9.
28. Tatro DS, ed. *Drug Interaction Facts*. St. Louis: Facts and Comparisons Divisions, J. B. Lippincott Co; 1993.
29. Feldman M, Burton ME. Histamine$_2$-receptor antagonists. Standard therapy for acid-peptic diseases (first of two parts). *N Engl J Med* 1990 Dec; 323 (24): 1672–80.
30. McCarthy DM. Sucralfate. *N Engl J Med* 1991 Oct; 325 (14): 1017–25.
31. Gibaldi M, Grundhofer B, Levy G. Effect of antacids on pH of urine. *Clin Pharmacol Ther* 1974; 16: 520–5.
32. Rubin W. Medical treatment of peptic ulcer disease. *Med Clin N Am* 1991 Jul; 75 (4): 981–98.
33. Glaxo will proceed with OTC Zantac but timetable uncertain, company tells analysts; ranitidine bismuth citrate for peptic ulcer set for 1994 filing. *FDC Reports* 1991 Dec 23: 6–7.
34. Adams MH, Ostrosky JD, Kirkwood CF. Therapeutic evaluation of omeprazole. *Clin Pharm* 1988; 7: 725–45.
35. Bettarello A. Anti-ulcer therapy: past to present. *Dig Dis Sci* 1985; 30 (suppl 11): 36S–42S.
36. Kitchin LI, Castell DO. Rationale and efficacy of conservative therapy for gastroesophageal reflux disease. *Arch Intern Med* 1991 Mar; 151: 448–54.
37. Garris RE, Kirkwood CF. Misoprostol: a prostaglandin E_1 analogue. *Clin Pharm* 1989 Sep; 8: 627–44.
38. Graham DY, Agrawal NM, Roth SH. Prevention of NSAID-induced gastric ulcer with misoprostol: multicentre, double-blind, placebo-controlled trial. *Lancet* 1988 Dec; 2: 1277–80.
39. Marshall BJ. The use of bismuth in gastroenterology. *Gastroenterology* 1991; 86 (1): 16–25.
40. Katz KD, Hollander D. Practical pharmacology and cost-effective management of peptic ulcer disease. *Am J Surg* 1992 Mar; 163: 349–59.
41. Kurata JH, Haile BH. Epidemiology of peptic ulcer disease. *Clin Gastroenterol* 1984 May; 13 (2): 289–307.
42. Berardi RR. Peptic ulcer disease and Zollinger-Ellison syndrome. In: Depiro JT, Talbert RL, Hayes PE, et al., eds. *Pharmacotherapy: A Pathophysiologic Approach*. Salem, Mass: Elsevier Science Publishing Co, Inc; 1989: 418–36.
43. Katz J. The course of peptic ulcer disease. *Med Clin N Am* 1991 Jul; 75 (4): 831–40.

44. Greenberger NJ, Toskes PP, Isselbacher KJ. Diseases of the pancreas. In: Braunwald E, Isselbacher KJ, Petersdorf RG, eds. *Harrison's Principles of Internal Medicine.* 11th ed. New York: McGraw-Hill, Inc; 1987: 1372–5.
45. Brooks FP. The pathophysiology of peptic ulcer disease. *Dig Dis Sci* 1985 Nov; 30 (suppl 11): 15S–29S.
46. Caldwell SH, McCallum RX. Peptic ulcer disease and *Campylobacter pylori*: new insights into an old disease. *Triangle* 1988; 27 (4): 165–77.
47. Lewis JH. Treatment of gastric ulcer. What is old and what is new. *Arch Intern Med* 1983 Feb; 143: 264–74.
48. Hixson LJ, Kelley CL, Jones WN, et al. Current trends in the pharmacotherapy for peptic ulcer disease. *Arch Intern Med* 1992 Apr; 152: 726–32.
49. O'Riordan T, Mathai E, Tobin E, et al. Adjuvant antibiotic therapy in duodenal ulcers treated with colloidal bismuth subcitrate. *Gut* 1990; 31: 999–1002.
50. Graham DY, Lew GM, Evans DG, et al. Effect of triple therapy (antibiotics plus bismuth) on duodenal ulcer healing: a randomized controlled trial. *Ann Intern Med* 1991 Aug; 115: 266–9.
51. Peterson WL, Sturdevant RA, Frankl HD, et al. Healing of duodenal ulcer with an antacid regimen. *N Engl J Med* 1977; 297: 341–5.
52. Sewing K. Efficacy of low-dose antacids in the treatment of peptic ulcers: pharmacological explanation. *J Clin Gastroenterol* 1991; 13 (suppl 1): S134–S138.
53. Kumar N, Vij JC, Anand BS. Controlled therapeutic trial to determine the optimum dose of antacids in duodenal ulcer. *Gut* 1984; 25: 1199–1202.
54. Weberg R, Berstad A, Lange O, et al. Duodenal ulcer healing with four antacid tablets daily. *Scand J Gastroenterol* 1985; 20: 1041–5.
55. Nauert C, Caspary WF. Duodenal ulcer therapy with low-dose antacids: a multicenter trial. *J Clin Gastroenterol* 1991: 13 (suppl 1): S149–S154.
56. McCarthy DM. Duodenal ulcer: is there a role for chronic prophylactic therapy? In: Barkin JS, Rogers AL, eds. *Difficult Decisions in Digestive Diseases.* Chicago: Year Book Medical Publishers, Inc. 1989: 95–107.
57. Graham DY, Lew GM, Klein PD, et al. Effect of treatment of *Helicobacter pylori* infection on the long-term recurrence of gastric or duodenal ulcer. *Ann Intern Med* 1992 May; 116 (9): 705–8.
58. Walsh JH. *Helicobacter pylori*: Selection of patients for treatment. *Ann Intern Med* 1992 May; 116 (9): 770–1.
59. Bardhan KD, Hunter JO, Miller JP, et al. Antacid maintenance therapy in the prevention of duodenal ulcer relapse. *Gut* 1988; 29: 1748–54.
60. Hui WM, Lam SK, Lok ASK, et al. Maintenance therapy for duodenal ulcer: a randomized controlled comparison of seven forms of treatment. *Am J Med* 1992 Mar; 92: 265–74.
61. Agrawal NM, Dajani EZ. Options in the treatment and prevention of NSAID-induced gastroduodenal mucosal damage. *J Rheumatol* 1990; 17 (suppl 20): 7–11.
62. Graham DY, Lidsky MD, Cox AM, et al. Long-term nonsteroidal antiinflammatory drug use and *Helicobacter pylori* infection. *Gastroenterology* 1991; 100: 1653–57.
63. Drugs for treatment of peptic ulcers. *Med Lett Drugs Ther* 1991 Nov; 33 (858): 111–3.
64. Englert EJ, Freston JW, Graham DY, et al. Cimetidine, antacid, and hospitalization in the treatment of benign gastric ulcer. *Gastroenterology* 1978; 74 (2, part 2): 416–25.
65. Berstad A, Weberg R. Antacids for peptic ulcer: do we have anything better? *Scand J Gastroenterol* 1986; 21 (suppl 125): 32–6.
66. Orlando RC. Reflux esophagitis. In: Yamada T, Alpers DH, Owyang C, eds. *Textbook of Gastroenterology.* Philadelphia: J. B. Lippincott Co; 1991; 1.
67. Lieberman D. Diagnosis and treatment of gastroesophageal reflux disease. *Compr Ther* 1991 Apr; 17 (4): 43–50.
68. Richter JE. Gastroesophageal reflux: diagnosis and management. *Hosp Pract* 1992 Jan 15; 59–66.
69. Holloway RH, Dent J. Pathophysiology of gastroesophageal reflux. Lower esophageal sphincter dysfunction in gastroesophageal reflux disease. *Gastroenterol Clin N Am* 1990 Sep; 19 (3): 517–35.
70. Welage LS. Gastroesophageal reflux. In: DiPiro JT, Talbert RL, Hayes PE, et al. *Pharmacotherapy: A Pathophysiologic Approach.* Salem, Mass: Elsevier Science Publishing Co, Inc; 1989: 409–36.
71. Traube M. The spectrum of the symptoms and presentations of gastroesophageal reflux disease. *Gastroenterol Clin N Am* 1990 Sep; 19 (3): 609–17.
72. Kozarek RA. Complications of reflux esophagitis and their medical management. *Gastroenterol Clin N Am* 1990 Sep; 19 (3): 713–31.
73. Lanza F, Smith V, Page-Castell J, et al. Effectiveness of foaming antacid in relieving induced heartburn. *South Med J* 1987; 79: 327–30.
74. Stanciu C, Bennett JR. Alginate/antacid in the reduction of gastro-oesophageal reflux. *Lancet* 1974 Jan; 1: 109–11.
75. Castell DO, Dalton CB, Becker D. Alginic acid decreases postprandial upright gastroesophageal reflux. Comparison with equal-strength antacid. *Dig Dis Sci* 1992 Apr; 37 (4): 589–93.
76. Hixson LJ, Kelley CJ, Jones WN, et al. Current trends in the pharmacotherapy for gastroesophageal reflux disease. *Arch Intern Med* 1992 Apr; 152: 717–23.
77. Hetzel DJ, Dent J, Reed WD, et al. Healing and relapse of severe peptic esophagitis after treatment with omeprazole. *Gastroenterology* 1988; 95 (4): 903–12.
78. Weinstein WM. Gastritis. In: Sleisinger J, Fordtan JS, eds. *Gastrointestinal Disease.* 3rd ed. Philadelphia: W. B. Saunders, Co; 1983: 559–64.
79. Graham DY, Davis RE. Acute upper-gastrointestinal hemorrhage. New observations on an old problem. *Dig Dis Sci* 1978 Jan; 23 (1): 76–84.
80. McGarrity TJ, Jeffries GH. Gastritis: is it a distinct clinical entity? In: Barkin JS, Rogers AI, eds. *Difficult Decisions in Digestive Diseases.* Chicago: Year Book Medical Publishers, Inc; 1989: 74–88.
81. Guslandi M. Gastric cytoprotection. What does it really mean for the prescriber? *Drugs* 1991; 41 (4): 507–13.
82. Marshall BJ. *Campylobacter pylori*: its link to gastritis and peptic ulcer disease. *Rev Infect Dis* 1990 Jan-Feb; 12 (suppl 1): S87–S93.
83. Parsonnet J, Friedman GD, Vandersteen YC, et al. *Helicobacter pylori* infection and the risk of gastric carcinoma. *N Engl J Med* 1991 Oct; 325: 1127–31.
84. Nomura A, Stemmermann GN, Chyou PH, et al. *Helicobacter pylori* infection and gastric carcinoma among Japanese Americans in Hawaii. *N Engl J Med* 1991 Oct; 325: 1132–6.
85. Veldhuyzen van Zanten SJO, Tytgat KMA, Jalali S, et al. Can gastritis symptoms be evaluated in clinical trials? An overview of treatment of gastritis, nonulcer dyspepsia and campylobacter-associated gastritis. *J Clin Gastroenterol* 1989 May; 11 (5): 496–501.
86. Wylie FA. *Helicobacter pylori*: current perspectives. *J Clin Gastroenterol* 1991; 13 (suppl 1): S114–S124.
87. Guslandi M. Comparison of sucralfate and ranitidine in the treatment of chronic nonerosive gastritis. *Am J Med* 1989 Jun; 86 (suppl 6A): 45–8.
88. Warndorff DK, Knottnerus JA, Huijnen LGJ, et al. How well do general practitioners manage dyspepsia? *J R Coll Gen Pract* 1989 Dec; 39: 499–502.
89. Fries JF, Miller SR, Spitz PW, et al. Identification of patients at risk for gastropathy associated with NSAID use. *J Rheumatol* 1990; 17 (suppl 20): 12–9.
90. Larkai EN, Smith JL, Lidsky MD, et al. Gastroduodenal mucosa and dyspeptic symptoms in arthritic patients during chronic

90. nonsteroidal anti-inflammatory drug use. *Am J Gastroenterol* 1987; 82: 1153–8.
91. Armstrong CP, Blower AL. Non-steroidal anti-inflammatory drugs and life-threatening complications of peptic ulceration. *Gut* 1987; 28: 527–37.
92. Paulus HE. FDA Arthritis Advisory Committee Meeting: serious gastrointestinal toxicity of nonsteroidal anti-inflammatory drugs. *Arthritis Rheum* 1988 Nov; 31 (11): 1450–1.
93. Soll AH, Weinstein WM, Kurata J, et al. Nonsteroidal anti-inflammatory drugs and peptic ulcer disease. *Ann Intern Med* 1991 Feb; 114: 307–19.
94. Sievert W, Stern AI, Lambert JR, et al. Low-dose antacids and nonsteroidal anti-inflammatory drug-induced gastropathy in humans. *J Clin Gastroenterol* 1991; 13 (suppl 1): S145–S148.
95. McCarthy DM. Nonsteroidal antiinflammatory drug-induced ulcers: management by traditional therapies. *Gastroenterology* 1989 Feb; 96 (2): 662–74.
96. Gerber LH, Rooney PJ, McCarthy DM. Healing of peptic ulcers during continuing antiinflammatory drug therapy in rheumatoid arthritis. *J Clin Gastroenterol* 1981; 3: 7–11.
97. O'Laughlin JC, Silvoso GK, Ivey KJ. Resistance to medical therapy of gastric ulcers in rheumatic disease patients taking aspirin. A double-blind study with cimetidine and follow-up. *Dig Dis Sci* 1982; 27 (11): 976–80.
98. Talley NJ, Phillips SF. Non-ulcer dyspepsia: potential causes and pathophysiology. *Ann Intern Med* 1988 Jun; 108: 865–79.
99. Greenberg RE, Bank S. The prevalence of *Helicobacter pylori* in nonulcer dyspepsia. Importance of stratification according to age. *Arch Intern Med* 1990 Oct; 150: 2053–55.
100. Shaffer EA. Nonulcer dyspepsia. A complex spectrum of disorders. *Can Fam Physician* 1992 Mar; 38: 466, 470–1.
101. Dobrilla G, Comberlato M, Steele A, et al. Drug treatment of functional dyspepsia. A meta-analysis of randomized controlled clinical trials. *J Clin Gastroenterol* 1989 Feb; 11 (2): 169–77.
102. Kang JY, Tay HH, Guan R, et al. Effect of colloidal bismuth subcitrate on symptoms and gastric histology in non-ulcer dyspepsia. A double blind placebo controlled study. *Gut* 1990; 31: 476–80.
103. Talley NJ, Ormand JE, Carpenter H, et al. Triple therapy for *Helicobacter pylori* in nonulcer dyspepsia. *Am J Gastroenterol* 1991 Jan; 86 (1): 121–3.
104. Gotthard R, Bodemar G, Brodin U, et al. Treatment with cimetidine, antacid, or placebo in patients with dyspepsia of unknown origin. *Scand J Gastroenterol* 1988; 23: 7–18.
105. Lagarde SP, Spiro HM. Non-ulcer dyspepsia. *Clin Gastroenterol* 1984 May; 13 (2): 437–46.
106. FDA changes approach to hangovers. *NDMA Executive Newsletter* 1992 Jan 3; 1–92: 1–2.
107. Mayo M, Middleton RK. Calcium carbonate in hyperphosphatemia. *DICP, Ann Pharmacother* 1991 Sep; 25: 945–7.
108. Wasan SM. Phosphate binders in hyperphosphatemia of chronic renal failure. *DICP, Ann Pharmacother* 1991 Sep; 25: 942–5.
109. Sperber AD, Zuili I, Bearman JE, et al. The effect of an antacid containing aluminum hydroxide on plasma cholesterol and lipoproteins. *Curr Ther Res* 1988; 77: 986–90.
110. D. P. Hamacher & Associates. Antacids and antidiarrheals. *NARD J* 1989 Nov: 145–6.
111. Stewart RB, Hale WE, Marks RG. Antacid use in an ambulatory elderly population. *Dig Dis Sci* 1983 Dec; 28 (12): 1062–9.
112. Holt PR. Approach to gastrointestinal problems in the elderly. In: Yamada T, Alpers DH, Owyang C, eds. *Textbook of Gastroenterology*. Philadelphia: J. B. Lippincott Co; 1991; 1: 882–99.
113. Griffin MR, Ray WA, Schaffner W. Nonsteroidal anti-inflammatory drug use and death from peptic ulcer in elderly persons. *Ann Intern Med* 1988 Sep; 109 (5): 359–63.
114. Day JP, Richter JE. Medical and surgical conditions predisposing to gastroesophageal reflux disease. *Gastroenterol Clin N Am* 1990 Sep; 19 (3): 587–607.
115. Lieberman DA, Melnyk CS. Gastrointestinal hemorrhage. In: Gitnick G, ed. *Principles and Practice of Gastroenterology and Hepatology*. New York: Elsevier Science Publishing Co, Inc; 1988: 1542–63.
116. A new standard for antacids. *FDA Consumer* 1974 Jul–Aug; 25–8.

CHAPTER 12

Emetic and Antiemetic Products

Gary M. Oderda and Jenifer C. Jennings

Questions to ask in patient assessment and counseling

Emetics

- *Do you want the emetic for immediate or possible future emergency use?*
- *If for immediate use, have you spoken to a poison control center?*
- *For whom is the medication? How old is the patient? What substance was taken? How long ago did the ingestion occur? How much was taken?*
- *Has the patient already been given something for the ingestion?*
- *What symptoms is the patient showing?*
- *Does the patient have any chronic or acute illnesses that may affect the poisoning?*
- *Is the patient taking any nonprescription or prescription medications?*

Antiemetics

- *Do you know what caused the nausea and vomiting?*
- *For whom is the medication?*
- *How old is the patient?*
- *Is the patient pregnant?*
- *Is the patient diabetic?*
- *How long has the nausea or vomiting been present?*
- *Have you noted blood in the vomitus that is bright red or resembles coffee grounds?*
- *Have you noted other symptoms such as abdominal pain, headache, or diarrhea?*
- *What medications is the patient currently taking?*
- *Is the patient receiving or has the patient recently received radiation therapy or cancer chemotherapy?*
- *What other medical problems does the patient have?*

Editor's Note: This chapter is based in part on the chapter with the same title that appeared in the 9th edition but was written by Gary M. Oderda and Barbara H. Korberly.

Severe nausea and the realization that one is about to vomit are two of the more unpleasant symptoms an individual may experience. However disagreeable the sensation, vomiting (emesis) is an important defense mechanism by which the body attempts to rid itself of a variety of toxins and poisons; vomiting can also be caused by travel (i.e., motion sickness) or pregnancy.

Nonprescription emetic drugs are used to induce vomiting, primarily in the treatment of poisoning. Nonprescription antiemetics have been used to prevent or control the symptoms of nausea and vomiting primarily due to motion sickness, pregnancy, and mild infectious diseases. Some nonprescription antiemetics are promoted for the relief of such vague symptoms as "upset stomach," indigestion, and distention associated with food indulgence; however, their value in treating these complaints is not well documented.

Nausea and vomiting associated with radiation therapy; cancer chemotherapy; and serious metabolic, central nervous system (CNS), gastrointestinal (GI), and endocrine disorders, which are not appropriate conditions for self-medication, are not covered in this chapter because they require physician referral and management.

The Vomiting Process

Vomiting is a complex process involving both the CNS and the GI systems. Nausea, which is an unpleasant sensation that is vaguely associated with the epigastrum and abdomen, usually precedes vomiting. Retching is a strong, involuntary effort to vomit.

The vomit reflex is mediated by a "vomiting center" located in the medulla of the brain. The vomiting center itself does not carry out the function of vomiting; rather, it coordinates the activities of other neural structures to produce a patterned response. The vomiting center receives stimuli from peripheral areas, such as the gastric mucosa, in addition to areas within the CNS itself. Stimulation of the chemoreceptor trigger zone (CTZ), which is the afferent pathway to the vomiting center, is responsible for its activation and may be involved in eliciting nausea and vomiting from a variety of causes.[1,2] Centrally acting emetics (e.g., codeine, morphine) work primarily by stimulating the CTZ whereas centrally active antiemetics (e.g., phenothiazines) inhibit it. In addition to stimuli from the CTZ, the vomiting center also receives impulses from the GI tract and the labyrinth apparatus in the ear. Stimuli then are sent via a cranial nerve to the abdominal musculature, stomach, and esophagus to initiate vomiting.

Vomiting begins with a deep inspiration, the closing of the glottis, and the depression of the soft palate. A forceful contraction of the diaphragm and abdominal musculature occurs, producing an increase in intrathoracic and intra-abdominal pressure that compresses the stomach and raises esophageal pressure. The body of the stomach and the esophageal musculature relax. The positive intrathoracic and intra-abdominal pressure moves stomach contents into the esophagus and mouth. Regurgitation is the casting up of stomach contents without oral expulsion. Several cycles of reflux into the esophagus occur before actual vomiting begins.[3] Vomitus is expelled from the esophagus by a combination of increased intrathoracic pressure and reverse peristaltic waves.[3,4] Normally, the glottis closes off the trachea and prevents the vomitus from entering the airway; however, aspiration of the vomitus can occur in patients with CNS depression or an absent or impaired gag reflex.

Overstimulation of the labyrinth (inner ear) apparatus produces the nausea and vomiting of motion sickness. The three semicircular canals on each side of the head in the labyrinth are responsible for maintaining equilibrium. Postural adjustments are made when the brain receives nervous impulses initiated by the movement of fluid in the canals. Motion sickness may be produced by unusual motion patterns in which the head is rotated on two axes simultaneously. Mechanisms other than stimulation of the semicircular canals are also important. Erroneous interpretation of visual stimuli by stationary subjects, such as occurs when one watches a film taken from a roller coaster or an airplane doing aerobatics or when one simply extends one's head upward while standing on a rotating platform, can produce motion sickness. Some individuals are more tolerant than others to the effect of a particular type of motion, but no one is immune. Moreover, it appears that individuals can vary in their susceptibility to various kinds of motions, such as flying and boat riding.[5] But regardless of the type of stimulus-producing event, motion sickness is much easier to prevent than to treat once it has already begun.

One-half of all pregnant women experience nausea, and about one-third suffer vomiting.[3] However, the mechanism of vomiting or "morning sickness" associated with pregnancy has not been established. Increased levels of chorionic gonadotropin have been implicated as a cause of morning sickness because levels of this hormone are highest during early pregnancy when nausea and vomiting are most common.[6] Other research suggests that there is no relationship between chorionic gonadotropin levels and morning sickness.[7] Nausea and vomiting due to pregnancy are difficult symptoms to treat. In part, this is because no agent seems to be completely effective, but, more important, it is because the potential for teratogenic effects dictates that drug use during pregnancy be restricted whenever possible.[6]

Acute transient attacks of vomiting in association with diarrhea are very common. This symptom is often observed with viral gastroenteritis, a common acute infectious disease that is usually a harmless, self-limiting disorder and that may affect any age group.[8]

Vomiting is a symptom produced not only by benign processes but also by serious illnesses. The practitioner should be aware that patients may be using nonprescription antiemetics to self-treat the early stages of a serious illness. Knowledge of the patient's drug history is also important in assessing the cause of nausea and vomiting. These symptoms are common side effects of most oral medications and some parenteral and topical drugs. They may also be caused by cancer chemotherapy or may indicate such diverse disorders as those listed in Table 1. Frequent vomiting, particularly in young women, may indicate an eating disorder associated with ipecac abuse and should be evaluated by a physician. Vomiting may produce complications that include dehydration, aspiration, malnutrition, and electrolyte and acid–base abnormalities.

Emetics

Emetics induce vomiting and are used to remove potentially toxic agents from the stomach. Emetics are used most commonly to treat poisoning.

Incidence of Poisoning

Unintentional poisonings occur most frequently in children under 5 years of age and are a leading cause of injury-related hospitalizations in preschoolers even though fatalities have declined significantly over the past 30 years. During 1990, 72 poison centers throughout the United States, serving a population of 191.7 million, submitted 1,713,462 cases to the American Association of Poison Control Centers' data collection system.[9] Included in these cases were 612 fatalities.[9] However, mortality data alone do not adequately describe the problem because many poisonings result in significant morbidity and mortality that are not reported to poison centers.

Baseline Information for Poison Management

It is often difficult to decide whether a patient should be referred directly to an emergency treatment facility or given a nonprescription emetic and managed at home. Obtaining a reliable history, identifying the agent, and accurately assessing the patient's condition are critical in making this decision. Knowing the telephone number of the nearest poison control center is extremely important. All ingestions in which moderate to severe toxicity is possible must be referred to an emergency treatment facility. If minimal toxicity (no serious or life-threatening symptoms) is anticipated, the administration of a nonprescription emetic at home by a competent adult may be all that is necessary. Many ingestions reported to poison control centers fall into this category. For example, a child who ingests aspirin at 150–300 mg/kg of body weight can usually be treated at home by emesis induced with syrup of ipecac and appropriate follow-up.

Of the 1,713,462 cases reported to the American Association of Poison Control Centers' data collection system during 1990, 104,731 used ipecac syrup.[9] Approximately half of these were in health care facilities; the rest primarily in the home. To determine whether administration of a nonprescription emetic in the home is appropriate or whether the patient should be referred to a health care facility, the following information must be obtained.

Name of Product Ingested

From the name of the ingested product, the pharmacist can determine the identity and the amount of each ingredient.

TABLE 1	Primary causes of nausea and vomiting
System/category and pathophysiology	**System/category and pathophysiology**

Primary central nervous system disease
Elevated intracranial pressure
    Neoplasm
    Infection
Epilepsy
Vascular diseases
    Arteriosclerosis
    Embolism
    Vasculitis
    Migraine
Psychologic suggestion
 	
Metabolic and endocrine disease
Diabetic ketoacidosis
Lactic acidosis
Starvation ketosis
Hypothyroidism
Uremia
Adrenal insufficiency
 	
Chemical and drug-induced toxicity
Direct effect on chemoreceptor trigger zone
    Opiates
    Digitalis glycosides
    Cancer chemotherapy
    Radiation sickness
    Food poisoning
    Other drug toxicity or withdrawal
Direct effect on stomach
    Drug-induced gastritis
    Irradiation enteritis
    Ethanol toxicity or withdrawal
	Gastrointestinal disease
	Peptic ulcer
	Reflex esophagitis
	Biliary tract disease
	Hepatic disease
	Gastroenteritis
	Appendicitis
	Functional disorders
	    Aerophagia
	    Pyloroduodenal spasm
	    Mechanical or paralytic obstruction
	
	Genitourinary disease
	Endometritis
	Parametritis
	Salpingitis
	Obstructive uropathy
	Pyelonephritis
	Renal calculi and stones
	
	Labyrinthine disease
	Infection
	Vascular disturbance
	Meniere's disease
	Motion sickness

Adapted from Mellencamp E, Wang RIH. The patient with nausea: I. Causes. *Drug Ther* (Hosp) 1977; 2: 62–9.

The potential toxicity of each ingredient must be investigated. The product label or container, if available, may also list ingredients, as well as the name of the manufacturer.

Amount Ingested
The amount ingested is often difficult to determine. For example, a child may be found with an empty bottle of medication, and the parent may be unable to determine how full the bottle was before ingestion. Parents often underestimate the amount consumed or provide unreliable information. For example, a parent reports that a child has taken only two digoxin tablets and bases that estimation on the fact that the child was alone for only a short period or that the tablets have an unpleasant taste.

Drugs can be both therapeutic agents and poisons, depending on the dose. Thus, a 2-year-old who takes two iron-containing multiple vitamin tablets would require no treatment; the same child who takes 15 adult ferrous sulfate tablets may be severely poisoned.

Time Since Ingestion
The time since ingestion is important to know because an emetic is useful only if a substantial amount of the ingested substance remains in the stomach. Thus, an emetic is not recommended if several hours have elapsed after ingestion of quickly absorbed agents, yet its use may be appropriate several hours after ingestion of agents that are slow to leave the stomach. Drugs that slow gastric emptying and GI motility include anticholinergics, such as atropine and scopolamine, as well as drugs that have anticholinergic activity, such as antihistamines, antidepressants, and phenothiazines.

Symptoms
Certain symptoms contraindicate the use of emetics. For example, if CNS depression or other significant symptoms such as lethargy, somnolence, ataxia, hallucinations, or seizures are present, a nonprescription emetic at home should not be used because it could have serious toxic effects such as convulsions or respiratory depression. Patients with those

symptoms must be referred to a physician or emergency room for immediate medical evaluation and treatment.

Illnesses or Other Drugs
It is important to consider the impact of preexisting illnesses or of therapeutic prescription or nonprescription medications on the toxicity expected or on recommendations for therapy. For example, patients with a preexisting seizure disorder, particularly if it is not well controlled, would not be good candidates for ipecac syrup use at home. Patients chronically taking theophylline would be at higher risk from an additional theophylline ingestion and would need to be referred to an emergency department after ingesting lower doses than would individuals taking the same single acute dose of theophylline.

Patient's Age and Weight
Information on the toxicity of an agent is generally provided on a dose per body weight (mg/kg) basis. Thus, knowledge of the patient's weight is often needed to determine appropriate treatment. The patient's age may also help to determine the appropriateness and dose of an emetic.

Prior Treatment
The practitioner must determine if any first aid or other procedure has been performed. Some procedures, such as the use of salt water as an emetic, may actually cause toxicity, resulting in such conditions as hypernatremia and convulsions. Such effects would influence further treatment recommendations.

Name and Location of Patient
If talking with the patient or caretaker by phone, the practitioner should ask for the patient's name, location, and telephone number in case the call is cut off. This also allows for follow-up by the pharmacist or poison control center staff.

Appropriate information should also be sought to help answer the following questions: Is an emetic indicated? Are there any contraindications to using an emetic? Can the emetic be administered safely outside an emergency treatment facility? Poison control centers are available to help pharmacists answer these questions or handle referrals. Pharmacists should be prepared to contact the nearest poison control center if the need arises. A list of certified regional centers is printed in the appendix at the end of this chapter.

Treatment of Poisoning

Treatment of poisoning depends primarily on basic management principles, including prevention of absorption and provision of supportive care. Support of vital functions, especially respiratory and cardiovascular, is critical. Treatment of specific symptoms such as seizures is also important, as are other specific treatments, including emptying the stomach and administering agents such as adsorbents, cathartics, or antidotes. Stomach contents may be emptied by mechanical lavage or removed by administration of an emetic such as syrup of ipecac. Both techniques are most effective if used shortly after the ingestion. However, these treatments do not replace the need for symptomatic and supportive care, and many patients will detoxify themselves and survive with *only* care of that nature.

Gastric Lavage
Gastric lavage is a procedure in which a tube is placed into the stomach through the mouth or nose and the esophagus. Fluid is then instilled into the tube, allowed to mix with stomach contents, and removed through suction or aspiration.

Syrup of Ipecac
Syrup of ipecac is the emetic of choice. It is prepared from ipecac powder, a natural product derived from *Cephaelis ipecacuanha* or *acuminata*, and contains approximately 2.1 g of powdered ipecac per 30 mL. Vomiting is probably produced by both a local irritant effect on the GI mucosa and a central medullary effect (stimulation of the CTZ).[10] The central effect is probably caused by emetine and cephaeline, two alkaloids present in ipecac.

When a patient asks to purchase syrup of ipecac, the pharmacist should determine whether it is to be used immediately to treat a poison ingestion or kept in the home as a first-aid measure. If the purchase is for immediate use, the pharmacist should determine whether that use is appropriate and whether the local poison center or other medical advisor has been contacted. If the answer is no in either case, the pharmacist should contact the poison center to alert it of the problem and to receive instructions on how to manage the ingestion and instruct the purchaser.

If the ipecac is being purchased should an ingestion occur in the future, the pharmacist should discuss poison prevention with the patient, distribute poison prevention materials, and provide the telephone number of the nearest poison control center. Additionally, the purchaser should be advised that, whenever possible in poisoning emergencies, syrup of ipecac should not be given without first consulting a poison control center, pharmacist, or physician.

Dosages For children 1 year of age and older, the recommended dose of syrup of ipecac is 15 mL (1 tbsp), and this dose can be repeated once if vomiting has not occurred within 20 minutes. Children under 1 year of age may be given 5–10 mL (1 to 2 tsp). Although home use of ipecac in children under 1 year of age is controversial, a recent study has shown that this practice is both safe and effective.[11] For adolescents and adults, the initial dose is 15–30 mL and it can be repeated once, if necessary. Syrup of ipecac is virtually 100% effective when 15 mL or more are given.[12]

Recommended Procedure Ipecac does not work as well if the stomach is nearly empty. Therefore, it is recommended that at least 6–8 oz of a fluid be given to children and 12–16 oz be given to adults immediately after the ipecac dose to partially distend the stomach. One study of adult volunteers given a 15-mL ipecac dose suggests that the time needed to induce vomiting is longer when milk is given with the ipecac than when other fluids are used.[13] However, two studies of overdosed children given either milk or water with ipecac showed no difference in time for vomiting to occur.[14,15] Thus, the use of clear fluid is preferred because administration of milk offers no apparent advantages over that of clear fluid, and milk may obscure examination of the vomitus for evidence of tablets and capsules. Vomiting should occur within 15–20 minutes. If it has not, the initial dose of syrup of ipecac should be repeated.

Whether fluids are given before or after ipecac or whether the fluids are tepid (104°F or 40°C) or cold (50°F or 10°C) does not appear to affect the time for vomiting to occur in adults.[16] Although no scientific evidence exists, patients who are ambulatory seem to vomit more quickly than those who are not; therefore, children should be encouraged to play quietly rather than recline, and adults should be encouraged to move around.

If the patient is to be brought to an emergency facility or physician's office for follow-up, the patient should vomit into a bucket or other container and that container should be brought to the treatment facility so the vomitus can be inspected for evidence of the poison. It is not necessary or advisable to wait for the patient to vomit before setting out. A container should be taken along in case the patient vomits en route to treatment.

Ipecac Toxicity Toxicity following syrup of ipecac administration is rare. After therapeutic doses, diarrhea and slight CNS depression are common; mild GI upset may last for several hours following emesis. Clinical experience has shown that ingestion of 30 mL of syrup of ipecac (the largest amount available without a prescription in a single unit of purchase) is safe in children over 1 year of age. (The death of a 14-month-old child following administration of less than 30 mL of ipecac syrup given for an ingestion of amaryllis leaves was not a direct result of the pharmacologic effects of ipecac but rather was due to a congenital anomaly.)[17] In larger doses, ipecac is cardiotoxic and may cause hypotension, bradycardia, atrial fibrillation, ventricular fibrillation, and death.[10,18]

Several cases of chronic ipecac poisoning by proxy have been reported; in these cases, parents have repeatedly given ipecac syrup and have sought medical attention for repeated vomiting.[19] This has been described as a form of Münchausen's syndrome by proxy.[19] Most patients demonstrate recurrent GI effects, including grossly bloody stools, and other effects such as cardiac myopathy.[19]

Fluidextract of ipecac is 14 times stronger than syrup of ipecac and should no longer be found in any pharmacy. Severe toxicity and death have occurred when fluidextract of ipecac was given by mistake.[20–22]

Pharmacists must be aware that syrup of ipecac is used inappropriately by some bulimic patients to remove food from the stomach and to lose weight. This practice is particularly dangerous because it brings about a drug-induced fluid and electrolyte imbalance and cardiotoxicity. However, the abuse problem does not warrant removing 1-oz (30-mL) bottles of syrup of ipecac from nonprescription status.[23,24] Pharmacists should question any person buying syrup of ipecac regularly to be certain it is being purchased for its appropriate use, and they should view with suspicion frequent purchases by the same person.

Expired Ipecac Using drugs beyond their stated expiration date is not recommended as a general rule. If, however, parents have an expired container of ipecac syrup and it is the only ipecac available, should it be used? A recent study demonstrated no difference in the percentage of patients who vomited or in the time lapsed before vomiting when ipecac was used either within the expiration date or beyond it.[25] The ipecac used in this study ranged from 1 month to 16 years beyond the expiration date.

Drug Interactions The only potential drug interaction with syrup of ipecac involves activated charcoal. Activated charcoal is used as an adsorbent in many poisoning cases. When it is administered with ipecac, the concern has been that the ipecac may be adsorbed by the charcoal, thus delaying or preventing emesis. In addition, the adsorptive capacity of the charcoal could be reduced. However, a recent prospective study disproved these concerns.[26] In fact, there is no scientific evidence that administering ipecac syrup either after or at the same time as activated charcoal inhibits vomiting. However, although use of activated charcoal and ipecac may be an appropriate combination regimen in an emergency room, it is not currently recommended for use at home.

Ipecac Versus Lavage Several studies have compared the efficacy of ipecac treatment and lavage in removing gastric contents. One study found ipecac to be superior in removing salicylates from 20 patients 12–20 months of age;[27] another found it superior in removing a toxic dose of aspirin from two adults.[28] A third study determined that ipecac was three times as effective as lavage when treatment was delayed.[29] However, a prospective study using thiamine as a marker in overdosed patients found that lavage was superior to induced emesis.[30–32] Concerns relating to methodology leave findings of various studies unresolved.[33]

Generally speaking, ipecac syrup, when used with appropriate instruction and follow-up, is the only safe and effective in-home method of induced emesis. Not only can it prevent emergency room visits, but in those cases when treatment in the hospital is necessary, it also allows for earlier administration and vomiting. In the hospital setting, however, both induced emesis and lavage are frequently used. Some hospitals prefer lavage over ipecac, particularly for adults; others have stopped using GI decontamination in favor of activated charcoal alone. Further discussion of the merits of this latter approach is provided below.

Activated Charcoal

Activated charcoal is an effective adsorbent for most drugs and chemicals. It is usually administered as a water slurry (60–100 g for adults and 15–30 g for children in 250 mL of water). The slurry can be prepared by adding water to the container and shaking it. Because measuring the correct amount of charcoal is difficult, preweighed packages are available in glass or polyethylene containers.

Activated charcoal preparations with a higher surface area (e.g., Superchar®) have been developed and are approximately three times as effective as traditional activated charcoal. Products premixed with water, the cathartic sorbitol, or water and carboxymethylcellulose are commercially available. When multiple doses of activated charcoal are given, a cathartic should be given only with the first dose. Pharmacists should check premixed charcoal products to see if they contain sorbitol; if they do, other cathartics should not be given and the sorbitol-containing product should be given only once.

Optimally, activated charcoal should be given as soon as possible after ingestion; however, in some cases, it has been shown to be effective even when administration has been delayed by several hours. There is no systemic toxicity or maximum dose limit. Repeat doses of activated charcoal are recommended to interrupt enterohepatic recycling and to bind agents secreted into the GI tract (e.g., phenobarbital, cyclic antidepressants, or theophylline).

Contrary to popular belief, burnt toast is not a substitute for activated charcoal and is not indicated in the treatment of poisoning.

Although not effective for all ingestions, activated charcoal can reduce absorption of many poisons such as analgesics (e.g., salicylates, acetaminophen, or propoxyphene), sedatives, hypnotics, and tricyclic antidepressants (see Table 2). Previously, a "universal antidote" mixture of activated charcoal, magnesium oxide, and tannic acid was used. This combination is ineffective, however, because the adsorptive capacity of the charcoal is diminished as some of the tannic acid is adsorbed by the charcoal. The remaining tannic acid may produce significant dose-related toxicity.

Following ingestion of activated charcoal that does not contain sorbitol, a single dose of a saline cathartic such as magnesium sulfate may be administered—if bowel sounds are present—to speed elimination of the charcoal–drug complex.

The possible benefits of gastric emptying over activated charcoal in preventing absorption from the GI tract and toxicity are unclear. Studies have compared various combinations of induced gastric emptying with charcoal and cathartics.[34–37] Two studies used near-therapeutic doses or simulated overdoses in human volunteers.[35,36] Two other studies used a clinic trial prospective design of overdose patients treated in an emergency room.[36,37] Both pairs of studies showed no added benefit of induced GI emptying over charcoal alone in hospital-treated patients. In the home, however, activated charcoal is not a viable substitute for syrup of ipecac because it is difficult for parents to administer a therapeutic dose to children successfully.

Other Methods To Induce Emesis

Vomiting may be induced in numerous ways. Syrup of ipecac, however, is the only safe and effective nonprescription emetic. Home remedies (emetics) other than ipecac produce erratic and unpredictable results, are often ineffective, and are sometimes dangerous.

Liquid dishwashing detergent, which contains anionic and nonionic surfactants, has been studied as an emetic agent.[38] Almost all patients who drank most of the administered solution vomited, although many patients refused to drink any or all of it. Administration of liquid dishwashing solution should not replace the use of syrup of ipecac. However, when ipecac cannot be obtained quickly, liquid dishwashing detergent can be considered. The pharmacist must be aware that the ingredients in liquid dishwashing detergent are subject to frequent reformulation and that toxic ingredients may be included in the future. For this reason, it would be appropriate to check with a poison control center or manufacturer before recommending a given product. It should also be noted that automatic dishwasher products and laundry detergents contain caustic ingredients and must *never* be used as emetics.

Salt water is an unpalatable, unreliable, and potentially dangerous emetic. Salt solutions may be quite toxic because of sodium absorption; in fact, using salt as an emetic has produced fatalities in children and adults.[39,40] If vomiting is not produced, severe hypernatremia may result. It is estimated that 1 tbsp (15 mL) of salt contains about 250 mEq of sodium. If retained and absorbed,

TABLE 2 Compounds known to be effectively bound by activated charcoal in man or animals

Oral-activated charcoal inhibits absorption of the following chemicals from the gastrointestinal tract[a]

Acetaminophen	Methyl salicylate
Aconitine	Nadolol
d-Amphetamine	Nicotine
Aspirin	Nortriptyline
Atropine	Paraquat
Barbital	Pentobarbital
Benzene	Phencyclidine
Carbamazepine	Phenobarbital
Chlordane	Phenylbutazone
Chloroquine	Phenylpropanolamine
Chlorpheniramine	Phenytoin
Chlorpromazine	Propantheline
Chlorpropamide	Propoxyphene
Digoxin	Quinine
Doxepin	Salicylamide
Ethchlorvynol	Secobarbital
Ethylene glycol	Sodium salicylate
Glutethimide	Sodium valproate
Hexachlorophene	Strychnine
Kerosene	Theophylline
Malathion	Tetracycline
Mefenamic acid	Tolbutamide
Mercuric chloride	Yohimbine

Multiple oral doses of activated charcoal accelerate body clearance of the following drugs[b]

Carbamazepine	Phenobarbital
Dapsone	Phenylbutazone
Digitoxin	Theophylline
Nadolol	

[a]Based on controlled experimental investigations in man or experimental animals.
[b]Not necessarily clinically significant.

Adapted with permission from Ellenhorn M, Barceloux D, eds. *Medical Toxicology: Diagnosis and Treatment of Human Poisoning*. 1st ed. New York: Elsevier Science Publishing; 1988: 59.

this amount could raise the serum sodium level by 25 mEq/L in a healthy 3-year-old child with an estimated total body water of 10 L. Thus, salt water should *not* be used under any circumstances.

Mustard water is also an unreliable and unpalatable emetic that should not be routinely recommended.

Copper and zinc sulfate have been used as emetics. They act by producing direct gastric irritation that leads to reflex stimulation of the vomiting center. Copper sulfate is usually given in a dose of 150–250 mg dissolved in 30–60 mL of water. Based on the available data, copper sulfate is an effective emetic;[41] however, appropriate concerns about copper absorption and its potential toxicity[41,42] preclude recommendation of this agent to induce emesis.

Apomorphine, an opiate analog, produces rapid emesis; however, it is available only by prescription and must be given parenterally. Apomorphine may produce or worsen CNS and respiratory depression. Naloxone given intravenously can usually reverse these effects. In several cases, however, significant respiratory and/or CNS depression unresponsive to naloxone has developed in patients given apomorphine.[43]

Finally, vomiting can be mechanically induced by giving the patient fluids and then manually stimulating the gag reflex at the back of the throat with either a blunt object or a finger. The percentage of persons who vomit following this procedure is low, however, and the mean volume of vomitus is small compared with that induced by syrup of ipecac.[44] Thus, lack of efficacy and potential injury to the patient make mechanically induced vomiting a poor choice.

Contraindications to Use

CNS Depression or Seizures
Efforts to induce vomiting should not be attempted in patients who are lethargic or comatose because these patients are at high risk of aspirating gastric contents while vomiting. There is also a high risk of aspiration if vomiting occurs while a patient is experiencing a seizure. Emetics are generally not recommended when patients have taken agents that may produce a rapid decrease in level of consciousness (e.g., antidepressants) or may rapidly produce seizures (e.g., camphor or amphetamines). The stimulation of vomiting may also produce seizures if the patient has taken a poison that may cause seizures.

Caustic Ingestions
Patients who have ingested a caustic substance should *not* be made to vomit. Caustic agents are strong acids or bases that can produce severe burns of the mucous membranes of the GI tract, including the mouth, esophagus, and stomach. Should vomiting occur, the esophagus and oral cavity would be reexposed to the caustic agent and more damage could occur. In addition, if the esophagus is already damaged, the force of vomiting could cause esophageal or gastric perforation.

When ingestion of a caustic agent is suspected, the patient, if conscious and able to drink, should immediately be given water or milk to dilute the caustic agents. Attempts to neutralize the caustic agent using an acid or base would generate heat and produce more serious injury and must therefore be avoided. Most patients who have ingested a caustic agent should be immediately referred to a medical facility.

Controversial Areas

Antiemetic Drug Ingestion
Emetic use in cases of acute overdose of antiemetic medications is controversial. Concern exists that if an emetic is not given soon after an antiemetic has been ingested, a significant emetic failure rate may result. Two limited studies suggest, however, that this is not a problem clinically.[45,46] If an emetic is given and vomiting does not occur, gastric lavage may be necessary to remove the ingested antiemetic substance.

Hydrocarbon Ingestion
Patients who have ingested aliphatic hydrocarbons (e.g., kerosene, gasoline, or furniture polish) traditionally have not been given emetics because induced vomiting has been thought to increase the likelihood of aspirating the hydrocarbon into the lungs, leading to alveolar irritation and pneumonitis. Even though studies have shown that aspiration is not likely to occur when vomiting is induced, emptying the stomach of aliphatic hydrocarbons is generally not necessary. This is because the systemic toxicity caused by these agents does not appear to be directly related to their absorption. However, when a potentially dangerous chemical such as a pesticide is dissolved in a hydrocarbon base, emptying the stomach may be necessary, and the use of syrup of ipecac is generally considered appropriate.

A retrospective study revealed that, of patients who had ingested petroleum distillates, a lower percentage developed aspiration pneumonitis when vomiting was induced with ipecac than when lavage was used or vomiting occurred spontaneously.[47] Other research has shown that aspiration pneumonitis is less likely to occur in ipecac-treated patients than in those who were lavaged and is less severe in the former group when it does occur.[48] Based on these findings, it is suggested that ipecac be used instead of gastric lavage for alert patients who have ingested a hydrocarbon and for whom gastric removal is necessary. Use of ipecac syrup in aliphatic hydrocarbon ingestions is generally not recommended outside of a hospital setting, however.

Antiemetics

Nausea and vomiting are symptoms common to many minor as well as serious disorders. Most minor nausea and vomiting, such as that which occurs with motion sickness or overeating, is self-limiting and requires minimal therapy.

Although many patients choose to self-medicate their nausea and vomiting with various nonprescription products to avoid visiting a physician, the pharmacist should be cautious about recommending self-medication for these symptoms and should question the patient to determine whether referral to a physician is indicated.

Evaluation

In assessing the patient's complaint, the pharmacist should determine:

- Age of the patient;
- Onset and duration of symptoms;
- Description of precipitating factors;
- Complete history of recent medication use;
- Symptoms other than nausea and vomiting;
- Current chronic or acute medical conditions.

Symptoms or medical conditions associated with nausea and vomiting that necessitate physician referral include:

- Blood in the vomitus;

- Abdominal pain or distention;
- Prolonged nausea and vomiting (> 24–48 hours), especially for children under 1 year of age, or projectile vomiting;
- Dehydration;
- Weight loss of more than 5% of body weight;
- Fever;
- Severe headache;
- Change in behavior or alertness;
- Pregnancy;
- Presence of diabetes or other medical conditions that may be affected by lack of nutritional intake or missed doses of oral medications;
- Recent trauma, particularly a significant head injury.

The following are some of the more important considerations in determining whether an antiemetic should be used.

Age of Patient

Vomiting in newborns results from a number of serious abnormalities, including obstruction of the GI tract, neurologic disorders, and neuromuscular control disorders, and it may lead to acid–base disturbances and dehydration. Dehydration and electrolyte disturbances occur more often in children and, if not appropriately managed, may result in death. Thus, physician referral is recommended for further evaluation of any vomiting in newborns.

Regurgitation or spitting up, in which milk appears to spill gently from the mouth, is common in infants. Often the causes are simple, such as overfeeding, too rapid feeding, ineffective burping, laying the infant down after feeding, and immaturity of the esophageal sphincters. Regurgitation generally should not cause concern and does not require physician referral.

One of the more common causes of vomiting in children is acute viral gastroenteritis. However, acute onset of vomiting in children can also be secondary to head trauma, toxic ingestion, CNS infection, and GI obstruction. Treatment of gastroenteritis is directed primarily at preventing and correcting dehydration and electrolyte disturbances. Fluid loss should generally be replaced within 24 hours. Oral rehydration solutions may be used in mild cases. If severe diarrhea or vomiting persists for more than 24–48 hours, the child should be referred to a physician for evaluation and for parenteral fluid and electrolyte replacement.[49] Antiemetic studies have included primarily adult patients. Some clinicians question the wisdom and value of treating children with antiemetics in an acute, self-limiting disorder. It is suggested that vomiting in gastroenteritis is a host defense process that sheds the pathogen and should therefore not be suppressed. However, recurrent or protracted vomiting can lead to marked dehydration and electrolyte imbalance that cannot be ignored, especially in small children.

Pregnancy

Nausea, with or without vomiting, may be one of the earliest symptoms of pregnancy. A woman who experiences nausea and vomiting, and who has no other symptoms except a missed menstrual period and perhaps weight gain, should be referred for a pregnancy test and follow-up. Women who report nausea and vomiting during pregnancy generally suffer these symptoms in the early part of the day—hence the term "morning sickness." However, some pregnant women experience these symptoms in the afternoon or evening, and a small number of women experience morning sickness throughout the day.

Nausea and vomiting during the first trimester of pregnancy are real and often worrisome to the patient. These symptoms, which may be mild to severe, should be taken seriously and the patient reassured. However, because teratogenicity is a major consideration during pregnancy, most physicians are reluctant to prescribe any medication for a pregnant woman unless it is absolutely necessary. Indications for nonprescription antiemetics approved by the Food and Drug Administration (FDA) do not include the treatment of nausea and vomiting associated with pregnancy. Instead, health care professionals most often recommend nonpharmacologic approaches such as eating small, frequent meals; lowering the fat content of meals; ingesting crackers before arising in the morning; lying down; and avoiding precipitating factors. If nausea and/or vomiting continue despite such measures, patients should be referred to their physician.

Motion Sickness

Motion sickness occurs when visual and vestibular stimuli are not in accord. The symptoms consist of pallor, yawning, restlessness, nausea, and then vomiting. Although anyone can experience motion sickness, some individuals are more likely to be affected than others, and susceptibility appears to vary with age. Infants are generally least likely to experience it whereas young children aged 2–12 years are more likely to do so. In young children, motion sickness associated with car travel may be minimized by placing the child in a car seat. The resulting elevation and position is sufficient to allow vision out of the front window and may prevent the disorder. Antihistamines are the primary nonprescription agents used to prevent or control motion sickness.

Overeating

For complaints associated with excessive or disagreeable food or beverage intake, avoidance or moderation of consumption may prove beneficial. Otherwise, antacids or bismuth-containing products are indicated for the relief of heartburn, indigestion, and upset stomach associated with dietary overindulgence.

Current Medication Use

Many medications, such as cancer chemotherapeutic agents, narcotics, antibiotics, and estrogens, are known to cause nausea and vomiting as an adverse side effect. Other medications, such as digitalis or theophylline, may produce nausea and vomiting as a sign of toxicity. In these situations, nonprescription antiemetics are not indicated, and referral to a physician is appropriate.

Other Medical Problems

Bulimia (binge–purge behavior) is a psychologic disorder in which patients attempt to control weight by repeated vomiting and the chronic use of emetics (most commonly syrup of ipecac), and such patients should be referred for medical and psychologic management of the underlying problems.[50] Patients with other chronic medical conditions, such as diabetes, which could be affected by lack of nutritional intake or missed doses of medication, should also be referred to their physician. In addition, any patient who exhibits severe nausea, vomiting, and abdominal pain or who has forceful, bloody, or protracted vomiting should be seen by a physician immediately, as should adults in whom vomiting persists for more than 2 days.

Ingredients in Nonprescription Products

Antacids

Antacids neutralize gastric acidity, thereby increasing the pH of the stomach and duodenum. Antacids are therefore indicated for the symptomatic relief of upset stomach associated with hyperacidity. This includes complaints of heartburn, gastroesophageal reflux, and acid indigestion. For relief of these symptoms, 15 mL of most antacids should be taken 20–40 minutes after meals and at bedtime. Because antacids may impair the absorption of many drugs, patients may be counseled not to take certain other oral medications within 1 to 2 hours of the antacid dose. The available nonprescription antacid products contain various combinations of drugs such as magnesium hydroxide, aluminum hydroxide, calcium carbonate, and magnesium carbonate. (See Chapter 11, "Antacid Products," for a thorough review of antacid pharmacotherapy.)

Antihistamines

Antihistamines are the primary nonprescription agents used as antiemetics. These agents depress labyrinth excitability and therefore are effective, to varying degrees, for the prevention and control of motion sickness. The available nonprescription antihistamine preparations that are classified as safe and effective for the prevention and treatment of nausea, vomiting, or dizziness associated with motion sickness include meclizine (Bonine®), cyclizine (Marezine®), dimenhydrinate (Dramamine®), and diphenhydramine (Benadryl®). The FDA has stated, however, that the effectiveness of all nonprescription antiemetic agents for the treatment of nausea and vomiting not associated with motion sickness has not been determined.

Meclizine and cyclizine are members of the piperazine group of antihistamine compounds. Dosages of meclizine for adults are 25–50 mg once a day. The drug has a relatively long duration of action and may be administered every 24 hours. The initial dose should be taken 1 hour prior to travel, if possible. Meclizine is not recommended for children under 12 years of age. Adult dosages of cyclizine are 50 mg every 4–6 hours, not to exceed 200 mg in 24 hours. Pediatric dosages for children 6–12 years of age are 25 mg every 6–8 hours, not to exceed 75 mg in 24 hours; cyclizine is not recommended for children under 6 years of age. Cyclizine has a shorter duration of action than meclizine and therefore requires more frequent dosing. The initial dose of cyclizine should be taken approximately 1 hour prior to travel.

In 1965, the FDA required that products containing meclizine and cyclizine carry a warning against their use during pregnancy. This warning was based on animal studies and anecdotal case reports, which suggested that the drugs might have teratogenic potential. However, subsequent epidemiologic studies of pregnant women have not shown an increase in fetal deaths or malformations with exposure to these drugs during the first trimester,[51] and the warning regarding possible teratogenic effects of these agents during pregnancy is no longer required. Still, these agents do not have an FDA-approved indication for the management of nausea and vomiting associated with pregnancy. Antihistamines appear to have a low risk of teratogenicity but should be reserved for pregnant women who have severe nausea and vomiting that is unresponsive to nonpharmacologic measures.[52] Pregnant women should always consult their physician before taking any medication.

Doxylamine is an antihistamine of the ethanolamine class. Doxylamine was in the combination product, Bendectin®, which the FDA had approved for the treatment of nausea and vomiting in pregnancy. This product was withdrawn from the market in 1983 because of the high cost of defending the manufacturer against lawsuits claiming birth defects in infants exposed to it. However, the ingredients, doxylamine and pyridoxine, are still available as nonprescription products, and many physicians continue to recommend these agents for control of nausea and vomiting in pregnancy that does not respond to nonpharmacologic management.

Dimenhydrinate, the 8-chlorotheophyllinate salt of the antihistamine diphenhydramine, is safe and effective for the prevention and treatment of nausea and vomiting associated with motion sickness. The usual adult dosage is 50–100 mg every 4–6 hours, not to exceed 400 mg in 24 hours. The dosage for children aged 2–6 years is 12.5–25 mg every 6–8 hours, not to exceed 75 mg in 24 hours. For children aged 6–12 years, the dose is 25–50 mg every 6–8 hours, not to exceed 150 mg in 24 hours.

Diphenhydramine, an antihistamine of the ethanolamine class, is also safe and effective for the prevention and treatment of motion sickness. The recommended dosage for adults is 25–50 mg every 4–6 hours, not to exceed 300 mg in 24 hours. The recommended dosage for children (> 20 lbs or 9.1 kg) is 12.5–25 mg every 4–6 hours, not to exceed 150 mg in 24 hours.

The antihistamines mentioned above should be taken 30–60 minutes before departure for travel and continued during travel to be effective in preventing motion sickness. Drowsiness with therapeutic doses of antihistamines can occur and is the most common side effect. Patients should be cautioned not to drive a vehicle, operate hazardous machinery, or engage in tasks requiring a high degree of mental alertness and physical dexterity while using these products. The effects are additive to those of other CNS depressants such as alcohol, tranquilizers, hypnotics, and sedatives. In large doses, these agents may also produce anticholinergic adverse effects including blurred vision, dry mouth, and urinary retention. Antihistamines should be used with caution in patients with asthma, narrow-angle glaucoma, obstructive disease of the GI or genitourinary tracts, or benign prostatic hypertrophy.

Pyridoxine

Pyridoxine (vitamin B_6) is a water-soluble B complex vitamin that is essential in the human diet. Uncontrolled studies in the 1940s suggested that pyridoxine might be effective in the treatment of nausea and vomiting associated with pregnancy. Although the American Medical Association

Council on Drugs stated in 1979 that there was no conclusive evidence that pyridoxine was effective for this indication, a more recent controlled study using 25 mg of pyridoxine given orally every 8 hours produced significant improvement in women who complained of severe nausea and vomiting during pregnancy.[53] As noted above, pyridoxine was included in the formulation of Bendectin® (10 mg pyridoxine and 10 mg doxylamine), which had FDA approval for the management of nausea and vomiting during pregnancy until it was withdrawn from the market in 1983.

Phosphorated Carbohydrate Solution

Phosphorated carbohydrate solution (Emetrol®, Calm-X®, Nausetrol®) is a mixture of levulose (fructose), dextrose (glucose), and phosphoric acid; phosphoric acid is added to adjust the pH of the commercial product to between 1.5 and 1.6. This hyperosmolar carbohydrate product is indicated for nausea and vomiting associated with upset stomach caused by intestinal flu, food indiscretions, and emotional upset. Theoretically, this mixture has the potential to inhibit gastric emptying and reduce gastric tone through the high osmotic pressure exerted by the solution of simple sugars. There are no clinical studies establishing the efficacy of this product; therefore, the FDA Advisory Review Panel on Over-the-Counter Antiemetic Products classified phosphorated carbohydrate as Category III (insufficient evidence to establish effectiveness).

The usual adult dosage of the phosphorated carbohydrate is 15–30 mL or 1 to 2 tbsp at 15-minute intervals until vomiting ceases. Doses should be limited to no more than five and should not be taken for more than 1 hour. The solution should not be diluted, and the patient should not consume other liquids for 15 minutes after taking a dose. If vomiting does not cease after five doses, a physician should be contacted. Large doses of fructose may cause abdominal pain and diarrhea. Practitioners should be aware of the product's high glucose content and of associated problems in persons with diabetes. Phosphorated carbohydrate should not be used by individuals with hereditary fructose intolerance.

Bismuth Salts

Bismuth salts have been used for centuries for various GI complaints such as upset stomach, indigestion, nausea, and diarrhea. Bismuth subsalicylate (Pepto-Bismol®) is available as a nonprescription suspension and chewable tablet for the relief of upset stomach associated with nausea, heartburn, and fullness (gas) caused by overindulgence of food and drink. The proposed mechanism of action is a coating effect of the bismuth preparation on the gastric mucosa. Bismuth salts appear to be poorly absorbed from the GI tract, although the large quantities of bismuth subsalicylate recommended in nonprescription preparations may allow for absorption of some salicylate. Patients should be counseled that the mouth, tongue, and stool may temporarily appear gray-black or black while bismuth-containing products are being used. Also, patients should avoid bismuth subsalicylate if they are taking medications that may interact adversely with salicylates. Other bismuth salts, such as bismuth subgallate, bismuth subcarbonate, and bismuth subnitrate, may also be found in nonprescription products marketed for GI complaints. Bismuth subsalicylate should *never* be recommended for children with viral influenza or chickenpox because of concern about development of Reye's syndrome.

Oral Rehydration Solutions

Dehydration secondary to vomiting and diarrhea is a result of a net loss of extracellular fluid that is composed of sodium, chloride, potassium, water, and bicarbonate. Replacement of fluid should mimic extracellular fluid losses. Active glucose absorption in the small bowel promotes sodium absorption. Therefore, oral rehydration therapy is based on the use of glucose to increase sodium absorption and allow for rapid replacement of extracellular fluid.[54] Oral electrolyte mixtures for rehydration include Pedialyte®, Lytren®, Ricelyte®, Infalyte®, Gastrolyte®, Rehydralyte®, Resol®, and Pediatric Maintenance Solution®. Although not as osmotically or chemically balanced, gelatin water, Gatorade®, fruit juices, and carbonated beverages can also be administered. These products are adequate energy sources but are too low in sodium, potassium, and chloride to produce a rapid and significant therapeutic response to severe dehydration with electrolyte depletion. Use of homemade sugar–water or salt–water solutions should be discouraged. If the child is vomiting, the fluid should be given very slowly, starting with 5 to 10 mL every 10 minutes. The quantity of fluid may be increased as tolerated. If vomiting and diarrhea have stopped after 24 hours of clear liquids, the child may gradually return to a regular diet over the next 2 or 3 days.[49]

Scopolamine

Some data indicate that scopolamine may be more effective as an antiemetic than some of the currently available antihistamines.[55-57] Scopolamine is available by prescription as a transdermal patch that can be easily applied and removed before and after travel but must be applied well in advance of motion that may cause nausea. Side effects are minimal and may include drowsiness and some anticholinergic effects such as blurred vision and dry mouth. Scopolamine may also result in dry eyes, which can pose a problem for contact lens wearers.

Summary

Nonprescription emetic and antiemetic products are intended to be used for the treatment of minor self-limiting conditions.

Emetics are useful in cases of poisoning to remove gastric contents and to prevent further absorption of the ingested agent. Syrup of ipecac is the safest and most effective nonprescription emetic for this purpose. It should be kept in all homes with young children (a 1-oz [30-mL] bottle for each child under 5 years of age) and used with the guidance of a poison control center or physician if an ingestion occurs. The pharmacist should ascertain why an emetic (syrup of ipecac) is being purchased and provide appropriate guidance in its use, suggesting referral if necessary.

Antiemetics are useful in limited situations, but should always be used with caution because of the potential danger of masking the symptoms of more severe disease. The pharmacist should ascertain why an antiemetic is being purchased and suggest referral if necessary. Chronic unsupervised use of antiemetics, especially for an upset stomach, should be discouraged, and the patient should be encouraged to seek additional medical evaluation for continuous discomfort. Overuse or misuse of nonprescription antiemetics may result in adverse effects, toxicity, or delayed diagnosis and treatment of serious medical conditions.

References

1. Borison HL, Wang L. Physiology and pharmacology of vomiting. *Pharmacol Rev* 1953; 5: 193–230.
2. Cummins AJ. Nausea and vomiting. *Am J Dig Dis* 1958; 3: 710–21.
3. Feldman M. Nausea and vomiting. In: Sleisenger MH, Fordtran JS, eds. *Gastrointestinal Disease: Pathophysiology, Diagnosis, Management*. 4th ed. Philadelphia: W. B. Saunders; 1989: 222–38.
4. Friedman LS, Isselbacher KJ. Anorexia, nausea, vomiting and indigestion. In: Wilson JD, Braunwald E, Isselbacher KJ, et al., eds. *Harrison's Principles of Internal Medicine*. 12th ed. New York: McGraw-Hill; 1991: 251–6.
5. Brand J, Perry W. Drugs used in motion sickness. *Pharmacol Rev* 1966; 18: 895–924.
6. Cunningham FG et al., eds. *Williams Obstetrics*. 18th ed. Norwalk, Conn: Appleton and Lange; 1989: 270–1.
7. Soules MR, Hughes CL, Garcia JA, et al. Nausea and vomiting of pregnancy: role of human chorionic gonadotropin and 17-hydroxyprogesterone. *Obstet Gynecol* 1980; 55: 696–700.
8. Kapikian AZ. Viral gastroenteritis. In: Wyngaarden JB, Smith LH, eds. *Cecil Textbook of Medicine*. 18th ed. Philadelphia: W. B. Saunders; 1988: 1768–72.
9. Litovitz TL et al. 1990 Report of the American Association of Poison Control Centers National Data Collection System. *Am J Emerg Med* 1991; 9: 461.
10. Klaassen CD. Principles of toxicology. In: Gilman AG, Rall TW, Nies AS, et al., eds. *The Pharmacological Basis for Therapeutics*. 8th ed. Elmsford, NY: Pergamon Press; 1990: 49–61.
11. Litovitz T et al. Safety and efficacy of ipecac administration in children younger than 1 year of age. *Pediatrics* 1985; 76: 761.
12. Robertson WO. Syrup of ipecac—a fast or slow emetic? *Am J Dis Child* 1972; 103: 58.
13. Varipapa RJ, Oderda GM. Effect of milk on ipecac induced emesis. *N Engl J Med* 1977; 296: 112.
14. Grbcich PA et al. Does milk delay the onset of ipecac induced emesis? *Vet Hum Toxicol* 1986; 28: 499.
15. Klein-Schwartz W et al. The effect of milk on ipecac-induced emesis. *J Toxicol Clin Toxicol* 1991; 29: 505–11.
16. Spiegel RW et al. The effect of temperature of concurrently administered fluid on the onset of ipecac induced emesis. *Clin Toxicol* 1979; 14: 281.
17. Robertson WO. Syrup of ipecac associated fatality: a case report. *Vet Hum Toxicol* 1979; 21: 87.
18. McLeod J. Ipecac intoxication—use of a cardiac pacemaker in management. *N Engl J Med* 1963; 268: 146.
19. Johnson JE et al. Hemorrhagic colitis and pseudomelanosis coli in ipecac ingestion by proxy. *J Ped Gastroenterol Nutr* 1991; 12: 501.
20. Speer JD et al. Ipecacuanha poisoning: another fatal case. *Lancet* 1963; 1: 475.
21. Bates T, Grunwaldt E. Ipecac poisoning. *Am J Dis Child* 1962; 103: 169.
22. Smith RR, Smith DM. Acute ipecac poisoning: report of a fatal case and review of the literature. *N Engl J Med* 1964; 265: 23.
23. Schiff RJ et al. Death due to chronic syrup of ipecac use in a patient with bulimia. *Pediatrics* 1986; 78: 412.
24. Litovitz T. In defense of retaining ipecac syrup as an over-the-counter drug. *Pediatrics* 1986; 82: 514.
25. Grbcich PA et al. Expired ipecac syrup efficacy. *Pediatrics* 1986; 78: 1085.
26. Freedman GE et al. A clinical trial using ipecac and activated charcoal concurrently. *Ann Emerg Med* 1987; 16: 164.
27. Boxer L et al. Comparison of ipecac induced emesis with gastric lavage in the treatment of acute salicylate ingestion. *J Pediatr* 1969; 74: 800.
28. Goldstein L. Emesis vs lavage for drug ingestion. *JAMA* 1969; 208: 2162.
29. Arnold F Jr et al. Evaluation of the efficacy of lavage and induced emesis in treatment of salicylate poisoning. *Pediatrics* 1959; 23: 286.
30. Auerbach PS et al. Efficacy of gastric emptying: gastric lavage vs emesis induced with ipecac. *Ann Emerg Med* 1986; 15: 692.
31. Vasquez TE et al. Efficacy of ipecac-induced emesis for emptying gastric contents. *Clin Nucl Med* 1988; 13: 638.
32. Tandberg D et al. Ipecac induced emesis vs gastric lavage: a controlled study in normal adults. *Am J Emerg Med* 1986; 4: 205.
33. Litovitz T. Emesis vs lavage for poisoning victims. *Am J Emerg Med* 1986; 4: 294.
34. Curtis RA et al. Efficacy of ipecac and activated charcoal/cathartic on salicylate absorption in a simulated overdose. *Arch Intern Med* 1984; 144: 48.
35. Neuvonen PJ et al. Comparison of activated charcoal and ipecac syrup in prevention of drug absorption. *Eur J Clin Pharmacol* 1983; 24: 557.
36. Kulig K et al. Management of acutely poisoned patients without gastric emptying. *Ann Emerg Med* 1985; 14: 562.
37. Merigian KS et al. *Am J Emerg Med* 1990; 8: 479.
38. Geiseker DR, Troutman WG. Emergency induction of emesis using liquid detergent product: a report of 15 cases. *Clin Toxicol* 1981; 18: 283.
39. Barer J et al. Fatal poisoning from salt used as an emetic. *Am J Dis Child* 1973; 125: 899.
40. DeGenaro F, Nyhan W. Salt—a dangerous antidote. *J Pediatr* 1971; 78: 1048.
41. Holtzman NA, Haslam HA. Elevation of serum copper following copper sulfate as an emetic. *Pediatrics* 1976; 42: 189.
42. Stein RS et al. Death after cupric sulfate. *JAMA* 1976; 235: 801.
43. Schofferman J. A clinical comparison of ipecac and apomorphine use in adults. *J Am Coll Emerg Phys* 1976; 5: 22.
44. Dabbous IA et al. The ineffectiveness of mechanically induced vomiting. *J Pediatr* 1965; 66: 952.
45. Manoguerra AS, Krenzelok EP. Rapid emesis from high dose ipecac syrup in adults and children intoxicated with antiemetics and other drugs. *Am J Hosp Pharm* 1978; 35: 1360.
46. Thoman ME, Verhulst HJL. *JAMA* 1966; 196: 433.
47. Molinas S. A note on the use of ipecac syrup by poison control centers. *National Clearinghouse for Poison Control Centers*. Washington, DC: U.S. Public Health Service; 1966.
48. Ng RC et al. Emergency treatment of petroleum distillate and turpentine ingestion. *Can Med Assoc J* 1974; 111: 537.
49. Brownlee HJ. Family practitioner's guide to patient self-treatment of acute diarrhea. *Am J Med* 1990; 88: 27S–29S.
50. Beumont PJV, George GCW, Smart DE. "Dieters" and "vomiters and purgers" in anorexia nervosa. *Psychol Med* 1976; 6: 617–22.
51. Shapiro S, Heinonen OP, Siskind V, et al. Antenatal drug

52. Leathem AM. Safety and efficacy of antiemetics used to treat nausea and vomiting in pregnancy. *Clin Pharm* 1986; 5: 660–8.
53. Sahakian V, Rouse D, Sipes S, et al. Vitamin B_6 is effective therapy for nausea and vomiting of pregnancy: a randomized, double-blind placebo-controlled study. *Obstet Gynecol* 1991; 78: 33–6.
54. Balisteri WF. Oral rehydration in acute infantile diarrhea. *Am J Med* 1990; 88: 30S–33S.
55. Clissold SP, Heel RC. Transdermal hyoscine (scopolamine): a preliminary review of its pharmacodynamic properties and therapeutic efficacy. *Drugs* 1985; 29: 189–207.
56. Noy S, Shapira S, Zilbiger A, et al. Transdermal therapeutic system scopolamine (TTSS), dimenhydrinate and placebo—a comparative study at sea. *Aviat Space Environ Med* 1984; 55: 1051–4.
57. Dahl E, Offer-Ohlsen D, Lillevold PE, et al. Transdermal scopolamine, oral meclizine, and placebo in motion sickness. *Clin Pharmacol Ther* 1984; 36: 116–20.

exposure to doxylamine succinate and dicyclomine hydrochloride (Bendectin) in relation to congenital malformations, perinatal mortality rate, birth weight, and intelligence quotient score. *Am J Obstet Gynecol* 1977; 128: 480–5.

Appendix: Major Poison Control Centers

Alabama

- Alabama Poison Center
  408-A Paul Bryant Drive
  Tuscaloosa, AL 35401
  205-345-0600
  800-462-0800 (Alabama only)

- Regional Poison Control Center
  Children's Hospital of Alabama
  1600 Seventh Avenue South
  Birmingham, AL 35233
  205-939-9201
  205-933-4050
  800-292-6678 (Alabama only)

Alaska

- Anchorage Poison Control Center
  Providence Hospital Pharmacy
  P.O. Box 196604
  Anchorage, AK 99519-6604
  907-261-3193
  800-478-3193

Arizona

- Arizona Poison and Drug Information Center
  Health Sciences Center
  1501 North Campbell, Room 3204K
  Tucson, AZ 85724
  602-626-6016 (Tucson)
  800-362-0101 (Arizona only)

- Samaritan Regional Poison Center
  Good Samaritan Medical Center
  1130 East McDowell, Suite A5
  Phoenix, AZ 85006
  602-253-3334

Arkansas

- Arkansas Poison and Drug Information Center
  College of Pharmacy-UAMS
  4301 West Markham Street, Slot 522
  Little Rock, AR 72205
  800-482-8948

California

- Fresno Regional Poison Control Center
  Fresno Community Hospital and Medical Center
  2823 North Fresno Street
  Fresno, CA 93721
  800-346-5922

- Los Angeles County Medical Association Regional Poison Center
  1925 Wilshire Boulevard
  Los Angeles, CA 90057
  213-484-5151
  800-777-6476

- San Diego Regional Poison Center
  UCSD Medical Center
  225 Dickinson Street
  San Diego, CA 92103-1990
  619-543-6000
  800-876-4766

- San Francisco Regional Poison Center
  San Francisco General Hospital
  1001 Potrero Avenue, Building 80, Room 230
  San Francisco, CA 94122
  415-476-6600
  800-523-2222

- Santa Clara Valley Medical Center
  Regional Poison Center
  751 South Bascom Avenue
  San Jose, CA 95128
  408-299-5112
  800-662-9886

- UC Davis Regional Poison Control Center
  2315 Stockton Boulevard, Room 1511
  Sacramento, CA 95817
  916-453-3692
  800-342-9293 (northern California only)

- University of California Irvine Medical Center
  Regional Poison Center
  101 The City Drive
  Route 78
  Orange, CA 92668
  714-634-5988
  800-544-4404 (southern California only)

Colorado

- Rocky Mountain Poison and Drug Center
  645 Bannock Street
  Denver, CO 80204-4507
  303-629-1123 (Colorado only)

Connecticut

- Connecticut Poison Control Center
  University of Connecticut Health Center
  309 Farmington Avenue
  Farmington, CT 06030
  800-343-2722

District of Columbia

- National Capital Poison Center
  Georgetown University Hospital
  3800 Reservoir Road, N.W.
  Washington, DC 20007
  202-625-3333
  202-784-4660 (TTY)

Florida

- Florida Poison Information Center
  The Tampa General Hospital
  Davis Islands
  P.O. Box 1289
  Tampa, FL 33601
  813-253-4444 (Tampa only)
  800-282-3171 (Florida only)

- St. Vincent's Medical Center
  1800 Barrs Street
  Jacksonville, FL 32203
  904-387-7500

- University Hospital of Jacksonville
  Clinical Toxicology Service
  655 West Eighth Street
  Jacksonville, FL 32209
  904-549-5000

Georgia

- Georgia Regional Poison Control Center
  80 Butler Street, S.E.
  Atlanta, GA 30335-3801
  404-589-4400
  800-282-5846 (Georgia only)

Hawaii

- Hawaii Poison Center
  Kapiolani Women's and Children's Medical Center
  1319 Punahou Street
  Honolulu, HI 96826
  808-941-4411

Illinois

- Chicago and Northeastern Illinois Regional
    Poison Control Center
  Rush-Presbyterian-St. Luke's Medical Center
  1653 West Congress Parkway
  Chicago, IL 60612
  312-942-5969
  800-942-5969 (Illinois only)

- Regional Poison Control Center for Central
  and Southern Illinois
  St. John's Hospital
  800 East Carpenter
  Springfield, IL 62769
  217-753-3330
  800-252-2022

Indiana

- Indiana Poison Center
  Methodist Hospital of Indiana, Inc.
  1701 North Senate Boulevard
  P.O. Box 1367
  Indianapolis, IN 46206
  317-929-2323
  317-929-2336 (TTY/TTD)
  800-382-9097 (Indiana only)

Iowa

- St. Luke's Poison Center
  St. Luke's Regional Medical Center
  2720 Stone Park Boulevard
  Sioux City, IA 51104
  712-277-2222
  800-352-2222 (statewide WATS)

- Variety Club Poison and Drug Information Center
  Iowa Methodist Medical Center
  1200 Pleasant Street
  Des Moines, IA 50309
  515-283-6254
  800-362-2327 (outside Des Moines)

Kansas

- Mid-America Poison Control Center
  Kansas University Medical Center
  Department of Pharmacy, Room B-400
  39th and Rainbow Boulevard
  Kansas City, KS 66103
  913-588-6633
  800-332-6633 (Kansas only)

Kentucky

- Kentucky Regional Poison Center of Kosair
     Children's Hospital
  315 East Broadway
  P.O. Box 35070
  Louisville, KY 40232
  502-629-7270
  800-722-5725 (Kentucky only)

Louisiana

- Terrebone General Medical Center
  936 East Main Street
  Houma, LA 70360
  504-873-4066

Maine

- Maine Poison Control Center
  Maine Medical Center
  22 Bramhall Street
  Portland, ME 04102
  207-871-2950
  800-442-6305 (Maine only)

Maryland

- Maryland Poison Center
  20 North Pine Street
  Baltimore, MD 21201
  410-528-7701
  800-492-2414 (Maryland only)

Massachusetts

- Massachusetts Poison Control System
  300 Longwood Avenue
  Boston, MA 02115
  617-232-2120 (Boston area)
  800-682-9211 (Massachusetts only)

Michigan

- Bixby Medical Center Poison Center
  818 Riverside Avenue
  Adrian, MI 49221
  517-263-0711

- Blodgett Regional Poison Center
  1840 Wealthy Street, S.E.
  Grand Rapids, MI 49506
  800-356-3232 (TTY)
  800-632-2727 (Michigan only)

- Bronson Poison Information Center
  252 East Lovell Street
  Kalamazoo, MI 49007
  616-341-6409
  800-442-4221 (Michigan only)

- Poison Control Center
  Children's Hospital of Michigan
  3901 Beaubien Boulevard
  Detroit, MI 48201
  313-745-5711 (Metro Detroit)
  800-462-6642 (rest of Michigan)

- Saginaw Regional Poison Center
  Saginaw General Hospital
  1447 North Harrison
  Saginaw, MI 48602
  517-755-1111
  800-451-4585

- University of Michigan Poison Information Center
  1500 East Medical Center Drive
  Ann Arbor, MI 48109
  313-764-7667

Minnesota

- Hennepin Regional Poison Center
  Hennepin County Medical Center
  701 Park Avenue South
  Minneapolis, MN 55415
  612-347-3141

- Minnesota Regional Poison Center
  St. Paul-Ramsey Medical Center
  640 Jackson Street
  St. Paul, MN 55101
  612-221-2113
  800-222-1222 (Minnesota only)

Mississippi

- Forrest General Hospital
  400 South 28th Avenue
  P.O. Box 16389
  Hattiesburg, MS 39402
  601-288-4235

Missouri

- Cardinal Glennon Children's Hospital
  Regional Poison Center
  1465 South Grand Boulevard
  St. Louis, MO 63104
  314-772-5200
  800-366-8888
  800-392-9111 (Missouri only)

- Children's Mercy Hospital
  24th at Gillham Road
  Kansas City, MO 64108
  816-234-3430

Nebraska

- The Poison Center
  8301 Dodge Street
  Omaha, NE 68114
  402-390-5555 (local)
  800-955-9119 (Nebraska only)
  800-228-9515 (surrounding states)

New Hampshire

- New Hampshire Poison Information Center
  Dartmouth-Hitchcock Medical Center
  2 Maynard Street
  Hanover, NH 03756
  603-646-8053
  800-562-8236 (New Hampshire only)

New Jersey

- New Jersey Poison Information
    and Educational System
  201 Lyons Avenue
  Newark, NJ 07112
  201-923-0764 (outside New Jersey)
  800-962-1253 (New Jersey only)

New Mexico

- New Mexico Poison and Drug Information Center
  University of New Mexico
  Albuquerque, NM 87131
  505-843-2551
  800-432-6866 (New Mexico only)

New York

- Central New York Poison Control Center
  750 East Adams Street
  Syracuse, NY 13210
  315-476-4766
  800-252-5655

- Ellis Hospital Poison Control Center
  1101 Nott Street
  Schenectady, NY 12308
  518-382-4039

- Finger Lakes Regional Poison Control Center
    at Life Line
  University of Rochester Medical Center
  601 Elmwood Avenue
  Box 777
  Rochester, NY 14642
  716-275-5151
  800-533-0542

- Hudson Valley Poison Center
  Nyack Hospital
  100 North Midland Avenue
  Nyack, NY 10960
  914-358-1000
  800-336-6997

- Long Island Regional Poison Control Center
  2201 Hempstead Turnpike
  East Meadow, NY 11554
  516-542-2323

- New York City Poison Center
  455 First Avenue, Room 123
  New York, NY 10016
  212-340-4494
  212-764-7667

- Western New York Poison Control Center
    at Children's Hospital of Buffalo
  219 Bryant Street
  Buffalo, NY 14222
  716-878-7654

North Carolina

- Duke Regional Poison Control Center
  Duke University Medical Center
  Box 3007
  Durham, NC 27710
  800-672-1697 (North Carolina only)

- Poison Control Center
  Catawba Memorial Hospital
  810 Fairgrove Road
  Hickory, NC 28602
  704-322-6649

- Triad Poison Center
  1200 North Elm Street
  Greensboro, NC 27401-1020
  919-379-4105 (local)
  800-722-2222 (North Carolina only)

North Dakota

- North Dakota Poison Center
  720 Fourth Street North
  Fargo, ND 58122
  701-234-5575
  800-732-2200 (North Dakota only)

Ohio

- Akron Regional Poison Center
  281 Locust Street
  Akron, OH 44308
  216-379-8562
  800-362-9922 (Ohio only)

- Bethesda Poison Control Center
  Bethesda Hospital
  2951 Maple Avenue
  Zanesville, OH 43701
  614-454-4221

- Central Ohio Poison Center
  700 Children's Drive
  Columbus, OH 43205
  614-228-1323
  800-682-7625

- Greater Cleveland Poison Control Center
  2074 Abington Road
  Cleveland, OH 44106
  216-231-4455

- Mahoning Valley Poison Center
  St. Elizabeth Hospital Medical Center
  1044 Belmont Avenue
  Youngstown, OH 44501
  216-746-2222
  216-746-5510 (TTD)
  800-426-2348

- Regional Poison Control System and Cincinnati Drug and Poison Information Center
  231 Bethesda Avenue, M.L. #144
  Cincinnati, OH 45267-0144
  513-558-5111
  800-872-5111 (Ohio only)

- Stark County Poison Control Center
  1320 Timken Mercy Drive, N.W.
  Canton, OH 44708
  800-722-8662

- Western Ohio Poison and Drug Information Center
  Children's Medical Center
  One Children's Plaza
  Dayton, OH 45404
  513-222-2227
  800-762-0727

Oklahoma

- Oklahoma Poison Control Center
  Children's Memorial Hospital
  940 N.E. 13th Street
  Oklahoma City, OK 73104
  405-271-5454
  800-522-4611 (Oklahoma only)

Oregon

- Oregon Poison Center
  Oregon Health Sciences University
  3181 S.W. Sam Jackson Park Road
  Portland, OR 97201
  503-494-8968
  800-452-7165 (Oregon only)

Pennsylvania

- Central Pennsylvania Poison Center
  University Hospital
  The Milton S. Hershey Medical Center
  Hershey, PA 17033
  717-531-6111
  800-521-6110

- Poison Control Center of the Greater Philadelphia Metropolitan Area
  One Children's Center
  34th and Civic Center Boulevard
  Philadelphia, PA 19104
  215-386-2100

- Hamot Poison Information Center
  Hamot Medical Center
  201 State Street
  Erie, PA 16550-0001
  814-870-6111
  814-870-6112 (TDD)
  800-221-5252 (Pennsylvania, Ohio, New York only)

- Keystone Region Poison Center
  Mercy Hospital of Altoona
  2500 Seventh Avenue
  Altoona, PA 16603
  814-946-3711

- Lehigh Valley Poison Center
  The Allentown Hospital Site
  17th and Chew Streets
  Allentown, PA 18102
  215-433-2311

- Northwest Regional Poison Control Center
  Saint Vincent Health Center
  232 West 25th Street
  Erie, PA 16544
  814-452-3232 (24-hour hotline)
  800-822-3232 (Pennsylvania, New York, and Ohio only)

- Pittsburgh Poison Center
  One Children's Place
  3705 Fifth Avenue at DeSoto
  Pittsburgh, PA 15213
  412-681-6669

- St. Joseph Hospital and Health Care Center
  250 College Avenue
  Lancaster, PA 17604
  717-291-8111

Rhode Island

- Rhode Island Poison Center
  593 Eddy Street
  Providence, RI 02903
  401-277-5727
  401-277-8062 (TDD)

South Carolina

- Palmetto Poison Center
  University of South Carolina
  College of Pharmacy
  Columbia, SC 29208
  803-765-7359
  800-922-1117 (South Carolina only)

South Dakota

- St. Luke's Midland Regional Medical Center
  305 South State Street
  Aberdeen, SD 57401
  605-229-3100

- McKennan Poison Center
  800 East 21st Street
  Sioux Falls, SD 57117-5045
  605-336-3894
  800-952-0123 (South Dakota only)
  800-843-0505 (Iowa, Minnesota, Nebraska, and North Dakota)

Tennessee

- Middle Tennessee Regional Poison Center
  1161 21st Avenue South
  501 Oxford House
  Nashville, TN 37232-4632
  615-322-6435
  800-288-9999

- Southern Poison Center, Inc.
  848 Adams Avenue
  Memphis, TN 38103
  901-528-6048

Texas

- Medical Center Hospital
  500 Medical Center Boulevard
  Conroe, TX 77304
  409-539-7700

- North Texas Poison Center
  P.O. Box 35926
  Dallas, TX 75043
  214-590-5000
  800-441-0040 (Texas only)

- Texas State Poison Center
  University of Texas Medical Branch
  Galveston, TX 77550-2780
  409-765-1420 (Galveston)
  713-654-1701 (Houston)
  512-478-4490 (Austin)
  800-392-8548 (Texas only)

Utah

- Intermountain Regional Poison Control Center
  50 North Medical Drive, Building 528
  Salt Lake City, UT 84132
  801-581-2151
  800-456-7707 (Utah only)

Vermont

- Vermont Poison Center
  Medical Center Hospital of Vermont
  111 Colchester Avenue
  Burlington, VT 05401
  802-658-3456

Virginia

- Blue Ridge Poison Center
  Blue Ridge Hospital
  Box 67
  Charlottesville, VA 22901
  804-924-5543
  800-451-1428 (Virginia only)

- Southwest Virginia Poison Center
  Roanoke Memorial Hospitals
  Belleview at Jefferson Street
  Roanoke, VA 24033
  703-981-7336

- Tidewater Poison Center
  DePaul Medical Center
  150 Kingsley Lane
  Norfolk, VA 23505
  804-489-5288
  800-552-6337 (Virginia only)

- Virginia Poison Center
  Virginia Commonwealth University
  Box 522 MCV Station
  Richmond, VA 23298-0522
  804-786-9123
  800-552-6337 (Virginia only)

Washington

- Central Washington Poison Center
  2811 Tieton Drive
  Yakima, WA 98902
  509-248-4400
  800-572-9176 (Washington only)

- Mary Bridge Poison Center
  317 South K Street
  Box 5299
  Tacoma, WA 98405-0987
  206-594-1414
  800-542-6319 (Washington only)

- Seattle Poison Center
  Children's Hospital and Medical Center
  4800 Sand Point Way, N.E.
  Seattle, WA 98105
  206-526-2121
  206-527-4859
  800-732-6985 (Washington only)

- Spokane Poison Center
  711 South Cowley
  Spokane, WA 99202
  509-747-1077
  800-572-5842 (Washington only)
  800-541-5624 (outside Washington)

West Virginia

- West Virginia Poison Center
  3110 MacCorkle Avenue, S.E.
  Charleston, WV 25304
  304-348-4211 (local)
  800-642-3625 (West Virginia only)

Wisconsin

- Green Bay Poison Control Center
  St. Vincent Hospital
  835 South Van Buren
  Green Bay, WI 54307-3508
  414-433-8100
  414-433-8101

- LaCrosse Area Poison Center
  700 West Avenue South
  LaCrosse, WI 54601
  608-784-0971

- Milwaukee Poison Center
  Children's Hospital of Wisconsin
  P.O. Box 1997
  Milwaukee, WI 53201
  414-266-2222

- University of Wisconsin Hospital Regional
    Poison Center
  600 Highland Avenue, E5/238 CSC
  Madison, WI 53792
  608-262-3702

Chapter 13

Antidiarrheal Products

R. Leon Longe

Questions to ask in patient assessment and counseling

- *How long have you had diarrhea (≥2 days)?*
- *Was the onset of diarrhea sudden?*
- *How often do the episodes of diarrhea occur?*
- *What is the character of the stool (i.e., its consistency, odor, and color)?*
- *Do your stools contain blood or mucus?*
- *Is the diarrhea associated with other symptoms such as fever, malaise, anorexia, vomiting, dizziness, rapid heart rate, gas, or abdominal pain?*
- *Have you tried any antidiarrheal treatments or products? Which ones? How effective were they?*
- *How old are you?*
- *How often do you normally have a bowel movement?*
- *Have other family members experienced similar symptoms?*
- *Have you changed your diet recently?*
- *Can you relate the onset of diarrhea to a specific cause such as a particular meal or food (e.g., milk product) or drug?*
- *Have you recently traveled to a foreign country or a border area of the United States?*
- *Have you recently consumed nonchlorinated water such as that from a river, pond, or lake?*
- *Are you currently taking or have you recently taken any prescription or nonprescription medications? Which ones?*
- *Do you have diabetes, heart or blood vessel disease, or any other chronic medical condition?*

The frequency of normal bowel movements varies with the individual. Some healthy adults may have as many as three well-formed stools a day; others may defecate once every 2 or more days.[1] Except for vegetarians, who consume a fiber-rich diet and thus may produce daily stools of more than 300 g, the mean daily fecal weight loss is 100–150 g. An increase to 200–300 g may be interpreted as diarrhea.

Diarrhea is a symptom that is characterized by an increased frequency of loose, watery stools during a limited period. It may be acute or chronic in nature. Its presence may signal either a gastrointestinal (GI) or non-GI disease. Most often diarrhea is due to an enteritis of noninfectious or infectious etiology. A major feature of diarrhea is the excretion of a relatively large volume of water normally reabsorbed from the gut. Disruption of intestinal water absorption of even a few hundred milliliters may bring on diarrhea. The approach to treatment depends on recognizing the cause of diarrhea.

Physiology of the Intestinal Tract

The intestinal tract, consisting of the small intestine and the large intestine (colon), is a long, hollow tube surrounded by layers of smooth muscle. These include a thick, circular layer on the mucosal side of the intestine; a thinner, longitudinal layer on the serosal side; and a third layer of both circular and longitudinal muscle fibers. Active contractions of the various muscles control intestinal tone. As a rule, this tone is maintained with little energy, so the intestinal musculature stays relatively free from fatigue and remains capable of performing normally.

The small intestine, a convoluted tube about 6.4 m long, has three sections: the duodenum, jejunum, and ileum. It begins at the pylorus of the stomach and ends at the cecum of the ascending branch of the colon. Although the digestive process begins in the mouth, the small intestine is the primary site of digestion, absorption of nutrients, and retention of waste material. These activities depend on normal musculature, neurologic innervation, muscular tone, and digestive enzymes.

A mucus layer protects and lubricates the walls of the intestines. Mucus is released from goblet cells interspersed among the columnar epithelial cells in the intestines. This secretion is increased by local irritation from foods or stimulant cathartics or by psychic trauma. The mucus is more viscous in the upper portion of the small intestine than in the colon, and it forms a protective physical barrier to the intestinal lining, thus reducing contact with irritating substances, bacteria, and viruses. The alkalinity of the mucus contributes further to protection of the intestinal lining as it neutralizes acidic dietary and bacterial products.

Normal intestinal motility and peristalsis are maintained by smooth muscles and intrinsic nerves. The vagus and parasympathetic pelvic nerves stimulate intestinal motility and secretion, whereas sympathetic innervation inhibits these activities. Extrinsic autonomic innervation influences the strength and frequency of intestinal movements and mediates reflexes by which activity in one part of the intestine influences another.

Eating causes the lumen of the small and large intestines to distend and the smooth muscle layers to

TABLE 1	Electrolyte and water content of normal and diarrheal feces	
Components	Normal	Diarrheal
Bicarbonate[a]	30	30–45
Chloride[a]	15	20–40
Potassium[a]	90	35–60
Sodium[a]	40	25–50
Water[b]	0.1–0.2	3–10

[a]mEq/L.
[b]L/24 hr.

Adapted from Longe RL, DiPiro JT. In: *Pharmacotherapy: A Pathophysiologic Approach*. New York: Elsevier Science Publishing; 1989.

contract. Normally, segmental contractions of the circular muscles are accompanied by a decrease in the propulsive activity of the gut. This process mixes and retains food in the lumen and increases the duration of its exposure to digestive elements, thus enhancing digestion and absorption.

Normally, about 9 L of digestive fluid enter the GI tract daily. Of these, approximately 8 L are reabsorbed in the small intestine. The large bowel reabsorbs about 850 mL of the remaining 1 L, leaving about 150 mL to be excreted in the stool each day.

Approximately 3–5 L of stomach fluid containing electrolytes and nutrients enter the small intestine every 24 hours. Reabsorption reduces the quantity that reaches the large intestine to an isotonic semiliquid substance, chyme, which consists primarily of unabsorbed, undigested food residue; nutrients; electrolytes; water; and bacteria. Ileal chyme has an average electrolyte content of 140 mEq/L of sodium, 70 mEq/L of bicarbonate, 8 mEq/L of potassium, and 60 mEq/L of chloride. Stool electrolyte content (mEq/L) is bicarbonate 30, chloride 15, potassium 90, and sodium 40.[2]

The colon, which is about 1.5 m long, is composed of the cecum, ascending colon, transverse colon, descending colon, sigmoid colon, and rectum. It has two primary functions: absorption and storage. The first two-thirds of the colon facilitates absorption, and the remaining third functions as a storage area. The proximal half (ascending and transverse parts) of the colon reduces chyme to a semisolid substance called feces, or stool. Stool is a 75% water and 25% solid material containing unabsorbed food residue and minerals, bacteria, desquamated epithelial cells, and a small quantity of electrolytes (Table 1). Stool is generally stored in the descending colon until defecation.

The colon is structured like the small intestine, with both circular and longitudinal muscles. The longitudinal muscles are shorter than the underlying colonic tissue and tend to draw the colon into sacs. The segments of the circular musculature further divide the colon into sausage-like units known as haustra. Through segmented contractions, the haustra help churn colonic contents and assist in the absorption of water. Should the frequency or intensity of these segmental contractions decrease, the predominance of propulsive forces of the longitudinal musculature may lead to diarrhea. Without circular muscle contractions, mass colonic movements may occur in which the colon contracts to half its normal length and resembles a smooth, hollow tube without segmented units. As noted above, colonic motor activity is increased by parasympathetic stimulation and inhibited by sympathetic stimulation.

Peristaltic waves propel feces to the rectum. Normal bowel movements begin with the stimulation of stretch receptors in the rectum by feces. The external anal sphincter controls voluntary defecation.

In the colon, bacteria produce enzymes necessary for degradation of waste products, synthesize certain vitamins, and generate ammonia. *Bacteroides* species and anaerobic *Lactobacillus* species comprise much of the colonic bacterial flora. Organisms such as Enterobacteriaceae species (e.g., *Escherichia coli*), hemolytic *Streptococcus*, *Clostridium* species, and yeasts may also be present in the colon but represent only a small portion of the normal flora. Many factors such as diet, pH, coexisting disease, and drugs may influence the relative proportion of these organisms. If these potential pathogens are allowed to overgrow, they may cause serious symptoms and complications.

Etiology of Diarrhea

Variability in the causes of diarrhea makes identification of the pathophysiologic mechanism difficult. A

TABLE 2	Classification of diarrhea		
Type	Mechanism	Typical Causes
Osmotic	Unabsorbed solute	Lactase deficit, magnesium antacid excess
Secretory	Increased secretion of electrolytes	*E. coli* infection, ileal resection, thyroid cancer
Exudative	Defective colonic absorption, outpouring of mucus and/or blood	Ulcerative colitis, Crohn's disease, shigellosis, leukemia
Motility disorder	Decreased contact time	Irritable bowel syndrome, diabetic neuropathy

TABLE 3 Pathophysiologic classification of chronic diarrhea

Decreased absorption

Small intestine
Generalized malabsorption
    Mucosal damage (celiac disease)
    Impaired intraluminal digestion
    (pancreaticinsufficiency)
    Bacterial overgrowth (bile salt deconjugation and mucosalinjury—scleroderma)
Specific malabsorption
    Enzyme deficiency (disaccharidases)
    Transport defect (chloridorrhea glucose–galactose malabsorption)
    Unabsorbed solute (magnesium, lactulose)

Colon
Idiopathic inflammatory bowel disease
    Ulcerative colitis
    Crohn's disease
Specific inflammatory bowel disease
    Amebiasis
    Ischemic colitis
    Radiation colitis

Increased secretion

Small intestine
Dumping syndrome
Gastric hypersecretion (Zollinger–Ellison syndrome)
Endogenous secretagogues (vasoactive intestinal peptide, prostaglandins, serotonin)

Colon
Unabsorbed fatty acids
Bile acids (failure of ileal reabsorption)
Unabsorbed carbohydrates (lactase deficiency)

Motility disturbances (decreased mixing activity)

Small intestine and colon
Carcinoid syndrome
Postvagotomy diarrhea
Hyperthyroidism
Diabetic visceral neuropathy
Scleroderma

Colon
Irritable bowel syndrome

Malabsorption syndromes

Failure of digestion
Decreased pancreatic enzymes
Impairment of bile acid micelle formation
Bacterial overgrowth
Inadequate mixing of food, bile, and pancreatic enzymes
Gastrojejunostomy

Failure of absorption
Inadequate absorptive surface
    Intestinal bypass surgery

Damaged absorbing surface
Celiac disease

Biochemical defect without anatomic alteration
Lactase deficiency

Infiltration of intestinal wall
Crohn's disease

Impaired lymph and blood flow
Developmental abnormality
Lymphatic obstruction
Tuberculosis
Mesenteric vascular insufficiency
Fluid-secreting tumor (large villose adenoma)

Adapted from Harvey et al. *The Principles and Practice of Medicine.* 22nd ed. San Mateo, Calif, and Norwalk, Conn: Appleton and Lange; 1988; 814, 823.

---

complete medical assessment, including clinical laboratory evaluation, may be required to identify the cause. The etiology may be psychogenic, neurogenic, surgical, endocrine, irritant, osmotic, dietary, allergenic, malabsorptive, infectious, or inflammatory (Figure 1).

Mechanisms of Diarrhea

The development of diarrhea may involve four general pathophysiologic mechanisms: decreased absorption, increased secretion, excessive exudation, and motility alterations (Tables 2 and 3). These mechanisms classify diarrhea into four clinical groups: osmotic, secretory, exudative, and motility disorder.

The gut normally maintains a balance between absorption and secretion of GI fluids. The intestine has a maximum rate at which it can absorb water and electrolytes. If challenged with excessive volume, the absorptive capacity is exceeded and diarrhea occurs. Simply stated, intestinal absorption must equal or exceed secretion. Normally, secretory processes are less active than absorptive processes.

Electrolyte fluxes, especially sodium, are handled by villi and crypt cells.[3] Villi are absorptive; crypt cells

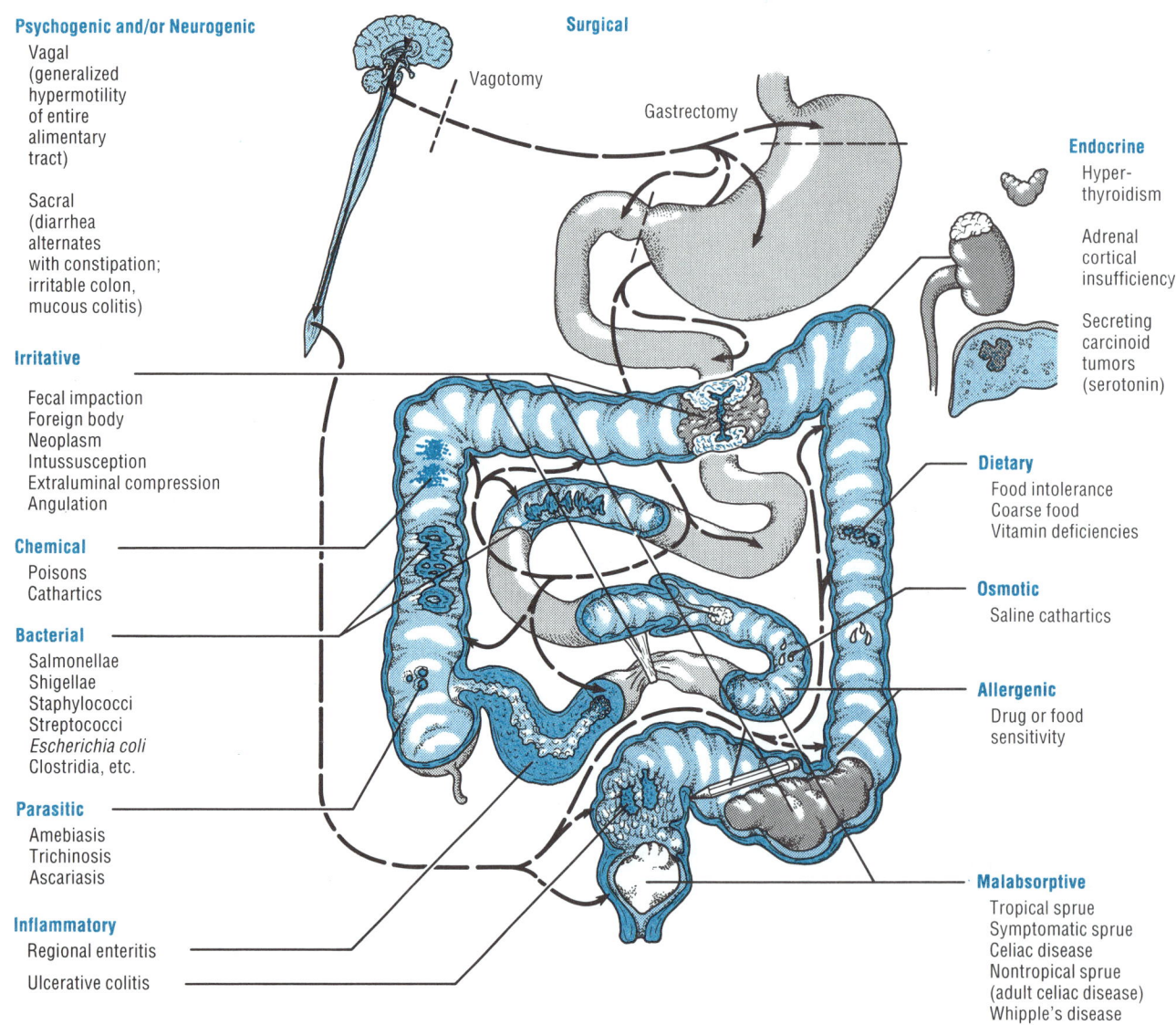

FIGURE 1 Etiology of diarrhea. Adapted from Netter, FN. *The Ciba Collection of Medical Illustrations,* vol. 1. New York: Ciba Pharmaceutical Co; 1962: 99.

are secretory in nature. Sodium is the primary ion absorbed by active mechanisms. In both secretion and absorption, sodium is exchanged for potassium. Also, sodium and chloride are transported by carrier mechanisms.

Water gains and losses are the essential controllers of diarrhea. As the semipermeable intestinal wall allows selective solvent and solute movements, water moves passively across it with sodium.

Intestinal transit time is under neuronal and hormonal control. Increased cholinergic activity promotes rapid transit throughout the gut and, if significant enough, may produce diarrhea. Excessive secretion of angiotensin, glucocorticoids, or vasopressin affects intestinal absorption and secretory mechanisms associated with the development of diarrhea.

Types of Diarrhea

Acute Diarrhea

Acute diarrhea is characterized by a sudden onset of abnormally frequent, watery stools accompanied by weakness, flatulence, pain, and possibly fever or vomiting.

Acute diarrhea may be infectious, toxic, drug induced, or dietary in origin. It may occur as the result of various acute or chronic illnesses. In the United States, infectious diarrhea is usually viral in origin, especially in children.

Food-Borne Diarrhea

Although the causative agent is often not readily identifiable, pathogens most commonly responsible for producing diarrhea in the United States are *Shigella* sp., *Salmonella* sp., *Campylobacter* sp., *Staphylococcus* sp., *Bacillus cereus*, and Norwalk viruses.[4] Some organisms cause diarrhea through an enterotoxin (toxigenic *E. coli* and *Staphylococcus aureus*). Others (*Shigella, Salmonella, Yersinia, Campylobacter jejuni*, and invasive *E. coli*) directly invade the mucosal epithelial cells. Patients with diarrhea caused by toxin-producing agents may present clinically with a cholera-like syndrome, which primarily involves the small intestine. Such patients experience an abrupt onset of large-volume watery stools, variable nausea, vomiting, cramps, and possibly a low-grade fever. If the large bowel is the site of attack, invasive organisms produce a dysentery-like syndrome. This syndrome is characterized by fever, abdominal cramps, tenesmus (straining), and the frequent passage of small-volume stools that may contain blood and pus.

An attentive and thorough history regarding food intake during the week prior to the onset of diarrhea is essential in identifying a probable cause. For example, staphylococci grow rapidly in food (especially salads, custard, sausage, ham, dairy products, and poultry), producing a toxin. Upon ingestion, the toxin quickly (within 1 to 2 hours) provokes an attack of vomiting with some diarrhea. In contrast, the incubation period for salmonellae, which are harbored on raw foods and particularly on eggs, is 12–24 hours. These microbes invade the mucosal layer to disrupt absorption–secretory mechanisms. Fever, malaise, muscle aches, and profound epigastric or periumbilical discomfort with severe anorexia suggest an infectious, inflammatory disease of the bowel. Severe periumbilical pain, vomiting, and possibly diarrhea may be experienced with viral gastroenteritis, and symptoms usually persist for 2 to 3 days before gradually subsiding.

Campylobacter species are another cause of acute bacterial diarrhea.[5] With an onset of 2–4 days, the diarrhea is usually limited to 1 week. If supportive therapy fails to manage symptoms, erythromycin may be used to eradicate the organism. *Yersinia enterocolitica* and *Yersinia pseudotuberculosis* are isolates of bacterial diarrhea, and symptoms of this self-limiting infectious process may persist for 1–3 weeks.

The acute diarrhea that may develop among tourists visiting foreign countries or U.S. border areas with warm climates and poor sanitation is usually caused by bacterial enteropathogens. Enterotoxigenic *E. coli* is the most common infecting organism in travelers' diarrhea, a secretory diarrhea acquired, for the most part, via contaminated food or water. After ingestion of the causative organism, usually found in foods such as fruits, vegetables, raw meat, seafood, and the local water (and ice cubes), the bacteria produces two plasmid-mediated enterotoxins known as heat-labile toxin and heat-stable toxin. These toxins cause a diarrheal disorder characterized by a sudden onset of loose stools (usually within 3–7 days of arrival), nausea, occasional vomiting, abdominal cramping, bloating, malaise, and possibly a low-grade fever. Travelers' diarrhea is also a self-limiting illness;[6] patients may experience between three and eight (or more) watery stools per day, and symptoms usually subside over 3–5 days, even if treated.

Infectious diarrhea may be treated with fluid and electrolytes. Often the illness is self-limiting, and normal function of the alimentary tract is restored with or without treatment in 24–72 hours. If the patient has a persistent case of infectious diarrhea, a specific anti-infective such as doxycycline, trimethoprim–sulfamethoxazole, or one of the fluoroquinolones may be indicated (Table 4). Prophylactic antibiotic use is controversial.

Food-Induced Diarrhea

Food intolerance can also provoke diarrhea. It may be caused by a food allergy or by ingestion of foods that are excessively fatty or spicy or that contain a high amount of roughage or many seeds.

Carbohydrates in the diet commonly include the disaccharides, lactose and sucrose, which are normally hydrolyzed to monosaccharides by the enzyme lactase. Infants born with a lactase deficiency and adults who develop one are intolerant of whole milk and milk-based products (e.g., ice cream). Milk and ice cream may be particularly problematic because of the lactose content. Enzymatic activity of lactase may be reduced in intestinal disorders such as infectious diarrhea and GI allergy. Acute viral diarrhea may cause a temporary milk intolerance at all ages. When disaccharides such as sucrose and lactose are not hydrolyzed, they pool in the lumen of the intestine, where they not only ferment but also produce an osmotic imbalance and pH change. The resulting hyperosmolarity draws fluid into the intestinal lumen, resulting in diarrhea.

Viral Diarrhea

Diarrhea is a common clinical problem in infants and young children. Although the etiology may be difficult to determine, the diarrhea is often caused by a viral infection of the intestinal tract.

Rotaviruses have been implicated as the cause of approximately 50% of all infantile diarrhea.[7] Children aged 6–24 months are most susceptible to this viral gastroenteritis. Respiratory illnesses such as otitis media or tonsillitis may occur concurrently. The peak infectious period is during the winter months. Spread is by the fecal–oral route. Clinical features include a 12- to 48-hour incubation period, vomiting, watery diarrhea, and a low-grade fever. The illness tends to be self-limiting, lasting 5–8 days, and treatment is usually restricted to symptomatic therapy.

Norwalk viruses have also been implicated in children and adults with signs and symptoms resembling those of rotaviruses. Norwalk is of the parvovirus group. The diarrhea is sudden and is often accompanied by a low-grade fever, malaise, mild nausea, and abdominal cramps. The diarrhea usually lasts 2 to 3 days. Like rotavirus

TABLE 4   Infectious diarrheas and their treatment

Type	History	Symptoms	Treatment	Prognosis
Bacterial				
Salmonella sp.	Ingestion of improperly cooked or refrigerated poultry and dairy products, immunocompromised host	Onset of 24–48 hours, diarrhea, fever, and chills	Fluid and electrolytes; no antibiotics	Self-limiting
Shigella sp.	Ingestion of contaminated vegetables or water, immunocompromised host	Onset of 24–48 hours, nausea, vomiting, diarrhea	Fluid and electrolytes; antibiotics (cotrimoxazole, ampicillin, ciprofloxacin/ norfloxacin)	Self-limiting
Enterotoxigenic *Escherichia coli* (Travelers' diarrhea)	Ingestion of contaminated food or water, recent travel outside the United States or to a U.S. border area	Onset of 8–72 hours, watery diarrhea, fever, abdominal cramps	Fluid and electrolytes; in moderate or severe cases, antibiotics (cotrimoxazole, fluoroquinolones)	Self-limiting
Campylobacter jejuni	Ingestion of contaminated water, fecal–oral route, immunocompromised host	Nausea, vomiting, headache, malaise, fever, watery diarrhea	Fluid and electrolytes; in severe or persistent diarrhea, antibiotics (erythromycin, fluoroquinolones)	Self-limiting
Clostridium difficile	Antibiotic-associated diarrhea	Watery or mucoid diarrhea, high fever, cramping	Water and electrolytes; discontinuation of offending agent; oral vancomycin, oral metronidazole, bacitracin, cholestyramine	Good, if treated

continued

infections, most outbreaks occur in the winter months. The virus is usually transmitted by contaminated water or food. Community-wide outbreaks may result when municipal water supplies become contaminated.

In children, particularly infants, acute diarrhea may cause severe and possibly dangerous dehydration and electrolyte imbalance; children under 2 years of age are most likely to suffer complications requiring hospitalization. In newborns, water may make up 75% of total body weight; water loss in severe diarrhea may be 10% or more of body weight. After 8–10 bowel movements within a 24-hour period, a 2-month-old infant could lose enough fluid to cause circulatory collapse and renal failure. Moderate to severe diarrhea in infants requires a physician evaluation. The pharmacist must be cautious in recommending treatment for any pediatric patient with diarrhea.[8]

Protozoal Diarrhea

Giardia lamblia and *Entamoeba histolytica* are protozoa associated with acute diarrhea. Giardiasis is an infection of the small intestine most commonly involving children, travelers, institutionalized patients, and hikers who drink from streams or ponds. Symptoms may be absent or mild. Following a 1- to 3-day incubation, symptoms may include sudden onset of watery stool, abdominal cramps, flatulence, and epigastric pain. Although quinacrine, 100 mg taken orally three times a day for 5–7 days, is effective therapy in most adults,[9] metronidazole (Flagyl®), 250 mg taken orally three times a day for 5–7 days, is equally effective and is better tolerated.

E. histolytica causes amebiasis in areas with poor sanitation and among institutionalized patients, travelers, and migrant workers. The illness is characterized by severe crampy pain, tenesmus, and dysentery within 3–10 days. Metronidazole, 750 mg taken orally three times a day for 10 days, is generally effective against this protozoan.

Drug-Induced Diarrhea

All antibiotics can produce adverse GI symptoms, but severity depends largely on the specific antibiotic, its spec-

TABLE 4 *continued*

Type	History	Symptoms	Treatment	Prognosis
Staphylococcus aureus	Ingestion of improperly cooked or stored food	Nausea, vomiting, watery diarrhea	Fluid and electrolytes; no antibiotics	Self-limiting
Protozoa				
Giardia lamblia	Ingestion of water contaminated with human or animal feces, travel outside the United States, immunocompromised host	Chronic watery diarrhea	Metronidazole, quinacrine, furazolidone	Good, if treated
Cryptosporidia	Travel outside the United States, AIDS, immunocompromised host	Chronic watery diarrhea	Fluid and electrolytes	Self-limiting, except in AIDS or other immunocompromised patients
Entamoeba histolytica	Travel outside the United States, fecal-soiled food or water, immunocompromised host	Chronic watery diarrhea	Fluid and electrolytes; metronidazole; iodoquinol	Good, except for immunocompromised patients
Viruses				
Rotaviruses	Infects infants, fecal–oral spread	Vomiting, fever, nausea, acute watery diarrhea	Vigorous fluid and electrolyte replacement; no antibiotics	Self-limiting
Norwalk	Infects all ages	"24-hour flu," vomiting, nausea, headache, myalgia, fever, watery diarrhea	Fluid and electrolytes; no antibiotics; bismuth subsalicylate; loperamide	Self-limiting

trum, and the dose and duration of therapy. Commonly prescribed antibiotics that have a broad spectrum of activity against aerobic and anaerobic organisms (e.g., ampicillin and numerous other penicillins, clindamycin, erythromycin, azithromycin, clarithromycin, lincomycin, neomycin, trimethoprim–sulfamethoxazole, the tetracyclines, the fluoroquinolones, and the cephalosporins) can produce diarrhea as a side effect.[10]

Antibiotic-associated diarrhea (AAD) may be caused by overgrowth of an antibiotic-resistant bacterial or fungal strain or of toxin-producing *Clostridium difficile*. Intestinal microorganisms other than *C. difficile* that tend to proliferate during antibiotic therapy include *S. aureus, Pseudomonas aeruginosa, Streptococcus faecalis, Candida albicans,* and selected species of *Salmonella* and *Proteus*. AAD may be self-limiting with antibiotic discontinuation.

C. difficile may also cause antibiotic-associated pseudomembranous colitis.[11] *C. difficile* produces at least two identified toxins (A and B). Because these can be spread to other persons, enteric isolation precautions are recommended. The diagnosis is suggested by a test for the toxins in the stool, although the toxins have been found in patients without AAD. The watery or greenish-mucoid diarrhea usually starts during antibiotic treatment, but it can begin up to 4 weeks after the antibiotic has been discontinued. The offending antibiotic must be discontinued and *C. difficile* eradicated. Relapses are common and can be treated with the same agent, if the microorganisms have been shown to be susceptible. Oral vancomycin (125–500 mg every 6 hours for 7–10 days) or oral metronidazole (1 to 2 g per day in divided doses for 7–10 days) are more often prescribed for adults.[12,13] Treatment in children is less well defined. Bacitracin may be used in treatment failure. Exchange resins, such as cholestyramine, bind the toxins but do not eradicate *C. difficile* and so are used to treat only mild cases.

Other drugs, such as stimulant cathartics, anticancer agents, quinidine, and colchicine, may irritate the intestinal mucosa and cause diarrhea. Drugs that cause the retention of electrolytes and water in the intestinal lumen may produce a hyperosmolar, osmotic diarrhea. Certain antacid preparations contain small quantities of magnesium to prevent the constipating effects of aluminum and calcium; depending on the dose taken and the individual's susceptibility, magnesium-containing antacid preparations may induce diarrhea. Drugs that affect the autonomic control of normal intestinal motility, such as certain antihypertensive agents with sympatholytic activity (e.g., guanethidine, methyldopa, and reserpine), may also cause diarrhea. And generalized cramping and diarrhea may follow the use of a parasympathomimetic (cholinergic) drug such as bethanecol or an antidopaminergic drug such as metaclopramide.

AIDS-Associated Diarrhea

Patients with acquired immunodeficiency syndrome (AIDS) and even asymptomatic individuals infected with human immunodeficiency virus (HIV) are known to be susceptible to many intestinal infections that produce diarrhea as one of their manifestations. An estimated 80% of AIDS patients will experience a diarrheal infection at some time in their illness.[14] These immunocompromised patients may be infected with bacteria, fungi, parasites, viruses, and protozoal organisms. Common stool isolates are *Cryptosporidium, C. difficile, Isospora belli, G. lamblia,* and *E. histolytica.*[15]

Following a 1- to 3-day incubation, fever and a sudden onset of explosive watery stool begin. Abdominal cramps also occur frequently. No currently available antimicrobial has been shown to be effective in diarrhea due to *Cryptosporidium. Isospora* infections are managed with trimethoprim–sulfamethoxazole. Quinacrine and metronidazole are the treatments of choice for proven *G. lamblia* diarrhea in adults and older children.[16] For empiric therapy of suspected giardiasis, metronidazole may offer advantages relative to its tolerability, side effect profile, and effects on other causes of persistent diarrhea. For managing giardiasis in small children, a pediatric liquid formulation of furazolidone is available.

E. histolytica infection, which produces acute amebic dysentery, is characterized by severe crampy pain, tenesmus, and dysentery within 3–10 days of infection. Metronidazole, 750 mg taken orally three times a day for 5–10 days, combined with iodoquinol, 650 mg taken orally three times a day for 20 days, is recommended therapy by the Centers for Disease Control and is generally effective.[16]

Chronic Diarrhea

Chronic diarrhea is the long-term (lasting more than 2 weeks), abnormally frequent passage of poorly formed or watery stools. Its etiology is often multifactorial and therefore may be difficult to diagnose (Table 3); however, chronic diarrhea is generally related to GI diseases. It may be caused by a disease of the small or large intestine or the stomach, or it may be a secondary manifestation of a systemic disease. Some clinicians differentiate chronic diarrhea into functional or organic groups. The pharmacist should refer patients with persistent or recurrent diarrhea to a physician; a definitive diagnosis can generally be made only after a physician carefully evaluates the patient's history, performs a physical examination, and orders and receives proper laboratory reports.

Diagnosing chronic diarrhea is often complicated by the fact that the condition does not always involve frequent daily passage of watery stools. The three categories of chronic diarrhea are (1) frequent, small, formed stools with tenesmus; (2) large, oily, malodorous, formed stools (suggestive of fat malabsorption); and (3) frequent, voluminous, loosely formed stools. The patient may complain of weight loss, fever, anxiety, depression, nausea, vomiting, or perianal tenderness.

Psychogenic factors are frequent causes of chronic diarrhea. Psychogenic diarrhea is related to emotional stress that may periodically increase the flow of parasympathetic impulses to the GI tract. It is usually characterized by small, frequent stools and abdominal pain. The stools may be watery and may follow a normal bowel movement or appear shortly after eating. The diarrhea may alternate with constipation. Patients complaining of chronic diarrhea that appears to be psychogenic in origin should be referred to a physician.

Many people believe that a daily bowel movement is essential for good health. This belief is seriously flawed and may lead to the abuse of laxatives (particularly irritant/stimulant laxatives), which itself may create a serious health problem due to iatrogenic chronic diarrhea. Chronic laxative use may result in serious fluid and electrolyte loss, protein wasting (hypoalbuminemia), and colitis. Recovery requires laxative withdrawal, bowel training, psychologic counseling, and, on rare occasions, hospitalization.

In recent years, chronic abuse of laxatives in poorly developed weight control programs has become a problem. However, the role of the inappropriate use of laxatives may not be discovered until other potential causes of the chronic diarrhea are ruled out. The laxative abuser usually complains of weight loss and diarrhea. Upon questioning, however, the patient may deny laxative abuse. A hospitalized patient's diarrhea may stop only to recur at home. To identify the laxative abuser, the practitioner must take a thorough drug history. The pharmacist should monitor for frequent laxative purchases. (See Chapter 15, "Laxative Products.")

Some patients who suffer from persistent diarrhea are aware of the cause and can manage the condition symptomatically. For example, many persons with diabetes who have evident neuropathy experience chronic diarrhea. (See Chapter 16, "Diabetes Care Products and Monitoring Devices.") However, individuals who experience persistent or recurrent diarrhea and are unaware of its cause should seek prompt medical attention. Conditions such as cancer of the stomach or colon or an endocrine tumor may be causing the diarrhea.[17] One of the seven danger signals of cancer is a change in bowel habits. In both sexes, cancer of the colon and rectum is frequently reported. The American Cancer Society estimates that three of every four patients with cancer of the GI tract could be saved by early diagnosis and proper treatment.

Evaluation

Evaluation of the patient's responses to the questions presented at the beginning of this chapter should enable the pharmacist to assess the patient's condition and recommend a proper course of action, which may include self-treatment or referral to a physician. This triage function requires the pharmacist to differentiate symptoms and make clinical judgments.

The pharmacist should acquire a history of the patient's present illness before recommending self-treatment. The following four groups of patients with either acute or chronic diarrhea should be referred to a physician for a complete diagnostic evaluation:

- Children under 3 years of age;
- Persons over 60 years of age who have multiple medical conditions;
- Persons with a medical history of chronic illness such as asthma, peptic ulcer, diabetes, or heart disease;
- Pregnant women.

Other medical conditions that generally suggest the need for physician referral include:

- The presence of bloody or mucoid stools;
- Moderate to severe abdominal tenderness or cramping;
- High fever (≥101°F or 38°C);
- Evidence of dehydration;
- Weight loss of greater than 5% of body weight;
- Diarrhea that has lasted 2 or more days.

Clinical judgment must be used in evaluating these patients. For example, access to medical treatment may not be readily available, and temporary self-treatment may be needed until a medical appointment can be arranged.

A properly conducted medication history may help detect drug-induced diarrhea. The pharmacist should determine the self-treatments that have been tried, the patient's age, the symptoms, the date of onset, and the characteristics of stools (number, consistency, odor, and appearance). When a drug is implicated as a cause of diarrhea, the pharmacist should refer the patient to a physician because the patient may need to continue taking the drug even though it is causing problems.

Alcohol abuse, diverticulitis, emotional problems, gastritis, irritable bowel syndrome, peptic ulcer disease, and ulcerative colitis or regional enteritis are some frequently reported past medical problems. Patients with a history of chronic GI disease should also be referred to a physician for care.

The patient needs to be monitored for signs of volume depletion. The early to intermediate signs of dehydration include sunken eyes, dry oral mucous membranes, low urine output, no tears in children when crying, and decreased skin turgor with tenting. The patient should be asked about vomiting, high and/or prolonged fever, the nature and amount of fluid intake, and decreased urine output.

Stool character gives valuable information about diarrhea. For example, undigested food particles in the stool suggest small bowel irritation; black, tarry stools may indicate upper GI bleeding; and red stools suggest possible lower bowel bleeding or perhaps simply the recent ingestion of red food such as beets or of drug products such as rifampin. Diarrhea originating from the small intestine is probably characterized by a marked outpouring of fluid high in potassium and bicarbonate. A pasty or semisolid loose stool suggests diarrhea associated with a colon disorder. Yellowish stool may indicate the presence of bilirubin and a potentially serious pathology of the liver.

Treatment

Treatment goals are to (1) prevent excessive fluid and electrolyte loss and acid–base disturbance; (2) identify and treat the cause, if possible; (3) manage secondary conditions causing diarrhea; and (4) provide symptomatic relief.

However, because diarrhea is a symptom, symptomatic relief must not be interpreted as a cure for the underlying cause. Symptomatic relief generally is adequate for simple functional diarrhea that is only temporary, self-limiting, and uncomplicated. Many nonprescription products are available to assist in managing diarrhea; however, the pharmacist should exercise caution in recommending their use. Certain diarrhea-producing diseases might be serious or treated more effectively with agents specific for the underlying cause. Table 4 summarizes the primary causes of diarrhea and some of the more standard approaches to treatment.

Prophylaxis and Management of Infectious (Travelers') Diarrhea

Travelers' diarrhea is caused by a variety of bacteria. Tap water used for brushing teeth or for ice in drinks may be a source of infection. Travelers to areas where hygiene and sanitation are poor may prevent diarrhea by eating only recently peeled and thoroughly cooked foods and by drinking only boiled or bottled water, bottled carbonated soft drinks, beer, or wine.

Many remedies have been tried to prevent travelers' diarrhea; antibiotics are the most effective drugs currently available. However, users should be cautious regarding the prophylactic use of antibiotics that may produce photosensitivity reactions (e.g., sulfonamides and tetracyclines) in travelers exposed to the sun. Doxycycline (100 mg daily) has been effective in preventing travelers' diarrhea. Trimethoprim–sulfamethoxazole (160–800 mg twice daily) has also been shown to prevent this disorder or to attenuate symptoms when the offending organism is enterotoxigenic *E. coli*, *Salmonella* sp., or *Shigella* sp.[18] Norfloxacin, ofloxacin, and ciprofloxacin may also be effective in preventing diarrhea although the therapy is expensive.[19] Generally, many infectious disease experts do not recommend drug prophylaxis but tell travelers to begin treatment at the first signs of symptoms.[20]

Travelers' diarrhea may be managed with fluid and electrolyte replacement. Antibiotics such as trimethoprim–sulfamethoxazole, norfloxacin, ciprofloxacin, and trimethoprim have been used successfully in therapy and are more effective than placebo. Loperamide (Imodium®, Imodium A-D®) has also been shown to be an effective treatment. For symptomatic management, loperamide (4-mg loading dose; then 2 mg taken orally after each loose stool, not to exceed 16 mg per day) plus a fluoroquinolone antibiotic (e.g., ciprofloxacin 500 mg taken twice daily, ofloxacin 300 mg taken twice daily, or norfloxacin 400 mg taken twice daily) may be effective.[21]

Bismuth subsalicylate (Pepto-Bismol®) has been shown to be effective in both prevention and treatment of symptoms of travelers' diarrhea,[22] because it appears to inhibit intestinal secretions. The adult prophylactic dosage is 60 mL or two tablets taken four times a day with meals and at bedtime during the first 2 weeks of travel. During acute illness in adults, 30–60 mL or two tablets should be taken every 30–60 minutes following each loose stool, not to exceed eight doses per 24-hour period. Package labeling should be consulted with regard to dosing pediatric patients.

The salicylate may be a problem, however, if patients are taking aspirin or other salicylate-containing drugs. Toxic levels of salicylate may be reached even if the patient follows dosing directions on the label for each drug. Thus, patients who are sensitive to aspirin should not use bismuth subsalicylate. This product may also interact adversely with oral anticoagulants, methotrexate, probenecid, and sulfinpyrazone or any other drug that potentially interacts with aspirin. Also, serum salicylate levels may exert an antiplatelet effect. Black-stained stool is commonly associated with use of bismuth subsalicylate and does not necessarily suggest the presence of occult blood in the feces. Mild tinnitus is a side effect that may be associated with moderate to severe salicylate toxicity.

Antiperistaltic agents such as diphenoxylate (Lomotil®) may prolong or enhance the severity of the symptoms of travelers' diarrhea and should be avoided. If the patient has fever or is passing blood because invasive bacteria are present in the intestine, opiate or opiate-like drugs should not be used.[19]

Fluid and Electrolyte Replacement

Replacement of fluid loss and correction of electrolyte imbalance are very important. The secretory and absorptive mechanisms appear to function separately; therefore, an oral sugar–electrolyte solution can be absorbed during diarrhea.[23] In mild to moderate diarrhea, oral fluids can be safely prescribed if the patient is not vomiting. In severe cases of diarrhea, fluid deficits must be replaced intravenously. This treatment has saved many lives in the Third World countries. Glucose is essential for the absorption of electrolytes. The World Health Organization (WHO) recommends an oral replacement fluid that contains, per liter, 20 g of glucose, 90 mEq of sodium, 80 mEq of chloride, 30 mEq of bicarbonate, and 20 mEq of potassium.[24] No commercial product currently available strictly fulfills WHO recommendations. In both developed and developing countries, commercial oral electrolyte replacement solutions, even though different from the WHO-recommended formulation, are more convenient and potentially safer because they are premixed and there is less chance of error in preparation (Table 5). Administering fluid without electrolytes is potentially dangerous because of the risk of inducing hyponatremia.

Mild acute diarrhea, which is sometimes accompanied by vomiting, is usually self-limiting. Proper dietary measures can help replace lost fluids and electrolytes and thus prevent dehydration. The following oral rehydration dietary management of mild diarrhea without high fever or vomiting has been recommended as treatment in cases of uncomplicated gastroenteritis:[25]

- Infants and young children under 5 years of age: An estimate of a patient's fluid requirement is based on body surface area (BSA); two methods for estimating a child's BSA are shown in Figure 2. Maintenance therapy is 1.5 L/m^2; maintenance plus replacement is 2.4 L/m^2.
- Older children and adults with mild to moderate fluid loss: Children 5–10 years of age should take 960–1,920 mL per day; children over 10 years of age and adults should take 1,920–2,880 mL per day.
- Children under 3 years of age who have diarrhea and adults with diarrhea who lose more than 5% of their body weight: Both groups should be promptly referred to their physicians.

TABLE 5 Oral rehydration solutions

	WHO-ORS[a]	Pedialyte®	Rehydralyte®	Ricelyte®	Resol®
Osmolarity (mOsm/L)	333	249	304	200	269
Carbohydrates (g/L)[b]	20	25	25	30[c]	20
Electrolytes (mEq/L)					
Sodium	90	45	75	50	50
Potassium	20	20	20	25	20
Chloride	80	35	65	45	50
Citrate	—	30	30	34	34
Bicarbonate	30	—	—	—	—
Calcium	—	—	—	—	4
Magnesium	—	—	—	—	4
Phosphate	—	—	—	—	5

[a]World Health Organization oral rehydration solution.
[b]Carbohydrate is glucose.
[c]Rice syrup solids.

Source: *Med Lett* 1991 Nov 15; 33: 107–10.

Oral rehydration products (e.g., Pedialyte®, Gastrolyte®, Ricelyte®, Rehydralyte®, and Resol®) are commonly used in the management of mild diarrhea and are available in pharmacies without a prescription. These solutions are termed oral rehydration therapy and are used in the above prescribed manner. However, in moderate (5–10% weight loss) to severe diarrhea (>10% weight loss) with severe vomiting, fluid and electrolytes must be given intravenously. Symptoms that suggest more serious diarrhea-induced pathology are increased thirst, decreased urine output, dry skin and mucous membranes, weight loss, and low blood pressure with tachycardia. If the child cannot retain fluid or if watery diarrhea persists, a physician should be contacted. As symptoms subside, a normal diet should be restarted slowly. If milk intolerance occurs, infants may receive soy-based formulas (e.g., Isomil®, Soyalac®, or ProSobee®).

Pharmacologic Agents

Some antidiarrheal drugs are directed against the symptoms of diarrhea, some are directed against the cause, and some are directed against the effects of the disease, such as loss of nutrients or electrolytes. The categories of drugs generally used are opiates, adsorbents, electrolytes, nutrients, anti-infectives, digestive enzymes, and anticholinergics. Many of these drugs are available only by prescription.

Loperamide, attapulgite, and polycarbophil are recognized as being safe and effective for nonprescription use. The Food and Drug Administration (FDA) concluded, however, that many active ingredients in nonprescription antidiarrheal products have not been proven to be safe and effective.[26] As of May 1991, the following drugs were to be removed from nonprescription antidiarrheal products: aluminum hydroxide, atropine sulfate, calcium carbonate, carboxymethylcellulose, glycine, homatropine methylbromide, hyoscyamine sulfate, *Lactobacillus acidophilus*, *Lactobacillus bulgaricus*, opium powder, opium tincture, paregoric, phenyl salicylate, scopolamine hydrobromide, and zinc phenosulfonate.

Antiperistaltic Agents

Opiates and opiate-like agents exert a direct musculotropic effect on and inhibit propulsive movements in the small intestine and colon. Hyperperistalsis is diminished and the passage of intestinal contents slows, allowing reabsorption of water and electrolytes. In the usual oral antidiarrheal dosages, addiction liability is low for acute diarrheal episodes because the opiate or opiate derivative is not well absorbed orally and is only used short term. The low dose given produces an effective action in the GI tract without causing analgesia or euphoria. However, acute overdose or chronic use, as in ulcerative colitis, increases the risk of physical dependency. Opiate derivatives are central nervous system (CNS) depressants, and excessive sedation may be a problem in patients taking other CNS depressants with the antidiarrheal medication. As mentioned, the FDA has removed opiates and opiate derivatives from nonprescription products.

Loperamide is emerging as a very effective antidiarrheal agent and is available without a prescription. Loperamide also possesses a more favorable side effect profile than opiate and opiate-like agents. It slows intestinal motility and produces a positive movement of electrolyte and water through the gut. Like other antiperistaltic drugs, it should be used for no more than 48 hours in acute diarrhea. Loperamide is supplied as 2-mg caplets or 1 mg per 5 mL palatable liquid. The usual nonprescription adult dosage is 4 mg initially, and then 2 mg after each loose bowel movement, not to exceed 8 mg a day. Package labeling should be consulted for dosage guidelines in pediatric patients. Loperamide is not recommended for children under 2 years of age.

Antiperistaltic drugs (e.g., diphenoxylate, opiate-derivatives, and loperamide) are effective in relieving cramps and stool frequency. They may worsen the effects of invasive bacterial infection, however, and may cause toxic megacolon in antibiotic-induced diarrhea. These drugs should be used with caution in patients presenting with fecal leukocytes, fever, or a recent history of antibiotic use, as well as in cases of diagnosed acute ulcerative colitis.

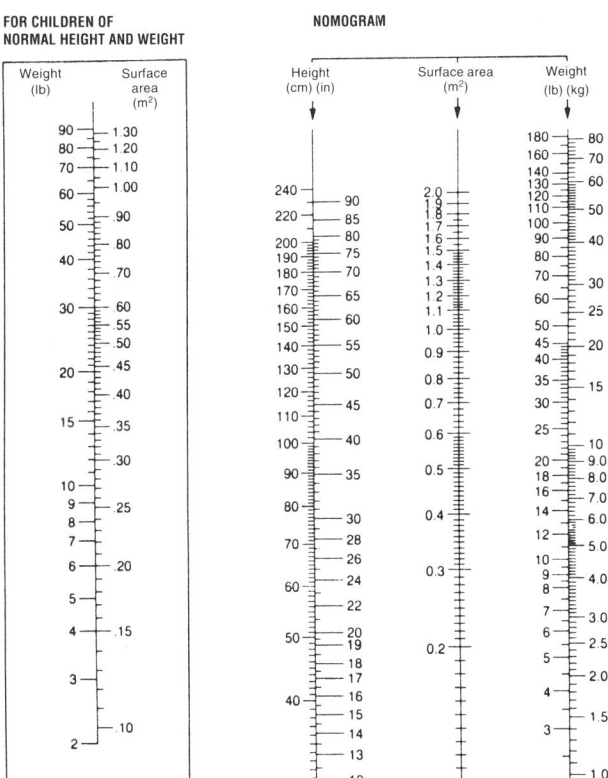

FIGURE 2 Methods for estimating body surface area of children. For children of average size, find weight and corresponding surface area on the boxed scale to the left. To use the nomogram on the right, lay a straightedge on the correct height and weight points for the child; then read the intersecting point on the surface area scale. Adapted with permission from *Nelson Textbook of Pediatrics.*, 14th ed. Philadelphia: W. B. Saunders; 1992.

Adsorbents

Adsorbents are the type of drug used most often in nonprescription antidiarrheal preparations. Because large doses are generally used, most commercially available products are formulated as flavored liquid suspensions to improve palatability. Adsorbents are generally used to treat mild nonspecific diarrhea.

Adsorption is not selective, and when adsorbents are given orally, they may adsorb nutrients and digestive enzymes as well as toxins, bacteria, and various noxious materials in the GI tract. They may also have the undesirable effect of adsorbing drugs in the GI tract. Although the systemic absorption of an orally administered drug from the GI tract is expected to be compromised during a diarrheal episode, it may be further hampered by the concomitant administration of an antidiarrheal adsorbent. A clinical judgment must be made regarding when the patient will take medications other than the antidiarrheal preparations. Depending on the medication involved, the usual rate and site of absorption, and the absolute necessity of getting specific and consistent blood levels of the drug, a change in the dose or the dosage interval may be required. Sometimes, it might be better to administer the drug parenterally (if available by injection) until the diarrheal episode is over and the adsorbent drugs are discontinued.

Following initial treatment, most antidiarrheal preparations containing adsorbents are taken after each loose bowel movement until the diarrhea is controlled or the maximum daily dosage is reached. The total amount of adsorbent taken may be quite large if the diarrheal episodes recur in rapid succession over several hours. Because there is negligible systemic absorption of the adsorbent drug, the most common side effect associated with adsorbents is constipation.

The GI adsorbents used clinically are activated charcoal, cholestyramine, attapulgite, polycarbophil, and pectin. Attapulgite is currently the primary active adsorbent ingredient in Kaopectate® and Donnagel®. Adsorbents used with ion-exchange resins such as cholestyramine combine their individual activities in relieving gastric distress and diarrhea. Adsorbents are inert and nontoxic except for possible interference with drug and nutrient absorption and a few mild side effects. Although seldom used as an antidiarrheal, activated charcoal has excellent adsorptive properties and is used for treating certain types of drug overdoses and poisonings.

Polycarbophil is a synthetic polyacrylic resin that acts as an absorbent. Because of its ability to absorb up to 60 times its original weight in water, it has been recommended in the treatment of both diarrhea and constipation. Polycarbophil is metabolically inert, and no systemic toxicity has been shown. Side effects, which are mild and infrequent, include dose-related epigastric pain and bloating. The effective adult oral antidiarrheal dose of polycarbophil is 4–6 g daily in divided doses. Adults should chew two 500-mg tablets four times a day, children 6–12 years of age should chew one 500-mg tablet three times a day, and children 3–6 years of age should chew one 500-mg tablet two times a day. Use in children under 3 years of age is not recommended without the advice of a physician.

Anticholinergics

The formulations of adsorbents have historically been fortified by the addition of one or more belladonna alkaloids (anticholinergics) in concentrations that make them prescription drugs. The primary effect of anticholinergic agents is relief of cramping through the reduction of contractile activity. However, their effectiveness in reducing diarrhea is negligible in doses typically found in nonprescription products. Therefore, manufacturers have voluntarily deleted most anticholinergics from nonprescription antidiarrheals.

Lactobacillus Preparations

A controversial form of diarrhea treatment has been the use of *Lactobacillus* organisms. Seeding or reseeding the bowel with viable *L. acidophilus* and *L. bulgaricus* has been suggested as effective treatment for selected intestinal disturbances, including diarrhea. These microorganisms are believed to successfully suppress the growth of pathogenic microorganisms and reestablish the normal intestinal flora. However, antibiotic therapy often disrupts the balance of intestinal microorganisms, resulting in abnormal intestinal function, and broad-spectrum, chronically administered antibiotics are the most troublesome. Overgrowth of nonsusceptible organisms may even produce diarrhea. The FDA reports that there are no adequately controlled studies documenting the safety or efficacy of lactobacillus preparations in treating diarrhea, drug induced or otherwise; these preparations were subsequently removed from the market. A diet of milk, yogurt, or buttermilk containing 240–400 g of lactose or dextrin appears to be just as effective in colonizing the intestine without supplemental lactobacilli.

Digestive Enzymes

For patients with lactase enzymatic deficiency, lactase enzymes are available as Lactaid®, Dairy Ease®, and Lactrase®. These preparations may be added to milk products or taken with milk at mealtimes to prevent osmotic diarrhea.

Product Selection Guidelines

The information obtained during the patient interview and from the family medication record must be assessed before a product is selected. Water–glucose–electrolyte products are extremely important to treatment planning. Antidiarrheal treatment choices include an adsorbent such as attapulgite–pectin mixture; an antiperistaltic such as loperamide, polycarbophil, or bismuth subsalicylate; or physician referral.

The pharmacist should assess the patient's previous response to treatments. A product that the patient has taken for the same condition and found satisfactory may be the best choice. Nonprescription antidiarrheal products can usually assist in managing mild to moderate acute nonspecific diarrhea. In mild to moderate acute noninfectious diarrhea, loperamide is effective when taken at a nonprescription dosage level. Severe acute nonspecific diarrhea and infectious diarrhea usually require physician referral. Aggressive fluid and electrolyte therapy and antibiotic therapy may be indicated. Cases of suspected antibiotic-associated pseudomembranous colitis should also be managed by a physician.

Uncomplicated acute diarrhea usually improves within 24 hours. If the condition remains the same, the pharmacist should recommend continuing treatment for another 24 hours with the same or a more potent product or should recommend that the patient consult a physician. If control of the symptoms is not accomplished with nonprescription drug therapy within 48 hours, a physician should be consulted. Immediate physician contact is required if the patient is an infant or a frail elderly person, or is chronically ill, hypotensive, or already volume depleted.

The pharmacist should review label contents to determine the appropriate dosage schedule based on the patient's age, the maximum number of doses per 24 hours, proper storage, and auxiliary administration information such as the need to shake the product before use. The patient must be informed of special precautions on the label such as contraindications to use and drug–drug interactions.

Adjunctive therapy includes rest, appropriate fluids, possible avoidance of milk and milk products, and maintenance of a proper diet. Additionally, the pharmacist should encourage the patient to rest in bed and limit intake of solid foods to allow the patient's GI tract to rest. Fluid loss and electrolyte and acid–base disturbances are primary concerns, especially in infants, young children, and elderly patients.

Patients with chronic medical conditions should be under a physician's care. Treatment of diarrhea should be based on managing the underlying cause and avoiding the ingestion of agents that contribute to the condition. Medications prescribed may include prescription-only drugs, such as antispasmodics and opiate or opiate-like agents, and nonprescription products, such as bulk formers.

Summary

Diarrhea is often treated casually, but it can be a symptom of a more serious underlying disease. The condition can be either acute or chronic. Acute diarrhea is characterized by a sudden onset of loose stools in a previously and otherwise healthy patient. Chronic diarrhea is characterized by persistent or recurrent episodes of loose stools accompanied by anorexia, weight loss, and weakness. Simple diarrhea can usually be treated by supportive care and/or a nonprescription drug or oral rehydration product.

The debilitating effect of persistent diarrhea is due largely to loss of water through excretion resulting in both fluid and electrolyte imbalance. The replacement of these important fluids and electrolytes is an integral part of diarrhea therapy, particularly in infants, children, and frail elderly persons. This replacement can be accomplished by appropriate intravenous fluids or oral sugar–electrolyte formulations.

Patients who appear volume depleted, weak, dizzy, or hypotensive should be referred to a physician. Similarly, all severely acute, uncontrolled, or chronic complaints involving the GI tract should be promptly referred to a physician for medical evaluation. For minor acute problems, however, such as food or drink intolerance, relief may be provided by a nonprescription product such as loperamide.

References

1. Connell AM, Hilton C, Irvine G. Variation of bowel habits in two population samples. *Br Med J* 1965; 2: 1095–9.
2. Diem K, Lenthner C. *Scientific Tables*. 7th ed. Basile, Switzerland: Ciba-Geigy Ltd; 1970: 657–8.
3. Field M, Rao MC, Chang EB. Intestinal electrolyte transport and diarrheal disease. *N Engl J Med* 1989 Sep 21; 321: 800–6.
4. Archer DL, Young FE. Contemporary issues: diseases with a food vector. *Clin Microbiol Rev* 1988; 1: 377–98.
5. Cover TL, Blaser MJ. The pathobiology of campylobacter infections in humans. *Annu Rev Med* 1989; 40: 269–85.
6. Levine MM. *Escherichia coli* that cause diarrhea: enterotoxigenic, enteropathogenic, enteroinvasive, enterohemorrhagic, and enteroadherent. *J Infect Dis* 1987; 155: 377–89.
7. Christensen ML. Human viral gastroenteritis. *Clin Microbiol Rev* 1989; 2 (1): 51–89.
8. Feld LG, Kaskel FJ, Schoeneman MJ. The approach to fluid and electrolyte therapy in pediatrics. *Adv Pediatr* 1988; 35: 497–536.
9. Sanford JP. *Guide to Antimicrobial Therapy 1992*. Dallas: Antimicrobial Therapy Inc; 1992: 76–7.
10. Gross MH. Management of antibiotic-associated pseudomembranous colitis. *Clin Pharm* 1985; 5: 304–10.
11. Qualman SJ, Petric M, Karmali MA, et al. *Clostridium difficile* invasion and toxin circulation in fatal pediatric pseudomembranous colitis. *Am J Clin Pathol* 1990; 94: 410–6.
12. Fekety R, Silva J, Kauffman C, et al. Treatment of antibiotic-associated *Clostridium difficile* colitis with oral vancomycin: comparison of two dosage regimens. *Am J Med* 1989; 86: 15–9.
13. Teasley OG, Gerdine ON, Olsen MM. Prospective, randomized study of metronidazole versus vancomycin for clostridium-associated diarrhea and colitis. *Lancet* 1983; 2: 1043–6.
14. Langhon BE, Druckman DA, Vernon A, et al. Prevalence of enteric pathogens in homosexual men with and without acquired immunodeficiency syndrome. *Gastroenterology* 1988; 94: 984–93.
15. Tanowitz HB, Simon D, Wittner M. Gastrointestinal manifestations. *Med Clin North Am* 1992; 76: 45–62.
16. Drug for parasitic infections. *Med Lett* 1992 Mar 6; 34 (865): 17–26.
17. Fedorak RH, Field M, Chang EB. Treatment of diabetic diarrhea with clonidine. *Ann Intern Med* 1985; 102: 197–9.
18. Ebert SC, Goodwin SK, Rybak MJ, et al. ASHP therapeutics guidelines on nonsurgical antibiotic prophylaxis. *Clin Pharm* 1990; 9: 423–45.
19. Ericsson CD, Johnson PC, DuPont HL, et al. Ciprofloxacin or trimethoprim-sulfamethoxazole as initial therapy for travelers' diarrhea. *Ann Intern Med* 1987; 106: 216–20.
20. Travelers' diarrhea. Consensus conference. *JAMA* 1985; 253: 2700–4.
21. Advice for travelers. *Med Lett* 1992 May 1; 34 (869): 41–4.
22. Gorbach SL. Pathophysiology of gastrointestinal infections: the role of bismuth subsalicylate. *Rev Infect Dis* 1990; 12: 53–119.
23. Pizarro D, Posada G, Sandi L, et al. Rice-based oral electrolyte solutions for the management of infantile diarrhea. *N Engl J Med* 1991; 324: 517–21.
24. Avery ME, Snyder JD. Oral therapy for acute diarrhea. *N Engl J Med* 1990; 323: 891–4.
25. Olin BR, ed. *Facts and Comparisons*. St. Louis, Mo: J. B. Lippincott Co; 1992: 17a.
26. *Federal Register* 1990 Nov 7; 55: 46914–21.

CHAPTER 14

Anthelmintic Products

Kathryn K. Bucci

Questions to ask in patient assessment and counseling

- *Who is the patient? (Who is this for?)*
- *Why do you think you or your child might have worms?*
- *Have you seen any worms in stools?*
- *Describe your symptoms. Have you had any nausea, diarrhea, abdominal pain, rectal itching, or weight loss? Do you become fatigued easily?*
- *How long have the symptoms been present?*
- *Are other members of your family or close contacts also affected?*
- *Have you seen a physician for this problem?*
- *Has the problem occurred in the past? How was it treated? Did the treatment work?*
- *If the patient is not an adult, what is the age and approximate weight of the patient?*
- *If the patient is female, is she pregnant or breast-feeding?*
- *Have you traveled out of the country? If so, where and when?*

Anthelmintics are used to treat worm (helminthic) infections. The incidence of helminthic infection may exceed 90% in areas where sanitation is insufficient, water is not clean, waste disposal is inefficient, rodents and insects are poorly controlled, economic conditions are poor, and preventive medicine practices are inadequate.[1] Increases in world travel and immigration have escalated the spread of helminthic infections. Use of immunosuppressive drugs and the spread of acquired immunodeficiency syndrome (AIDS) are resulting in infections by previously unfamiliar parasites in various settings. Worm infections are primarily parasitic and may produce serious health problems, particularly in tropical regions, and result in the general debilitation of large populations. These infections reduce resistance to disease, may impair physical development in children, and decrease occupational productivity.

Helminthic infections in the United States can be serious, but their impact is not generally widespread; therefore, they do not pose a major societal threat. Endemic nematode (roundworm) infections include enterobiasis (pinworms), ascariasis, whipworms, hookworms, anisakiasis,

and trichinosis. Other worms that parasitize humans are cestodes (tapeworms) and trematodes (flukes). Table 1 lists some human helminthic infections and their most common symptoms.

Intestinal parasitic infection during pregnancy requires special attention. Care of the mother and fetus is of major concern. Parasitic infections during pregnancy may (1) impair fertility, (2) injure the mother's health, (3) injure the fetus, (4) induce premature labor and/or delivery, and (5) infect the neonate. Care requires risk and benefit considerations for the mother and fetus.

Patient Assessment

The one nonprescription anthelmintic presently on the market (pyrantel pamoate) is indicated only for pinworms. The pharmacist is often the first person called upon when a patient suspects a helminthic infection. Most people find the thought of a worm infection extremely disturbing. The pharmacist should be aware of the signs, symptoms, and preferred treatment of common helminthic infections to appropriately counsel patients and refer them to a physician when indicated.

The first indication of a helminthic infection may be a worm passed with a stool; often, however, worms passed with a stool are not detected. The most common species of helminths in the United States are pinworms. Vegetable material, mucus strands, or other artifacts may look like worms. Patients should be advised to place a suspected worm in tap water and take it to a physician or laboratory for identification.

If children are showing any of the common signs of pinworm infection, parents should be advised to observe the skin of the child's perianal region at night for adult worms. If pinworms are observed in one child, the whole family should be treated and appropriate hygiene methods initiated.

Enterobiasis

Enterobiasis, or oxyuriasis, is commonly called pinworm, seatworm, or threadworm infection. The intestinal infection in humans is caused by *Enterobius vermicularis*. Unlike many helminthic infections, enterobiasis is not limited to rural and poverty-stricken areas, but occurs in both rural and urban communities and infects individuals from all socioeconomic strata. *Enterobius vermicularis* is most common in temperate climates but is widely distributed and is especially prevalent among schoolchildren. Pinworm infections are the most common helminthic infection in the United States.

This chapter is based in part on the chapter with the same title that appeared in the 9th edition but was written by John M. Kinsella.

TABLE 1 Common human helminthic infections in the United States

Class/Genus and species	Common name	Source of infection	Symptoms
Nematoda			
Ancylostoma duodenale, Necator americanus	Hookworm	Contact with contaminated soil; larvae are ingested or penetrate the skin on contact	Anemia caused by blood loss (0.15 mL per worm per day); indigestion, anorexia, headache, cough, vomiting, diarrhea, weakness, urticaria at the site of entry into the skin
Ascaris lumbricoides, Ascaris suum	Roundworm	Ingestion of eggs through contact with fecally contaminated soil	Mild cases may be asymptomatic; GI discomfort, pain, diarrhea; intestinal obstruction in severe cases; occasionally, bile or pancreatic duct may be obstructed; allergic reactions
Enterobius vermicularis	Pinworm, seatworm, threadworm, oxyurias	Ingestion of eggs by fecal contamination of hands, food, clothing, and bedding; reinfection is common; the most common worm infestation in the United States, especially in schoolchildren	Indigestion; intense perianal itching, especially at night, resulting in loss of sleep, irritability and fatigue in children; scratching may cause infection
Trichuris trichiura	Whipworm	Ingestion of eggs through contact with fecally contaminated soil	Mild cases may be asymptomatic; insomnia, loss of appetite, diarrhea, anemia; in severe cases, colitis, proctitis, prolapsed rectum
Anisakis and Pseudoterranova	None	Eating raw or poorly cooked fish	Tingling throat, abdominal pain, fever, nausea, vomiting, diarrhea
Cestoidea			
Taenia saginata	Beef tapeworm	Eating poorly cooked infected beef	No characteristic symptoms; digestive upset, diarrhea, anemia, dizziness vary with the degree of infestation
Taenia solium	Pork tapeworm	Eating poorly cooked infected pork	Similar to beef tapeworm infection; self-infection with eggs may lead to cysts in eye, brain, heart, other organs
Diphyllobothrium latum	Fish tapeworm	Eating raw or inadequately cooked fish	Similar to beef tapeworm infestation
Hymenolepis nana	Dwarf tapeworm	Eating food contaminated with human feces	Similar to beef tapeworm infestation

The female adult worm measures 8 to 13 mm in length; the adult male is about 2 to 5 mm in length. The adult worms inhabit the first portion of the large intestine. Pinworms seldom cause damage to the intestinal wall. The mature female usually stores eggs in her body until several thousand accumulate. She then migrates down the colon and out the anus, deposits 10,000 to 11,000 sticky eggs in the perianal region, and dies. Within a few hours, infective larvae develop within the eggs. If the eggs are then transferred to the mouth, most commonly on the fingers of a child who scratches the area, the cycle begins again. Within 15–43 days of egg ingestion, the larvae are released, they mature, and newly developed gravid females migrate to the anal area and again discharge eggs, and the cycle continues.

The most common ways of transmitting pinworm infection in children are probably direct anus-to-mouth transfer of eggs by contaminated fingers and ingestion of food that has been handled by soiled hands. Reinfection may occur readily because eggs are often found under the fingernails of infected children who have scratched the anal area. Eggs dislodged from the perianal region into the environment may survive for as long as 3 weeks and can be inhaled and swallowed if they become airborne.

Symptoms

Slight infections of enterobiasis may be asymptomatic. The most important and most frequent symptom is usually an irritating itching in the perianal and perineal regions. This itching normally occurs at night when the gravid female deposits her eggs in these areas. Scratching to relieve the itching may lead to a secondary bacterial infection of the area. Nervousness, inability to concentrate, lack of appetite, and unusual dark circles around the eyes are frequently observed in children infected with pinworms. Worms occasionally enter the female genital tract and become encapsulated within the uterus or fallopian tubules, or they may migrate into the peritoneal cavity, resulting in the formation of granulomas in these areas.

The physical symptoms are not the only misery-inducing effects of pinworms. Parents are often dismayed to find worms near the anus of a child, and this psychologic trauma or "pinworm neurosis" must also be considered one of the harmful effects of enterobiasis.[2] Patients need to be assured that pinworms are common and that no social stigma is attached to their occurrence.

Perianal itching is a symptom of many conditions and is often mistakenly attributed to pinworm infection.[3] Seborrheic dermatitis, atopic eczema, tinea cruris, psoriasis, lichen planus, and neurodermatitis may produce severe itching when the perianal region is involved. An allergic or contact dermatitis may result from soaps or ointments used by the patient in an attempt to alleviate the initial mild symptoms of pinworm infestation. Ointments containing local anesthetics are well-known sensitizers and should be suspected of contributing to the problem. Other parasitic infestations that induce itching, such as scabies and pediculosis pubis, may involve the perianal skin in addition to larger areas of the body. Candidiasis may be the cause of pruritus ani, especially in patients with diabetes mellitus or a suppressed immune system. Other causes of pruritus include excessive vaginal discharge and urinary incontinence in women and excessive sweating during hot weather. When mineral oil is used as a cathartic, it tends to leak and may produce increased moisture and perianal itching.

Treatment

Treatment of pinworm infection should begin with an accurate diagnosis. The presence of pinworms can be determined by either of two methods. One method is to cover the end of a cotton swab or tongue depressor with tape (sticky side out) and apply this end to the perianal area. The presence or absence of eggs is confirmed by examining the tape under the microscope. Collection of eggs can be done at home, but inspection and evaluation must be done in a laboratory or physician's office. Another method used frequently by parents is visual inspection of the anal area with a flashlight an hour or so after the child has gone to bed. Female pinworms can be seen emerging from the anus to deposit their eggs, an event that usually occurs at night.

In the past, gentian violet was the only nonprescription drug available for treatment of pinworm infections. Genetic toxicity data indicate that gentian violet interacts with deoxyribonucleic acid (DNA) in cultured cells, suggesting a potential carcinogenic effect. Even though the evidence is not conclusive, the Food and Drug Administration (FDA) has declared gentian violet a "nonmonograph ingredient." It is no longer marketed as an anthelmintic and should not be used.[4]

Pyrantel pamoate (e.g., Antiminth®, Pin-X®, Reese's Pinworm®) was first used in veterinary practice as a broad-spectrum drug for pinworms, roundworms, and hookworms. Because of its effectiveness and lack of toxicity, it became an important drug for treating certain helminthic infections in humans.[5] Pyrantel pamoate is a depolarizing neuromuscular agent that paralyzes and kills helminths.

The FDA accepted the recommendation to move pyrantel pamoate from prescription-only to nonprescription status when used for the treatment of pinworms.[6] Helminthic infections other than pinworms should be diagnosed and treated by a physician.

Guidelines for the proper use of pyrantel pamoate are as follows:

- Side effects are uncommon. If, however, a patient experiences abdominal cramps, nausea, vomiting, anorexia, diarrhea, headache, drowsiness, or dizziness after taking this drug, a second dose should not be taken without consulting with a pharmacist or physician. If any of these conditions persist, consult a physician.
- Patients who are pregnant or have liver disease should not take this product unless directed by a physician.
- For adults and children 2 years to under 12 years of age, a single dose of 5 mg/lb or 11 mg/kg is recommended, not to exceed 1 g. A dosage schedule by weight is included with the product.
- The drug may be taken at any time of the day, with or without meals.
- When one individual in a household has pinworms, the entire household should be treated at the same time. Infants under 2 years of age or children who weigh less than 25 pounds should not be treated without first consulting a physician.
- The liquid formulation, which contains 50 mg/mL, should be shaken well before the dose is measured. The measuring device provided with the package should be used.
- The recommended dosage should not be exceeded.
- Standard treatment tables recommend retreatment 2 weeks after the initial dose, even if symptoms have not recurred.
- If any worms other than pinworms are present before or after treatment, a physician should be consulted.

The following nondrug measures are recommended to prevent reinfections.

- Wash bed linens, bed clothes, towels, and underwear of the infected individual and the entire family. A daily morning shower is encouraged to remove eggs deposited in the perianal region during the night.
- Disinfectants should be used daily on toilet seats and bathtubs.
- Close-fitting shorts under one-piece pajamas should be worn at night to prevent migration of worms and harm from scratching.
- After an infected child goes to the bathroom, the child's fingers should be scrubbed with soap and a brush. The child's nails should be trimmed regularly to prevent harboring of eggs and hand-to-mouth reinfection (autoinoculation).
- Hands should be washed frequently, especially before meals and after using the toilet.

The prescription drug mebendazole (Vermox®) in a single dose of 100 mg for adults or children, repeated after 2 weeks, can also be used to treat pinworms.[7] Because mebendazole has been shown to be teratogenic in animal studies, pyrantel pamoate is the treatment of choice in pregnant women.[8] However, pregnant women who wish to self-medicate with pyrantel pamoate should do so under the direction of a physician.[8]

Ascariasis

Ascariasis is caused by *Ascaris lumbricoides*, also referred to as giant roundworm. This species is distributed worldwide and infects over 1.0 billion people. The adult ascarids are 15–35 cm long and live in the small intestine. The female lays eggs that are passed in the feces and develop into infective larvae in the soil. Although mature larvae in the shell remain viable in the soil for many months, the eggs do not hatch until they are ingested by humans. On ingestion, the larvae are released in the small intestine. They penetrate the intestinal wall, migrate via the bloodstream to the lungs, travel up the respiratory tree to the epiglottis where they are swallowed, and develop into male and female adults in the small intestine.

Although *A. lumbricoides* has been primarily a problem of the southeastern United States, recent information has shown that swine ascaris, *A. suum*, is also infective to humans. It occurs in northern states such as New Hampshire, Washington, and Montana.[9] *A. suum* is more common in children and usually does not develop to the egg-laying stage. Instead, the immature worm, which is about 15 cm long, is rejected and passed out with the stool. Because of the possible presence of *A. suum*, the use of pig manure in home gardens should be discouraged. Pharmacists should consider this type of infection if a patient mentions that a large worm has been passed.

Symptoms

The larvae and adults of ascarids are capable of extensive migration and therefore induce diverse symptoms involving the respiratory and gastrointestinal (GI) tracts. Although many infected patients are asymptomatic, the most common symptoms caused by ascarid infections are vague abdominal discomfort and abdominal colic.[10] Occasionally nausea, vomiting, bloating, diarrhea, or weight loss is present. Children characteristically have fever and may lose weight or fail to grow. The symptoms may mislead clinicians into suspecting that the patient has an abdominal tumor, peptic ulcer disease, or some other serious medical condition. Migration of the worms may cause an intestinal obstruction that may lead to intestinal perforation, suppurative cholangitis, cholecystitis, liver abscess, pancreatitis, appendicitis, or peritonitis. Patients with minor infestations may be asymptomatic, whereas severe infestations can cause symptoms that may be mistaken for a variety of respiratory and GI diseases.

Migration of the larvae through the lungs may cause a cough; in fact, the larvae may be coughed up and seen in the sputum. Fever and pulmonary infiltrate may also accompany this pulmonary syndrome.

Allergic reactions such as asthma, hay fever, urticaria, or conjunctivitis may also result from absorption of toxins from the worm.

Treatment

Nutritional supplementation is the first therapeutic step in treatment. The drugs of choice for treating ascarid infections are mebendazole (100 mg taken twice a day for 3 days) or pyrantel pamoate (11 mg/kg in a single dose, not to exceed 1.0 g).[7] Cure rates typically exceed 99% with drugs. Pyrantel pamoate is no longer marketed in the United States as a prescription drug. However, an approved indication for the nonprescription treatment of ascarid infections is not currently approved but is being considered. The treatment of swine ascariasis is unnecessary if the worm has already been passed, but the physician may prescribe a course of treatment for the patient's peace of mind in case more worms are present.

Hookworm Infection

Worldwide, 700 to 900 million people are infected by hookworms. In the United States, hookworm infection in humans is caused by *Necator americanus*. The adult worms, which are about 10 mm long, attach themselves to the small intestine. Their eggs are excreted in the feces, hatch in warm, moist soil, and develop into active filariform larvae. On contact with humans, the larvae rapidly penetrate the skin, enter the bloodstream, and are carried to the lungs. They then enter the alveoli, ascend the trachea to the throat, are swallowed, and pass into the small intestine, where they develop into mature adults.

Symptoms

When the larvae penetrate exposed skin, an erythematous maculopapular rash and edema with severe itching may persist for several days. The lesions most commonly occur on the feet, particularly between the toes, and have been termed "ground itch." Dog and cat hookworm larvae may also penetrate human skin and cause a similar condition, but they do not progress to the pulmonary or intestinal stages.

Severe infections may produce dyspnea, a cough, congestive heart failure, or fever when the larvae migrate through the lungs. Mild intestinal infections may be asymptomatic; moderately severe infections may result in indigestion, dizziness, headache, anemia, weakness, fatigue, palpitations, nausea, or vomiting. In advanced cases, there is epigastric pain, abdominal tenderness, chronic fatigue, and alternating constipation and diarrhea. The epigastric pain is relieved by eating foods high in bulk or fiber.[10] These symptoms, like those of ascariasis, may be mistaken for those of some respiratory and GI disorders.

A major clinical manifestation of hookworm infection is iron deficiency anemia resulting from the loss of blood (as much as 0.15 mL per worm each day), which the adult worm extracts while it is attached to the intestinal mucosa.[11] Malnourished children and some menstruating women are especially prone to anemia, depending on the severity of the infection. Even people with adequate iron intake may become anemic if the hookworm infection is severe enough to cause a blood loss that cannot be compensated for by the body's normal erythropoietic mechanisms.

Treatment

The correction of hookworm-induced anemia (if present) with oral iron supplements is strongly encouraged. Mebendazole (100 mg taken twice a day for 3 days) and pyrantel pamoate (11 mg/kg, not to exceed 1 g, taken once a day for 3 days) are the drugs of choice to treat hookworm infections.[7] However, it should be noted that the FDA considers treating this condition with pyrantel pamoate to be investigational.[7]

Whipworm

Whipworms (*Trichuris trichiura*) range from 30 to 50 mm in length; they are whip-shaped, with a threadlike anterior end and a thick posterior end. The anterior end is burrowed into the mucosa of the ileocecal area. Eggs excreted in the feces mature in warm, shady soil in about 21 days. When swallowed, the eggs hatch in the small intestine and the larvae enter the Lieberkühn's crypts. After molting, they reenter the lumen and migrate to the ileocecal area, maturing in about 3 month.

Symptoms

Infections of fewer than 100 worms rarely cause clinical symptoms. Trauma to the intestinal epithelium and submucosa caused by these worms can, however, cause a chronic hemorrhage, resulting in anemia. Secondary bacterial infection may result in colitis, proctitis, or, in extreme cases, prolapse of the rectum. Symptoms of whipworm infection include insomnia, loss of appetite, urticaria, flatulence, and prolonged diarrhea.[12]

Treatment

Mebendazole, 100 mg taken twice daily for 3 days, is the preferred drug and dose for treating trichuriasis (whipworms) in adults and children.[7] No nonprescription drugs are available for treating this infection.

Anisakiasis

Because of the recent popularity of raw fish dishes such as sushi, previously rare anisakid infections have become a growing problem in the United States, especially on the West Coast and in Hawaii.[13] Larval *Anisakis* nematodes, infective to marine mammals such as seals and sea lions, may cause moderate to severe intestinal problems when ingested by man. Pacific red snapper and Pacific salmon have a particularly high prevalence of infection by these nematodes.[14]

Symptoms

Larvae of some anisakid species do not invade the intestinal mucosa but wander into the oropharynx or esophagus, causing a tingling sensation. These larvae, which are up to 3 mm long, are often coughed up within 48 hours of ingestion, causing the patient considerable anxiety and fear. Other species penetrate the wall of the stomach or intestine, resulting in symptoms that mimic diseases such as acute appendicitis, ulcer, or cancer. Because no eggs are produced, stool examination is of no use and diagnosis of anisakiasis may depend on endoscopic examination or even laparotomy.[14]

Treatment

Anthelmintics are apparently ineffective in killing anisakid larvae. The only definitive treatment in severe cases is surgical resection of the inflamed intestine. Patients should be warned of the dangers of eating raw or poorly cooked fish, especially fish from areas where marine mammals are prevalent. Freezing fish at 1.4°F (-17°C) for 24 hours will kill any larvae present.

Cercarial Dermatitis

Cercarial dermatitis, or swimmer's itch, is caused by flukes of the genera *Trichobilharzia* and *Ornithobilharzia*, which are normally blood parasites of ducks and muskrats. Eggs of these worms, when released into water, infect various species of snails, which, in turn, release a free-swimming infective stage called a cercaria. These cercariae are capable of penetrating the skin of swimmers or waders, where they are rapidly killed by an immune reaction.

Symptoms

Inflammation resulting from the cercariae produces a local erythema, a minute macule at the site of penetration, and an intense itching. Because hundreds of cercariae may penetrate, the result is a generalized fiery rash. Cases usually occur in spring and summer in both freshwater and saltwater areas where migratory waterfowl and large snail populations are present.

Treatment

Treatment of swimmer's itch should be symptomatic because it generally subsides in 24–48 hours. Antihistamines and topical corticosteroids will reduce the local immune response, and warm baths are helpful in combating the itching.

Summary

The pharmacist should be familiar with common helminthic infections, their symptoms, and their treatment. Enterobiasis (pinworm) is the only helminthic infection that should be treated with a nonprescription drug, although pyrantel pamoate is a secondary drug in treating ascariasis (roundworm). Self-medication should be discouraged for all helminthic infections other than enterobiasis. The clinical manifestations of these parasitic diseases may be characteristic of so many other illnesses that attempting self-diagnosis is not only difficult but may result in neglect of a more serious condition. The availability of effective, relatively safe, easy-to-take prescription drugs that can eradicate many helminthic infections should be reason enough to avoid self-medication. The pharmacist should encourage the patient to consult a physician for treatment when helminths other than pinworms are suspected.

References

1. Schmidt GD, Roberts LS. *Foundations of Parasitology*. 2nd ed. St. Louis: C. V. Mosby; 1981: 2.
2. Garcia LS, Bruckner DA. *Diagnostic Medical Parasitology*. New York: Elsevier Science Publishers; 1988: 153.
3. Schrock TL. Diseases of the anorectum. In: Sleisinger MH, Fordtran JS, eds. *Gastrointestinal Disease*. Philadelphia: W. B. Saunders Co; 1978: 1882–4.
4. *Federal Register* 1980; 45: 59548.
5. Gilman AG, Rall TW, Nies AS, Taylor P, eds. *The Pharmacological Basis of Therapeutics*. 8th ed. New York: Pergamon Press, Inc; 1990: 969–70.
6. *Federal Register* 1986; 51: 27756.
7. Drugs for parasitic infections. *Med Lett Drugs Ther* 1992; 34: 17–26.
8. Butler CD. Treatment of intestinal parasites during pregnancy. *Facts and Comparison Drug Newsletter* 1990; 9: 41–3.
9. Lord WD, Bullock WL. Swine Ascaris in humans. *N Engl J Med* 1982; 306: 1113.
10. Brandborg LL. Parasitic diseases. In: Sleisinger MH, Fordtran JS, eds. *Gastrointestinal Diseases*. Philadelphia: W. B. Saunders Co; 1978: 1164–69.
11. Schmidt GD, Roberts LS. *Foundations of Parasitology*. 2nd ed. St. Louis: C. V. Mosby; 1981: 473.
12. Schmidt GD, Roberts LS. *Foundations of Parasitology*. 2nd ed. St. Louis: C. V. Mosby; 1981: 448.
13. Deardorff TL, Keyes SG, Fukumura T. Human anisakiasis transmitted by marine food products. *Hawaii Med J* 1991; 50: 9–16.
14. McKerrow JH, Sakanari J, Deardorff TL. Anisakiasis: revenge of the sushi parasite. *N Engl J Med* 1988; 319: 1228–9.

CHAPTER 15

Laxative Products

Clarence E. Curry, Jr., and Demetris Tatum-Butler

Questions to ask in patient assessment and counseling

- *Why do you feel you need a laxative?*
- *Are you experiencing or have you experienced abdominal discomfort or pain, bloating, weight loss, nausea, or vomiting?*
- *What other symptoms do you have?*
- *Are you currently being treated by a physician for any illness?*
- *Have you recently had abdominal surgery?*
- *Are you pregnant?*
- *How often do you normally have a bowel movement? Have you noticed a change in frequency?*
- *How would you describe your bowel movements? Has the nature of your bowel movements recently changed in any way?*
- *Has the appearance of your stools changed? In what way?*
- *How long has constipation been a problem?*
- *Have you attempted to relieve the constipation by eating more cereals, bread with a high fiber content, fruits, or vegetables?*
- *How much physical exercise do you get?*
- *How many glasses of water or other fluids do you drink each day?*
- *Have you previously used laxatives to relieve constipation?*
- *Are you using a laxative now? How often and how long have you used a laxative?*
- *Have you had any unwanted effects from laxatives, such as diarrhea or stomach pain?*
- *Are you currently taking any medication other than laxatives? If so, what prescription and nonprescription medications are you currently taking?*
- *Are you allergic to any medication?*

Extensive media advertising suggests that having clockwork-like bowel movements somehow enhances physical well-being and social acceptability. In 1991, overall sales of laxatives in chain pharmacies alone in the United States increased 5.6% over those of the previous year and accounted for more than $500 million in sales.[1]

By definition, a laxative facilitates the passage and elimination of feces from the colon and rectum. Despite numerous recognized indications for the use of laxatives, many people use them inappropriately to alleviate what they consider to be constipation. Constipation is generally defined as a decrease in the frequency of fecal elimination and is characterized by the difficult passage of hard, dry stools. It usually results from the abnormally slow movement of feces through the colon with a resultant accumulation in the descending colon.

Causes of Constipation

Causes of constipation are numerous (Tables 1–5). Idiopathic constipation often begins in childhood or adolescence. Elderly persons often suffer constipation owing to inappropriate diet, lack of exercise, or lack of muscle tone in the colon. Constipation of recent onset suggests a possible organic or drug-induced cause. Constipation is often a problem in patients with ulcerative colitis that is limited to the rectum: when such patients experience diarrhea, the use of antidiarrheal agents can result in colonic dilation and the accumulation of hard stool in an area of bowel not affected by disease.[2]

Constipation of organic origin may be caused by numerous pathologic conditions including hypothyroidism, megacolon, stricture, or lesions (benign or malignant). Laxatives are contraindicated in such cases; proper diagnosis and medical treatment should be obtained.

Physiology of the Gastrointestinal Tract

The digestive and absorptive functions of the gastrointestinal (GI) system involve the intestinal smooth muscle, visceral reflexes, and GI hormones (Figure 1). Nearly all absorption (>94%) occurs in the small intestine; relatively little occurs in the stomach or duodenum.

The function of the colon is to allow for the orderly elimination from the body of nonabsorbed food products, desquamated cells from the gut lumen, and detoxified and metabolic end products. The colon functions to conserve fluid and electrolytes so that the quantity that is eliminated represents about 10% of what was presented to it in a 24-hour period. In addition, the colon has the capacity (as does the kidney) to absorb certain electrolytes because of differences in osmotic pressure.[3] If approximately 6 L of fluid per day are ingested and supplied by

TABLE 1	Drugs that may induce constipation

Analgesics
Anesthetics
Antacids (calcium and aluminum compounds)
Anticholinergics
Anticonvulsants
Antidepressants
Barium sulfate
Bismuth
Diuretics
Drugs for parkinsonism
Ganglionic blockers
Hematinics (especially iron)
Hypotensives
Laxative addiction
Monoamine oxidase inhibitors
Metallic intoxication (arsenic, lead, mercury, phosphorus)
Opiates
Psychotherapeutic drugs (e.g., phenothiazines, butyrophenones)

Adapted with permission from Fordtran JS, Sleisenger M, eds. *Gastrointestinal Disease.* Philadelphia: W. B. Saunders; 1989: 336–8.

secretions of the GI tract, about 1.5%, or 90 mL, will be excreted with the feces.

Tonic contractions of the stomach churn and knead food, and large peristaltic waves start at the fundus and move food toward the duodenum. The rate at which the stomach contents are emptied into the duodenum is regulated by autonomic reflexes or a hormonal link between the duodenum and the stomach. Carbohydrates are emptied from the stomach most rapidly, proteins more slowly, and fats exhibit the slowest emptying rate. Vagotomy and fear tend to lengthen emptying time; excitement generally shortens it. Most factors that slow the emptying rate also inhibit secretion of hydrochloric acid and pepsin. When the osmotic pressure of stomach content is higher or lower than that of the plasma, the gastric emptying rate is slowed until isotonicity is achieved.

The mixing and passage of the contents of the small and large intestines are the result of four muscular movements: pendular, segmental, peristaltic, and vermiform. Pendular movements result from contractions of the longitudinal muscles of the intestine, which pass up and down small segments of the gut at the rate of about 10 contractions per minute. Pendular movements mix, rather than propel, the contents. Segmental movements result from contractions of the circular muscles and occur at about the same rate as pendular movements. Their primary function is also mixing. Pendular and segmental movements are caused by the intrinsic contractility of smooth muscle and occur in the absence of innervation of intestinal tissue.

Peristaltic movements propel intestinal contents by circular contractions that form behind a point of stimulation and pass along the GI tract toward the rectum. The contraction rate ranges from 2 to 20 cm per second. These contractions require an intact myenteric (Auerbach's) nerve plexus, which apparently is located in the intestinal mucosa. Peristaltic waves move the intestinal contents through the small intestine in about 3.5 hours. Vermiform (worm-like) movements occur mainly in the large intestine (colon) and are caused by the contraction of several centimeters of the colonic smooth muscle at one time. In the cecum and ascending colon, the contents retain a fluid consistency, and peristaltic and antiperistaltic waves occur frequently. However, the activity of the transverse, descending, and sigmoid segments of the colon is very irregular, and here, through further water absorption, the contents become semisolid.

Three or four times a day, a strong peristaltic wave (mass movement) propels the contents about one-third (38 cm) the length of the colon. When initiated by a meal,

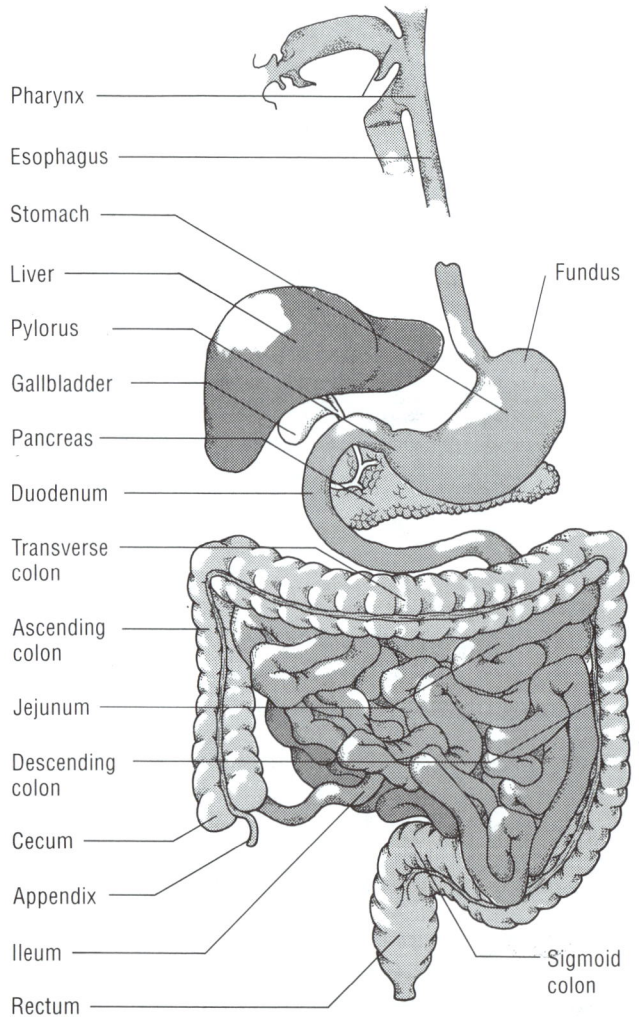

Note: portion of small intestine pulled aside for clarity.

FIGURE 1 Anatomy of the digestive system.

TABLE 2	Metabolic and endocrine disorders associated with constipation

Metabolic disorders
Diabetic ketoacidosis
Diabetic neuropathy
Hypokalemia
Porphyria
Type I (Portuguese) and II (Indiana) amyloid neuropathy; sporadic primary amyloidosis
Uremia

Endocrine disorders
Enteric glucagon excess
Hypercalcemia: pseudohypoparathyroidism, hyperparathyroidism, milk–alkali syndrome, carcinomatosis
Hypothyroidism
Panhypopituitarism
Pheochromocytoma

Adapted with permission from Fordtran JS, Sleisenger M, eds. *Gastrointestinal Disease*. Philadelphia: W. B. Saunders; 1989: 336–8.

TABLE 3	Conditions associated with neurogenic constipation

Peripheral
Aganglionosis (Hirschsprung's disease)
Autonomic neuropathy: paraneoplastic, pseudo-obstruction
Chagas' disease
Ganglioneuromatosis:
    Multiple endocrine neoplasia, type 2B
    Primary
    von Recklinghausen's disease
Hyperganglionosis
Hypoganglionosis

Central medulla
Cauda equina tumor
Meningocele (anterior or posterior)
Multiple sclerosis
Shy–Drager syndrome
Tabes dorsalis
Trauma to the medulla
Trauma to nervi erigentes

Brain
Cerebrovascular accidents
Parkinson's disease
Tumors

Reprinted with permission from Fordtran JS, Sleisenger M, eds. *Gastrointestinal Disease*. Philadelphia: W. B. Saunders; 1989: 337.

the mass movement is referred to as the gastrocolic reflex. This normal reflex seems to be associated with the entrance of food into the stomach and the subsequent distention of the stomach, and it is very strong in infants. The sigmoid colon serves as a storage place for fecal matter until defecation. The alimentary canal normally functions involuntarily in a coordinated manner.

The act of defecation involves multiple physiologic processes, but it is basically the rectal passage of accumulated fecal material. The fecal material from the sigmoid colon is propelled into the rectum by a mass peristaltic movement, which often occurs at breakfast time in persons with normal eating habits. This movement results in a desire to defecate because somatic impulses are sent to the defecation center in the sacral spinal cord. The defecation center then sends impulses to the internal anal sphincter, causing it to relax; this causes intra-abdominal pressure to increase as the muscles of the abdominal wall tighten, and a Valsalva maneuver forces the stool down. Voluntary relaxation of the external anal sphincter occurs, followed by elevation of the pelvic diaphragm, which lifts the anal sphincter over the fecal mass, allowing the mass to be expelled. Defecation, a spinal reflex, either is voluntarily inhibited by keeping the external sphincter contracted or is facilitated by relaxing the sphincter and contracting the abdominal muscles. Children usually defecate after meals; in adults, however, habits and cultural factors may determine the "proper" time for defecation.

Pathophysiology of the Lower Gastrointestinal Tract

Alteration in motor activities is responsible for various disorders in the small intestine. Distention or irritation of the small intestine can cause nausea and vomiting; the duodenum is most sensitive to irritation. Motility in the small intestine is intensified when the mucosa is irritated by bacterial toxins, chemical or physical irritants, and mechanical obstruction.

Pain from various causes, including gallbladder disease, appendicitis, and regional ileitis, may inhibit GI reflexes. As a result, functional obstruction may occur in the small intestine and with it, symptoms of acute intestinal blockage.

Large masses of fecal material tend to accumulate in a greatly dilated rectum. This is especially true in older individuals. The loss of tonicity in the rectal musculature may be caused by ignoring or suppressing the urge to defecate. It also may be caused by degeneration of nerve pathways concerned with defecation reflexes.

Painful lesions of the anal canal, such as ulcers, fissures, and thrombosed hemorrhoidal veins, impede defecation by causing a spasm of the sphincter and promoting voluntary suppression of defecation to avoid pain. The normal rectal mucosa is relatively insensitive to cutting or burning. However, when it is inflamed, it becomes highly sensitive to all stimuli, including those acting on the receptors mediating the stretch reflex. A constant urge to defecate in the absence of appreciable material in the rectum may occur with an inflamed rectal mucosa.[4]

TABLE 4	Diseases of the large intestine (colon) associated with constipation

Lesions of the colon

Stenotic obstruction
Extraluminal
    Chronic volvulus
    Hernias
    Tumors
Luminal
    Chronic amebiasis
    Corrosive enemas
    Diverticulitis
    Endometriosis
    Ischemic colitis
    Lymphogranuloma venereum
    Strictures
    Surgery
    Syphilis
    Tuberculosis
    Tumors

Muscular abnormalities
Dermatomyositis
Diverticular disease
Myotonic dystrophy
Segmental dilatation of the colon
Systemic sclerosis

Lesions of the rectum
Internal rectal prolapse
Rectocele
Surgical stricture (EEA anastomosis)
Tumors
Ulcerative proctitis

Lesions of the pelvic floor
Descending perineum syndrome

Lesions of the anal canal
Anal fissure
Anterior ectopic anus
Mucosal prolapse
Stenosis

Reprinted with permission from Fordtran JA, Sleisenger M, eds. *Gastrointestinal Disease.* Philadelphia: W. B. Saunders; 1989: 338.

TABLE 5	Dietary issues related to the development of constipation

Insufficient intake of fluid
Low fiber content of the diet
Excessive ingestion of foods (e.g., processed cheese) that harden stools

Symptoms of Constipation

If constipation does occur, symptoms of varying degrees of severity may develop. Typical symptoms include anorexia, dull headache, lassitude, low back pain, abdominal distention, and lower abdominal distress. Abdominal discomfort and an inadequate response to an increasing variety and dosage of laxatives are frequent complaints. The frequency of bowel movements in humans generally ranges from three times a day to three times a week.[5] Individuals in the latter category are usually symptom free and do not have any specific abnormality related to their individual pattern of defecation. Therefore, constipation cannot be defined solely in terms of the number of bowel movements in any given period. Regularity is what is "regular" or typical for the individual who experiences none of the classic symptoms of constipation.

Treatment of Constipation

Constipation that does not have an organic etiology can often be alleviated without a laxative product. The pharmacist should stress the importance of a high-fiber diet, adequate fluid consumption, and exercise. However, treatment may require recommendation of a laxative.

Pharmacologic Agents

The ideal laxative would (1) be nonirritating and nontoxic; (2) act only on the descending and sigmoid colon; and (3) produce a normally formed stool within a few hours, after which its action would cease and normal bowel activity would resume. Because a laxative that meets these criteria is not currently available, proper selection of a laxative depends on the etiology of the constipation.

Laxative drugs have been classified according to their chemical structure, site of action, intensity of action, or mechanism of action. The most meaningful classification is the mechanism of action, whereby laxatives are classified as bulk forming, emollient, lubricant, saline, hyperosmotic, and stimulant (Table 6).

Bulk-Forming Laxatives

Because they most closely approximate the physiologic mechanism in promoting evacuation, bulk-forming products are the recommended choice as initial therapy for most forms of constipation. These laxatives are natural and semisynthetic hydrophilic polysaccharides and cellulose derivatives that dissolve or swell in the intestinal fluid, forming emollient gels that facilitate passage of the intestinal contents and stimulate peristalsis. They are usually effective in 12–24 hours but may require as long as 3 days in some individuals. This type of laxative may be indicated for people on low-residue diets that cannot be corrected as well as for postpartum women; elderly patients; and patients with colostomies, irritable bowel syndrome, or diverticular disease.

The hydrophilic colloid bulk laxatives are not absorbed systemically but do not seem to interfere with the absorption of nutrients. When given as a powder or as granules, bulk laxatives should be mixed with pleasant-tasting fluids and administered with a full (8-oz) glass of fluid. Most people prefer juices, sugar-free fruit drinks, or soft drinks to water because such fluids help mask the gritty tastelessness of some bulk-forming laxatives, although some newer formulations have been introduced that claim to have no gritty taste. Because failure to consume sufficient fluid with a bulk laxative decreases drug efficacy and may result in intestinal or esophageal obstruction, bulk-forming laxatives may be inappropriate for persons who must severely restrict their fluid intake, such as those with significant renal dysfunction.

Esophageal obstruction has occurred in elderly persons, in patients who have difficulty swallowing, and in patients with strictures of the esophagus, following ingestion of a bulk laxative that has been chewed or taken in dry form. Symptoms of esophageal obstruction include chest pain, vomiting, excessive salivation, and an inhibited swallowing reflex that may precipitate choking. In addition, there have been reports of acute bronchospasm associated with the inhalation of dry hydrophilic mucilloid,[6] as well as of hypersensitivity reactions including swollen, watery eyes and skin rash. Because of the danger of fecal impaction or intestinal obstruction, the bulk-forming laxatives should not be taken by individuals with intestinal ulcerations, stenosis, or disabling adhesions. Diarrhea, abdominal discomfort, flatulence, and excessive loss of fluid can also occur. However, when taken properly, these agents have few systemic side effects because they are not absorbed.

Bulk-forming laxatives are derived from agar, plantago (psyllium) seed, kelp (alginates), and plant gums including tragacanth, chondrus, and karaya (*Sterculia*). The synthetic cellulose derivatives—methylcellulose and carboxymethyl cellulose sodium—are being used more often, and many preparations that contain these drugs also contain stimulant and/or fecal-softening laxative drugs (e.g., docusate). These synthetic colloidal materials have a high degree of uniformity and can be readily compressed into tablets.

Calcium polycarbophil, the calcium salt of a synthetic polyacrylic resin, has a marked capacity for binding water. It is often used to treat constipation associated with irritable bowel syndrome and diverticular disease. The maximum calcium content of this agent is approximately 150 mg (7.6 mEq) per tablet. Ingestion of the recommended therapeutic dosages may increase the risk of hypercalcemia in susceptible patients; however, the maximum daily dosage limit for calcium adopted by the Food and Drug Administration (FDA) is considerably higher than the 1,800 mg of calcium contained in the maximum daily dosage of 12 calcium polycarbophil tablets.

Another bulk-forming laxative, malt soup extract, is obtained from barley and contains maltose protein and potassium as well as amylolytic enzymes. An interesting aspect of this agent is that it reduces fecal pH, which may contribute to its laxative activity.

A mixture of cellulose and pectin (Phybrex®) appears to be equivalent to psyllium as a bulk laxative. This agent has the added advantage of not gelling when mixed with liquids, which allows its usage in baked foods, sauces, drinks, stews, and other recipes. Because of its wider range of methods of consumption, this agent may ensure better compliance over long periods of time.

Choosing among the different bulk products is a matter of personal preference. It is more important that each dose be taken with a full glass of fluid (at least 240 mL, or 8 oz). The dose should be adjusted as directed until the required effect has been obtained. In addition to being relatively safe, bulk-forming laxatives are appropriate for long-term therapy. However, the dextrose content of some of the commercial products should be evaluated for usage by diabetic patients and other patients on carbohydrate-restricted diets.

Emollient Laxatives

Docusate, formerly known as dioctyl sodium sulfosuccinate, is an anionic surfactant that, when administered orally, increases the wetting efficiency of intestinal fluid and facilitates admixture of aqueous and fatty substances to soften the fecal mass. It is commonly known as a stool softener. Other fecal-softening laxatives are docusate calcium and docusate potassium (both anionic surfactants). In many cases of fecal impaction, a solution of docusate is added to the enema fluid. Docusate does not retard absorption of nutrients from the intestinal tract.

Of little or no value in treating long-term constipation in progress, especially in elderly and debilitated patients, orally administered emollient laxatives are best suited to prevent the development of constipation. Thus, their value when used in proper doses is more prophylactic than therapeutic. Emollient laxatives should be used only for short-term therapy (less than 1 week without physician consultation) where hard fecal masses are present. Primary indications are in cases of acute perianal disease to soften and inhibit painful elimination of stool or when avoidance of straining at the stool is desirable (e.g., rectal surgery, abdominal surgery, after labor and delivery, and myocardial infarct). Emollient laxatives do not stimulate bowel movements when used alone, but do achieve this purpose when combined with stimulant laxatives. Fecal-softening emollient laxatives are usually effective in 1 to 2 days but may take as long as 3–5 days in some individuals. Liquid formulations may be more palatable if mixed with juices or milk. Fluid intake should be increased to facilitate softening of stools.

By facilitating the absorption of other poorly absorbed substances such as mineral oil, emollient laxatives, concomitantly administered, may increase the toxicity of those substances.[7] Docusate and its congeners are claimed to be nonabsorbable, nontoxic, and pharmacologically inert. However, it has been postulated that the detergent (surfactant) properties of docusate facilitate transport of other substances across cell membranes. Consequently, an FDA advisory panel recommended that these laxatives carry the following warning statement: "Do not take this product if you are presently taking a prescription drug or mineral oil."[8]

Patients with abdominal hernia, severe hypertension, or cardiovascular disease should not strain to defecate; neither should patients who are immediately postpartum, or who are about to undergo or have undergone surgery for hemorrhoids or other anorectal disorders. An emollient or fecal-softening laxative is indicated in such cases, but its use should be avoided if nausea and vomiting, symptoms of appendicitis, or undetermined abdominal pain exist.

TABLE 6 Classification and properties of laxatives

Agent	Dosage form	Daily dosage range Adult	Daily dosage range Pediatric (age in yr)	Site of action	Approximate time required for action	Systemic absorption
Bulk-forming						
Methylcellulose	Solid	4–6 g	1–1.5 g (>6)	Small and large intestines	12–72 hr	No
Carboxymethyl cellulose sodium	Solid	4–6 g	1–1.5 g (>6)	Small and large intestines	12–72 hr	No (laxative) Yes (sodium)
Malt soup extract	Solid, liquid, powder	12–64 g	6–32 oz (1 mo–2 yr)	Small and large intestines	12–72 hr	—
Polycarbophil	Solid	1–6 g	0.5–1.0 g (<2) 1–1.5 g (2–5) 1.5–3.0 g (6–12)	Small and large intestines	12–72 hr	No
Plantago seeds	Solid	2.5–30 g	1.25–15 g (>6)	Small and large intestines	12–72 hr	No
Emollient						
Docusate calcium	Solid	0.05–0.36 g	0.025 g (<2) 0.05–0.150 g (≥2)	Small and large intestines	12–72 hr	Yes
Docusate sodium	Solid	0.05–0.36 g	0.02–0.05 g (<2) 0.05–0.15 g (≥2)	Small and large intestines	12–72 hr	Yes
	Liquid	50–240 mg	10–40 mg (<3) 20–60 mg (3–6) 40–120 mg (6–12)	—	—	—
Docusate potassium	Solid	100–300 mg	100 mg (≥6) at bedtime	Colon	2–15 min	—
Lubricant						
Mineral oil	Liquid (oral)	14–45 mL	10–15 mL (>6)	Colon	6–8 hr	Yes, a minimal amount
Saline						
Magnesium citrate	Liquid	240 mL	0.5 ml/kg	Small and large intestines	0.5–3 hr	Yes
Magnesium hydroxide	Liquid	15–40 mL	0.5 ml/kg	Small and large intestines	0.5–3 hr	
Magnesium sulfate	Solid	10–30 g	2.5–5.0 g (2–5) 5.0–10.0 g (≥6)	Small and large intestines	0.5–3 hr	Yes
Dibasic sodium phosphate	Solid (oral) Solid (rectal)	1.9–3.8 g 3.8 g	1/4 adult dose (5–10) 1/2 adult dose (≥10) 1/2 adult dose (>2)	Small and large intestines Colon (rectal)	0.5–3 hr 2–15 min	Yes
Monobasic sodium phosphate	Solid (oral)	8.3–16.6 g	1/4 adult dose (5–10) 1/2 adult dose (≥10)	Small and large intestines	0.5–3 hr	Yes
	Solid (rectal)	16.6 g	1/2 adult dose (>2)	Colon	2–15 min	
Sodium biphosphate	Solid (oral)	9.6–19.2 g	1/4 adult dose (5–10) 1/2 adult dose (≥10)	Small and large intestines	0.5–3 hr	Yes
	Solid (rectal)	19.2 g	1/2 adult dose (>2)	Small and large intestines	2–15 min	—

continued

TABLE 6 continued

Agent	Dosage form	Daily dosage range — Adult	Daily dosage range — Pediatric (age in yr)	Site of action	Approximate time required for action	Systemic absorption
Hyperosmotic						
Glycerin	Solid (rectal)	3 g	1–1.5 g (<6)	Colon	0.25–1 hr	—
	Liquid (rectal)	Not recommended	1–1.5 g/kg or 40 g/m^2	—	—	—
Stimulant						
Anthraquinones	Solid	0.12–0.25 g	Not recommended (<6)	Colon	8–12 hr	Yes
Aloe			0.04–0.08 g (6–8)			
Cascara sagrada	Fluidextract (aromatic)	0.5–1.5 mL		Colon	6–8 hr	Yes
	Fluidextract	2–6 mL	1/4 adult dose (<2)	—	—	—
	Bark	0.3–1.0 g				
	Extract	0.2–0.4 mL	1/2 adult dose (2–12)	—	—	—
	Casanthranol	0.03–0.09 mL				
Senna	Solid	0.5–2.0 g	1/8 adult dose (>2)	Colon	6–10 hr	Yes
	Fluidextract	2.0 mL				
	Syrup	8.0 mL	1/4 adult dose (1–6)			
	Fruitextract	3.4–4.0 mL	1/2 adult dose			
	Suppository	1 at bedtime	1/2 adult dose (children over 60 lb)			
Calcium salt of sennosides A and B	Solid	12–24 mg	20 mg (≥6) at bedtime	Colon	6–10 hr	Yes
Diphenylmethane stimulants						
Bisacodyl	Solid (oral)	10–30 mg	5–10 mg (>6)	Colon	6–10 hr	Yes
	Solid (rectal)	10 mg	5 mg (<2)	Colon	15–60 min	Yes
			10 mg (≥2)			
Phenolphthalein	Solid	0.03–0.27 g	Not recommended (<2)	Colon	6–8 hr	Yes
			0.015–0.020 g (2–6)			
			0.03–0.06 g (>6)			
	Liquid	60–194 mg at bedtime	1 mg/kg or 30 mg/m^2	—	—	—
Miscellaneous						
Castor oil	Liquid	15–60 mL	1–5 mL (<2)	Small intestines	2–6 hr	Yes
			5–15 ml (2–12)			

Lubricant Laxatives

Liquid petrolatum (mineral oil) and certain digestible plant oils such as olive oil soften fecal contents by coating them, thus preventing colonic absorption of fecal water. Emulsified products are used to increase palatability. There is little difference in their cathartic efficacy, although emulsions of mineral oil penetrate and soften fecal matter more effectively than nonemulsified preparations. Liquid petrolatum is beneficial when used judiciously in cases requiring the maintenance of a soft stool to avoid straining (e.g., when there has been hernia, aneurysm, hypertension, myocardial infarct, or cerebrovascular accident, or after a hemorrhoidectomy or abdominal surgery). However, routine use of liquid laxatives in these cases is probably not indicated; instead, stool softeners such as docusate sodium are probably better agents for preventing constipation.

The side effects and toxicity of mineral oil are associated with repeated and prolonged use. Significant absorption of mineral oil may occur, especially if emulsified products are used. The oil droplets may reach the mesenteric lymph nodes and may also be present in the intestinal mucosa, liver, and spleen, where they elicit a typical foreign-body reaction.

Lipid pneumonia may result from the oral ingestion and subsequent aspiration of mineral oil, especially when the patient reclines. The pharynx may become coated with the oil, and droplets may reach the trachea and the posterior part of the lower lobes of the lungs. Because aspiration into the lungs is possible, mineral oil should not be administered at bedtime or to very young, elderly, or debilitated patients.

The role of mineral oil in impairing the absorption of fat-soluble nutrients is uncertain. Mineral oil may impair the absorption of vitamins A, D, E, and K; impaired vitamin D absorption may affect the absorption of calcium and phosphates. Mineral oil should not be taken with meals because it may delay gastric emptying. Additionally, it should not be given to pregnant patients because it can decrease the availability of vitamin K to the fetus. Patients taking oral anticoagulants should use mineral oil with caution because potentially decreased absorption of vitamin K may increase the blood-thinning property of the anticoagulant.

When large doses of mineral oil are taken, the oil may leak through the anal sphincter and produce anal pruritus (pruritus ani), hemorrhoids, cryptitis, and other perianal conditions. This leakage can be avoided by reducing or dividing the dose, or by using a stable emulsion of mineral oil. Prolonged use should be avoided. Because surfactants tend to increase the absorption of otherwise "nonabsorbable" drugs, mineral oil should not be taken with emollient fecal softeners.

Saline Laxatives

The active constituents of saline laxatives are relatively nonabsorbable cations and anions such as magnesium and sulfate ions. Sulfate salts are considered to be the most potent of this category of laxatives. The wall of the small intestine, acting as a semipermeable membrane to the magnesium, sulfate, tartrate, phosphate, and citrate ions, retains the highly osmotic ions in the gut. The presence of these ions draws water into the gut, causing an increase in intraluminal pressure. The increased intraluminal pressure exerts a mechanical stimulus that increases intestinal motility.

However, different mechanisms independent of the osmotic effect may be partially responsible for the laxative properties of the salts. Saline laxatives produce a complex series of reactions, both secretory and motor, on the GI tract. For example, the action of magnesium sulfate on the GI tract is similar to that of cholecystokinin–pancreozymin. There is evidence that this hormone is released from the intestinal mucosa when saline laxatives are administered.[9] This release in turn favors intraluminal accumulation of fluid and electrolytes.

Saline laxatives are indicated for use only when acute evacuation of the bowel is required (e.g., to prepare for endoscopic examination or to eliminate drugs in suspected poisonings) and when conditions such as hepatic coma necessitate ridding the gut of blood. Saline laxatives have no place in the long-term management of constipation.

In some cases of food or drug poisoning, saline laxatives are used in purging doses. Magnesium sulfate is recommended except in cases of depressed central nervous system (CNS) activity or renal dysfunction. Liquid preparations may be more palatable if they are chilled prior to administration, but that is not possible in acute medical emergencies.

In some cases, the choice of a saline laxative may result in serious side effects. As much as 20% of the administered magnesium ion may be absorbed from magnesium salts. If renal function is normal, the absorbed ion can be eliminated without consequence. However, if renal function is markedly impaired, or if the patient is a newborn or is elderly, toxic concentrations of the magnesium ion could accumulate with resulting intoxication.[10] Hypotension, muscle weakness, and electrocardiographic changes may indicate a toxic effect of magnesium. In addition, excessive serum magnesium levels exert a depressant effect on the CNS and neuromuscular activity. Other adverse effects include abdominal cramping, excessive diuresis, nausea, vomiting, and dehydration.

Phosphate salts are available in oral and rectal dosage forms. The typical oral dose contains 96.5 mEq of sodium and therefore should be administered with caution to patients on sodium-restricted diets. When phospate salts are given as an enema, up to 10% or more of the sodium content may be absorbed. The rectal use of phosphates is indicated in barium enema preparations and in elimination of fecal impaction. However, cathartics containing sodium may be toxic to individuals with edema, congestive heart disease, or renal failure; phosphates will accumulate with impaired renal function and should be avoided in such patients. The use of phosphate salts in children under 2 years of age can result in hypocalcemia, tetany, hypernatremia, dehydration, and hyperphosphatemia. Because dehydration may occur with the repeated use of hypertonic solutions of saline cathartics, phosphate salts should not be used by those who cannot tolerate fluid loss. Phosphates should be followed by at least one full glass of water in normal patients to prevent dehydration.

Hyperosmotic Laxatives

Glycerin has been available for many years in suppository form to be used for lower bowel evacuation. Its laxative capability is caused by the combination of glycerin's osmotic effect with the local irritant effect of sodium stearate. Rectal irritation may occur with its use.

Use of glycerine suppositories in infants and adults usually produces a bowel movement within 30 minutes. In infants, the physical manipulation and insertion of a solid rectal mass will usually initiate the reflex to defecate. Adverse reactions and side effects from glycerin suppositories are minimal.

The customary rectal dosages of glycerin considered to be safe and effective for adults and for children older than 6 years of age is 3 g as a suppository or 5–15 mL as an enema. For infants and for children under 6 years of age, the dose is 1–1.5 g as a suppository or 2–5 mL as an enema.[8]

Stimulant Laxatives

Stimulant laxatives, such as castor oil and bisacodyl, are often used before radiologic examination of the GI tract and before GI surgery, when thorough evaluation of the bowel is crucial. Bisacodyl may be administered orally or rectally and used instead of an enema for emptying the colon before proctologic examination.

It has long been believed that stimulant laxatives act to increase the propulsive peristaltic activity of the intestine by local irritation of the mucosa or by a more selective action on the intramural nerve plexus of intestinal smooth muscle, thus increasing motility. More recently, it has been suggested that these laxative products stimulate secretion of water and electrolytes in either the small or large intestine or both, depending on the specific laxative.[11] Intensity of action is proportional to dosage, but individually effective doses vary. All stimulant laxatives may produce griping, colic, increased mucus secretion, and, in some people, excessive evacuation of fluid. Listed doses and dosage ranges are only guides in determining the optimal individual dose.

Stimulant laxatives should be used with caution when symptoms of appendicitis (abdominal pain, nausea, and vomiting) are present, and they should not be used at all when the diagnosis of appendicitis is made.

Major hazards of stimulant laxative use are severe cramping, electrolyte and fluid deficiencies, enteric loss of protein, malabsorption resulting from excessive hypermotility and catharsis, and hypokalemia. Stimulant laxatives are effective but should be recommended cautiously; because the intensity of their activity is proportional to the dose used, a large enough dose of any stimulant laxative can produce unwanted and sometimes dangerous side effects. Unfortunately, of all the laxative products available, stimulant laxatives are the most widely abused.[12] Chronic abuse can lead to "cathartic colon," a poorly functioning colon.

In general, stimulant laxatives are not recommended as initial therapy in patients with constipation, and they should never be used for more than 1 week of regular treatment. The dose should be within the recommended dosage range (Table 6).

Stimulant laxatives are conveniently classified according to their chemical structure and pharmacologic activity.

Anthraquinone Stimulants Anthraquinone laxatives include aloe, cascara sagrada, casanthranol, senna, aloin, danthron, rhubarb, and frangula. The drugs of choice in this group are the cascara, casanthranol, and senna compounds. Rhubarb, aloe, and aloin, which are very irritating, should not be recommended. The properties of each anthraquinone laxative vary somewhat, depending on the anthraquinone content and the speed with which the active principles are liberated. The anthraquinones are hydrolyzed by colonic bacteria into active compounds.

The precise mechanism by which peristalsis is increased is unknown. The cathartic activity of anthraquinones is limited primarily to the colon. Anthraquinones usually produce their action 8–12 hours after administration but may require up to 24 hours.

The active principles of anthraquinones are absorbed from the GI tract and subsequently appear in body secretions, including human milk. However, the practical significance of this event in nursing infants is poorly defined. After taking a senna laxative, postpartum patients have reported a brown discoloration of breast milk and subsequent catharsis by their nursing infants. A study with constipated postpartum breast-feeding women receiving a senna laxative reported that 17% of their infants experienced diarrhea.[13]

Chrysophanic acid, a component of rhubarb and senna excreted in the urine, colors acidic urine yellowish-brown and colors alkaline urine reddish-violet. The pharmacist should warn patients that a number of prescription and nonprescription medications and some foods produce either alkaline or acidic urine and may result in this effect.

The prolonged use of anthraquinone laxatives, especially cascara sagrada, can result in a harmless, reversible melanotic pigmentation of the colonic mucosa, which is usually found on sigmoidoscopy or rectal biopsy.

The liquid preparations of cascara sagrada are more reliable than the solid dosage forms. Aromatic cascara fluidextract is less active and less bitter than cascara sagrada fluidextract, as is reflected by the recommended dosages (Table 6). Magnesium oxide, used in the preparation of the aromatic cascara fluidextract, removes some of the bitter and irritating principles from the crude drug.

Preparations of senna are more potent than those of cascara and produce considerably more abdominal cramping.

In 1987, the FDA announced the total recall of a formerly popular stimulant laxative known as danthron. Danthron, a breakdown product of the glycosides of senna, is an anthraquinone with actions similar to those of the natural anthraquinones. It was withdrawn from the market because of reports of its tendency to produce liver tumors in rats.[14]

Diphenylmethane Stimulants The most commonly used diphenylmethane laxatives are bisacodyl and phenolphthalein.

The tablet and suppository combination of bisacodyl has been recommended for cleaning the colon before surgery and before GI X-ray examination. Bisacodyl is effective in patients with colostomies, and it may reduce or eliminate the need for irrigations.

Bisacodyl acts in the colon on contact with the mucosal nerve plexus. Stimulation is segmented and axonal, producing contractions of the entire colon. Bisacodyl's action is independent of intestinal tone, and the drug is minimally absorbed systemically (approximately 5%).[15] Action on the small intestine is negligible. A soft, formed stool is usually produced 6–10 hours after oral administration and 15–60 minutes after rectal administration.

Side effects, which come with chronic, regular use (abuse), include metabolic acidosis or alkalosis, hypocalcemia, tetany, loss of enteric protein, and malabsorption. The suppository form may produce a burning sensation in the rectum. No systemic or adverse effects on the liver, kidney, or hematopoietic system have been observed following administration.

Enteric-coated bisacodyl tablets prevent irritation of the gastric lining and therefore should not be broken, crushed, chewed, or administered with alkaline materials such as antacid products or with histamine II antagonists.

Phenolphthalein is effective in small doses and is tasteless, making it desirable for use in candy, wafer, and chewing gum dosage forms. When ingested, it passes through the stomach unchanged and is dissolved by the bile salts and the alkaline intestinal secretions. As much as 15% of the dose is absorbed; the rest is excreted unchanged in the feces.

This drug exerts its stimulating effect primarily on the colon. Although the exact mechanism of action is not known, phenolphthalein appears to alter multiple steps of the absorptive process. It is usually active 6–8 hours after administration.

Part of absorbed phenolphthalein is secreted back into the intestinal tract along with bile. The resulting enterohepatic cycle may prolong the action of phenolphthalein for 3 or 4 days. Because bile must be present for it to be effective, phenolphthalein is ineffective in relieving constipation associated with obstructive jaundice.

Phenolphthalein is usually nontoxic. However, at least two types of allergic reactions may follow its use. In susceptible individuals, a large dose may cause diarrhea, colic, cardiac and respiratory distress, or circulatory collapse. The other reaction is a polychromatic rash that ranges from pink to deep purple. The eruptions may be as small as a pinhead or as large as the palm of the hand. Itching and burning may be moderate or severe. If the rash is severe, it may lead to vesication and erosion, especially around the mouth and genital areas. Patients should be advised to report any rash to the physician or the pharmacist. Other skin reactions, including toxic epidermal necrosis and bullous eruptions, may occur and appear to be related to sunlight exposure.[12]

Osteomalacia caused by impaired absorption of vitamin D and calcium is one untoward effect that has been attributed to excessive phenolphthalein ingestion.[16] Phenolphthalein abuse can mimic Bartter's syndrome by inducing juxtaglomerular cell hyperplasia with secondary hyperaldosteronism. This is characterized by hypokalemic alkalosis and marked renin increase in the absence of hypertension.[17]

Some of the absorbed drug appears in the urine, which is colored pink to red if it is sufficiently alkaline. Similarly, the drug excreted in the feces causes a red coloration if the feces are sufficiently alkaline. This effect may be alarming, so the patient should be forewarned.

Castor Oil   Castor oil is used in situations requiring a thorough evacuation of the GI tract; it is seldom used routinely for constipation. Castor oil's laxative action is produced by ricinoleic acid, which is produced when castor oil is hydrolyzed in the small intestine by pancreatic lipase. Its mechanism of action is unknown. However, its laxative effect appears to depend primarily on cyclic adenosine monophosphate–mediated fluid secretion and not an increased peristalsis caused by the irritant effect of ricinoleic acid.

Castor oil, a glyceride, may be absorbed from the GI tract and is probably metabolized like other fatty acids. Because the main site of action is the small intestine, its prolonged use may result in excessive loss of fluid, electrolytes, and nutrients.

Castor oil is most effective when administered on an empty stomach, and it produces an evacuation within 2–6 hours after ingestion. Because a laxative effect occurs quickly, the drug should not be given at bedtime. The most commonly used products containing castor oil are the more palatable emulsions. When plain castor oil is used, it may be administered with fruit juice or a carbonated beverage to mask its unpleasant taste.

Laxative Dosage Forms

Laxative products are available in a wide array of dosage forms, most of them for oral use. This variety probably yields the most benefits for pediatric and geriatric patients. Many of the dosage forms enhance patient acceptability and perhaps make laxative use more pleasant. However, laxatives available as chewing gum, wafers, effervescent granules, and chocolate tablets may not be thought of as drug products and thus are more likely to be misused and abused.

Enemas and suppositories are dosage forms often used for laxative administration. Enemas are used routinely to prepare patients for surgery, child delivery, and radiologic examination and to treat certain cases of constipation. The enema fluid determines the mechanism by which evacuation is produced. Tap water and normal saline create bulk by an osmotic volume effect; vegetable oils lubricate, soften, and facilitate the passage of hardened fecal matter; soapsuds produce defecation by their irritant action. However, prolonged rectal irritation may occur after soap enemas, which have also led to reports of anaphylaxis, rectal gangrene, and serious fluid loss secondary to acute colitis.[18] Therefore, soap enemas are not recommended for use.

The popular sodium phosphate–sodium biphosphate enemas (e.g., Fleet®) fall into the category of saline laxatives. They are usually effective evacuants in preparing patients for surgical, diagnostic, or other procedures involving the bowel. These agents are more efficient and effective than tap water, soapsuds, or saline enemas. Because they can alter fluid and electrolyte balance significantly if used on a prolonged basis, chronic use of these products is not warranted in the control of constipation.

A properly administered enema cleans only the distal colon, most nearly approximating a normal bowel movement. Proper administration requires that the diagnosis, the enema fluid, and the technique of administration be correct. Improperly administered, an enema can produce fluid and electrolyte imbalances. Enema fluids have caused mucosal changes or spasm of the intestinal wall. Water intoxication has resulted from the use of tap water or soapsud enemas in the presence of megacolon. A misdirected or inadequately lubricated nozzle may cause abrasion of the anal canal and rectal wall or colonic perforation.

Patients should be advised to follow all directions carefully when using these products. To administer an enema properly, the patient should lie or be placed on the left side with knees bent or in the knee–chest position. If the patient is in a sitting position, use of an enema clears only the rectum of fecal material. The solution should be allowed to flow into the rectum slowly; if the patient is uncomfortable, the flow is probably too fast. One pint (500 mL) or less of properly introduced fluid usually produces adequate evacuation if it is retained until definite lower abdominal cramping is felt. As long as 1 hour may be needed for the entire procedure.

Bisacodyl suppositories are promoted as replacements for enemas when cleaning the distal colon is required. Suppositories that contain bisacodyl are promoted for postoperative, antepartum, and postpartum care and are adequate in the preparation for proctosigmoidoscopy. Although bisacodyl suppositories are prescribed and used more often than others, some clinicians still prefer enemas as agents for cleaning the lower bowel.

Pediatric Laxative Use

Laxatives are often given to children in accordance with what the parents believe normal bowel habits should be. As a result, indiscriminate use of laxatives may occur. Stool patterns vary widely in children, and constipation can be a complex problem that is often difficult to detect and manage. Parents should observe their child for stool frequency, difficulty in passing stools, pain experienced during bowel movements, and the child's withholding of stools. Any deviation from the child's normal pattern should be noted. Infants and children appear to show a decreasing frequency of stools with increasing age. Normally, neonates may pass more than four stools a day during the first week of life. This declines to approximately 1.2 stools a day by 4 years of age. Constipation can occur in infants who pass one to two stools daily and is often unrecognized as such. Infants whose stool frequency is less than average in the first weeks of life may be prone to develop chronic constipation in later years.[19-21]

A number of factors can alter a child's bowel habits, including emotional distress; febrile illness; family conflict; dietary changes (e.g., human to cow's milk); or environmental changes, which might include a move or recent travel. Such factors must be considered to determine whether constipation exists.

As with adults, increasing both fluids and the bulk content of the child's diet may improve bowel habits and decrease frequency of constipation. Simply increasing the amount of fluid or sugar in the formula may be corrective in the first few months of life. After this age, better results are obtained by adding or increasing the amounts of high-fiber cereal, vegetables, and fruits. Sugar–water solutions (fruit juice or soda) often diminish the child's appetite for solid foods and should be administered in moderation. The child should be encouraged to drink water, and excessive milk intake should not be considered a substitute. Unbuttered popcorn is a good bulk-containing snack for children.

If medications are indicated in children under 5 years of age, glycerin suppositories may initiate the defecation reflex with an onset usually within 15–60 minutes. Malt soup extract is relatively safe for infants under 2 months of age. Dark corn syrup (one to two teaspoons per feeding) or milk of magnesia (beginning with one-half teaspoon) may be useful for fecal impaction. Bisacodyl may be used for moderate to severe constipation. In general, stimulants should probably be avoided, as should excessive use of enemas.[22] Enemas are not usually recommended for children under 2 years of age. Senna and mineral oil should be administered only on the advice of a physician. In cases when successful bowel evacuation cannot be achieved with oral supplementation or enemas, pediatricians may prescribe a balanced polyethylene glycol–electrolyte solution (e.g., Golytely® or Colyte®) to be administered orally. Children may find that such a solution is more palatable if it is chilled.

A child's age should always be considered when recommending laxative products. The route of administration and the taste of oral products may be especially significant in children. The use of laxatives in older children may be avoided if the children are encouraged to establish a regular pattern of bowel movements and adhere to suggested dietary guidelines.

Geriatric Laxative Use

Constipation is a common complaint of many elderly persons. It may progress with age, and prolonged and excessive laxative use is not uncommon in this population. Many elderly persons have been laxative-dependent for many years. However, because of the physiologic effects of chronic laxative use on the intestine, laxative dependency is often difficult to manage. Thus, proper education about laxative products and advice on product selection and use are particularly crucial for the elderly patient.

It has been suggested that the three primary causes of constipation in elderly persons are (1) failure to establish a time habit; (2) insufficient fluid and/or bulk intake; and (3) abuse of stimulant laxatives, which usually results from a patient's attempt to regulate bowel activity.[23] Constipation in this population is often associated with a prolonged transit time through the colon and a decreased perception of the need to defecate.[24,25] Elderly patients often strain to pass hard stools, which may predispose them to serious complications, including cardiovascular problems and hemorrhoids. In addition, geriatric patients tend to have multiple diseases and take multiple drugs, including sedative/hypnotics, antipsychotics, tricyclic antidepressants, and various medications with anticholinergic properties, which might contribute to the development of constipation.

Laxative preparations can increase the rate at which other drugs pass through the GI tract by increasing GI motility; this could result in the decreased absorption of other drugs. Thus, concurrent administration of laxatives with other medications may decrease the latter's effectiveness.

Elderly patients are particularly sensitive to shifts in fluid with the accompanying shifts in electrolytes. Use of any laxative that alters fluid and electrolyte balance, particularly saline-type laxatives, may be inappropriate in certain elderly patients.

In geriatric patients without a history of constipation, a thorough investigation should be conducted to determine whether acute cases of constipation have resulted from new or old diseases or from the use of medications. Many geriatric patients have a colon that lacks normal tone. This may produce an overreliance on oral laxatives or enemas for bowel movements.

A low-residue diet, a diet consisting mainly of soft foods, or the poor chewing of food may cause constipation in this age group. If any of these factors exists, the pharmacist should consider corrective action in the patient's lifestyle or current drug therapy before recommending a laxative.

It has been suggested that an acute episode of constipation should be treated with plain water or saline enemas.[24-26] Soapsud enemas should be avoided because they can be irritating and may produce serious complications.[25,27] Sodium phosphate and biphosphate enemas are effective.[28] Polyethylene glycol–electrolyte solutions, commonly used as bowel preparations for GI procedures, have been safely used for acute management of constipation in elderly patients suffering from cardiac or renal disease.[24,25] Dietary fiber should be increased by including bran, fruits, and vegetables in the diet (Table 7). Pharmacists should advise patients that increasing bran in the diet may lead to erratic bowel habits, flatulence, and abdominal discomfort during the first few weeks. It is suggested that excess bran be avoided in patients with hypocalcemia or low serum iron and in patients confined to bed.[24–26]

For elderly patients requiring laxatives, bulk-forming agents are generally preferred; onset is usually in 2 to 3 days. Sugar-free products (e.g., Konsyl®, Serutan®, SF Metamucil®) are recommended for diabetic patients.[25] Glycerin suppositories and orally administered lactulose are safe and have been used successfully in elderly patients;[25] lactulose may be of particular benefit to those who are bedridden.[25] Some physicians may recommend chronic stimulant laxative use for certain elderly patients, but such use should not be generally recommended for all elderly patients.

Caution should be exercised when using magnesium-containing cathartics in elderly patients because of the potential risks of hypermagnesemia in those with renal failure and of sodium overload in those with cardiovascular disease. The use of mineral oil should be discouraged because of possible malabsorption of fat-soluble vitamins or possible aspiration.

Recommendations of laxative products for geriatric patients should be individualized because these patients are vulnerable to medications and complicating pathology. Even though bulk-forming agents are often successfully used in this population, a complete and thorough history should provide the information needed to make appropriate individual recommendations.

Self-Medication in Pregnancy

Constipation is common in pregnancy, often because the increasing size of the uterus causes compression of the colon. However, the primary reason is probably a reduction in intestinal muscle tone, which contributes to a decrease in peristalsis.[29] In addition, prenatal vitamin and mineral supplements that contain iron and calcium tend to be constipating.

One study showed a 31% incidence of constipation in pregnancy, with 65% of these women self-treating with either diet or laxatives and without professional advice.[13] Most types of laxatives appear to be effective in pregnancy. However, because of such adverse effects as possible loss of vitamin absorption caused by mineral oil, premature labor brought on by the irritant effects of castor oil, or possible dangerous electrolyte imbalances with osmotic agents, pregnant women should probably use only bulk-forming or emollient laxatives.[30] Although stimulant laxatives should generally be avoided during pregnancy, at least one report indicates that some stimulants may be acceptable for use during the lactation period if precautions are taken.[31] Senna and related anthraquinones have been used during breast-feeding despite a lack of information regarding their concentration in breast milk. Bisacodyl appears in breast milk in trace amounts but may not pose problems for the infant.[31] If these products are used, the infant should be carefully observed for diarrhea. Saline cathartics should probably be avoided during pregnancy and lactation because appreciable GI absorption can occur in the mother. Toxicity occurring from excessive use of a saline cathartic such as magnesium sulfate could be significant, considering that such toxicity could result in diarrhea, drowsiness, hypotonia, and respiratory difficulty.

Pregnant women should be counseled on proper diet, adequate fluid intake, and reasonable exercise.[29] If these measures do not alleviate or prevent the development of constipation, a laxative preparation may be appropriate. In some instances, the pharmacist should consult with the woman's physician, especially if any doubt exists regarding the physician's desire for the patient to have a laxative. Laxatives may also have to be administered postpartum to reestablish normal bowel function that may have been lost because of perineal pain, ileus secondary to colonic dilatation in a decompressed abdomen, laxness of the anal sphincter and abdominal musculature, low fluid intake, and administration of enemas during labor. In addition, hemorrhoids in the period after delivery may be aggravated, if not caused, by constipation.

Laxative Abuse

Routine, chronic use of most laxative preparations is considered laxative abuse and should be avoided if at all possible. Although we often have a stereotypic view of the laxative abuser, that person is not always elderly. For example, some adolescents, college students, and young adults use laxatives for weight control.[32,33] Such abuse is often part of a pattern of "purging behavior," which also may include self-induced vomiting. These persons may suffer from bulimia nervosa.

Excessive use of laxatives can cause diarrhea and vomiting, leading to fluid and electrolyte losses, especially hypokalemia, which may result in a general loss of tone of smooth and striated muscle. Clinical features of laxative abuse include:

- Factitious diarrhea;
- Electrolyte imbalance (e.g., hypokalemia, hypocalcemia, and hypermagnesemia);
- Osteomalacia;
- Protein-losing enteropathy;
- Steatorrhea;
- Cathartic colon;
- Liver disease.

Cathartic colon, which develops after years of laxative abuse, is difficult to diagnose. In a study of seven hospitalized female patients, 26–65 years of age, the chief admitting complaints were abdominal pain and diarrhea, the number of hospital admissions ranged from 2 to 11, and the total number of days spent in the hospital ranged from 58 to 202.[34] The diagnosis of laxative abuse was difficult because the patients invariably denied taking laxatives, and none of the colonic tissue characteristics usually associated with excessive laxative use was observed on sigmoidoscopy or radiologic examination. However, excessive laxative use was later revealed.

Diarrhea can be a serious consequence of the overuse of laxative products, especially irritant laxatives. The prolonged misuse of laxatives can produce morbid anatomic changes in the colon. In a study of 12 chronic stimulant laxative users, the primary anatomic changes

TABLE 7　Provisional dietary fiber table

Food	Analytical method[a]	Fiber (g) per 100 g	Calories per 100 g	Serving size	Fiber (g) per serving	Calories per serving
Breakfast cereals						
All-Bran	1	29.9	249	1/3 c (1 oz)	8.5	71
Bran Buds	1	27.7	258	1/3 c (1 oz)	7.9	73
Bran Chex	1	16.2	319	2/3 c (1 oz)	4.6	91
Cheerios-type	1	3.8	391	1 1/4 c (1 oz)	1.1	111
Corn Bran	1	19.0	346	2/3 c (1 oz)	5.4	98
Cornflakes	1	1.1	389	1 1/4 c (1 oz)	0.3	110
Cracklin' Bran	1	15.1	382	1/3 c (1 oz)	4.3	108
Crispy Wheats n' Raisins	1	4.6	349	3/4 c (1 oz)	1.3	99
40% Bran-type	1	13.4	325	3/4 c (1 oz)	4.0	93
Frosted-Mini Wheats	1	7.6	359	4 biscuits (1 oz)	2.1	102
Graham Crackos	1	6.1	361	3/4 c (1 oz)	1.7	102
Grape-Nuts	1	4.8	357	1/4 c (1 oz)	1.4	101
Heartland Natural Grain, plain	1	4.7	434	1/4 c (1 oz)	1.3	123
HoneyBran	1	11.1	341	7/8 c (1 oz)	3.1	97
Most	1	12.4	337	2/3 c (1 oz)	3.5	95
Nutri-Grain, barley	1	5.8	372	3/4 c (1 oz)	1.7	106
Nutri-Grain, corn	1	6.2	381	3/4 c (1 oz)	1.8	108
Nutri-Grain, rye	1	6.4	359	3/4 c (1 oz)	1.8	102
Nutri-Grain, wheat	1	6.3	360	3/4 c (1 oz)	1.8	102
Oatmeal, regular, quick, and instant, cooked	4,5	0.9	62	3/4 c (1 oz)	1.6	108
100% Bran	1	29.6	269	1/2 c (1 oz)	8.4	76
100% Natural Cereal, plain	1	3.7	470	1/4 c (1 oz)	1.0	133
Raisin Bran-type	1	11.3	312	3/4 c (1 oz)	4.0	115
Rice Krispies	1	0.2	395	1 c (1 oz)	0.1	112
Shredded Wheat	1	9.3	359	2/3 c (1 oz)	2.6	102
Special K	1	0.8	390	1 1/3 c (1 oz)	0.2	111
Sugar Smacks	1	0.9	373	3/4 c (1 oz)	0.4	106
Tasteeos	1	3.5	393	1 1/4 c (1 oz)	1.0	111
Total	1	7.2	352	1 c (1 oz)	2.0	100
Wheat 'n' Raisin Chex	1	6.6	343	3/4 c (1 1/3 oz)	2.5	130
Wheat Chex	1	7.4	367	2/3 c (1 1/3 oz)	2.1	104
Wheat germ	1	14.3	386	1/4 c (2 oz)	3.4	108
Wheaties	1	7.0	349	1 c (1 oz)	2.0	99
Fruits						
Apple (w/o skin)	2,3,4	2.1	57	1 med	2.7	72
Apple (w/skin)	2	2.5	59	1 med	3.5	81
Apricot (fresh)	2,3	1.7	48	3 med	1.8	51
Apricot (dried)	6	8.1	238	5 halves	1.4	42
Banana	2,4	2.1	92	1 med	2.4	105
Blueberries	2	2.7	51	1/2 c	2.0	39
Cantaloupe	3	1.0	24	1/4 melon	1.0	30
Cherries, sweet	2,3	1.2	72	10	1.2	49
Dates	3,4	7.6	275	3	1.9	68
Grapefruit	2,3,4	1.3	32	1/2	1.6	38
Grapes	3,4	1.3	63	20	0.6	30
Orange	2,4	2.0	47	1	2.6	62
Peach (w/skin)	4	2.1	43	1	1.9	37
Peach (w/o skin)	2,3	1.4	43	1	1.2	37
Pear (w/skin)	4	2.8	59	1/2 large	3.1	61

continued

TABLE 7 *continued*

Food	Analytical method[a]	Fiber (g) per 100 g	Calories per 100 g	Serving size	Fiber (g) per serving	Calories per serving
Pear (w/o skin)	2,3,4	2.3	59	1/2 large	2.5	61
Pineapple	2,3	1.4	49	1/2 c	1.1	39
Plums, Damsons	2,4	1.7	60	5	0.9	33
Prunes	3,4	11.9	239	3	3.0	60
Raisins	3,4	8.7	300	1/4 c	3.1	108
Raspberries	3,4	5.1	57	1/2 c	3.1	35
Strawberries	2,3	2.0	30	1 c	3.0	45
Watermelon	2	0.3	26	1 c	0.4	42
Juices						
Apple	2	0.3	47	1/2 c (4 oz)	0.4	56
Grape	2	0.5	51	1/2 c (4 oz)	0.6	64
Grapefruit	2	0.4	41	1/2 c (4 oz)	0.5	51
Orange	2	0.4	45	1/2 c (4 oz)	0.5	56
Papaya	2	0.6	57	1/2 c (4 oz)	0.8	71
Vegetables						
Cooked						
Asparagus, cut	2,3	1.5	20	1/2 c	1.0	15
Beans, string, green	2,3,4	2.6	25	1/2 c	1.6	16
Broccoli	2,4	2.8	26	1.2 c	2.2	20
Brussel sprouts	2,3	3.0	36	1/2 c	2.3	28
Cabbage, red	4	2.0	20	1/2 c	1.4	15
Cabbage, white	4	2.0	20	1/2 c	1.4	15
Carrots	2,3,4	3.0	31	1.2 c	2.3	24
Cauliflower	3,4	1.7	22	1/2 c	1.1	14
Corn, canned	2,3	2.8	83	1/2 c	2.9	87
Kale, leaves	3	2.6	34	1/2 c	1.4	22
Parsnip	3,4	3.5	66	1/2 c	2.7	51
Peas	2,3,4	4.5	71	1/2 c	3.6	57
Potato (w/o skin)	3,4	1.0	93	1 med	1.4	97
Potato (w/skin)	4	1.7	93	1 med	2.5	106
Spinach	2,4	2.3	23	1/2 c	2.1	21
Squash, summer	2,4	1.6	14	1/2 c	1.4	13
Sweet potatoes	2,3	2.4	141	1/2 med	1.7	80
Turnip	3,4	2.2	23	1/2 c	1.6	17
Zucchini	4	2.0	12	1/2 c	1.8	11
Raw						
Bean sprout, soy		2.6	46	1/2 c	1.5	13
Celery, diced	3,4	1.5	8	1/2 c	1.1	10
Cucumber	3,4	0.8	15	1/2 c	0.4	8
Lettuce, sliced	3,4	1.5	12	1 c	0.9	7
Mushrooms, sliced	3	2.5	28	1/2 c	0.9	10
Onions, sliced	3,4	1.3	23	1/2 c	0.8	33
Pepper, green, sliced	3,4	1.3	23	1/2 c	0.5	9
Tomato	3,4	1.5	22	1 med	1.5	20
Spinach	2	4.0	26	1 c	1.2	8
Legumes						
Baked beans, tomato sauce	3	7.3	121	1/2 c	8.8	155
Dried peas, cooked	3,4	4.7	115	1/2 c	4.7	115
Kidney beans, cooked	3	7.9	118	1/2 c	7.3	110
Lentils, cooked	3	3.7	97	1/2 c	3.7	97
Lima beans, cooked/canned	2	5.4	75	1/2 c	4.5	64
Navy beans, cooked	6,3	6.3	118	1/2 c	6.0	112

continued

TABLE 7 continued

Food	Analytical method[a]	Fiber (g) per 100 g	Calories per 100 g	Serving size	Fiber (g) per serving	Calories per serving
Breads, pastas, and flours						
Bagels	1	1.1	264	1 bagel	0.6	145
Bran muffins	1	6.3	263	1 muffin	2.5	104
Cracked wheat	1	4.1	246	1 sl	1.0	62
Crisp bread, rye	1	14.9	376	2 crackers	2.0	50
Crisp bread, wheat	1	12.9	376	2 crackers	1.8	50
French bread	1	2.0	291	1 sl	0.7	102
Italian bread	1	1.0	278	1 sl	0.3	83
Mixed grain	1	3.7	235	1 sl	0.9	59
Oatmeal	1	2.2	253	1 sl	0.5	63
Pita bread (5")	1	0.9	273	1 piece	0.4	123
Pumpernickel bread	1	3.2	207	1 sl	1.0	66
Raisin bread	1	2.2	267	1 sl	0.6	67
White bread	1,4	1.6	279	1 sl	0.4	78
Whole wheat bread	1,4	5.7	243	1 sl	1.4	61
Pasta and rice (cooked)						
Macaroni	1,5	0.8	111	1 c	1.0	144
Rice, brown	3,5	1.2	119	1/2 c	1.0	97
Rice, polished	1,4,5	0.3	109	1/2 c	0.2	82
Spaghetti (regular)	1,5	0.8	111	1 c	1.1	155
Spaghetti (whole wheat)	1,5	2.8	111	1 c	3.9	155
Flours and grains						
Bran, corn	4	62.2				
Bran, oat	3	27.8				
Bran, wheat	1,3,4,5	41.2				
Rolled oats	4,5	5.7				
Rye flour (72%)[b]	4	4.5	350			
Rye flour (100%)[b]	4	12.8	335			
Wheat flour:						
Brown (85%)[b]	3,4	7.3	327			
White (72%)[b]	3,4	2.9	333			
Wholemeal (100%)[b]	3,4	8.9	318			
Nuts						
Almonds	4	7.2	627	10 nuts	1.1	79
Filberts	3	6.0	634	10 nuts	0.8	90
Peanuts	3	8.1	568	10 nuts	1.4	105

Dietary fiber values are averages compiled from literature sources. Users of the table are advised to read the accompanying manuscript to understand fully the derivation and meaning of the values.

[a]The numbers in this column refer to the analytical method used to obtain the mean dietary fiber value, as follows:
1. Neutral detergent fiber
2. Neutral detergent fiber plus water-soluble fraction
3. Southgate procedure
4. Total dietary fiber procedure
5. Englyst, nonstarch polysaccharide (NSP)

[b]The number in parentheses refers to the extraction rate of the flour. White-type breads and household flour are made with 72% flour; 85% extraction flour was consumed in the United States before World War II.

Reprinted from Lanza E, Butrum RR. *J. Am. Dietetic Assoc* 1986; 86: 732.

were mucosal inflammation, loss of intrinsic innervation, atrophy of smooth muscle coats, and pigmentation of the colon.[35] Most users had been taking laxatives regularly for 30–40 years. In such cases, the transverse colon is often pendulous, the sigmoid section is highly dilated, and the muscle layers are thin and contain excess adipose tissue, indicating some tissue atrophy.

Laxative abuse can usually be classified as either habitual or surreptitious. The habitual abuser often believes that a daily bowel movement is a necessity and uses a laxative to accomplish this end. Such patients may freely admit to this practice because they believe regular laxative use to be entirely correct and natural. On the other hand, surreptitious abuse is similar to other illnesses. Surreptitious abusers tend to manifest various psychiatric disturbances. Confronting this type of abuser does not usually help resolve the problem, and psychiatric intervention should be encouraged. To assess the abuser, the diagnostic process must include effective detection methods. Urine samples may be analyzed for the presence of the most commonly used laxatives.[36]

Once the abuse has been adequately substantiated, it may be possible to wean the patient off the laxative before permanent bowel damage occurs and to regularize the patient's bowel habits with a high-fiber diet supplemented by bulk-forming laxatives as needed. After an abuser is withdrawn from one or more laxatives, several months may be required to retrain the bowel to work in regular, unaided function. Affected patients should be educated about laxative abuse. The information provided should describe types of laxatives and their harmful effects. Patients should be advised that constipation, weight gain, bloating, or abdominal distention may occur following the end of laxative abuse. These persons should be encouraged to exercise, increase dietary fiber, and maintain adequate fluid intake. The pharmacist should also encourage them to discuss their attitudes about laxative abuse and should be prepared to answer questions that arise in such discussions.

Patient Assessment

The pharmacist should obtain as much lifestyle and clinical information as possible before making any recommendations for preventing or treating constipation. Appropriate information allows the pharmacist to make rational recommendations based on knowledge of the patient, the problem, and the product, as well as on the pharmacist's own judgment and experience. Because laxative products are both widely used and abused, the pharmacist can also provide a valuable service by educating patients about the appropriate use of laxatives.

A fundamental question is for what purpose the patient intends to use a laxative product. Not all people purchasing a laxative are constipated. A laxative might be needed to evacuate the bowel prior to an upcoming radiologic examination of the colon, or it may be purchased for a friend or a relative. It is important to know why the patient feels a laxative product is necessary.

If symptoms have persisted for more than 2 weeks or have recurred after previous dietary or lifestyle changes or laxative use, the patient should be referred to a physician. Any patient who has an established disease affecting the GI tract presents particular concern because laxative products very possibly may affect their condition adversely. The pharmacist should obtain accurate information regarding all comorbidity and should refer the patient to a physician when insufficient information or any doubt exists regarding disease status.

As previously noted, the "normal" population experiences from three bowel movements a day to three bowel movements a week, and individuals who fall outside this range might be classed as unusual but not always abnormal. Thus, the frequency of bowel movements may not be the most relevant concern; consistency of the stool, difficulty in elimination, and accompanying symptoms are also important characteristics of constipation.

The pharmacist should always inquire about the patient's current and past use of laxative products. The patient may already be using one or more such products, and improper use may be either preventing the desired effect or producing laxative dependency. The possibility of laxative abuse should also be considered. An in-depth knowledge of the patient's history of laxative use provides the pharmacist with information about the frequency and severity of constipation, prior patterns of drug use, effective or ineffective products, and the use of home remedies. Depending on the pharmacist's findings, referral to a physician may be necessary.

The pharmacist should exercise caution when recommending laxatives for patients who are receiving prescription drug products. Laxative preparations may interact adversely with other drugs that pass through the GI tract; the resulting effect could be decreased absorption of those other drugs. Drugs with constipating side effects (e.g., calcium- or aluminum-containing antacids, narcotic analgesics, and drugs with anticholinergic activity) may counteract the therapeutic effects of laxatives or require their use. Tricyclic antidepressants and certain calcium channel blockers are two frequently used groups of prescription drugs that have persistently caused constipation in many patients. A clinical condition known as the narcotic bowel syndrome is characterized by chronic abdominal pain, nausea and vomiting, abdominal distention, constipation, and at least one occurrence of intestinal pseudo-obstruction.[37] When narcotics are discontinued and narcotic bowel syndrome does not abate, patients may require continuous subcutaneous infusions of metoclopramide.[38] Such a condition might occur in a cancer patient or in other patients who require chronic administration of large doses of narcotics. Some drugs, such as magnesium-containing antacids, prostaglandins (e.g., misoprostol), and antiadrenergic drugs, may produce laxative side effects (e.g., diarrhea). Pharmacists must assess all drug use and foster the rational selection of appropriate laxatives.

In some cases, treatment for another medical condition may relieve symptoms of constipation. In perianal disease, for example, constipation is usually the result of the patient's unwillingness to defecate because of the pain encountered. When medical or surgical treatment is provided, the barrier to normal defecation is removed. Similarly, conditions such as hypothyroidism or depression may be responsible for constipation, which can be eliminated if these underlying medical conditions are treated successfully.

Product Selection Guidelines

The fact that normal defecation empties only the descending and sigmoid branches of the colon should be remembered when the use of any preparation in a suspected situation of constipation is being considered. The preparation chosen should duplicate the normal physiologic process as nearly as possible. Clearly, most stimulant products act more widely than other types of laxatives, given that they foster emptying of the entire colon. However, the laxative user who is unaware of this effect may take another laxative dose on the first or second postlaxative day, thereby maintaining a completely empty colon. Thus, when it is necessary to use a laxative to treat constipation, the recommended initial choice is most often a bulk-forming product.

Primary indications for self-treatment with a nonprescription laxative include preparation for diagnostic GI procedures and acute constipation. A physician should supervise the use of laxatives during treatment for perianal disease (pre- or postoperatively), during conditions in which straining is undesirable (e.g., postoperative or postmyocardial infarct), or for chronic constipation. Because defecation has been found to alter hemodynamics, straining to defecate may result in blood pressure surges or cardiac rhythm disturbances and has resulted in death from emboli, ventricular rupture, and cardiogenic shock in patients who had previously experienced a myocardial infarct.

The pharmacist should also recognize the situations in which laxative use is inappropriate. For example, laxatives are not recommended to treat constipation associated with intestinal pathology or secondary to laxative abuse unless bowel retraining has been successful. Laxatives also are not a cure for functional constipation and therefore are of only secondary importance in treating this condition. Attention should be directed first to questions relating to diet, fluid intake, physical activity, and underlying pathology that may be producing constipation as a symptom.

Laxative products containing more than 15 mEq (345 mg) of sodium, more than 25 mEq (975 mg) of potassium, or more than 50 mEq (600 mg) of magnesium in the maximum daily dose should not be used if kidney disease, heart failure, hypertension, or other conditions requiring sodium, potassium, or magnesium restriction are present. Any product containing dextrose should be used with caution in labile diabetic patients because of the possibility of loss of glycemia control.

Consultation Information

The most useful approach in counseling the person who requests a laxative product for self-treatment should first include a discussion of dietary habits (adequate fiber and fluids), physical exercise, the ability to respond to the urge to defecate, and general emotional well-being. Although it is well recognized that these factors may be largely responsible for problems associated with constipation, people may not understand how these factors may affect the development of constipation and how they can return a person to a relatively normal state of bowel function without laxative intervention.

A diet consisting of plenty of fluids (four to six 8-oz glasses a day) and high-fiber foods will help prevent chronic constipation. Caution regarding fluid intake must be used in patients on fluid restriction. Dietary fiber is that part of whole grain, vegetables, fruits, and nuts that resists digestion in the GI tract (Table 7). Food fiber content, which is expressed in terms of crude fiber residue after treatment with dilute acid and alkali, has a significant effect on bowel habits. Because fiber holds water, stools tend to be softer, bulkier, and heavier in persons with a higher fiber intake, and probably pass through the colon more rapidly.

Along with a high-fiber diet, the pharmacist may encourage regular, mild exercise such as walking, provided the patient's cardiovascular system is healthy and mild exercising presents no apparent health risk owing to other pathology. Exercise in any form improves muscle tone, but exercise using the abdominal muscles is the most beneficial in maintaining or improving intestinal muscle tone.

The patient should be advised not to ignore the urge to defecate and should allow adequate time for elimination. A relaxed, unhurried atmosphere can be very important in aiding elimination. The patient should be encouraged to set a regular pattern for bathroom visits. Having a specific time set aside for elimination may help the body adjust itself to producing a regular stool.

In counseling the patient on rational laxative use, the pharmacist should stress the following points:

- Laxative agents should not be used regularly; more natural methods such as diet, exercise, and fluid intake should be used to foster regular bowel movements.
- The use of a laxative to treat constipation should be only a temporary measure; once regularity has returned, laxative use should be discontinued.
- Laxatives are not designed for long-term use; if they are not effective after 1 week, a physician should be consulted.
- If a skin rash appears after the patient has taken a laxative containing phenolphthalein, the product should be discontinued and a physician should be contacted.
- Saline laxatives should not be used daily, nor should they be administered orally to children under 6 years of age or rectally to infants under 2 years of age.
- Mineral oil should not be given to children under 6 years of age or in conjunction with emollient laxatives; it should not be used during pregnancy, and it should be avoided in elderly patients and in patients taking anticoagulants.
- Castor oil should not be used to treat constipation.
- Enemas and suppositories must be administered properly to be effective.
- Laxatives should not be used in the presence of abdominal pain, perianal lesions, nausea, vomiting, bloating, or cramping without consulting a physician.
- Laxatives containing phenolphthalein or senna may discolor urine; laxatives containing phenolphthalein may discolor feces and urine pink to red, depending on the alkalinity.

Summary

The widespread misuse and abuse of nonprescription laxatives is evidence of the need for professional consultation and patient education. Successful treatment of constipation depends on careful identification of the cause. To determine whether referral to a physician or self-therapy is indicated, the pharmacist needs to know the case history and current symptoms. If the case history discloses a sudden change in bowel habits that has persisted for 2 weeks, the pharmacist should refer the patient to a physician immediately. However, if the constipation can be treated without physician intervention, knowledge of the many available products is essential.

For most cases of simple constipation, proper diet, exercise, and adequate fluid intake will be helpful. Therapy with any laxative product should be limited in most cases to short-term use (1 week). If no relief has been achieved after 1 week of proper laxative therapy, use of the product should be discontinued and a physician consulted.

References

1. *Drug Store News* 1992; 2 (4): 43.
2. Jacknowitz AI. Ulcerative colitis and its treatment. *Am J Hosp Pharm* 1980; 37: 1635.
3. Carey WD. Colon physiology: a review. *Cleve Clin* 1977; 44: 73.
4. Netter FH. *The Ciba Collection of Medical Illustrations.* Vol. 3, part II. Summit, NJ: Ciba Pharmaceuticals; 1962: 98.
5. Connell AM, Hilton C, Irvine G, et al. Variation of bowel habit in 2 population samples. *Br Med J* 1965; 2: 1095.
6. Gross R. Acute bronchospasm associated with inhalation of psyllium hydrophilic mucilloid. *J Am Med Assoc* 1979; 241: 1573.
7. Safety of stool softeners. *Med Lett Drugs Ther* 1977; 19: 45.
8. Proposed monograph of the Panel on the Safety and Efficacy of Laxatives, Antidiarrheals, Antiemetics and Emetics. *Federal Register* 1975; 40 (56): part II.
9. Harvey RR, Read AE. Saline purgatives act by releasing cholecystokinin. *Lancet* 1973; 2: 185.
10. Mofenson HC, Caraccio TR. Magnesium intoxication in a neonate from oral magnesium hydroxide laxatives. *J Toxicol Clin Toxicol* 1991: 29 (2): 215–22.
11. Moriarty KJ, Silk DBA. Laxative abuse. *Dig Dis* 1988; 6: 15–29.
12. Pietrusko RG. Use and abuse of laxatives. *Am J Hosp Pharm* 1977; 34: 291.
13. Greenhalf JO, Leonard HS. Laxatives in the treatment of constipation of pregnant and breast feeding infants. *Practitioner* 1973; 210: 259.
14. Gilbertson WE, Lessing M. Danthron alarm, FDA response: crucial OTC drug control. *Milit Med* 1988; 153: 487–8.
15. Brunton LL. Agents affecting gastrointestinal water flux and motility, digestants and bile acids. In: Gilman AG, Rall TW, Nies AS, et al., eds. *The Pharmacological Basis of Therapeutics.* 8th ed. New York: Pergamon Press; 1990: 921.
16. Frame B, Guiang HL, Frost HM, et al. Osteomalacia induced by laxative (phenolphthalein) ingestion. *Arch Intern Med* 1971; 128: 794.
17. Fleisher N, Brown H, Graham DY, et al. Chronic laxative-induced hyperaldosteronism and hypokalemia stimulating Bartter's syndrome. *Ann Intern Med* 1969; 70: 791.
18. Pike BF, Phillippi PJ, Lawson EH, et al. Soap colitis. *N Engl J Med* 1971; 285: 217.
19. Pettei MJ. Chronic constipation. *Pediatr Ann* 1987; 16 (10): 796–800, 804–6, 811–3.
20. Lemoh JN. Frequency and weight of normal stools in infancy. *Arch Dis Child* 1979; 54: 719.
21. Weaver LT. The bowel habits of young children. *Arch Dis Child* 1984; 59: 649.
22. Liebmann WM. Disorders of defecation in children: evaluation and management. *Postgrad Med* 1979; 66: 105.
23. Castle SC. Constipation: a pressing issue. *Arch Intern Med* 1987; 147 (10): 1702–4.
24. Brandt LJ. Constipation in the elderly. *Pract Gastroenterol,* 1987 Mar/Apr; 11 (2): 31–6.
25. Rosseau P. Treatment of constipation in the elderly. *Postgrad Med* 1988; 83 (4): 339–40, 343–5, 349.
26. Brandt LJ. *Gastrointestinal Disorders of the Elderly.* New York: Raven Press; 1984: 261–367.
27. Rosseau P. No soapsuds enemas. *Postgrad Med* 1988; 83 (4): 352–3.
28. Brocklehurst JC. The gastrointestinal system: the large bowel. In: Brocklehurst JC, ed. *Textbook of Geriatric Medicine and Gerontology.* New York: Longman (Churchill-Livingstone); 1985: 534-56.
29. Biggs JSG, Vesey EJ. Treatment of gastrointestinal disorders of pregnancy. *Drugs* 1980; 19: 70.
30. Hart LH. Constipation and diarrhea. In: Young LY, Koda-Kimble MA, eds. *Applied Therapeutics: The Clinical Use of Drugs.* 4th ed. Vancouver, Wash: Applied Therapeutics, Inc; 1989: 112.
31. Chaplin S, Sanders GL, Smith JM, et al. Drug excretion in human breast milk. *Adv Drug React* 1982; 1: 255.
32. Vanin JR, Saylor KE. Laxative abuse: a hazardous habit for weight control. *J Am Coll Health* 1989 Mar; 37 (5): 227–30.
33. Halmi KA, Falk JR, Schwartz E. Binge-eating and vomiting: a survey of a college population. *Psychol Med* 1981; 11 (4): 697–706.
34. Babb RR. Constipation and laxative abuse. *West J Med* 1975; 122: 93.
35. Smith B. Pathologic changes in the colon produced by anthraquinone purgatives. *Dis Colon Rectum* 1973; 16: 455.
36. deWolff FA. A screening method for establishing laxative abuse. *Clin Chem* 1981; 27: 914.
37. Sandgren JE, McPhee MS, Greenberger NJ. Narcotic bowel syndrome treated with clonidine. *Ann Intern Med* 1984; 101: 331–4.
38. Bruera E, Brenneis C, Michaud M, et al. Continuous sc infusion of metoclopromide for the treatment of narcotic bowel syndrome. *Cancer Treat Rep* 1987; 71: 1121–22.

CHAPTER 16

Diabetes Care Products and Monitoring Devices

John R. White, Jr., and R. Keith Campbell

Questions to ask in patient assessment and counseling

- *When were you last tested for diabetes? What were the results of those tests?*
- *How long have you had diabetes?*
- *Is there a history of diabetes in your family?*
- *How do you feel about having diabetes? Do members of your family understand the condition and the factors that affect control?*
- *Do you belong to the local diabetes association? Do you carry or wear special identification regarding the fact that you are diabetic?*
- *How long has it been since you discussed your diabetes treatment program with your physician? Pharmacist? Dietitian? Nurse educator? Physical therapist?*
- *What drugs have been prescribed for you? Are you taking anything for diabetes?*
- *Do you use insulin? What type do you use? What brand do you use? How do you store your insulin?*
- *If you use insulin, how do you draw it into the syringe? Where do you inject it? How much do you inject? Do you rotate the sites of injection? How often do you rotate sites? How do you dispose of your needles and syringes?*
- *Are you taking any other medicines, such as pain killers, cough medicines, decongestants, or appetite suppressants?*
- *Are you allergic to sulfa drugs? Are you allergic to beef or pork insulin?*
- *Do you test your blood glucose? If so, how often do you do the testing? Do you compare the strips visually or do you use a meter? Do you keep track of all your blood glucose readings? Do you show your blood glucose records to your physician or pharmacist?*
- *Do you test your urine for glucose at home? If so, how often do you do the testing? Which test do you use? Do you keep track of all your urine glucose readings? Do you report abnormal urine glucose test results to your physician or pharmacist?*
- *Do you test your urine for ketones? If so, how often do you do the testing? Which test do you use? Do you keep track of all your urine ketone readings? Do you report all positive urine ketone test results to your physician?*
- *Explain how you test your urine using TesTape®, Clinitest® tablets, Diastix®, Clinistix®, or Chemstrip uG®.*
- *What kind of diet has your physician prescribed? Do you have any trouble following the diet?*
- *Do you use any of the current popular "fad" diets? If so, which one? Who recommended the diet to you?*
- *Have you worked with a dietitian to help plan meals and snacks?*
- *Do you have a regular schedule for exercise? Do you check your blood glucose before and after exercise? What do you do if your blood glucose is low? What do you do if your blood glucose is high?*
- *How much alcohol (including wine and beer) do you drink in a week? What have you been told about alcohol consumption and your diabetes?*
- *Do you visit an ophthalmologist regularly? When was your last eye exam? What did the doctor tell you?*
- *Do you visit a dentist regularly? When was your last checkup?*
- *Do you ever see a podiatrist? When? What special foot care procedures do you practice?*
- *What do you think has affected the control of your diabetes? Are you eating differently? Are you exercising more or less? Have you had any infections? When? What was the location of the infection? Is anything emotionally upsetting you?*

Editor's Note: This chapter is based in part on the chapter with a similar title that appeared in the 9th edition but was written by L. M. Evenson-St. Amand and R. Keith Campbell.

Approximately 8 million persons with diabetes (PWDs) are being treated in the United States, while approximately 6 million individuals have undiagnosed diabetes (with mild symptoms or none at all).[1] The prevalence of diagnosed diabetes increased by about 17% in the 1980s.[2] Currently, another 5 million individuals will develop diabetes at some time during their lives. The incidence of diabetes in the U.S. population is about 5%. Roughly 25% of the population (approximately 50 million people) either have diabetes, will develop diabetes, or have a relative with diabetes.

Diabetes is the number one cause of new blindness in individuals between 25 and 74 years of age. More than half of all heart attacks are related to diabetes. Diabetic kidney disease is one of the leading causes of end-stage renal disease. Neurologic complications, both autonomic and peripheral, occur frequently. Complications of pregnancy due to diabetes are well recognized. More than 40,000 amputations a year are performed owing to diabetes-related complications in the foot and leg. Patients with diabetes are two to three times more likely to suffer from macrovascular disease than their nondiabetic counterparts. Overall, diabetes and its complications are responsible for approximately 8% of hospital admissions[3,4] and represent the third leading cause of death in the United States.

Women are 50% more likely to have diabetes than men; non-Whites are 20% more likely to have diabetes than Whites; and the chance of developing diabetes doubles with every 20% of excess weight and every decade of life[5]. Approximately 50% of the diabetic population is over the age of 55.[1]

The estimated annual cost of diabetes care in the United States is more than $20 billion. Economic costs are about 13% higher for insulin-dependent patients than for noninsulin-dependent patients.[6] The average cost of diabetes care products is estimated to be about $4 per day. Frequently, the patient is neglected by manufacturers of pharmaceuticals, health and beauty aids, food, drinks, and candy, who instead offer a bewildering selection of products that are improperly formulated or poorly labeled (i.e., lacking the adequate patient education and comprehensive instructions essential to optimal self-care).

The pharmacist has an excellent opportunity to assist the patient by reiterating instructions and pointing out warning signs, assessing the patient's ability to engage in self-care, providing patient education related to self-care measures, and verifying that the patient understands the information provided. The pharmacist can also serve as a consultant to both the physician and the patient concerning the disease as well as drugs, devices, and monitoring systems used in its treatment.

Carbohydrate Metabolism

Normal Carbohydrate Metabolism

Under normal conditions, the body maintains a balance among glucose, fatty acids, and ketone bodies in the tissue cells and blood to keep plasma glucose levels within a relatively narrow range and provide adequate glucose to the central nervous system. Insulin is stored in pancreatic beta cells as granules, which are released in response to changes in the concentration of plasma glucose. An initial, rapid insulin release in response to an increase in plasma glucose is followed by a slower, sustained release, which gradually increases. Insulin, which is needed to facilitate glucose transport into the fat or muscle tissue, stimulates glucose uptake and use. It also stimulates increases in muscle and liver glycogen levels, and in the synthesis of fatty acids and triglycerides; decreases in hepatic glucose output, lipolysis, and the production of ketone bodies; and enhanced incorporation of amino acids into proteins. Insulin is rapidly cleared by the liver, which allows changes in insulin secretion to compensate for fluctuations in blood glucose levels. Together with glucagon, somatostatin, growth hormone, corticosteroids, epinephrine, and other hormones, insulin maintains the blood glucose between 50 and 150 mg/100 mL (mg%) at all times. Any increase or decrease in hormones or other chemicals that affects insulin activity (such as occurs in drug therapy) can cause a person to become diabetic or a patient who has diabetes to lose glycemia control.

Diabetic Carbohydrate Metabolism

Type I Diabetes

In Type I diabetes, there is a gross lack of insulin release in response to increased blood glucose levels after a meal or a snack and hyperglycemia is the result. To compensate for the missing insulin to provide glucose to the glucose-deficient tissue, amino acids are converted into glucose by gluconeogenesis, and liver glycogen is converted into glucose by glycogenolysis. However, without insulin, the dependent tissues cannot use this glucose either, and the hyperglycemia becomes even more pronounced.

The blood glucose level at which glucose first appears in the urine is referred to as the renal threshold for glucose. Normally, glucose is found in the urine when venous blood glucose exceeds 180 mg/100 mL. In PWDs and in patients of advanced age, the threshold level for glucose may be higher.

The increased osmotic load in the kidney draws body water with it and is responsible for the excretion of large amounts of urine (polyuria), a loss of fluid, and dehydration. This osmotic diuresis may initially cause dry mouth and could progress to significant hypovolemia, electrolyte loss, and cellular dehydration. A compensatory increase in thirst (polydipsia) occurs. Additionally, tissue cells cannot use the circulating blood glucose because of a lack of insulin, and the nervous system signals the person to eat (polyphagia). Eating continues to increase the blood glucose level.

Insulin also has a direct inhibitory effect on the enzyme lipoprotein lipase, which mobilizes body fat (lipolysis). Other hormones, such as glucocorticoids and epinephrine, enhance lipolysis. A lack of insulin results in enhanced lipase activity, and fat is converted into free fatty acids. Because fats, rather than carbohydrates, are being metabolized, weight loss occurs over a period of time. The acidic ketone bodies that result from the breakdown of free fatty acids eventually induce metabolic acidosis in the absence of insulin. This ketoacidosis can lead to deep and labored breathing, sometimes called air hunger or Kussmaul's respiration. The breath will have a fruity acetone odor. Ketones can also depress the central nervous system, resulting in coma and death if insulin is not administered. Ketones in the urine (ketonuria) suggest ketoacidosis.

Figure 1 shows the clinical manifestations that result in a patient with untreated Type I diabetes. The insulin deficiency results in abnormal urine and blood values that can be monitored and used to determine how well the patient's diabetes is being controlled.

TABLE 1 Classification of diabetes and glucose intolerance

Current names	Old names
Clinical Categories	
Type I: Insulin-dependent diabetes mellitus (IDDM)	Juvenile diabetes Juvenile-onset diabetes Ketosis-prone diabetes Growth-onset diabetes Brittle diabetes

Type II: Noninsulin-dependent diabetes mellitus (NIDDM)
    Type a: nonobese
    Type b: obese
	Adult-onset diabetes
	Maturity-onset diabetes
	Ketosis-resistant diabetes
	Stable diabetes
	Maturity-onset diabetes of youth

Diabetes mellitus associated with other conditions or syndromes	Secondary diabetes (drug-induced diabetes; impaired glucose tolerance due to other hormonal irregularities)
Impaired glucose tolerance	Asymptomatic diabetes Chemical diabetes Subclinical diabetes Borderline diabetes Latent diabetes
Gestational diabetes	Gestational diabetes
Statistical Risk	
Previous abnormality of glucose tolerance	Latent diabetes Prediabetes
Potential abnormality of glucose tolerance	Potential diabetes Prediabetes

Reprinted with permission from *Diabetes* 1979; 28 (12): 1039.

Type II Diabetes

Whereas Type I diabetes typically has a rapid onset with the usual signs of polyuria, polyphagia, polydipsia, weakness, weight loss, dry mouth, and ketonuria or ketoacidosis, Type II diabetes is frequently unaccompanied by any symptoms. Type II diabetes is detected most often when glucose is found in the urine (glucosuria) or when elevated blood glucose is found on a routine examination. Figure 2 provides a flow diagram that reveals the pathogenesis of Type II diabetes. Careful study of the older, obese group of patients reveals glucosuria, proteinuria (protein in the urine), postprandial hyperglycemia, microaneurysms, and even retinal exudates.

Nonobese Type II patients may have low, normal, or high blood insulin levels, depending on a number of factors. Obese Type II patients usually have normal or elevated blood insulin levels. Glucose is transported into muscle and fat cells, so these patients are not ketosis-prone and seldom develop ketoacidosis except during periods of significant stress. However, because of their high blood glucose levels, they may develop hyperglycemic, hyperosmolar, nonketotic coma. Increased obesity in patients may cause high levels of insulin in the blood (hyperinsulinemia), resulting in a downregulation of insulin receptors and thus producing the clinical finding of hyperglycemia. Weight reduction to an ideal body weight will often be accompanied by a return to normal blood glucose levels.

Classification of Diabetes Mellitus

Diabetes mellitus is not a single disease but rather a syndrome composed of several specific diseases, all of which are characterized by hyperglycemia and a tendency toward the development of macro- or microvascular disease and neuropathy. Several types of diabetes have been identified. Table 1 summarizes the current classification system. Table 2 classifies the two major clinical types of diabetes according to their distinguishing features. Approximately 10% of

TABLE 2 Distinguishing features of the two major types of diabetes mellitus

	Insulin-dependent Type I (IDDM)	Noninsulin-dependent Type II (NIDDM)
Age of onset	Usually, but not always, during childhood or adolescence	Frequently > 35
Type of onset	Abrupt	Usually gradual
Prevalence	0.5%	2–4%
Incidence	< 10%	> 75%
Family history of diabetes	Frequently negative	Commonly positive
Primary cause	Pancreatic beta cell deficiency	End organ (insulin receptors) unresponsiveness to insulin action
Nutritional status at time of onset	Usually thin with weight loss	Usually obese
Postglucose plasma or serum insulin[a], mcU/mL	Absent or minimal	Normal or elevated
Symptoms	Polydipsia, polyphagia, and polyuria	Maybe none
Hepatomegaly	Rather common	Uncommon
Stability	Blood sugar fluctuates widely in response to small changes in insulin dose, exercise, and infection	Blood sugar fluctuations are less marked
Possible etiologic factors include:		
Inheritance	Associated with specific HLA[b] tissue types, but only 40–50% concordance in twins	95–100% concordance in twins, but not associated with specific HLA[b] tissue types
Autoimmune disease	50–80% circulating islet cell antibodies	Negative; < 10% circulating islet cell antibodies
Viral infections	Coxsackie, mumps, influenza	No evidence
Proneness to ketosis	Frequent, especially if treatment program is insufficient in food and/or insulin	Uncommon except in the presence of unusual stress or moderate to severe sepsis
Insulin defect	Defect in secretion; secretion is impaired early in disease; secretion may be totally absent late in disease	Insulin deficiency present in some patients; others are insulin resistant
		Insulin deficiency—in most patients, insulin secretion fails to keep pace with inordinate demands caused by obesity; this defect may appear initially as a failure to respond to glucose alone, suggesting an impairment in the glucoreceptor of the pancreatic beta cell
		Insulin resistance—in some patients, there is a defect in tissue responsiveness to insulin and evidence of hyperinsulinemia; in such patients, insulin resistance may be mediated by a decreased number of insulin receptors in target cells
		Increased hepatic glucose production in response to altered cellular glucose uptake

continued

TABLE 2   continued

	Insulin-dependent Type I (IDDM)	Noninsulin-dependent Type II (NIDDM)
Plasma insulin (endogenous)	Negligible to zero	Plasma insulin response may be either adequate but delayed, so that postprandial hypoglycemia may be present when diabetes is discovered, or diminished but not absent
Vascular complications of diabetes and degenerative changes	Infrequent until diabetes has been present for ~ 5 years	Frequent
Usual causes of death	Degenerative complications in target organs (e.g., renal failure due to diabetic nephropathy)	Accelerated atherosclerosis (e.g., myocardial infarct); to lesser extent, microangiopathic changes in target tissues (e.g., renal failure)
Diet	Mandatory in all patients	If diet is used fully, hypoglycemic therapy may not be needed
Insulin	Necessary for all patients	Necessary for 20–30% of patients
Oral agents	Rarely efficacious	Often efficacious

[a]Normal response is between 50 and 135 mcU/mL at 60 minutes and less than 100 mcU/mL at 120 minutes after 100 g of oral glucose.
[b]Human leukocyte antigen.

PWDs in the United States are classified as having Type I or insulin-dependent diabetes mellitus (IDDM); the remaining 90% have Type II or noninsulin-dependent diabetes mellitus (NIDDM).

Within the Type II classification are two distinct categories of patients. Approximately 10% of patients with NIDDM are nonobese; the other 90% are obese. Nonobese Type II diabetes often occurs in patients during youth and is inherited in an autosomal dominant pattern. Obese Type II diabetes often occurs in adults over the age of 40.

Etiology

Factors associated with the development of diabetes include heredity, obesity, age, stress, hormonal imbalance, vasculitis of the vessels supplying the beta cells of the pancreas, and viruses affecting the autoimmune responses of the body.

Type I diabetes (IDDM) is characterized by an absence of functioning, insulin-secreting pancreatic islet cells. The abnormal cells may be affected by intrinsic factors such as (1) genetic defects in the production of certain macromolecules necessary for proper insulin synthesis, packaging, or release; or (2) inability of beta cells to recognize endogenous glucose levels or replicate normally.[7] Extrinsic factors that have been identified as adversely affecting beta cell function include viruses such as mumps or Coxsackie B4, de-

TABLE 3   Harmful effects of hyperglycemia (blood glucose ≥ 150 mg/dL)

Increased capillary basement membrane thickening

Glucose metabolized via polyol pathway, leading to increased levels of sorbitol

Increased plasma viscosity

Faulty lipid metabolism, leading to higher levels of fat and possibly accelerating atherosclerosis

Abnormally high levels of glycosylated hemoglobin

Impairment of phagocytosis and subsequent ability to fight infection

Increased neonatal morbidity and mortality

Reprinted from Pharmaceutical services for patients with diabetes. *Am Pharm* (module 4) 1986 May; NS26 (5): 7.

structive cytotoxins and antibodies released by sensitized lymphocytes, or autodigestion in the course of an inflammatory disorder involving the adjacent exocrine pancreas. Cells have many different antigen types. Specific human leukocyte antigen (HLA) genes may increase susceptibility to a diabetogenic virus, or certain immune-response genes may predispose patients to a destructive autoimmune response against their own islet

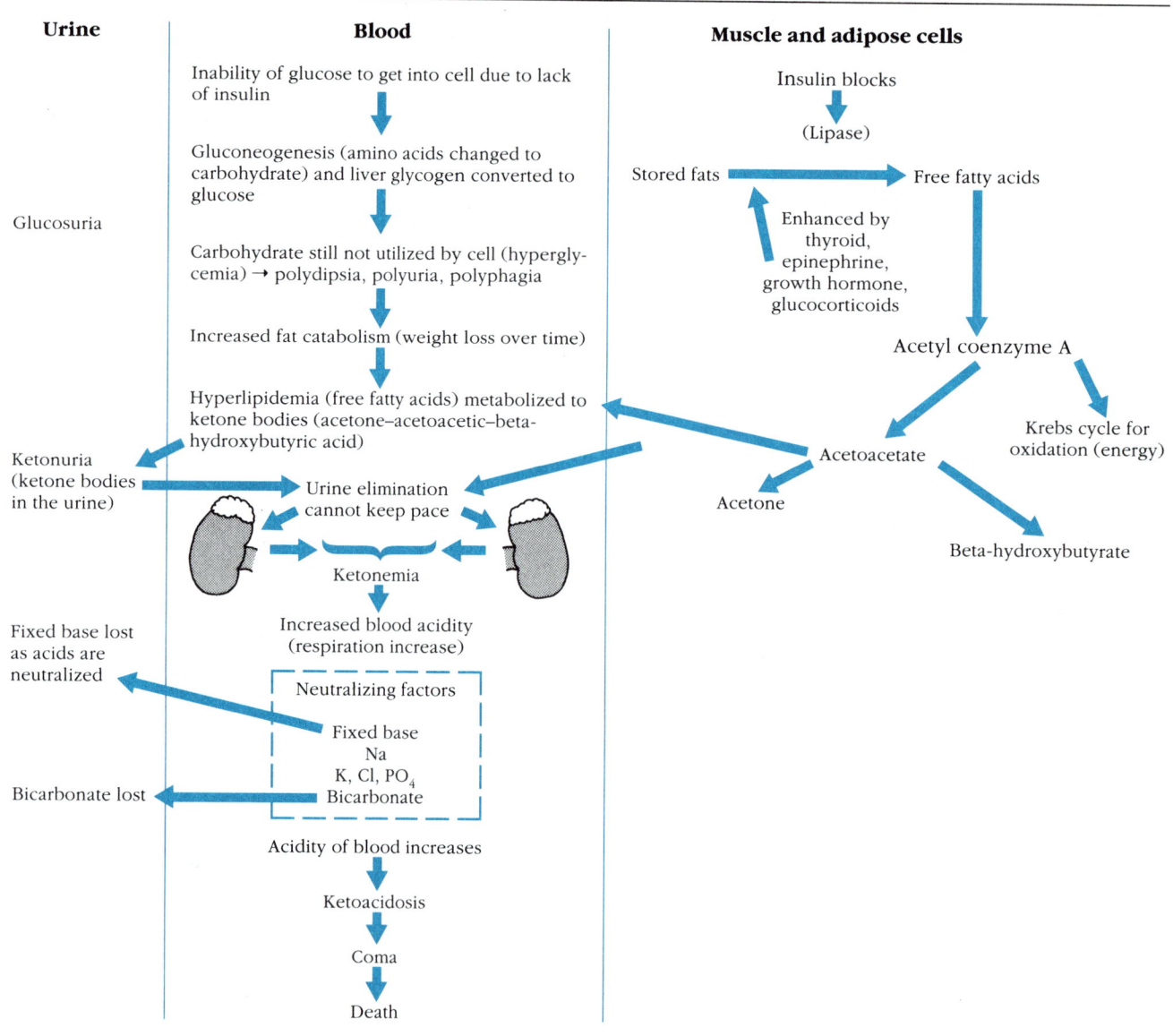

FIGURE 1 Clinical manifestations of Type I insulin-dependent diabetes mellitus.

cells. In the severe form of Type I diabetes, circulating islet cell antibodies have been detected in as many as 80% of cases in the first few weeks of disease onset.[7,8] Type II patients, like those with severe Type I diabetes, may inherit a response to a viral infection that causes a beta cell defect as a consequence of viral stress.

In patients with Type II diabetes (NIDDM) who have excess insulin and are obese, hyperinsulinism and insulin resistance may be correlated with a decrease in insulin receptors.[9,10] Moreover, studies have shown that the tissues of insulin-resistant, obese patients exhibit reduced insulin binding. The reduced number of insulin receptors is the basic, and often reversible, defect in insulin-resistant patients.[9,10]

Resistance to insulin's action also appears to result from an impairment in the target cell's response to insulin due to a defect in postreceptor binding. In Type II patients with severe hyperglycemia, both a decreased insulin receptor number and a postreceptor defect may exist in combination.[10]

Consequences of Diabetic Disease

All major physiologic systems are adversely affected by chronic hyperglycemia (Tables 3 and 4). Patients with diabetes often develop kidney failure (e.g., nephropathy), lesions of the eye (e.g., retinopathy), macrovascular disease, and peripheral and autonomic neuropathy. The molecular and biochemical mechanisms leading to these late complications of diabetes have not been conclusively established.

A number of events have been suggested as possible contributors to diabetic complications. For example, glucose, when present in abnormally high concentrations,

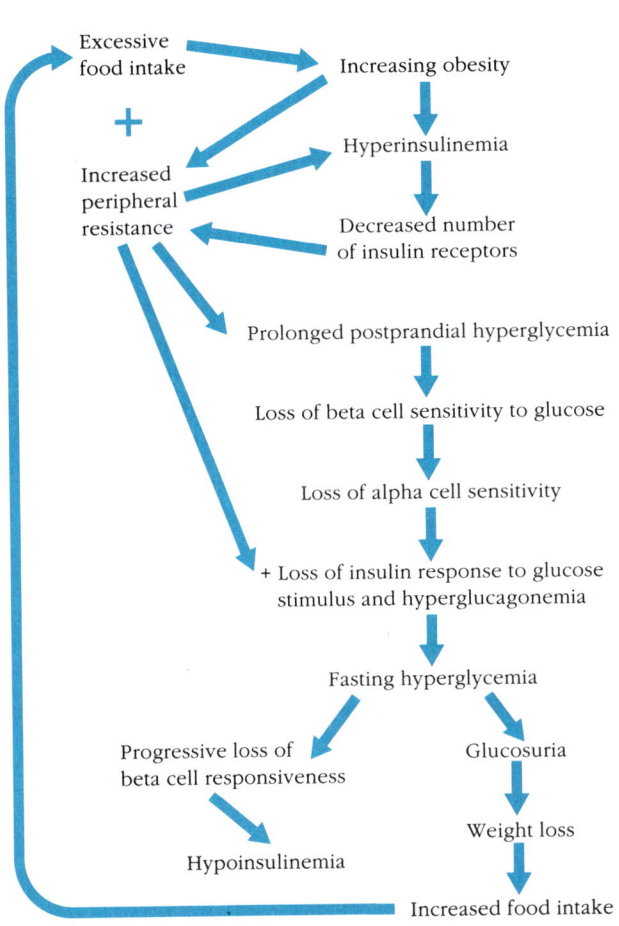

FIGURE 2 Pathogenesis of Type II noninsulin-dependent diabetes mellitus.

promotes the production of highly reactive glycosylated proteins, which interact to form advanced glycosylation end products. These products form covalent bonds with amino groups on other proteins, resulting in cross-linking and accumulation and thickening in the basement membrane.[11] Glucose is also present in high concentrations in noninsulin-dependent tissues, such as the lens of the eye and some neurons, when serum glucose levels are elevated. In these cell types, the enzymes normally involved in the polyol pathway metabolize the excess glucose, thus increasing sorbitol and fructose concentrations. Increased amounts of both sorbitol and fructose have been found in the lens and nerves of hyperglycemic diabetic animals. The accumulation of these polyols could produce osmotic injury to these cells. The elimination of hyperglycemia by insulin prevents or delays the development of diabetic neuropathy and cataracts in experimental diabetic animals. In addition, it has been demonstrated that, when acutely elevated blood glucose levels in PWDs are normalized, symptoms of neuropathy may be more severe and then may disappear.[12] Sorbinil (Pfizer) and tolrestat (Ayerst) are aldose reductase inhibitors. These agents, which are currently being evaluated in clinical trials, hold promise as medications that may help prevent or reduce the severity of several diabetic complications resulting from excess sorbitol.

Other abnormalities of glycoprotein metabolism have been found in both Type I and Type II patients. These findings include increased levels of a minor hemoglobin component, hemoglobin A_{1c}, which is used clinically to monitor diabetes control. Hemoglobin A_{1c} levels reflect mean blood glucose concentration over a period of weeks and are sensitive in assessing chronic control of hyperglycemia.

There is substantial evidence to support the concept that the microvascular complications of diabetes are decreased by a reduction of blood glucose concentrations.[13] These findings have prompted a renewed emphasis on strict, but reasonable, control to prevent severe diabetic complications.

Atherosclerotic lesions in persons with diabetes appear to be the same as those in persons without diabetes, but they tend to develop earlier, occur more often, and be more severe.[14] Atherosclerosis contributes to the twofold increase in cardiovascular mortality and morbidity that occurs in PWDs. Less clear is how much atherosclerosis contributes to the development of microvascular disease.[12] Hyperglycemia causes damage to the intimal cells of the arteries, and this is probably the initial lesion in atherosclerosis. It has been suggested that lower than normal levels of plasma high-density lipoprotein cholesterol and elevated levels of low-density lipoprotein cholesterol contribute to cholesterol deposition and plaque formation.[15,16] Atherosclerotic lesions produce symptoms in various areas. PWDs may suffer from occlusive vascular changes in the lower extremities as a result of both atherosclerosis and damage to smaller arteries (microangiopathies). Peripheral lesions, alone or in combination with hemorrheologic factors, may cause increased intermittent claudication, gangrene, and impotence. Widespread disease of small vessels is common. Cardiomyopathy, cardiovascular neuropathy, and silent myocardial infarct may also occur in diabetic patients.

Hyperglycemia may impair the phagocytic activity of the body's white blood cells. Most chronic adverse conditions in PWDs can be traced to an inadequate blood supply to the area. Besides the vascular and nerve changes and prolonged hyperglycemia that can take place, PWDs often experience difficulty in eradicating bacterial infections.[17] Because glucose levels in saliva are increased in patients with noncontrolled diabetes, these patients experience a higher incidence of dental caries and gum disease. Pharmacists should encourage good oral hygiene and regular dental examinations.

Symptoms of Diabetes

The pharmacist should obtain a careful patient history before attempting an evaluation. In addition to the more common symptoms of diabetes (e.g., polydipsia, polyphagia, polyuria, fatigue, nocturia [nighttime urination], blurred vision, ketosis, and dry mouth), there are several other symptoms the pharmacist should be aware of in assessing potential PWDs and in monitoring diagnosed PWDs for blood glucose control. Pharmacists who detect these symptoms and conditions should refer the patient to a physician.

TABLE 4 Potential complications of diabetes mellitus and its treatment

Body location	Description	Treatment
Eyes	Retinopathy, cataract formation, glaucoma, and periodic visual disturbances due to microvascular disease and other metabolic complications such as increased sorbitol; leading cause of new blindness	Strict control of blood glucose to avoid need for treatment (e.g., laser photocoagulation, vitrectomy)
Mouth	Gingivitis, increased incidence of dental cavities and periodontal disease	Strict control of blood glucose and daily hygiene; see dentist regularly
Reproductive system (pregnancy)	Increased incidence of large babies, stillbirths, miscarriages, neonatal deaths, and congenital defects due to metabolic abnormalities	Strict control of blood glucose before and during pregnancy
Nervous system	Motor, sensory, and autonomic neuropathy leading to impotence, neurogenic bladder, paresthesias, gangrene, altered gastrointestinal motility, and cardiovascular problems	Strict control of blood glucose, daily foot care, surgery, and antidepressants and phenothiazines when indicated
Vascular system	Large vessel disease resulting in atherosclerosis and microvascular disease leading to retinopathy, nephropathy, and decreased peripheral perfusion	Strict control of blood glucose
Skin	Numerous infections and specific lesions such as skin spots, diabetic bullae, lipodystrophies, and necrobiosis lipoidica diabeticorum due to small vessel disease, increased lipids in blood, and pruritus	Strict control of blood glucose, daily hygiene
Kidneys	Diabetic glomerulosclerosis causing nephropathy	Strict control of blood glucose; eventually, diet low in proteins. Prednisone, dialysis, and renal transplantation if necessary.
Reticuloendothelial system (infections)	Cystitis, tuberculosis, skin infections, difficulty in overcoming infections, and moniliasis in diabetic women	Strict control of blood glucose and aggressive anti-infective therapy when indicated

Adapted from Pharmaceutical services for patients with diabetes. *Am Pharm* (module 4) 1986 May; NS26 (5): 8.

Weight Loss

Losing weight while consuming regular meals may be an indication of diabetes. In PWDs, the pharmacist must evaluate dietary restriction versus loss of blood glucose control as the primary reason for weight loss. Other conditions associated with weight loss include hyperthyroidism, cancer, and anorexia nervosa.

Recurrent Monilial Infections

Monilial infections, especially fungal infections of the vulva and anus in women, are common in PWDs. Recurrent monilial vaginal infections may be the first indicator of increased blood glucose levels in females. PWDs may also experience loss of blood glucose control whenever they have infections and may require close monitoring and alterations in their treatment regimen. Chronic skin infections, carbuncles, furuncles, and eczema are also common in patients with this disease. Any recurrent or abnormally slow healing infections should be evaluated by a physician for cause.

Gout

The percentage of patients with gout who have diabetes (5–10%) is higher than the norm. Thus, patients with gout should be screened for diabetes.

Prolonged Wound Healing

Minor cuts and scratches may take approximately twice as long to heal in a PWD. They are also more likely to become infected if not properly treated. All patients at risk of having diabetes, as well as those who have diabetes, should be instructed in proper wound care. Wounds that do not heal properly or that become infected should be evaluated by a physician.

Visual Disturbances

Patients who wear glasses may notice that increasingly stronger lenses are required at relatively short time intervals. Ophthalmologists detect a large number of PWDs. Cataracts and open-angle glaucoma in older patients are common. Research suggests that the increased frequency of cataracts seen in PWDs may be due to an increased level of sorbitol, which accumulates in certain tissues when hyperglycemia is present. Sorbitol accumulation, reduced nucleotide levels, and increased ketone levels contribute to various pathologic changes in diabetes mellitus. Cataract formation appears to be associated with the high sugar alcohol concentration in the lens, which produces an influx of water and the eventual disruption of lens fiber membranes and protein deposits.

Psychologic Changes

Some of the first symptoms of hypoglycemia affecting the nervous system are irritability, nervousness, and anxiety. Generalized fatigue and depression occur more often in PWDs. Frequent emotional flare-ups may signal abnormal biochemistry that may be due to diabetes.

Screening for Diabetes

The pharmacist's role in promoting and supporting diabetes detection programs cannot be overstated. The accessibility and professional competency of the pharmacist provides an excellent opportunity to screen patients for diabetes. Individuals suspected of having diabetes can then be referred to a physician for a complete physical examination, history, and laboratory analysis. Patients already known to have diabetes can also be monitored by the pharmacist for compliance and blood glucose control. During the screening program, as well as at other times, the pharmacist should be able to answer patients' questions concerning diabetes.

If all pharmacists set aside 1 day each month to screen patients for diabetes, they would have a substantial impact on detecting the more than 5 million undiagnosed PWDs in the United States. The actual screening itself requires alcohol swabs, lancets, literature, blood test strips, and a glucose meter to test the strip's color changes. One screening program involves taking a blood sample from the subject's finger and analyzing it using a blood glucose meter. In some states, however, only licensed medical technicians, registered nurses, or physicians may legally withdraw blood from patients.

Also available are urine dipstick screening tests that are highly sensitive, simple, and fast and can provide early detection of glucosuria. As noted previously, however, the renal threshold level for glucose in the urine usually correlates with a blood glucose level of 180 mg/dL or higher. Thus, urine screening will not detect mild to moderate elevations in blood glucose. Also, some urine screening tests are largely qualitative whereas others are quantitative. Pharmacists interested in developing or participating in diabetes screening programs or patient education can find assistance from the resources listed under "Information for Pharmacists" in Appendix 1.

Several selection criteria may be used in a screening program. Patients with a variety of cardiac problems, including high blood pressure, stroke, congestive heart failure, and angina, have a higher incidence of diabetes. Diabetes is also more common in patients who have suffered from hyperthyroidism, Addison's disease, or Cushing's syndrome or who have been on long-term steroid therapy. At least 75% of all PWDs have relatives with diabetes. Approximately 80% of patients aged 40–65 are overweight and approximately 40% of the diabetic population is over the age of 65.

If a patient has glucose in the urine, higher than normal glucose in the blood, or one or more of the symptoms of diabetes, the physician should administer an appropriate screening test. Patients with borderline oral glucose tolerance tests should be rechecked periodically, especially if they become symptomatic. Other tests used as diagnostic or screening tests for diabetes include fasting blood sugar, the 2-hour postprandial blood glucose test, and the hemoglobin A_{1c}.

Nondiabetic causes of glucose intolerance include liver disease, prolonged physical inactivity, acute stress, fever, trauma, surgery, heart attack, starvation, a deficiency of potassium in the blood (hypokalemia), renal disease, certain endocrine diseases, and selected drugs (Table 5). A positive test for glucose in the urine is not necessarily diagnostic for diabetes, but it is an indication for more definitive testing. Glucosuria generally occurs when the blood glucose level is at least 180 mg/dL, although studies have shown it to occur from 54 to 180 mg/dL. The renal threshold for glucose may rise to more than 300–400 mg/dL with age and decreasing renal function so that older and severely renally impaired PWDs may not demonstrate glucosuria despite high blood glucose levels.[18] Glucosuria without hyperglycemia may occur in pregnancy or impaired renal function.

TABLE 5 — Drugs that may cause hypoglycemia or hyperglycemia

Hypoglycemia	Hyperglycemia
Acetaminophen	Acetazolamide
Alcohol (acute)	Albuterol
Amitriptyline	Alcohol (chronic)
Anabolic steroids	Amiodarone
Beta blockers	Amoxapine
Biguanides	Antimicrobial (pentamidine, rifampin, sulfasalazine, nalidixic acid)
Chloroquine	Asparaginase
Chlorpromazine	Caffeine
Clofibrate	Calcium channel blockers
Disopyramide	Chlorpromazine
Fenfluramine	Chlorthalidone
Fluphenazine	Corticosteroids
Haloperidol	Cyclosporine
Imipramine	Diazoxide
Insulin	Droperidol
Lithium	Encainide
Monoamine oxidase inhibitors	Epinephrine-like drugs (phenylephrine, phenylpropanolamine, and pseudoephedrine)
Norfloxacin	Estrogens
Oxytetracycline	Ethacrynic acid
Pentamidine	Fentanyl/Furosemide
Perphenazine/Amitriptyline	Guanethidine
Phenobarbital	Indapamide
Prazosin	Indomethacin
Propoxyphene	Interferon alpha
Quinine	Lactulose
Salicylates in large doses	Levadopa
Sulfonamide antibiotics	Loxapine
Sulfonylurea agents	Morphine
Tetrahydrocannabinol	Niacin and nicotinic acid
	Nicotine
	Nifedipine
	Oral contraceptives
	Phenytoin
	Probenecid
	Rifampin
	Sugars (dextrose, fructose, mannitol, sorbitol, sucrose)
	Sympathomimetic amines
	Terbutaline
	Theophylline
	Thiazide diuretics
	Thyroid preparations
	Tricyclic antidepressants

Diagnostic criteria from the American Diabetes Association for nonpregnant adult diabetes mellitus are as follows:[19]

- A random plasma glucose level of at least 200 mg/dL, in addition to classic and overt symptoms including polydipsia, polyphagia, polyuria, and/or weight loss;
- A fasting plasma glucose of at least 140 mg/dL on at least two separate occasions;
- A fasting plasma glucose below 140 mg/dL plus at least two oral glucose tolerance tests that yield 2-hour plasma glucose levels of at least 200 mg/dL and one intervening value (at 30, 60, or 90 minutes) of at least 200 mg/dL.

Diagnostic criteria for children and pregnant women are different from those for nonpregnant adults and are also available from the American Diabetes Association.

Treatment

The basic objectives in the treatment of diabetes, in order of importance, are to:

- Relieve and prevent diabetic symptoms (polyuria, polydipsia, polyphagia, weight loss, fatigue, recurrent infections, ketoacidosis, or hyperosmolar nonketotic episodes);

- Prevent hypoglycemic reactions;
- Maintain optimal weight;
- Maintain blood glucose levels close to euglycemia (between 50 and 150 mg/dL) to prevent or slow progression of chronic complications;
- Promote normal growth and development in children;
- Eliminate or minimize all other cardiovascular risk factors;
- Integrate the patient into health care through intensive education.

These objectives can only be met through the combined efforts of the physician, pharmacist, nurse, dietitian, patient, and possibly other caregivers.

Key elements in the treatment of diabetes can be easily remembered with the five DEEDS: Diet, Exercise, Education, Drugs, and Self-monitoring of blood glucose. Sulfonylureas or insulin, diet, and exercise are used to control hyperglycemia, and nonprescription products formulated especially for use by the patient are helpful adjuncts.

Diet, exercise, and insulin must be delicately balanced in Type I diabetes. Caloric restrictions and increased physical activity should be a part of the treatment plan for both types of diabetes. Intensive insulin therapy using multiple daily injections or an insulin infusion pump improves glycemia control with few complications in Type I patients. Self-monitoring of urine and blood glucose has made it possible for the patient to adjust medication, diet, and exercise carefully to maintain blood glucose levels near normoglycemia. Strict control of blood glucose levels may delay or decrease the severity of some late complications of diabetes.[19,20]

Drug Therapy

Although this chapter deals primarily with nonprescription products used in diabetes, the pharmacist must understand the proper use of all drugs used to control diabetes. These drugs can be categorized into two broad areas: oral hypoglycemic agents and insulin.

Oral Hypoglycemic Agents

The use of oral hypoglycemic agents has been controversial from the standpoint of effectiveness and long-term side effects. However, when used properly, they are both safe and effective. Pharmacists should monitor patients using these agents for drug interactions that may cause either hypoglycemia or hyperglycemia (Table 5).

The mechanism by which the first- and second-generation sulfonylureas correct defects in insulin action is not completely understood. It is known that sulfonylureas initially stimulate pancreatic insulin secretion and possibly increase the number of insulin receptors on target tissues. It is also believed that the sulfonylureas decrease liver glycogen conversion to glucose and somehow correct or improve the postreceptor defect.[21] The seven specific oral sulfonylureas prescribed in the United States are presented in Table 6. The differences in metabolism of each account for their clinical differences in onset and duration of action.

The most common side effect associated with the sulfonylureas is hypoglycemia (blood glucose < 50–70 mg/dL). Numerous drug–drug interactions may interfere with diabetes control by interfering either with blood glucose levels themselves or with the pharmacotherapeutics and pharmacokinetics of the oral sulfonylureas (Table 5).

Chlorpropamide, the longest acting sulfonylurea, has the highest incidence of adverse effects (5–8%). Chlorpropamide is not recommended as a drug of choice in elderly patients or in patients with renal failure because they may suffer severe hypoglycemia due to decreased elimination. In Type II diabetes, diet is the main method of treatment, accompanied by regular exercise whenever possible; sulfonylureas should be used only when both diet and exercise fail.

Not all Type II diabetes patients are candidates for oral agents. Patients for whom oral antidiabetic agents are usually contraindicated or are not recommended routinely include those who:

- Are under 30 years of age;
- Have gestational diabetes;
- Are pregnant or lactating;
- Are prone to ketosis;
- Have or are prone to having symptoms of acidosis;
- Have Type I diabetes mellitus;
- Need rapid control of their blood glucose levels;
- Have Type II diabetes and have not tried diet control;
- Have severe infections;
- Are undergoing major surgery (during and immediately after);
- Are allergic to sulfa or sulfonylurea compounds.

Controversial candidates include underweight Type II patients, and patients with fasting plasma glucose concentrations greater than 200 mg/dL.

No treatment plan will succeed, however, if the patient has not been thoroughly educated about the importance of all aspects of therapy, including self-monitoring. Pharmacists dispensing sulfonylureas should tell the patient the brand and generic name of the drug, and they should explain that the medication is to be used long term to treat diabetes and that it must be taken regularly and exactly as prescribed. If the patient develops an adverse drug reaction to a sulfonylurea, such as hypoglycemia, sore throat, fever, mouth sores, water retention, or dark-colored urine, the physician should be contacted. The pharmacist should advise the patient to avoid using alcoholic beverages and drugs containing salicylates or to use such products cautiously. The importance of using an oral hypoglycemic agent in conjunction with a prescribed diet and exercise should be stressed.

Approximately 60–80% of Type II patients treated with sulfonylureas respond to initial therapy. The secondary failure rate ranges from 3 to 10% per year of treatment. This failure rate tends to increase each year for patients experiencing initial satisfactory control, perhaps because the patient develops a type of tolerance to the drug. Patients who experience decreased control with a first-generation agent may benefit from a change to a second-generation agent. The second-generation sulfonylureas are the preferred agents for initial therapy, however, as they are more potent, produce fewer side effects, have less drug interaction potential, can usually be given once a day, and produce more predictable responses than some first-generation oral sulfonylureas. If the oral sulfonylureas fail and if diet and exercise alone cannot control the hyperglycemia, insulin therapy will be required.

Insulin

Although insulin is prescribed by a physician, pharmacists are often the health care professionals who are consulted

TABLE 6 Selected characteristics of the oral sulfonylureas

Drug	Equivalent therapeutic dose (mg)	Usual minimum and maximum daily dose	Mean half-life (hr)	Duration of activity (hr)	Metabolism and excretion
First-generation sulfonylureas					
Acetohexamide (Dymelor®)	500	0.25–1.5 g single or divided doses	1.5 parent; 6 metabolites	12–18+	Metabolite's activity greater than parent drug. Metabolite excreted, in part, via kidney
Chlorpropamide (Diabinese®)	250	0.1–0.5 g single dose	35	24–72	Extensively metabolized to compounds with unknown activity; 20% excreted unchanged (may vary widely)
Tolazamide (Tolinase®)	250	0.1–1.0 g single or divided doses	7	12–18+	Some metabolites have weak activity; excreted via kidney
Tolbutamide (Orinase®)	1,000	0.5–3.0 g divided doses	7	6–12	Totally metabolized to compounds with negligible activity
Second-generation sulfonylureas					
Glyburide- nonmicronized (DiaBeta®, Micronase®)	5	1.25–20 mg single or divided doses	10	24	Metabolized to weak active metabolites
Glyburide- micronized (Glynase PresTab®)	3	0.75–12 mg single or divided doses	4	24	Metabolized to weak active metabolites
Glipizide (Glucotrol®)	10	2.5–40 mg single or divided doses	4	10–16	Metabolized to inactive compounds

about problems. Therefore, pharmacists should be highly knowledgeable about insulin products and the pharmacotherapy of insulin.

Type I diabetic patients must be treated with exogenous insulin. Generally, persons who require insulin initially tend to be younger than 30 years of age at diagnosis and are lean, prone to developing ketoacidosis, and markedly hyperglycemic, even in the fasting state. Insulin is also indicated for Type II PWDs who do not respond to diet and exercise therapy alone or to therapy with oral hypoglycemic drugs, or who have fasting plasma glucose concentrations of greater than 200 mg/dL. Insulin therapy is also necessary in some Type II patients who are subject to situational stresses such as infection, pregnancy, or surgery. Type II patients must receive intensive education concerning diet when they start on insulin because increased hunger and a resultant weight gain can be major problems for them. Patients who are receiving parenteral nutrition, who require large-calorie supplements to meet increased energy needs, or who have drug-induced diabetes may require insulin exogenously on a short-term or intermittent basis to maintain normal glucose levels. By combining the appropriate modification of diet, exercise, and variable mixtures of short- and longer-acting insulins with self-monitoring, these patients can achieve acceptable control of blood glucose. To normalize blood glucose, intensified insulin regimens using multiple daily injections or insulin pumps are usually required.

All classes of PWDs should be trained to inject themselves with insulin. Children with diabetes should begin giving themselves their own insulin injections at about 6–9 years of age. Parents should administer one or two injections each week to stay in practice, to ensure that injection sites are rotated, and to inject in areas that are difficult for the child to reach.[22]

Use in Ketoacidosis Diabetic ketoacidosis (DKA) constitutes an acute medical emergency, necessitating immediate diagnosis and therapy. It accounts for less than 1% of the deaths occurring in the diabetic population; however, the mortality

TABLE 7   Insulin time–action profile

Type	Insulin preparation	Onset (hr)	Peak activity (hr)	Duration of action (hr)
Short-acting	Regular	0.5–1.0	3–4	6–8
	Semilente	1.0–1.5	6–10	12–15
Intermediate-acting	NPH	1.0–1.5	6–12	18–24
	Lente	1.0–2.5	8–14	18–24
Long-acting	PZI	4.0–8.0	12–24	~36
	Ultralente	4.0–8.0	12–30	~36–42

associated with acute episodes is 5–15%. The physician can diagnose DKA rapidly by assessing urinary glucose and ketones, arterial blood pH, blood gases, and serum ketone and glucose values. Pharmacists should refer patients with high blood glucose levels and urine glucose and ketones to their physicians immediately for evaluation and treatment.

Shock and cerebral edema are among the complications encountered in DKA. Treatment is directed at plasma volume expansion, electrolyte replacement, correction of hypotension, reversal of acidosis and severe ketosis, and control of plasma glucose levels. Low-dose intravenous (IV) insulin regimens are recommended to treat DKA and hyperosmolar nonketotic coma.

Regular human insulin is usually administered to the patient in DKA as an initial IV bolus of 0.1 U/kg, followed by a continuous infusion of about 0.1 U/kg per hour. Concurrently, IV fluids with appropriate electrolyte concentrations should also be administered.[23,24]

Insulin Preparations   A multitude of insulin products are available in the United States. For ease of discussion, insulins may be categorized based on the species source, type, strength, and purity.

The source from which insulin is derived and its antigenicity can influence its effect on blood glucose control, insulin resistance, and sensitivity.[25,26] Commercially available, animal-derived insulins are a mixture of beef and pork, pure beef, or pure pork. Beef insulin has greater antigenicity because it differs in structure from human insulin by three amino acids; pork differs by only one amino acid. Biosynthetic human insulin is now available from two manufacturers in the United States: Eli Lilly and Novo-Nordisk. Each species source of insulin has a distinct time–action profile. Human insulin has a more rapid onset and a shorter duration of action than pork insulin, which has a more rapid onset and a shorter duration of action than beef insulin. Patients who are switched from one species to another require medical supervision.

Insulins may be divided into three groups according to promptness, duration (e.g., short acting, intermediate acting, or long acting), and intensity of action following subcutaneous (SC) injection. Rapid or short-acting insulins include semilente and regular insulin. Intermediate-acting insulins include neutral protamine hagedorn (NPH) and lente insulin suspensions. The long-acting insulins are protamine zinc insulin (PZI) and ultralente insulin suspensions. Fixed-dose mixtures of insulin at a ratio of 70% NPH to 30% regular and a ratio of 50% NPH to 50% regular are also available. For information concerning the time–action profiles of these insulins, refer to Table 7. Many factors such as injection site, species source, and ambient temperature affect the time–action profiles of insulins; therefore, the values listed in Table 7 are given in ranges and are subject to a degree of variability. Another factor that can affect the clinical use of insulin preparations is their route of administration. Regular insulin injected intramuscularly (IM) provides faster absorption with a greater initial drop in plasma glucose levels than does injection by the SC route. IV regular insulin produces the highest pharmacologic level of insulin in the least time. Insulin suspensions (e.g., PZI, NPH, semilente, lente, and ultralente) are never administered IM or IV.

Insulin absorption is also affected by exercise. Leg exercise accelerates absorption from the leg; arm or abdominal injections avoid this response during leg exercise and reduce exercise-induced hypoglycemia. Thus, a PWD whose day includes a hard game of tennis might do well to inject that day's insulin into the abdomen rather than into the arm or leg. If more than 60 U of insulin are injected at one site, there is potential for erratic absorption. Thus, patients receiving large doses of insulin should split the doses, inject in two different sites, and be monitored closely.

Methods used to increase the duration of action of regular insulin include the addition of zinc and protein molecules. NPH and PZI are examples of insulins in which zinc and proteins have been added. Protamine is a fish protein that slows insulin absorption from the site of injection. The amount of protamine and the zinc content differ among insulin products. The lente insulins have variable durations of action depending on the amount of zinc present.

In March 1980, the Food and Drug Administration (FDA) decertified U-80 insulin, leaving two strengths of insulin—U-40 and U-100—available for diabetic patients. In 1990, the FDA decertified U-40 insulin. Unfortunately, the insulin that is usually available in non–English-speaking countries is U-40. Thus, patients traveling abroad need to be encouraged to carry extra insulin and corre-

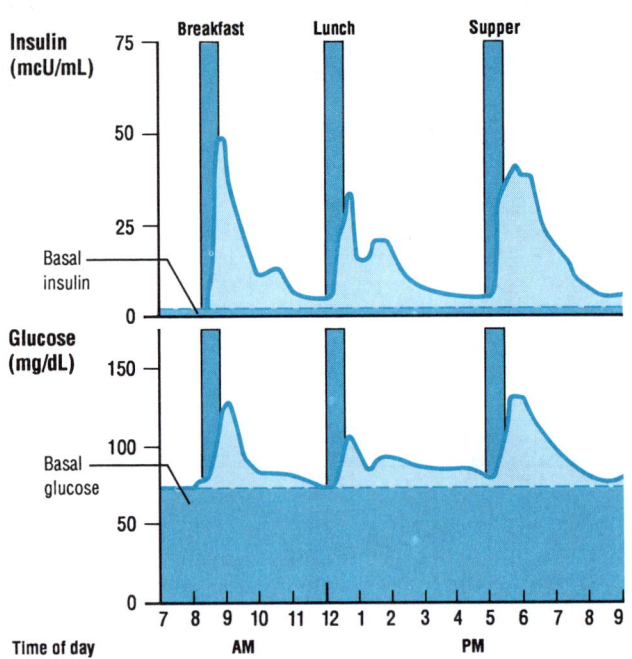

Intensive insulin therapy regimens

	7 AM	11 AM	4-5 PM	Bedtime
1. 2 doses, intermediate	X		X	
2. 2 doses, regular and intermediate	Reg. & intermed.		Reg. & intermed.	
3. 3 doses, regular or regular and intermediate	Reg. & intermed.	Reg.	Reg. & intermed.	
4. 4 doses, regular and long acting	Reg.	Reg.	Reg.	Long acting

Note: Many other regimens are used as "intensive" therapy plans. The therapy is individualized to the responses of the diabetic patient.

FIGURE 3 Relationship between insulin and glucose. Adapted with permission from *U.S. Pharmacist* 1988; 13 (11) (suppl): 41.

sponding insulin syringes to prevent problems or errors.[25] U-500 regular insulin is available from Eli Lilly as a prescription-only product for insulin-resistant patients who use more than 100–200 U per injection.

Newer methods of purifying insulin now ensure that all commercially available insulins are highly purified. The average content of proinsulin, arginine insulin, esterified insulin, and glucagon has been decreased, resulting in fewer insulin-sensitivity reactions. High purification of pork semisynthetic human insulin is important in reducing insulin allergy and dose, lipoatrophy (SC concavities caused by a wasting of the lipid tissue), and insulin binding. All insulin preparations available in the United States are now relatively highly purified and contain between 0 and 10 ppm of proinsulin. Humulin® has 0 ppm of proinsulin. Novo-Nordisk's human insulins (Novolin®, Velosulin®, and Insulatard®) have less than 1 ppm of proinsulin. The purified pork insulins have 1 ppm whereas beef or beef–pork insulins have 10 ppm of proinsulin. Highly purified insulin is less antigenic and allows use of lower insulin doses.

Insulin Regimens The insulin regimen is a key element of the overall treatment plan for diabetes. Pharmacists should be familiar with the different types of insulin regimens prescribed by physicians.

Intensified insulin regimens that help maintain blood glucose levels that approximate euglycemia consist of multiple daily injections or the use of an infusion pump. Normalization of blood glucose via an intensified insulin regimen can be achieved while the patient is allowed to continue the activities of daily living without an interruption of lifestyle. In fact, some of these intensive programs actually increase lifestyle flexibility. For example, pump patients can more easily adjust insulin doses to accommodate changes that occur in the activities of daily living.

For those patients willing to use multiple injections, various combinations of insulins can be used, depending on the individual's response pattern (see Table 7 and Figure 3). For example, regular insulin can be injected before meals, and an intermediate-acting insulin can be injected at bedtime to cover blood glucose levels during the sleeping hours. Another alternative would be to inject long-acting (ultralente) and regular insulin before breakfast, regular insulin before lunch, and regular and ultralente again before dinner. The pain and inconvenience of multiple injections may be helped by using the Button Infuser®, a flexible catheter inserted SC. Doses of insulin can be injected through the proximal end. Blood glucose monitoring at least four times a day is essential for patients who use multiple injections.

Many studies have evaluated the effectiveness of combination insulin–sulfonylurea therapy in patients with Type II diabetes; these studies have been reviewed in the literature.[27,28] Many patients are able to reduce insulin doses after adding a sulfonylurea. Currently, however, combination therapy is only suggested for patients with poor glycemic control (fasting plasma glucose > 200 mg/dL) who are receiving twice-daily injections of insulin in dosages greater than 70 U per day, or for patients who are secondary failures to maximum-dose sulfonylurea therapy.[29] There are no long-term (> 12 month) studies evaluating combination therapy, and it is considered by many to be an experimental form of therapy.

As the purity of insulins has improved, the problem of stability in mixing insulins has decreased. Regular insulin may be mixed with NPH insulin in any proportion desired;[27,28] the resultant combination is stable for approximately 1 month at room temperature and 3 months when refrigerated. Lente insulin binds with regular insulin when the two are mixed, thus decreasing the action of the regular insulin. This reaction occurs within minutes and continues for up to 24 hours. Patients mixing regular and lente insulin should either inject the mixture immediately or allow it to stand for 24 hours and then inject it. The manufacturers of insulin will not guarantee the sterility of prefilled syringes produced by the pharmacist or in the home; thus, patients should be given the smallest possible number of prefilled syringes at any one time. Novo-Nordisk's Velosulin® and Lilly's Humulin BR® should not be mixed with any lente preparation. Semilente, lente, and ultralente insulins may be combined with one another in any ratio desired at any time. Mixtures are stable in any proportion for 18 months if refrigerated although sterility is not guaranteed.

Regular insulin may be mixed in any proportion with normal saline for use in an infusion pump, but the combination should be used within 2 to 3 hours after mixing because changes in the pH and dilution of the buffer may adversely affect stability. Regular insulin may be mixed with Lilly's Insulin Dilution Fluid® in any proportion, and it will be stable indefinitely. Patients using infusion pumps may use either normal saline or Lilly's Insulin Dilution Fluid® to dilute the insulin used in the pump. However, the mixture is more stable using insulin-diluting fluid than using normal saline. Because regular insulin may form crystal deposits in the tubing of insulin pumps, the manufacturers of Humulin BR® and Velosulin® have added phosphate buffer to help limit or prevent this reaction.

Because insulin is a heat-labile protein, all preparations must be stored carefully to maintain potency and maximum stability. Regular insulin's potency may decline by as much as 1.5% per month if the insulin is stored at room temperature (59–85°F, 15–29°C); however, some studies have indicated that all commercially available insulins are stable for several months at room temperature. Color changes may be associated with denaturation of protein and should be interpreted as evidence of potency loss. With regular insulin, the rate of potency loss increases as the temperature increases. At 100°F (38°C), all insulins lose a significant amount of potency within 1 to 2 months. The lente forms of insulin retain their potency when stored at room temperature for 24 months, but signs of loss of potency such as discoloration and clumping may occur after 30 months. With NPH and PZI, loss of potency does not occur at room temperature for up to 36 months. Thus, many insulins are stable in unrefrigerated areas for long periods. Patients may keep vials of insulin currently in use out of the refrigerator because the vials contain bacteriostatic agents, but the insulin should be used within 1 to 2 months and should be stored away from radiators or sunny windows. However, the pharmacist should advise patients to keep any extra bottles of insulin in the refrigerator (36–46°F, 2–8°C) but not the freezer. Freezing insulin does not necessarily affect potency, but it may cause aggregation, precipitation, and clumping.[29] When patients are traveling for prolonged periods in warm climates, they can ensure the stability and potency of their insulin by storing it in an insulated container with ice, "blue ice," or some other form of cooling agent or in a Medical Insulin Protector®, or by packing it between several layers of clothing in a suitcase. Insulin should never be stored in the glove compartment or trunk of an automobile or in uninsulated backpacks or cycle bags.

Higher temperatures may also cause the suspensions of insulin to aggregate, precipitate, or clump. Potency may not necessarily be lost, but there may be a problem in drawing up the correct dose when clumping has occurred. Injection of insulin at room temperature is recommended because refrigerator-temperature insulin produces more pain.

All insulins are produced at a near-neutral pH of 7.4. Regular insulin is a clear solution. If it looks cloudy or has become tinted, it may be contaminated and should not be dispensed or used. All other available insulins are cloudy suspensions that will settle out after standing. If a suspension clumps or discolors, or if a crystal-like glaze or frost forms on the sides of the vial or a white flocculation develops in any of the insulins, the insulin may be contaminated and should not be dispensed or used.

Changing attitudes concerning how to administer insulin (i.e., once a day versus multiple times daily, or multiple intermittent injections versus continuous infusions by pump) and which insulin to use at what time have created confusion. Table 7 presents information that can be used to compare insulins.

It is important that the patient understand how to mix insulin properly within the syringe. The technique generally recommended is as follows:

- Inspect vials for signs of contamination or degradation.
- Wash the hands with soap and water.
- Make sure the proper insulin is used—that is, the correct insulin in the correct strength from the source normally used.
- Agitate the insulin thoroughly. All insulins, except regular insulin, are suspensions and must be shaken before they are withdrawn from the vial. New, unused vials may require prolonged, relatively gentle agitation to loosen the sediment on the bottom.
- Before using bottles, wait until any foam that has formed from agitation subsides. Otherwise, gently roll the vial between the palms of the hands or repeatedly invert it until the suspension is evenly distributed. To avoid generating air bubbles in the insulin, do not shake the bottle.
- Wipe off the top of the vial with an alcohol swab or a cotton ball moistened with alcohol, and be sure that no cotton or cloth fibers remain on the rubber stopper.
- Remove the clean syringe from storage. Touch only the hub of the plunger and the barrel of the syringe; avoid touching the hub of the needle.
- Inject an amount of air equivalent to the insulin dose needed into the intermediate-acting insulin vial.
- Inject an amount of air equivalent to the insulin dose needed into the regular insulin vial.
- Withdraw the appropriate number of units of insulin from the regular insulin vial.
- Repeat the above step with the vial of intermediate-acting insulin.
- When the correct number of units of insulin (without air bubbles) has been measured, withdraw the needle.
- Holding the syringe with the needle upright, draw an air bubble into the syringe, invert the syringe, and roll the bubble through to mix.
- Tap the barrel of the syringe briskly two or three times to remove any tiny air bubbles that may have clung to the barrel.
- Expel the air bubble and recap the needle, or lay the syringe on a flat surface such as a table or shelf with the needle over the edge to avoid contamination.
- Check the administration site and administer the insulin to the patient.
- Some insulins may also be premixed in a vial in the proper short-, intermediate-, and long-acting proportions.

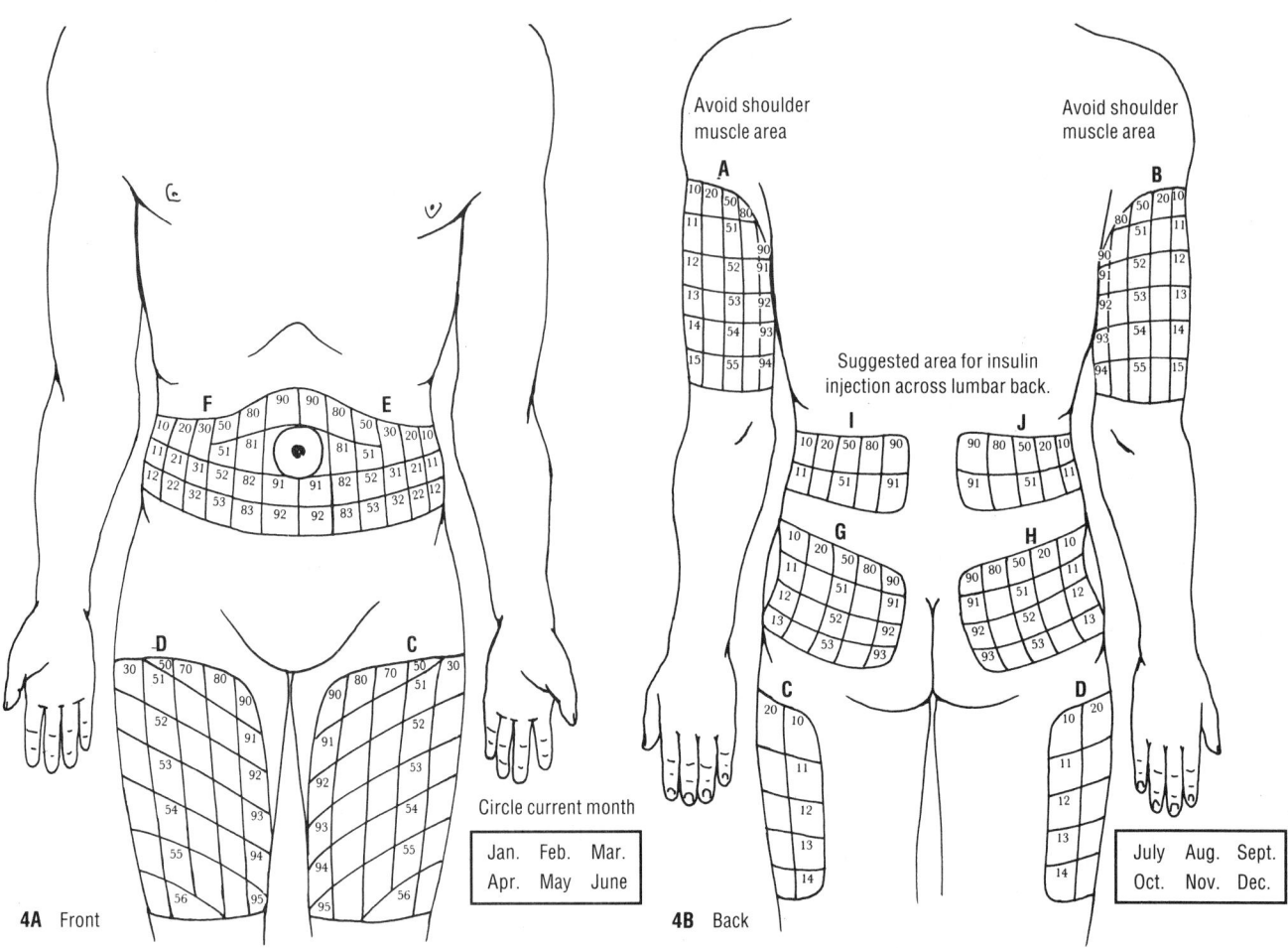

FIGURE 4 Body map of subcutaneous insulin injection sites. This body map is designed to record insulin injection sites systematically. The diagram is for both hospital and home use; the numbers printed in the squares are mainly for hospital recording of insulin injection sites on each patient's chart. The numbers may be used at home, but a simpler method of recording would be to write the date of each injection in the corresponding square on the map at the time of injection. With continued use, this diagram will facilitate the rotation of insulin injection sites over the entire body and thereby avoid injection too often in a single location. Adapted with permission from "The Body Map." Birmingham, Ala: the Baptist Hospitals Foundation.

Pharmacists should also make sure that PWDs know the correct way to inject insulin. The following procedure is recommended:

- After properly preparing the insulin dose, check the record to confirm where the insulin was injected previously. Injection sites should be rotated (see Figure 4).
- Clean the injection site with an alcohol swab or a cotton ball moistened with alcohol.
- Pinch a fold of skin with one hand. With the other hand, hold the syringe like a pencil, place the needle on the skin with the beveled edge up, and push the needle quickly through the fold of skin at a 45–90° angle, depending on the degree of obesity. Before injecting the insulin, draw back slightly on the plunger (aspirate) to be sure a blood vessel has not been penetrated. If blood appears in the syringe barrel, withdraw the needle and repeat the injection in another spot (see Figure 5).
- Inject the insulin by pressing the plunger in as far as it will go.
- Withdraw the needle quickly, and press on the injection site with the swab or cotton ball moistened with alcohol.
- When injection is completed, dispose of the syringe and needle properly.
- Record the injection site.

Patients should be taught that insulin is to be injected deep into SC tissue. The technique for injection may need to be altered with each individual, depending on the amount of SC fat present. For many, a 60° angle or more with the skin stretched will accomplish the deep SC injection needed (see Figure 5). For a thin person, a 45° angle with the skin pinched up may be required to

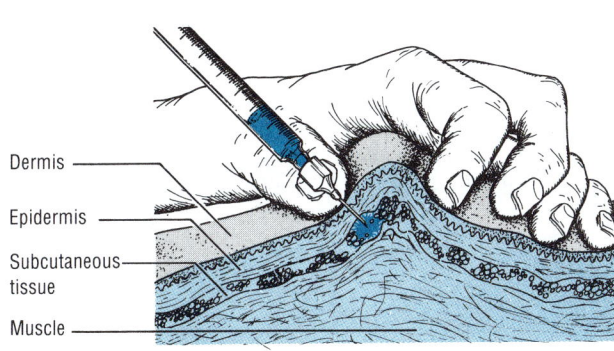

FIGURE 5 Correct method of subcutaneous insulin injection. Avoid areas already fibrotic or atrophic. Prevent fibrosis or atrophy by injecting in one site at no less than 10-day intervals. Properly injected insulin leaves only the needle puncture dot to show the injection site. Several techniques are good; the one illustrated serves well because the needle penetrates the skin at its thinnest area (dimple) and must enter the subcutaneous space. The needle angle should be 45° or more.

avoid penetrating the muscle. The purpose of pinching is to lift the fat off the muscle and thus avoid IM or IV injection, which may result in a more rapid onset of action and severe hypoglycemia. Properly injected insulin leaves only the needle puncture dot to show the injection site.

Pharmacists should stress to patients the importance of rotating injection sites to prevent local irritation, tissue reactions, and lipodystrophy. The site of the injection is one of many factors that can influence the rate at which insulin is absorbed. Injection sites, in decreasing order of degree of absorption, include the abdomen, upper arms (deltoid region), thighs, and hips (see Figure 4). Massaging or exercising the injection area will increase the rate of absorption from that site. Patients who exercise regularly should be advised to avoid injecting into the thigh on days when they will be running or working their legs excessively and to avoid the deltoid on days when they will be using their arms extensively as in playing tennis and lifting weights. Injection into a site where the SC tissue has atrophied or thickened will produce erratic absorption. A patient who is experiencing erratic control might consider confining the injection site rotation to a specific area of the body such as the abdomen. Fibrosis and atrophy can be prevented by injection into the same site at no less than 14-day intervals. Deep IM injections will produce a much more rapid onset of action because the absorption rate from the injection site is increased. Fever, exercise, extremely hot weather, or a sauna or Jacuzzi can increase peripheral blood flow, which speeds insulin absorption. Conversely, cold packs, cold extremities, or a hypothermal blanket may slow the onset of action because the absorption rate is decreased.

If insulin leaks through the puncture in the skin, a longer needle should be used, inserted at a right angle to the skin.

Adverse Reactions Associated with Insulin Therapy Adverse reactions to insulin include insulin resistance, insulin allergy, lipodystrophies, and hypoglycemia, the most common complication of insulin therapy. Factors predisposing the patient to insulin reactions include insufficient food intake (e.g., skipping meals, vomiting, diarrhea), excessive exercise, drug interactions, inaccurate measurement of insulin dose, concomitant intake of hypoglycemic drugs, very tight glycemia control, or termination of diabetogenic conditions.

In PWDs, the counterregulatory hormones (glucagon, epinephrine, cortisol, and growth hormone), which serve to protect people from hypoglycemia, may not respond appropriately to the hypoglycemic stimuli.[30] Symptoms of hypoglycemia include a parasympathetic response (nausea, hunger, and flatulence), diminished cerebral function (confusion, irritability, agitation, lethargy, and personality changes), sympathetic responses (tachycardia, sweating, and tremor), coma, and convulsions. Ataxia and blurred vision are common. Put more succinctly, the profile of the hypoglycemic patient is characterized by pale moist skin, nervousness, excitability, irritability, mental confusion, hunger, headache, normal to rapid breathing, and a tongue that may be numb or tingling.

Patients using intensive insulin therapy who manifest an altered counterregulatory hormone response to hypoglycemia are at high risk for undetected severe hypoglycemic reactions. They may no longer experience the warning signs that normally occur in response to hypoglycemia or hyperglycemia in the morning (see next paragraph), or their first symptom may be cerebral dysfunction. In elderly patients with decreased nerve function, diabetic patients with advanced neuropathy, or patients receiving nonselective beta blockers, the symptoms of hypoglycemia are sometimes lacking and the reaction may go undetected and untreated until it is advanced.

A pattern of hyperglycemia in the morning (the Somogyi phenomenon) has been shown to be a result of asymptomatic nocturnal hypoglycemia in patients who were otherwise well controlled on current intensive insulin regimens. These patients may present with confusion or be unconscious without any other signs or symptoms of hypoglycemia, and appropriate therapy may not be administered. If their normal hormonal defenses do not respond to increased blood glucose, they will continue to be hypoglycemic until the injected insulin dissipates. These patients must monitor their blood glucose levels at least four times a day, and occasionally between 2:00 AM and 3:00 AM to ensure normoglycemia. They should record the results along with any changes in their diet and activities. They should be instructed as to how to interpret the results and how to make adjustments in their therapy. All manifestations of hypoglycemia are relieved rapidly by glucose administration.

Because of the potential danger of insulin reactions progressing to hypoglycemic coma, diabetic patients should always carry packets or cubes of table sugar, a candy roll, or glucose tablets and should eat 2 tsp (10 g) or two cubes of sugar, five to six Lifesavers®, or two glucose tablets at the onset of mild hypoglycemic symptoms (e.g., sweating, hunger, weakness, nausea, dizziness, and mood changes). Patients may also drink at least one-half cup of orange juice, one-third cup of apple juice, or 6–12 oz of any sugar-containing carbonated beverage. The treatment may be repeated in 15 minutes if glucose concentration remains below 60 mg/dL. A snack consisting of one to two cups of milk, a piece of fruit, or cheese and soda crackers is generally enough to treat mild hypoglycemia if mealtime is not imminent. Blood glucose should be monitored frequently to ensure adequate levels and prevent recurrent hypoglycemia.

If symptoms are intermediate and consist of confusion, poor coordination, headache, and double vision, more aggressive administration of glucose and a sugar load may be required. A glucagon emergency kit containing an ampule of glucagon (1 mg), a syringe of diluent, and clearly illustrated directions should be provided to every insulin-dependent diabetic in case of hypoglycemia-associated unconsciousness. Glucagon should be reconstituted with the accompanying solvent, and 0.25–1.0 mg should be administered in the same manner as insulin. Normally, the patient will regain consciousness within 5–10 minutes and be able to swallow some sweetened water. If there is no response after 5–10 minutes, a second injection may be given. Glucagon injection may cause nausea and vomiting 2–4 hours after injection; care should be taken to prevent aspiration of gastric contents.[31] If the response is still insufficient, the patient should be taken to an emergency room or a physician immediately.

If a hypoglycemic person is mistakenly thought to be hyperglycemic and given insulin, severe hypoglycemia and subsequent brain damage may result. When there is doubt about whether a PWD is hypoglycemic or hyperglycemic, sugar should be given initially until the condition can be evaluated accurately.

PWDs who demonstrate a sensitivity to insulin usually develop redness at the injection site. When a patient first begins taking animal-source insulin, such a reaction may be common and may occur over several weeks before gradually subsiding. The reactions may be treated with diphenhydramine chloride (Benadryl®) or hydroxyzine. Newly diagnosed PWDs requiring insulin are now started routinely on human insulin, and reactions are very rare.

Insulin resistance, a state requiring more than 200 U a day of insulin for more than 2 days in the absence of ketoacidosis or acute infection, occurs in about 0.001% of PWDs. These patients almost invariably have high titers of insulin-neutralizing immunoglobulin G antibodies and should be switched to human insulin. If this switch does not resolve the problem, glucocorticoids are indicated.

Another potential complication of insulin therapy is insulin lipodystrophy. Lipodystrophy occurs in two forms: lipoatrophy (the breakdown of SC fatty tissue, leaving hollowed areas under the skin) and lipohypertrophy (the hyperdevelopment of fatty tissue, causing bulges under the skin). Lipodystrophic changes are usually unattractive and may be difficult for the patient to accept. Lipoatrophy improves in most patients when human insulin is substituted; this is because the condition may be due to an immune response to a more antigenic insulin preparation. Lipohypertrophy is generally seen in patients who use the same sites for repeated insulin injection. Because this condition may decrease insulin absorption from the affected site, it represents one of the primary reasons for rotating injection sites.

Nondrug Therapy

One objective in controlling diabetes is maintaining normal weight. The pharmacist should stress the importance of proper exercise and diet. Patients who need help adjusting their diet or complying with the prescribed exercise program should be referred to a dietitian or physical therapist who deals with PWDs.

Exercise

Although exercise is now nearly always recommended by physicians as part of the treatment of diabetes, it was rarely considered a vital part of treatment in the past and was seldom prescribed. With the advent of specialized training in the area of exercise physiology, diabetes management, and certification of physical therapists as diabetes educators, more physicians are referring PWDs for individualized exercise training. The physical therapist is trained in the physiology of exercise and its effects on glucose levels and overall glycemia control. He or she can work with the patient, physician, and dietitian to develop an exercise program tailored to the patient's age, activity level, disability, response of blood glucose levels, and daily glucose variations to help ensure compliance and decrease the risk of hypoglycemia (see Table 8). The physical therapist can determine the optimal mode and intensity of exercise for the patient's individual lifestyle and diagnosis.

Daily aerobic exercise as prescribed by the physical therapist aids in lowering blood glucose levels by allowing glucose to penetrate the muscle cells and be metabolized without the assistance of insulin. Exercise also improves circulatory function, an important factor in diabetic management; helps maintain ideal body weight; aids in breathing, digestion, and metabolism; and improves the cardiovascular endurance of the individual. Exercise has varying effects on plasma glucose levels: it may cause hyperglycemia if there is inadequate insulin available when the patient begins to exercise, or it may cause hypoglycemia if the patient's blood glucose concentration is normal or low just before exercise and proper precautions are not observed.

Patients are encouraged to participate in activities that use the large muscle groups at submaximal levels; swimming, running, and biking are highly recommended. Activities that require heavy straining, such as weight lifting, are discouraged because of the risk of damage to the smaller optic capillaries.

Consistency with exercise is a key component. Patients should maintain a daily exercise program to complement the insulin dose and avoid extremes in blood glucose levels. Consistent exercise is more difficult for the juvenile PWD, so parents must play an integral role in their child's exercise program.

Patients must be trained to monitor their blood glucose levels before, during, and after exercise, and to adjust their diet and insulin injections accordingly. Those who monitor their own blood glucose become motivated to exercise because they easily see the beneficial effects of exercise on maintaining a favorable blood glucose profile and controlling weight. An exercise log may help the patient maintain a regular daily schedule. The pharmacist should encourage the patient to follow the prescribed exercise plan as part of the total treatment plan and should monitor the blood glucose log to ensure that hypoglycemia is not occurring. If it appears there is a problem, the pharmacist should check to ensure that the patient is ingesting carbohydrates before exercise, is injecting insulin at nonexercised sites, is participating in prescribed physical activities at the appropriate time of day with regard to peak insulin activity and food intake, recognizes the symptoms of hypoglycemia, carries a sugar source as well as a glucagon emergency kit, and wears a medical identification necklace or bracelet. Patients may need to be encouraged to tell friends, teachers, or neighbors that they are diabetic; should a PWD experience a hypoglycemic event and be unable to self-treat, others must know what is happening so the patient can receive appropriate treatment as swiftly as possible.

TABLE 8	Guidelines for managing and monitoring PWDs who exercise conscientiously

1. Test blood glucose concentrations before, during, and after exercise.

2. For moderate exercise (e.g., bicycling or jogging for 30–45 minutes), decrease the preceding dose of regular insulin by 30–50%. If glucose concentration is normal or low before exercise, supplement the diet with a snack containing 10–15 g of carbohydrate.

3. To avoid increased absorption of regular insulin by exercise, inject into the abdomen or exercise 30 minutes to 1 hour following injection.

4. Use caution in the case of individuals with low glycogen stores who may be predisposed to the hypoglycemic effects of exercise. These individuals include alcoholics, fasting individuals, and patients on diets that are extremely hypocaloric (< 800 cal) and low in carbohydrates (< 10 g per day).

5. Watch for postexercise hypoglycemia. Individuals who exercise during the day should increase their carbohydrate intake and test their blood glucose concentration during the night to detect nocturnal hypoglycemia. (Hypoglycemia can occur 8–15 hours following exercise.) Patients taking insulin are more susceptible to hypoglycemia than those taking sulfonylureas. Patients with Type II diabetes treated with diet are unlikely to develop hypoglycemia.

6. Do not exercise if the glucose concentration exceeds 240–300 mg/dL. This level indicates severe insulin deficiency. These patients are predisposed to hyperglycemia secondary to exercise.

7. If severe proliferative retinopathy or retinal hemorrhage is present, avoid jarring exercise or exercise that involves moving the head below the waist.

Adapted from *Applied Therapeutics: The Clinical Use of Drugs.* Vancouver, Wash: Applied Therapeutics, Inc.; 1992: 1697.

Diet

Diet is the most critical element in the treatment of Type II diabetes and, in combination with exercise and insulin, is also necessary in treating Type I diabetes. However, diet therapy often fails, creating feelings of frustration, pessimism, failure, and anger, which may, in turn, result in inadequately motivated patients. Pharmacists can help provide patient education on proper diet and nutrition, and can assist the patient in understanding the need to comply strictly with the prescribed diet and in monitoring his or her own diet and blood glucose. The pharmacist can also refer the patient to a registered dietitian for education and training regarding basic nutrition; food selection and preparation; daily food plans; and plans to meet needs during special times, such as on holidays, when traveling, or when eating out.

Factors in Dietary Control Successful diet programs require education, clear goals, motivation, and behavior modification on the part of the patient. PWDs may benefit from being referred to a registered dietitian who is trained in diet management and can help develop an individualized diet for the patient. A team approach to education, counseling, and planning that includes the PWD as an integral member should be used. Each patient should be able to discuss the reasons for the diet, set dietary goals, participate actively in developing a meal plan to fit his or her lifestyle, and include foods that are acceptable while meeting nutritional and caloric needs. Failure to consider patient food preferences, ethnic or religious restraints, and lifestyle factors may cause diet therapy to fail. The dietitian can also inform the patient about eating patterns, food exchanges, and variations on meal plans to meet social needs such as parties, eating out, and holidays. Dietary education and counseling must be a continuing process that is conducted in an understanding and nonjudgmental manner and that considers psychological, physical, and socioeconomic factors in developing each individual's daily food plan. If the patient has a role in planning and selecting the diet and understands the diet's importance in the overall treatment of diabetes, and if the diet is tailored as much as possible to meet the patient's needs, diet therapy may be more successful.

To help PWDs modify their eating behaviors, they should be encouraged to keep a diet log similar to the exercise log. They should record (for 4–10 days) each time they eat, what they eat, how much they eat, and why they eat (e.g., social pressure, loneliness, depression, nervousness, time of day, or hunger). Once eating patterns are defined and understood, modifications can be made and dietary behaviors changed.

When diet therapy is begun, the dietitian and physician must consider the patient's activity level and dose level of medication. Overtreatment with insulin or oral hypoglycemics is probably the most common cause of inadequate diabetic control and weight gain. Diabetic patients should be evaluated to determine whether they are consuming food up to the level of insulin present. It is known that insulin causes an increased uptake of free fatty acids and conversion to triglycerides, resulting in increased hunger and weight gain in some patients. In patients using insulin, it is important to time peak insulin activity to food intake and activity levels;

any adjustment in medication timing must correlate with activity and meal changes. Patients who use multiple insulin injections each day and eat on a more liberal time schedule have to be sure they use their insulin properly to avoid periods of hyper- or hypoglycemia. These individuals need to monitor their blood glucose levels more often and must be reminded of the hazards of quick snacks that may enable them to put off eating a meal but may also add significant calories that are not accounted for in their basic meal plan.

Goals of Diet Therapy One goal of dietary treatment of diabetes is to improve the overall health of the patient by controlling weight, lipid levels, and blood glucose levels while attaining and maintaining optimal nutrition to prevent vascular complications. The dietary treatment prescribed should also provide for the normal physical growth of children and meet the needs of pregnant and lactating women. It is also important to maintain consistency in timing meals and snacks to prevent swings in blood glucose levels for patients using medication as part of the treatment plan.

Because about 75% of the deaths among PWDs are due to cardiovascular disease compared with 50% of deaths in the general population, diabetic patients should avoid dietary risk factors such as animal fats, which have been shown to be associated with hyperlipidemia, increased atherosclerosis, and cardiovascular disease. The American Diabetes Association recommends a diet that contains 55–60% carbohydrates, 10–15% protein or 0.8 g/kg of body weight, no more than 30% fat, and calories that will achieve and maintain a desirable body weight. Cholesterol is also restricted to fewer than 300 mg per day, and sodium intake should not exceed 1,000 mg/l,000 kcal, or 3,000 mg per day. Simple and refined sugars are also contraindicated for all PWDs because of the stress they put on the patient.

Many PWDs believe that, because diabetes results in increased blood glucose levels, carbohydrates in general should be avoided. But whereas simple carbohydrates produce a rapid increase in blood glucose and add stress on the pancreas, complex carbohydrates require smaller quantities of insulin. The glycemic index is shedding new light on which carbohydrates cause blood glucose levels to increase rapidly. However, clinical trials have shown that an increased proportion of complex dietary carbohydrates (bread, potatoes, pasta, or rice and not simple sugars) does not cause a deterioration of diabetic control as long as the total calories are limited to maintain or achieve ideal body weight.

A high-fiber diet is valuable in the diabetic patient. Studies have indicated that increased proportions of dietary carbohydrates that are high in fiber, especially of the soluble variety (e.g., whole grain cereals, oat bran, fruit, vegetables, lentils, and soluble-fiber supplements), rather than of the more highly refined carbohydrates, appear to offer some improvement in carbohydrate metabolism, lower total cholesterol, and lower low-density lipoprotein cholesterol. These carbohydrates also have other beneficial effects, which the insoluble fibers (e.g., wheat bran) may not have. Adequate dietary roughage reduces intraluminal pressure in the bowel and decreases the absorption rate of saccharides. When guar and pectin, components of dietary fiber, were added to a carbohydrate meal, the postprandial rise of blood glucose was shown to be delayed significantly.[32] Fiber does not have miraculous weight-controlling properties; it simply makes it easier for a person to take in fewer calories without feeling hungry. Patients changing to a high-fiber diet should be warned to do it gradually. A sudden large increase may cause temporary flatulence and bloating. The amount of fiber in the diet necessary to achieve a maximum benefit has not been determined, but a maximum daily intake of 50 g appears to be reasonable.

Diabetic patients who follow their diet therapy and maintain near-normoglycemic blood glucose levels are generally able to keep their triglyceride and serum cholesterol levels within the normal range. Several companies are investigating indigestible sucrose polyesters, which may eventually replace a significant amount of oils and fats used in food preparation. The indigestible fat may be used in cooking and in frozen desserts that now rely heavily on animal or vegetable oils and fats. The only major side effect of the indigestible fat, when consumed in large quantities, is diarrhea. Restriction of saturated fats and avoidance of pie, cake, sugar, syrup, candy, alcoholic beverages, and sweetened soft drinks is advised for all PWDs. Calories should also be restricted to help maintain ideal body weight, control blood glucose levels, and decrease the occurrence or progression of complications associated with hyperglycemia.

Use of Alternative Sweeteners In general, food may be adapted or prepared for the PWD in two ways: (1) by restricting the sugar content, and (2) by restricting both the sugar content and the caloric value. When special foods are being prepared, sucrose should be omitted and other sweetening agents substituted. The term *alternative sweeteners* has replaced the term *artificial sweeteners* because some of the sweeteners used are now derived from natural sources.

Sweeteners are classified as nonnutritive or nutritive by the FDA. The term *nonnutritive* refers to sweeteners without calories, such as saccharin or cyclamates. *Nutritive* refers to sweeteners with calories, such as aspartame, fructose, sorbitol, and mannitol. The use of various nutritive and nonnutritive sweeteners is acceptable in the management of diabetes, although the safety of some of these substitutes has been questioned.

Saccharin, which is 400 times as sweet as sucrose, is a common sucrose substitute in the United States. Because it has been implicated in causing malignant tumors in rats consuming exaggerated quantities, the FDA requires a warning on all products containing saccharin. The FDA also requires all retail establishments selling saccharin-containing products to display a warning statement concerning saccharin.

The use of sorbitol and fructose is discouraged because their caloric contribution is significant and may undermine efforts to lose weight and control blood glucose levels. Sorbitol, a glucose alcohol that is 60% as sweet as sugar, is absorbed slowly from the gut, converted to glucose, and metabolized. Sorbitol is one of the end products of the polyol pathway of glucose metabolism that results in some of the late complications of diabetes. Although it is generally without side effects, large quantities of sorbitol may produce osmotic effects leading to diarrhea and abdominal discomfort. Similarly, the amount of sorbitol in foods is not considered to be a risk factor to PWDs unless very large amounts are consumed. The energy value of sorbitol (4 cal/g) must be counted by patients for whom weight control is necessary. Foods containing sorbitol are often labeled "not for weight control purposes" because they may have more calories than other sweeteners.

Fructose is another sucrose substitute that is found naturally in fruits, honey, and other sources. It is also an end product of glucose metabolism by insulin-independent pathways and has some potential for adding to the late complications of diabetes. Fructose has the same caloric content as table sugar. PWDs planning to use fructose as a substitute sweetener should first consult with their physician or dietitian. The daylong quantitative reduction of hyperglycemia that may result from substantial substitution of sorbitol, fructose, and xylitol for glucose and sucrose in the diabetic diet and the long-term effectiveness and safety of these agents when they are ingested in substantial quantities have not been conclusively established.

The G. D. Searle Company manufactures aspartame, which is a combination of two naturally occurring amino acids. Aspartame is classified as a nutritive sweetener by the FDA because technically it has calories. The agent is 200 times sweeter than sugar and yields only 0.1 cal/tsp. Because of this, aspartame has been classified as a noncaloric sweetener. It is commonly found in diet soft drinks, other drink mixes, candies, and cereals, and it is available in a crystal form for use. It is heat labile and cannot be used in cooking. Some physicians do not recommend its use in very young children.

The Hoechst Company has received FDA approval to market a new artificial sweetener, acesulfame potassium, or Sunette®, for use in gum and dry food products and for sale in packets and tablets. Sunette® is similar to saccharin in that it has no calories, but it differs in that it has no aftertaste and, unlike aspartame, does not lose potency after heating or long-term storage. Hoechst is also seeking FDA approval to market Sunette® for use in candies, liquids, and baked goods.

Any PWD who ingests an excessive amount of any sweetener requires nutritional counseling and assessment of needs. Limitations on intake of sweeteners have been established in most cases; however, intake should be individualized, the use of other sweeteners considered, and the overall diet and nutritional adequacy considered.

Pharmacists have a supportive and educational role to play in all phases of diet therapy. They should encourage diabetic patients to follow the prescribed diet, discourage prolonged fasting or use of fad diets to lose weight, and help the patient understand the vital importance of diet therapy in the overall treatment plan. Pharmacists can also help PWDs establish a self-monitoring program that will let the patient see the effect of food intake on blood glucose control beginning in the initial or survival phase and continuing throughout the rest of the training and adjustment period. Patients should be encouraged to obtain dietitian or physician approval for any change in dietary habits.

Pharmacists should also encourage patients to read the labels of all foods marked "dietetic" because such labeling does not mean "diabetic" and the foods may not be sugarless or even intended for PWDs. Better labeling is needed to inform PWDs about the specific individual sweeteners and the amount (in grams or milligrams) contained per serving. Some dietetic foods actually have more calories than regular food. Pharmacists should be familiar with all products that are directed at diet therapy. They should know which ingredients are acceptable for use by the PWD, how much fat the product will contribute to the diet, and which products should be avoided by diabetic patients and why. This will assist the patient in selecting the right products for his or her individual situation.

Use of Alcohol and Alcohol-Containing Products

Precautions regarding the use of alcohol that apply to the general public apply to PWDs. Alcohol burns like fat; alters insulin response; changes the manufacture, storage, and release of glycogen; and can cause impaired judgment, coordination, and a host of other adverse effects. However, avoidance is not always possible or desired, and PWDs should be assessed individually to determine if the advantages of ingesting alcohol (e.g., reducing emotional tension, relieving anxiety, and stimulating appetite) outweigh the potential adverse effects on blood glucose control. Alcohol consumed as dry wine in moderate quantities (no more than the equivalent of two alcoholic beverages once or twice a week) has been advocated by some diabetologists as part of the therapy.

Either hyper- or hypoglycemia may develop in patients who ingest alcohol. Hypoglycemia is the most common effect, and it is believed to be due to either increased early endogenous insulin response to glucose or inhibition of hepatic gluconeogenesis. Relatively small quantities of alcohol (48 mL of 100 proof) may cause hypoglycemia. If a diabetic patient is fasting and consumes alcohol, hypoglycemia may be severe. But if that patient has adequate amounts of glucose in the blood, the alcohol produces a less significant hypoglycemic effect.

Although tolbutamide and chlorpropamide have been reported to interact with alcohol, resulting in a disulfiram-like reaction, the other available oral sulfonylureas (see Table 6) are not as likely to cause this reaction.

The additive hypoglycemic effect of high-level alcohol intake with insulin has produced severe hypoglycemia, resulting in coma, brain damage, and even death. PWDs who are well-fed and consume alcoholic beverages may eventually develop hyperglycemia.

Alcohol is one of the most readily oxidizable food substances known and, unlike sugar, can be metabolized readily without insulin participation. Several studies have shown that PWDs who are on a diabetic diet alone or in conjunction with insulin or a sulfonylurea can consume up to 2 oz (60 mL) of dry wine daily without any significant alteration in blood glucose values. In fact, there is little evidence to support concern over consumption of small (temperate) amounts of any alcohol. However, if ethyl alcohol—regardless of source (wine, beer, or distilled spirits)—is consumed in excess, ketosis may arise.

One equivalent of liquor is equal to the amount of alcohol in a 1.5-oz shot of distilled beverage, a 4-oz glass of wine, or 12 oz of beer. A typical 4-oz serving of dry table wine contains 90–100 cal with a sugar content generally averaging 400 mg. Rosé wines tend to be sweeter; a 4-oz serving contains about 1.3 g of sugar. Champagne contains about 1.4 g of sugar. The sweeter white wines may contain as much as 5 g of sugar per 4-oz serving. The caloric intake of fortified wines is about twice that of an equal volume of dry wine. The sugar content may be as high as 6 g per 2-oz serving of sweet sherries, ports, and muscatels. Thus, light beer and dry wine may be better choices because of the lower carbohydrate and caloric content than regular beer or wine.

Alcoholic beverages should always be consumed with food. Four ounces of dry wine could be consumed with the evening meal without difficulty as long as no food is omitted in the Type I diabetes meal plan and there are no other contraindications for use. For individuals with Type II diabetes, alcohol may be substituted for fat exchanges because it is metabolized like fat (1 oz = two fat exchanges). PWDs prone to alcohol abuse should be discouraged from using alcohol at any time.

More individualized guidelines for alcohol use in diabetic patients have been established. Alcohol is generally contraindicated in PWDs with neuropathies, alcoholism, or proliferative retinopathy; in Type I patients who are prone to hypoglycemia or are pregnant; and in Type II patients who have experienced the chlorpropamide–alcohol flush. Additional guidelines for alcohol use in PWDs include:

- Discussing the use of alcohol with a physician to ensure that no other contraindications exist;
- Drinking in moderation;
- Eating first and spacing drinks apart;
- Not drinking if an alcoholic, if overweight or pregnant, or if diabetic control is unstable;
- Avoiding mixes that contain sugar;
- Using only dry drinks and avoiding beer, ale, cordials, and sweet wines;
- Calculating the alcohol in the diet schedule and decreasing fat intake;
- Considering that alcohol promotes hypoglycemia the "morning after."

Use of Caffeine

The response to caffeine is highly variable among patients. Caffeine intake may need to be considered in patients who tend toward hyperglycemic episodes at specific times of the day. The caffeine contained in coffee, tea, soft drinks, and other products, if consumed in large amounts, may cause an increase in blood glucose because of increased liver glycogen breakdown. Large amounts of caffeine can also alter the patient's perception of hyperglycemia and affect its management.

Use of Vitamins and Minerals

The diet of a PWD should meet the standard recommended requirements for vitamins and minerals. There is no evidence that diabetic patients have a unique or special need for specific vitamin or mineral supplementation above the recommended daily allowance unless the patient is on a very low calorie diet or other special circumstances exist. For example, supplementation of calcium may be necessary for a patient who is pregnant, lactating, or on a calcium-poor diet.

Preventing Complications

The complications of diabetes include microangiopathy, macroangiopathy, dermopathy, retinopathy, neuropathy, nephropathy, and a decreased ability to overcome infections. Prevention of complications through good glycemia control is the ultimate goal. That entails self-monitoring as part of the overall therapy plan.

Patients must be careful using products that affect their diabetes. For instance, the ingestion of large quantities of aspirin or even of ascorbic acid (vitamin C) may influence urine tests and affect diabetic control. Decongestant nasal sprays; asthma, allergy, and hay fever medications containing decongestants; and cold and cough preparations that contain sympathomimetic amines should be used with caution, especially in patients with poorly controlled diabetes. Patients should also avoid medications that contain sugar or alcohol. Antihistamines or other products that produce drowsiness and decrease mental acuity may result in skipped insulin doses.

Diabetic patients have a greater incidence of atherosclerosis that can be detected earlier in life than do nondiabetic patients; the disease appears to progress at an accelerated rate among PWDs and is more extreme. Patients considering the use of niacin or nicotinic acid to control or prevent hypercholesterolemia without their physician's knowledge should be warned of the many adverse effects of the drug, and self-medicating should be strongly discouraged.

Areas in which specific measures can be taken to prevent problems that require special attention in diabetic patients include general hygiene, foot care (see Chapter 37, "Foot Care Products"), dental care (see Chapter 23, "Oral Health Products"), and eye care (see Chapter 20, "Ophthalmic Products").

General Hygiene

Diabetic patients are more susceptible to bacterial infection, and particularly to monilial infection, than is the general population. The most easily infected part of the body is the skin. Infections in PWDs with vascular disease or periods of hyperglycemia heal slowly. Minor cuts and scratches should be cleansed thoroughly with soap and water. Any patient with a serious cut, burn, or puncture wound should see a physician immediately.

Monilial infections of the vagina and anus are much more common in patients with glycosuria. A product found useful in treating pruritus contains three parts Amphogel®, one part kaolin powder, and one part Unibase®. Application of this mixture to the anal area reduces itching and irritation but is not curative because the mixture has no antifungal activity. Daily bathing with thorough drying is recommended; patients should use mild soaps and avoid all harsh chemicals including caustic powders, iodine-containing preparations, astringents, and any other products that may produce or exacerbate vascular or neurologic complications.

Patients should inspect their bodies daily, starting at the top of their head and working down to the feet and toes. They should check for any signs of dry or cracked skin, chafing or irritation, infections, injuries, and areas that may be altered owing to increased pressure from clothing or shoes. Patients should also ensure that any problem areas already identified are being cared for and are healing properly. Any new complications noted or any old complications not resolving properly should be brought to the attention of a physician as soon as possible.

Pharmacists should know which products the physicians in their area prefer to use or avoid, and why. This ensures a better working relationship and health care partnership among the pharmacist, the patient, and the physician. Pharmacists should discuss with the patient the appropriate use of nonprescription topical antimicrobial products and should refer the patient to a physician when further medical attention is indicated.

Foot Care

Gangrene has been reported to occur 50 times more often in PWDs over 40 years of age than in nondiabetic patients over 40 years of age. Before the advent of antibiotics, leg amputations were performed on 9 of 10 patients undergoing surgery for gangrene of the foot (see color plates, photograph 1). Even with the discovery of antibiotics, approximately 50% of major leg amputations (40,000 a year) are performed on PWDs.

Diabetic patients are predisposed to infection of the lower extremities because of vascular changes resulting in poor blood supply. If feet are exposed to minor trauma or infection, the thick-walled vessels become obliterated more easily. This results in decreased perfusion of tissue; increased relative tissue hypoxia; decreased delivery of immune system components to the area; decreased removal of cellular waste; and increased risk of severe ulcerations, gangrene, osteomyelitis, and systemic infections.

To prevent foot problems, diabetic patients must learn how to optimize glycemia control and care properly for their feet. Widespread application of good foot care and patient education among PWDs can markedly reduce the amputation rate. Other measures in addition to those described in Chapter 37, "Foot Care Products," include:

- With the aid of a mirror, inspect feet and lower legs daily (especially between toes and pressure areas) for cuts, scratches, cracks, fissures, changes in color, excessive dryness, and excessive moisture.
- Rub dry feet thoroughly with vegetable oil, lanolin, or an appropriate commercial product to keep them soft and prevent dryness. Excessively dry skin may crack and fissure, allowing infection to enter.
- If feet become too soft and tender, rub them with alcohol once a week. Feet that are too soft and overly moist are more susceptible to skin infections such as athlete's foot.
- Never treat athlete's foot with acidic or astringent preparations. A specific antifungal drug should be used.
- Avoid going barefoot in areas where there is a risk of foot trauma (e.g., sticker, splinter, or cut).
- Cut toenails to follow the contour of the toe and never shorter than the underlying soft tissue; never cut the corner of the nails.
- Never cut corns or calluses.
- Avoid corn medications, all of which contain keratolytic agents.
- Prevent exercise-induced callus formation under the ball of the foot. Finish each step on the toes and not on the ball of the foot. Wear shoes that fit well and do not have excessively high heels.
- Avoid extremes in temperatures and never apply heat of any kind to the diabetic foot.
- Never step into a bathtub before checking the temperature first.
- Have shoes professionally fitted and break new shoes in slowly.
- Change shoes often and inspect them daily (inside and out).
- Never wear tight stockings.
- Do not sit with crossed legs; this posture constricts the circulation and promotes pressure on certain nerves.
- Have feet evaluated by a physician or podiatrist at every clinic or office visit.
- Select a diabetologist, general physician, or podiatrist familiar with diabetic foot problems.
- See a physician or podiatrist immediately if any type of foot problem is noted.

It is recommended that diabetic patients abstain from using tobacco products. This is because components of tobacco can cause vasoconstriction in the extremities and represent an important risk factor in the development of coronary artery disease.

The pharmacist can play an active role in preventive foot care by asking patients at risk of diabetic foot ulcers about any neuropathic symptoms, history of claudication or resting pain, history of prior orthopedic foot problems or surgeries, and social history of smoking habits and alcohol intake. Patients who are overweight, especially males, also have a higher risk of foot pathology. Patients with any of the above risk factors should be instructed in the appropriate care of their feet and monitored closely. Pharmacists should also know which foot care products are not recommended for use by PWDs and be available to assist patients in making appropriate decisions as to which products to buy and when to seek additional medical attention.

Dental Care

Gingivitis and dental caries occur at an increased rate in diabetic patients. Occult abscesses of the teeth are common in hyperglycemic patients and may contribute to poor blood glucose control. Patients should have their teeth checked at least twice each year; they should brush and floss their teeth at least twice daily and should massage their gums with a brush, a Water Pik®, or their fingers. Because uncontrolled diabetes seems to predispose to the various stages of periodontal disease, patients should consult a dentist at the first sign of abnormal conditions of the gums. They should inform their dentist that they have diabetes and then discuss appropriate dental care products.

Pharmacists should ensure that PWDs use sugar- and alcohol-free dental products, know which toothbrush has been recommended, and know how to floss correctly. Patients should be monitored closely for changes in oral health and referred to their dentist when appropriate.

Eye Care

Diabetes is the leading cause of blindness in the United States. Some cases of blindness can be avoided or significantly reduced if (1) retinopathy is detected early and the retina is photocoagulated with laser therapy, and (2) glaucoma is detected and treated early. Pharmacists should encourage PWDs to evaluate the status of their vision and have their eyes examined at least once each year. Pharmacists can also educate PWDs concerning good vision and good blood glucose control. As mentioned earlier, glucose is metabolized to sorbitol during hyperglycemic episodes. Sorbitol accumulates in the lens as well as in other tissues, and it can result in a water influx into the lens and in the swelling or precipitation of protein, which may then lead to cataract formation. Pharmacists should monitor medications so that those that might affect the retina, optic nerve, pupil, and ciliary muscle can be avoided. Parasympatholytic drugs, including anticholinergics, antidepressants, antihistamines, and ganglionic blockers, can alter the pupil and ciliary muscles and result in blurred vision. Patients should be discouraged from using any topical ophthalmic preparations unless such products are recommended or prescribed by their physician, ophthalmologist, or optometrist. Patients who note any change in vision or develop any irritation of the eye should see their doctor immediately.

TABLE 9 Drugs of abuse that impair diabetes management

Alcohol

Impairs judgment

Is metabolized similarly to fat and alters insulin response when taken with carbohydrates

Promotes hypoglycemic attacks

Impairs the manufacture, storage, and release of glycogen

Interacts with other drugs (e.g., chlorpropamide)

Can cause precipitous drop in blood glucose in alcoholic persons who have stopped eating

Can increase blood glucose when used with sugar-containing mixers or in "sweet drinks"

Nicotine (smoking)

Is a potent vasoconstrictor

Causes a 1 to 2°F drop in skin temperature with one cigarette

Significantly alters oral and intravenous glucose tolerance tests

Is a risk factor in etiology of diabetic nephropathy

May decrease subcutaneous absorption of insulin

May increase insulin requirements by as much as 15–20%

Caffeine (coffee, tea, colas)

In large amounts, increases blood glucose levels

Marijuana

Alters time perception, which may affect control

May cause "munchies"

Impairs short-term memory in intoxicated state

Causes a highly dose-related effect, which is dangerous because patient may not know tetrahydrocannabinol content

Yields profound impairment when used with alcohol

With heavy use, impairs glucose tolerance, causing hyperglycemia

Central nervous system stimulants (amphetamines, sympathomimetics, decongestants, anorectics, cocaine, and psychedelics)

Increase blood glucose levels

Increase liver glycogen breakdown, which causes hyperglycemia

Alter time perception, which may affect management steps

May cause anorexia, which increases blood glucose levels

Sedatives and hypnotics

Impair thinking and thus self-control

Opiates (heroin, morphine)

Cause euphoria, which may affect management and increase blood glucose levels

Reprinted from Pharmaceutical services for patients with diabetes. *Am Pharm* (module 4) 1986 May; NS26 (5): 4.

TABLE 10	Drugs that could cause peripheral neuropathies
Antimicrobials	Nitrofurantoin, ethambutol, isoniazid, colistin, streptomycin, metronidazole, amphotericin B
Anticonvulsants	Phenytoin
Antirheumatics	Indomethacin, colchicine, penicillamine, gold compounds
Cytotoxics	Vincristine, procarbazine, cytarabine, chlorambucil
Cardiovascular drugs[a]	Hydralzine, clofibrate, disopyramide
Miscellaneous agents	Cimetidine, ergotamine, methysergide, amitriptyline, amphetamines

[a]Nitroglycerin can cause postural hypotension in diabetics with autonomic neuropathy.
Adapted from Pharmaceutical services for patients with diabetes. *Am Pharm* (module 4) 1986 May; NS26 (5): 5.

As stated earlier, pharmacists have a major role in monitoring drug use in PWDs. They need to be familiar with drugs that may affect blood glucose control by themselves or by interacting with sulfonylureas or insulin, and to recognize which drugs could cause or exacerbate peripheral neuropathy, retinopathy, and nephropathy (see Tables 9–11).

Product Selection Guidelines

Pharmacists should be able to advise the PWDs on the purchase of various diabetes care products. Injection aids are available for patients with a fear of needles or with handicaps such as impaired vision. Several syringe types are available, including those using prefilled and premixed cartridges and insulin pumps that provide high-intensity dosing of insulin without multiple daily injections. There are also a large number of different methods for monitoring blood and urine glucose. Special products have recently been made available for patients who travel or spend a lot of time away from home and carry their insulin with them.

The pharmacist should be aware of any effects that other nonprescription and prescription products may have on the diabetic patient, as well as of which drugs will interfere with testing methods for urine and blood glucose. Because PWDs are more prone to certain types of infection than other people, the pharmacist should recommend appropriate products to be kept in the home medicine cabinet and the use of strict skin hygiene measures. Some pharmacists have developed diabetes care centers to actively assist PWDs. This effort is both professionally and financially rewarding. Several publications listed in Appendix 1 provide useful information to pharmacists interested in developing a diabetes care center.

Syringes and Needles

Pharmacists are responsible for ensuring that the PWD is purchasing the proper type of insulin and syringe. Problems with insulin use occur when patients use the wrong insulin or syringe. The problems with administering the wrong insulin (either the wrong type or from the wrong source) were discussed previously. Problems with using the wrong syringe occur when there is no correspondence to the strength of the insulin. Insulin is administered in units and not in milliliters; therefore, syringes are calibrated in units. The calibration of the syringe should correspond to the concentration of the insulin used (e.g., U-100 syringes with U-100 insulin).

Two types of syringes are available: glass (reusable) and plastic (disposable). Almost all patients use plastic insulin syringes. However, plastic syringes are more expensive than glass ones. The advantages of disposable syringes and needles include ensured sterility and ease of penetration because of a 25% less angle in the needle bevel, thinner metal, and a wide bore. The needles are finer (27, 28, and 29 gauge), sharper, and silicone coated for ease of insertion. There is less pain associated with the smaller (28- or 29-gauge) needles, and there is virtually no

TABLE 11	Drugs that may induce nephropathics

Penicillamine, gold salts, nonsteroidal analgesics (large doses over time)

Aminoglycoside antibiotics (neomycin, kanamycin, gentamicin, tobramycin)

Cephaloridine, rifampin, cyclophosphamide, heroin, methotrexate, and methysergide

Adapted from Pharmaceutical services for patients with diabetes. *Am Pharm* (module 4) 1986 May; NS26 (5): 5.

"dead space"—that is, the measurable space in the needle and at the hub of the needle and syringe. Dead space is a potential source of error when two different fluids are drawn, measured, and mixed in the same syringe. Needles are available in 1/2-in. and 5/8-in. lengths; the longer needle is used for obese patients and when back leakage of insulin occurs.

Disposable syringes with the capacity of 0.3 cc (30 U) and 0.5 cc (50 U), called low-dose syringes, and those with the capacity of 1.0 cc (100 U) may be used with U-100 insulin only. The low-dose syringes have a smaller caliber barrel so that the highly concentrated U-100 insulin can be measured in 1-U increments, yielding a more accurate dose. The 1.0 mL syringes, on the other hand, are graduated in 2-U increments. Thus, patients who require less than 30–50 U of U-100 insulin per injection may use the low-dose syringes to measure the dose more accurately. The 1.0 mL syringes resemble the tuberculin syringes but should not be interchanged with them because of differences in labeling.

Several researchers have reported the reuse of insulin syringes. One study revealed that plastic disposable syringes can be reused for at least 3 days with safety and patient satisfaction, whereas another indicated that patients reused syringes for an average of 4 days and that dullness was a major reason for changing to a new syringe.[33,34] Patients have been reported to place transparent tape over the barrel of the syringe to keep the numbers from rubbing off, refrigerate their syringes between uses, and wipe their needles with alcohol before reusing. There have not been any reports of an increased rate of infection at the site of injection in these patients, but there have not been any large, long-term, well-controlled prospective studies to confirm this. In general, reuse of disposable plastic syringes is not recommended. However, patients who have been following this practice without problems for several years should not be discouraged. Those PWDs who are not at increased risk for developing infection and who are capable of safely recapping the syringe may be allowed to reuse syringes.[35] It is important to ensure that any patient who reuses a syringe and needle pay close attention to aseptic technique and carefully replace the cap over the needle without touching the needle. The needles should probably not be cleaned with alcohol because this removes the silicon coating. Syringes that are to be reused over a few days may be stored at room temperature.

Injection Aids for the Visually Impaired

Pharmacists should be familiar with the many products available to assist the diabetic patient in filling the syringe and self-injecting. They should also be aware of any special adapter or product needs associated with the specific aids, as well as of the type and amount of product training available to both them and the patient.

A variety of products are available, including "drawing aids" that hold the syringe and vial, align the needle, and help draw up the insulin and can be used with magnifier devices if necessary. Magnifiers enlarge the calibrations on an insulin syringe to twice their normal size. There are "dose gauges" that allow doses to be dialed in, have audible dose selectors, come in Braille with raised numbers, or have prefilled syringes that are disposable after multiple dose use. Jordan's Count-a-Dose® holds two vials of insulin for those who need to take mixed doses.

There are currently several different types of insulin injection devices or automatic injectors designed for patients who have an aversion to self-injections. These products include insertion aids, insulin pens, jet injectors, and infusers. An insertion aid is usually a jacket that fits over a filled syringe, is spring-loaded, and guides the needle into the skin. The needle may or may not be visible to the patient, depending on the design of the injector. Some injectors adjust the depth and angle of skin penetration. The size of the automatic injectors varies depending on type. The syringe may be prefilled and carried until ready to use. The insulin pens look like writing pens; use disposable cartridges filled with 150 U of human insulin (regular, NPH, or a 30:70 mix); can deliver preset or dial-in doses, depending on the type; and require only one hand for injection. There are also needleless injectors called jet injectors, which allow the insulin to be delivered as a tiny liquid stream that is forced through the skin under pressure. The injected insulin disperses into a very thin spray as it enters the SC tissue. Patients who are using this type of device for the first time may have to adjust the insulin dose because the increased tissue contact may cause the insulin to be absorbed faster than when injected with a needle. Patients who do not have enough fat tissue may actually inject insulin into muscle tissue with a jet injector. Jet injector devices cause less lipoatrophy and inflammation than customary needle administration; they also facilitate reaching and rotating the injection sites.

All the above devices have maximum dose-delivery limitations that must be considered when advising a patient. For patients who use the syringe and needle for injection but dislike sticking themselves, there is a small flexible catheter (the Button Infuser®) that can be inserted SC, usually in the abdomen, and anchored at the site. It allows the patient to give multiple doses of insulin by simply attaching a syringe to the portal and injecting. The syringe is then disconnected from the SC catheter portal, which is "plugged" until the next dose is administered. The catheter can remain in place for 24–72 hours, and the patient may inject insulin several times a day through the catheter. The Button Infuser® is not as complicated as an insulin pump and is often more acceptable than the individual needle and syringe to patients requiring multiple daily injections. The patient must be instructed on how to prepare the site before insertion and how to care for the site while the catheter is in place to prevent infection. If the patient is not instructed in the proper use of these devices, the insulin may be delivered IM or IV, improper doses may be drawn or injected, or only part—or none—of the dose may be injected.

Several other adapter and injector devices are being tested, including a new needle design called the sprinkler needle. This needle has a sealed end hole and 14 small holes in the side walls to allow insulin to be sprinkled into the SC tissue instead of being deposited into a single reservoir. This is supposed to lead to more rapid absorption of the short-acting insulin, thereby allowing patients to inject themselves immediately before eating rather than 30 minutes before eating.

Insulin Infusion Pumps

Intensified insulin therapy to achieve tight control of blood sugar requires either multiple daily injections or continuous insulin pump infusion that allows a small (basal infusion) amount of insulin (usually 0.5–1.0 U per hour) to continuously infuse SC and a bolus of insulin to be injected before meals and snacks. The use of portable, battery-driven, open-loop continuous infusion pumps to administer insulin to some Type I PWDs has gained support. These pumps are referred to as open-loop devices because the regulation of insulin is not automatically controlled by the blood glucose level and they do not include an artificial pancreas. It is up to the patient to self-monitor blood glucose at least four times a day and to determine how much insulin should be injected and at what dosing interval. Some pumps can be programmed to change basal rates automatically at different times of the day; this allows the insulin therapy to be tailored to the patient's lifestyle, prevents the early morning rise in blood sugar, and thus enables the patient to maintain blood glucose levels that approximate euglycemia. Many physicians and diabetic patients support the idea that tight control and close monitoring of blood glucose will help prevent or delay the late complications of diabetes mellitus.

There are numerous pumps available to administer SC insulin. Some have electronic control systems, but most are basically microcomputers that use rechargeable batteries. All currently available pumps sound an alarm when the battery is running low, the infusion line is occluded, or the insulin reservoir is almost empty. Most of these pumps use a syringe filled with diluted regular insulin and a motorized device that is programmed to push the plunger of the syringe a set distance forward; this forces the insulin through a plastic tube (infusion line) attached to a 27-gauge, 5/8-in. needle or flexible cannula, which is inserted SC and taped in place. Some pumps have special storage containers or reservoirs that contain insulin and use different pumping mechanisms to push the insulin through the infusion line. The infusion line can be disconnected from the syringe when the patient is swimming, showering, or involved in intimate activities or when the infusion line is occluded. (Buffered insulin such as Humulin BR® or Velosulin® appear to be less likely to precipitate in the insulin pump and cause blockage of insulin flow.) Most patients should change the infusion line and cannula sites every 2 days to prevent soreness and infection. When the syringe or reservoir is empty, it must be replaced. Some pumps continue to have "runaway" alarms that sound if a runaway should occur. However, most manufacturers say that runaways are so unlikely that such an alarm is not necessary.

The pump is programmed to provide an individualized, continuous basal amount of SC insulin throughout a 24-hour period, and it will handle fluctuations in blood glucose when the patient is not eating. Guidelines for adjusting doses to account for food, exercise, and the results of self-monitoring of blood glucose are established when the patient begins using the pump. Before eating, the patient pushes several buttons on the pump to deliver a predetermined bolus amount of insulin to handle what is consumed during the meal. Problems at the SC site include the variability in insulin absorption, local skin reactions, and possible infection.

The pumps differ with regard to size, alarm systems, need for insulin dilution, simplicity of dosing, supplementary dosing features, cumulative dose, manufacturer dependability, cost, life of the battery, durability, water resistance, and availability of syringes or reservoirs and infusion sets (cannulas and tubing) used with the pump. The smallest pump is about the size of a credit card and half an inch thick. Other pumps are about the size of a deck of cards or larger. A number of auxiliary pump devices can be purchased by the diabetic patient using insulin infusion pumps; these devices include infusion tubing (12–42 in.), batteries and battery rechargers, syringes or reservoirs that fit specific pumps, tape (Micropore®, Ensure®, Tagaderm®, or OpSite®), tape adhesive remover, surgical soap, skin conditioner, diluting fluid for insulin, blood testing supplies, and logbooks.

Blood glucose self-monitoring is essential for pump users, and many studies have shown that various metabolic parameters can be normalized using insulin pumps. Some problems with pump use are related to the fact that (1) some patients can go into a ketotic phase within a matter of hours, should an interruption of the flow of insulin occur; (2) many patients do not experience the normal symptoms of hypoglycemia; and (3) injection sites must be carefully monitored to prevent infections.

Not all diabetic patients are candidates for insulin pump therapy. At present, Type II patients and children with diabetes are not encouraged to use an insulin pump. PWDs who are candidates for the insulin pump therapy include the following:

- Pregnant patients;
- Patients with complications;
- Patients with a renal transplant;
- Brittle (difficult to control) patients;
- Motivated Type I patients.

The objectives of insulin pump therapy include the following:

- Normalization of blood glucose values (70–150 mg/dL);
- Maintenance of blood glucose values under 200 mg/dL;
- Normalization of glycosylated hemoglobin values;
- Prevention or reversal of diabetic complications;
- Maintenance of daily activities;
- Increased lifestyle flexibility (pump patients can more easily adjust to eating, sleeping, and exercise schedules);
- Avoidance of weight gain by maintenance of a well-planned diabetic diet;
- Avoidance of infection and complications with pump procedures;
- Achievement of a sense of well-being.

Success in the use of insulin infusion devices is directly correlated with patient characteristics. Patients selected for insulin pump therapy must be highly motivated, capable of being educated, responsible for keeping records, willing and able to follow specific procedures, and willing to perform and log blood tests daily.

The role of these open-loop systems in delivering insulin to the PWDs will gain significance in the next few years. Closed-loop systems are also being studied and are in initial clinical trials as an investigational method for insulin delivery. Unlike the open-loop systems, closed-loop systems can monitor serum glucose levels and deliver programmed amounts of insulin in response to a particular level of serum glucose. Such systems include implantable devices and the artificial pancreas. The implantable pumps being tested are primarily constant-rate, vapor-powered Infusaid® devices that deliver insulin IV or intraperitoneally. The programmable implantable medication system, which allows remote programming and interrogation by radio telemetry or telephone communication, is also being investigated. There have been several problems with the implantable pumps, including flow stoppage due to tissue blockage and formation of insoluble aggregates of insulin in the pump reservoirs due to prolonged exposure to body heat and movement. The implantable glucose sensors have also produced inconsistent results. An alternative route for insulin delivery is nasal mucosal absorption. Pharmacists should review the literature closely and remain current with new products that are available or in development.

Blood and Urine Testing and Record Keeping

The pharmacist's role in emphasizing the importance of testing for and recording urine and blood glucose levels, as well as keeping records of medications, doses, diet, and exercise, is significant in improving the patient's diabetic control. Urine testing for glucose is only indicated for those PWDs who are unable or unwilling to perform blood glucose self-monitoring. Pharmacists should assist patients in selecting and using urine glucose and ketone test kits and in interpreting color changes. They should be able to explain to patients why it is necessary to keep accurate records, and they should be able to discuss concurrent drug interferences with each urine monitoring method. Pharmacists should also help the patient to select and use blood monitoring equipment and should make samples of testing products available in the pharmacy's diabetic center so that patients can practice techniques and demonstrate their ability to test urine or blood properly. Pharmacists should also encourage diabetic patients to bring in their logbook, which contains records of blood or urine tests, body weight, activities, diet, and medication use, to determine how well the patient's diabetes is being controlled.

Proper urine or blood testing for glucose and ketones, as well as adequate records of daily control, is essential. Blood glucose testing lets the diabetic patient know whether the treatment program is successful. It also allows the patient to learn what effect exercise, various foods, various medications, illness, and emotional stress have on blood glucose levels. Urine testing does not indicate the current blood glucose level but gives the patient an idea of what that level has been in the past several hours. Changes in urine glucose or ketone test results, especially when those results go from negative to positive, may signal the patient to monitor the blood glucose more often. Ketones in the urine, combined with elevated blood glucose, are the first indicators of DKA. The pharmacist should monitor the patient's drug therapy for drugs that interfere with either the copper reduction or glucose oxidase methods of testing for glucose.

Factors in Selection of Test Method

Proper blood and urine testing is especially important to the PWD who is using insulin and must adjust the daily dose according to test results. Several studies have indicated that many PWDs either do not perform glucose tests properly or do not interpret the color changes properly. Insulin doses should almost never be adjusted based on urine glucose testing because the test indicates only that there has been a blood glucose increase (but not a decrease) in the past and that sugar spilled over into the urine when the blood glucose level exceeded the renal threshold. Blood glucose values are essential to rational and optimal dosing of insulin. Blood glucose monitoring that uses available home blood glucose tests results in reliable indicators of diabetes control, and when used alone or in combination with urine glucose and ketone testing, should provide the patient with the information needed to make good decisions concerning therapy changes, and should improve the overall control of blood sugar.

In ambulatory PWDs who have a relatively normal renal threshold for glucose (160–200 mg/100 mL), testing urine glucose is one way to determine diabetic control. The renal glucose threshold varies from individual to individual; in older patients, it increases. Conditions other than diabetes that may cause glucosuria are pheochromocytoma, acute pancreatitis, ingestion of very large amounts of glucose and other reducing sugars (fructose, lactose, and galactose), acromegaly, and Cushing's syndrome. Factors that may lead to unreliable urine glucose determinations include residual urine (prostate hypertrophy) and neurogenic bladder, which is a complication of diabetes that prevents the collecting of urine specimens at the correct time.

To repeat, urine glucose testing as the only method for self-monitoring is recommended only for patients who cannot or will not monitor their blood glucose. This includes individuals who refuse to lance themselves, cannot be taught the proper technique, or are otherwise unreliable and noncompliant. Blood glucose monitoring is considered the most accurate way for ambulatory patients to determine diabetic control. The tests do not depend on the renal glucose threshold, are relatively easy to perform, and accurately indicate the blood glucose level at the time the test is performed. It must be remembered the blood glucose levels are approximately 15% lower than whole blood levels reported by laboratories. Testing for urine ketones is advised for all PWDs who use insulin. The urine should be tested whenever blood glucose levels are greater than 200–250 mg/dL and during periods of illness or stress. The presence of ketones on two or more consecutive urine tests should be reported to the physician.

Numerous factors need to be considered in selecting a product to test the urine or blood of a PWD. These factors are discussed below.

Diabetes Category

The type of diabetes is a major factor in determining which method of blood glucose self-monitoring to recommend. Patients who are brittle obviously need to test more often than stable Type II patients.

Patients' Ability and Motivation

Patients who are unable or unwilling to perform the more complex tests should be tested with simple tests, even though the simpler tests may not be as quantitative. Patient willingness to learn and perform the more complicated tests (the more complex drop method of Clinitest® versus the strip method of TesTape® or Diastix®) should also be taken into account. Willingness and ability to learn and perform the tasks associated with using strips and a glucose monitor are also factors in the selection of home blood glucose tests.

Physical Handicaps

Patients with trembling hands cannot perform the Clinitest® test accurately. Patients with poor vision, which is common in PWDs, may be unable to see the Clinitest® drops and therefore would have difficulty both performing the tests and interpreting the color changes on the visually read blood glucose monitoring strips. Few visually impaired PWDs are able to match the strips accurately to the corresponding color chart, especially if lighting is poor. Visually impaired PWDs who perform the color match using single-source direct lighting (a table lamp) are more accurate. Special kits are available for the visually impaired PWD, who may also be able to use blood glucose meters that have audio components.

Patients who are ketosis-prone should be advised to test their urine and blood for glucose; those who show positive results should also test their urine for ketones. All patients should periodically test their urine for protein as an indication of nephropathy. Protein in the urine can be easily determined by using Albustix®, Combistix®, Chemstrip GP®, or Uristix®.

Blood Glucose Tests

The ability to achieve and maintain normal blood glucose levels helps prevent or delay the complications of diabetes, particularly retinopathy and nephropathy. Speculation concerning the benefits of tight control is supported by research with patients who self-monitor their blood glucose daily. Evaluations of these patients have shown the following:

- The frequent checking of blood glucose at home increased patients' motivation to maintain their blood glucose within normal range and thus to regulate their daily lives.
- The method encouraged patients to become more involved in dietary control.
- More information on diabetic control became available, which facilitated proper insulin dosage and allowed dosage to be adjusted with confidence.
- Abnormal blood glucose levels were normalized more quickly.

Maintenance of blood glucose control is impossible without measurement, and blood glucose monitoring is the most accurate method a patient can use to determine the level of management needed to control the diabetes condition. Moreover, because it is convenient and less costly for the patient to self-monitor, that approach is highly recommended for all types of PWDs. Even though a few PWDs are not candidates for self-monitoring, others enthusiastically follow protocol if sophisticated, intelligent training is provided. Eventually, most patients will test their own blood glucose levels. Proper education of the patient concerning methods for self-monitoring and the differences between individual meters, the importance of multiple daily tests, and interpretation of test results may motivate more patients to self-monitor their blood glucose levels. The following types of PWDs should be strongly encouraged to self-test their blood glucose:

- Patients with abnormal or unstable renal threshold;
- Patients with renal failure;
- Patients who are unstable and insulin-dependent;
- Patients with impaired color vision;
- Patients who have trouble with urine testing;
- Patients who have difficulty recognizing true hypoglycemia;
- Patients who are pregnant;
- Patients who are using nontraditional methods of injecting insulin;
- Patients who prefer to monitor their own blood glucose.

Calibrated Blood Glucose Tests

Most blood glucose monitoring systems use reagent strips that are impregnated with glucose oxidase. There are no known medications that cause false readings while blood glucose is being tested using the glucose oxidase reagent strips.

The strips can be divided into two types. The first type is read visually. The patient places a drop of blood on the strip and waits 30–60 seconds before wiping or washing off the blood; then, after waiting about a minute longer, the patient compares the color on the strip with those colors on a color meter chart or on the color chart on the side of the bottle containing the strips. If the patient placed the blood properly and waited the correct amount of time, a highly accurate result can easily be achieved. Visually read strips are listed in the product reference tables.

Several PWDs have reported that they prefer knowing the specific blood glucose level rather than a range, which is what the visually read strips provide. Many patients begin by reading visually and then go to a meter. Thus, the second method of self-monitoring blood glucose involves using the strips in conjunction with a blood glucose meter. Several strips can be placed into a corresponding meter with a resulting visual (or audio) readout of the blood glucose. (Some monitoring systems that use strips do not require that the blood be removed from the strip before the glucose level can be determined.) All of the available meters provide a digital readout of the blood glucose level; several have memories for later recall of recent blood glucose levels; and some can give a printout of the retained data. The meters can be compared with regard to size, timing devices, calibration, accuracy, ease of use, memory/data management and printout features, battery types, need for cleaning, accessories required, audio capabilities, teaching materials or training available, price, and manufacturer dependability and availability. Whatever blood glucose monitoring method is recommended to the patient, however, must be flexible and capable of being easily incorporated into the patient's daily lifestyle or routine. If the meter selected is too complex or requires more dexterity than the patient is capable of, it will not be useful. Patients should be allowed to try several meters before selecting one for home use.

When blood glucose monitoring equipment is used properly, calibrated frequently, and interpreted correctly, accuracy is ±10%. Test strips should be stored at room temperature. Bottle caps should be replaced immediately and tightly after a strip is removed.

In addition to these test devices, patients should also purchase alcohol swabs or cotton balls and alcohol, blood lancets and lancet holders, and other accessories. Cost may be a factor for some patients; however, most insurance companies, under the provisions of major medical plans, will reimburse patients for all or part of the cost of home glucose monitoring devices. Pharmacists should ensure that patients using such devices are properly trained. Pharmacists can become distributors of the blood testing devices and require the training needed to assist patients in their use. Manufacturers are very helpful in providing education and training materials.

Urine Glucose Tests

There are two methods of testing for glucose in the urine: copper reduction tests (Clinitest®) and glucose oxidase tests (also called dip-and-read tests). In the qualitative copper reduction tests, cupric sulfate (blue) in the presence of glucose yields cuprous oxide (green to orange). Copper reduction tests are not specific for glucose and may detect the presence of other reducing substances in the urine. Care must be exercised when using copper reduction test materials. The tablets and solutions are very caustic, and handling or splashing should be avoided. The tablets can also be quite dangerous if accidentally ingested, so they must be kept out of the reach of children. Moreover, this method of testing has a "pass-through phenomenon"; this means that, if there is greater than 2% glucose in the urine, the reaction may go past green to orange very quickly and then fade back to a brown. Because such a reaction may be erroneously interpreted as less than 2%, the patient must watch the reaction develop.

A second qualitative method is based on the enzyme glucose oxidase. Glucose in the urine, in the presence of glucose oxidase, yields gluconic acid and hydrogen peroxide (H_2O_2), which, in the presence of o-toluidine, results in a color change. The glucose oxidase test is more convenient and less expensive to use than the copper reduction tests, although the test strips can be affected by humidity and are not as easily read. Patients must be specifically trained to use any of the urine testing products, and the pharmacist may have the patient demonstrate his or her technique to ensure accuracy and proficiency. Patients must consider the accuracy, sensitivity, range, ease of testing and timing, cost, availability of tests, and advantages or disadvantages of multitest kits versus individual test kits when considering which urine test kit to purchase.

Patients who are taking drugs that can interfere with urine glucose testing methods (see Tables 12–15) should be instructed to test their urine using both methods. If the test results differ, there is a strong possibility that a drug is interfering with the test results. Table 16 summarizes the disadvantages of urine glucose testing compared with self-monitoring of blood glucose.

The Biotel/Diabetes Home Screening Test® (Ameri-

TABLE 12 Substances that interfere with glucose oxidase tests

False-positive

Chloride	Hydrogen peroxide
Glucose hypochlorite	Peroxide

False-negative

Alcaptonuria	Homogentisic acid
Ascorbic acid	5-Hydroxyindoleacetic acid
Aspirin	5-Hydroxytryptamine
Bilirubin	5-Hydroxytryptophan
Catalase	L-Dopamine
Catechols	Levodopa
Cysteine	Meralluride injection
3,4 Dihydroxy-phenyl-acetic acid	Methyldopa (Aldomet®)
	Sodium bisulfate
Epinephrine	Sodium fluoride
Ferrous sulfate (Feosol®)	Tetracycline (Tetracyn®, Achromycin®) with vitamin C
Gentisic acid	Uric acid
Glutathione	

Adapted from *Contemp Pharm Pract* 1980; 3: 224–5.

can Diagnostics) is an extremely sensitive test used to detect glucose in the urine; however, it is not a conclusive test for diabetes. The detection of glucose is based on the glucose oxidase–peroxidase–chromogen reaction. The test strips contain a control pad, which should not change color, and a test pad. Color fields on the container correspond to ranges of glucose concentrations. Patients are instructed to report positive results to their physicians. The primary source of error for this test is a large amount of ascorbic acid in the urine; antibiotics may also lead to lower or false-negative results. False-positive results may be caused by a residue of cleansing agents containing peroxide.

Tests for Urinary Ketones

Because ketones in the blood overflow into the urine, urinary ketone levels can be tested to detect whether ketoacidosis is occurring. All PWDs should be counseled on the proper way to test for ketones in the urine. The basis for the test is that sodium nitroprusside alkali turns lavender in the presence of acetone or acetoacetic acid.

Acetest® reagent tablets are specific for acetoacetic acid and acetone. Acetest® will not react with beta-hydroxybutyric acid in 100 mL of urine. In serum, plasma, or whole blood, Acetest® will detect 10 mg of acetoacetic acid in 100 mL. Acetest® can be tested for reliability by using nail polish remover that contains acetone.

Ketostix®, Chemstrip K®, and other tests will detect 5–10 mg of acetoacetic acid in 100 mL of urine. These tests are easier to perform than Acetest®, and no dropper is required. However, the new, improved Ketostix® only tests for acetoacetic acid and thus shows a false-negative result if the patient produces acetone or beta-hydroxybutyric acid. It is also difficult to find a substance at home to test the reliability of the Ketostix®.

TABLE 13 — Minimal concentrations of chemicals that produce false glucose oxidase reactions

Chemical	Concentration in urine (mg/mL)	False-positive or false-negative
Homogentisic acid	0.05	False-negative
L-Dopamine	0.6	False-negative
Levodopa	2.5	False-negative
Methyldopa	5.0	False-negative
5-Hydroxytryptophan	1.0	False-negative
5-Hydroxytryptamine	1.0	False-negative
Cysteine	9.0	False-negative
Glutathione	9.0	False-negative
Sodium bisulfate	5.0	False-negative
Glucuronic acid conjugates	20.0	False negative
Glucose hypochlorite		False-positive
Chlorine		False-positive
Peroxide		False-positive
Hydrogen peroxide		False-positive
Ascorbic acid	0.08	False-negative
Gentisic acid	0.05	False-negative
5-Hydroxyindole-acetic acid	0.25	False-negative

Reprinted from *Contemp Pharm Pract* 1980; 3: 224–5.

TABLE 14 — Substances that interfere with copper-reduction tests to give false-positive results

Ascorbic acid	Levodopa
Cephalosporins	Metaxalone (Skelaxin®) metabolite
Dilute urine	Methyldopa
Aspirin	Penicillin
Glucuronic acid conjugates	Probenecid (Benemide®)
Homogentisic acid	Reducing sugars
Isoniazid	Salicylates
Lactose in pregnant women	Streptomycin

From *Contemp Pharm Pract* 1980; 3: 224–5.

Tests for Other Chemicals

Several products are available to test urine for pH, protein, glucose, acetone, bilirubin, blood, and urobilinogen. Although these tests are more commonly used in physicians' offices, PWDs may be instructed in the use of these reagents to test for various chemicals in the urine that may indicate the degree of diabetic control. Fresh urine is required in all tests. Urine may be refrigerated for a short time (up to 4 hours before testing), but the actual test must be performed with the urine at room temperature.

Identification Tags

All PWDs should wear identification bracelets, necklaces, or tags and carry identification cards. This identification may be lifesaving if hypoglycemia or ketoacidosis occurs. If a patient becomes unconscious through an accident or a hypoglycemic or hyperglycemic coma, medications that must be taken regularly may be missed. Moreover, because a hypoglycemic (insulin) reaction may be confused with drunkenness, there have been reports of hypoglycemic patients being jailed rather than given medical care.

An identification tag that can be seen easily on any PWD should indicate that the person is diabetic and receiving medication. A diabetic identification card should include the person's name, address, and telephone number; the amount and type of medication used; the name of the patient's physician; and the number where the physician can be contacted.

The MedicAlert® identification bracelet can be obtained from MedicAlert Foundation, P.O. Box 1009, Turlock, CA 95381.

Recommendations for Travel

Diabetic patients should always take enough supplies for the entire trip plus 1 week. They should always carry an extra vial of insulin to ensure that they have insulin derived from the same source. If traveling abroad, diabetic patients should be sure they have an adequate number of syringes because U-40 syringes are the most common type available in foreign countries. They should control their diets carefully, allow time for physical activity, and carry candy or sugar to combat possible hypoglycemic attacks. They should not travel with prefilled syringes because the syringes may be accidentally jarred and the dose wasted. Patients should carry one or two glucagon kits and instructions for use.

All PWDs, and especially those who travel, should carry an identification card and wear an identification bracelet, necklace, or tag that indicates they have diabetes and, in the event that a hypoglycemic attack occurs, are not intoxicated. Many organizations recommend that patients traveling in countries where English is not the dominant language carry the names of English-speaking physicians in each city they will be visiting; organizations are available that help locate physicians abroad. PWDs traveling to foreign countries must

TABLE 15	Minimal concentrations of chemicals that produce false copper-reduction reactions		
Chemical		Concentration in urine (mg/mL)	False-positive or false-negative
Isoniazid		5	False-positive
Streptomycin		5	False-positive
Cephaloridine		5	False-positive
Cephalothin		5	False-positive
Fructose		10	False-positive
Galactose		10	False-positive
Lactose		10	False-positive
Maltose		10	False-positive
Penicillin		10,000 U/mL	False-positive

From *Contemp Pharm Pract* 1980; 3: 224–5.

be able to communicate their medical needs. Although most metropolitan hotels have English-speaking employees, it is recommended that PWDs carry cards with some key phrases, such as "I am diabetic," "Please get me a doctor," and "Sugar or orange juice, please," written in the dominant language of the countries to be visited. They should also carry a letter from a physician stating that they have diabetes and noting other major medical problems, current medications by both brand and generic names, and information concerning medical insurance.

PWDs changing time zones should carefully plan a diet, exercise, and insulin adjustment. As a rule, changes in time zones of 2 hours or more will require adjustments of the insulin dose. The diabetic traveler heading west may use this formula to make a one-time adjustment:

New NPH/lente dose = usual NPH/lente dose × (1 + number of time zones crossed/24).

If the PWD is headed east, the formula is:

New NPH/lente dose = usual NPH/lente dose × (1 − number of time zones crossed/24).

Patients using a mixture of insulins or intensive therapy may not be able to use these formulas. Frequency of blood glucose monitoring should be increased to ensure control.

Because PWDs will probably need to monitor their blood glucose more often owing to changes in diet, activity, and meal schedules, they should also take extra batteries and strips for the glucose meter, a bottle of strips that can be read visually, alcohol wipes, cotton balls, and lancets. Even if the patient does not usually monitor his or her urine for ketones, it is advisable to do so while traveling.

The sale of syringes in various states differs. Some states have no regulations governing it; in others, syringes must be sold by a pharmacist. Certain states require a prescription for the purchase of syringes and needles. The patient should be aware that procedures may be different and take the appropriate precautions.

Nonprescription Products Affecting Diabetes

Reading the label on all food and drug products is essential to maintaining diabetic control. PWDs should develop this habit early to avoid potential adverse effects and complications in managing diabetes.

Sugar-Containing Products

A list of sugar-free pharmaceutical preparations is useful so that the pharmacist may suggest a suitable sugar-free product for diabetic patients. (See Appendix 2, "Sugar-Free Preparations by Therapeutic Category.") Cough preparations that contain simple syrup could have a clinically significant effect on a brittle insulinopenic diabetic. However, the amount of extra sugar ingested to relieve a cough would not be significant in most well-controlled cases of diabetes. To put this in perspective, the difference between a large and small orange could include more sugar than would be found in 2 tsp of most cough syrups.

Many companies are promoting a number of dietary products that are sugar-free and contain aspartame. These products are usually low in calories and fat. Each product must be evaluated individually, and if a patient chooses to include it in the diet, it must be accounted for in the overall meal plan.

PWDs should read labels carefully to ensure that the dietetic product will fit into their diet plan. Many dietetic products cost much more than their nondietetic counterparts and actually have as many, if not more, calories.

TABLE 16	Disadvantages of urine glucose tests

1. Inability to detect low blood sugar (hypoglycemia)
2. Many possible drug interferences
3. Patient variance with reference to renal threshold for glucose
4. Lack of correlation between urine and blood glucose levels
5. In some patients, difficulty in reading and performing tests
6. More privacy required than blood testing
7. Inability to detect how high blood glucose really is

Sympathomimetic Amines

Ephedrine, pseudoephedrine, phenylpropanolamine, phenylephrine, and epinephrine increase blood glucose and cause increased blood pressure by vasoconstriction. These substances should be used cautiously in diabetic patients. Sympathomimetic amines do not have as potent an effect on blood glucose as does epinephrine, which can stimulate glycogenolysis. Hyperglycemia, acetonuria, and glycosuria have been reported in three nondiabetic children who received therapeutic oral doses of phenylephrine. The major problem would occur in unstable Type I PWDs.

Salicylates

Aspirin products do not bear a warning statement for PWDs. However, aspirin in these patients may cause hypoglycemia, possibly by stimulating general cellular metabolism. In Type I patients, the degree of hypoglycemia resulting from large doses of aspirin (5 or 6 g) could stimulate a hypoglycemic reaction. However, the clinical significance of aspirin is questionable if a diabetic patient is monitoring for diabetes control. In addition, aspirin may cause misleading results in urine tests for glucose, but it is a dose-related phenomenon. False-negative glucose oxidase readings have been associated with doses of aspirin of approximately 2.5 g. Similar doses of aspirin can also cause false-positive glucosuria readings when the copper reduction test method is used.

Diabetic Patient Monitoring

The therapeutic goal of diabetes treatment (drug, diet, exercise, education, and self-monitoring) is to control the patient's blood glucose. Diabetic patients vary considerably in their responses to therapy and in their adherence to prescribed instructions. The pharmacist can assist the patient in adhering to the prescribed regimen and in monitoring medications that may impair thinking, affect blood glucose levels, interfere with urine testing, or induce or contribute to complications. The pharmacist can also verify whether the patient has been thoroughly educated in self-care and self-monitoring. And the pharmacist is in a strategic position to develop a network of health care professionals whose specialty is diabetes. Then, because diabetic patients frequently see the pharmacist more often than they do any other health care professional, the pharmacist may be the "gatekeeper" for the rest of the medical community—that is, the first health care professional to detect a problem related to an aspect of the diabetic patient's care and the one who refers the patient to other health care professionals for treatment and follow-up.

Figures 6 and 7 represent a patient profile checklist designed to monitor the drug therapy of the diabetic patient. The checklist enables the pharmacist to gather pertinent information about the patient such as blood and urine glucose test results; prescribed therapy (special diet and therapy for concurrent diseases); and the patient's drug therapy, including insulin types, dosage, and dosage changes. The checklist may be used as the sole patient profile or in conjunction with existing profiles.

Behavioral and Psychosocial Issues in Diabetes

Despite continuing gains in understanding diabetes, the state of knowledge remains insufficient to prevent the disease, cure it, or provide diabetic patients with optimally effective treatment. The search for a means of prevention and cure continues. However, there is also a need to focus energies on improving the quality of life for PWDs and their families. And this entails finding a better way to control blood glucose; food that tastes better and is noncaloric; and a health team that understands the varied emotional states of the diabetic patient and cares enough to provide honest, helpful, and informed information.

To be successful in the treatment program of PWDs, each health team member must be sensitive to the patients' emotional problems. Anxiety and depression are major emotions these patients experience. In a several-hour or even several-day program of diabetic education, the patient is often exposed to a learning process that includes the causes and complications of diabetes, food types, diet exchanges, urine testing, blood testing, effects of exercise, insulin mixing and injection, rotation of injection sites, foot care, treatment of insulin reactions, travel tips, what to do during sick days, and miscellaneous ancillary products. The patient may feel confused and have a high level of anxiety about understanding the treatment issues and the daily regimen to be followed. These emotions may be partially overcome, however, by empathetic teachers.

Many PWDs live with fear because of the serious health implications of the disease. Fear of an early death, apprehension about suffering from diabetic complications, and embarrassment over bizarre behavior during a hypoglycemic reaction may strongly affect a PWD's adjustment and decrease good diabetic control. For instance, patients who have suffered a serious insulin reaction often keep their blood glucose high to avoid a repeat episode.

Some patients may try to "beat the odds" or "live each day to the fullest" and not fully comply with the treatment regimen. They may overindulge themselves and rationalize that having a chocolate shake, for example, will not cause a medical emergency, pain, or any other acute symptom. However, bad habits such as overeating are easily formed and difficult to break, leading to chronically poor diabetic control.

Often, patients feel guilty when they are noncompliant with the prescribed treatment protocol. However, if that protocol is too stringent, it can cause frustration. There is seldom positive feedback as to whether the PWD is following the proper procedures to maintain control and avoid complications. This is one reason why blood glucose self-monitoring is one of the most significant advances in diabetes care in the past 40 years. With proper patient education, blood glucose self-testing allows the PWD to monitor blood glucose closely and regulate diet, exercise, and medications.

Living with the fear of complications, in addition to the daily demands of a rigorous medical regimen, is very stressful, not only for the PWD but also for the entire family. Many patients are subject to powerful, unpredictable mood and behavioral changes caused by metabolic imbalance. Moreover, there are also chronic, nonmetabolic stresses associated with the disease; these include the need for diet management, rigid meal schedules, blood testing, various

Patient

Name _____ Home phone (_____) _____

Present address (street, city, zip) _____

History

Is there diabetes in your family?	☐ Yes	☐ No	Relationship	What type?

When was the last time the nondiabetic members of your family were tested?

How long have you had diabetes?

How do you feel about having diabetes?

Do members of your family understand the conditions and factors that affect control?   ☐ Yes   ☐ No

Is there anything that is upsetting you emotionally?   ☐ Yes   ☐ No

Do you belong to a diabetes association?   ☐ Yes   ☐ No

Physician/Laboratory Test Results

When was your last glucose tolerance test?   What was your last blood glucose level?

When was it conducted?

What test was used (e.g., random, glucose tolerance)?

Medication

Are you taking anything for diabetes?	☐ Yes	☐ No	Where do you inject your insulin?			
If "Yes," what?			Do you rotate injection sites?	☐ Yes	☐ No	
			How much do you inject?			
Do you take insulin?	☐ Yes	☐ No	How often?			
If "Yes," what kind?						
			Are you allergic to any drugs?	☐ Yes	☐ No	
			If "Yes," which one(s)?			

Personal Observation

What do you think has adversely affected the control of your diabetes?

Complications

Have you had any infections?   ☐ Yes   ☐ No

Any other problems?

Diet

What kind of diet has your doctor prescribed?

Do you use "fad" diets?	☐ Yes	☐ No
If "Yes," which one(s)?		
Do you use alcohol?	☐ Yes	☐ No
How much?		
Are you eating differently?	☐ Yes	☐ No

Exercise

Do you have a regular schedule for exercise?   ☐ Yes   ☐ No

Type of exercise?   Frequency of exercise?

Are you exercising more or less?   ☐ More   ☐ Less

Testing

Do you test your urine?	☐ Yes	☐ No	If "Yes," how?	
	Which product?		How often?	
What do you test for?	☐ Sugar	☐ Ketones	☐ Protein	
Do you test your own blood for glucose?	☐ Yes	☐ No	If "Yes," how?	
	Which product?		How often?	

FIGURE 6 Diabetic condition analysis form. Adapted from Pharmaceutical services for patients with diabetes. *Am Pharm* (module 4) 1986 May; NS26 (5): 10, 11.

Adverse Episodes		Dates	Severity–Outcome
Hypoglycemia	☐		
Hyperglycemia	☐		
Glucosuria	☐		
Ketoacidosis	☐		

Drug Interaction Guide (see Table 5)

Prescription Drugs Currently Taken

Medication						
Date						
Rx #						
Prescriber						
Directions						
Route						
Quantity						
Refills						
Price						
Comments						

Nonprescription Drugs (taken on a regular basis)   ☐ None

	Category	Name of Product	How Often Used
1.			
2.			
3.			
4.			

Patient Education

Date _____

Subjects _____

FIGURE 6 *continued*

Patient's name _____	☐ Insulin-dependent ☐ Non–insulin-dependent	Year of onset _____

Address _____ Tel. # _____ Date of birth _____
_____

Insurance _____

Physician _____ Tel. # _____

Physician _____ Tel. # _____

Responsible person/ _____ Tel. # _____
Emergency
Relationship to patient _____

HISTORY

Known Allergies/Sensitivities

Causative Agent	Occurrence Date	Treatment	Outcome
1.			
2.			

Concurrent Diseases	Date Diagnosed	Treatment
1.		
2.		
3.		

ANTIDIABETES THERAPY

Diet: Calories _____ Sweetener _____

Oral: Sulfonylureas

Agent _____

Date					
Strength					
Frequency					

Insulin

Type _____

Date					
Units					
Frequency					

Type _____

Date					
Units					
Frequency					

Syringe size _____ Needle size _____

Monitoring   Urine ☐   Ketones ☐   Blood glucose ☐

Test or Kit   _____   _____   _____

FIGURE 7 Diabetic patient record form. From Pharmaceutical services for patients with diabetes. *Am Pharm* (module 4) 1986 May; NS26 (5): 9.

daily therapeutic decisions, insulin injections (if required), and alterations in lifestyle. These stresses often result in significant emotional disequilibrium and occasionally in clinical psychiatric disorders. Impaired self-esteem is common. Denial, anxiety, hostility, and depression also occur and may impair interpersonal relationships at various levels.

Patient Education

Patient education is one of the critical keys to success in controlling diabetes. Some diabetologists insist that the patient know as much about diabetes from the practical management aspect as the physician.

Education, periodic reeducation, and support systems from friends and family members are essential in fighting the burdens accompanying diabetes. Because diabetes is a particularly difficult disease for children and adolescents, it is especially important that positive steps be taken to help young PWDs understand their emotions. Diabetes is the only disease in which the young patient and his or her parents are expected to make independent therapeutic decisions based on daily clinical observations. But although this day-to-day control of the disease depends on the efforts of the patient and family members, it has been repeatedly demonstrated that an understanding of the disease and mastery of the necessary skills are inadequate in a large proportion of diabetic patients and their families. Although improved understanding leads to improved care and health outcome, there continues to be a need for accessible and well-designed educational programs. These issues affect not only the patient but also the patient's family, friends, teachers, employers, and entire community. Clearly, the emotional, social, economic, and public health problems of diabetes are enormous. The pharmacist plays a significant role in helping to overcome some of these problems.

Diabetic patients live with their disease 24 hours a day, so it is essential that they understand the condition and know when they are in trouble and need to call for help. Every diabetic patient should know:

- What diabetes is and why treatment is necessary;
- How to select the proper foods at each meal;
- How to test urine for sugar and acetone;
- How to test blood for glucose;
- How to administer and store insulin;
- What the symptoms are of uncontrolled diabetes and ketosis;
- What the symptoms are of hypoglycemia;
- What the emergency treatment is for hypoglycemia;
- When to return for follow-up;
- How to contact the attending physician, pharmacist, or emergency department;
- What precautionary measures to take while traveling;
- How to modify treatment for exercise or illness;
- How to care for the feet;
- What dose and time is best for administration of oral agents, if appropriate.

A team approach to patient education is essential. After diagnosing the condition and classifying the patient's type of diabetes, the physician explains the disease and the treatment objectives. The dietitian emphasizes the importance and methods of reaching and maintaining an ideal body weight. The diabetes nurse specialist may train the patient in using syringes and needles, mixing insulins, and injecting insulin SC; the nurse may also give advice on proper personal hygiene, foot care, urine testing techniques, and record keeping. The physical therapist teaches the patient how to incorporate exercise into daily life, develops strategies to avoid the complications of exercise, and instructs the patient in the many benefits related to regular physical exercise.

The pharmacist plays a special role in patient education with regard to mixing, storing, and injecting insulin. In addition, the pharmacist is often called upon to reinforce education and training provided by the physician, nurse, dietitian, and physical therapist. Thus, the pharmacist should be able to answer questions about the disease, blood and urine testing, record keeping, foot care, diet, treatment of cuts and scratches, the use of antihistamines and decongestants, products safe to use in weight control, and the alcohol and sugar content of both prescription and nonprescription drugs.

The pharmacist's role in patient education is significant. The challenge of understanding diabetic products and teaching patients how to use them properly has many benefits. Diabetes information sources for pharmacists and their patients are listed in Appendix 1. With the aid of this information, pharmacists should be prepared to discuss the following topics with patients:

- The relationship among diet, exercise, and insulin;
- The strength, dose, times of administration, and types of insulin;
- The correct use of insulin syringes and needles, and how to avoid dead space;
- The diabetic diet and prescribed caloric level;
- Injection sites and proper site rotation;
- The proper technique for preparing the syringe (withdrawing insulin) and mixing insulin;
- The pharmacotherapy of oral hypoglycemic agents;
- The availability and use of insulin infusion devices;
- Blood and urine testing methods and techniques;
- Urine testing times;
- The proper interpretation of testing results and record keeping;
- The symptoms of possible hypoglycemic and hyperglycemic reactions;
- The appropriate treatment of hypoglycemic and hyperglycemic reactions;
- Proper identification, including diabetic information cards and MedicAlert® jewelry or emblems;
- Skin care, foot care, and personal hygiene.

Diabetic Care Center

To emphasize to PWDs that the pharmacist is truly concerned and interested in serving their needs, a clearly identified diabetes section may be established in the pharmacy. This diabetic care center should include a complete line of diabetic products, including sugar-free food and drink products, nonprescription products that are safe for diabetic patients to use, booklets about diabetes, and information about available diabetic products and services. An area may also be established in which patients can practice testing their urine or blood and using syringes properly. Appendix 1 lists several publications that provide information to pharmacists interested in developing a diabetes care center.

Diabetic Detection Programs

Free diabetes testing kits may be distributed to pharmacy patrons. The American Diabetes Association may be helpful in providing information on how to set up a detection program. Some pharmacists set aside 1 to 2 days each month when patrons can be tested for diabetes in the pharmacy.

Communication

Team effort and coordination are vital in patient education, and communication must be part of that effort. Pharmacists concerned about diabetes control should become involved in their local diabetes association or local Juvenile Diabetes Foundation. In addition, they should become familiar with community physicians who treat diabetes and develop a working relationship with them.

A system for communication with PWDs may be developed. Using a drug-monitoring checklist for diabetic patients or merely a series of questions allows the pharmacist to show concern for the patient and gather information that may be helpful in monitoring the condition.

Summary

Diabetes control requires a team effort on the part of the physician, pharmacist, dietitian, nurse, physical therapist, podiatrist, and patient. The pharmacist plays an important role by monitoring patient therapy and remaining informed about all aspects of the disease. Patient consultation should reinforce the patient's understanding of diabetes and emphasize the importance of testing and controlling blood and urine glucose levels, eating properly, exercising, and keeping accurate records. Concerned pharmacists should join their local diabetes associations and consult recent literature to keep their knowledge current.

References

1. Garrelts L. *U.S. Pharmacists' Guide to Diabetes Management* 1988; 13(11) (suppl): 4.
2. *ADA Vital Statistics*. Washington, DC: American Diabetes Association; 1990.
3. Harris MI, Hamman RF. *Diabetes in America*. Pub. No. 85NIH. Bethesda, Md: U.S. Department of Health and Human Services; 1985: 1468.
4. Foster DW. In: Braunwald E, Isselbacher KJ, Petersdorf RG, et al., eds. *Harrison's Principles of Internal Medicine*. 11th ed. New York: McGraw-Hill; 1987: 1778–96.
5. *Fact Sheet*. New York: Juvenile Diabetes Foundation; 1977.
6. Bonheim R. *Diabetes Forecast* 1985; 3: 32, 38.
7. Karam JH. In: Krumpp MA, Chatton, MJ, eds. *Current Medical Diagnosis and Treatment*. Los Altos, Calif: Lange Medical; 1980: 749.
8. Bennett RW. Understanding diabetes. *U.S. Pharmacists' Guide to Diabetes Management* 1991; 16 (suppl).
9. Hepp KD. *Diabetologia* 1977; 13: 177.
0. Kolterman OG, Gray RS, et al. *J Clin Invest* 1981; 68: 957.
11. Brownlee M, Cerami A, et al. *N Engl J Med* 1988; 319: 1315–21.
12. Motlich ME. *Postgrad Med* 1989; 85: 182.
13. Ungar RH. *Med Clin North Am* 1982; 66: 1317.
14. Colwell JA, Lopes-Virella MF, Mayfield RK, et al. *Metabolism* 1985; 34 (suppl).
15. Crepaldi G, Manzato E. *Postgrad Med* 1988; 64 (suppl): 10–2.
16. Betteridge DJ. *Br Med Bull* 1989; 45: 285–311.
17. Rayfield EJ. *Am J Med* 1982; 72.
18. Koda-Kimble MA, Rotblatt MD. In: Young LY, Koda-Kible MA, eds. *Applied Therapeutics for Clinical Pharmacists*. 4th ed. Vancouver, Wash: Applied Therapeutics Inc.; 1988: 1662–1742.
19. Goldline JE. Diabetes mellitus. *Med Clin North Am* 1988; 72: 1271–84.
20. Raskin P, Pietri AO, Unger R, et al. *N Engl J Med* 1983; 309: 1546.
21. Gerich JE. *N Engl J Med* 1989; 321: 1232–45.
22. Eastman DG, Guthrie RA, Hare JW, et al. *Patient Care* 1975; 19.
23. Androgue HJ, et al. *Hosp Pract* 1981 Feb.
24. Sanson TH, Levine S. *Drugs* 1989; 38: 2.
25. Campbell RK. *Prac Diab* 1988 Jan/Feb; 15–17.
26. Krosnick A. In: Bergman M, ed. *Principles of Diabetes Management*. New Hyde Park, NY: Medical Exam Publishing Co; 1986.
27. Anderson JHY, Campbell RK. *Diabetes Educator* 1990; 16.
28. White J, Campbell RK. *Hosp Pharm* 1991; 26: 12.
29. Waife SO. *Diabetes Mellitus*. 8th ed. Indianapolis, Ind: Lilly Research Laboratories; 1980; 169.
30. Cryer PE, Gerich JE. *N Engl J Med* 1985; 313: 232.
31. Alberti KGMM. *Br Med Bull* 1989; 45: 242–63.
32. Jenkins DJA, Goff DV, Leeds AR, et al. *Lancet* 1976; 172.
33. Crouch M, Jones A, Kleinbeck E, et al. *Diabetes Care* 1979; 2: 418.
34. Aziz S. *Diabetes Care* 1984; 7: 118.
35. *Diabetes Care: Clin Pract Rev*. 1991; 14 (suppl 2).

Appendix 1: Diabetes Information Sources

Information for Pharmacists and Patients

- American Diabetes Association, Inc.
  1660 Duke Street
  Alexandria, VA 22314
  703-549-1500
  Numerous publications on all aspects of diabetes. Monthly magazine for members.

- The American Dietetic Association
  216 West Jackson Boulevard
  Suite 800
  Chicago, IL 60606-6995
  312-899-0040
  Numerous publications on diabetes education.

- Becton Dickinson and Company
  Becton Dickinson Consumer Products
  One Becton Drive
  Franklin Lakes, NJ 07417
  201-847-7100
  Pharmacists: numerous diabetes education products.
  Patients: numerous publications on diabetes education and management.

- Boehringer Mannheim Diagnostics
  9115 Hague Road
  Indianapolis, IN 46250
  800-858-8072
  Numerous publications on diabetes education.

- Chronomed
  13911 Ridgedale Drive
  Suite 250
  Minnetonka, MN 55305
  800-876-6540
  Numerous publications, including slides and audio cassettes, on diabetes education and management.

- *Diabetes Self-Management*
  Subscription Department
  P.O. Box 51125
  Boulder, CO 80321-1125
  800-234-0923
  Bi-monthly publication.

- Diagnostics Division/Miles, Inc.
  P.O. Box 3115
  Elkhart, IN 46515
  219-264-8410
  Pharmacists: several publications and CE programs related to diabetes education.
  Patients: numerous publications on diabetes management.

- Eli Lilly and Company
  Lilly Corporate Center
  Indianapolis, IN 46285
  317-276-2000
  Numerous publications on diabetes management.

- Herc Publishing
  P.O. Box 30090
  Lincoln, NE 68503
  402-476-2221
  Diabetes—Living and Learning, a book for the adult with Type I or Type II diabetes, 1988.
  Diabetes—Stuff and More Stuff, a book for children with diabetes and their parents, 1988.

- Hoechst-Roussel Pharmaceuticals, Inc.
  Medical Information
  Route 202-206 North
  P.O. Box 2500
  Somerville, NJ 08876-1258
  800-445-4774
  Numerous publications on diabetes education.

- International Diabetes Center
  5000 West 39th Street
  Minneapolis, MN 55416
  612-927-3393
  Numerous publications on diabetes education and management.

- The Joslin Diabetes Center
  One Joslin Place
  Boston, MA 02215
  617-732-2400
  Numerous publications on diabetes education and management.

- The Juvenile Diabetes Foundation
  432 Park Avenue South
  New York, NY 10016-8013
  212-889-7575
  Pharmacists: numerous diabetes education products.
  Patients: numerous publications on diabetes education.

- Lifescan, Inc.
  A Johnson & Johnson Company
  1051 South Milpitas Boulevard
  Milpitas, CA 95035
  800-227-8862
  "Blood Glucose Monitoring: For the Phases of Your Life," published for LifeScan, Inc., by Health Education Technologies.

- MedicAlert Foundation, International
  P.O. Box 1009
  Turlock, CA 95381-1009
  800-432-5378
  MedicAlert Emergency Medical Identification necklace or bracelet engraved with the patient's specific health problem and a wallet card. The patient's medical history is computerized and is available to emergency personnel 24 hours a day via a collect phone call to the MedicAlert Foundation.

- National Institute of Child Health and Human Development
  Building 31, Room 2A32
  9000 Rockville Pike
  Bethesda, MD 20892
  301-496-5133
  "Understanding Gestational Diabetes: A Practical Guide to a Healthy Pregnancy," D. Thomas-Doberson et al., 1989.

- Novo-Nordisk Pharmaceuticals Inc.
  100 Overlook Center, Suite 200
  Princeton, NJ 08540
  800-727-6500
  Numerous publications on diabetes education and management.

- Pfizer Inc.
  235 East 42nd Street
  New York, NY 10017
  212-573-2323
  Pharmacists: numerous diabetes education products.
  Patients: numerous publications on diabetes education and management.

- *U.S. Pharmacist*
  Jobson Publishing Corporation
  352 Park Avenue South
  New York, NY 10010
  212-274-7000
  Annual diabetes supplement to *U.S. Pharmacist*.

- The Upjohn Company
  7000 Portage Road
  Kalamazoo, MI 49001
  616-323-4000
  Numerous publications on diabetes education.

Additional Suggested Reading

The pharmacist should contact the local diabetes association for information to provide diabetic patients about membership and activities.

Appendix 2: Sugar-Free Preparations by Therapeutic Category

The following list of sugar-free nonprescription preparations was developed by searching APhA's database for products that the manufacturers have designated–or "flagged"–as "sugar free." It is not, nor can it be, a comprehensive list. Some manufacturers did not flag their products, the *Handbook* is subject to space limitations, and limitations of the database precluded us from reporting all flags marked for all products. In this list, we have included the therapeutic categories that we hoped would be most helpful to pharmacists.

It is very important that each health care provider using this list realize that the manufacturers of these products frequently change the ingredients. It is thus *critical* that patients be instructed to read labels carefully and not assume that a product that was once sugar-free will always be sugar-free. In addition, patients should be instructed to look for sugar substitutes that are calorigenic. Just because a product is labeled as "dietetic" or "sugar-free" does not mean that it is intended for use by a patient with diabetes. Many dietetic products are free of sucrose but contain dextrose, fructose, or sorbitol. Patients should also read labels of products to check for alcohol content.

Patients with diabetes who are ill are usually under stress and thus should be instructed to monitor their blood sugar glucose levels more frequently. While the amount of sugar in a given dose of most medication is not enough to significantly change the treatment protocol, the following list contains sugar-free nonprescription medications that are less likely to affect blood glucose levels.

Antacid Products
Aluminum Hydroxide, Concentrated
Banacid
Calcium Carbonate
Calglycine
Dimacid
Maalox HRF
Maalox Caplets
Maalox Plus, Extra Strength
Mag-Ox 400
Maox
Marblen
Nephrox
Neutralin
Riopan
Riopan Plus
Riopan Plus 2 Mint or Cherry Flavor
Titralac Extra Strength Antacid
Titralac Plus Tablets
Titralac Plus Liquid Antacid
Titralac Antacid
Uro-Mag

Antidiarrheal Products
Kaolin Pectin Suspension
K-C
Kao-Spen
Loperamide Hydrochloride Solution

Antiemetic Products
Bonine
Dramamine
Dramamine II

Antipyretic Products
Acetaminophen Oral Solution USP, cherry
Acetaminophen Oral Solution USP, lime
Actamin Extra
Actamin
Actamin Super
Addaprin
Aminofen Max
Aminofen
Arthritis Pain Formula Caplets
Aspercin Extra
Aspercin
Aspermin Extra
Aspermin
Aspirtab Max
Aspirtab
Bayer Aspirin, Maximum
Bayer Aspirin, Genuine
Bayer Children's Chewable Aspirin
Bayer Extended Release 8-Hour Aspirin
Bayer Select Ibuprofen Pain Reliever/Fever Reducer
Buffinol Extra
Buffinol
Buffasal Max
Buffasal
Buffaprin Extra
Buffaprin
Cama In-Lay Tablets
Cama Arthritis Pain Reliever
Dapa-500
Dapa
Dapa, Extra Strength
Emagrin
Motrin IB
Myapap Drops
Panadol Children's Chewable Tablets
Panadol Children's Liquid
Panadol Children's and Infants' Drops
Panadol Caplets, Maximum Strength
Panadol Maximum Strength
St. Joseph Aspirin-Free For Children And Infants
Tempra 3 Chewable Tablets
Tempra 3 Chewable Tablets, Double Strength
Tempra 1 Drops
Tempra 2 Syrup
Tri-Pain
Tylenol Children's Fruit Flavor

Tylenol Children's Grape Flavor
Tylenol Children's Suspension Liquid
Tylenol Infants'
Tylenol Extra Strength Caplets
Tylenol Extra Strength Gelcaps
Tylenol Extra Strength Tablets
Tylenol Infants' Suspension Drops
Tylenol Junior Strength Fruit Chewable Tablets
Tylenol Junior Strength Grape Chewable Tablets
Tylenol Junior Strength Swallowable
Tylenol Regular Strength Caplets
Tylenol Regular Strength Tablets
Ultraprin
Valorin Extra
Valorin
Valorin Super
Valprin
Vanquish Caplets

Appetite Suppressant Products

Acutrim Late Day
Acutrim II Maximum Strength
Acutrim 16 Hour Steady Control
Dexatrim Maximum Strength Extended Duration
Dexatrim Caffeine Free Maximum Strength with Vitamin C
Thinz Back-To-Nature

Asthma Inhalant Products

Broncho Saline
Bronitin Mist
Bronkaid Mist
Primatene Mist
Primatene Mist Suspension

Calcium Products

Biocal 250
Biocal 500
Bone Meal With Vitamin D
Calci-Mix
Calcium Oyster Shell
Calcium Carbonate
Calcium 600
Calel-D
Caltrate, Jr.
Cal-Sup
Caltrate 600 + D
Caltrate 600 + Iron
Caltrate
Calcium With Vitamin D
De-Cal
Florical
Gerimed
Nephro-Calci
Oystercal 500
Posture D
Posture
Scooby-Doo Calcium
Super Calcium 1200
Super Calci Caps

Cold, Cough, and Allergy Products

Actifed With Codeine
Alamine
Benylin DM Pediatric Cough Syrup
Breonesin
Bron Kote
Fedahist Expectorant Pediatric
Fedahist Expectorant
Naldecon Senior DX
Naldecon Senior EX
Naldecon DX Pediatric Drops
Noratuss II Expectorant
PediaCare Night Rest Cough-Cold Formula
Phanatuss Cough
Ryna-C
Ryna-CX
Ryna
Silexin
Tolu-Sed DM
Tricodene
Tricodene Sugar Free
Trind
Trind-DM
Tussar-SF (Sugar Free)
Tuss Kote

Dentrifice Products

Mouth Kote Toothpaste
Perigel Oral Care System
Revelation
Viadent Fluoride
Viadent Original
Viadent Fluoride Gel

Food Supplement Products

Casec
Criticare HN
Fibersource
Fibersource HN
Impact
Impact with Fiber
Isocal HCN
Isocal
Isosource
Isosource HN
Lonalac
MCT Oil
Moducal
Stresstein
Tolerex
Vivonex T.E.N.

Formula Products for Infants and Children

Isomil SF
RCF

Internal Analgesic Products

Acetaminophen Oral Solution USP, cherry
Acetaminophen Oral Solution USP, lime
Actamin Extra

Actamin
Actamin Super
Addaprin
Allerest Headache Strength
Allerest, No Drowsiness
Allerest, Sinus Pain Formula
Aminofen Max
Aminofen
Arthriten
Arthritis Pain Formula Caplets
Arthriten PM
Aspercin Extra
Aspercin
Aspermin Extra
Aspermin
Aspirtab Max
Aspirtab
Bayer Aspirin, Maximum
Bayer Children's Aspirin
Backaid Pills
Back-Quell
Backaid PM Pills
Bayer Aspirin, Genuine
Bayer Children's Chewable Aspirin
Bayer Extended Release 8-Hour Aspirin
Bayer Select Ibuprofen Pain Reliever/Fever Reducer
Bayer Select Maximum Strength Headache
Buffinol Extra
Buffinol
Buffasal Max
Buffasal
Buffaprin Extra
Buffaprin
Cope
Dapa Extra Strength Capsules
Dapa
Doan's Extra Strength
Doan's Original
Dolanex
Dyspel
Emagrin
Ibufen-200
Ibuprin Tablets
Lurline PMS Tablets
McNess Pain Tablets
Midol Menstrual, Maximum Strength
   Multisymptom Formula
Midol PM, Nighttime Pain Reliever/Sleep Aid Caplets
Midol Menstrual, Regular Strength Multisymptom Caplets
Migranol
Midol PMS Capsules
Momentum
Motrin IB
Myapap Drops
Panadol Children's Chewable Tablets
Panadol Children's Liquid
Panadol Children's and Infants' Drops
Panadol Caplets, Maximum Strength
Panadol Maximum Strength
Sinarest, No Drowsiness
Synabrom

Tempra 3 Chewable Tablets
Tempra 3 Chewable Tablets, Double Strength
Tempra 1 Drops
Tempra 2 Syrup
Tri-Pain Caplets
Tranquil Plus
Tylenol Children's Fruit Flavor
Tylenol Children's Grape Flavor
Tylenol Children's Suspension Liquid
Tylenol Infants'
Tylenol Extra Strength Caplets
Tylenol Extra Strength Gelcaps
Tylenol Extra Strength Tablets
Tylenol Infants' Suspension Drops
Tylenol Junior Strength Fruit Chewable Tablets
Tylenol Junior Strength Grape Chewable Tablets
Tylenol Junior Strength Swallowable
Tylenol Regular Strength Caplets
Tylenol Regular Strength Tablets
Ultraprin
Valorin Extra
Valorin
Valorin Super
Valprin
Vanquish Caplets

Iron Products

Chel-Iron Pediatric
Chel-Iron
Fer-In-Sol Iron Capsules
Ferro-Sequels Tablets
Hytinic
Irospan
Nephro-Fer
Niferex
Slow Fe
Stresstabs 600 With Iron
Theragran Stress Formula
Vitron-C Plus

Laxative Products

Adlerika
Agoral
Agoral Plain
Ceo-Two
Doxidan
Doxinate
Emulsoil
Espotabs
Fiberall, Orange
Fiberall, Natural
Fiberall
Fleet Laxative Suppositories
Fleet Flavored Castor Oil Emulsion Oral
   Stimulant Laxative
Fleet Babylax
Fleet Glycerin Suppositories Laxative Child Size
Fleet Glycerin Suppositories Laxative Adult Size
Fleet Mineral Oil Oral Lubricant Laxative
Garfields Tea

Ex-Lax Gentle Nature, Natural Laxative
Haleys M-O
Herb-Lax
Hydrocil Instant
Innerclean Herbal
Kondremul
Konsyl
Liqui-Doss
Mag-Ox 400
Metamucil Instant Mix, Lemon Lime Flavor
Metamucil Orig. Text., Effervescent/Sugar Free/Lemon-Lime
Metamucil, Orange Flavor, Instant Mix
Milk Of Magnesia USP
Milkinol
Milk Of Magnesia-Cascara Suspension, Concentrated
Naturlax Sunlax Citrus Sugar Free
Naturlax Sunlax Orange Sugar Free
Purge Evacuant
Surfak 240mg
Therac Plus
Therevac-SB
Unilax
Uro-Mag
Zymenol

Lozenge Products
Cylex Sugar Free
Larynex
Mycinettes
Thorets

Menstrual Products
Addaprin
Aqua-Ban
Aqua-Ban Plus
Arthritis Pain Formula Caplets
Diurex Timed-Release Water Caplets
Diurex MPR Tablets
Diurex PMS Tablets
Diurex-2 Water Pills
Dyspel
Femcaps
Humphrey's No. 11
Lurline PMS Tablets
Midol For Cramps, Maximum Strength Caplets
Midol Menstrual, Maximum Strength Multisymptom Formula
Midol 200
Midol PM, Nighttime Pain Reliever/Sleep Aid Caplets
Midol Menstrual, Regular Strength Multisymptom Caplets
Midol Regular Strength
Midol PMS Capsules
Panadol Jr.
Ultraprin
Valprin

Mouth Pain, Cold Sore, and Canker Sore Products
Amosan
Anbesol
Anbesol, Maximum Strength
Anbesol Gel, Baby, Grape and Original
Babee Teething Lotion
Blistex Lip Ointment
Cylex Sugar Free
Dr. Hand's Teething Gel
Dr. Hands Teething Lotion
Hurricane
Kank-A Liquid Professional Strength
Lip Medex
Mouth Kote-OR
Mouth Kote-PR
Orabase-B With Benzocaine
Orabase Baby
Orabase Plain
Orabase Lip Healer
Peroxyl Mouthrinse
Peroxyl Oral Spot Treatment Gel
Rid-A-Pain Dental Drops
Tanac
Zilactin Medicated Gel
Zilactin-L Liquid
ZilaDent

Multiple Vitamin Products
Bugs Bunny Childrens Chewable Tablets
Bugs Bunny With Extra C, Children's
Bugs Bunny Plus Iron Chewable Tablets
Bugs Bunny Vitamins And Minerals
Beelith Tablets
Bo-Cal
Cal-Prenal Improved Tablets
Centrum Silver Gel-Tabs
C & E Capsules
Certagen
Chelated Calcium Magnesium Tablets
Chelated Calcium Magnesium Zinc Tablets
Daylets Plus Iron Filmtabs
Dolomite Tablets
Ecee Plus
Filibon
Flintstones Complete
Gerimed
Geriplex-FS Kapseals
Gevral T
Herbal Cellulex
Herpetrol
Ibex Therapeutic
K L B6 Complete
K L B6 Softgels
Mag-Cal
Multi-Mineral
Multi-Vita With Iron
Multi Vit
Multi-Vita
Mucoplex
Myadec
Natabec Kapseals
Neo Vadrin B-Complex 50
Neo Vadrin B-Complex 100

Nestabs
Nova-Dec
OcuCaps
One-A-Day Plus Extra C
One-A-Day Essential
One-A-Day Stressgard
One-Tablet-Daily With Iron
Optivite For Women
Osteogard
Oxi-Freeda
Poly-Vi-Sol with Iron Vitamin Drops
Poly-Vita Drops
Poly-Vi-Sol Vitamin Drops
Preventamine Multivitamin Mineral Complex (Iron-free)
Preventamins Multivitamin Mineral Complex (with Iron)
Sunkist Multis Complete
Sunkist Multis Plus C
Sunkist Multis Plus Iron
Sunkist Multis Regular
Stresstabs Advanced Formula
Stresstabs 600 Plus Zinc
Thera-Combex H-P Kapseals
Theragran Stress Formula
Tri-Vita Drops
Tri-Vi-Sol Vitamins A,D+C Drops
Tri-Vi-Sol With Iron Vitamin A,D+C Drops
Ultra Freeda
Vi-Daylin Multi-Vitamin Plus Iron
Vi-Daylin Multi-Vitamin
Vi-Daylin ADC Vitamins Plus Iron
Vi-Daylin ADC Vitamins
Vita-Lea
Ze Caps
Ze Caps Plus

Oral Rinse Products
Chloraseptic Mouthwash/Gargle
Larylgan
Listerine Coolmint
Listerine
Listermint With Fluoride
Ora Fresh (Cinnamon)
Peroxyl Mouthrinse
Plax Original Flavor
Plax Softmint
Sucrets Maximum Strength Mouthwash/Gargle
Viadent Oral Rinse

Sleep Aid Products
Tranquil Plus

CHAPTER 17

Nutritional Products

Loyd V. Allen, Jr.

> **Questions to ask in patient assessment and counseling**
>
> - *Why do you think you need a vitamin, mineral, or nutritional supplement?*
> - *What are your symptoms? Have they appeared suddenly or gradually?*
> - *What is your age and weight?*
> - *Do you eat meats, vegetables, dairy products, and grain products every day?*
> - *Are you dieting or do you have any type of dietary restrictions?*
> - *Do you participate regularly in sports or do you have a job requiring physical activity?*
> - *Do you have any chronic illness (diabetes, peptic ulcer, ulcerative colitis, or epilepsy)?*
> - *Are you currently taking any prescription or nonprescription medications?*
> - *Are you taking or have you recently taken any vitamins, minerals, or nutritional supplements?*
> - *Do you donate blood? How often? When did you last donate blood?*
> - *Do you smoke or are you around smokers daily?*
> - *Do you drink alcohol? How often and how much?*
> - *Are you pregnant?*
> - *Do you take oral contraceptives (birth control pills)?*

Vitamins are potent organic compounds (exclusive of protein, carbohydrate, and fat) that are essential in small quantities for the specific body functions of growth, maintenance, and reproduction. Vitamins are classified as fat soluble or water soluble. Because most vitamins (with the exception of vitamin D) cannot be synthesized by the body in sufficient quantities to meet metabolic needs, they must be supplied by food or supplementation. Vitamins are widely consumed by the American public, accounting for annual sales in excess of $3 billion.[1]

In most cases, the typical American diet does not need supplementation. Nutrition experts agree that foods, not supplements, are the preferred source of vitamins and minerals and that most individuals can easily meet their requirements by eating a balanced diet. There is less agreement, however, about the extent to which the U.S. population consumes a balanced diet. There are those who believe that most Americans receive adequate levels of vitamins and minerals from their usual diet; the lack of symptoms of deficiency supports this position. But some segments of society (e.g., elderly persons, smokers, nursing home patients, and teenagers) are less likely to consume the recommended dietary allowances (RDAs) of all vitamins and minerals. The issue of who would benefit from supplements is complex. Primary attention should be directed toward improving the diet; under some circumstances, however, a supplement is appropriate.

One of the greatest dangers of food fads, high-potency supplements, and large doses of single vitamins is that they are sometimes used in place of sound medical care. The false hope of superior health or freedom from disease may attract desperate or uninformed individuals who have cancer, heart disease, arthritis, or other serious illnesses and may place them at great risk because it causes them to delay seeking and receiving appropriate medical attention.

Guidelines for optimum nutrition are provided by two organizations: the Food and Nutrition Board of the National Academy of Sciences–National Research Council and the Food and Drug Administration (FDA).

Recommended Dietary Allowances

RDAs are the levels of daily intake of essential nutrients that, based on scientific knowledge, the Food and Nutrition Board judges to be adequate to meet the known nutrient needs of most healthy persons (Table 1). The RDA is two standard deviations above the minimal daily requirement, which is the minimal amount of a vitamin necessary to prevent deficiency of that vitamin in the U.S. population. RDA values are periodically updated based on new information, and they are set high enough to allow for variations in individual requirements caused by minor illnesses. In the Food and Nutrition Board's recommendations, an "estimated safe and adequate daily dietary intake" of other nutrients for which human requirements are not quantitatively known has also been promulgated (Table 2). These data should be used merely as guidelines for nutritional assessment.

RDAs have certain applications and limitations. Their applications include:

- Evaluating the adequacy of the national food supply;
- Establishing standards for menu planning;

Editor's Note: This chapter is based in part on the chapter with a similar title that appeared in the 9th edition but was written by Marianne Ivey and Gary Elmer.

TABLE 1 Food and Nutrition Board, National Academy of Sciences–National Research Council recommended dietary allowances (RDA),[a] revised 1989

Category	Age (yr) or condition	Weight[b] (kg)	(lb)	Height[b] (cm)	(in)	Protein (g)	Fat-soluble vitamins Vitamin A (mcg RE)[c]	Vitamin D (mcg)[d]	Vitamin E (mg α–TE)[e]	Vitamin K (mcg)	Vitamin C (mg)	Thiamine (B_1) (mg)
Infants	0.0–0.5	6	13	60	24	13	375	7.5	3	5	30	0.3
	0.5–1.0	9	20	71	28	14	375	10	4	10	35	0.4
Children	1–3	13	29	90	35	16	400	10	6	15	40	0.7
	4–6	20	44	112	44	24	500	10	7	20	45	0.9
	7–10	28	62	132	52	28	700	10	7	30	45	1.0
Males	11–14	45	99	157	62	45	1,000	10	10	45	50	1.3
	15–18	66	145	176	69	59	1,000	10	10	65	60	1.5
	19–24	72	160	177	70	58	1,000	10	10	70	60	1.5
	25–50	79	174	176	70	63	1,000	5	10	80	60	1.5
	51+	77	170	173	68	63	1,000	5	10	80	60	1.2
Females	11–14	46	101	157	62	46	800	10	8	45	50	1.1
	15–18	55	120	163	64	44	800	10	8	55	60	1.1
	19–24	58	128	164	65	46	800	10	8	60	60	1.1
	25–50	63	138	163	64	50	800	5	8	65	60	1.1
	51+	65	143	160	63	50	800	5	8	65	60	1.0
Pregnant						60	800	10	10	65	70	1.5
Lactating	1st 6 months					65	1,300	10	12	65	95	1.6
	2nd 6 months					62	1,200	10	11	65	90	1.6

[a]The allowances, expressed as average daily intakes over time, are intended to provide for individual variations among most normal persons as they live in the United States under usual environmental stresses. Diets should be based on a variety of common foods in order to provide other nutrients for which human requirements have been less well defined.
[b]The use of these figures does not imply that the height-to-weight ratios are ideal.
[c]RE = retinol equivalents. One RE = 1 mcg retinol or 6 mcg beta carotene. One IU = 0.3 mcg retinol or 0.6 mcg beta carotene.

- Establishing nutritional policy for public institutions/organizations and hospitals;
- Evaluating diets in food consumption studies;
- Developing materials for nutritional education;
- Establishing labeling regulations;
- Setting guidelines for food product formulation.

RDAs have limitations because:

- They are too complex for direct consumer use;
- They do not state ideal or optimal levels of intake;
- The allowances for some categories are based on limited data;
- The data on some nutrients in foods are limited;
- They do not evaluate nutritional status;
- They do not apply to seriously ill or malnourished patients.

Lack of knowledge prevents RDAs from being set for all known nutrients. Further, the application of RDAs to individuals may require adjustment owing to climate, strenuous physical activity, and the presence of a disease state.

The FDA publishes a less comprehensive set of values to be used for labeling purposes. These values, known as the U.S. recommended daily allowances (U.S. RDAs), are included in Table 3. Pharmacists may find U.S. RDA values useful for patient discussions because all vitamin and mineral product potencies are expressed as percentages of the adult U.S. RDA values. However, the U.S. RDAs should not be used in place of the RDAs for planning diets.

RDAs provided in this chapter are primarily for infants, children, adult men and women, and pregnant and lactating women (Table 1). Resource information is available from several standard textbooks and reference books in nutrition and pharmacy.[2–8] The availability of dosage forms is primarily limited to those items for nonprescription oral administration.[9–10]

Nutritional Assessment

Assessment of nutritional status is difficult in the ambulatory environment. Clinical impressions about nutrition are often erroneous because the stages between well-nourished and poorly nourished states are not readily evident. There are guidelines, however, which may help to provide a more objective impression of a patient's nutritional status. Pharmacists should know which population groups are most often poorly nourished, should exercise good observational skills, and should know which questions yield helpful information.

Water-soluble vitamins					Minerals						
Ribo-flavin (B₂) (mg)	Niacin (B₃) (mg NE)ᶠ	Pyri-doxine (vitamin B₆) (mg)	Folic Acid (folate) (mcg)	Cyano-cobalamin (vitamin B₁₂) (mcg)	Cal-cium (mg)	Phos-phorus (mg)	Mag-nesium (mg)	Iron (mg)	Zinc (mg)	Iodine (mcg)	Sele-nium (mcg)
0.4	5	0.3	25	0.3	400	300	40	6	5	40	10
0.5	6	0.6	35	0.5	600	500	60	10	5	50	15
0.8	9	1.0	50	0.7	800	800	80	10	10	70	20
1.1	12	1.1	75	1.0	800	800	120	10	10	90	20
1.2	13	1.4	100	1.4	800	800	170	10	10	120	30
1.5	17	1.7	150	2.0	1,200	1,200	270	12	15	150	40
1.8	20	2.0	200	2.0	1,200	1,200	400	12	15	150	50
1.7	19	2.0	200	2.0	1,200	1,200	350	10	15	150	70
1.7	19	2.0	200	2.0	800	800	350	10	15	150	70
1.4	15	2.0	200	2.0	800	800	350	10	15	150	70
1.3	15	1.4	150	2.0	1,200	1,200	280	15	12	150	45
1.3	15	1.5	180	2.0	1,200	1,200	300	15	12	150	50
1.3	15	1.6	180	2.0	1,200	1,200	280	15	12	150	55
1.3	15	1.6	180	2.0	800	800	280	15	12	150	55
1.2	13	1.6	180	2.0	800	800	280	10	12	150	55
1.6	17	2.2	400	2.2	1,200	1,200	320	30	15	175	65
1.8	20	2.1	280	2.6	1,200	1,200	355	15	19	200	75
1.7	20	2.1	260	2.6	1,200	1,200	340	15	16	200	75

ᵈAs cholecalciferol; 10 mcg cholecalciferol = 400 IU of vitamin D.
ᵉα-TE = alpha-tocopherol equivalents. 1 mg D-alpha tocopherol = 1 mg α-TE = 1.49 IU.
ᶠNE = niacin equivalent, equal to 1 mg of niacin or 60 mg of dietary tryptophan.
Adapted with permission from Food and Nutrition Board, National Research Council–National Academy of Sciences. *Recommended Dietary Allowances.* 10th ed. Washington, DC: National Academy Press; 1989.

Undernourished groups in the United States often include infants, preschoolers, lactating or pregnant women, elderly persons, alcoholics, the homeless, and the impoverished. Other populations at risk are people on restricted diets, people with certain intestinal diseases that lead to nutritional deficits, people taking certain drugs that may adversely affect nutrient absorption, and women of childbearing age who have regular blood loss. Epidemiologic surveys have shown that schoolchildren, factory workers, businesspersons, and farmers are less likely to be poorly nourished.

The pharmacist should observe the patient's physical condition but must realize that only severe dietary deficiencies are likely to be reflected physically. A thorough nutritional assessment includes a determination of weight loss or gain, fat (measured by triceps and subscapular skinfold thickness), somatic protein or muscle mass (measured by midarm muscle circumference, creatinine height index, hair pluckability, and myoderma), and visceral protein markers (measured by serum albumin, prealbumin, transferrin, retinol levels, skin antigen response, and pitting time). Although these assessment measures are beyond the scope of routine pharmacy practice, some observations may be made on the status of the patient. For example, a patient's fingernails may indicate malnutrition if they lose their luster and become dark at the upper ends. The texture, amount, and appearance of the hair may indicate the patient's nutritional status. The eyes, particularly the conjunctiva, may indicate vitamin A and iron deficiencies, and the mouth may show stomatitis, glossitis, or hypertrophic or pale gums. The number and general condition of the teeth may reflect the patient's choice of food. Visible goiter, poor skin color and texture, obesity or thinness relative to bone structure, and the presence of edema may also be indications of malnutrition.

The more specific the information obtained from the patient, the more helpful the pharmacist can be in determining the need for nutritional supplementation. Questions regarding foods generally not included in the diet and previous treatment of similar symptoms may also be important.

Just as nutritional deficiencies may lead to disease, disease may lead to nutritional deficiencies. It is the pharmacist's responsibility to refer patients with a suspected serious illness to a physician. Epidemics of vitamin deficiency do not occur in the United States; however, patients may present with one or more deficiencies, which may be very difficult to diagnose. Such patients are usually seriously ill or malnourished because of alcoholism, food faddism, or poverty. Guidelines for the clinical appraisal of nutritional status include evaluation of growth, development, fitness, and medical and dietary history;

TABLE 2	Estimated safe and adequate daily dietary intakes of selected vitamins and minerals[a]							
		Vitamins		Trace elements[b]				
Category	Age (yr)	Biotin (mcg)	Panto-thenic acid (mg)	Copper (mg)	Manganese (mg)	Fluoride (mg)	Chromium (mcg)	Molybdenum (mcg)
Infants	0–0.5	10	3	0.4–0.6	0.3–0.6	0.1–0.5	10–40	15–30
	0.5–1	15	3	0.6–0.7	0.6–1.0	0.2–1.0	20–60	20–40
Children and adolescents	1–3	20	3	0.7–1.0	1.0–1.5	0.5–1.5	20–80	25–50
	4–6	25	3–4	1.0–1.5	1.5–2.0	1.0–2.5	30–120	30–75
	7–10	30	4–5	1.0–2.0	2.0–3.0	1.5–2.5	50–200	50–150
	11+	30–100	4–7	1.5–2.5	2.0–5.0	1.5–2.5	50–200	75–250
Adults		30–100	4–7	1.5–3.0	2.0–5.0	1.5–4.0	50–200	75–250

[a]Because there is less information on which to base allowances, these figures are not given in Table 1 and are provided here in the form of ranges of recommended intakes.
[b]Because the toxic levels for many trace elements may be only several times the usual intakes, the upper levels for the trace elements given in the table should not be habitually exceeded.
Adapted with permission from Food and Nutrition Board, National Research Council–National Academy of Sciences. *Recommended Dietary Allowances*. 10th ed. Washington, DC: National Academy Press; 1989: 284.

observation of signs consistent with deficiencies; and biochemical assessment. Rarely in the United States do pharmacists encounter patients with severe deficiencies resulting in diseases such as scurvy, pellagra, or kwashiorkor. However, milder forms of malnutrition may be seen. The evolution of vitamin deficiency may include several stages (Table 4).[11]

Malnutrition

The primary causes of malnutrition include starvation, disease-related factors, and food faddism. In elderly persons, the causes of nutritional deficiency may be related to disease, malabsorption, physiologic changes of the gastrointestinal (GI) tract, mastication difficulty, or loss of perception (taste, smell, or sight). Other factors include social isolation, fear for personal safety, lack of knowledge about an adequate diet, poverty, alcoholism, and drug abuse.

The incidence of vitamin deficiency due to inadequate dietary intake is approximately 10% in the homebound elderly population. Elderly people have a 34–88% reduction in circulating levels of one or more vitamins.

Poor nutrition increases the risks of cancer and infection, as well as of surgery and chemotherapy. Wound-healing time and mortality may be increased. The conditions associated with severe malnutrition include marasmus, kwashiorkor, and mixed malnutrition. Marasmus is caused by inadequate total dietary intake and presents as decreased fat deposits, decreased muscle mass, and cachexia, primarily in infants or children. Kwashiorkor is caused by inadequate dietary intake of protein and is characterized by edema, decreased serum protein levels, and hypoalbuminemia. Mixed malnutrition is caused by inadequate dietary intake of calories and protein and exhibits features of both marasmus and kwashiorkor.

The Pharmacist's Role in Vitamin and Mineral Use

By being familiar with daily RDAs of the various vitamins and minerals and by knowing which natural food sources provide these RDAs, the pharmacist should be able to recognize overt but nonspecific symptoms of vitamin and mineral deficiencies where prompt physician referral may be crucial. By asking key questions, the pharmacist may also detect cultural, physical, environmental, and social conditions that may suggest inadequate vitamin intake. Emphasis should be on educating the patient and improving the diet so that nutritional requirements are met through food. If a supplement is needed, the pharmacist can recommend a product that will provide appropriate levels of the needed vitamins at a reasonable price.

The average American consuming an average diet does not need vitamin supplementation. Although some claim that everyone would benefit from supplements, the general lack of knowledge concerning the risks and benefits of megadose vitamin therapy leads others to argue that vitamin supplements are unnecessary and that megavitamin therapy is even dangerous. The truth probably lies closer to the second claim. Some segments of the population may benefit from supplemental multivitamins, but most others do not. And although there are specific situations in which high doses of specific vitamins have been reported to be of therapeutic benefit, the exaggerated claims of the megavitamin enthusiasts have not been confirmed. Furthermore, prolonged ingestion of vitamins has not been tested for safety; and some vitamins, such as A, D, niacin, and pyridoxine, are known to be toxic in high doses. Thus, the consumer should be cautioned against initiating high-dose self-medication with vitamins. Chronic ingestion of large doses of any drug, including vitamins, for relief of a relatively

TABLE 3 U.S. recommended daily allowances (U.S. RDAs) for labeling purposes

	Unit	Infants	Children under age 4	Adults and children aged 4 or older	Pregnant and lactating women
Vitamin A	IU	1,500	2,500	5,000	8,000
Vitamin D	IU	400	400	400	400
Vitamin E	IU	5	10	30	30
Ascorbic acid	mg	35	40	60	60
Folic acid	mg	0.1	0.2	0.4	0.8
Thiamine	mg	0.5	0.7	1.5	1.7
Riboflavin	mg	0.6	0.8	1.7	2.0
Niacin	mg	8	9	20	20
Pyridoxine	mg	0.4	0.7	2	2.5
Cyanocobalamin	mcg	2	3	6	8
Biotin	mg	0.05	0.15	0.3	0.3
Pantothenic acid	mg	3	5	10	10
Calcium	g	0.6	0.8	1.0	1.3
Phosphorus	g	0.5	0.8	1.0	1.3
Iodine	mcg	45	70	150	150
Iron	mg	15	10	18	18
Magnesium	mg	70	200	400	450
Manganese[a]	mg	0.5	1.0	4.0	4.0
Copper	mg	0.6	1.0	2.0	2.0
Zinc	mg	5	8	15	15
Protein	g	—	20(28)[b]	45(65)[b]	—

[a]Proposed U.S. RDA.
[b]Values in parentheses are U.S. RDAs when the protein efficiency ratio (PER) is less than that of casein; the other values are used when the PER is equal to or greater than that of casein. No claim may be made for a protein with a PER equal to or less than 20% that of casein.

mild and self-limiting condition such as the common cold should be discouraged.

Vitamins are used both as dietary supplements and as therapeutic agents to treat deficiencies. As dietary supplements, vitamins usually use 50–150% of the U.S. RDA. As therapeutic agents, they are used to treat clinical deficiencies or other pathologic conditions. Therapeutic use should be recommended only by physicians according to specific medical indications. The therapeutic dose should not exceed 2–10 times the RDA, depending on the vitamin.

Multivitamin Therapy

Although health authorities agree that a balanced diet and adequate caloric intake obviate the necessity for supplemental vitamins for most individuals, certain segments of the population known to be at risk for vitamin deficiencies may benefit from special attention to diet or vitamin supplements. Such an approach is indicated in the following situations:

- *Iatrogenic situations*: for example, oral contraceptive and estrogen users, patients on prolonged broad-spectrum antibiotics, or patients on prolonged parenteral nutrition;
- *Inadequate dietary intake*: for example, alcoholics, the impoverished, the aged, or patients on severe caloric-restricted diets or fad diets;
- *Increased metabolic requirements*: for example, pregnant or lactating women; infants; children undergoing periods of accelerated growth; or patients with major surgery, cancer, severe injury, infection, or trauma;
- *Poor absorption*: for example, the aged, or patients with such conditions as prolonged diarrhea, severe GI disorders and malignancy, surgical removal of a section of the GI tract, celiac disease, obstructive jaundice, or cystic fibrosis.

The pharmacist should counsel patients on appropriate multivitamin selection. In general, an inexpensive supplemental preparation that supplies close to 100% of the RDA for each vitamin will meet the needs of most patients requiring or desiring supplements. The need for expensive high-potency vitamins is rare.

"Natural" Vitamins

Because the body cannot distinguish between a vitamin molecule derived from a synthetic source and one derived from a natural source, synthetic vitamins are absorbed and used

TABLE 4	Stages in the evolution of a vitamin deficiency
Stages	**Effects**
Preliminary	Decreased tissue stores, decreased urinary excretion
Biochemical	Reduced enzyme activity, negligible urinary excretion
Physiologic	Malaise, weight loss, insomnia, impaired psychologic functions
Clinical	Increased nonspecific symptoms, appearance of clinical signs
Anatomic	Clear specific symptoms, pathologic tissue changes that may be fatal

to the same extent as the more expensive natural vitamins. Frequently, natural vitamins are supplemented with the synthetic vitamin. For example, the amount of ascorbic acid that can be acquired from rose hips (the fleshy fruit of a rose) is relatively small, and synthetic ascorbic acid is added to prevent too large a tablet size. However, this addition may not be noted on the label, and the price of the partially natural product is often considerably higher than that for the completely synthetic but equally effective product.

Fat-Soluble Vitamins

Vitamins A, D, E, and K are the fat-soluble vitamins. They are soluble in lipids and are usually absorbed along with chylomicrons into the lymphatic system of the small intestine, where they pass into the general circulation. Their absorption is facilitated by bile. Deficiencies of these vitamins occur when fat intake is limited or fat absorption is compromised. Drugs that affect lipid absorption, such as cholestyramine (which binds bile acids and thereby hinders lipid emulsification) and mineral oil (which increases fecal elimination of lipids), may precipitate such a deficiency. These vitamins are stored in body tissues when excessive quantities are ingested, and they may be toxic, especially when taken in megadoses.

Vitamin A
Description The designation "vitamin A" refers to a group of compounds essential for vision, growth, cellular differentiation and proliferation, and reproduction and integrity of the immune system. There are a number of names and forms of vitamin A, including the retinoids (e.g., retinol and retinoic acid) and the carotenoids (e.g., beta carotene). The term *retinoid* is also used to refer to this very large group of compounds, some of which are without vitamin A activity. Additionally, more than 500 of the carotenoids, which are precursors of vitamin A, are found naturally but only about 50 are precursors of retinol. Biochemical changes occur in the retinoids and carotenoids during absorption in the intestine to form active compounds.

More than 90% of the body's supply of vitamin A is stored in the liver, and these reserves are usually sufficient for several months to a year. Infants and young children are more susceptible to vitamin A deficiency because they have not established the necessary reserves.[12]

The primary dietary source of vitamin A is the carotenoids, which are synthesized by plants and converted in the body into vitamin A. Vitamin A is measured in international units (IU); 1 IU equals 0.3 mcg of retinol, 0.6 mcg of beta carotene, or 1.2 mcg of other carotenoids. The retinol equivalent (RE) has been recommended by the Food and Nutrition Board as a way to determine the amount of absorption of the carotenes as well as their degree of conversion to vitamin A in the body. In the RE system, 1 RE equals 1 mcg of retinol, 6 mcg of beta carotene, and 12 mcg of other carotenoids. This system is appropriate because retinol is assumed to be completely absorbed from the GI tract whereas carotenes are only about one-third absorbed. Because only about half of the absorbed beta carotene is converted to retinol, only one-sixth of the intake is actually used. One-fourth of the other carotenoids is converted to retinol, so only one-twelfth of the intake is available. (The carotenes are split in the intestinal mucosa to form retinaldehyde, which is reduced to form retinol.)

Because vitamin A and carotenoids are fat soluble, they are found mainly in fatty foods. Good sources are fish, butter, cream, eggs, milk, and organ meats. Carotenoids are the yellow-orange pigments of carrots, squash, and pumpkin; they are also present in many dark, leafy vegetables. However, the color intensity of a vegetable is not a reliable indicator of its vitamin A content.

Indications Vitamin A is essential for normal growth and reproduction, normal skeletal and tooth development, and the proper functioning of most organs of the body, notably the specialized functions involving the conjunctiva, retina, and cornea of the eye. It is thus indicated in the prevention and treatment of symptoms of vitamin A deficiency, such as dry eye (xerophthalmia) and night blindness (nyctalopia). The synthesis of the glycoproteins necessary to maintain normal epithelial cell mucous secretions requires vitamin A, which is also vital to the body's defense against bacterial infections in the upper respiratory system.

Vitamin A deficiency is rare in well-nourished populations and develops slowly because the body has available stores of fat-soluble vitamins. Serum levels usually remain normal until the liver reserve becomes highly depleted. Deficiency occurs when vitamin A plasma levels fall below 10 mcg/dL. (Normal blood levels range from 20 to 80 mcg/dL.) It is most common in poorly nourished children under 5 years old. Conditions such as cancer, tuberculosis, pneumonia, chronic nephritis, urinary tract infections, and prostate disease may cause excessive excretion of vitamin A. Conditions in which there is fat malabsorption, such as celiac disease, short gut syndrome, obstructive jaundice, cystic fibrosis, and cirrhosis of the liver, may impair vitamin A absorption. Neomycin or cholestyramine may cause significant malabsorption of vitamin A and other fat-soluble vitamins and may precipitate deficiencies with long-term use. In the United States, vitamin A deficiency occurs more often because of diseases of fat malabsorption than because of malnutrition.

One of the earliest symptoms of vitamin A deficiency is night blindness, caused by failure of the retina to obtain adequate supplies of retinol for the formation of rhodopsin. If the situation is not reversed, it may be rapidly followed by structural changes in the retina and xerosis of the conjunctiva. Bitot's spots (small patches of bubbles that resemble tiny drops of meringue) may appear. The conjunctiva may look dry and opaque, and photophobia (light sensitivity) may occur. If the deficiency continues, xerosis of the cornea occurs, followed by corneal distortion. The loss of continuity of the surface epithelium, with formation of a noninflammatory ulcer and infiltration of the stroma, can lead to softening of the cornea, alteration of the iris, and permanent loss of vision.

Other characteristic clinical findings in a deficiency disorder include increased susceptibility to infection, follicular hyperkeratosis, loss of appetite, impaired taste and smell, impaired equilibrium, and an increase in cerebrospinal fluid pressure. Some of these findings may be masked by concurrent deficiencies of other nutrients. Notable, however, is the drying and hyperkeratinization of the skin, which predisposes patients to infections. The integrity of epithelial tissues depends on vitamin A activity.

One of the most encouraging developments in vitamin research has been the discovery that vitamin A analogs show promise in the prevention and treatment of certain cancers and in the treatment of certain skin disorders. It has long been known that vitamin A deficiency in animals leads to hyperkeratosis and metaplasia (preneoplastic conditions) of epithelial tissues. Systemic administration of high doses of vitamin A may retard the development of these precancerous lesions. Experimental results also suggest that certain systemic retinoids may be useful in treating acne, psoriasis, and other skin conditions characterized by hyperkeratosis. Topical retinoic acid (Retin-A®) and systemic isotretinoin (Accutane®) are currently used to treat acne vulgaris, although not without side effects.

Dose/RDA The usual requirements for vitamin A are supplied by an adequate diet. The use of supplemental vitamin A would be appropriate in treating vitamin A deficiency and as prophylaxis in at-risk patients during times of increased requirements (e.g., infancy, pregnancy, or lactation). Dietary intake of vitamin A should be estimated when determining the dosage for administration. Vitamin A is usually administered orally.

The RDA values published by the Food and Nutrition Board express the potency of vitamin A in terms of an RE. Thus, the RDA in adult men and women is 1,000 and 800 mcg RE, respectively. The U.S. RDA still retains the IU as a measure of potency, so the U.S. RDA for adults is 5,000 IU, which is equivalent to 1,000 RE. This is increased to 8,000 IU for pregnant and lactating women, and decreased to 1,500 IU for infants and to 2,500 IU for children under 4 years of age (Table 3). If the pharmacist determines that a vitamin A supplement is appropriate, a nonprescription multiple vitamin that contains no more than the RDA of vitamin A should be recommended. High-dose vitamin A therapy should be undertaken only with close medical supervision. There does not appear to be a special requirement for vitamin A for the elderly. Tables 1, 2, and 3 show the requirements for children; it is interesting to note that the 11- to 14-year-old group is separated by sex because of differences in lean body mass that occur during this period.

Adverse Effects/Drug Interactions An excessive intake of vitamin A may result from overzealous prophylactic vitamin therapy and prolonged self-medication. Because vitamin A is stored in the body, high doses of it can lead to a toxic syndrome known as hypervitaminosis A. The incidence of hypervitaminosis A is increasing because of publicity regarding the potential application of vitamin A in cancer and in skin disorders. Toxicity in the form of bulging fontanelles or hydrocephalus has occurred in infants given doses 10 times the RDA for several weeks. Fatigue, malaise, and lethargy are also common symptoms. Abdominal upset, bone and joint pain, throbbing headaches, insomnia, restlessness, night sweats, loss of body hair, brittle nails, exophthalmos, rough and scaly skin, peripheral edema, and mouth fissures may also occur. Severe constipation, menstrual irregularity, and emotional lability have been reported in some cases. A single dose (2,000,000 IU, or 400,000 RE) may precipitate acute toxicity 4–8 hours after ingestion. Headache is a predominant symptom, but it may be accompanied by diplopia, nausea, vomiting, vertigo, hypercalcemia, or drowsiness. Chronic daily ingestion of at least 25,000 IU of vitamin A, a dose readily available to the public, has resulted in toxicity in children. Treatment consists of discontinuing vitamin A supplementation, and the prognosis is good. Carotene does not produce toxicity rapidly because the rate at which it converts to vitamin A is slow. However, eating large amounts of carrots daily may result in carotenemia, which can produce a yellow skin hue.

Large doses of vitamin A may increase the hypoprothrombinemic effect of warfarin. Cholestyramine and mineral oil may reduce the absorption of vitamin A. Oral contraceptive use may increase plasma levels of vitamin A.

The recommended dosage of vitamin A supplements should not be exceeded, and prolonged use of cholestyramine or mineral oil should be avoided while using supplements. Pregnant women or women of childbearing age who are not using contraception should avoid vitamin A doses above the RDA.

Vitamin D (Calciferol)

Description A number of chemicals are associated with vitamin D activity; Table 5 lists the structurally similar chemicals and their metabolites for which vitamin D is a collective name. Cholecalciferol (vitamin D_3) is the natural form of vitamin D. It is synthesized in the skin from endogenous or dietary cholesterol on exposure to ultraviolet radiation (sunlight). Ergocalciferol, which differs structurally only slightly from cholecalciferol, is of dietary importance. Ergocalciferol and cholecalciferol are equipotent.

Vitamin D requires activation involving both the liver and the kidney. One metabolite, 25-hydroxycholecalciferol, is formed by the liver and then hydroxylated by the kidney to its most active form, 1,25-dihydroxycholecalciferol. This explains the observation of hypocalcemia in patients with renal failure, and the failure of some patients to respond even to massive doses of vitamin D_3. Administration of 1,25-dihydroxycholecalciferol (available as calcitriol) to these patients has been successful.

TABLE 5 Chemicals that have vitamin D activity

Activity ratio	Name	Synonyms	
1	Vitamin D_3	Cholecalciferol	Calciol
2–5	25-Hydroxyvitamin D_3	25-Hydroxycholecalciferol	Calcifediol
10	1,25-Dihydroxyvitamin D_3	1,25-Dihydroxycholecalciferol	Calcitriol
1	Vitamin D_2	Ergocalciferol, Ergocalciol	Ercalciol
2–5	25-Hydroxyvitamin D_2	25-Hydroxyergocalciferol	Ercalcidiol
10	1,25-Dihydroxyvitamin D_2	1,25-Dihydroxyergocalciferol	Ercalcitriol

Vitamin D, which has properties of both hormones and vitamins, is necessary for the proper formation of the skeleton and for mineral homeostasis. It is closely involved with parathyroid hormone, phosphate, and calcitonin in the hemostasis of serum calcium.

Milk and milk products are the major source of preformed vitamin D in the United States, given that milk is routinely supplemented with 400 IU of vitamin D per quart. Eggs and animal livers are also rich in vitamin D, and fish, beef, and butter are additional natural sources. Vitamin D is stable, and normal food processing does not appear to alter its activity.

Indications A deficiency of vitamin D may be due to dietary deficiency; GI disorder (hepatobiliary disease, malabsorption, or chronic pancreatitis); acidosis; chronic renal failure; hereditary disorders of vitamin D metabolism; phosphate depletion; renal tubular disorders; poisoning from lead, cadmium, or outdated tetracycline; and prolonged parenteral nutrition without proper vitamin D supplementation.

The signs and symptoms of vitamin D deficiency diseases are reflected as calcium abnormalities, specifically those involved with bone formation. The classic deficiency state is rickets. Vitamin D increases calcium and phosphate absorption from the small intestine, mobilizes calcium from bone, permits normal bone mineralization, improves renal absorption of calcium, and maintains serum calcium and phosphorus levels. As serum calcium and inorganic phosphate decrease, compensatory mechanisms attempt to increase the calcium. Parathyroid hormone secretion increases, possibly leading to secondary hyperparathyroidism. If physiologic mechanisms fail to make the appropriate adjustments in levels of calcium and phosphorus, demineralization of bone will ensue to maintain essential plasma calcium levels. During growth, demineralization leads to a failure of bone matrix mineralization, and in adults, it may lead to severe osteomalacia. The epiphyseal plate may widen because of the failure of calcification combined with weight load on the softened structures during growth. As a result, rickets is manifested by soft bones and deformed joints. The diagnosis is made radiologically by observing the bone deformities. The lack of adequate calcium in muscle tissue results in tetany.

Although the incidence of rickets in the United States is low, the increasing popularity of vegetarian diets has led to rickets in some children who abstain from milk and in infants breast-fed by mothers who do not drink milk, fail to take prenatal vitamins, or otherwise receive inadequate intake of vitamin D. A deficiency of vitamin D may also result in liver disease and myopathy because of decreased muscle phosphate.

Osteomalacia may develop in elderly persons owing to vitamin D deficiency (malabsorption syndromes, inadequate diet or sunlight, gastrectomy, laxative abuse, and pancreatic insufficiency); anticonvulsant, cholestyramine, or glucocorticoid therapy; liver disease; chronic renal failure; hypoparathyroidism; postmenopausal endocrine changes; and/or cadmium and strontium toxicity. In adults, bone fractures may result from the bone loss that accompanies hypocalcemia.

Dose/RDA Most persons obtain the RDA (Tables 1 and 3) of vitamin D from dietary sources and exposure to sunlight. People exposed regularly to sunlight will generally have no dietary requirement for vitamin D. However, a substantial part of the U.S. population is exposed to very little sunlight, especially during the winter.

If a patient asks for a vitamin D supplement and the pharmacist determines that the need is based on poor dietary intake or on indoor confinement, a multivitamin supplement containing no more than 100 IU of vitamin D may be recommended. Liquid preparations that contain vitamin D should be measured carefully, particularly when given to infants. Patients who request therapeutic doses of vitamin D should be referred to a physician; those using a prescription vitamin D product should be encouraged to see their physician regularly.

Large doses of vitamin D (1,000–4,000 IU) are prescribed for treatment of rickets. For adults with osteomalacia caused by renal disease, 0.25–1 mcg of calcitriol is often prescribed. Dihydrotachysterol, a synthetic analog that does not require kidney activation, may also be used.

Vitamin D is included in most multivitamin preparations and is also available alone in various strengths as tablets, capsules, and drops. Two active metabolites, 25-hydroxycholecalciferol (calcifediol) and 1,25-dihydroxycholecalciferol (calcitriol), are available by prescription for use in patients with hypocalcemia associated with renal failure. The former compound has a longer half-life but is less potent. Dihydrotachysterol, which is available by prescription, is also useful in renal failure because it does not require metabolic activation by the kidneys.

Adverse Effects/Drug Interactions Taking five or more times the RDA of vitamin D may lead to adverse effects, including hypercalcemia, hypercalciuria, polyuria, nephrocalcinosis, renal failure, metastatic calcification, and kidney stones. Doses exceeding 400 IU (25 mcg of cholecalciferol) are not advisable. In infants, as little as 1,800 IU of vitamin D per day may inhibit growth.

The more common symptoms of hypervitaminosis D are anorexia, nausea, weakness, weight loss, polyuria, constipation, vague aches, stiffness, soft tissue calcification, nephrocalcinosis, hypertension, anemia, hypercalcemia, acidosis, and irreversible renal failure. If a recent blood test has not been taken to measure serum calcium, a physician should be consulted.

Concurrent drug therapy must be closely monitored because vitamin D may interact with other drugs. Phosphate in chronically used drugs, such as certain laxatives, may lower the calcium level and contribute to a vitamin D deficiency. Patients who have such a deficiency because of renal problems should use caution in taking antacids. Patients with severe renal problems should be advised to select antacids for the specific ingredients they contain. Aluminum-containing antacids may be chosen because they bind phosphates, and calcium-containing antacids may be used to help increase serum calcium levels; however, magnesium-containing antacids should be avoided because magnesium tends to accumulate to toxic levels in renal disease. Cholestyramine and mineral oil may reduce the amount of vitamin D absorbed, so their prolonged use should be avoided. Phenytoin or barbiturates may decrease the half-life of vitamin D.

Vitamin E (Tocopherol)
Description Vitamin E is present in all cell membranes, and it functions to prevent oxidation of polyunsaturated fatty acids. The term *vitamin E* refers to a series of eight compounds. The tocopherols and the tocotrienols are naturally occurring compounds in plants. Alpha-tocopherol, the most active of these compounds, is used to calculate the vitamin E content of food.

The following equivalents can be used to estimate the total alpha-tocopherol equivalents (α-TEs) of diets containing only natural forms of vitamin E. To use the table below, the number of milligrams of vitamin E in the diet should be multiplied by the number in the factor column to estimate the total α-TEs. One α-TE equals 1.49 IU.

Item	Factor
beta-tocopherol	0.5
gamma-tocopherol	0.1
alpha-tocotrienol	0.3
all-rac-alpha-tocopherol	0.74

Its metabolic roles are not completely understood, but vitamin E functions primarily as an antioxidant in protecting cellular membranes from oxidative damage or destruction. This process may be aided by selenium and ascorbic acid. Vitamin E may also have a more specific coenzyme role in heme biosynthesis, steroid metabolism, and collagen formation.

Foods rich in vitamin E include vegetable oils, margarines (made from plant oils), green vegetables, nuts, wheat germ, and whole grains. Refining grains to produce white flour removes much of the vitamin, and bleaching grains further depletes it. Meats, fruits, and milk contain very little vitamin E.

Indications Vitamin E deficiency is extremely rare but apparently occurs in two population groups: premature, very low birthweight infants; and patients who do not absorb fat normally, such as children with cystic fibrosis. The primary signs of vitamin E deficiency are reproductive failure and neurologic abnormalities. Symptoms include increased hemolysis of red blood cells, creatinuria, and smooth muscle deposits of brown pigment.

A deficiency syndrome involving premature infants who were fed a vitamin E–depleted formula has been noted. Symptoms include edema, hemolytic anemia, reticulocytosis, and thrombocytosis, which clears upon supplementation with vitamin E. In adults, chronic ingestion of a vitamin E–depleted diet resulted only in an increased propensity for erythrocyte hemolysis. Evidence for deposition of ceroid (age) pigments, creatinuria, altered erythropoiesis, and myopathy has been found in patients with vitamin E deficiency secondary to steatorrhea. Neurologic abnormalities responsive to supplemental vitamin E have been reported in some patients with biliary disease and cystic fibrosis. Patients with these conditions should receive vitamin E supplements.

Dose/RDA The average daily diet contains approximately 3–15 mg of vitamin E; therefore, large doses (i.e., ≥ 100 mg per day) are not necessary unless the patient is experiencing malabsorption. Doses of 300–400 mg per day have been prescribed for claudication, angina, and diabetes, with inconclusive results.

Requirements for vitamin E may vary in proportion to the amount of polyunsaturated fatty acids in the diet. Although the polyunsaturated fatty acid content of the U.S. diet has increased in recent years, the plant oils responsible for the increase are rich in tocopherol. It has been theorized that, with the increasing oxidant insult to the environment in the form of atmospheric pollutants, the intake of vitamin E should be increased. However, the lack of evidence of deficiency at the present intake supports the current adult RDA of 8–10 mg per day.

Adverse Effects/Drug Interactions Vitamin E is relatively nontoxic. Most adults tolerate 100–1,000 IU daily without adverse effects. But the hazards of long-term, high-dose therapy are unknown. Nevertheless, the enhancement of warfarin anticoagulation has been reported. The pharmacist should caution patients taking oral anticoagulants to avoid vitamin E in large doses. Nor should vitamin E be taken at the same time as iron. Studies with supplementation of infant formulas containing iron and vitamin E show that blood tocopherol levels do not increase.

Vitamin K
Description Phytonadione (vitamin K_1) was first isolated from alfalfa and is present in many vegetables. Menaquinone (vitamin K_2), which was produced from putrefied fishmeal, is a product of bacterial metabolism, and the colonic bacteria may be able to synthesize about 2 mcg/kg of body weight per day of the vitamin. Menadione (vitamin K_3) is a synthetic compound that is two to three times as potent as the natural vitamin K. There are at least five proteins in the body, in addition to prothrombin, that depend upon vitamin K.

Sources of the vitamin include pork liver and vegetables such as spinach, kale, cabbage, and cauliflower.

Food composition tables and product labels may not list vitamin K content because it is not precisely known.

Indications Deficiency may be caused by breast-feeding of newborns; severe liver disease; malabsorption syndromes; biliary obstruction; regional enteritis; blind loop syndrome; ulcerative colitis; and chronic, broad-spectrum antibiotic therapy. A deficiency may be assessed by determining the prothrombin time.

Deficiencies do not readily occur because normal U.S. diets contain 300–500 mcg of vitamin K daily, so there is a low incidence of deficiency among healthy, well-nourished individuals. Moreover, microbiologic flora of the normal gut synthesize enough menaquinones to supply a significant part of the body's requirement for vitamin K. However, because the absorption of vitamin K requires bile in the small intestine, anything that interferes with bile production or secretion may contribute to a vitamin K deficiency. Malabsorption syndromes and bowel resections may decrease vitamin K absorption. Liver disease may also cause symptoms of vitamin K deficiency if hepatic production of the prothrombin clotting factor is decreased.

Vitamin K deficiencies are almost always associated with severe pathologic conditions in which the patient is receiving intensive medical care. The only evident symptom of a deficiency state is defective blood coagulation; hemorrhage is the most common symptom of clinical deficiency.

Dose/RDA The 1989 RDA values include vitamin K for the first time: 65 mcg daily for adult women and 80 mcg daily for adult men. For minor bleeding, 1–5 mg of vitamin K is given daily; for a major hemorrhage, 20 mg is given. The cause of the deficiency and the severity of bleeding will determine whether oral administration is adequate. Vitamin K (phytonadione) is routinely given to neonates at birth (one dose of 1 mg) to prevent hemorrhaging. This is necessary because placental transport of vitamin K is low and the neonate has yet to acquire the intestinal microflora that produce the vitamin.

Only a small number of available nonprescription products contain vitamin K.

Adverse Effects/Drug Interactions Even in large amounts over an extended period, vitamin K does not produce toxic manifestations. Administration of menadione (but not of phylloquinone) may cause hemolytic anemia, hyperbilirubinemia, and kernicterus in the newborn owing to interaction with sulfhydryl groups.

In addition to agents such as cholestyramine resins and mineral oil, which interfere with the absorption of all fat-soluble vitamins, the oral anticoagulants are antagonists of vitamin K. Although dietary amounts of vitamin K (near the RDA value) do not usually interfere with coumarin anticoagulant activity, an interaction with the 5-mg therapeutic dose of warfarin sodium (Coumadin®) may be significant. Conversely, 2.5–25 mg of oral or parenteral vitamin K may be used to counteract an overdose of coumarin anticoagulant.

Long-term, broad-spectrum antibiotic therapy may initiate a vitamin K deficiency by decreasing gut flora; however, this interaction is not usually seen if dietary intake is normal. Vitamins A and E, in large quantities, may interfere with the absorption or metabolism of vitamin K.

Water-Soluble Vitamins

Ascorbic Acid (Vitamin C)

Description Ascorbic acid is the most easily destroyed of all the vitamins. A relatively simple compound, it is a powerful reducing agent that serves to protect the capillary basement membrane. As a nutrient, ascorbic acid is necessary to form collagen and to serve as a water-soluble antioxidant. Humans must ingest it, however, because it is not produced by the body.

Ascorbic acid is necessary for the biosynthesis of hydroxyproline, a precursor of collagen, osteoid, and dentin. It also assists in the absorption of nonheme iron from food by reducing the ferric iron in the stomach and by combining in complex formation with ions that remain solubilized in the alkaline pH of the duodenum.

Ascorbic acid has been promoted for prevention of the common cold and attenuation of symptoms should a cold occur, but these claims are largely unsupported by well-designed and controlled clinical studies. It has been suggested that a decreased recovery time from cold sores, an increased healing rate of pressure sores, and a decreased incidence of rectal polyps may occur following administration of ascorbic acid. There is conflicting and equivocal data, however, concerning the ability of ascorbic acid to lower cholesterol levels in nonascorbatic, hypercholesterolemic patients.

Ascorbic acid has been called the "fresh-food" vitamin, and most of the daily intake is derived from the vegetable and fruit groups. Sources relatively high in vitamin C content include green and red peppers, collard greens, broccoli, spinach, tomatoes, potatoes, strawberries, oranges, and other citrus fruits. Meat, fish, poultry, eggs, and dairy products contain some vitamin C, but it is generally absent in grains.

Indications Characteristics of ascorbic acid deficiency include malaise, weakness, capillary hemorrhages and petechiae, hyperkeratotic follicles (corkscrew hairs), petechiae–ecchymoses, swollen hemorrhagic gums, and bone changes. A deficiency may also impair wound healing and reopen old wounds. A profound dietary deficiency can eventually lead to scurvy and produce widespread capillary hemorrhaging and a weakening of collagenous structures.

Scurvy, the classical deficiency state, is rare in the United States. It develops only when there is chronically inadequate nutritional consumption of ascorbic acid. Infants who are fed artificial formulas without vitamin supplements may develop symptoms of scurvy. In adults, scurvy would not occur for 3–5 months after all ascorbic acid consumption was stopped.

Several other uses of ascorbic acid are worthy of mention. For example, marginal ascorbic acid deficiencies have been reported in institutionalized elderly patients. Ascorbic acid supplementation in these patients may measurably improve their general health and well-being. It may also benefit smokers and women taking oral contraceptives, in whom lower than normal levels of ascorbic acid (and several other vitamins) have been noted. Ascorbic acid can also be used to increase iron absorption because it can form a soluble iron chelate and can inhibit the oxidation of ferrous to ferric iron.

Dose/RDA Pharmacists are rarely confronted with overt symptoms of ascorbic acid deficiency. Only 10 mg per day of ascorbic acid prevents scurvy; a normal diet containing fresh fruits and vegetables contains many times this amount. The RDA of ascorbic acid for most adults is 60 mg per day. The apparent average daily intake of vitamin C in the United States is about 77 mg for women and 109 mg for men, although losses during cooking may decrease the actual amount ingested. About 200 mg per day will saturate the body; most of a dose above this level will be excreted. Most multivitamin supplements contain 60–100 mg of ascorbic acid, an appropriate level to consume if supplements are required. Doses of more than 200 mg are rarely indicated. In patients with a severe vitamin C deficiency, as evidenced by clinical signs of deficiency, 300 mg of ascorbic acid per day is recommended to replenish body stores. Infants who do not have ascorbic acid supplements in their formula should receive 35–50 mg per day; those who are breast-fed by well-nourished mothers will receive a sufficient amount. The Food and Nutrition Board recommends that smokers ingest at least 100 mg of supplemental vitamin C per day to compensate for increased ascorbic acid metabolism and lower levels of ascorbic acid in the body. If a supplement is warranted, a multivitamin product containing 60–100 mg of ascorbic acid may be recommended.

Ascorbic acid tablets should be stored in a sealed container and kept away from heat and moisture to maintain potency. Ascorbic acid and its various salt forms are available in 25- to 500-mg regular and chewable tablets, 500- to 1,500-mg timed-release capsules and tablets, 60-mg lozenges, crystal (4 g/tsp), powder (4 g/tsp), solution (100 mg/mL), and syrup (500 mg/5 mL) dosage forms, as well as in numerous combination products.

Adverse Effects/Drug Interactions The pharmacist is urged to weigh the relative risks and benefits of ascorbic acid therapy. The incidence of toxicity with ascorbic acid is low. Short-term use to promote healing, for example, or for serious disorders such as rectal polyps may warrant a trial of ascorbic acid with medical supervision. Megadoses, however, may be harmful in certain circumstances, and the expense and potential risks of long-term ingestion of large quantities of the vitamin may be questionable for a seemingly minor beneficial effect on the common cold, a self-limiting condition. Thus, the pharmacist must consider the risks when advising patients on supplements. Ascorbic acid toxicity may increase oxalate excretion, produce nephrolithiasis, and lead to hemolysis in patients deficient in glucose 6-phosphate dehydrogenase.

Urine glucose tests are affected by large quantities of ascorbic acid in the urine: the TesTape® and Clinistix® urine glucose tests may give false-negative readings, whereas Benedict's solutions and Clinitest® tablets may give false-positive readings. The pharmacist should instruct the patient on testing procedures to minimize the interaction between tape tests and ascorbic acid.

Crystalluria may result from the simultaneous administration of sulfonamides and ascorbic acid because sulfonamide solubility is decreased in the acidified urine. The clinical significance of the effects of ascorbic acid on the reabsorption and elimination of acidic and basic drugs is controversial because the ascorbic acid-induced decrease in urine pH has been shown to be small. Nevertheless, patients should be monitored if they are on acidic or basic medications eliminated by renal excretion and if they initiate megadose ascorbic acid therapy.

Ascorbic acid (0.5–2.0 g every 4 hours) has been used to acidify urine in patients taking methenamine compounds for urinary tract infections. The lower pH of the urine facilitates hydrolysis of methenamine to the antibacterial product, formaldehyde. When the urine is acidified, acidic drugs are reabsorbed more readily from the tubules, resulting in higher, more prolonged blood levels. On the other hand, basic drugs such as tricyclic antidepressants and amphetamines may be excreted more rapidly from acidified urine and their effect reduced by ascorbic acid therapy.

There have been isolated anecdotal reports of oxalate urinary tract stone formation, possible ascorbate-mediated destruction of dietary vitamin B_{12}, and rebound scurvy upon sudden withdrawal of ascorbic acid. This last effect was detected in infants whose mothers took megadoses of vitamin C during pregnancy. Ascorbic acid may increase the serum levels of estrogens and reduce the anticoagulant action of warfarin.

Cyanocobalamin (Vitamin B_{12})

Description Cyanocobalamin contains a single atom of cobalt and is the most complex vitamin molecule. It is available in the body as methylcobalamin, hydroxycobalamin, and adenosylcobalamin, all designated as "cobalamins." The term *vitamin B_{12}* refers to all cobalamins that have vitamin activity in humans. Cyanocobalamin, the common pharmaceutical form of the vitamin, is one of two commercially available forms and is the most stable; however, it is present in only small amounts in the body.

Vitamin B_{12} is active in all cells, especially those in the bone marrow, the central nervous system (CNS), and the GI tract. It is also involved in fat, protein, and carbohydrate metabolism. A cobalamin coenzyme functions in the synthesis of deoxyribonucleic acid (DNA) and in the synthesis and transfer of single-carbon units such as the methyl group in the synthesis of methionine and choline. Vitamin B_{12} participates in methylation reactions and cell division, usually in concert with folic acid. It is necessary for the metabolism of folates; therefore, a folate deficiency may be observed as a feature of vitamin B_{12} deficiency. Vitamin B_{12} is also necessary for the metabolism of lipids, the maintenance of sulfhydryl groups in the reduced state, and the formation of myelin.

Vitamin B_{12} is produced almost exclusively by microorganisms, which accounts for its presence in animal protein (meats, oysters, and clams). It may also be found in small amounts in the root nodules of legumes and in selected vegetables and fruits, again because of the presence of microorganisms.

Indications In healthy individuals who have not restricted their diets, cyanocobalamin levels are maintained by the body. Vitamin B_{12} deficiency may be caused by poor absorption or utilization, or by an increased requirement or excretion of this vitamin. Because vitamin B_{12} is conserved by the body, it generally requires approximately 3 years for the deficiency to develop. In patients with malabsorption (ileal diseases or resection), the reabsorption phase of the enterohepatic cycle is affected, and the deficiency may occur much earlier.

Some people lack the glycoprotein (intrinsic factor) necessary for the absorption of vitamin B_{12}, resulting in pernicious anemia. Because of the lack of vitamin B_{12} in vegetables, vegetarians who consume no animal products are at risk for developing a vitamin B_{12} deficiency, several cases of which have been reported in infants breast-fed by vegetarian mothers. Strict vegetarians should consider taking vitamin B_{12} supplements or adjust their diet to include fermented foods, such as soy sauce, that contain the vitamin.

The symptoms of a vitamin B_{12} deficiency mimic those of a folate deficiency and are manifested in organ systems with rapidly duplicating cells. Thus, one effect of such a deficiency on the hematopoietic system is macrocytic anemia. The GI tract is also affected, with glossitis and epithelial changes occurring along the entire digestive tract. Because vitamin B_{12} is necessary to the maintenance of myelin, deficiency states produce many neurologic symptoms, such as paresthesia (manifested as tingling and numbness in the hands and feet), unsteadiness, poor muscular coordination, mental confusion, agitation, optic atrophy, hallucinations, and overt psychosis.

The clinical manifestations of a cyanocobalamin deficiency include megaloblastic anemia, macrocytic anemia, atrophic gastritis, achlorhydria, glossitis, neurologic degeneration, and dementia.

The pharmacist should caution patients that an accurate diagnosis of the causes of a suspected anemia is essential in selecting effective treatment. For example, anemia due to a folic acid deficiency should be treated with folic acid, pernicious anemia should be treated with vitamin B_{12}, and iron deficiency anemia should be treated with iron. The use of "shotgun" antianemia preparations containing multiple hematinic factors should be discouraged.

Dose/RDA The RDA for vitamin B_{12} is 2 mcg for adults. Requirements increase to 2.2 mcg during pregnancy and to 2.6 mcg during lactation.

Past treatment of vitamin B_{12} deficiency involved crude liver extracts administered orally or parenterally. Crystalline vitamin B_{12} is now available. Cyanocobalamin is available for oral use as 25-, 50-, 100-, and 250-mcg tablets and as a 400-mcg/0.1-mL unit of nasal gel. Oral forms can be used if the deficiency is nutritionally based; intramuscular or subcutaneous administration is necessary for deficiencies due to malabsorption.

Hydroxycobalamin is a longer acting form equal in hematopoietic effect to cyanocobalamin. Because it is more extensively bound to proteins at the site of injection and to plasma proteins, renal excretion is slower and the vitamin remains in the body for a longer period.

Adverse Effects/Drug Interactions Excessive doses have not resulted in toxicity, nor has any benefit been reported from nondeficient patients taking large quantities of the vitamin.

Certain drugs such as neomycin may impair absorption of vitamin B_{12}. Absorption is further decreased if colchicine is a part of the therapy.

Folic Acid (Pteroylglutamic Acid, Folacin)

Description The term *folacin* is used as a generic term to designate folic acid, pteroylglutamic acid, and other similar-acting compounds. Current guidelines for terminology are that folate and folic acid are preferred synonyms for pteroylglutamate and pteroylglutamic acid. Because folates can be used in a generic sense referring to the above, the term *folacin* should not be used.

Folates are reduced in vivo to the bioactive form, tetrahydrofolic acid, through a complex process and are involved in the biosynthesis of purine, pyrimidine, serine, methionine, and choline. Folic acid is further biotransformed in the body and is involved in DNA synthesis and maturation and cell production activities. In its function in the body, folic acid is closely related to vitamin B_{12}. A folic acid deficiency can occur as a consequence of a vitamin B_{12} deficiency.

Folates are present in nearly all natural foods. Primary sources of folates in the diet include liver, lean beef, veal, yeast, leafy vegetables, legumes, some fruits, eggs, and whole-grain cereals. The diet should include some foods that require little cooking, however, because folates are heat labile and the folic acid content of food is subject to destruction depending on how the food is processed. Canning, long exposure to heat, and extensive refining may destroy 50–100% of the naturally occurring folic acid.

Indications Causes of folic acid deficiency include alcoholism, malabsorption, food faddism, pregnancy, and liver disease.

A deficiency of folic acid results in impaired cell division and protein synthesis. The requirements for folic acid are related to the metabolic rate and cell turnover. Thus, increased amounts of folic acid are needed during infancy, pregnancy, and lactation, as well as for infection, hemolytic anemias and blood loss (in which red blood cell production must be increased to replenish blood supply), and hypermetabolic states such as hyperthyroidism. Rheumatoid arthritis may also increase folic acid requirements.

Symptoms of folic acid deficiency are similar to those of vitamin B_{12} deficiency and include sore mouth, diarrhea, and CNS symptoms such as irritability and forgetfulness. The most common laboratory feature of folic acid deficiency is megaloblastic anemia.

Because vitamin B_{12} is essential for metabolism of folates, a megaloblastic anemia responsive to folic acid administration is a feature of pernicious anemia. Folic acid given without vitamin B_{12} to patients with pernicious anemia will correct the anemia but will have no effect on the more insidious damage to the CNS. Symptoms of CNS damage include lack of coordination, impaired sense of position, and various behavioral disturbances. Because of the potential for folic acid to mask the signs of pernicious anemia, which is caused by a vitamin B_{12} deficiency, products containing more than 0.8 mg of folic acid per dose are available only by prescription. Pharmacists should refer all patients with suspected anemias for medical consultation.

Dose/RDA The RDA for folic acid is 200 mcg for most adult men and 180 mcg for most adult women, increasing to 400 mcg during pregnancy.

The oral dose of folic acid for correction of a deficiency is usually 1 mg daily, particularly if the deficiency occurs with conditions that may increase the folate requirement or suppress red blood cell formation (e.g., pregnancy, hypermetabolic states, alcoholism, and hemolytic anemia). Doses larger than 1 mg daily are not necessary except in some life-threatening hematologic diseases. Maintenance therapy for deficiencies may be stopped after 1–4 months if the diet contains at least one fresh fruit or vegetable daily. For chronic malabsorption diseases, folic acid treatment may be lifelong and parenteral doses may be required.

Adverse Effects/Drug Interactions Folic acid toxicity is virtually nonexistent because of folic acid's water solubility and rapid excretion. Up to 15 mg have been given daily without toxic effect.

Several drugs taken chronically may increase the need for folic acid. Phenytoin and possibly other related anticonvulsants may inhibit folic acid absorption, leading to megaloblastic anemia. This problem is further complicated by the fact that folic acid supplementation may decrease serum phenytoin levels and complicate seizure control. The pharmacist should note when folic acid is prescribed to patients whose medication records indicate concurrent phenytoin therapy.

Trimethoprim may act as a weak folic acid antagonist in humans. Megaloblastic anemia may be precipitated in patients who possess a relatively low folic acid level at the onset of trimethoprim therapy; however, this problem is rarely seen in most patients using trimethoprim. Pyrimethamine, which is related to trimethoprim, may induce megaloblastic anemia in large doses. The mechanism of pyrimethamine's folic acid antagonism is inhibition of active tetrahydrofolate production. Methotrexate is also a folic acid antagonist.

Niacin (Nicotinic Acid)

Description The physiologically active form of niacin is nicotinamide. Niacin and niacinamide (nicotinic acid amide) are constituents of the coenzymes nicotinamide adenine dinucleotide and nicotinamide adenine dinucleotide phosphate. These coenzymes are electron transfer agents (i.e., they accept or donate hydrogen in the aerobic respiration of all body cells). Niacin is unusual as a vitamin in that humans can synthesize it from dietary tryptophan, with about 60 mg of tryptophan being equivalent to 1 mg of niacin. Most individuals receive about 50% of their niacin requirement from tryptophan-containing proteins and the rest as preformed niacin or niacinamide. In high doses, niacin will lower triglycerides and low-density lipoprotein cholesterol by mechanisms unrelated to its function as an essential micronutrient.

Niacin is present in most foods, including lean meats, fish, liver, cold cereals, whole grains, green vegetables, and legumes.

Indications Clinical findings of niacin deficiency include the three "Ds" of *d*ermatitis, *d*iarrhea, and *d*ementia, often accompanied by neuropathy, glossitis, stomatitis, and proctitis. The classical niacin deficiency state is pellagra. The pellagra syndrome involves dermatitis, diarrhea, dementia, and neurologic changes (e.g., mild tremor, depression, and peripheral neuropathy).

Pellagra is rare, occurring most often in alcoholics, poorly nourished elderly persons, and individuals on bizarre diets. It also occurs in areas where much corn is eaten; this is because the niacin in corn is bound to undigestible constituents, making it unavailable. The main body systems affected are the CNS, the skin, and the GI tract. Symptoms involving the CNS include peripheral neuropathy, myelopathy, and encephalopathy. Mania may occur. Seizures and coma precede death. Before the cause of CNS manifestations of niacin deficiency was discovered, many psychiatric admissions were due to the symptoms of niacin deficiency. Both niacin and niacinamide are effective in treating pellagra.

There is a characteristic rash in niacin-deficient patients. The skin over the face and on pressure points may become thickened or hyperpigmented, or may appear burned. Secondary infections may occur in such lesions. The entire GI tract is generally affected, with angular fissures around the mouth, atrophy of the epithelium, a beefy-red color of the tongue, and hypertrophy of the papillae. Inflammation of the small intestine may be associated with episodes of occult bleeding and/or diarrhea.

An individual's niacin status can be estimated by measuring the urinary levels of niacin metabolites. Low values together with symptoms point to a diagnosis of pellagra.

Dose/RDA The RDA of niacin is 19 mg for most adult men and 15 mg for most adult women. A niacin equivalent is 1 mg of niacin or 60 mg of dietary tryptophan.

Niacin requirements are increased during acute illness; during convalescence after a severe injury, infection, or burns; when either caloric expenditure or dietary caloric intake is substantially increased; or when the patient has a low tryptophan intake (e.g., a low-protein diet or a high intake of corn as a staple in the diet).

Treatment of pellagra involves the ingestion of 300–500 mg of niacinamide daily in divided doses. Because other nutritional deficiencies may be present, treatment may include the other B vitamins, vitamin A, and iron.

Niacin has been used in daily dosages of 1 to 2 g three times per day, up to 8 g per day, to treat hyperlipidemias and hypercholesterolemia. Niacin treatment increases beneficial high-density lipoprotein cholesterol and decreases levels of potentially harmful triglycerides, total cholesterol, and low-density lipoprotein cholesterol. In the Coronary Drug Project, niacin treatment correlated with a decrease in nonfatal recurrent myocardial infarct and, upon long-term follow-up, a decrease of 11% in mortality from all causes. This beneficial effect was evident 9 years after cessation of both the study and the niacin therapy. Niacin treatment of hyperlipidemias requires close medical supervision for evidence of effectiveness and manifestations of drug-induced toxicity.

Niacin and niacinamide are available as tablets and capsules in strengths ranging from 25 to 500 mg, both as regular and timed-release products. It is also available in elixir form (50 mg/5 mL) as well as in many combination products. Prenatal multivitamins may contain up to 20 mg of niacin.

Adverse Effects/Drug Interactions Niacin toxicity can involve GI symptoms (e.g., nausea, vomiting, and diarrhea), hepatotoxicity, skin lesions, tachycardia, hypertension, and flushing. High doses of niacin may cause significant and potentially serious adverse effects. Doses in excess of 1 g per day may result in flushing and burning sensations. Chronic high-dose usage may also lead to hyperkeratotic pigmented skin lesions.

Because of the adverse effects on the GI tract, high doses of niacin are contraindicated in patients with gastritis or peptic ulcer disease. Niacin can provoke the release of histamine, so its use in patients with asthma should be undertaken carefully. Niacin may also impair liver function, as evidenced by cholestatic jaundice, and it can disturb glucose tolerance and cause hyperuricemia. If niacin and niacinamide are used in high doses, laboratory parameters suggested by the potential side effects should be followed.

Patients should be forewarned that niacin may cause flushing and a sensation of warmth, especially around the face, neck, and ears. This reaction, which many people experience especially upon initiation of therapy, may be diminished if they take 325 mg of aspirin or 200 mg of ibuprofen 30 minutes before the niacin dose, provided there are no contraindications. Itching or tingling and headache may also occur. All these effects will usually subside or decrease in intensity with continued therapy. If niacin causes GI upset, it should be taken with meals.

Niacinamide does not produce the discomforting flushing associated with therapeutic doses of niacin; however, it also does not have a beneficial lowering effect on plasma lipids.

Pantothenic Acid

Description Pantothenic acid is a water-soluble vitamin of the B-complex family. Only the dextrorotatory isomer of pantothenic acid has biologic activity; however, pantothenic acid is a precursor of coenzyme A, a product that is active in many biologic reactions and that plays a primary role in cholesterol, steroid, and fatty acid synthesis. Pantothenic acid is important for acetylation reactions and the formation of citric acid for the Krebs cycle, and it is crucial in the intraneuronal synthesis of acetylcholine. It is also important in gluconeogenesis; the synthesis and degradation of fatty acids; the synthesis of sterols, steroid hormones, and porphyrins; the release of energy from carbohydrates; and acylation reactions. In addition, it has been used to eliminate burning feet syndrome.

Pantothenic acid is widely distributed in plant and animal tissues. Sources include meat, liver, milk, eggs, vegetables, cereal grains, and legumes.

Indications Because pantothenic acid is contained in many foods, deficiency states are rare and hard to detect. In malabsorption syndromes, it is difficult to separate pantothenic acid deficiency symptoms from symptoms of other deficiencies. Symptoms of pantothenic acid deficiency include somnolence, fatigue, headache, paresthesia of hands and/or feet followed by hyperreflexia and muscular weakness in the legs, cardiovascular instability, GI complaints, changes in disposition, and increased susceptibility to infections. Administration of pharmacologic doses of pantothenic acid reverses these symptoms.

Dose/RDA The Food and Nutrition Board does not list an RDA value for this vitamin but estimates a safe and adequate daily intake to be 4–7 mg for adults. Pantothenic acid is available as calcium pantothenate in 25-, 100-, 250-, and 500-mg tablets and in multivitamin products.

Adverse Effects/Drug Interactions Pantothenic acid is generally considered nontoxic, even in large doses. Doses as high as 10 g of calcium pantothenate daily have been given to young men for 6 weeks with no toxic symptoms. However, ingestion of more than 20 g has been reported to result in diarrhea and water retention. Dexpanthenol may prolong bleeding time in hemophiliacs and should be used with extreme caution.

Pyridoxine (Vitamin B_6)

Description Pyridoxine serves as a cofactor for more than 60 enzymes, including decarboxylases, synthetases, transaminases, and hydroxylases. It is important in heme production and in the conversion of oxalate to glycine.

This water-soluble vitamin exists in three forms: pyridoxine (vitamin B_6), pyridoxal, and pyridoxamine. Although all three forms are equally effective in nutrition, pyridoxine hydrochloride is the form most often used in vitamin formulations.

Foods rich in pyridoxine include meats, cereals, lentils, nuts, and some fruits and vegetables such as bananas, avocados, and potatoes. Cooking destroys some of the vitamin. The average U.S. diet provides slightly less than the RDA; certain restricted diets may result in low pyridoxine intake. Infant formulas are required to contain pyridoxine hydrochloride.

Indications Causes of pyridoxine deficiency include alcoholism, severe diarrheal syndromes, food faddism, drugs (isoniazid, hydralazine, penicillamine, and cycloserine), malabsorption syndromes, and genetic diseases (cystathioninuria and xanthinuric aciduria). Serious deficiency symptoms include convulsions, peripheral neuritis, and sideroblastic anemia.

The symptoms of severe pyridoxine deficiency in infants are convulsive disorders and irritability. Treatment with pyridoxine hydrochloride (2 mg daily for infants) generally brings the electroencephalogram back to normal and resolves clinical symptoms. Symptoms in adults whose diets are deficient in pyridoxine or who have been given a pyridoxine antagonist are difficult to distinguish from symptoms of niacin and riboflavin deficiencies. These symptoms include pellagra-like dermatitis; scaliness around the nose, mouth, and eyes; oral lesions; peripheral neuropathy; and dulling of mentation.

Dose/RDA The RDA is 2 mg for most adult men and 1.6 mg for most adult women. This requirement should be increased to 2.2 mg during pregnancy and to 2.1 mg during lactation.

Treatment of sideroblastic anemia requires 50–200 mg per day of pyridoxine hydrochloride to aid in the production of hemoglobin and erythrocytes. At least five pyridoxine-dependent inborn errors of metabolism have been shown to respond to large doses of pyridoxine. Pyridoxine (100 mg taken three times daily) for at least 11 weeks has been reported to relieve paresthesia and pain in the hands of patients with carpal tunnel syndrome, but the value of such therapy has not been clearly and objectively determined. Pyridoxine is available as 25-, 50-, and 100-mg tablets, in 100-mg timed-release tablets, and in combination products.

Adverse Effects/Drug Interactions Pyridoxine is toxic in high doses. A severe sensory neuropathy, similar to that observed with the deficiency state, has been reported when gram quantities were taken to relieve symptoms of premenstrual syndrome (PMS). Similar symptoms have been reported in women taking doses as small as 50 mg a day for PMS. Recovery occurred upon withdrawal of pyridoxine but was slow.

High daily doses of pyridoxine (200–600 mg) have been shown to inhibit prolactin. Prenatal vitamins contain 1–10 mg per dosage unit and do not appear to have a significant antiprolactin effect. Large doses of pyridoxine may also increase the activity of plasma aminotransferase, but the consequences of this effect are unknown.

Several drugs interact with pyridoxine use, and pyridoxine affects the action of several drugs. Isoniazid and cycloserine (antitubercular drugs) antagonize pyridoxine; hydralazine appears to have this effect as well. Perioral numbness resulting from peripheral neuropathy is a clinical manifestation of this antagonism. Psychotic behavior and seizures, both produced by cycloserine, may be prevented with increased pyridoxine intake. To overcome the antagonism, 50 mg per day of pyridoxine hydrochloride with isoniazid and as much as 20 mg per day with cycloserine should be used routinely. Another recommended dosage is 10 mg of pyridoxine per 100 mg of isoniazid. Penicillamine may bind with pyridoxine hydrochloride, causing pyridoxine-responsive neurotoxicity. Pyridoxine may reduce the clinical effects of phenobarbital and phenytoin by reducing their serum levels.

Pyridoxine is intimately involved in amino acid metabolism, particularly that of tryptophan. Low pyridoxine levels result in the appearance of excess xanthurenic acid, a tryptophan metabolite, in the urine. In fact, pyridoxine status is assessed by quantitation of urinary xanthurenic acid following administration of a loading dose of tryptophan. Estrogens seem to increase xanthurenic acid production significantly, and women taking oral contraceptives may show laboratory signs of pyridoxine deficiency. Supplementation with pyridoxine (2–40 mg) returns the tryptophan metabolic pattern to normal. The pathologic consequences of these events are not known; however, a depressive syndrome occasionally experienced by women on oral contraceptives has responded to daily pyridoxine supplementation of 20–100 mg. Levels of other vitamins are marginally lower in some oral contraceptive users. Women who take oral contraceptives should consider improving their diet. For some, a multivitamin supplement may be indicated.

Pyridoxine hydrochloride antagonizes the therapeutic action of levodopa because it facilitates the transformation of levodopa to dopamine before the former can cross into the CNS. The pharmacist should inform patients taking levodopa of the interaction and should advise them to avoid supplemental pyridoxine hydrochloride. On the other hand, pyridoxine hydrochloride may be useful in treating patients who have overdosed on levodopa. A multivitamin product (Larobec®) does not contain pyridoxine hydrochloride and has been formulated for parkinsonian patients taking levodopa. Sinemet®, the combination product containing levodopa and carbidopa, a peripherally acting dopa decarboxylase inhibitor, does not appear to be affected by the concurrent administration of pyridoxine hydrochloride.

Riboflavin (Vitamin B_2)

Description Riboflavin occurs in the free state in foods or in combination with phosphates or with both phosphates and proteins. The free riboflavin is released and absorbed during digestion.

Riboflavin, a constituent of two coenzymes, flavin adenine dinucleotide and flavin mononucleotide, is involved in numerous oxidation and reduction reactions, including the cytochrome P-450 reductase enzyme system involved in drug metabolism. Cellular growth cannot occur without riboflavin.

Primary sources of riboflavin include meats; poultry; fish; dairy products; enriched and fortified grains, cereals, and bakery products; and green vegetables such as broccoli, turnip greens, asparagus, and spinach.

Indications Riboflavin deficiency, in a pure, uncomplicated form, is probably not encountered alone in patients but rather is accompanied by other nutrient deficiencies. Early signs of riboflavin deficiency may involve ocular symptoms as the eyes become light sensitive and easily fatigued. Also, blurred vision, itching, watering, sore eyes, and increased capillarization may develop in the cornea with a bloodshot appearance of the eye. Later clinical findings of deficiency include stomatitis, glossitis, seborrheic dermatitis, and magenta tongue.

Dose/RDA The RDA for riboflavin is 1.7 mg for most adult men and 1.3 mg for most adult women. The need for riboflavin appears to increase during periods of increased cell growth, such as during pregnancy and wound healing.

Riboflavin is poorly soluble. If oral absorption is poor, 25 mg of the soluble riboflavin salt may be injected intramuscularly. Riboflavin may also be given intravenously as a component of an injectable multivitamin, but the dose is relatively low (about 10 mg). Riboflavin is available as 25-, 50-, and 100-mg tablets and in various combination products in various strengths.

Adverse Effects/Drug Interactions Surveys have revealed lower than anticipated riboflavin levels in women taking oral contraceptives; however, the pathologic consequences are unknown. Marginal riboflavin deficiencies have also been detected in vegetarians, alcoholics, and some inner-city youths. Riboflavin deficiency usually accompanies other vitamin deficiencies attributable to an inadequate diet. The use of riboflavin may cause a yellow-orange fluorescence or discoloration of the urine. Patients should be reassured if they report this adverse effect.

Thiamine (Vitamin B_1)

Description Thiamine is a water-soluble vitamin. Its active form, thiamine pyrophosphate (formerly known as cocarboxylase), plays a vital role in the oxidative decarboxylation of pyruvic acid; in the formation of acetyl coenzyme A (CoA), which enters the Krebs cycle; and in other important biochemical conversion cycles.

Thiamine hydrochloride is necessary for several critical functions in carbohydrate metabolism, and the amount of vitamin that is required increases with increased caloric consumption. Additionally, thiamine is essential in neurologic function.

The most familiar natural thiamine source is the hull of rice grains. Other sources are pork, beef, fresh peas, and beans.

Indications Several genetic diseases respond to the administration of thiamine. These fall into the category of vitamin-responsible inborn errors of metabolism and generally are attributable to a defect in the binding of enzyme and cofactor. Large daily doses of vitamins (5–100 mg in the case of thiamine) saturate the enzyme system(s) and usually obviate the pathology. Examples of thiamine-responsive inborn metabolic errors are lactic acidosis due to defective pyruvate carboxylase, branched-chain aminoacidopathy due to defective branched-chain amino acid decarboxylase, and some cases of the Wernicke–Korsakoff syndrome due to defective transketolase. These disorders justify rational use of megadose thiamine therapy.

The primary causes of thiamine deficiency are generally related to inadequate diet, alcoholism, malabsorption syndromes, prolonged diarrhea, increased use (pregnancy), or food faddism.

Thiamine deficiency in the United States is found primarily in alcoholics, in patients with chronic diarrhea, and in patients maintained on a high carbohydrate diet. In fact, among alcoholics, thiamine deficiency is common. Not only is the alcoholic's diet often nutritionally deficient and imbalanced, but alcohol ingestion further impairs thiamine absorption and transport across the intestine and increases the rate of destruction of thiamine diphosphate.

The neurologic signs of thiamine deficiency (Wernicke's encephalopathy) are particularly evident. Nystagmus occurs when the patient is asked to gaze up and down along a vertical plane or from side to side along a horizontal plane. Damage to the cerebral cortex may occur in patients who survive severe thiamine deficiency, and the deficiency may lead to Korsakoff's psychosis. The symptoms of the psychosis are impaired retentive memory and cognitive function; the patient commonly confabulates when given a piece of information or when asked a question. Irreversible neurologic damage and death may ensue if severe thiamine deficiency is left untreated. High-dose, parenteral thiamine is commonly given to patients who are admitted to hospitals for alcohol detoxification and treatment. A vitamin supplement containing thiamine is often prescribed for the alcoholic patient. Fortification of alcoholic beverages with thiamine has been suggested as a means of preventing this disorder.

A diet consisting chiefly of unenriched white rice and white flour, or situations in which low dietary levels of thiamine are accompanied by the consumption of large amounts of raw fish with thiaminase containing intestinal microbes, may also produce a thiamine deficiency. Individuals subsisting on a diet of 0.2 to 0.3 mg of thiamine per 1,000 calories (slightly less than the thiamine requirement) may gradually become depleted of thiamine and develop peripheral neuropathy. If the patient has been subsisting on substantially less than 0.2 mg of thiamine per 1,000 calories, deficiency will be more severe.

Symptoms of thiamine deficiency may become evident in 3 weeks after thiamine intake is stopped. The deficiency causes cardiac dysfunction, possibly accompanied by edema; tachycardia on only minimal exertion; enlarged heart; and electrocardiographic abnormalities. The patient may have pain in the precordial or epigastric areas. Neuromuscular symptoms include paresthesia of the extremities, weakness, and atrophy.

If severe and prolonged, thiamine deficiency may result in either dry beriberi (evidenced by polyneuropathy, muscle weakness, symmetrical paresthesia, wrist-foot drop, and encephalopathic stages—i.e., Korsakoff's and Wernicke's syndromes) or wet beriberi (evidenced by the more common high-output cardiac failure, lactic acidosis–vasodilation, and/or the less common low-output cardiac failure). Beriberi literally means "I cannot," stemming from the fact that people affected have difficulty walking. Beriberi may develop in infants whose mothers are on a polished rice diet in regions where thiamine hydrochloride supplements are not used. The symptoms of infantile beriberi are also neurologic. Aphonia, or silent crying, may occur, and the signs of meningitis may be mimicked. Death will ensue if thiamine treatment is not initiated. Today, beriberi caused by nutritional deficiency rarely occurs in the Western world.

Dose/RDA The RDA for most adult men and women is 1.5 and 1.1 mg, respectively.

The treatment of beriberi is 25 mg of thiamine two or three times daily for 5 days, followed by a daily dose of 5 mg taken orally. For severe malabsorption, 5 mg daily is given parenterally.

The dosage of thiamine for treating the symptoms of heart failure caused by this deficiency is 5–10 mg taken three times a day. At this dosage, the heart failure is rapidly corrected but the neurologic signs correct much more slowly. The daily dosage of thiamine for neurologic deficits is 30–100 mg given parenterally for several days or until an oral diet can be started. Thiamine is available as 50-, 100-, 250-, and 500-mg tablets and is included in several strengths in combination products. If it is mixed in a solution, the solution should be acidic because thiamine is labile at an alkaline pH.

Adverse Effects/Drug Interactions The kidney easily clears excessive thiamine intake, and oral doses of 500 mg have been found to be nontoxic. There may be some toxicity from large doses given parenterally, however, with symptoms of itching, tingling, and pain. In rare instances, anaphylactic reactions are possible.

Vitamin-Like Compounds and Pseudovitamins

Bioflavonoids (Vitamin P)

The term *bioflavonoids* has been used to designate flavones and flavonols. The early extract apparently contained several flavonoids, chemically related substances derived from phenol. Because this work was not confirmed, it was recommended that the term *vitamin* be discontinued in this context and the word *bioflavonoids* be used to designate flavonoids with biologic activity.

These flavonoids are widely distributed in plants and are concentrated in the skin, peel, and outer layers of fruits and vegetables. As there is no known bioflavonoid deficiency condition, bioflavonoids have no accepted preventive or therapeutic role in human nutrition.

The average daily dietary intake of flavonoids is approximately 1,000 mg. Consequently, dietary supplementation using 20- to 30-mg tablets would not be significant.

Bioflavonoids are available as capsules and tablets and in combination products (both regular and sustained release) as tablets, capsules, and wafers.

Biotin (Vitamin H)

Description Biotin, a member of the B-complex group of vitamins, is required for various metabolic functions such as gluconeogenesis, lipogenesis, fatty acid biosynthesis, propionate metabolism, and the catabolism of branched-chain amino acids. There are now nine known biotin-dependent enzymes, including six carboxylases, two decarboxylases, and a transcarboxylase; four carboxylases occur in human tissues and include those for acetyl-CoA, propionyl-CoA, beta-methylglutaconyl-CoA, and pyruvate. Biotin plays an important role in fat, amino acid, and carbohydrate metabolism.

Biotin is widely distributed in animal tissue and is thus present in the diet. Sources include liver, egg yolk, cauliflower, salmon, carrots, bananas, soy flour, and yeast. Colonic flora probably contribute to the amount of biotin in the body.

Indications Deficiency states of biotin are rare but have been associated with nausea, vomiting, lassitude, muscle pain, anorexia, and depression. Dermatitis and glossitis may also be among the physical findings, and hypercholesterolemia and cardiac abnormalities may occur.

Biotin deficiency in humans can be caused by the ingestion of a large number of raw egg whites. Raw egg white contains avidin, a protein that binds biotin, preventing its absorption. Avidin causes a dermatitis, a grayish color of the skin, anorexia, anemia, hypercholesterolemia, and lassitude. Biotin deficiency symptoms have also been noted in patients on parenteral nutrition without biotin supplements. In pregnant women, blood biotin levels decrease as gestation progresses.

Individuals undergoing a rapid weight loss program with intense caloric restriction or those with malnutrition may not be obtaining adequate biotin and should receive supplementation.

Dose/RDA Although biotin is known to be necessary for carboxylation reactions in the body, the nutritional requirements for this vitamin are imprecise and no RDA has been determined for it. However, 100–200 mcg per day is generally considered safe and adequate. Biotin has been included in several multivitamin preparations.

Adverse Effects/Drug Interactions Side effects and drug interactions have not been reported with biotin therapy.

L-Carnitine (DL-Carnitine)

Description Carnitine, a vitamin-like molecule, can be synthesized from lysine and methionine in the liver and kidney; thus, it is considered an essential nutrient but not necessarily a vitamin. A number of actions are attributed to carnitine, including oxidation of fatty acids, promotion of certain organic acid excretions, and enhancement of the rate of oxidative phosphorylation.

L-Carnitine is required to transport long-chain fatty acids in mitochondria, which is prerequisite to their beta oxidation and to maintenance of energy production. Although carnitine is biosynthesized adequately by adults, newborns have a low capacity for carnitine synthesis from lysine and methionine and may be further compromised if fed soy formulas or maintained on total parenteral nutrition with no supplemental carnitine.

Dietary sources and synthesis in the liver and kidney satisfy the primary need for carnitine. Food sources include dairy products and meat, especially red meat.

Indications Carnitine deficiency may be evidenced by muscle weakness, cardiomyopathy, abnormal hepatic function, decreased ketogenesis, and hypoglycemia during fasting. Lipids may accumulate between muscle fibers.

Dose/RDA Human carnitine deficiency has been documented, but no RDA has been established. Therapy for carnitine deficiency should include a pharmaceutical supplement and a high-carbohydrate, low-fat diet. L-Carnitine is available as 250-mg capsules, 330-mg tablets, and a liquid containing 100 mg/mL, and it is present in several strengths in various combination products.

Adverse Effects/Drug Interactions L-Carnitine is without appreciable adverse effects in normal adults, and doses of 15 g per day have been well tolerated.

Choline

Description Choline is contained in most living cells and in foods. It is usually present in the form of phosphatidylcholine, commonly known as lecithin, and in several other phospholipids found in cell membranes. Intestinal mucosal cells and pancreatic secretions contain enzymes capable of splitting phospholipids to release choline. Choline is also found in sphingomyelin and is highly concentrated in nervous tissue.

Choline is a precursor in the biosynthesis of acetylcholine, and it is an important donator of methyl groups used in the biochemical formation of other substances in vivo. It can be biosynthesized in humans by the donation of methyl groups from methionine to ethanolamine. Additionally, choline and inositol are considered to be lipotropic agents (agents involved in the mobilization of lipids). They have been used to treat fatty liver and disturbed fat metabolism, but their efficacy has not been established.

Although choline is found in egg yolks, cereal, fish, and meat, it is also synthesized in the body; therefore, it is doubtful that choline is a vitamin. Choline is obtained from the diet as either choline or lecithin.

Indications A deficiency state has not been identified in humans, possibly because choline is readily available in the diet.

Dose/RDA An average diet will furnish 200–600 mg of choline daily. Choline is available as 250-, 300-, 500-, and 650-mg tablets; as a powder; and in combination products in various strengths.

Adverse Effects/Drug Interactions The administration of large doses of lecithin has been associated with sweating, GI distress, vomiting, and diarrhea. Most humans, however, tolerate up to 20 g per day and some tolerate as much as 30 g per day with no adverse effects.

Essential Fatty Acids (Vitamin F)

The essential fatty acids are involved in the proper development of various biomembranes; they are also important as precursors of prostaglandins, leukotrienes, and various hydroxy fatty acids. The polyunsaturated fatty acids regulate cell permeability to a significant degree because they are constituents of phospholipids. Linoleic acid, the 18-carbon fatty acid with two double bonds, cannot be synthesized in the body and must be present in the diet. It is rapidly converted to arachidonic acid, a functioning polyunsaturated fatty acid that is physiologically important.

Linolenic acid has some essential fatty acid properties, but its biochemical role is not well defined. It is not a substitute for linoleic acid.

Linoleic and linolenic acids are essential in human nutrition but do not meet the definition of a vitamin. They are considered macronutrients. The typical Western diet, with its heavy polyunsaturated fat and oil content, provides ample essential fatty acids.

Linoleic acid deficiency symptoms can include scaly skin, hair loss, and impaired wound healing. If the total dietary calories consist of 1 to 2% linoleic acid, biochemical and clinical evidence for deficiencies do not occur.

Inositol

Inositol is a hexitol found in large amounts in muscle and brain tissues. It is widely distributed in nature and is synthesized in the body. Inositol seems to be necessary for amino acid transport and for the movement of potassium and sodium, but its value in human nutrition has not been well documented. Like choline, it is considered a lipotropic agent of unproven therapeutic value.

Inositol is a sweet, water-soluble substance occurring in fruits, vegetables, whole grains, meats, and milk. Its significance in human nutrition has not been completely established, but its physiologic role partially resembles that of choline. Inositol is present in cells as a phosphatide, and inositol lipids appear to be involved in the calcium-mediated control of cell functions, in cell proliferation, and in the attachment of enzymes to the plasma membrane.

A normal dietary intake is approximately 1 g per day, derived primarily from plant sources. The human requirement has not been established. Inositol is available in 250-, 500-, and 650-mg tablets and in a powder.

Laetrile (Amygdalin, Vitamin B_{17})

Laetrile occurs naturally in almond, apricot, and peach pits and in apple seeds. It consists of 6% cyanide by weight; it is made up of two parts glucose, one part benzaldehyde, and one part cyanide. When spelled with a capital "L", it refers to a synthetic substance that was never marketed; when spelled with a small "l", it refers to amygdalin, the product marketed by laetrile promoters as a cancer cure, and is a synonym for cyanogenetic glycosides. Many toxic reactions have been reported worldwide with the ingestion of cyanogenetic glycosides; cyanide poisoning has occurred with some laetrile products.

Although it is called vitamin B_{17}, laetrile contains no vitamin activity and has no nutritional or therapeutic value and no approved medical use. Moreover, no physiologic or biochemical abnormalities develop when the diet is deficient in laetrile. Thus, the term *vitamin B_{17}* is erroneous, misleading, and fraudulent, and it should not be used. Use by desperate and uninformed individuals may lead to critical delays in seeking and receiving appropriate medical attention.

Pangamic Acid (Vitamin B_{15})

Pangamic acid is an uncharacterized extract of the Prunus family. The unsupported claim has been that the extract was a preparation for the immunization of toxic products present in the human or animal system to produce symptomatic relief and immunity to persons afflicted with asthma, eczema, arthritis, neuritis, painful nerve and joint affections, and numerous other conditions. Pangamic acid is described as a poorly defined mixture of dimethylglycine and sorbitol. No studies have shown it to have any efficacy in treating any medical disorder, and its safety is questionable. Pangamic acid has been categorized as a pseudovitamin, and it has no nutritional or therapeutic value.

Taurine (Aminoethanesulfonate)

Along with carnitine, choline, and inositol, taurine has been referred to as a vitamin-like compound. It is now considered important enough to be included in human infant formulas and some parenteral nutritional solutions.

A unique chemical aspect of taurine is that it contains a sulfonic acid group that replaces the carboxyl group of what would otherwise be glycine. It is not incorporated into peptides, but it does participate in a few biochemical reactions. Taurine is present in most cells and exhibits a wide range of activity. Some of the physiologic functions that are affected by taurine include retinal photoreceptor activity, bile acid conjugation, white blood cell antioxidant activity, CNS neuromodulation, platelet aggregation, cardiac contractility, sperm motility, growth, and insulin activity.

Taurine is important in many metabolic activities and is normally biosynthesized in adequate amounts. Plasma taurine levels normally range from 50 to 220 mcmol/L, and any excess is excreted in the urine.

Even though it is not known whether taurine is essential for humans, some concern has been expressed about the risk of taurine insufficiency in formula-fed infants—especially if born prematurely—as compared with breast-fed infants. Cow's milk contains lower levels of taurine than does human milk. No RDA is established at this time.

Minerals

Minerals constitute about 4% of body weight. The major mineral content of the skeleton consists of calcium and phosphorus in a ratio of approximately 2:1. Any change of one may be reflected in changes of the other.

Minerals are present in the body in a diverse array of organic compounds such as phosphoproteins, phospholipids, hemoglobin, and thyroxine; in inorganic compounds such as sodium chloride, potassium chloride, calcium, and phosphate; and as free ions. Different body tissues contain different quantities of different elements. For example, bone has a high content of calcium, phosphorus, and magnesium; soft tissue has a higher quantity of potassium. Minerals function as constituents of enzymes, hormones, and vitamins. They are involved in regulating cell membrane permeability, osmotic pressure, and acid–base and water balance.

A well-balanced diet is required to maintain proper mineral balance. Calcium and iron are two elements that may require particular dietary attention from normal individuals. Optimal mineral intake values for humans are still imprecise, and only estimated ranges are available for minerals such as chromium, fluoride, copper, manganese, and molybdenum. These ranges are based on the mineral content of the average diet. Similarly, the possible adverse effects of long-term ingestion of high-dose mineral supplements are unknown, and high doses of one mineral can decrease the bioavailability of other minerals and even of vitamins.

Unlike vitamins, minerals exist in plants in varying amounts, according to the composition of the soil in which the plant is grown. This, in turn, affects the mineral content of local livestock. Mineral intake varies considerably from region to region, although the use of foods delivered from diverse geographic locations tends to minimize intake variations. Marginal deficiencies of minerals have been reported only in certain segments of the population, but the increasing use of highly refined foods, which are low in minerals, may contribute to these deficiencies.

Mineral deficiency is often difficult to evaluate. Hair analysis has received attention in recent years, and its noninvasiveness is advantageous. However, a number of factors such as distance from the scalp where the sample was obtained, color of the hair, and the use of shampoos, sprays, and conditioners, can adversely influence the accuracy of results. The analysis for zinc and toxic minerals such as arsenic, mercury, and lead has provided interesting results, but accepted normal values have not been established in routine nutritional assessment.

Calcium

Description

The most abundant cation in the body is calcium (about 1,200 g); about 99% of calcium is present in the skeleton and the remaining 1% is present in the extracellular fluid, intracellular structures, and cell membranes. Calcium is a major component of bones and teeth. The calcium content in bone is continuously undergoing a process of resorption and formation. In elderly people, the resorption process predominates over formation, and a decrease in calcium absorption efficiency results in a gradual loss of bone (osteoporosis). This effect can be minimized by ensuring an optimal calcium intake during the formative years to develop optimal bone mass.

Calcium is important because it activates a number of enzymes (e.g., pancreatic lipase, adenosine triphosphatase, and some proteolytic enzymes), is required for acetylcholine synthesis, increases cell membrane permeability, aids in Vitamin B_{12} absorption, regulates muscle contraction and relaxation, and catalyzes several blood-clotting steps. It is also necessary for the functional integrity of many cells, especially those of the neuromuscular and cardiovascular system.

The average blood level of calcium in the body is about 9.0–10.5 mg/dL. There are three forms of calcium in the blood and body fluids; these forms include ionized calcium, calcium complexes with organic acids, and protein-bound calcium.

The small intestine controls calcium absorption. Patients ingesting relatively low amounts of calcium absorb proportionately more, and some patients taking large amounts of calcium excrete more as fecal calcium. Calcium requirements may increase as the consumption of protein increases.

Rich dietary sources of calcium include milk and other dairy products. Teenagers experiencing rapid growth and bone maturation need to consume adequate calcium via dairy products, especially milk, or nutritional supplements in tablet or capsule form. Adults can easily meet calcium RDA levels by incorporating dairy products (especially low-fat and nonfat milk) into their diets. Nonfat milk contains about 300 mg of calcium per 8 oz. As an alternative, calcium supplements are essentially free of adverse effects in daily doses of less than 2 g of calcium.

Dietary factors that increase calcium absorption include certain amino acids such as lysine and arginine, vitamin D, and lactose. Dietary factors that decrease the efficiency of calcium absorption include foods with high phosphate content (e.g., unpolished rice, hexaphosphoinositol in bran, and wheat meal) and foods high in oxalate content (e.g., cocoa, soybeans, kale, and spinach). Vitamin D deficiency may also reduce the absorption and use of calcium.

Indications

Decreased calcium levels may have profound and diverse consequences, including convulsions, tetany, behavioral and personality disorders, mental and growth retardation, and bone deformities, the most common being rickets in children and osteomalacia in adults. Common causes of hypocalcemia and associated skeletal disorders are malabsorption syndromes; hypoparathyroidism; vitamin D deficiency; renal failure with impaired activation of vitamin D; long-term anticonvulsant therapy (with increased breakdown of vitamin D); and decreased dietary intake of calcium, particularly during periods of growth, pregnancy, and lactation and in elderly individuals.

Low serum calcium levels or lowered parathyroid function can result in tetany, characterized by uncontrolled muscle contractions and increased excitability of nerves, and may lead to osteomalacia. Changes that occur in osteomalacia include softening of bones, rheumatic-type pain in the bones of the legs and lower back, general weakness with difficulty walking, and spontaneous fractures.

Dose/RDA

To maximize bone mass before the inevitable decline that occurs after menopause, the RDA values have been set at 1,200 mg per day for both women and men aged 11–24. The RDA for adults over 24 years of age is 800 mg per day. Some suggest that, for women, about 1,100 mg daily before menopause and 1,500 mg daily after menopause is advantageous; during pregnancy and lactation, 1,200 mg daily is recommended. Exercise is also very important in maintaining bone mass, and any program to decrease the risk for osteoporosis should include regular exercise.

Calcium is available in many salt forms and strengths as tablets (regular, chewable, and effervescent), capsules, powders, and liquids, as well as in combination products. The calcium salts available without a prescription are the carbonate, citrate, lactate, gluconate, and phosphate salts, which vary in the amount of calcium contained per gram from 9% for the gluconate to 40% for the carbonate. Calcium carbonate and calcium phosphate salts are insoluble and should be taken with meals to enhance absorption, which depends on a low pH in the stomach. Patients requiring supplementation who have low levels of gastric hydrochloric acid (achlorhydria) or are on histamine II (H_2) antagonists or omeprazole should probably take a soluble salt (e.g., calcium citrate, calcium lactate, or calcium gluconate). Bone meal (mostly a calcium phosphate matrix) and oyster shell products (calcium carbonate matrix) are insoluble and require an acid pH for absorption. Some products do not disintegrate as well as others, which further limits the amount of calcium available for absorption.

Adverse Effects/Drug Interactions

Calcium in doses greater than 2 g per day can be harmful. Large amounts taken as dietary supplements or antacids can lead to high levels of calcium in the urine and to renal stones; the latter development may result in renal damage. Hypercalcemia, with associated anorexia, nausea, vomiting, constipation, and polyuria, is also possible, particularly in patients taking high-dose vitamin D preparations. Hypercalcemia can also result in increased deposition of calcium in soft tissue and can also occur in individuals who ingest excessive vitamin D independent of calcium supplements.

High calcium intake levels may inhibit the absorption of iron, zinc, and other essential minerals. Corticosteriods inhibit calcium absorption from the gut, and their use has been associated with increased bone fractures and osteoporosis. The excessive ingestion of aluminum-containing antacids has been shown to result in negative calcium balances. Several other drugs, including phosphates, calcitonin, sodium sulfate, furosemide, magnesium, cholestyramine, estrogen, and some anticonvulsants, also lower calcium serum levels. Thiazide diuretics, on the other hand, increase serum calcium levels.

Magnesium

Description

Magnesium, which is essential for all living cells, is the second most plentiful cation of the intracellular fluids and the fourth most abundant cation in the body. About 2,000 mEq of magnesium are present in an average 70-kg adult, with about 50% of this in bone, about 45% as an intracellular cation, and 1–5% in the extracellular fluid. Magnesium is required for normal bone structure formation and the proper functioning of more than 300 enzymes, including those involved with adenosine triphosphatase–dependent phosphorylation, protein synthesis, and carbohydrate metabolism. Extracellular magnesium is critical to both the maintenance of nerve and muscle electrical potentials and the transmission of impulses across neuromuscular junctions.

Magnesium tends to mimic calcium in its effects on the CNS and skeletal muscle. Magnesium deficiency blunts the normal response of the parathyroid glands to hypocalcemia. Thus, tetany due to a lack of calcium cannot be corrected with calcium unless the magnesium deficiency is also corrected.

Individuals consuming natural diets should not develop magnesium deficiency because all unprocessed foods contain magnesium, albeit in widely varying amounts. Vegetables are a good source of magnesium; whole seeds such as nuts, legumes, and unmilled grains contain the highest concentrations. Processing, which leads to removal of the germ and outer layers of cereal grains, results in a loss of more than 80% of the magnesium.

Indications

Deficiency states are usually due to GI tract abnormalities, renal dysfunction, general malnutrition, alcoholism, and iatrogenic causes.

Magnesium deficiency causes apathy, depression, increased CNS stimulation, delirium, and convulsions. Magnesium deficiencies are rarely noted in the normal adult population because magnesium is present in most foods. Deficiencies have been observed, however, in individuals with alcoholism, diabetes, chronic diarrhea, and renal tubular damage and in patients receiving long-term intravenous feedings without magnesium supplementation.

Hypomagnesemia may result from diarrhea and steatorrhea, chronic alcoholism, prolonged total parenteral nutrition therapy with magnesium-free solutions, hemodialysis, diabetes mellitus, pancreatitis, diuretic-induced electrolyte imbalance, renal tubular damage, and primary aldosteronism. Hypomagnesemia may also be associated with hypokalemia and hypocalcemia. Symptoms of hypomagnesemia may include nausea, muscle weakness, irritability, behavioral changes, and myographic changes.

Hypermagnesemia is characterized by muscle weakness, CNS depression, hypotension, and confusion. Excess magnesium intake may also decrease bone decalcification. Because excess magnesium has a direct, depressive effect on skeletal muscle, magnesium sulfate may be used to block the seizures of eclampsia. However, hypermagnesemia can occur with overzealous use of magnesium sulfate (epsom salts) or magnesium hydroxide (milk of magnesia) as a laxative, or even with use of magnesium-containing antacids in patients with severe renal failure.

Dose/RDA

The RDA values of magnesium for men and women over 18 years of age are 350 and 280 mg daily, respectively. Magnesium is available in numerous strengths and salt forms as tablets, capsules, and liquids and in various combination products.

Adverse Effects/Drug Interactions

No evidence is available to suggest that oral intake of magnesium is harmful to individuals with normal renal function. Hypermagnesemia, if it should occur, may be accompanied by nausea, vomiting, hypotension, bradycardia, cutaneous vasodilatation, electrocardiographic changes, hyperreflexia, and CNS depression. Eventually, respiratory depression, coma, and cardiac arrest may occur.

Phosphorus

Description

Phosphorus is present throughout the body. Approximately 85% of the body's store is located in bone. About 1% of body weight, or one-fourth of the total mineral content in the body, is phosphorus. Plasma levels of inorganic phosphate range between 2.5 and 4.4 mg/dL.

Phosphorus is essential for many metabolic processes. As calcium phosphate, it serves as an integral structural component of the bone matrix and a functional component of phospholipids, carbohydrates, nucleoproteins, and high-energy nucleotides. Accordingly, plasma phosphate levels are under tight biologic control involving parathyroid hormone, calcitonin, and vitamin D. The DNA and ribonucleic acid (RNA) structures contain sugar–phosphate linkages. Cell membranes contain phospholipids, which regulate the transport of solutes into and out of the cell. Many metabolic processes depend on phosphorylation. The storage and controlled release of energy, the adenosine diphosphate–adenosine triphosphate system, involves phosphorus compounds.

And an important buffer system of the body consists of inorganic phosphates.

There is a reciprocal relationship between calcium and phosphorus. Both minerals are regulated partially by parathyroid hormone. Secretion of parathyroid hormone stimulates an increase in calcium levels through increased bone resorption, gut absorption, and reabsorption in renal tubules. Parathyroid hormone causes a decrease in resorption of phosphate by the kidney. Thus, when serum calcium is high, serum phosphate is generally low, and vice versa.

Phosphorus is present in nearly all foods, especially protein-rich foods and cereal grains. Milk, meat, poultry, and fish contain about half the dietary phosphorus in the U.S. diet. Other rich sources of phosphorus include seeds, nuts, and eggs.

Indications

Because nearly all foods contain phosphorus, deficiency states do not usually occur unless induced. For example, patients receiving aluminum hydroxide as an antacid for prolonged periods may exhibit weakness, anorexia, malaise, pain, and bone loss. This is because aluminum hydroxide binds phosphorus, making it unavailable for absorption because of the formation of insoluble and poorly absorbed complexes.

In patients with diabetic ketoacidosis, phosphorus deficiency may result from increased tissue catabolism, impaired glucose use and cellular phosphorus uptake, and increased renal excretion of phosphorus caused by metabolic acidosis. The opposite situation, hyperphosphatemia (along with hypocalcemia and hypermagnesemia), may occur with acute renal failure, as renal phosphorus elimination is decreased in the face of continued release of phosphorus from tissues.

Dose/RDA

The RDA for phosphorus is 800 mg for adults over the age of 24, 1,200 mg for those aged 11–24, 800 mg for children aged 1–10, and 1,200 mg for women during pregnancy and lactation. In addition to being used to alleviate the deficiency state, phosphates have been used to increase tissue calcium uptake in osteomalacia and to decrease serum calcium levels in hypercalcemia. Sodium and potassium phosphate salts are available without a prescription for those requiring supplements. Products available include different salt forms and strengths of phosphorus in tablet, capsule, powder, and liquid dose forms, as well as in numerous combination products.

Trace Elements

Trace elements, which are present in minute quantities in plant and animal tissue, are considered essential for numerous physiologic processes. "Ultratrace minerals" have been defined as those elements with an estimated dietary requirement of usually less than 1 mcg/g; these include arsenic (E), boron (E), bromine (NE), cadmium (NE), chromium (E), fluorine (NE), lead (NE), lithium (PE), molybdenum (E), nickel (E), selenium (E), silicon (E), tin (NE), and vanadium (PE). The designation "E" represents essential, "PE" means probably essential but further study is required, and "NE" means not essential because the evidence for essentiality is inadequate. Based on the amount of trace elements in the average diet, a range of intake values for those elements thought to be safe and adequate has been published by the Food and Nutrition Board (Table 2).

Chromium

Description

About 5 mg of chromium is present in the normal adult, and levels decline with age. Higher concentrations occur in the hair, spleen, kidney, and testes, and lesser concentrations are present in the heart, pancreas, lungs, and brain.

Chromium functions to maintain normal glucose use. Chromium is a component of glucose tolerance factor, a dietary organic chromium complex that appears to facilitate the glucose utilization that is apparently essential for the efficient use of insulin. Fatty acid stimulation and cholesterol synthesis are attributed to chromium as is the possible role of RNA in protein synthesis.

Significant amounts of chromium are present in liver, fish, whole grains, and milk. There is concern that the increasing consumption of refined foods may lead to a marginal chromium deficiency in the population.

Indications

Deficiency of trivalent chromium, the chemical form present in diets, is manifested by glucose intolerance, elevated circulating insulin, glycosuria, fasting hyperglycemia, elevated serum cholesterol and triglycerides, neuropathy, and encephalopathy. Impaired glucose tolerance may be a manifestation of chromium deficiency, especially in older persons and protein-calorie malnourished infants.

Low chromium concentrations have been associated with juvenile diabetes and coronary artery disease. However, evaluation of chromium-deficient patients is difficult because of problems associated with total chromium analysis.

Dose/RDA

Chromium intake in the United States is low (about 50 mcg per day) compared with that of other countries. The estimated safe and adequate dietary intake for adults has been set at 50–200 mcg per day. Chromium has a relatively high margin of safety. Chromium is available in 1-mg tablets.

Adverse Effects/Drug Interactions

The oral administration of trivalent chromium has not been reported to be toxic. However, the hexavalent forms of chromium can be toxic and carcinogenic. These forms, which are encountered through industrial exposure, may enter the body through inhalation or absorption through the skin.

Cobalt

Cobalt is an essential component of vitamin B_{12}, but ingested cyanocobalamin is metabolized in vivo to form the B_{12} coenzymes. No deficiency state is reported to exist in humans. No RDA exists for cobalt.

Large doses of cobalt may result in goiter, myxedema, and congestive heart failure. Cardiomyopathy has also been described. Cyanosis and coma may result from accidental ingestion by children.

Copper

Description
Copper ions exist in two states, the cuprous and the cupric (the potent oxidizing agent). Copper is similar to zinc in the complexes it forms with a number of the same chelating agents. Copper is found in virtually all tissues of the body, but concentrations are highest in the liver, brain, heart, and kidney.

Copper is essential for the proper structure and function of the CNS, and it plays a major role in iron metabolism. Ceruloplasmin, one of the copper metalloenzymes, is especially important in the conversion of absorbed ferrous iron to transported ferric iron. Other copper-containing enzymes are cytochrome oxidase, dopamine beta-hydroxylase, and superoxide dismutase.

Food sources for copper include organ meats (especially liver), shellfish, chocolate, whole-grain cereals, legumes, and nuts.

Indications
Deficiency of copper is uncommon in humans even though many individuals may have lower than recommended intake. Copper deficiencies have been observed in premature infants; in severely malnourished infants fed milk-based, low-copper diets; and in patients receiving parenteral nutrition with inadequate copper. Contemporary diets provide about 0.9 mg of copper per day for women and 1.2 mg per day for men, which is somewhat less than the estimated safe and adequate range of 1.5–3.0 mg.

One of the prominent features of copper deficiency is impaired iron absorption. This is most likely caused by the loss of activity of the copper metalloenzymes, ferroxidase and ceruloplasmin (a protein–copper complex), which results in hypochromic anemia. In copper-deficient animals, bone cortices are fragile and thin owing to the failure of collagen cross-linking. Spontaneous rupture of major vessels may also be observed in deficiency states.

Wilson's disease is an inborn error of metabolism resulting in failure to eliminate copper. The result is CNS, kidney, and liver damage. Acute symptoms of copper toxicity include nausea, vomiting, diarrhea, hemolysis, convulsions, and GI bleeding. Symptoms respond to treatment with penicillamine.

Dose/RDA
Adults can safely take 2 to 3 mg of copper per day; 0.7–2.5 mg per day is suggested for children. Copper is available in different salt forms.

Adverse Effects/Drug Interactions
Copper administered orally has an emetic action, with doses in excess of 250 mg of copper sulfate producing vomiting. Molybdenum, zinc, and cadmium are antagonistic to copper, and large amounts of ascorbic acid impair copper absorption. Oral contraceptives have been shown to increase serum copper at the expense of tissue levels.

Fluorine

Description
Available therapeutic forms of fluorine include sodium fluoride and acidulated phosphate fluoride, both of which are available for oral and topical administration; sodium monofluorophosphate; and stannous fluoride. Sodium fluoride contains about 45% fluoride ion, and stannous fluoride contains about 24% fluoride ion.

Fluoride occurs normally in bones and tooth enamel as a calcium salt. Intake of small amounts has been shown to markedly reduce tooth decay, presumably by making the enamel more resistant to the erosive action of acids produced by bacteria in the oral cavity. Fluoride has also been used in women with osteoporosis at a dose of 50 mg daily. However, this treatment may have adverse effects, so the patient must be carefully monitored.

Fluoride is present in soil and water, but the content varies widely from region to region. Most municipal water supplies are fluoridated to 1 ppm of fluoride, a level that has been shown to be safe and to reduce caries in children by about 50%.

Dose/RDA
The safe and adequate estimated range for children is 0.5–2.5 mg per day and for adults, 1.5–4.0 mg per day. Fluoride is a normal constituent of the diet, given that it occurs in soils, water supplies, plants, and animals. Fluoride supplements should be routinely administered to children who consume water that is low in fluoride ion. Sodium fluoride is available by prescription as oral tablets and solutions, topical solutions, and gels, as well as in combination products. Nonprescription products include topical rinses containing 0.01 to 0.02% fluoride, such as sodium fluoride.

Adverse Effects/Drug Interactions
Excess fluoride can be toxic. Acute toxicity should not result from the low levels present in drinking water but may result from the administration of excessive doses of fluoride supplements. It has been recommended that sodium fluoride tablets used as dietary supplements be dispensed in containers containing less than 264 mg of sodium fluoride (120 mg of fluoride ion). In unit-dose containers, the limit of 300 mg per package is acceptable.

Because acute toxicity affects the GI system and the CNS, it can be life-threatening. Symptoms include salivation, abdominal pain, nausea, vomiting, diarrhea, dehydration, thirst, urticaria, muscle weakness, tremors, and (rarely) seizures. Because of the calcium-binding effect of fluoride, symptoms of calcium deficiency, including tetany, may be seen. The patient may exhibit mental irritability. Eventually, respiratory and cardiac failure may occur. The dose that causes acute toxicity in adults is approximately 5 g. Death has occurred after ingestion of as little as 2 g, but much larger overdoses have been treated successfully. In children, as little as 0.5 g of sodium fluoride may be fatal. Treatment includes precipitation of the fluoride by using gastric lavage with 0.15% calcium hydroxide solution, administration of intravenous glucose and saline for hydration, and treatment with calcium to prevent tetany.

Chronic fluoride toxicity is manifest as changes in the structure of bones and teeth. Bones become more dense and may be afflicted with disabling disease. Tooth enamel acquires a mottled appearance consisting of white, patchy plaques occurring with pitting brown stains. Prolonged ingestion of water that contains more than 2 ppm of fluoride has resulted in a significant incidence of mottling. Extremely large doses (e.g., 20–80 mg daily) have resulted in chalky, brittle bones that tend to fracture easily, a condition known as skeletal fluorosis.

Iodine

Description
The thyroid gland contains about one-third of the iodine in the body, stored in the form of a complex glycoprotein, thyroglobulin. The only known function of thyroglobulin is to provide thyroxine and triiodothyronine. These hormones regulate the metabolic rate of cells and therefore influence physical and mental growth, nervous and muscle tissue function, circulatory activity, and the use of nutrients.

Iodine is required to synthesize thyroxine and triiodothyronine and is an essential micronutrient. Although in high concentrations iodine inhibits the release of these hormones, in its absence thyroid hypertrophy occurs, resulting in classic goiter. However, iodine is usually present as the iodide in food and water, and it is sometimes organically bound to amino acids. The consumption of foods from diverse sources and the addition of iodide to table salt have essentially eliminated goiter as a health problem in the United States.

The primary dietary source of iodine is iodized salt, which contains 1 part of sodium or potassium iodide per 10,000 parts (0.01%) of salt. A dose of about 95 mcg of iodine can be obtained from about one-fourth of a teaspoon of salt (1.25 g). In the United States, most of the table salt sold is iodized; however, that used in food processing and for institutional use is not. Additional dietary sources of iodine include saltwater fish and shellfish. Seacoast soils used for raising vegetables produce vegetables with higher iodide content because plants extract iodine from the soil.

Dose/RDA
The iodine content of typical diets in the United States has been slowly declining but is still well above the RDA value of 0.15 mg for adults. Iodine supplements are unwarranted for most individuals. Potassium iodide is available as a tablet and solution and is included in various combination products.

Adverse Effects/Drug Interactions
Symptoms of chronic iodide intoxication (iodism) include an unpleasant taste and burning in the mouth or throat along with soreness of the teeth or gums. Increased salivation, sneezing, irritation of the eyes, and swelling of the eyelids commonly occur. Some individuals are sensitive to iodide or to organic preparations containing iodine.

Iron

Description
Iron is widely available in the U.S. diet. Iron absorption from the intestinal tract is controlled by the body's need for iron, intestinal lumen conditions, and the food content of the meal. Although iron-deficient persons may absorb about 10–20% of dietary iron, persons with normal iron stores absorb about 5–10%.

Iron plays an important role in oxygen and electron transport. In the body, it is either functional or stored. Functional iron is found in hemoglobin, myoglobin, heme-containing enzymes, and transferrin, the transport form of iron. The hemoglobin of red blood cells represents the major body store of iron, containing 60–70% of total body iron. The rest is stored primarily in the form of ferritin and hemosiderin; storage sites are the intestinal mucosa, liver, spleen, and bone marrow.

Normally, adult men have iron stores of about 50 mg/kg of body weight; women have about 35 mg/kg of body weight. The normal hemoglobin level in adult men is about 14–17 g/100 mL of blood; in adult women it is 12–14 g/100 mL of blood.

Dietary iron is available in two forms. Heme iron is found in meats and is reasonably well absorbed. Nonheme iron constitutes most of the dietary iron and is poorly absorbed. Therefore, the published values of the iron content of foods are misleading because the amount absorbed depends on the nature of the iron. To gain an accurate assessment of the iron available in a meal, the composition of the meal must be considered in detail. About half of the iron in meats is heme iron, which is about 25% absorbed. The amount of absorbable nonheme iron contributed by vegetables and grains in the diet varies greatly.

The available iron content of foods is calculated by assuming that only 10% of the total iron (heme plus nonheme) is absorbable if no iron deficiency exists. In the iron-deficient state, iron absorption improves so that as much as 20% may be absorbed and used from an average diet. As Americans appear to be moving away from a "red meat" diet, it will be increasingly important to monitor the population for iron status.

Nonheme-ingested iron, which is mostly in the form of ferric hydroxide, is solubilized in gastric juice to ferric chloride, reduced to the ferrous form, and chelated to substances such as ascorbic acid, sugars, and amino acids. Chelates have a low molecular weight and can be solubilized and absorbed before they reach the alkaline medium of the distal small intestine, where precipitation may occur. In the plasma, iron is oxidized to the ferric state and bound to a beta globulin to form transferrin. When released at the spleen, liver, bone marrow, intestinal mucosa, and other iron storage sites, the iron is combined with apoferritin to form ferritin or hemosiderin. Iron is used in all cells of the body; however, most of it is incorporated into the hemoglobin of red blood cells. Iron is lost from the body by the sloughing of skin cells and GI mucosal cells; by hemorrhagic loss; by menstruation; and by excretion of urine, sweat, and feces.

Indications
Early symptoms of iron deficiency are vague. Easy fatigability, weakness, and lassitude cannot in themselves be easily related to iron deficiency. Other symptoms of anemia include pallor, split or "spoon-shaped" nails, sore tongue, angular stomatitis, dyspnea on exertion, palpitation, and a feeling of exhaustion. Coldness and numbness of extremities may also be reported. Small red blood cells and low

hemoglobin concentrations (microcytic, hypochromic anemia) characterize iron deficiency.

There are three general stages of iron deficiency:

- Iron depletion, in which iron stores are depleted and associated with plasma ferritin levels that are below 12 mcg/L;
- Iron-deficient erythropoiesis, in which red cell protoporphyrin levels are elevated, but the hemoglobin levels are within the 95% reference range;
- Iron deficiency anemia, in which the total blood hemoglobin levels are below normal levels.

Iron deficiency anemia is a widespread clinical problem and the most common form of anemia in the United States. Although it causes few deaths, it contributes to the poor health and suboptimal performance of many people. Furthermore, it is possible that less severe iron deficiencies (those resulting not in overt anemia but rather in more subtle clinical manifestations) may be quite common.

Iron deficiency results from inadequate diet, malabsorption, pregnancy and lactation, or blood loss. The four life periods during which iron deficiency is most common are:

- From 6 months to 4 years of age, because of the low iron content in cow's milk;
- During early adolescence, when rapid growth entails an expanding red cell mass and the need for iron in myoglobin;
- During the female reproductive years, owing to menstrual iron losses;
- During pregnancy, owing to the expanding blood volume of the mother, the demands of the fetus and placenta, and blood losses during childbirth.

Because normal excretion of iron through the urine, feces, and skin is small, iron deficiency caused by poor diet or malabsorption may develop very slowly and be manifested only after several years. The differential diagnosis in adults or postmenopausal women should rule out iron deficiency due to excess blood loss associated with hiatal hernia, peptic ulcer disease, esophageal varices, diverticulitis, intestinal parasites, regional enteritis, ulcerative colitis, and cancer. Pharmacists should be aware that anemia may indicate an illness more serious than iron deficiency.

Drug-induced blood loss may occur because of irritating effects on the gastric mucosa or an indirect effect on the GI tract. Drugs implicated include salicylates, nonsteroidal anti-inflammatory drugs (NSAIDs), reserpine, corticosteroids, and most drugs used to treat neoplasms.

Menstruation normally results in a loss of 60–80 mL of blood per month and of about 1.4 mg of iron in addition to that normally lost. The daily amount required for replacement is about 0.7–2.3 mg of absorbed iron. The average U.S. diet contains about 5–7 mg of iron per 1,000 calories, but only about 10% of iron in food is absorbed. If the menstrual blood loss exceeds 60–80 mL, supplemental iron may be desirable because the dietary requirement may be as high as 40 mg per day.

The donation of 500 mL (one pint or unit) of blood produces a loss of approximately 250 mg of iron. This is not a significant problem in healthy, well-nourished adults with adequate iron stores; however, some blood donors, especially those who donate frequently, may benefit from short-term iron replacement following blood donation.

Despite fortification of flour and educational efforts, iron deficiency remains a problem for certain segments of the population, especially inner-city children and menstruating and pregnant women. Iron supplements are routinely recommended as a component of prenatal care.

The pharmacist may ascertain the cause of the patient's condition by consulting the medication record. The patient may have been treated for ulcers or hemorrhoids, conditions that could cause blood loss. Chronic use of drugs such as NSAIDs, reserpine, corticosteroids, or warfarin might yield another reason for blood loss. Medications such as aspirin or ibuprofen may cause blood loss but may not be included on a medication record if they were bought without a prescription. Thus, the pharmacist should routinely question the patient regarding the use of nonprescription drugs.

A patient who reports blood loss should be referred to a physician immediately. Abnormal blood loss may be indicated by (1) vomiting blood ("coffee ground" vomitus); (2) bright red blood in the stool or black, tarry stools; (3) large clots or an abnormally heavy flow during the menstrual period; or (4) cloudy or pink-red urine (assuming that dyes in drugs that may cause urine discoloration have been ruled out).

Blood loss, particularly through the stool, is not always obvious. Even when abnormal blood loss occurs, the patient may not notice it and the blood loss may not be reported. Periodic testing using home occult blood test kits may be considered.

The pharmacist should also ascertain whether the patient's problem is chronic, whether self-treatment has been tried, and whether medical care has been sought or received. The pharmacist should appreciate the fact that the presence of anemia in patients other than those who are pregnant, lactating, menstruating, or on a restricted diet may be a symptom of a more serious medical disorder, and these individuals should be strongly encouraged to seek a medical diagnosis.

Dose/RDA

The RDA for iron is 10 mg for adult men, 15 mg for adult women, and 30 mg for pregnant women. Most healthy individuals who self-medicate, including menstruating females, will absorb adequate iron from one 325-mg ferrous sulfate tablet per day. In a 325-mg ferrous sulfate tablet, 20% (about 60 mg) is elemental iron. In patients with iron deficiencies, 20% of the elemental iron (12 mg) may be absorbed. Because 36–48 mg of iron daily are enough to support maximum incorporation into red blood cells (0.3 g of hemoglobin per 100 mL of blood) and replace iron stores, the usual therapeutic dose of two to four tablets daily for 3 months is probably reasonable in treating a deficiency. If the patient has an inadequate response after this period, a physician should be consulted. In cases of severe or chronic iron deficiency and when serious medical conditions have been ruled out, continuous low-maintenance doses of three to four tablets daily for approximately 3–6 months should normalize hemoglobin and replace iron stores, provided there is no ongoing bleeding and the diet is adequate.

If iron supplementation is appropriate, the pharmacist must determine which iron product is best. The choice of an iron preparation should be based on how well it is absorbed and tolerated, as well as on its price. Because ferrous salts are more efficiently absorbed than ferric salts, an iron product of the ferrous group is usually appropriate. Ferrous sulfate is the standard against which other iron salts (e.g., ferrous succinate, ferrous lactate, ferrous fumarate, ferrous glycine sulfate, ferrous glutamate, and ferrous gluconate) are compared. Ferrous citrate, ferrous tartrate, ferrous pyrophosphate, and some ferric salts are not well absorbed.

Ferrous salts may be given in combination with ascorbic acid. At a ratio of 200 mg of ascorbic acid to 30 mg of elemental iron, the increased amount of iron absorbed validates this practice. Other agents that may help increase absorption include sugars and amino acids. Chemicals that may decrease iron absorption include phosphates in eggs, phytates in cereals, carbonates, oxalates, and tannins.

Iron is available in numerous salt forms as tablets, capsules, liquids, and controlled-release products. It is also available in various strengths in combination products. The enteric-coated and delayed-release products are more expensive but may cause fewer symptoms of gastric irritation. Because progressively less iron is absorbed as it moves from the duodenum (the site of maximum absorption) to the ileum of the small intestine, overall iron absorption is decreased by delaying the time of release.

Adverse Effects/Drug Interactions

All iron products tend to irritate the GI mucosa and may produce nausea, abdominal pain, and diarrhea. These adverse effects may be minimized by reducing the dose or by giving iron with meals. However, because food may decrease the amount of iron absorbed by as much as 50%, physicians may recommend iron with instructions for between-meal dosing. It is advantageous for absorption if the patient is able to tolerate iron taken in this manner. But if nausea or diarrhea is intolerable, it is usually better to take the iron with food or decrease the number of tablets taken per day than to stop taking iron supplements entirely.

A frequent side effect of iron therapy is constipation. This adverse effect has prompted the formulation of iron products that also contain a stool softener (e.g., docusate).

During iron therapy, stools may become black and tarry, usually owing to unabsorbed iron. Black, tarry stools may also indicate GI blood loss and a serious GI problem. Medical referral is indicated if an underlying GI condition is suspected or if there is a history of peptic ulcer disease, Chrohn's disease, ulcerative colitis, or ulcerogenic or antiprothrombinemic medication use. If the stool does not darken somewhat during iron therapy, the iron product may not have disintegrated properly or released the iron.

Accidental poisoning with iron occurs most often in children, who are attracted to the sugar-coated, colored tablets. An accidental poisoning could also occur from overingestion of chewable multivitamins containing iron. Such poisoning is considered a medical emergency. As few as fifteen 325-mg ferrous sulfate tablets have been lethal to children; however, recovery has followed the ingestion of as many as 70 such tablets. The clinical outcome depends on the speed of treatment.

Toxic ingestion of iron may be life-threatening and should be referred to a poison control center or emergency medical facility immediately. Symptoms of acute iron poisoning include pain, vomiting, diarrhea, electrolyte imbalances, and shock. In later stages, cardiovascular collapse may occur, especially if the cause has not been properly recognized and treated as a medical emergency. Treatment of iron toxicity may begin immediately at home by giving ipecac syrup to induce vomiting. (See Chapter 12, "Emetic and Antiemetic Products.")

A more insidious toxicity may occur during prolonged therapy with iron. In the treatment of refractory anemia, oral iron may be excessively absorbed, leading to iron overload. Certain alcoholic patients may also become overloaded with iron because wine contains iron and alcohol increases ferric iron absorption. Patients with chronic liver or pancreatic disease absorb more iron than normal from the gut. Iron overload also may occur if individuals who do not require long-term iron supplementation take iron for prolonged periods. The pharmacist should discourage the chronic use of iron supplements if no clinical evidence indicates its need.

Iron is chelated by many substances. Its interaction with antacids may be clinically significant. The mechanism of this interaction is probably related to the relative alkalinization of the stomach contents by an antacid. The chelate of iron with an antacid is more insoluble in the alkaline medium. Iron appears to chelate with several of the tetracyclines, resulting in decreased tetracycline and iron absorption. If simultaneous administration of an iron salt and a tetracycline is medically necessary, patients should take tetracycline 3 hours after or 2 hours before iron administration. Allopurinol should not be given with iron unless recommended by a physician.

Manganese

Description

Manganese is required for glucose utilization, synthesis of the mucopolysaccharides of cartilage, steroid biosynthesis, and the biologic activity of pyruvate carboxylase. Manganese can apparently substitute for magnesium in selected enzymes involved in oxidative phosphorylation.

Manganese is widely available in the diet in vegetables and fruits. Nuts, legumes, and whole-grain cereals are particularly good sources.

Indications

In animals, poor reproductive performance, growth retardation, congenital malformations, abnormal bone and cartilage formation, and impaired glucose tolerance are related to manganese deficiency. Only one case has been reported of human manganese deficiency with symptoms involving the hair, nails, nausea/vomiting, decreased serum phospholipids and triglycerides, and moderate weight loss.

Dose/RDA

Even though manganese is poorly absorbed after oral administration (3%), sufficient quantities are present in the average diet to maintain appropriate levels. A dose or dietary intake of 2–5 mg per day is considered safe and adequate. Manganese is available as different salt forms, primarily as 20- and 50-mg tablets and in various combination products.

Adverse Effects/Drug Interactions

Toxicity is rare for orally administered manganese. It has been observed, however, from inhalation of dust and industrial fumes containing manganese.

There is a possible antagonistic effect between manganese and iron, resulting in less iron absorption. Also, low iron levels may result in enhanced manganese absorption and possible toxicity.

Molybdenum

Description

Molybdenum can readily change its oxidation state and act as an electron transfer agent in oxidation–reduction reactions. It may also function as an enzyme cofactor.

The molybdenum content of food varies and is dependent on the growth environment. Milk, organ meats, beans, breads, and cereals appear to contribute the most dietary molybdenum.

Indications

Molybdenum is a cofactor for several flavoprotein enzymes and is found in xanthine oxidase. Because xanthine oxidase is involved in the oxidation of xanthine to uric acid, high molybdenum intake has been associated with goutlike symptoms. Parenteral nutrition without molybdenum has resulted in an acquired molybdenum deficiency, which has been treated with ammonium molybdate.

Dose/RDA

It appears that the human molybdenum requirement is low (about 75–250 mcg per day for adults) and is easily furnished by the average diet. A safe and adequate daily dietary intake of 150–500 mcg has been estimated.

Adverse Effects/Drug Interactions

Molybdenum is relatively nontoxic. When consumed in excess, however, it may be antagonistic to copper, resulting in symptoms of copper deficiency.

Nickel

Divalent and trivalent forms of nickel are important in biologic systems. The absorption of nickel may be related to iron, but only a very low percentage is absorbed, most of it being lost in the feces. Nickel is found in highest concentrations in chocolate, nuts, dried beans, peas, and grains.

It has been speculated that nickel is involved in specific metalloenzymes, but its actual activity has not been clearly delineated, even though it is essential. Symptoms of a deficiency state have not been documented in humans.

Selenium

Description

Selenium is present in all tissues. Many selenium compounds are analogous to sulfur compounds. Glutathione peroxidase, a selenoenzyme, is important in the destruction of inflammatory hydroperoxides.

Selenium is generally incorporated into organic compounds involving amino acids such as methionine or cysteine. Selenium compounds are about 80% absorbed. The highest concentrations are found in the kidneys and liver; the lowest are in the lungs and brain. The kidney is the primary route of excretion.

Dietary sources of selenium include meat, seafoods, and some cereal grains. Vegetables and fruits contain little of this element. The selenium content of foods depends on the soils in which the plants are grown.

Indications

Selenium is an essential trace element in humans, but deficiencies are not common in the general population. Selenium deficiency has been reported in patients with alcoholic cirrhosis, probably owing to an insufficient diet or the altered metabolism of selenium. It has been rarely reported in patients on long-term parenteral nutrition. Epidemiologic studies suggest that cancer and heart disease may be common in areas of low selenium availability.

Limited evidence in humans suggests that deficiency results in cardiomyopathy, muscle pain, and abnormal nail beds. Keshan disease (a disorder characterized by abnormalities of the myocardium) has been shown to respond to selenium.

Dose/RDA

The RDA for selenium has been set at 70 mcg for adult men and 50–55 mcg for adult women. Selenium is included in some multivitamin and mineral preparations. It is available as 50-mcg tablets and in various strengths in combination products. Doses in excess of 0.2 mg per day are not recommended.

Adverse Effects/Drug Interactions

Toxic effects reported include loss of hair and nails, skin lesions, and CNS and teeth involvement. Selenium toxicity may be evidenced by growth retardation, muscular weakness, infertility, focal hepatic necrosis, dysphagia, dysphonia, bronchopneumonia, and respiratory failure.

Silicon

Description

Little is known about the absorption, distribution, metabolism, and excretion of silicon. It apparently functions in the development and maintenance of connective tissue, and it is required for collagen biosynthesis and for the mineralization process in bone calcification.

Silicon is obtained in diets primarily from foods of plant origin, especially cereal products, root vegetables, and unrefined grains of high fiber content. The role of silicon in human nutrition is speculative.

Indications

Silicon deficiency states in humans have not been described.

Dose/RDA

The daily requirement of silicon has not been established. The best dosage form of silicon administration has not been determined.

Adverse Effects/Drug Interactions

When taken orally, silicon is essentially nontoxic. This is evidenced by the administration of silicon-containing magnesium trisilicate, a nonprescription antacid taken for more than 40 years without apparent toxic effects, and the ingestion of simethicone, a common antigas ingredient in many nonprescription antacids. The absorption and metabolism of silicon may be altered by fiber, molybdenum, magnesium, and fluoride.

Tin

Tin may be involved in growth and reproductive functions, but the evidence of its requirement is lacking. A deficiency state for tin has not been described in humans. Adequate quantities of tin are apparently obtained from the diet.

Vanadium

The most important forms of vanadium in biologic systems are the tetravalent and pentavalent states. The tetravalent form easily complexes with other substances such as transferrin or hemoglobin to stabilize it against oxidation. Vanadium may be involved in functions related to growth and reproduction; however, the evidence of its necessity is not well established.

Vanadium is presumed essential, but a deficiency state has not been confirmed. It is obtained in sufficient quantities in the diet. Shellfish, mushrooms, parsley, and some spices (e.g., dill seed and black pepper) are rich in vanadium.

Toxicity can occur through excessive dietary intake. Symptoms include diarrhea, anorexia, depressed growth, and neurotoxicity. Vanadium toxicity may be diminished by administration of ascorbic acid, ethylenediaminetetraacetic acid, chromium, protein, ferrous iron, chloride, and possibly aluminum hydroxide.

Zinc

Description

Zinc is an integral part of at least 70 metalloenzymes, including carbonic anhydrase, lactic dehydrogenase, alkaline phosphatase, carboxypeptidase, aminopeptidase, and alcohol dehydrogenase. It is also a cofactor in the synthesis of DNA and RNA, and it is involved in the mobilization of vitamin A from the liver and in the enhancement of follicle-stimulating hormone and luteinizing hormone. It is essential for normal cellular immune functions and for spermatogenesis and normal testicular function, and it is important in the stabilization of membrane structure.

The divalent ion is most commonly found and used in the body. Zinc has a relatively rapid turnover rate, and the body pool appears to be about 2 to 3 g. Zinc is efficiently regulated in the body.

Most dietary zinc (about 70%) is derived from animal products. Good sources of zinc include oysters; liver; high-protein foods such as beef, lamb, pork, legumes, and peanuts; and whole-grain cereals.

Indications

Symptoms of zinc deficiency include growth retardation, loss of appetite, skin changes, and immunologic abnormalities. Additional symptoms of deficiency may include delayed sexual maturation, hypogonadism and hypospermia, alopecia, behavioral disturbances, night blindness, impaired taste and smell, and impaired wound healing. Although such deficiencies are not widespread in the United States, marginally low zinc values have been associated with growth retardation in children, slow wound healing in adults, birth defects, and problems in childbirth. Malabsorption syndromes, infection, myocardial infarct, major surgery, alcoholism, liver cirrhosis, high-fiber diets rich in phytate, pregnancy, and lactation predispose an individual to a suboptimal zinc status. Zinc depletion is relatively rare but may be seen in patients on long-term parenteral nutrition.

Zinc deficiencies adversely affect DNA, RNA, carbohydrate, and protein metabolism. Iron supplements decrease zinc absorption just as zinc supplements decrease iron absorption, probably owing to competition for the same transport system. If these minerals are taken with a meal, the adverse interaction is less pronounced. Vegetarian diets, despite their high fiber content, do not result in low plasma zinc levels. In patients with impaired wound healing, zinc supplementation may be marginally beneficial.

Dose/RDA

The RDA for zinc is 15 mg and 12 mg for adult men and women, respectively. The RDA for infants is 5 mg and for children, 10 mg. Typical Western diets supply 10–15 mg of zinc per day. Because zinc is only 10–40% absorbed from the GI tract, ingestion of 220-mg dose form of zinc sulfate (50 mg of elemental zinc) will supply 5–20 mg of zinc. Treatment of suspected deficiencies usually involves administration of 150 mg of elemental zinc in three divided doses daily. At these dosages, copper deficiency may be induced, so it has been suggested that the zinc dose be limited to 40 mg daily if therapy with zinc is going to be chronic.

If parenteral nutrition is continued longer than 3–5 days, zinc should be added to the regimen unless otherwise indicated. Patients with large GI losses via fistulas, ostomies, or stool require larger supplemental doses of zinc. Zinc is available in various salt forms as capsules, generally ranging in strength from 1.5 to 50 mg of elemental zinc, and in numerous combination products in various strengths. Chronic ingestion of more than 15 mg per day is not recommended without adequate medical supervision.

Adverse Effects/Drug Interactions

The ingestion of 2 g or more of zinc sulfate has resulted in GI irritation and vomiting. Zinc is toxic, although the emetic effect that occurs after consumption of large amounts may minimize problems with accidental overdose. Reported signs of zinc toxicity in humans include vomiting, dehydration, muscle incoordination, dizziness, and abdominal pain. Copper levels may be adversely affected by high intake of zinc, and zinc may decrease tetracycline absorption. Because zinc may cause GI upset, it can be taken with food. However, dairy and bran products, as well as foods high in calcium, phosphorus, or phytate, may decrease absorption of zinc.

Nutritional Supplements

Supplemental nutritional products should be used as adjuncts to a regular diet and not as substitutes for food. Often, persons who request a nutritional supplement have self-diagnosed their condition. However, although dietary supplements can be obtained without a prescription, they are complex agents with specific indications, and medical assessment should precede their use. The pharmacist should not be reluctant to consult a dietitian or physician concerning nutritional supplementation and should refer patients when necessary.

Patients purchasing a nonprescription dietary supplement should be instructed on its proper use and storage, including dilution and preparation techniques. In addition, the pharmacist should offer to discuss with the patient possible adverse side effects such as diarrhea.

Enteral Nutrition

Advances in supplements specifically designed for enteral use and the availability of sophisticated formulas, small-bore nasogastric tubes, and constant-infusion delivery systems have lead to a resurgence of interest in enteral nutrition.

Supplemental protein-calorie formula products are to be used only as adjuncts to a regular diet because they are not nutritionally complete. Some products (Mull-Soy® and Nutramigen®) are milk-free and can be used by individuals who have a milk allergy and lactose malabsorption. One product (Controlyte®) with a low protein and electrolyte content may be appropriate for patients with acute or chronic renal failure.

Complete formulas can be used orally or as tube feedings and may be used as sole dietary intake (if the patient's electrolytes are monitored) or as supplementation. These products may contain ingredients that make them appropriate for special needs. Several such products (Instant Breakfast®, Sustacal®, and Meritene®) are milk based; others (Compleat-B® and Gerber Meat Base Formula®) have a mixed-food base. A third type supplies protein in the form of crystalline amino acids or protein hydrolysate, carbohydrate in the form of oligosaccharides or disaccharides, and vitamins and minerals in the form of individual chemicals. These last products are chemically defined diets known as "elemental diets"; examples include Vivonex® and Jejunal®. Some other complete products (Precision LR® and Portagen®) are only partly chemically defined.

Nearly all elemental diets have low-fat content and contain electrolytes, minerals, trace elements, and water- and fat-soluble vitamins. All chemically based products require little or no digestion, are absorbed over a short distance in the small intestine, and have low residue. These attributes mean that the number and volume of the stools are reduced, making these products appropriate for patients who had ileostomies or colostomies and who wish to decrease fecal output. The low-residue products may also facilitate the care of elderly patients with stool incontinence or patients with brain damage from strokes, congenital defects, or retardation. Because of the ease of absorption and the low fecal residues, these products are often used in postoperative care, in treating GI disease, and in treating neoplastic disease, in which tissue breakdown is extensive.

Supplemental and complete formulas are available in several forms, including powders that must be diluted with water or milk, liquids that must be diluted, and liquids and puddings that are ready to use. The extent of dilution is based on the amount of nutrients needed and the amount that can be tolerated. Adults will not generally tolerate preparations of more than 25% weight per volume (w/v), which generally delivers 1.0 cal/mL. The maximum concentration for infants is 12% w/v, which generally delivers 0.5 cal/mL. Infants should generally be started on a concentration of 7–7.5% w/v, increasing to 12% over 4 to 5 days as tolerated. For children over 10 months of age, 15% w/v formulas may be initiated, with gradual increases to 25%. Higher concentrations may cause osmotic diarrhea.

If the preparations are taken orally, 100–150 mL should be ingested at one time. Over the course of a day, 2,000 mL of most preparations provide about 2,000 cal. If the patient is tube fed, 40–60 mL of the product per hour may be given initially. Once opened, the container should be kept cold to prevent bacterial growth, and all prepared products remaining after 24 hours should be discarded. Tubing should be rinsed three times a day with water. If diarrhea, nausea, or distention occur, the diet should be withheld for 24 hours and then gradually resumed. For elderly or unconscious persons or for patients who recently had surgery, elevating the head of the bed is advisable during administration to avoid aspiration.

Pharmacists should store supplemental formula products at temperatures under 75°F (23.8°C). Expiration dates should be checked before dispensing.

Patients must be monitored for biochemical abnormalities, electrolyte values, and adequate nutrition and hydration. Urine and blood glucose concentrations can be monitored. Persons with diabetes may require increased insulin doses. Edema may be precipitated or aggravated in patients with protein-calorie malnutrition or cardiac, renal, or hepatic disease because of the relatively high sodium content of the elemental diets. Some commercially available nutritional products (e.g., Ensure® and Ensure Plus®) are a source of vitamin K supplementation, which may interfere with oral anticoagulant therapy. Tube feedings have been shown to interfere with the absorption of phenytoin administered via the tube. This interaction can be avoided by flushing the tube with saline (or water) before and after phenytoin and waiting 15 minutes both before and after the dose is given.

Specialty formulations include puddings (Sustacal Pudding®), predigested/hydrolyzed formulas (Criticare HN®), low-carbohydrate formulas (Pulmocare®), high-carbohydrate polymers (Exceed®), low-protein formulas (Amin-Aid®), isotonic formulas (Osmolite®), clear liquid formulas (Citrotein®), nutrient-dense products, and modular products (Moducal®).

In addition to the various vitamins and minerals previously discussed in this chapter, the bulk volume/weight of these supplements consists primarily of proteins, carbohydrates, and lipids (fats, oils). The reader is referred to Chapter 18, "Infant Formula Products," for detailed information on infant nutrition.

TABLE 6 Selected information useful in counseling patients about nutritional supplements

1. Labels on all vitamin or vitamin and mineral preparations should be read carefully before supplements are taken. The contents and the amounts of vitamins and minerals should be compared with those in the RDAs.
2. Doses of vitamins and minerals higher than the RDAs should be taken with caution. All vitamins and minerals have adverse effects that are dose related.
3. High doses of vitamins or minerals may be dangerous and should not be taken indiscriminately. It is best to not exceed the RDA. Label directions should be followed carefully.
4. Vitamins or vitamin and mineral supplements should be taken with meals if their use is associated with GI symptoms. Iron and other supplements may cause less stomach upset if taken with meals.
5. Patients should not self-medicate if they suspect a vitamin deficiency but should instead consult their physician or pharmacist.
6. For proper nutrition, foods from all the basic food groups (meats, fruits and vegetables, dairy products, and grains) should be eaten. Vitamin supplements are not a substitute for a well-balanced diet.
7. Liquid vitamin and mineral supplements may be mixed with food (fruit juice, milk, baby formula, or cereal).
8. Iron supplements or vitamins with iron may turn stool black. This occurrence is not a cause for alarm unless it is associated with other symptoms involving the GI tract.
9. Some vitamin supplements have a special coating and should be swallowed whole. The physician or pharmacist should inform a patient if this is the case.
10. Like any medicine, vitamin and combination vitamin and mineral supplements should be stored out of the reach of children, especially if the product contains iron.
11. Children's vitamins are not candy. Children should be taught that vitamins are drugs, should be respected as drugs and potential poisons, and cannot be taken indiscriminately.
12. Niacin-containing products may cause a flushing sensation, which should decrease in intensity with continued therapy.
13. Riboflavin-containing products may cause a yellow fluorescence in the urine.

Summary

Pharmacists can significantly contribute to improving the nutritional status of the population by becoming familiar with these basics of nutrition, observing patients, and listening to their requests and providing general nutritional counseling. Much misinformation is being disseminated, and pharmacists can dispel myths, downplay exaggerated claims, and provide objective facts on nutritional agents such as vitamins, minerals, and nutritional supplements. Selected patient information useful in educating and counseling patients is included in Table 6.

References

1. Ehrlich FJ. Drugstores and nutrition: played right, a winning combination. *Drug Topics* 1985 Feb 4; 129: 28–31.
2. Food and Nutrition Board, National Research Council. *Recommended Dietary Allowances*. 10th ed. Washington, DC: National Academy of Sciences; 1989.
3. Shils ME, Young VR, eds. *Modern Nutrition in Health and Disease*. 7th ed. Philadelphia: Lea and Febiger; 1988.
4. Robinson CH, Lawler MR, Chenoweth WL, et al. *Normal and Therapeutic Nutrition*. 17th ed. New York: Macmillan; 1990.
5. Goodman AG, Rall TW, Nies AS, et al. *The Pharmacological Basis of Therapeutics*. 18th ed. New York: Pergamon Press; 1990.
6. *American Hospital Formulary Service 1992*. Bethesda, Md: American Society of Hospital Pharmacists; 1992.
7. *U.S. Dispensing Information*. 12th ed. Bethesda, Md: U.S. Pharmacopoeial Convention; 1992.
8. Billups NF, Billups SM. *American Drug Index*. 35th ed. St. Louis, Mo: J. B. Lippincott Co; 1991.
9. Olin BR, ed. *Facts and Comparisons*. St. Louis, Mo: Facts and Comparisons; 1992.
10. Brin M. Erythrocyte as a biopsy tissue for functional evaluation of thiamine adequacy. *JAMA* 1964; 187: 762–6.
11. Hsu JM, David RL, eds. *Handbook of Geriatric Nutrition*. Park Ridge, NJ: Noyes; 1981: 163.
12. Marcus R, Coulston AM. In: Goodman AG, Rall TW, Nies AS, et al. *The Pharmacological Basis of Therapeutics*. 18th ed. New York: Pergamon Press; 1990: 1554.

Chapter 18

Infant Formula Products

Rosalie Sagraves, Claudia Kamper, and Judi Doerr

> **Questions to ask in patient assessment and counseling**
>
> - What is your baby's age and weight?
> - Is your baby under a physician's care?
> - Are you breast-feeding your baby or has your physician recommended an infant formula?
> - Is your baby allergic or sensitive to milk? Does your baby have other dietary restrictions or health problems?
> - Are you giving your baby a multivitamin product? Was it recommended by your physician?
> - Is your baby receiving fluoride supplementation?
> - Does your baby have diarrhea, constipation, or vomiting?
> - Does your baby have a fever, a loss of appetite, or fewer wet diapers?
> - Do you understand how your baby's formula should be prepared?

Breast-feeding is the desired method for feeding infants from birth to at least 4–6 months of age because human milk provides a nutritional source that is physiologically sound and because breast-feeding tends to facilitate a close mother–child relationship.[1] It also decreases the incidence of infant allergy and illness. Breast-feeding women can decrease the amount of time they spend in nutrition preparation, lower the cost of feeding their infants, and decrease their postpartum recovery time.[2–4]

However, some women do not want to breast-feed or are unable to do so, and, in industrially developed nations, commercially prepared infant formulas offer an excellent alternative to breast-feeding. The use of infant formulas is less desirable in developing countries, where inadequate sanitation, lack of refrigeration, and the inability of illiterate mothers to follow formula preparation instructions increase the risk of infant morbidity and mortality.[4]

Infant formulas have evolved to their present quality over the past century. Before the 20th century, 80–90% of infants not suckled by mothers or wet nurses died during their first year of life. Substitute milk feedings were made possible by discoveries in biology and medicine in the late 19th century, and technical advances in the early 20th century decreased infant mortality and helped to popularize artificial milk feedings. Between 1930 and 1960, evaporated milk was the product most used for infant formula preparation, but by 1978 fewer than 5% of formula-fed infants received evaporated milk formulas.[5]

In the 1970s, a greater acceptance of breast-feeding resulted in a change in infant feeding patterns in the United States. Between 1971 and 1984, breast-feeding at the time of hospital discharge increased from 24.7 to 59.7%, and the incidence of breast-feeding at age 5 to 6 months increased from 5.5 to 25.7%.[6,7] However, in 1989 the incidence of breast-feeding at the time of hospital discharge was 52.2% and the incidence at 6 months of age was 18.1%. Declines in breast-feeding occurred in all groups surveyed but were more likely to occur among young African-American women who had less than a high school education; who were enrolled in the Special Supplemental Food Program for Women, Infants, and Children (WIC) at the time surveyed; who worked outside the home; who lived in states other than western states; and who had low-birthweight (LBW) infants.[8] It must be noted that many of the women enrolled in WIC at the time of the survey did not do so until after the birth of their infants. Therefore, these women did not benefit from information on breast-feeding offered by WIC. This may, in part, account for the lower number of breast-feeding WIC mothers.

The WIC program is intended to give infants a better nutritional start in life. WIC serves one-third of all infants in the United States, providing either infant formula or supplemental food for the infants' breast-feeding mothers.[9] In 1989, 1.2 million infants enrolled in the WIC program, each consuming approximately 28 cans of formula monthly. Some of the cost of the WIC infant feeding program is covered through manufacturers' rebates. Pharmacists can find out more about WIC from local health department employees.

Advances in uniformity, convenience, nutritional quality, and safety have established infant formulas as an alternative way to feed infants.[10] The composition of commercial infant formulas conforms with guidelines based on extensive assessments of infant nutritional needs. Variations among formulas allow for the selection of a product that will meet a particular infant's nutritional requirements. However, these variations produce differences in palatability, digestibility, sources of nutrients, and convenience of administration. The pharmacist, in consultation with the infant's physician, should be able to evaluate indications, advise on the selection of an infant formula, and help ensure appropriate use of an infant formula.

Pharmacists should be knowledgeable about infant nutritional requirements, commercially prepared infant for-

---

This chapter is based in part on the chapter with the same title that appeared in the 9th edition but was written by Michael W. McKenzie, Kenneth J. Bender, and A. Jeanece Seals.

mulas, differences in formula composition, and specific uses for therapeutic formulas. Pharmacists also should be able to help educate women about breast-feeding and should refer women with questions about breast-feeding to organizations such as the La Leche League.

Infant Physiology and Growth

Physiology

The physiology of the infant's gastrointestinal (GI) and renal systems is crucial in infant nutrition. In early infancy, only liquid nutrition is appropriate until the infant can coordinate complex tongue movements and swallowing reflexes mature. Frequent feedings are necessary because the stomach capacity of a full-term infant (38–42 weeks' gestation and birthweight greater than 2,500 g) is only 20–90 mL at birth but increases rapidly to 90–150 mL by the time the infant is 1 month of age.[11]

Stomach acid and pepsin secretion peak in the newborn infant by day 10, decrease between days 10 and 30, and then gradually increase over the first year of life. A full-term infant can digest most carbohydrates because the intestinal enzymes lactase, sucrase, maltase, isomaltose, and glucomylase are sufficiently mature at birth.[12] Sucrase, maltase, and isomaltose usually are fully active in preterm infants (gestational period less than 38 weeks), but lactase activity may be immature. Lactose intolerance is clinically uncommon in infants because of postnatal adaptive responses to ingested carbohydrates. Lactase activity may decline in African-American and Asian children starting at 3 years of age. Pancreatic amylase activity and glucose transport are low in both full-term and preterm infants at birth and may not fully develop until the child is several years old.[12]

Newborn infants exhibit low lipase concentrations and slow rates for bile salt synthesis, which are important determinants for efficient fat absorption from the small intestine.[12] Breast-fed infants have a compensatory mechanism, bile salt–stimulated lipase, that helps ensure adequate dietary fat intake.[13,14] Long-chain saturated fatty acids (butterfat) are not absorbed as well as unsaturated fatty acids (vegetable oils), but fat absorption improves as the infant matures.

Protein digestion does not differ appreciably between infants and adults, even though infants digest a smaller quantity on an hourly basis.[15] Amino acids produced by protein digestion are absorbed by active transport mechanisms that reach adult levels by 14 weeks of age.[11] Because infants can readily absorb antigenic proteins, they are at an increased risk for developing food allergies later in life.[12]

The renal solute load is composed of soluble waste products that must be eliminated by the kidneys. Such solutes include nitrogenous waste and excess electrolytes and minerals. These are also excreted through the skin (in sweat), lungs (in water vapor), and GI tract. The potential renal solute load (PRSL) is defined as the solute load that is derived from dietary ingestion that would be excreted renally if amino acids from protein digestion were not

TABLE 1. Recommended dietary allowances of nutrients for full-term infants

Nutrient	RDA 0–6 mo	RDA >6–12 mo
Energy (kcal/kg/d)	108	98
Protein (gm/kg/d)	2.2	1.6
Essential fatty acids		
Linoleic acid (% of kcal)[a]	2.7	2.7
Vitamins		
Vitamin A (mcg)[b]	375	375
Vitamin D (mcg)[c]	7.5	10
Vitamin E (mg)[d]	3	4
Vitamin K (mcg)	5	10
Vitamin C (mg)	30	35
Thiamine (mg)	0.3	0.4
Riboflavin (mg)	0.4	0.5
Vitamin B6 (mg)	0.3	0.6
Vitamin B12 (mcg)	0.3	0.5
Niacin (mg)[e]	5	6
Folate (mcg)	25	35
Pantothenic acid (mg)[f]	2	3
Biotin (mcg)[f]	10	15
Minerals		
Calcium (mg)	400	600
Phosphorus (mg)	300	500
Magnesium (mg)	40	60
Iron (mg)	6	10
Iodine (mcg)	40	50
Zinc (mg)	5	5
Copper (mg)[e]	0.4–0.6	0.6–0.7
Manganese (mg)[f]	0.3–0.6	0.6–1
Fluoride (mg)[f]	0.1–0.5	0.2–1
Chromium (mcg)[f]	10–40	20–60
Selenium (mcg)	10	15
Molybdenum (mcg)[f]	15–30	20–40

[a]No specific recommendations for linolenic acid have been identified by the NRC, Food and Drug Administration, or CON/AAP.

[b]Retinol equivalents (REs); 1 RE = 3.33 IU of vitamin A activity from retinol.

[c]Cholecalciferol; 10 mcg of cholecalciferol equals 400 IU of vitamin D.

[d]Alpha-tocopherol equivalents (TEs); 1 mg of delta-alpha-tocopherol = 1 alpha-TE. The activity of alpha-tocopherol is 1.49 IU/mg.

[e]Niacin equivalents (NEs); 1 NE = 1 mg of niacin or 60 mg of dietary tryptophan.

[f]Estimated safe and adequate daily dietary intakes. Because there is less information on which to base allowances, some figures are provided as ranges of recommended intakes.

Reprinted with permission from Food and Nutrition Board, Commission on Life Sciences, National Research Council. *Recommended Dietary Allowances.* 10th ed. Washington, DC: National Academy Press; 1989.

TABLE 2 Nutritional recommendations for full-term infants (per 100 kcal)

Nutrient	FDA regulations Minimum	FDA regulations Maximum
Protein (g)	1.8	4.5
Fat		
(g)	3.3	6.0
(% calories)	30.0	—
Essential fatty acids		
Linoleic acid (g)	0.3	—
Vitamins		
Vitamin A (IU)	250.0	750.0
Vitamin D (IU)	40.0	100.0
Vitamin K (g)	4.0	—
Vitamin E (IU)	0.7	—
Vitamin C (mg)	40.0	—
B_1 (thiamine) (mcg)	40.0	—
B_2 (riboflavin) (mcg)	60.0	—
B_6 (pyridoxine) (mcg)	35.0	—
B_{12} (mcg)	0.15	—
Niacin (mcg)[a]	2.5	—
Folic acid (mcg)	4.0	—
Pantothenic acid (mcg)	300.0	—
Biotin (mcg)[b]	1.5	—
Choline (mg)[b]	7.0	—
Inositol (mg)	4.0	—
Minerals		
Calcium (mg)	60.0	—
Phosphorus (mg)	30.0	—
Magnesium (mg)	6.0	—
Iron (mg)	0.15	3.0
Iodine (mcg)	5.0	7.5
Zinc (mg)	0.5	—
Copper (mcg)	60.0	75.0
Manganese (mcg)	5.0	—
Sodium (mg)	20.0	60.0
Potassium (mg)	80.0	200.0
Chloride (mg)	55.0	150.0

[a]Includes nicotinic acid and niacinamide.
[b]Required only for non-milk–based infant formulas.
Reprinted from *Federal Register* 1985; 50: 45106.

used for growth or were not eliminated by nonrenal routes.[16]

The following equation can be used to calculate PRSL for breast milk or various infant formulas:

$$\text{PRSL (mOsm)} = \text{grams of protein}/0.175 + \text{sodium} + \text{chloride} + \text{potassium} + \text{phosphorus},$$

where sodium, chloride, potassium, and phosphorus are expressed in millimoles per unit volume.[10] Renal solute load will be discussed in greater depth later in this chapter.

Growth

The human body exhibits standard growth and development patterns. Birthweight is determined primarily by maternal prepregnancy and pregnancy weight and weight changes. The average birthweight for a full-term infant is approximately 3,500 g (about 7 1/2 lb); infants born prematurely may weigh less than 1,500 g (about 4 1/4 lb).[17]

After birth, a 6–10% weight loss usually occurs; this weight loss is primarily due to fluid loss. Weight gain then generally proceeds at a rate of 20–25 g per day in the first 4 months and 15 g per day in the next 8 months. Most infants can be expected to double their birthweight by 4 months and triple it by 12 months. In the second year of life, weight increase is equal to slightly less than the birthweight. Thereafter, a fairly constant growth rate of about 5 lb per year occurs until 9 or 10 years of age when growth velocity increases. At adolescence a major growth spurt occurs. Height shows a pattern similar to weight; most infants increase their length by 50% in the first year, 100% in the first 4 years, and 300% by age 13.

Changes in body composition accompany height and weight changes. Most notably, total body water decreases as adipose tissue increases. Total body water accounts for approximately 70% of total body weight at birth and declines to 60% by 1 year of age.[18]

Normal values of weight, height, and growth for infants and children are expressed in terms of percentiles for age; the majority of children fall between the 5th and 95th percentile. Most children stay within the same percentile as they grow, but spurts and plateaus are common. If growth is not progressing as expected, particularly in the first year of life when the expected growth rate is rapid, the energy and nutrient content of an infant's diet should be evaluated.

Nutritional Standards

Acceptable growth is achieved through an adequate intake of energy, protein, carbohydrates, minerals, and vitamins. The Food and Nutrition Board of the National Research Council (NRC) established recommended dietary allowances (RDAs) designed to meet the needs of most healthy infants. These general guidelines were last revised and published in 1989 (Table 1).[19] Table 2 contains the Food and Drug Administration (FDA) recommendations for nutrition for infants.

Energy requirements vary with age. Total energy requirements are a combination of basal energy needs, specific dynamic action of food, and activity and growth. The infant's energy requirement is large in relation to the child's body size but declines over time. The accepted RDA for infants from birth to 6 months is 108 kcal/kg per day, whereas infants 6–12 months of age require a somewhat lower intake of 98 kcal/kg per day, although there is some disagreement over direct energy expenditure measurements.[19] No significant differences in energy requirements have been noted between males and females younger than 10 years of age.

TABLE 3 Estimated amino acid requirements for infants and young children (mg/kg/d)

Amino acid	Infants (3–4 months old)	Children (≈ 2 years old)
Histidine	28	—
Isoleucine	70	31
Leucine	161	73
Lysine	103	64
Methionine + cystine	58	27
Phenylalanine + tyrosine	125	69
Threonine	87	37
Tryptophan	17	12.5
Valine	93	38

Fluid

Water is a particularly important component of the infant's diet because water makes up a larger proportion of infants' body composition than of older persons'. Water intake in the first 6 months of life is primarily derived from breast milk or formula. Both contain adequate amounts of water so that the normal, healthy infant should not need supplemental water. From 6 months to 12 months of age, when solid foods are introduced, water intake remains high; most children's foods contain 60–70% or more water.[20] Output is predominantly in renal excretion, evaporation from skin and lungs, and, to a lesser extent, feces. Increases in water loss caused by diarrhea, fever, or unusually rapid breathing, particularly in concert with decreased water intake, may result in significant dehydration and may be accompanied by an imbalance of electrolytes. Maintenance water or fluid needs in infancy are estimated to be approximately 100 mL/kg per day for the first 10 kg of body weight plus 50 mL/kg per day for each kilogram between 10 and 20 kg. Additional losses caused by conditions such as diarrhea, fever, and rapid breathing should be offset by fluids in excess of maintenance levels.

Carbohydrates

Although there is no RDA for carbohydrates, under normal circumstances an infant can efficiently use 40–50% of total calories from a carbohydrate source.[21] A carbohydrate-free diet is not desirable because such a diet leads to metabolic modifications favoring fatty acid breakdown, tissue protein and cation loss, and dehydration. Fiber intake is of considerable interest, due to associations made between high-fiber diets and the prevention of diseases such as diverticular disease, colon cancer, and coronary heart disease. The Committee on Nutrition of the American Academy of Pediatrics (CON/AAP) favors adequate fiber intake to ensure regular stool frequency but has not made a specific recommendation.[22] Lactose is the primary carbohydrate source in human milk and milk-based formulas. It is hydrolyzed by acids and the enzyme lactase to glucose and galactose. Disaccharide hydrolysis may be incomplete in a newborn, and because lactase activity develops late in fetal life, infants born during the seventh or eighth month of gestation may be unable to hydrolyze the same amount of lactose that a full-term infant can hydrolyze. Preterm infants are especially prone to lactose intolerance, which may be manifested by diarrhea, abdominal distention, and cramping.

Secondary lactase deficiency is a temporary reduction in intestinal lactase caused by gastroenteritis or malnutrition. Congenital lactase deficiency is a rare type of milk intolerance in infants that results from an inborn error of metabolism. Because of low levels of lactase in the GI tract, infants with congenital lactase deficiency and LBW infants may be unable to metabolize the quantity of lactose found in breast milk or infant formulas. Formulas with nutrient sources other than cow milk may be used when lactose intolerance or hypersensitivity is suspected.

Protein and Amino Acids

The accepted average RDA for protein is 2.2 g/kg per day from birth to age 6 months and 1.6 g/kg per day from age 6 months to 1 year.[19] Body protein increases by an average of 3.5 g per day in the first 4 months of life and by 3.1 g per day over the next 8 months, representing an overall change in body protein composition from 11–15%.[17]

Not only is overall protein intake important, but the amino acid composition of the protein is equally important. Amino acids can be classified as essential, nonessential, and conditionally essential. Nine amino acids (histidine, isoleucine, leucine, lysine, methionine, phenylalanine, threonine, tryptophan, and valine) are considered essential in adults because the body cannot synthesize them from precursors. Nonessential amino acids can be synthesized from precursors. Conditionally essential amino acids (e.g., cysteine and tyrosine) are nonessential ones that become essential because the synthesis process is impaired. This impairment may occur in preterm infants with immature enzyme systems.[19]

Estimates of specific amino acid requirements from the World Health Organization and others (Table 3) have been accepted by the NRC.[19] Despite similar amino acid densities and milk intakes, serum amino acid patterns in formula-fed infants tend to exceed those in infants fed human milk; however, the growth of such infants is normal.[23] Although the protein content of human milk adjusts to a growing infant's needs, the high protein needs of preterm infants have been shown not to be met by early human milk.[24] Fortification has been shown to produce reasonable plasma amino acid profiles and helps an infant meet expected intrauterine growth rates.[25]

Histidine is found in both human and cow milk in quantities larger than the estimated requirements. Synthesis of this amino acid becomes adequate by 2 to 3 months of age. Histidine deficiency results in poor nitrogen balance and growth. Supplemental tyrosine and cystine, as well as histidine, may be needed in the first weeks of life for the preterm infant.[19,26]

Taurine is an amino acid found in abundant quantities in breast milk.[27] Taurine is not an energy source, nor is it used for protein synthesis. It is considered a conditionally essential nutrient. Taurine deficiency can result in adverse changes such as retinal dysfunction, slow development of auditory brain stem–evoked response in preterm infants, and poor fat absorption in preterm infants and in children with cystic fibrosis (CF). These conditions can be improved with taurine supplements. Taurine serves a major nutritional role as a protector of cell membranes by attenuating toxic substances (e.g., oxidants, secondary bile acids, and excess retinoids) and by acting as an osmoregulator.[28] Taurine is now added to many infant formulas to provide the same margin of physiological safety that is provided by human milk, although disagreement still exists as to the necessity of taurine supplements even in LBW infants.[29]

In evaluating the adequacy of an infant's protein intake, one must consider not only the absolute amount of protein ingested, but also the growth rate of the child, the nonprotein calories and other nutrients necessary for protein synthesis, and the quality of the protein itself. Some authors have suggested that amino acid and protein requirements are more meaningful when expressed in terms of calories; therefore, requirements or supplementation levels may appear in grams per 100 kcal. In such cases, direct comparisons with RDAs expressed in grams per kilogram of body weight per day are not easily made.

Fat and Essential Fatty Acids

Fat is the most dense source of calories in the diet (9 kcal/g versus 4 kcal/g for protein and carbohydrates). It supplies approximately 40–50% of the energy intake of infants in developed countries.[17] Although there is concern in the adult population about dietary fat intake, the AAP recommends that the current recommendations of the American Heart Association and the National Institutes of Health Consensus Panel on Lowering Blood Cholesterol to Prevent Heart Disease "be followed with moderation" for children. The AAP says that 30–40% of calories from fat "seems sensible for adequate growth and development."[30] The FDA recommends a minimum fat intake of 3.3 g/100 kcal (30% of calories) and a maximum of 6 g/100 kcal (60% of calories).[31]

The diet must contain small amounts of the polyunsaturated fatty acid linoleic acid, which has been proven to be an essential nutrient. Linoleic acid and its derivatives, including arachidonic acid, enable optimum caloric intake and proper skin composition.[32] Linoleic acid deficiency manifests as increased metabolic rate, drying and flaking of the skin, hair loss, and impaired healing of wounds. Manifestations of essential fatty acid deficiency are generally delayed; however, rapid onset may occur in newborns with delayed provision of fat in their diets.[33] Linoleic acid represents the bulk of polyunsaturated fatty acids in infant formulas. Generally, an intake of linoleic acid equal to 1 to 2% of total dietary calories is adequate to prevent biochemical and clinical evidence of deficiency; 4 to 5% is thought to be optimal.[17] The AAP recommends linoleic acid intakes of 300 mg/100 kcal, or approximately 3% of total calories.[31] Linolenic acid, a polyunsaturated fatty acid found in plant foods, is thought by some to be essential; however, a specific deficiency state in humans has not been defined. No specific RDAs for fat have been established.

Micronutrients

RDAs for vitamins and minerals, including trace elements, are shown in Table 1. Precise needs are difficult to define and depend on energy, protein, and fat intakes and absorption. Infant formulas are generally supplemented with adequate amounts of vitamins and minerals to meet the needs of full-term infants.

Vitamins A, D, E, and K are classified as fat soluble. Vitamin A and the carotenoids that are vitamin A precursors are essential for vision, growth, and cellular function. Deficiency is found most often in young children with dietary insufficiencies;[19] however, deficiency in vitamin A and its precursors is uncommon in the United States. Vitamin A activity from food sources is expressed in retinol equivalents (REs); 1 RE is equal to 1 mcg of all-*trans*-retinol, 6 mcg of all-*trans*-beta-carotene, or 12 mcg of other provitamin A carotenoids.[19] Vitamin A needs for rapidly growing infants and children exceed the maintenance levels required by adults; therefore, RDA values change little as the growth rate decreases. Toxicity can occur with acute or chronic ingestion of exceedingly high doses. Sustained daily intakes of 6,000 mcg retinol by infants or young children may cause toxic manifestations—headache, vomiting, diplopia, alopecia, desquamation, bone abnormalities, liver damage, and dryness of the mucous membranes.[19] The breast milk of well-nourished women in this country contains adequate amounts of vitamin A and the carotenoids that supply about 10% of total vitamin A activity to prevent deficiencies in infants.[19]

Vitamin D is essential in mineral homeostasis and bone mineralization and is particularly important in infancy. Severe deficiency states in infancy can cause rickets. Adequate amounts of vitamin D can be synthesized with sufficient exposure to sunlight or artificial ultraviolet light.[19] Cow milk and infant formulas should be fortified with 400 IU vitamin D per quart.[19] Excessive intake (as little as five times the RDA) in children may result in toxicity with hypercalcemia, hypercalciuria, soft tissue calcium deposition, and irreversible calcium deposition in the kidneys and heart.[19]

Vitamin E serves an important role in muscular and neurologic function. The most potent and common form, alpha-tocopherol, is also an efficient antioxidant. Premature infants and children with fat malabsorption due to CF or other causes are prone to deficiency. Tocopherol levels should be proportional to the oxidants (iron) and oxidizable substrate (polyunsaturated fatty acids [PUFA]) in the diet. Most infant formulas are supplemented to provide 0.8 IU/g of polyunsaturated fatty acids because cow milk is low in linoleic acid (it has 20–25% as much as human milk).[19] The RDAs of 3 mg per day for infants 0–6 months of age and 4 mg for infants older than 6 months should be met in human milk or formula.

Compared with full-term infants, preterm infants are born with disproportionately small body stores of vitamin E and a reduced capacity for intestinal vitamin E absorption.[34] Hemolytic anemia has been reported in preterm infants who received iron-fortified formulas that contained high levels of PUFA.35 The additional oxidant activity of iron (≥ 8 mg/kg) increases the risk for hemolytic anemia in preterm infants who have insufficient tocopherol levels.

To avoid hemolytic anemia in preterm infants, the ratio of vitamin E intake to PUFA (E/PUFA) should not be less than 0.4 where E/PUFA is:36

$$\frac{\text{(vitamin E per unit volume (IU of alpha-tocopherol)}}{\text{PUFA per unit volume (grams of linoleic and arachidonic acid)}}$$

It has therefore been suggested that up to 17 mg of vitamin E may be required as an oral supplement until 3 months of age.19

Vitamin K and vitamin K–active compounds are essential in the formation of prothrombin and other proteins responsible for coagulation of the blood. Vitamin K activity is supplied by dietary sources and intestinal bacteria. Because intestinal flora are limited in the newborn, most hospital-born infants receive vitamin K prophylaxis at birth. Deficiency states are manifested primarily by prolonged clotting times. Milk-based formulas contain sufficient quantities of vitamin K to prevent deficiency. Furthermore, the bacterial flora generated by milk-based formulas in healthy infants contributes to an adequate supply of vitamin K.

Water-soluble vitamins are generally present in both breast milk and formulas in quantities adequate to prevent deficiency states.

Biotin, Choline, and Inositol

Biotin is an integral component of enzyme systems in humans and is considered an essential vitamin. Biotin deficiency in infants younger than 6 months has been reported to be manifested by seborrheic dermatitis, which can be reversed with supplementation.37 The recommended intake is 10–15 mcg per day.19 Choline and *myo*-inositol are both components of cell membrane and phospholipids or lipoproteins. The nutritional requirements for choline and inositol are currently unknown.

Minerals

Calcium and Phosphorus

Calcium and phosphorus are crucial to the development and maintenance of the human skeleton. In addition, phosphorus is an integral component of many biochemical reactions. Calcium requirements are affected by protein and phosphorus intake because of these nutrients' interactions with renal tubular reabsorption of calcium. The recommended ratio of calcium to phosphorus is 1.3:1 for infants between birth and 6 months of age and 1.2:1 for infants older than 6 months. A high phosphate intake has been associated with hypocalcemic tetany.38,39

For preterm and LBW infants, additional calcium and phosphorus in special infant formulas are necessary for normal bone growth and mineralization, and breast milk may need supplementation.40 Formulas designed for full-term infants are deficient in calcium and phosphorus relative to the needs of the LBW or preterm infant.

Table 1 contains RDAs for minerals for full-term infants.

Iron

Because iron is a component of hemoglobin and several enzymes, it is considered essential. A large portion of iron is found in storage forms in the liver, spleen, and bone marrow. Intestinal absorption is the primary method of regulating iron sufficiency. The FDA recommends that all formulas contain at least the lower level of iron found in human milk (0.5 mg/L) and that iron be in a bioavailable form. Infants at risk for iron deficiency should be given formulas supplemented with 1 to 2 mg/100 kcal (approximately 6–12 mg/L) of iron. Most iron-supplemented formulas contain 12 or 13 mg/L. Iron availability may be less in formulas with higher protein concentrations; iron deficiency is more common in infants fed 2.4% protein (3.6 g/100 kcal) than in those fed 1.5% protein (2.3 g/100 kcal) in a milk formula.41

Formulas for LBW infants contain less than or equal to 3 mg of iron per liter. Conservative levels of iron are used because iron supplementation in LBW infants up to 2 months of age has been associated with an increased risk of hemolytic anemia because of iron's interference with vitamin E metabolism. These formulas do not supply enough iron to meet the normal intrauterine accretion rate of iron. The decision to supplement iron in infants fed LBW formulas should be made by the physician.

Zinc, Copper, and Manganese

Full-term infants who are entirely breast-fed should meet their zinc requirements (approximately 2 mg per day for an infant 1 month of age) through breast milk and liver stores. Zinc is less bioavailable in formulas; therefore, the RDA for formula-fed infants is 5 mg per day.19 Less zinc may be absorbed from soy-protein formulas because of the presence of phytate in soy protein.42 The AAP recommendation for copper in infant formulas is 60 mcg/100 kcal.19 The requirement for manganese is currently unknown; the provisional recommendations are 0.3–0.6 mg per day for infants 0–6 months old and 0.6–1 mg per day in infants 6 months to 1 year of age.19

Vitamin and Mineral Supplements

There is no evidence that vitamin and mineral supplementation is necessary for formula-fed full-term infants or for normal, breast-fed infants of well-nourished mothers.43 However, iron and vitamin D supplementation has been recommended for breast-fed full-term infants.43

Vitamin and mineral supplementation may be needed for preterm and LBW infants and infants whose mothers are inadequately nourished. These infants and those with other nutritional deficiencies, malabsorptive and other chronic diseases, rare vitamin dependency conditions, inborn errors of vitamin or mineral metabolism, or deficiencies related to the intake of drugs will need vitamin and mineral supplementation directed by a physician.43 Table 4 gives guidelines for supplementation.

Breast-Fed Full-Term Infants

Vitamin D is recommended as a supplement for breast-fed infants as a protective measure against rickets.44,45 However, rickets caused by vitamin D deficiency has been reported in relatively few breast-fed infants in the United States. The vitamin D–fortified foods in the diets of most

TABLE 4 Guidelines for the use of vitamin and mineral supplements in healthy infants

	Multivitamin/ multimineral	Vitamin D	Vitamin E[a]	Folate	Iron[b]
Full-term infants					
Breast-fed	0	±	0	0	±
Formula-fed	0	0	0	0	0
Preterm infants					
Breast-fed[c]	+	+	±	±	+
Formula-fed[c]	+	+	±	±	+
Older Infants (>6 mo)					
Normal	0	0	0	0	±
High-risk[d]	+	0	0	0	±

Key:
+ means a supplement is usually indicated; ± means a supplement is possibly or sometimes indicated; 0 means a supplement is not usually indicated.
Vitamin K for newborn infants and fluoride in areas where there is insufficient fluoride in the water are not shown.
[a]Vitamin E should be in a form that is well absorbed by small, preterm infants. If this form of vitamin E is present in formulas, it need not be given separately to formula-fed infants. Infants fed breast milk are less susceptible to Vitamin E deficiency.
[b]Iron-fortified formula and/or infant cereal is a more convenient and reliable source of iron than a supplement.
[c]Multivitamin supplements (plus added folate) are needed primarily when calorie intake is below approximately 300 kcal per day or when the infant weights 2.5 kg; vitamin D should be supplied at least until 6 months of age in breast-fed infants. Iron should be started by 2 months of age.
[d]Multivitamin–multimineral preparations including iron are preferred to supplements containing iron alone.
Adapted from *Pediatrics* 1980; 66: 1017.

---

mothers reduce the risk of vitamin D deficiency. If the mother's diet has been inadequate in vitamin D, supplements of 400 IU of vitamin D may be administered.[46] Mothers should be encouraged to maintain a balanced diet and to drink five to six 8-oz glasses of milk a day while breast-feeding. If the mother cannot tolerate milk due to lactose intolerance, products that aid in lactose digestion are available (e.g., Lactaid®, Dairy Aid®, Lactogest®, or Dairy Ease®). If she wishes not to drink milk, she should be encouraged to increase her calcium intake from other dietary sources or to supplement her dietary calcium intake with calcium tablets.

Vitamin A deficiency rarely occurs in breast-fed infants; therefore, vitamin A may be omitted from supplements designed to provide vitamin D for infants.

Vitamin B12 deficiency has been reported in breast-fed infants of strict vegetarian mothers.[47] This deficiency is relatively rare in the United States. A malnourished nursing mother and her infant should receive multivitamin supplements to prevent megaloblastic anemia.

The concentration of iron in human milk averages about 0.3 mg/L.[15] Iron is well absorbed from human milk (i.e., 50% of the iron is absorbed).[48] Breast-fed infants rarely develop iron deficiency anemia before 4–6 months of age because neonatal stores of iron are adequate. After 6 months of age, neonatal stores may be depleted; consequently, in normal, breast-fed full-term infants, the addition of an iron supplement (2 mg/kg of ferrous sulfate) may be desirable. An iron supplement is preferable to iron-fortified cereal. Cereal diluted with milk or formula provides about 7 mg of elemental iron per 100-g serving. A 4% absorption of iron from a 50-g serving of cereal yields only 0.14 mg or 20% of the requirement.[7]

The bioavailability of the electrolyte iron powder used to fortify infant cereals has not been studied in human subjects. Because cereals contain potent inhibitors of iron absorption, they are questionable sources of iron. Iron-fortified wet-packed cereal and fruit combinations marketed in jars offer no exposure of the iron sulfate to oxygen until the jar is opened; therefore, oxidative rancidity is not a problem. These products may be better sources of dietary iron supplementation than dry cereals.[7] Products that require reconstitution of dehydrated flakes with water to produce instant baby foods appear to be nutritionally equivalent to the wet-packed foods.[7]

The CON/AAP states that fluoride supplements can be initiated shortly after birth in breast-fed infants if deemed necessary by a physician.[49,50] Since its statement in 1979, the committee has changed its view on fluoride supplements for breast-fed infants because infants who are totally breast-fed do not appear to develop caries at a higher rate than bottle-fed infants. Therefore, fluoride supplements may not be necessary if the breast-fed infant lives in an area where the water is fluoridated. If the physician wishes the infant to receive a supplement, Table 5 can be used to determine the proper fluoride supplementation; the level of supplementation should not be sufficient to cause enamel fluorosis. In fluoridated areas where breast-fed infants receive a diet supplemented by additional food and water, fluoride supplementation is not advised because of the risk of mild enamel fluorosis.[50]

Formula-Fed Full-Term Infants

Full-term infants who consume adequate amounts of an iron-fortified commercial milk-based formula do not need vitamin and mineral supplementation in the first 6 months of life.[51] An iron-fortified formula is preferred because of the concern for adequate iron stores for growing infants. Studies have shown that infants fed iron-fortified formulas do not demonstrate a difference in stool consistency, fussiness, colic, or regurgitation compared with infants fed nonfortified formulas.[52,53]

In a 1985 study, infants 7–12 months of age who were fed formula and solid foods had a more balanced intake of nutrients than infants fed cow milk and solid foods.[54] The table foods that were fed to infants on cow milk were high in protein, sodium, and potassium and low in iron and linoleic acid. Thus, the overall diet of infants fed cow milk and supplemental solid foods contained 52% of the RDA for iron.

Vitamin and mineral supplements are not needed for infants older than 6 months of age who receive a diet of formula, mixed feedings, and increased amounts of table food. A multivitamin with minerals may be needed if the infant is at special nutritional risk. If a powdered or concentrated formula is used, fluoride supplements should be administered only if the community's drinking water contains less than 0.3 ppm of fluoride. Ready-to-use formulas are manufactured with defluoridated water and contain less than 0.3 ppm of fluoride. Therefore, if an infant fed ready-to-use formula does not drink water or juice or eat solid foods, the physician may recommend a fluoride supplement.

Preterm Infants

Preterm infants, either breast-fed or formula-fed, need vitamin and mineral supplementation. Their nutrient needs are proportionately greater than those of full-term infants because of their more rapid growth rate, inability to ingest an adequate volume of formula or breast milk, and decreased intestinal absorption.[35,40] Until these infants can consume about 300 kcal per day or until they reach a body weight of 2.5 kg, a multivitamin supplement should be administered to provide the equivalent of the RDAs for full-term infants.

Because breast-fed preterm infants may develop rickets, they should receive a special preterm infant formula that contains appropriate amounts of calcium, phosphorus, and vitamin D.[40]

A multivitamin supplement should include vitamin E in a form well absorbed by preterm infants. Because of conflicting data from clinical studies, it may be prudent to monitor vitamin E serum concentrations and to maintain serum concentrations of 1–3 mg/dL.[55]

Folic acid deficiency has been reported in preterm infants.[56] The instability of folic acid precludes its use in commercial liquid multivitamin and mineral preparations. Folate can be added to a multivitamin preparation to provide the RDA (Table 1). The shelf life of folate is 1 month, and the label should read "shake well."[35]

Iron supplements should be withheld until the preterm infant is several weeks old to minimize the possibility of hemolytic anemia occurring in infants with insufficient vitamin E absorption. Iron is required at a dosage of 2 mg/kg per day starting by at least 2 months of age because the iron stores of preterm infants may become depleted earlier than those of full-term infants. Iron-fortified formulas supply sufficient iron to prevent iron deficiency in preterm infants.[35]

Calcium, phosphorus, and vitamin D supplementation in preterm infant formulas is necessary to ensure adequate bone mineralization and to prevent osteopenia and rickets.[35,40] The prevention of severe bone disease in preterm infants appears to depend on both high oral intakes of calcium and phosphorus and the intake of at least 500 IU of vitamin D per day.[35,40] (See Chapter 17, "Nutritional Products.")

Content of Various Milks

Comparison of Human Milk and Cow Milk

Cow milk is the nutrient source for commercially prepared milk-based infant formulas. Both human and cow milk are intricate liquids that contain more than 200 ingredients in the fat-soluble and water-soluble fractions. Nutrients contained in pooled human milk and in homogenized milk that meets minimum federal standards are listed in Table 6.

The two types of milk differ significantly in the quantity and availability of the nutrients. Mature human milk is more effective than cow milk in meeting the nutritional requirements of the human infant. Differences in milk composition reflect the different needs of the human infant and the calf. Both milks provide similar amounts of water and approximately the same quantity of energy. However, the nutrient sources for energy (i.e., calories) are different. Protein supplies approximately 7% of the calories in

TABLE 5 Supplemental fluoride dosage schedule (mg per day)

Age	Concentration of fluoride in drinking water (ppm)[a]		
	<0.3	0.3–0.7	>0.7
2 wk–2 yr	0.25	0	0
2–3 yr	0.50	0.25	0
3–16 yr[b]	1.00	0.50	0

[a]2.2 mg sodium fluoride contains 1 mg fluoride.
[b]The American Academy of Pediatrics recommends 16 as the termination age. The American Dental Association recommends 13 as the termination age.
Excerpted from *Am J Dis Child* 1980; 134: 866.

TABLE 6 Composition of mature human milk and cow milk

Composition	Human milk	Cow milk
Water (ml/100 ml)	87.1%	87.2%
Energy (kcal/100 ml)	69	66
Protein (g/100 ml)	0.9	3.1
(% of protein)		
Casein	40%	80%
Whey	60%	20%
(g/100mL)		
Alpha-lactalbumin	0.2–0.3	0.11
Beta-lactoglobulin	—	0.36
Lactoferrin	0.1–0.3	trace
Secretory IgA	0.05–0.1	trace
Albumin	0.05	0.04
Fat (g/100 ml)	4.0	3.8
Carbohydrate (g/100 ml)		
Lactose	6.8	4.9
Electrolytes (per liter)		
Calcium (mg)	340	1,200
Phosphorus (mg)	150	920
Calcium/phosphorus	2:1	1.2:1
Sodium (mg)	160	506
Potassium (mg)	530	1,570
Chloride (mg)	400	1,028
Magnesium (mg)	41	120
Sulfur (mg)	140	300
Minerals (per liter)		
Chromium (mcg)	4	2
Manganese (mcg)	4	20–40
Copper (mcg)	60	110
Zinc (mg)	0.5	3–5
Iodine (mcg)	200	80
Selenium (mcg)	20	5–50
Iron (mg)	0.5	0.5
Vitamins (per liter)		
Vitamin A (IU)	1,898	1,025
Thiamine (mcg)	150	370
Riboflavin (mcg)	380	1,700
Niacin (mcg)	1,700	900
Pyridoxine (mcg)	130	460
Pantothenate (mg)	2.6	3.6
Folic acid (mcg)	85	68
Vitamin B_{12} (mcg)	0.5	4
Vitamin C (mg)	43	17
Vitamin D (IU)	40	14
Vitamin E (mg)	3.2	0.4
Vitamin K (mcg)	34	170

Information extracted from from P. Pipes. *Nutrition in Infancy and Childhood.* 4th ed. St. Louis: Times Mirror/Mosby College Publishing: 1989: 89 and A.F. Williams. *Textbook of Paediatric Nutrition.* 3rd ed. London: Churchill Livingstone; 1991: 26–27.

human milk and 20% of the calories in cow milk. The low protein content of human milk is compensated by its higher protein quality (i.e., larger amounts of essential amino acids).[57] The carbohydrate lactose supplies approximately 42% of the calories in human milk and 30% of the calories in cow milk.[15] The percentage of calories provided by fat, approximately 50%, is similar in both milks. This percentage is higher than the 30% recommended for children older than 2 years, but there is a well-documented need for a higher dietary fat content for young infants with developing nervous systems.[30,57]

Carbohydrates

The carbohydrate percentage in cow milk is lower than the percentage in human milk, and carbohydrate supplementation is necessary for milk-based formulas. Honey and other unrefined foods are not recommended for carbohydrate supplementation because they may contain spores of *Clostridium botulinum*.[15] Lactose is the carbohydrate source in both cow milk and human milk. Lactose is absorbed into the brush border of the small intestine and is cleaved by the enzyme lactase into galactose and glucose. These sugars are then actively absorbed against concentration gradients.

Protein

Cow milk contains more than three times the ash (mineral residue) and protein normally found in human milk (3.5 g/100 mL of protein in cow milk versus 0.9 g/100 mL of protein in human milk).[15] This difference reflects the calf's more rapid growth rate and proportionate demand for protein and minerals. Although cow milk is usually administered to human infants diluted with water and carbohydrates, the solute load requiring renal excretion generally remains larger than the load from human milk.

Not only does cow milk contain a higher percentage of protein than human milk, but the protein differs in composition. This difference in protein composition alters digestibility and can create a milk sensitivity that may induce problems in the digestion of a milk-based formula or elicit an allergic response to milk protein. Milk proteins are defined broadly as either whey or casein. Human milk has an approximate whey-to-casein ratio of 60:40.[58] Cow milk, with a whey-to-casein ratio of 20:80, contains six to seven times more casein than does human milk. The whey protein in cow milk contains alpha-lactalbumin, beta-lactoglobulin, lactoferrin, serum albumin, lysozyme, and immunoglobulins A, G, and M (IgA, IgG, and IgM); human milk contains all of these proteins and immunologic factors except beta-lactoglobulin. Casein is relatively insoluble and is found in milk as a "tough" curd, whereas whey protein is highly soluble.[58] The large amount of casein in cow milk mixes with hydrochloric acid in the stomach to produce curds. This action slows the gastric emptying rate and may cause GI distress. Processing cow milk by acidification, boiling, or treatment with enzymes reduces curd tension and makes the milk more digestible. Because of its lower casein content, human milk forms a soft, flocculent, easy-to-digest curd.

Sensitivity to cow milk differs from milk allergy. Sensitivity may be relieved by altering the casein-to-lactalbumin ratio; however, an allergic reaction requires that all animal milk protein be eliminated from the diet. Although heating cow milk may increase its digestibility, it will not alter its antigen activity.

The amino acid content of cow milk is inappropriate for the neonate's immature enyzme system. The newborn has a limited ability to metabolize phenylalanine to tyrosine; human milk has low concentrations of these amino acids. High concentrations of these amino acids in cow milk have been associated with metabolic abnormalities.[57] Taurine and cystine are present in higher concentrations in human milk than in cow milk. In addition, cystathionase, an enzyme necessary for the transulfuration of methionine to cystine, is present in low concentrations in the neonate, which may explain the higher cystine content of human milk.[15]

Fat

Human milk and cow milk have similar total fat contents. Human milk contains 3–4.5% fat that consists of triglycerides (98 to 99% of total milk fat), phospholipids, and cholesterol. The fat composition of human milk changes during lactation; triglyceride concentrations rise and phospholipid and cholesterol concentrations decrease during the transition from colostrum to mature milk. When human milk is mature, the fat composition remains constant.[14]

Linoleic acid supplies an average of 7% (depending on the maternal diet) of the calories in human milk, but only 1% of the calories in cow milk. Most commercially prepared infant formulas contain more than 10% linoleic acid. Essential fatty acids should provide approximately 3% of the total caloric intake.[59] The cholesterol content varies in both milks, from 20 to 47 mg/100 mL in human milk and from 7 to 25 mg/100 mL in cow milk.[15]

The fat found in cow milk differs from that found in human milk in two ways. First, the triglycerides in cow milk contain primarily short- and long-chain fatty acids, whereas human milk fat contains medium-chain but not short-chain fatty acids. In addition, human milk contains primarily monounsaturated fatty acids, whereas the fat in cow milk (butterfat) consists principally of saturated fatty acids. Commercially prepared milk-based formulas incorporate the highly digestible unsaturated medium-chain triglycerides (MCTs) by replacing butterfat with vegetable oil and special MCT oils.

Both cow milk and human milk contain lipoprotein lipase, but human milk contains an additional lipase that contributes significantly to the higher percentage of absorption of human milk fat.[15] However, infants fed milk-based formula can efficiently digest fat from vegetable oil because of gastric enzyme activity.

Electrolytes and Minerals

The mineral content of cow milk is several times greater than that of human milk. Cow milk and human milk differ in absolute and proportionate amounts of calcium and phosphorus. The total calcium and phosphorus content of cow milk is approximately three and seven times that of human milk, respectively. Cow milk provides less calcium relative to phosphorus than does human milk. In cow milk–based formulas, the total concentration of calcium and phosphorus has been greatly reduced, but the calcium-to-phosphorus ratio imbalance persists and infants receive a relative phosphorus load that occasionally results in neonatal hypocalcemic tetany.[60] Calcium to phosphorus ratios are 2.4:1 in human milk, 1.3:1 in cow milk, and 1.3–1.4:1 in commercially prepared formulas.[60] The effect of differences in the calcium-to-phosphorus ratio on calcium absorption is not clear because of the interrelation of additional factors, such as vitamin D, fat absorption, and active transport.

The iron content of human milk decreases from 0.5 to 0.3 mg/L when the infant is between 2 weeks and 5 months of age. Levels of iron in cow milk remain at 0.5 mg/L throughout the time that the calf is nourished.[15] Because iron in human milk is more bioavailable, a nursing infant should be able to absorb approximately 50% of the iron from human milk (versus only 10% from cow milk).[48]

The zinc content of human milk is lower than that of cow milk, but it is more bioavailable (approximately 59% versus 42–50%).[61] Zinc binds strongly to casein in cow milk, whereas binding in human milk is minimal.

Cow milk contains more sodium, potassium, and chloride than does human milk. These higher electrolyte and mineral concentrations, when combined with the high protein content of cow milk, result in a smaller margin of safety against hyperosmolar dehydration. The larger renal solute load of cow milk, in combination with higher environmental temperatures or the presence of fever, vomiting, or diarrhea, can place an infant at risk for severe dehydration.

Reduced-Fat Cow Milk

Reduced-fat milks, such as skim milk (0.1% fat) and 2% milk (2% fat), have been used in an attempt to prevent obesity and atherosclerosis and to provide a "healthy diet."[62,63] The low-fat diet recommended for adults, when imposed on children younger than 2 years, puts them at risk for failure to thrive.[62] The CON/AAP does not recommend skim or 2% milks during the first 12 months of life.[51] Most dietitians and other nutrition experts agree that fat restriction is not recommended for young children.[63]

Infants who receive a major percentage of their caloric intake from reduced-fat milks such as skim or 2% milk may receive an exceedingly high protein intake and an inadequate intake of essential fatty acids. The maximum concentration of protein allowed in infant formulas is 4.5 g/100 kcal, but skim milk provides approximately 10 g of protein per 100 kcal and 2% milk provides nearly 7 g of protein per 100 kcal. Thus, a disadvantage of using reduced-fat milks as the only dietary source for infant nutrition is the unbalanced percentage of calories supplied from protein, fat, and carbohydrates.

It is important to recognize that, per unit volume, skim milk has a slightly higher PRSL than does whole cow milk (WCM) (Table 7). The solute concentration is further increased by water loss during boiling.[51] Reduced-fat milks are not recommended for the treatment of diarrhea because of the possibility of hypertonic dehydration.

Whole Cow Milk

The age at which it is appropriate to introduce unheated WCM into an infant's diet is controversial. Because the concentration and bioavailability of iron in WCM are low, WCM has been associated with iron-deficiency anemia.[51]

TABLE 7	Potential renal solute loads (PRSLs) of selected milks and infant formulas	
	PRSL	
	mOsm/L	mOsm/100 kcal
Human milk	93	14
Milk-based formula	135	20
Soy-based formula	177	26
Whole cow milk	308	46
Skim cow milk	326	93
FDA upper limit for PRSL	277	41

Adapted from Ziegler EE, Fomon SJ. Potential renal solute load of infant formulas. *J Nutr* 1989; 119 (suppl): 1785–8.

In the past decade, convincing evidence has accumulated that indicates that iron deficiency impairs psychomotor development and cognitive function in infants. This impairment has been observed even with relatively mild anemia. Through unknown mechanisms, WCM can also cause occult bleeding from the GI tract.[64] Milk-protein intolerance and/or allergy (estimated to affect 0.5–7.5% of the infant population in the first 2 years of life) poses another potential complication for the use of WCM.[64,65]

More research is needed to establish a time frame for the introduction of WCM. In 1976, the CON/AAP recommended that non–breast-fed infants receive an iron-fortified formula during the first 12 months of life. In 1983, the committee reversed its previous recommendation and concluded, "If breast feeding has been completely discontinued and infants are consuming one-third of their calories as supplemental foods consisting of a balanced mixture of cereal, vegetables, fruits, and other foods, whole milk may be introduced."[64,66] When WCM is fed together with solid food (beikost), infants receive unnecessarily high intakes of protein and electrolytes, resulting in a high renal solute load.[67] Also, infants fed an infant formula for the first year of life are less likely to develop iron deficiency.[7] The current position of the CON/AAP is that iron-fortified infant formula is the only acceptable alternative to breast milk. WCM and low-iron formulas are not recommended during the first year of life.[68]

Evaporated Milk

Evaporated milk is a sterile, convenient source of cow milk that has standardized concentrations of protein, fat, and carbohydrate. When ingested, evaporated milk produces a smaller, softer curd than that formed from boiled whole milk. Vitamin D is typically added to evaporated milk during processing, but evaporated milk formulas fail to meet recommendations for ascorbic acid, vitamin E for preterm infants, and essential fatty acids.[51,69,70]

Goat Milk

Goat milk is commercially available in powdered and evaporated forms. It contains primarily medium- and short-chain fatty acids and may be more easily digested than cow milk. Unfortified goat milk is deficient in folate and low in iron and vitamin D. The evaporated form of Meyenberg® goat milk is supplemented with vitamin D and folic acid. Powdered Meyenberg® goat milk is supplemented with folic acid only and is recommended for infants older than 1 year. Because the powder formulation is not a complete formula for infants, the manufacturer recommends supplementation with vitamins.

Breast-Feeding

The initial human breast milk is called colostrum. It is a clear, yellowish fluid that has a high protein content but lower fat and lactose concentrations than are found in mature human milk. It also has high concentrations of various immunologic factors. Within 1 week after delivery, human milk changes in its composition, at which time it is referred to as transitional milk. Approximately 3 weeks later breast milk is considered mature. Mature breast milk is the standard against which most commercially prepared infant formulas are compared.

During lactation a nursing mother may experience dramatic physiologic changes (e.g., increased cardiac output and increased blood flow to the breasts, intestinal tract, and liver). Blood flow to the breasts may be 500 times higher than the volume of milk (600–1,000 mL) produced daily. Maximum milk production occurs in the early morning hours (approximately 6 AM); the lowest production occurs between 6 AM and 10 PM. Thus, milk volume appears to be controlled by diurnal variation.[71] Some medications (e.g., vasoconstrictors) reduce blood flow to the breasts and thus decrease milk volume. Similarly, maternal stress and anxiety decrease milk production, as does the return of menses. The latter does this by reducing blood flow to the breasts.[71,72]

Although not bacteriologically sterile, human milk provides certain advantages over the use of cow milk, goat milk, and infant formulas. However, pharmacists should not issue dire warnings to mothers who cannot or do not wish to breast-feed; normal growth and development are possible without human milk.

Reported benefits of breast-feeding include protection against infections such as gastrointestinal illness and respiratory infection. Studies have shown that breast-fed infants have a lower incidence of gastroenteritis, fewer episodes of diarrhea, and infrequent hospitalizations for GI illness.[3] This lower rate may be particularly notable in infants born in nonindustrialized nations.

Conflicting results have been reported regarding breast-feeding and a low rate of respiratory infection. However, respiratory infections in breast-fed infants are likely to be of less severity.[3] Overall, the advantages of breast-feeding in lessening respiratory tract infections are most notable in the first 6 months of life.[3] Protective effects of breast-feeding also have been shown to decline in proportion to the degree of supplementation with formula or cow milk.

A review of the literature identifies studies that present conflicting data about other claimed advantages of breast-feeding.[73] Conditions on which conflicting data exist include sudden infant death syndrome, otitis media, urinary tract infections, bacteremia and meningitis, allergic disease, obesity, anemia, and childhood cancer.

Many questions about the apparent protective effect of breast-feeding remain to be answered. What is the duration of protection after breast-feeding is discontinued? What effect does change in age have on the protective effect? How great is the interactive effect of social and demographic variables? How does the addition of solid foods to the diet of a breast-fed infant influence the protective effect? What consequence does partial bottle-feeding have on the protective effect of breast-feeding? Better designed studies are needed to answer these questions and to document the protective effects of breast-feeding against a variety of infections.

Potential Problems with Breast-Feeding

Hyperbilirubinemia

One minor problem associated with human milk is the presence of increased levels of nonesterified fatty acid, caused by abnormal lipolytic activity, in the breast milk of some women.[74] This condition results in the inhibition of uridine diphosphate glucuronyl transferase and leads to a prolonged unconjugated hyperbilirubinemia in infants. However, breast-feeding need not be stopped in most cases of breast-milk jaundice;[75] the jaundice subsides even if breast-feeding is continued. If the infant appears in danger from hyperbilirubinemia itself, a temporary pause in breast-feeding for 1–3 days usually reduces the bilirubin to a safe level and can help determine the cause of bilirubin elevation. Formula feeding during this interval appears to increase stool volume and overall bilirubin elimination. Breast-feeding can then be resumed, although slight elevations or rebounds in serum bilirubin are often observed and may persist for several weeks.[76] No detrimental effects have been reported in infants as a result of breast-milk jaundice.

Human Immunodeficiency Virus

Although the risk of transmitting the human immunodeficiency virus (HIV) in breast milk appears to be low, there have been reports of such transmission.[77] Therefore, the Committee on Infectious Diseases of the AAP recommends that women in the United States who are HIV-infected should not breast-feed, nor should they donate breast milk to milk banks.[78] These recommendations may not be appropriate for women in developing countries, where infants may not receive adequate nutrition except from breast milk.[77]

Medications in Breast Milk

Oral Contraceptives Whether maternal use of an oral contraceptive while breast-feeding significantly affects lactation is debated. Some studies have found decreased milk production, changes in breast-milk protein composition, caloric deficits, and decreased weight gain in infants whose mothers used combination (estrogen- and progestogen-containing) oral contraceptives (COCs) while breast-feeding.[79–82]

Studies that have specifically addressed maternal use of COCs that contain 30–50 mcg of ethinyl estradiol or 50–100 mcg of mestranol have demonstrated that lactation is not inhibited after the immediate postpartum period. However, suppression of the quantity of milk produced and the duration of lactation may occur.[83,84] The use of COCs during lactation has not been clearly related to changes in milk composition. A study on the effects of two COCs and one progestogen-only oral contraceptive reported that milk volume and composition varied even in the absence of steroidal contraception but that changes remained within the normal ranges.[81]

Studies that address the use of progestogen-only oral contraceptives have shown no consistent alteration in breast milk composition, milk production, or lactation duration.[79,83] A study performed by the World Health Organization addressed the effects of a low-estrogen COC, a progestogen-only oral contraceptive, depot medroxyprogesterone acetate, and a nonhormonal birth control method. Women who used a COC had decreased milk volume, but their infants grew appropriately.[83]

AAP recommendations state that low-dose COCs or progestogen-only contraceptives are not contraindicated during breast-feeding as long as milk production has been established.[85,86]

Other Medications Health care personnel need to make decisions about the safety of drugs used by lactating mothers that might be ingested by a breast-feeding infant. Anderson's review of drug use during breast-feeding[87] and the textbook *Drugs in Pregnancy and Lactation*[79] are excellent sources of information.

Most medications are transferred from maternal blood to breast milk by passive diffusion, with the exception of water-soluble compounds of low-molecular weight (such as ethanol) that gain access to breast milk through water-filled pores. The transfer of a drug into breast milk is also dependent on a variety of other factors. Maternal factors include the dose of medication, route of administration, and pharmacokinetics of the drug. The pharmacokinetics may vary from the immediate postpartum period to a time several weeks after delivery when the physiologic changes of pregnancy wane. Alterations in renal function during pregnancy may affect drug clearance. These functions return to prepregnancy levels with time and thus may affect drug clearance. Blood flow to the breasts increases postpartum. Therefore, drug concentrations in the serum and milk of women several weeks or months postpartum may not be applicable to the early postpartum period. In addition, changes in breast milk composition from the immediate postpartum period through the weaning process may markedly affect drug excretion into breast milk.

Breast factors that affect a drug's ability to cross into breast milk include the quantity of blood flow to the breasts, pH differences between breast milk and maternal plasma, drug ionization, protein binding in breast milk, drug metabolism in breast milk, and possible reabsorption of a drug and/or its metabolites from breast milk into maternal blood.

Drug characteristics that affect passage into breast milk include molecular weight, plasma protein binding, lipid solubility, pKa, and maternal plasma pH versus breast milk pH. Most drugs can gain access to breast milk based on molecular weight; only drugs with high molecular weights (e.g., heparin) are unable to gain access. Typically, a low-molecular weight, un-ionized, basic compound that is lipid soluble and has a low plasma protein binding can easily cross into breast milk. In addition, when a weak base gains access to human milk, a shift in the ratio of un-ionized to ionized drug can occur in the relatively acidic breast milk and drug trapping results that inhibits passage back into maternal plasma.

Infant factors that must be considered include the infant's sucking pattern, time spent nursing during each feeding, milk volume consumed during feeding, the number of daily feeding periods, GI absorption of the drug by the infant, and the pharmacokinetics of the drug in infants. To determine the theoretical amount of drug that might be ingested by a breast-feeding infant, the reader is referred to the articles by Atkinson and colleagues.[88,89]

To help minimize an infant's intake of a medication via breast milk, the following strategies should be followed when possible:

- A drug should be selected from a class of drugs that is the least likely to be distributed into breast milk.
- A *nonoral* route that minimizes systemic absorption should be selected for maternal medication administration.
- Recommend a drug that can be taken as one daily dose.
- When multiple doses are needed, feedings should coincide with trough rather than peak drug concentrations.
- If there is concern about toxicity to the infant, the infant should be monitored and, if possible, serum or urine drug concentrations should be obtained.
- If the mother needs a short course of a drug that is not recommended during breast-feeding, breast-feeding may be interrupted for 4 to 5 half-lives. During this time, the infant should be given previously expressed breast milk or an infant formula and the woman should pump her breasts to prevent engorgement.
- If the breast-feeding infant is to be weaned soon, the mother could delay beginning a medication, if this option is medically acceptable.[90]

Medications listed in Table 8 are contraindicated during breast-feeding, should be used cautiously by nursing women, or require a temporary interruption of breast-feeding.[86,91]

Commercial Infant Formulas

Recommendations to standardize the nutrient composition of infant formulas were first published by the CON/AAP in 1967.[92] These recommendations were adopted by the FDA in 1971 and were revised by the AAP in 1976. The FDA published rules concerning the provision of nutrients in infant formulas in 1985.[93]

In 1978, two soy-based formulas were marketed that later were discovered to be deficient in chloride. Some children who received these formulas experienced a hypochloremic metabolic alkalosis and some failed to grow appropriately. Follow-up studies have shown that these children may be at risk for learning disabilities and language deficits.[94,95] As a result of this incident, the U.S. Congress passed an amendment to the Federal Food, Drug, and Cosmetic Act (Infant Formula Act of 1980) that gave the FDA authority to establish quality control, require adequate labeling, and revise nutrient levels.[93,96]

TABLE 8	Medications of concern to breast-feeding women

Medications contraindicated for breast-feeding[a]

Bromocriptine	Gold salts
Cimetidine	Lithium
Cyclophosphamide	Methimazole
Cyclosporine	Methotrexate
Doxorubicin	Phenindione
Ergotamine	

Medications to be used cautiously under medical supervision

Aspirin	Salicylazosulfapyridine
Phenobarbital	

A medication that requires temporary stopping of breast-feeding

Metronidazole

[a]In addition, all drugs of abuse (e.g., amphetamines, cocaine, heroin, marijuana, nicotine, and phencyclidine) are contraindicated for use during breast-feeding.

Manufacturers of infant formulas must follow regulations and quality control measures to ensure that infant formulas contain appropriate amounts of nutrients. Suppliers of ingredients used in infant formulas must provide "needed ingredients within rigid tolerance limits of quality" and comply with "good manufacturing practice."[10] Manufacturers may alter a formulation in response to changes in the availability of ingredients or modifications in recommended nutritional allowances, but such changes should not adversely affect the quality or consistency of the formula.[10] An accurate listing of the current ingredients and their quantities for a given formula may be obtained by direct communication with the manufacturer.

Microbiologic Safety

Guidelines of the Infant Formula Council (a voluntary nonprofit trade association composed of companies that manufacture and market infant formulas) require liquid formulations to be free of all viable pathogens, their spores, and other organisms that may cause product degradation. To ensure that this requirement is met, liquid formulas are usually sterilized by heat treatment and are incubated while samples are analyzed. Quality control measures help to ensure the production of a sterile product that is free of microbial effects as long as the container remains intact.[10] Powdered formulas are cultured to ensure that coliforms and other pathogens are absent and that the level of other microorganisms is below the acceptable level set by government standards. The heating required during the final preparation of the infant formula (as indicated on label directions) destroys most microorganisms.[10] If microbiologic contamination occurs, the infant ingesting such a formula could develop diarrhea with subsequent fluid and electrolyte losses.

Physical Characteristics

Infant formulas are emulsions of edible oils in aqueous solutions, but the separation of fat rarely occurs. If separation occurs, the fat can usually be redispersed by shaking the container, unless the separation occurred because of a lack of stabilizers or because the formula was stored beyond its shelf life.

Protein agglomeration may occur if storage time is excessive. This agglomeration may range from slight, grainy development through increased viscosity and formation of gels to eventual protein precipitation. Agglomeration and separation do not affect the safety or nutritional value of a formula; however, the appearance is a deterrent to its use.

Liquid infant formulas may contain thickening agents, stabilizers, and emulsifiers to provide uniform consistency and to prolong stability. Carrageen is a stabilizing agent found in many infant formulas.

Caloric Density
The RDA for energy is 108 kcal/kg per day for infants from birth to 6 months of age and 98 kcal/kg per day from age 6 months to 1 year.[19] A full-term infant should have no difficulty in consuming enough diluted formula (20 kcal/oz or 67 kcal/100 mL) to meet these caloric needs, but a preterm or LBW (less than 2,500 g) infant has a higher caloric need and may require as much as 130 kcal/kg per day.[59] An infant recovering from illness or malnutrition also requires more calories.[97] Infant formulas with caloric densities significantly lower or higher than 67 kcal/100 mL are regarded as therapeutic formulas to be used for the management of special clinical conditions and should be used only under medical supervision.

Osmolarity and Osmolality
The osmolarity of an infant formula may be expressed as the concentration of a solute per unit of total volume of solution or as the number of milliosmoles of solute per liter of solution (mOsm/L). Osmolarity cannot be measured but must be calculated using the osmolality value for the solution in question.[98] The osmolarity of human milk is approximately 273 mOsm/L. The CON/AAP recommends that formulas for normal infants have osmolarities no higher than 400 mOsm/L; formulas with higher osmolarities should have a warning statement on the label.[99] Infant formulas with 67 kcal/100 mL or 80 kcal/100 mL that are routinely used to feed preterm infants have osmolalities less than or equal to 300 mOsm/kg and pose no apparent increased risk of GI mucosal injury.[100] Hyperosmolar formulas have been implicated in the etiology of necrotizing enterocolitis.[20]

Osmolality may be expressed as the number of milliosmoles of solute per kilogram of solvent (mOsm/kg). "The osmolality of a formula is directly related to the concentration of molecular or ionic particles in a solution and is inversely proportional to the concentration of water in the formula."[101] The osmolality of human milk is approximately 290 mOsm/kg.[102] Osmolality is related to the carbohydrate and mineral content of the formula. For dilute solutions, there is little difference between osmolality and osmolarity. However, because infant formulas are relatively concentrated solutions, osmolarity may be only 80% of the osmolality.[101] Osmolality is the preferred term for reporting the osmotic activities of infant formulas because osmotic activity is a function of a solute–solvent relationship. However, manufacturers report both osmolality and osmolarity.

The relationship between osmolality and caloric density is reasonably linear in formulas with caloric densities of 44–90 kcal/100 mL, the range of caloric concentrations usually fed to infants.[101] If the osmolality of a 67 kcal/100 mL formula is known, the osmolality of a formula with a caloric density between 44 and 90 kcal/100 mL can be calculated, assuming a direct proportion between osmolality and caloric density. The osmolality of a formula increases with increasing caloric content.

There is no meaningful difference in the osmolalities of the commonly used ready-to-use formulas that provide 67 kcal/100 mL. The osmolalities of reconstituted concentrated products when diluted to provide 67 kcal/100 mL are not considerably different from the osmolalities of the corresponding ready-to-use products. Directions for diluting concentrated formulas must be followed exactly to prevent harmful hyperosmolar states, such as diarrhea and dehydration. Soy-protein formulas have lower osmolalities than the milk-based formulas because of differences in carbohydrate sources (milk-based formulas usually contain lactose; soy-protein formulas contain sucrose or corn syrup solids).

Renal Solute Load
Renal solute load is related to the protein, electrolyte, and mineral content of an infant formula. It represents the water-soluble substances that must be removed by the kidneys. (See "Infant Physiology and Growth" for more information on renal solute load.) Table 7 lists PRSLs for various milks and infant formulas and provides a comparison with the FDA upper limits for PRSL set for infant formulas.[16]

The renal solute load is important because it determines the quantity of water that is excreted by the kidneys. Infants have less ability to concentrate their urine than do older children and adults. Most infants can concentrate their urine to between 900 and 1,100 mOsm/kg, but some cannot concentrate to even 900 mOsm/kg. Thus, feeding an infant a formula that is too concentrated may produce a hypertonic urine that may cause dehydration because of increased renal losses. Under normal conditions, 67 kcal/100 mL infant formulas supply 1.5 mL of water per kilocalorie, an amount that provides adequate water for all losses, including urinary excretion. If an infant has a decreased water intake or an excessive loss, a diet that has a high renal solute load may stress the limited capacity of the infant's renal reabsorptive system. It has been suggested that the upper limit for protein in infant formulas be lowered from 4.5 to 3.2 g/100 kcal, which is the estimated protein requirement for an infant, and that the upper limit for phosphorus be less than 3 mOsm/100 kcal (93 mg/100 kcal). Such changes in two of the primary determinants of PRSL would enable an infant to maintain an adequate water balance and decrease the possibility of

TABLE 9 Indications for the use of therapeutic infant formulas

Problem	Suggested formula/product	Comments
Allergy or sensitivity to milk protein or soy protein	Protein hydrolysate formula (e.g., Alimentum, Nutramigen, or Pregestimil)	Protein allergy or sensitivity to cow milk
Biliary atresia	Portagen	Impaired digestion and absorption of long-chain fats
Carbohydrate intolerance	RCF, 3232A	Formulas are carbohydrate free; a source of carbohydrate that the patient can tolerate can be added
Cardiac disease	Enfamil, SMA, PM 60/40	Whey-predominant; low electrolyte content
Celiac disease	Pregestimil or Nutramigen, followed by a soy formula, and then a cow milk formula	Advance to more complete formula as intestinal epithelium returns to normal
Constipation	Routine formula, increase sugar	Mild laxative effect
Cystic fibrosis	Portagen, Pregestimil	Impaired digestion and absorption of long-chain fats
Diarrhea Chronic nonspecific Intractable	Routine formula or soy formula Pregestimil, Alimentum	Appropriate distribution of calories; impaired digestion of intact protein, long-chain fats, and disaccharides
Failure to thrive (e.g., when intestinal damage is suspected)	Pregestimil, Alimentum	Advance to more complete formula as intestinal epithelium returns to normal
Gastroesophageal reflux	Routine formula	Thicken with cereal (1 tbsp/oz of formula); try small frequent feedings
Homocystinuria	Low Methionine Analog XMET	Low content of methionine
Hepatitis Without liver failure With liver failure	Routine formula Portagen	Impaired digestion and absorption of long-chain fats
Lactose intolerance	Soy formula	Impaired digestion and utilization of lactose
Maple syrup urine disease	MSUD Diet Powder, Analog MSUD	Low content of leucine, isoleucine, and valine
Necrotizing enterocolitis (with resection)	Pregestimil (when oral feeding resumed)	Impaired digestion
Phenylketonuria	Lofenalac, Analog XP	Low content of phenylalanine
Prematurity (in those < 34 weeks gestational age)	Preterm infant formulas	Whey-predominant; easily digestible carbohydrates and fats; appropriate vitamin and mineral content
Renal insufficiency	Similac PM 60/40	Low phosphate content; low renal solute load

Supplemental information extracted from Walker WA, Hendricks KM. *Manual of Pediatric Nutrition*. 2nd ed. St. Louis: Mosby; 1990: 80.

hypernatremic dehydration secondary to a high PRSL (i.e., greater than or equal to 39 mOsm/100 kcal).[16]

Types, Uses, and Selection of Commercial Infant Formulas for Full-Term Infants

Formulas for full-term infants are milk-based or milk-based with added whey protein (whey-predominant). These formulas meet the minimum requirements for various nutrients per 100 kcal as required by the FDA and deemed appropriate by the CON/AAP. Other infant formulas are available for specific needs, but they should be used only on the advice of a physician.

Milk-Based Formulas

A milk-based formula is prepared from nonfat cow milk, vegetable oils, and added carbohydrate (lactose). The added carbohydrate is necessary because the ratio of carbohydrates to protein in nonfat milk solids from cow milk is less than is desirable for infant formulas. Protein provides approximately 9% of calories and fat furnishes 48–50% of calories.[100] The most widely used vegetable oils are corn, coconut, safflower, and soy. Replacement of the butterfat with vegetable oils allows for better fat absorption. Vitamins and minerals are added in accordance with the guidelines established by the FDA. Milk-based formulas are available as iron-fortified (approximately 1.8 mg/100 kcal) or low-iron (approximately 0.16 mg/100 kcal) formulas. Similac® is an example of a milk-based formula.

Milk-Based with Added Whey Protein

When whey is added in proper amounts to nonfat cow milk, the ratio of whey proteins to casein can be made to approximate that of human milk. The ratio of 60% whey to 40% casein in human milk differs considerably from the ratio in cow milk, in which casein accounts for approximately 80% of the protein and whey for only 20%.[59] Minerals are removed from whey by electrodialysis or ion-exchange processes and then are re-added to the formula to approximate the mineral content of human milk. Formulas containing partially demineralized whey proteins are not nutritionally superior to milk-based formulas. The high nutritional quality and relatively low renal solute load of these formulas are assets in the therapeutic management of ill infants. Enfamil® and SMA® are examples of whey-predominant formulas.

Therapeutic Formulas

Therapeutic infant formulas are used on an individual basis for infants being treated by medical specialists for conditions that require dietary adjustment. Table 9 lists indications for using various therapeutic infant formulas; Table 10 lists formulas for infants who have a variety of metabolic disorders. Therapeutic formulas include soy-protein formulas, casein-based formulas, casein or whey hydrolysate–based formulas, low-sodium formulas, a variety of formulas needed for specific medical problems, and formulas for LBW infants or for specific age groups.

Soy-Protein Formulas

Soy-protein formulas contain methionine-fortified isolated soy protein.[51] Vegetable oils provide the fat content, and corn syrup solids and/or sucrose supply the carbohydrate in these formulas. Vitamin K is added to provide a concentration of 15 mcg/100 kcal. Other vitamins, taurine, and carnitine (necessary for optimal oxidation of fatty acids) are also added. Carnitine supplementation of soy-protein formulas is necessary because of carnitine's low concentrations in foods of plant origin compared with foods of animal origin.[103]

About 15% of infants fed formulas receive soy-protein formulas such as Isomil®, Nursoy®, ProSobee®, Soyalac®,

TABLE 10 Formulas for infants with metabolic diseases

Disease	Product
Glutaric aciduria type 1	Analog XLYS, TRY
Homocystinuria	3200K-Low Methionine Diet Powder Analog XMET
Hypercalcemia	Calcilo XD
Hypermethioninemia	Analog XMET
Leucine catabolism disorders	Analog XLEU
Maple syrup urine disease	MSUD Powder Analog MSUD
Methylmalonic acidemia	80056-Protein Free Diet Powder Analog XMET, THRE, VAL, ISOLEU
Phenylketonuria	Lofenalac Analog XP
Propionic acidemia	80056-Protein Free Diet Powder Analog XMET, THRE, VAL, ISOLEU
Tyroseinemias	3200 AB-Low Phe/Tyr Diet Powder Analog XPHEN, TYR Analog XPHEN, TYR, MET

Adapted from:
Pediatric Products Handbook. Evansville, Ind: Mead Johnson Nutritionals; 1990.
Ross Laboratories Product Handbook. Columbus, Ohio: Ross Laboratories; 1990.

and I-Soyalac®.7 These formulas differ in amounts of ingredients, source of carbohydrates, and constituents of the fat source. The fat source in Soyalac® and I-Soyalac® is soy oil; Isomil® contains soy and coconut oils; ProSobee® contains soy, coconut, palm, and sunflower oils; Nursoy® contains safflower, soy, and coconut oils.

The carbohydrate source is an important factor in product selection. Isomil® and Soyalac® contain corn syrup solids and sucrose; Nursoy® and I-Soyalac® contain only sucrose; ProSobee® contains only corn syrup solids. Consequently, infants who are sensitive to corn and corn products and who cannot tolerate a milk-based formula may benefit from a corn-free soy-protein formula. Caution is advised, however, when the type of formulation is selected. The powdered formulation of Nursoy® contains corn syrup solids; the liquid concentrate and ready-to-use formulations do not.

Soy-protein formulas are lactose free and therefore can be used for infants with primary lactase deficiency (e.g., galactosemia) and for those with secondary lactose intolerance resulting from enteric infection or other causes of mucosal damage.[51] Resumption of a cow milk formula is generally possible 2–4 weeks after cessation of diarrhea.[97] Soy-protein formulas are also a nutritional source for infants whose parents are vegetarians.

RCF® (Ross Carbohydrate Free) soy-protein formula does not contain a carbohydrate source. This formula may be used in the dietary management of infants unable to tolerate the type or amount of carbohydrates in cow milk or other infant formulas. A physician may select a carbohydrate source (sucrose, dextrose, fructose, or glucose polymers) that can be added before feeding. RCF® is for use only under medical supervision.

Some infants with gastroenteritis develop intolerance to lactose and sucrose because of secondary lactase and sucrase deficiency. Isomil SF® and ProSobee® contain corn syrup solids (hydrolyzed corn starch, a glucose polymer) as the carbohydrate source and can thus be used in this situation.

Food allergy occurs in infants because the immature digestive and metabolic processes may not be completely effective in converting dietary proteins into nonantigenic amino acids. The incidence of cow milk allergy in the first 2 years of life is estimated to be 0.5–7.5%.[104] The diagnosis of cow milk allergy is defined as symptomatology involving the respiratory tract, skin, or GI tract that disappears when cow milk is removed from the diet and reappears on two separate challenges when cow milk is given during a symptom-free period. Rechallenge must be done with caution.[105]

Soy-protein formulas are promoted for use in the management of allergy to cow milk or for infants suspected of having milk allergy. However, the CON/AAP recommends that protein hydrolysate formulas rather than soy-protein formulas be used for infants with documented clinical allergy to cow milk and/or soy protein.[7,103] This recommendation is based on the concern that infants with severe allergy to cow milk—such as severe diarrhea, vomiting, laryngeal edema, urticaria, or wheezing—have intestinal mucosal damage sufficient to expose them to higher concentrations of foreign protein in soy-protein formulas. Such infants have demonstrated severe allergic manifestations when fed soy-protein formulas.[106,107] Most infants suspected of having adverse reactions to milk-based formulas have not experienced life-threatening manifestations and appear to tolerate soy-protein formulas, which are less expensive, better tasting, and have been more extensively studied than protein hydrolysate formulas.[7]

For infants who have a family history of atopy but who have not shown clinical manifestations of allergy, a soy-protein formula may be used with caution.[103] These infants should be monitored closely for allergy to soy protein.

The soy-protein source in these formulas provides an alternative for vegetarian families who do not wish to use animal protein formulas.

Soy-protein formulas should not be used for the routine feeding of preterm and LBW infants. In addition, soy-protein formulas are not recommended for infants with CF because these children do not adequately utilize soy protein, will lose substantial amounts of nitrogen in their stools, and may develop hypoproteinemia or even anasarca. Formula-fed infants with CF appear to do best nutritionally when given an easily utilized formula that contains predigested protein and MCTs (e.g., a casein hydrolysate–based formula).

Casein Hydrolysate-Based Formulas

Casein hydrolysate–based formulas are effective in the nutritional management of infants with a variety of severe GI abnormalities in which intolerance to enteral feeding and the malabsorption of standard forms of protein, fat, and carbohydrate are common. Indications for use include severe or intractable diarrhea, severe food allergies, sensitivity to intact protein, transition from parenteral feeding to normal diet, disaccharidase deficiency, intestinal resection, dysfunctional malabsorption, steatorrhea, CF, protein-calorie malabsorption, and severe protein-calorie malnutrition.

Use of these formulas for allergy prophylaxis remains controversial. Studies indicate that prolonged breast-feeding or extended use of hypoallergenic formulas and delayed introduction of solids helps prevent allergic disease in infancy, but other studies challenge these findings.[108] To date, the effectiveness of dietary and environmental regimens in the prevention of allergic disease have not been conclusively proven in prospective studies. Infants with documented clinical allergic symptoms to cow milk may benefit from a protein hydrolysate formula because approximately 15–50% of these infants also react to soy protein.[109]

There appear to be few data to support an association between colic and infant formula ingestion.[110] In selected situations, improvement occurs when cow milk or soy protein is eliminated and a hydrolysate formula is introduced. For this reason, some experts have suggested decreasing cow milk protein and/or soy protein in the diets of children with moderate to severe colic.[111] However, in the vast majority of infants, symptoms of colic persist after formula changes. In cases where improvement was noted, it was difficult to definitely attribute the improvement to a formula change.[110,111] Currently, no evidence exists that supports the use of hydrolysate formulas for treating colic, restlessness, or irritability.[108] These are common symptoms in infants but they rarely occur as a result of immune-mediated reaction to cow milk protein.

Extensively hydrolyzed casein protein makes formulas less palatable. However, infants usually accept the feedings satisfactorily. If the formula is rejected when first offered, it may be tried again after a few hours. These products are designed to provide a sole source of nutrition for infants up to 4–6 months of age and to provide a primary source of nutrition through 12 months of age when indicated. Extended use of hydrolysate formulas as a sole source of nutrition in children older than 6 months requires physician monitoring on a case-by-case basis.[112]

Pregestimil®, Nutramigen®, Alimentum®, and 3232A® are formulas with enzymatic hydrolysates of casein as the protein source. They contain nonantigenic polypeptides with less than 1,200 molecular weight;[108] therefore, they can be fed to infants who are sensitive to intact milk protein or other foods. These formulas differ from other formulas in that alpha-amino nitrogen is supplied by enzymatically hydrolyzed charcoal-treated casein rather than whole protein. Casein hydrolysate formulas are supplemented with three amino acids—L-cystine, L-tyrosine, and L-tryptophan—because the concentrations of these amino acids are reduced during charcoal treatment.

The carbohydrate sources in these formulas vary. Nutramigen® contains corn syrup solids and modified corn starch; Pregestimil® contains corn syrup solids, dextrose, and modified corn starch; Alimentum® contains sucrose and modified tapioca starch; and 3232A® contains tapioca starch as a stabilizer and no other source of carbohydrate.

Glucose polymers in corn syrup solids or modified corn starch are particularly useful in infants with malabsorption disorders, who are frequently intolerant to lactose, sucrose, and glucose. Glucose polymers are more easily digested and tolerated by infants whose capacity to handle lactose and sucrose may be impaired.[59] In addition, glucose polymers are a low-osmolar form of carbohydrate and contribute little to the total osmolar load. This is an advantage in infants with intestinal disorders who cannot tolerate the osmolar load of disaccharide- or glucose-containing elemental diets.

MCTs and corn oil are the fat sources found in 3232A®. Pregestimil® contains the same types of fat and also contains high-oleic safflower oil. Nutramigen® contains only corn oil, and Alimentum® contains safflower and soy oil (sources of linoleic acid) in addition to MCTs. MCTs do not require emulsification with bile and are more easily hydrolyzed than long-chain fats. Shorter chain fatty acids and MCTs are directly absorbed into the portal system. In addition, MCTs enhance the absorption of long-chain triglycerides. Formulas in which 40% of the fat consists of MCTs have been shown to relieve steatorrhea, promote weight gain, and improve calcium absorption in LBW infants.[113–115] Formulas in which at least 80% of the fat consists of MCTs improve calcium absorption[115] and increase magnesium absorption.[59,114] A possible adverse effect of MCT malabsorption from overfeeding or intestinal mucosal disease is diarrhea.[59]

Pregestimil® Pregestimil® is an effective nutritional source for infants with massive bowel resection (short-gut syndrome), severe diarrhea, protein-calorie malnutrition, milk and soy-protein intolerance, transition from intravenous parenteral nutrition, GI immaturity, or CF. Pregestimil® is also effective in the intractable diarrhea syndrome of infancy. Pregestimil® is not to be used routinely as a nutrient source for highly stressed LBW infants because of the increased risk of GI complications.[112]

Nutramigen® Nutramigen® is nutritionally effective for infants with severe diarrhea or GI disturbances and for infants who are allergic or intolerant to intact proteins of cow milk and other foods. In cases of galactosemia, a relatively rare disorder resulting from a deficiency of galactose-*l*-phosphate uridyltransferase or galactokinase, it is necessary to eliminate dietary lactose so that the body may convert glucose to the amount of galactose it requires. Infants with galactosemia may be fed formulas without lactose or sucrose (Nutramigen®, Pregestimil®, Alimentum®, or ProSobee®).

Alimentum® Alimentum® is composed of hydrolyzed casein supplemented with free amino acids and a blend of medium- and long-chain triglycerides. The addition of long-chain triglycerides improves the palatability but increases the allergenic potential for infants with cow milk allergy.[116] Alimentum® contains two carbohydrates (sucrose and modified tapioca starch) in lower concentrations than are found in other hydrolysate formulas. These carbohydrates are digested and absorbed by separate mechanisms (principally glucoamylase and sucrase-alpha-dextrinase). This formula can be used for infants with protein sensitivity, pancreatic insufficiency (e.g., that caused by CF), or intractable diarrhea.

3232A® The fat source in 3232A®, a monosaccharide- and disaccharide-free formula base, is 87% MCTs and 13% corn oil. Tapioca starch is used as a stabilizer and is the only carbohydrate in the formula base. The physician selects the carbohydrate source (e.g., sucrose, dextrose, fructose, or glucose polymers). The formula base is iron fortified and contains all essential vitamins and minerals. It can be used for infants with disaccharidase deficiencies, impaired glucose transport, or intractable diarrhea.

Sodium Caseinate Formula

Portagen® is a sodium caseinate formula. It contains corn syrup solids and sucrose as its carbohydrate sources. MCTs account for 87% of its fat. It also contains higher concentrations of both lipid- and water-soluble vitamins than are found in casein hydrolysate formulas. Higher concentrations of MCTs and vitamins in Portagen® compensate for their impaired digestion or absorption from conventional foods. Portagen® has been effective in feeding infants with pancreatic insufficiency (e.g., that caused by CF), bile acid deficiency, intestinal resection, lymphatic anomalies, and celiac disease. It can be used, on a physician's recommendation, as a sole dietary source for both infants and older children, or as a beverage to be consumed with each meal.

Whey Hydrolysate–Based Formulas

Casein hydrolysate formulas have been used for many years for infants with defects in protein digestion and adverse reactions to intact cow milk protein. Recently, heat-treated whey protein has been used as the protein source for an infant formula (Carnation Good Start H.A.®) for similar purposes. Enzymatic hydrolysates of whey contain some peptides with molecular weights greater than 2,000; these can increase the antigenicity of the product.[108] Anaphylactic-type reactions have been reported in patients with severe milk allergy who received hydrolysate formulas.[117] Therefore, whey hydrolysate–based formulas should not be used for infants with documented IgE-mediated allergy to cow milk protein.[104] The effectiveness of whey hydrolysate formula in infants with GI intolerance to cow milk but who are not allergic to cow milk suggests that it may be an acceptable alternative to milk-based and soy-protein formulas. This product is promoted as having a pleasant taste, smell, and appearance, and it may be better accepted than casein-hydrolysate formulas, which mothers and infants find noticeably different from milk-based and soy-protein formulas in appearance and taste.

Low Sodium Formulas

Infants with congestive heart failure, hypertension, nephrosis, or acute nephritis often require a formula with an increased caloric concentration because these infants may tire during feeding before they have consumed an adequate volume of formula. In addition, an excessive renal load needs to be avoided in these patients. The relatively low renal solute load and adequate caloric intake of whey-predominant milk formulas (SMA®, Similac PM 60/40®, and Enfamil®) permit their use in the long-term management of infants who require sodium restriction. Of these formulas, SMA® contains the smallest amount of sodium (15 mg/100 mL, equivalent to the sodium concentration found in breast milk).

Metabolic Formulas

Infants with inherited metabolic disorders require specific formulas tailored to their particular conditions. Table 10 lists various metabolic diseases and formulas available to treat them.

Low Birthweight and Preterm Formulas

LBW infants (infants weighing less than 2,500 g) and preterm infants (less than 38 weeks gestation, but especially those less than 34 weeks), because of their increased caloric needs and decreased ability to consume an adequate volume of formula, may need formulas that offer a higher caloric concentration for growth. For very-low-birthweight (VLBW) infants, human milk is insufficient in protein, phosphorus, and calcium.[118] The nutritional goal for preterm infants is to achieve postnatal growth that approximates the in-utero growth of a normal fetus at the same postconception age. No commercially available formula is completely satisfactory for LBW or VLBW infants; however, improvements in special formulas permit individualization of dietary regimens for these infants. Examples of special formulas that may be beneficial are Enfamil® Premature Formula®, Preemie SMA®, Similac® Special Care®, and Similac PM 60/40®. These formulas share common features, such as whey-predominant proteins; carbohydrate mixtures of lactose, corn syrup solids, and glucose polymers; and fat mixtures containing combinations of MCTs and long-chain triglycerides. They may differ in electrolyte, vitamin, mineral, and caloric content. Each formula has been shown to be associated with adequate growth and metabolic stability in preterm infants. An isotonic osmolality (approximately 300 mOsm/kg of water) is maintained at a dilution of 24 kcal/oz or 80 kcal/100 mL.[100]

Preterm and LBW infants are especially susceptible to iron deficiency anemia because they have lower iron stores. Without supplemental iron, body stores of iron in these infants will be depleted by 2 months of age, in contrast to depletion at 4–6 months of age in full-term infants.[19] Therefore, iron supplementation at 2 mg/kg per day is recommended by the CON/AAP for infants older than 2 months.[19] Iron supplementation before 2 months of age must be accompanied by ample vitamin E and PUFA additions to the diet to reduce the possibility of hemolytic anemia from vitamin E deficiency. Furthermore, a formula without iron is preferable for VLBW infants in the first 2–4 postnatal weeks to prevent decreased vitamin E serum concentrations.[119]

Human Milk Fortifiers

Commercial products have been developed to enhance the nutrient content of human milk. Enfamil® Human Milk Fortifier is a powder that can add nutrients to human milk without displacing volume, which allows for a higher intake of human milk. Similac Natural Care® is a liquid that may be given alternately with human milk or mixed in various ratios with human milk. Both products are made from cow milk with a whey-to-casein ratio of 60:40 and a carbohydrate mixture of lactose and glucose polymers. Enfamil® Human Milk Fortifier contains little fat and Similac Natural Care® contains a mixture of medium- and long-chain triglycerides. Studies support adequate weight gain and nutrient retention in infants when either human milk with fortifier or preterm commercial formulas are ingested.[120–122]

Whether human milk provides optimal nutrition for VLBW infants is a controversial issue. Mothers who deliver preterm produce milk that is higher in protein, sodium, potassium, and possibly other nutrients than is the milk of mothers who deliver at term. However, it is thought that these nutrients gradually decline to levels found in mature milk at 4–8 weeks postdelivery.

Most of the mineral content for an infant's development is delivered through the placenta during the last 2 months of gestation. During the third trimester, the fetus receives 125–150 mg of calcium per day and 65–80 mg of phosphorus per day, which is primarily deposited in bone. Human milk, preterm or mature, cannot supply the amount of calcium and phosphorus needed for the prevention of osteopenia of prematurity.[120]

Concentrated Formulas

A child with special nutritional needs that exceed normal requirements may be given concentrated formula under medical supervision. Concentrated ready-to-use formulas made from cow milk are available in concentrations of 24 kcal/oz; some are available in concentrations of 27 kcal/oz. Various concentrations can be prepared from liquid concentrates or powdered products by varying the amount of water added. (Tables 11 and 12). When concentrated formulas are used, the resulting increase in protein and electrolytes and decrease in fluid require careful monitoring of the infant's fluid intake and output, weight, serum electrolytes, blood urea nitrogen, and urine specific gravity and osmolality.[97]

Modular components are available as an alternative to formula concentration. Carbohydrates can be added in liquid or powdered form. Protein powder is available, but it should be used with caution because its use may increase the renal solute load. Fat may be added as MCTs (MCT Oil) for infants with fat malabsorption or intolerance. Microlipid, made from safflower oil, is also available as an emulsion that mixes well with formula.

Formula for Children Aged 1–6 Years

PediaSure® is a nutritionally complete, isotonic, lactose-free enteral formula designed for young children who cannot tolerate a normal diet or eat solid food. PediaSure® has a pleasant taste and can be used as a supplement to increase caloric intake. It contains adequate amounts of calcium, phosphorus, iron, and vitamin D for this age group; the amounts contained in adult nutritional enteral products are typically inadequate for children aged 1–6 years. PediaSure® with Fiber will soon be available.

Possible Problems with Infant Formulas

Diarrhea

Infants are particularly susceptible to dehydration because of their high metabolic rate and ratio of surface area to weight and height. Fluid volume depletion by diarrhea may quickly (within 24 hours) produce severe dehydration with fluid and electrolyte imbalances, shock, and possible death. A common cause of diarrhea is the improper dilution of a concentrated liquid or powdered formula.

If diarrhea is a problem, the pharmacist should ascertain the severity and duration of the diarrhea, frequency of stools, and method of preparing the infant formula. If the diarrhea is serious (many more stools per day than normal) or has continued for 48 hours or if the infant is clinically ill (with fever, lethargy, anorexia, irritability, dry mucous membranes, decreased urine output, or weight loss), the infant should be referred to a physician. (See Chapter 13, "Antidiarrheal Products.")

Mild diarrhea of short duration may resolve without medical measures, but the infant should be observed closely. Although improper digestion of the infant's formula may initiate diarrhea, continuation of a formula while diarrhea persists may yield only marginal nutrient absorption. A temporary (24-hour) discontinuation of usual dietary intake may be helpful. Oral electrolyte replacement solutions (e.g., Lytren®, Pedialyte®, Ricelyte®, or Infalyte® Powder) may be used cautiously for short-term management of fluid and electrolyte loss. However, these solutions should not be used when parenteral rehydration is required, nor should they be used to provide adequate nutrition. A solution such as Pedialyte® should not replace infant formula for the baby after diarrhea has ceased. A nutritionally adequate formula should be resumed under a physician's direction.

There are various recommendations for resuming formula. Formula may be resumed at half strength for 24 hours and then increased to full strength over a 48-hour period. If diarrhea resumes when formula is reintroduced, a lactose-free formula such as one of the soy-protein formulas may be used at half strength for 24 hours or resumed at full strength; then full-strength soy-protein formula may be used for 1–3 weeks (length of time is dependent on the severity of the diarrhea); finally, a milk-based formula may be resumed.[11]

Other Gastrointestinal Problems

Adverse effects of formula on an infant's GI tract range from mechanical obstruction (inspissated milk curds), diarrhea, and dehydration from a hyperosmolar formula to a hypersensitivity from specific milk protein. Intolerance to cow milk is associated most frequently with inability to digest lactose or milk proteins. It is estimated that approximately 15% of infants in the United States are fed soy-protein formulas because of concerns about cow milk allergy or sensitivity.[7]

Hyperosmolar formulas may adversely affect LBW infants during the early neonatal period and may be a potential cause of necrotizing enterocolitis.[20] Appropriately prepared formulas for LBW infants (20–24 kcal/oz) are isotonic, with osmolalities less than or equal to 300 mOsm/kg; other infant formulas in concentrations of 20–24 kcal/oz have osmolalities of less than or equal to 400 mOsm/kg.[100]

Tooth Decay

Baby bottle tooth decay can occur in children who bottle-feed beyond the typical weaning period and is especially prevalent in children who sleep with their bottles after 1 year of age. Caries are seen in children younger than 2 years and may involve the maxillary incisors, maxillary and mandibular first molars, or maxillary and mandibular canines.[123]

Nutritional Deficiencies

Generally, infant formulas have proven to be nutritionally adequate and safe. A number of past nutritional deficiencies associated with infant formulas have been corrected with appropriate supplementation procedures and technological advances in processing infant formulas. Some deficiencies that have occurred include the following:

- Vitamin K deficiency occurred in infants who were fed certain soy or non–milk-based formulas.[43,124,125]
- Vitamin E deficiency and hemolytic anemia were reported in LBW infants who received iron-fortified formulas with high concentrations of PUFA.[35]
- Thiamine deficiency developed in infants fed soy-protein formulas low in thiamine.[126]
- Convulsions occurred in infants who received pyridoxine-deficient formulas.[127]
- Goiters were observed in infants who were fed soy-protein formulas that were not supplemented with iodine.[128]
- Metabolic alkalosis developed in infants fed soy-protein formulas that contained low concentrations of chloride.[129] Some children who received these formulas failed to grow appropriately. These children may be at an increased risk for learning disabilities and deficits in language skills.[94,95]

In a more recent problem, rickets occurred in VLBW infants who received a soy-protein formula; this condition was caused by poor absorption of the calcium, phosphorus, and vitamin D contained in the formula.[130,131]

A new potential problem is possible vitamin D over- or undersupplementation of infant formulas and fortified milk. Researchers who measured the vitamin D content of five brands of infant formulas (10 samples) determined that none of the samples had vitamin D concentrations within 20% of the labeled content. None contained less than the amount of vitamin D stated on the label, but 70%

TABLE 11	Dilution of concentrated liquid infant formulas[a]	
Desired caloric concentration (kcal/oz)	Amount of liquid formula concentrate (oz)	Amount of water to add (oz)
10	1	3
20	1	1
24	3	2
26–27	3	1.5
28–29	5	2

[a]Commercial infant formula concentrates that contain 40 kcal per fluid ounce before dilution with water.

Adapted from Walker WA, Hendricks KM. *Manual of Pediatric Nutrition*. 2nd ed. St. Louis: Mosby; 1990: 86.

of the samples contained more than 200% of the labeled amount. One formula contained 419% of the labeled vitamin D content. This study also found inconsistency in the vitamin D content of fortified milk: 26 of 42 milk samples (62%) contained less than 80% of the labeled amount of vitamin D. In skim milk samples, 3 of 14 samples contained no detectable vitamin D. The authors concluded that better monitoring of vitamin D fortification is needed.[132]

Recently there has been concern about possible aluminum contamination of infant formulas, especially if such formulas are ingested by infants who have immature or impaired renal function. Infants fed soy formulas have been shown to have serum aluminum concentrations similar to those found in breast-fed infants, who have lower aluminum intakes. However, serum concentrations may not accurately reflect the body aluminum load because aluminum may be deposited in tissue as well as in the blood.

The highest concentrations of aluminum (455–2,346 mcg/L) have been reported in soy-based formulas.[133] Human milk typically contains less than 5–45 mcg of aluminum per liter and cow milk–based formulas have concentrations of 14–565 mcg/L. Formulas containing plant proteins, such as soy, appear to have higher aluminum concentrations because plants receive high aluminum concentrations from soil. The CON/AAP has stated that daily elemental aluminum doses in infants and children with underlying renal disease should not exceed 300,000 mcg/kg. The Joint Expert Committee on Food Additives of the Food and Agricultural Organization of the United Nations has set the maximum aluminum intake for infants, children, and adults at 7,000 mcg/kg.[133]

Formula Preparation

The preparation of infant formula requires careful technique. For all formulas, including special dilutions of therapeutic formulas and other modified formulas, the directions on the product container should be followed closely. If bottles with disposable plastic liners are used, the formula should not be mixed in the liner but should be prepared before the formula is poured into the liner; the measurements on the bottle are only approximate.

Infant formulas are available in three types: liquid ready-to-use, liquid concentrate, and powdered concentrate. Ready-to-use formulas do not require the addition of water and, as the name implies, are ready for use. Concentrated liquid and powdered formulations require the addition of water. Mixing equal amounts of water and concentrated liquid formula (e.g., 4 oz water to 4 oz formula) provides the desired 20 kcal/oz or 67 kcal per 100 mL formula (Table 11). Most powdered formulas require the addition of 1 packed level measure (1 tbsp) of powder for every 2 oz water to obtain a concentration of 20 kcal/oz (Table 12).[15,134]

McJunkin and colleagues reported that 11% of formulas (133 samples) provided and classified by mothers as either ready-to-use or concentrates were either hypoconcentrated (6%) or hyperconcentrated (5%).[135] Haschke et al. stated that 11–21% of formulas prepared from powdered concentrates by 88 women were hyperosmolar because of improper reconstitution.[136] Failure to properly dilute a concentrated formula can result in a hypertonic solution, precipitating diarrhea and dehydration. In extreme cases, the ingestion of overly concentrated formula has produced renal failure, disseminated intravascular coagulation, gangrene of the legs, and coma resulting from hypernatremic dehydration and metabolic acidosis.[15,137]

Overdiluting infant formulas or substituting water for milk may lead to water intoxication, which may result in irritability, hyponatremia, coma, or brain damage.[15] Such a situation may occur when a parent or caregiver misunderstands the instructions for preparing a concentrated formula, dilutes a ready-to-use formula, or tries to make a formula last longer by diluting it further.[15]

Because infants are susceptible to infection, various methods (e.g., the aseptic method and the terminal heating

TABLE 12	Dilution of concentrated powdered infant formulas[a]	
Desired caloric concentration (kcal/oz)	Amount of powdered formula concentrate (tbsp)[b]	Amount of water to add (oz)
10	1	4
20	1	2
24	3	5
28	7	10

[a]Powdered infant formulas that contain 40 kcal per level, packed tablespoonful before dilution. Because the powder displaces water and makes the volume larger and the formula more dilute, water should be added to the powder to equal the volume expected if a large volume of formula is to be prepared.
[b]1 tablespoonful = 1 scoop.

Adapted from Walker WA, Hendricks KM. *Manual of Pediatric Nutrition*. 2nd ed. St. Louis: Mosby; 1990: 86.

TABLE 13 Methods for infant formula preparation

Aseptic Method

(For the preparation of infant formulas from concentrated liquid or powder formulas and ready-to-use formulas)

For all types:
- Wash hands before preparing formula and again if interrupted during preparation. Wash all needed equipment (e.g., glass measuring cup, spoons, bottles, nipples, rings, and discs) with hot water and detergent. Rinse well with hot running water.
- Boil all needed equipment for 5 minutes in a covered pan or sterilizer in enough water to cover all items. Let the pan cool. Remove all items from the pan or sterilizer with tongs and place them on a clean towel.

For concentrated liquid or powder:
- While the equipment is being cleaned, boil water for formula preparation in a clean covered pan or teakettle for 5 minutes.
- Remove the boiled water from the stove and allow it to cool with the lid left in place.

For concentrated liquid:
- Let boiled water cool to almost room temperature.
- Wash the top of the can with hot water and detergent, rinse in hot running water, and dry. Shake the can, open it with a clean punch-type can opener, and mix appropriate amounts of concentrated liquid and sterilized water. The amounts of concentrated liquid and sterilized water added to the bottle(s) depend on the amount of formula needed per feeding. All measurements should be made with a measuring cup for accuracy, carefully following product instructions.
- Pour the formula into the sterilized bottles. Place nipples, rings, and discs on the bottles. Bottles can be stored in the refrigerator for up to 48 hours.
- Tightly cover any remaining concentrated liquid; store in the refrigerator for up to 48 hours.

For concentrated powder:
- Let boiled water cool to approximately 100°F (38°C).
- Wash the top of the can with hot water and detergent, rinse in hot running water, and dry. Open the can and mix appropriate amounts of powder and sterilized water. The amounts of powder and sterilized water added to the bottle(s) depend on the amount of formula needed per feeding. All measurements should be made with a measuring cup for accuracy, carefully following product instructions.
- Pour the formula into the sterilized bottles. Place nipples, rings, and discs on the bottles. Bottles can be stored in the refrigerator for up to 24 hours.
- Cover can with remaining powder with its plastic top. Store in a cool, dry place for up to 1 month.

For ready-to-use:
- Wash the top of the can with hot water and detergent, rinse in hot running water, and dry. Shake the can and open it with a clean punch-type can opener. Add amount of formula needed per feeding to a sterilized bottle. DO NOT ADD WATER. Place nipple and ring on the bottle.
- Tightly cover any formula remaining in the can. Store in the refrigerator for up to 48 hours.

For all types of formula:
- Warm the bottle to the desired temperature and shake well before feeding. After feeding, discard any formula left in the bottle and rinse the bottle and nipple in cool water immediately.

Terminal Heating Method

(For the preparation of infant formula from concentrated liquid formulas only)

- Wash hands before preparing formula and again if interrupted during preparation. Wash all needed equipment (e.g., glass measuring cup, spoon, bottles, nipples, rings, and discs) with hot water and detergent. Rinse well with hot running water.
- Wash the top of the can with hot water and detergent, rinse in hot running water, and dry. Shake the can and open it with a clean punch-type can opener.
- Measure the needed amount of concentrated formula and correct amount of water in a glass measuring cup. Mix well, using a clean spoon, and then pour specified amount of formula into each bottle and attach nipples, discs, and rings. Apply rings loosely.
- Place filled bottles on a rack in a deep pan or sterilizer that contains approximately 3 inches of water. Heat water to boiling and then allow it to boil gently for 20 minutes while covered. Remove pan from the stove.
- After the sides of the pan have cooled enough to be touched comfortably, remove the bottles. Tighten the nipple rings and store bottles in the refrigerator until needed. Use bottles within 48 hours.
- Warm the bottle to the desired temperature and shake well before feeding. After feeding, discard any formula left in the bottle and rinse the bottle and nipple in cool water immediately.

Adapted from *How to Prepare Your Baby's Infant Formula*. Evansville, Ind: Mead Johnson Nutritionals; 1991.

---

method; Table 13) have been recommended for the preparation of infant formula.[134] The Committee on the Fetus and the Newborn of the AAP does not recommend the use of unsterilized equipment and hot tap water to prepare formula but recommends that some method of sterilization be used.[138]

The heating of infant formulas, warming of breast milk, or thawing of frozen breast milk in a microwave oven is a questionable practice. Some of the hazards associated with the use of microwave ovens are scald injuries and palatal burns in infants and exploding containers. Glass bottles get much hotter than plastic bottles, and the tem-

TABLE 14	Number of daily feedings, according to age
Age	Average number of daily feedings
Birth–1 wk	6–9
1 wk–1 mo	6–8
1–3 mo	5–6
3–4 mo	4–5
4–8 mo	3–4
8–12 mo	3

Adapted from Barness LA. Nutrition and nutritional disorders: nutritional requirements. In: Behrman RE, ed. *Nelson Textbook of Pediatrics.* 14th ed. Philadelphia: W.B. Saunders Co.; 1992: 105–30.

perature of the milk may be uneven.[139] It also appears that microwaving can have detrimental effects on the anti-infective factors found in breast milk. When breast milk was microwaved at temperatures of 162–208°F (72–98°C), marked decreases in anti-infective factors (e.g., total IgA, specific secretory IgA, and lysozymes) occurred; significant decreases in IgA specific for *Escherichia coli* serotype 06 and lysozymes were noted even at temperatures between 68 and 77°F (20 and 25°C).[140]

Although it is not recommended by the AAP, some parents use the clean technique for formula preparation.[15] In this method, one bottle is prepared for each feeding. The person preparing the formula washes his or her hands carefully. Then all equipment for formula preparation (including cans of concentrated formula, bottles, and nipples) is washed thoroughly with detergent and hot water. The formula is then prepared, the opened can of concentrated formula is refrigerated, and the prepared formula is heated. Formula remaining in the bottle after feeding should be discarded. Studies have shown that the clean method of formula preparation is as safe as terminal sterilization if the water supply used for formula preparation is safe (i.e., if municipal water is available).[141,142]

Ready-to-use formula in bottles requires no preparation. Bottles can be stored at room temperature and warming of the formula before feeding is not required. The protective cap needs to be removed and a sterile nipple screwed onto the bottle before feeding. The bottle should be shaken to allow for adequate formula mixing. After feeding, the bottle and any unused formula should be discarded.[134] Ready-to-use formula in cans also needs no preparation. The top of the can should be washed with soap and hot water, shaken to allow for formula mixing, and then opened with a clean punch-type opener. Formula is then added to one bottle for a single feeding or to the bottles needed for a full day's feeding. If the latter is done, the bottles should be covered and refrigerated until needed. Formula remaining in the can may be covered and stored in the refrigerator for as long as 48 hours.

Formulas have specific instructions for preparation and most formulas have symbols on cans of concentrated formula, ready-to-use formula, and powders that can be used as guidelines in formula preparation. Formula containers should be checked for expiration dates and dents. Parents should store unopened formula where it will not be subjected to extreme temperature changes.[134]

Infant Feeding

The frequency of feeding for a newborn infant will vary from every 2 hours to every 4 hours. Smaller infants usually require more frequent feedings because they have lower stomach capacities and shorter stomach emptying times. Breast-fed infants desire more frequent feedings than do bottle-fed infants. Infants usually lengthen the interval between feedings to 4 hours by the time they are 3 to 4 weeks old. Typically, infants begin to stop nighttime feedings by the age of 3–6 weeks.[69] Average numbers of daily feedings for infants of different ages are shown in Table 14.

By the end of the first week of life, full-term infants increase the volume of their feedings from 30 mL to between 80 and 90 mL. The amount of formula offered to a bottle-fed infant should be consistent with the RDA for energy based on age and weight. The infant should be fed on demand and should not be forced to take more formula than is desired at any one feeding. If the infant finishes a bottle and still seems hungry, another bottle should be offered. An infant who is not losing weight by 7 days of age and who is gaining weight by 2 weeks of age appears to be receiving an appropriate amount of formula.[69] Thereafter, growth curves (weight, height, and head circumference) are used to determine whether an infant is growing appropriately. Table 15 lists typical quantities of feedings by age.

Product Selection Guidelines

For healthy full-term infants without the need for a therapeutic formula, either a milk-based formula or a milk-based formula with added whey protein is indicated. When

TABLE 15	Quantity of milk ingested per feeding, according to age
Age	Average quantity of milk per feeding (oz)
Birth–2 wk	2–3
3 wk–2 mo	4–5
2–3 mo	5–6
3–4 mo	6–7
5–12 mo	7–8

Adapted from Barness LA. Nutrition and nutritional disorders: nutritional requirements. In: Behrman RE, ed. *Nelson Textbook of Pediatrics.* 14th ed. Philadelphia: W.B. Saunders Co.; 1992: 105–30.

recommending a type of formula, the pharmacist should consider the method of preparation, the parents' ability to follow directions, the parents' attitudes and preferences, and the sanitary conditions and refrigeration facilities available.

For many parents, cost may be a critical factor in selecting an infant formula. Concentrated liquids and powdered formula preparations are less expensive than ready-to-use products. Convenience is also a consideration. The preparation of powdered and concentrated liquid formulas requires more manipulative functions and more attention to aseptic technique. The formula selected should be one that is well tolerated by the infant, convenient for the parents to prepare, and priced to fit the family's budget.

References

1. Garza C, Hopkinson J. Physiology of lactation. In: Tsang RC, Nichols BL, eds. *Nutrition During Infancy.* St. Louis: C. V. Mosby Co; 1988: 20–32.
2. Lawrence RA. Breastfeeding and medical disease. *Med Clin North Am* 1989; 73: 583–603.
3. Cunningham AS, Jelliffe DB, Jelliffe EF. Breast-feeding and health in the 1980s: a global epidemiological review. *J Pediatr* 1991; 118: 659–66.
4. Jason J. Breast-feeding in 1991 [editorial]. *N Engl J Med* 1991; 325: 1036–8.
5. Cone TE Jr. Infant feeding redux. *Pediatrics* 1990; 86: 473–4.
6. Martinez GA, Krieger FW. 1984 milk-feeding patterns in the U.S. *Pediatrics* 1985; 76: 1004–8.
7. Fomon SJ. Reflections on infant feeding in the 1970s and 1980s. *Am J Clin Nutr* 1987; 46 (suppl 1): 171–82.
8. Ryan AS, Rush D, Krieger FW, et al. Recent declines in breast-feeding in the U.S., 1984 through 1989. *Pediatrics* 1991; 88: 719–27.
9. Batten S, Hirschman J, Thomas D. Impact of the Special Supplemental Food Program on infants. *J Pediatr* 1990; 117 (suppl): S101–9.
10. Hansen JW, Cook DA, Cordano A, et al. Human milk substitutes. In: Tsang RC, Nichols BL, eds. *Nutrition During Infancy.* St. Louis: C. V. Mosby Co; 1988: 378–98.
11. Jones EG. In: Kelts DG, Jones EG, eds. *Manual of Pediatric Nutrition.* Boston: Little, Brown and Co; 1984: 17–34.
12. Hamilton JR. Gastrointestinal tract: normal digestive tract phenomena. In: Behrman RE, ed. *Nelson Textbook of Pediatrics.* 14th ed. Philadelphia: W. B. Saunders Co; 1992: 935–40.
13. Watkins JB. Lipid digestion and absorption. *Pediatrics* 1985; 75 (suppl): 151–6.
14. Hamosh M, Bitman J, Wood L, et al. Lipids in milk and the first steps in their digestion. *Pediatrics* 1985; 75 (suppl): 146–50.
15. Pipes PL. Infant feeding and nutrition. In: Pipes PL, ed. *Nutrition in Infancy and Childhood.* 4th. ed. St. Louis: Times Mirror/Mosby College Publishing; 1989: 86–119.
16. Ziegler EE, Fomon SJ. Potential renal solute load of infant formulas. *J Nutr* 1989; 119 (suppl): 1785–8.
17. Pipes PL. Nutrition: growth and development. In: Pipes PL, ed. *Nutrition in Infancy and Childhood.* 4th ed. St. Louis: Times Mirror/Mosby College Publishing; 1989: 1–38.
18. Fomon SJ, Haschke F, Ziegler EE, Nelson SE. Body composition of reference children from birth to age 10 years. *Am J Clin Nutr* 1982; 35: 1169–75.
19. Food and Nutrition Board, Commission on Life Sciences, National Research Council. *Recommended Dietary Allowances.* 10th ed. Washington, DC: National Academy Press; 1989.
20. Kliegman RM, Behrman RE. The fetus and neonatal infant: the digestive system. In: Behrman RE, ed. *Nelson Textbook of Pediatrics.* 14th ed. Philadelphia: W. B. Saunders Co; 1992: 474–81.
21. Pipes PL. Nutrient needs of infants and children. In: Pipes PL, ed. *Nutrition in Infancy and Childhood.* 4th ed. St. Louis: Times Mirror/Mosby College Publishing; 1989: 29–57.
22. Committee on Nutrition, American Academy of Pediatrics. Plant fiber intake in the pediatric diet. *Pediatrics* 1981; 67: 572–5.
23. Picone TA, Benson JD, Moro G, et al. Growth, serum biochemistries, and amino acids of term infants fed formulas with amino acid and protein concentrations similar to human milk. *J Pediatr Gastroenterol Nutr* 1989; 9: 351–60.
24. Sanchez-Pozo A, Lopez J, Pita ML, et al. Changes in the protein fractions of human milk during lactation. *Ann Nutr Metab* 1986; 30: 15–20.
25. Polberger SKT, Axelsson IE, Raiha NCR. Amino acid concentrations in plasma and urine in very low birthweight infants fed protein-unenriched or human milk protein-enriched human milk. *Pediatrics* 1990; 86: 909–15.
26. Gaull G, Sturman JA, Raiha NCR. Development of mammalian sulfur metabolism: absence of cystathionase in human fetal tissues. *Pediatr Res* 1972; 6: 538–47.
27. Rassin DK, Sturman JA, Gaull GE. Taurine and other free amino acids in milk of man and other mammals. *Early Hum Dev* 1978; 2: 1–13.
28. Gaull GE. Taurine in pediatric nutrition: review and update. *Pediatrics* 1989; 83: 433–42.
29. Michalk DV, Tittor F, Ringeisen R, et al. The development of heart and brain function in low-birth-weight infants fed with taurine-supplemented formula. *Adv Exp Med Biol* 1987; 217: 139–45.
30. Committee on Nutrition, American Academy of Pediatrics. Prudent life-style for children: dietary fat and cholesterol. *Pediatrics* 1986; 78: 521–5.
31. Committee on Nutrition, American Academy of Pediatrics. Commentary on breast-feeding and infant formulas, including proposed standards for formulas. *Pediatrics* 1976; 57: 278–85.
32. Schlenk H. Odd numbered and new essential fatty acids. *Fed Proc* 1972; 31: 1430–5.
33. Friedman ZA, Danon A, Stahlman MT, Oates JA. Rapid onset of essential fatty acid deficiency in the newborn. *Pediatrics* 1976; 58: 640–9.
34. Gross S, Melhorn DK. Vitamin E, red cell lipids and red cell stability in prematurity. *Ann N Y Acad Sci* 1972; 203: 141–62.
35. Committee on Nutrition, American Academy of Pediatrics. Nutritional needs of low-birth-weight infants. *Pediatrics* 1977; 60: 519–30.
36. Dicks-Bushnell MW, Davis KC. Vitamin E content of infant formulas and cereals. *Am J Clin Nutr* 1967; 20: 262–9.
37. Bonjour JP. Biotin in human nutrition. *Ann N Y Acad Sci* 1985; 447: 97–104.
38. Committee on Nutrition, American Academy of Pediatrics. Calcium requirements in infancy and childhood. *Pediatrics* 1978; 62: 826–34.
39. Mizrahi A, London RD, Gribetz D. Neonatal hypocalcemia—its causes and treatment. *N Engl J Med* 1968; 278: 1163–5.
40. Committee on Nutrition, American Academy of Pediatrics. Nutritional needs of low-birth-weight infants. *Pediatrics* 1985; 75: 976–86.
41. Dallman PR. Iron, vitamin E, and folate in the preterm infant. *J Pediatr* 1974; 85: 742–52.
42. Prasad AS, Oberleas D. Zinc deficiency in man. *Lancet* 1974; 1: 463–4.
43. Committee on Nutrition, American Academy of Pediatrics. Vitamin and mineral supplement needs in normal children in the United States. *Pediatrics* 1980; 66: 1015–21.
44. O'Connor P. Vitamin D–deficiency rickets in two breast-fed infants who were not receiving vitamin D supplementation. *Clin Pediatr* 1971; 16: 361–3.
45. Fomon SJ, Filer LJ, Anderson TA, Ziegler EE. Recommendations for feeding normal infants. *Pediatrics* 1979; 63: 52–9.

46. Bachrach S, Fisher J, Parks JS. An outbreak of vitamin D deficiency rickets in a susceptible population. *Pediatrics* 1979; 64: 871–7.
47. Higginbottom MC, Sweetman L, Nyhan WL. A syndrome of methylmalonic aciduria, homocystinuria, megaloblastic anemia and neurologic abnormalities in a vitamin B12–deficient breast-fed infant of a strict vegetarian. *N Engl J Med* 1978; 299: 317–23.
48. Saarinen UM, Siimes MA, Dallman PR. Iron absorption in infants: high bioavailability of breast milk iron as indicated by the extrinsic tag method of iron absorption and by the concentration of serum ferritin. *J Pediatr* 1977; 91: 36–9.
49. Committee on Nutrition, American Academy of Pediatrics. Fluoride supplementation: Revised dosage schedule. *Pediatrics* 1979; 63: 150–2.
50. Committee on Nutrition, American Academy of Pediatrics. Fluoride supplementation. *Pediatrics* 1986; 77: 758–61.
51. Committee on Nutrition, American Academy of Pediatrics. Formula feeding of infants. In: Forbes GB, Woodruff CW, eds. *Pediatric Nutrition Handbook*. Elk Grove Village, Ill: American Academy of Pediatrics; 1985: 16–27.
52. Oski FA. Iron-fortified formulas and gastrointestinal symptoms in infants: a controlled study. *Pediatrics* 1980; 66: 168–70.
53. Nelson SE, Ziegler EE, Copeland AM, et al. Lack of adverse reactions to iron-fortified formula. *Pediatrics* 1988; 81: 360–4.
54. Montalto MB, Benson JD, Martinez GA. Nutrient intakes of formula-fed infants and infants fed cow milk. *Pediatrics* 1985; 75: 343–51.
55. Hittner HM, Godio LB, Rudolph AJ, et al. Retrolental fibroplasia: efficacy of vitamin E in a double-blind clinical study of preterm infants. *N Engl J Med* 1981; 305: 1365–71.
56. Stevens D, Burman D, Strelling K, Morris A. Folic acid supplementation in low birthweight infants. *Pediatrics* 1979; 64: 333–5.
57. Benkov KJ, LeLeiko NS. A rational approach to infant formulas. *Pediatr Ann* 1987; 16: 225–6, 228, 230.
58. Raiha NC. Nutritional proteins in milk and the protein requirement of normal infants. *Pediatrics* 1985; 75 (suppl): 136–41.
59. Klish WJ. Special infant formulas. *Pediatr Rev* 1990; 12: 55–62.
60. Greer FR. Calcium, phosphorus, and magnesium: How much is too much for infant formulas? *J Nutr* 1989; 119 (suppl): 1846–51.
61. Milner JA. Trace minerals in the nutrition of children. *J Pediatr* 1990; 117 (suppl): S147–55.
62. Pugliese MT. Parental health beliefs as a cause of nonorganic failure to thrive. *Pediatrics* 1987; 80: 175–82.
63. Taras HL. Early childhood diet: recommendations of pediatric health care providers. *J Am Diet Assoc* 1988; 88: 1417–21.
64. Oski FA. Whole cow milk feeding between 6 and 12 months of age? Go back to 1976. *Pediatr Rev* 1990; 12: 187–9.
65. Woodruff CW. Milk intolerances. *Nutr Rev* 1976; 34: 33–7.
66. Committee on Nutrition, American Academy of Pediatrics. The use of whole cow's milk in infancy. *Pediatrics* 1983; 72: 253–5.
67. Ziegler EE. Milk and formulas for older infants. *J Pediatr* 1990; 117 (suppl): S76–9.
68. Committee on Nutrition, American Academy of Pediatrics. The use of whole cow's milk in infancy. *Pediatrics* 1992; 89: 1105–9.
69. Barness LA. Nutrition and nutritional disorders: nutritional requirements. In: Behrman RE, ed. *Nelson Textbook of Pediatrics*. 14th ed. Philadelphia: W. B. Saunders Co; 1992: 105–30.
70. Committee on Nutrition, American Academy of Pediatrics. Supplemental foods for infants. In: Forbes GB, Woodruff CW, eds. *Pediatric Nutrition Handbook*. 2nd ed. Elk Grove Village, Ill: American Academy of Pediatrics; 1985: 28–36.
71. Wilson JT. *Drugs in Breast Milk*. Sydney, Australia: ADIS Press; 1981.
72. Kirksey A, Groziak SM. Maternal drug use: evaluation of risks to breast-fed infants. *World Rev Nutr Diet* 1984; 43: 60–79.
73. Kovar MG, Serdula MK, Marks JS, Fraser DW. Review of the epidemiologic evidence for an association between infant feeding and infant health. *Pediatrics* 1984; 74 (suppl): 615–38.
74. Poland RL, Schultz GE, Garg G. High milk lipase activity associated with breast milk jaundice. *Pediatr Res* 1980; 14: 1328–31.
75. Poland RL. Breast-milk jaundice [editorial]. *J Pediatr* 1981; 99: 86–8.
76. Hopkinson JM, Garza C. Management of breastfeeding. In: Tsang RC, Nichols BL, eds. *Nutrition During Infancy*. St. Louis: C. V. Mosby Co; 1988: 298–313.
77. Ruff AJ, Halsey NA, Coberly J, Boulos R. Breast-feeding and maternal–infant transmission of human immunodeficiency virus type 1. *J Pediatr* 1992;121: 325–7.
78. Committee on Infectious Diseases, American Academy of Pediatrics. Summaries of infectious diseases: AIDS and HIV infections. In: Peter G, Lepow ML, McCracken GH, et al., eds. *Report of the Committee on Infectious Diseases*. 22nd ed. Elk Grove Village, Ill: American Academy of Pediatrics; 1991: 115–31.
79. Briggs GG, Freeman RK, Yaffe SJ. *Drugs in Pregnancy and Lactation*. 3rd ed. Baltimore: Williams & Wilkins; 1990.
80. Miller GH, Hughes LR. Lactation and genital involution effects of a new low-dose oral contraceptive on breast-feeding mothers and their infants. *Obstet Gynecol* 1970; 35: 44–50.
81. Lonnerdal B, Forsum E, Hambraeus L. Effect of oral contraceptives on composition and volume of breast milk. *Am J Clin Nutr* 1980; 33: 816–24.
82. Hull VJ. The effects of hormonal contraceptives on lactation: current findings, methodological considerations, and future priorities. *Stud Fam Plan* 1981; 12: 134–55.
83. World Health Organization Task Force on Oral Contraceptives. Effects of hormonal contraceptives on breast milk composition and infant growth. *Stud Fam Plan* 1988; 19: 361–9.
84. Koetsawang S. The effects of contraceptive methods on the quality and quantity of breast milk. *Int J Gynaecol Obstet* 1987; 25 (suppl): 115–27.
85. Committee on Drugs, American Academy of Pediatrics. Breast-feeding and contraception. *Pediatrics* 1981; 68: 138–40.
86. Committee on Drugs, American Academy of Pediatrics. Transfer of drugs and other chemicals into human milk. *Pediatrics* 1989; 84: 924–36.
87. Anderson PO. Drug use during breast-feeding. *Clin Pharm* 1991; 10: 594–624.
88. Atkinson HC, Begg EJ. Prediction of drug distribution into human milk from physicochemical characteristics. *Clin Pharmacokinet* 1990; 18: 151–67.
89. Atkinson HC, Begg EJ, Darlow BA. Drugs in human milk. Clinical pharmacokinetic considerations. *Clin Pharmacokinet* 1988; 14: 217–40.
90. R. Sagraves. Drugs in breast milk. In: Kuhn RJ, Piecoro JJ Jr., Shannon MC, eds. *Pediatric Pharmacotherapy*. Lexington, Ky: University of Kentucky; 1991. Module 28.
91. Briggs GG. Drugs in pregnancy and lactation. In: Young YL, Koda-Kimble MA, eds. *Applied Therapeutics: The Clinical Use of Drugs*. 5th ed. Vancouver, Wash: Applied Therapeutics Inc; 1992: 1–33.
92. Committee on Nutrition, American Academy of Pediatrics. Proposed changes in Food and Drug Administration regulations concerning formula products and vitamin-mineral dietary supplements for infants. *Pediatrics* 1967; 40: 916–22.
93. Food and Drug Administration. Nutrient requirements for infant formulas. *Federal Register* 1985; 50: 45106–8.
94. Silver LB, Levinson RB, Laskin CR, Pilot LJ. Learning disabilities as a probable consequence of using a chloride-deficient infant formula. *J Pediatr* 1989; 115: 97–9.
95. Malloy MH, et al. Hypochloremic metabolic alkalosis from ingestion of a chloride-deficient infant formula: outcome 9–10 years later. *Pediatrics* 1991; 87: 811–22.
96. Food and Drug Administration. Infant formula: labeling re-

quirements. *Federal Register* 1985; 50: 1833–40.
97. Chicago and Suburban Dietetics Association. Nutritional care of the high risk infant. In: *Manual of Clinical Dietetics.* Chicago: American Dietetics Association; 1988: 115–37.
98. Santeiro ML, Sagraves R, Allen LV Jr. Osmolality of small-volume i.v. admixtures for pediatric patients [published erratum *Am J Hosp Pharm* 1990; 47: 1978] *Am J Hosp Pharm* 1990; 47: 1359–64.
99. Anderson TA, Fomon SJ, Filer LJ. Carbohydrate tolerance studies with 3-day-old infants. *J Lab Clin Med* 1972; 79: 31–7.
100. *Comparison of Feeding of Infants and Young Children in the Hospital.* Columbus, Ohio: Ross Laboratories; 1990.
101. Tomarelli RM. Osmolality, osmolarity, and renal solute load of infant formulas. *J Pediatr* 1976; 88: 454–6.
102. Lifschitz CH. Carbohydrate needs in preterm and term newborn infants. In: Tsang RC, Nichols BL, eds. *Nutrition During Infancy.* St. Louis: C. V. Mosby Co; 1988: 122–32.
103. Committee on Nutrition, American Academy of Pediatrics. Soy-protein formulas: recommendations for use in infant feeding. *Pediatrics* 1983; 72: 359–63.
104. Merritt RJ, Carter M, Haight M, Eisenberg LD. Whey protein hydrolysate formula for infants with gastrointestinal intolerance to cow milk and soy protein in infant formulas. *J Pediatr Gastroenterol Nutr* 1990; 11: 78–82.
105. Gerrand JW, MacKenzie JWA, Goluboff N, et al. Cow milk allergy: prevalence and manifestations in an unselected series of newborns. *Acta Paediatr Scand* 1973; 234 (suppl): 1–21.
106. Goel K, Lifshitz F, Kahn E, Teichberg S. Monosaccharide intolerance and soy-protein hypersensitivity in an infant with diarrhea. *J Pediatr* 1978; 93: 617–9.
107. Powell GK. Milk- and soy-induced enterocolitis of infancy: Clinical features and standardization of challenge. *J Pediatr* 1978; 93: 553–60.
108. Committee on Nutrition, American Academy of Pediatrics. Hypoallergenic infant formulas. *Pediatrics* 1989; 83: 1068–9.
109. Sampson HA. Safety of casein hydrolysate formula in children with cow milk allergy. *J Pediatr* 1991; 118 (suppl): 520–5.
110. Barr RG, Kramer MS, Pless IB, et al. Feeding and temperament as determinants of early infant crying/fussing behavior. *Pediatrics* 1989; 84: 514–21.
111. Lothe L, Lindberg T. Cow's milk whey protein elicits symptoms of infantile colic in colicky formula-fed infants: a double-blind crossover study [published erratum *Pediatrics* 1989; 84: 17] *Pediatrics* 1989; 83: 262–6.
112. *Pediatric Products Handbook.* Evansville, Ind: Mead Johnson Nutritionals; 1990.
113. Andrews BF, Lorch V. Improved fat and CA absorption in L.B.W. infants fed a medium chain triglyceride containing formula [abstract]. *Pediatr Res* 1974; 8: 378.
114. Tantibhedhyangkul P, Hashim SA. Medium-chain triglyceride feeding in premature infants: effects on calcium and magnesium absorption. *Pediatrics* 1978; 61: 537–45.
115. Tantibhedhyangkul P, Hashim SA. Medium-chain triglyceride feeding in premature infants: effects on fat and nitrogen absorption. *Pediatrics* 1975; 55: 359–70.
116. Businco L, Cantani A, Longhi MA. Severe anaphylactic reactions following cow's milk protein hydrolysates (CMPHs) ingestion [abstract]. *Pediatr Res* 1987; 22: 222.
117. Businco L, Cantani A, Longhi MA, Giampietro PG. Anaphylactic reactions to a cow's milk whey protein hydrolysate (Alfa-Ré, Nestlé) in infants with cow milk allergy. *Ann Allergy* 1989; 62 333–5.
118. Forbes GB. Is human milk the best food for low birthweight babies? *Pediatr Res* 1978; 12: 434.
119. Dallman PR. Upper limits of iron in infant formulas. *J Nutr* 1989; 119 (suppl): 1852–4.
120. Thompson M, McClead RE. Human milk fortifiers. *J Pediatr Perinatal Nutr* 1987; 1 (Fall/Winter): 65–75.
121. Ehrenkranz RA, Gettner PA, Nelli CM. Nutrition balance studies in premature infants fed premature formula or fortified preterm human milk. *J Pediatr Gastroenterol Nutr* 1989; 8: 58–67.
122. Kashyap S et al. Growth, nutrient retention, and metabolic response of low-birth-weight infants fed supplemented and unsupplemented preterm human milk. *Am J Clin Nutr* 1990; 52: 254–62.
123. Johnsen D, Nowjack-Raymer R. Baby bottle tooth decay (BBTD): issues, assessment, and an opportunity for the nutritionist. *J Am Diet Assoc* 1989; 89: 1112–6.
124. Moss MH. Hypoprothrombinemic bleeding in a young infant: association with a soy protein formula. *Am J Dis Child* 1969; 117: 540–2.
125. Goldman HI, Amadio P. Vitamin K deficiency after the newborn period. *Pediatrics* 1969; 44: 745–9.
126. Cochrane WA, Collins-Williams C, Donohue WL. Superior hemorrhagic polioencephalitis (Wernicke's disease) occurring in an infant—probably due to thiamine deficiency from use of a soy bean product. *Pediatrics* 1961; 28: 771–7.
127. Molony CJ, Parmelee AH. Convulsions in young infants as a result of pyridoxine (vitamin B_6) deficiency. *JAMA* 1954; 154: 405–6.
128. Hydovitz JD. Occurrence of goiter in an infant on a soy diet. *N Engl J Med* 1960; 262: 351–3.
129. Roy S III, Arant BS Jr. Alkalosis from chloride-deficient Neo-Mull-Soy [letter]. *N Engl J Med* 1979; 301: 615.
130. Kulkarni PB, Hall RT, Rhodes PG, et al. Rickets in very low-birth-weight infants. *J Pediatr* 1980; 96: 249–52.
131. Finberg L. One milk for all—not ever likely and certainly not yet [editorial]. *J Pediatr* 1980; 96: 240–1.
132. Holick MF, Shao Q, Liu WW, Chen TC. The vitamin D content of fortified milk and infant formula. *N Engl J Med* 1982; 326: 1178–81.
133. Litov RE, Sickles VS, Chan GM, et al. Plasma aluminum measurements in term infants fed human milk or a soy-based infant formula. *Pediatrics* 1989; 84: 1105–7.
134. *How to Prepare Your Baby's Infant Formula.* Evansville, Ind: Mead Johnson Nutritionals; 1991.
135. McJunkin JE, Bithoney WG, McCormick MC. Errors in formula concentration in an outpatient population. *J Pediatr* 1987; 111: 848–50.
136. Haschke F, Pietschnig B, Vanura H. Infant formulas improperly prepared from powdered cow milk [letter]. *J Pediatr* 1988; 113: 163.
137. Owen GM, Kram KM, Garry PJ, et al. A study of nutritional status of preschool children in the United States, 1968–1970. *Pediatrics* 1974; 53 (suppl): 597–646.
138. Committee on the Fetus and the Newborn, American Academy of Pediatrics. Sterilization of milk-mixtures for infants. *Pediatrics* 1961; 28: 674–5.
139. Nemethy M, Clore ER. Microwave heating of infant formula and breast milk. *J Pediatr Health Care* 1990; 4: 131–5.
140. Quan R, Yang C, Rubinstein S, et al. Effects of microwave radiation on anti-infective factors in human milk. *Pediatrics* 1992; 89: 667–9.
141. Hughes RB, Sauvain KJ, Blanton LH, DeLoache WR. Outcome of teaching clean vs. terminal methods of formula preparation. *Pediatr Nurs* 1987; 13: 275–6.
142. Gerber MA, Berliner BC, Karolus JJ. Sterilization of infant formula. *Clin Pediatr* 1983; 22: 344–9.

CHAPTER 19

Weight Control Products

Glenn D. Appelt

Questions to ask in patient assessment and counseling

- *What is your age, height, and weight?*
- *How long have you had a weight problem?*
- *How many pounds overweight do you think you are?*
- *Is there a family history of obesity? Do either of your parents have a weight problem?*
- *Do you tend to eat excessively when you are anxious, nervous, or tired?*
- *Have you consulted a physician about the problem?*
- *Are you or have you been on a diet? If yes, which one(s)?*
- *What diet preparations have you used previously? Were they effective?*
- *In addition to dietary restriction, what efforts have you made to lose weight? Do you belong to a self-help group such as Weight Watchers®?*
- *Do you have a regular exercise program? Does your physician recommend that you exercise?*
- *Are you being treated for any chronic disease such as hypertension, angina, diabetes, or a thyroid condition?*
- *What medications are you currently taking?*

Obesity is a common condition in the developed countries of the world and certainly in the United States. It is most simply defined as the accumulation of fat in storage areas of the body exceeding the amount needed for optimal body function. From a quantitative and practical point of view, a body weight 20% over that stipulated in standard height–weight tables is arbitrarily considered obese (Table 1). However, although the term *obese* is often used interchangeably with the term *overweight*, they are not interchangeable. For example, a lean but heavily muscled person may be overweight according to standard tables but may not be obese.

Obesity is often classified as mild, moderate, or severe. Mild obesity is generally defined as 20–40% above the ideal body weight (IBW) contained in standard height–weight tables. Moderate obesity is considered to be 41–100% above IBW; severe (morbid) obesity includes all individuals weighing more than 100% above IBW. Various formulas may be employed to calculate IBW for use as a reference standard against which actual body weight (ABW) can be compared. Rather than use standard tables, IBW can be calculated using the following equations:

IBW (adult female) = 45 kg for first 152 cm of height + 0.9 kg for each cm > 152.

IBW (adult male) = 48 kg for first 152 cm of height + 1.1 kg for each cm > 152.

Degree of obesity (% IBW) is derived from the equation:

% IBW = (ABW/IBW) x 100.

Measurement of skinfold thickness has been suggested as a practical means of determining the extent of obesity. Initially, the triceps skinfold, as measured by calipers, was reported to be most representative of body fat. However, an expanded measuring system has been advocated using four sites: triceps, biceps, subscapular, and supraileac. Attempts have been made to measure subcutaneous fat thickness by X-rays, but this technique is less convenient than skinfold measurement and offers little compensating advantage. Ultrasound measures have been employed to estimate body fat, although circumference measurements of certain body parts using calibrated fiberglass tape may provide a better estimation. The waist-to-thigh ratio has been reported to be an appropriate index for upper and central body fat distribution, especially in women.

The fat distribution after puberty is characteristically different in men and women. Women tend to store fat in the breasts, hips, and thighs (gynecoid distribution) whereas men tend to accumulate fat in the abdomen (android distribution). However, some women have a relatively central (or android) fat distribution whereas some men exhibit a predominantly peripheral (or gynecoid) fat distribution. An android fat distribution may be more strongly associated with atherosclerosis, diabetes mellitus, and gouty arthritis than a similar amount of fat in a gynecoid distribution. Current interest extends to determining the proportion of abdominal fat that is subcutaneous or within the peritoneal cavity because growing evidence indicates that the amount of intra-abdominal fat rather than of subcutaneous fat located in the abdominal wall—that is, the distribution of fat rather than the total amount—is an important factor in the metabolic effects of obesity.

Daily caloric allowances for persons with moderate physical activity may vary with age and sex. As a general rule, an intake of 3,500 cal (kcal) over expenditure will produce a weight gain of approximately 0.454 kg (1 lb) whereas an expenditure of 3,500 calories over intake will result in a 0.454-kg (1-lb) loss of body fat. Daily caloric allowances for average males (weight, 70 kg or 154 lb; height, 1.78 m or 5'10") in a temperate climate range

TABLE 1	Metropolitan height and weight tables for men and women according to frame, ages 25–29							
	Men				**Women**			
Height[a]	Weight in Pounds[b]			Height[a]	Weight in Pounds[b]			
Inches	Small frame	Medium frame	Large frame	Inches	Small frame	Medium frame	Large frame	
62	128–134	131–141	138–150	58	102–111	109–121	118–131	
63	130–136	133–143	140–153	59	103–113	111–123	120–134	
64	132–138	135–145	142–156	60	104–115	113–126	122–137	
65	134–140	137–148	144–160	61	106–118	115–129	125–140	
66	136–142	139–151	146–164	62	108–121	118–132	128–143	
67	138–145	142–154	149–168	63	111–124	121–135	131–147	
68	140–148	145–157	152–172	64	114–127	124–138	134–151	
69	142–151	148–160	155–176	65	117–130	127–141	137–155	
70	144–154	151–163	158–180	66	120–133	130–144	140–159	
71	146–157	154–166	161–184	67	123–136	133–147	143–163	
72	149–160	157–170	164–188	68	126–139	136–150	146–167	
73	152–164	160–174	168–192	69	129–142	139–153	149–170	
74	155–168	164–178	172–197	70	132–145	142–156	152–173	
75	158–172	167–182	176–202	71	135–148	145–159	155–176	
76	162–176	171–187	181–207	72	138–151	148–162	158–179	

[a]Shoes with 1-in. heels.
[b]Indoor clothing weighing 5 lb for men and 3 lb for women.
Source of basic data: Society of Actuaries and Association of Life Insurance Medical Directors of America. *Build Study*. 1979. New York: Metropolitan Life Insurance Company; 1983.

from 3,200 cal at 25 years of age to 2,550 cal at 65 years of age. Corresponding figures for average females (weight, 58 kg or 128 lb; height, 1.63 m or 5'4") are 2,300 and 1,800 cal at ages 25 and 65, respectively. The daily caloric requirement for women increases slightly during pregnancy (300 cal) and significantly during lactation (500 cal for one child and 1,000 cal for twins).

Most obesity is associated with overeating, particularly of carbohydrates or fats. The calories ingested beyond those necessary for normal energy requirements usually are deposited and stored as fat. Because lack of food is rarely a problem in the United States, Americans must decide how much and what type of food to consume. Apparently, many people make unwise choices because obesity is estimated to occur in 30–45% of Americans over 30 years of age.

Clinical Considerations

Obesity is a subject of intense study. Many factors affect metabolic equilibrium. Appetite control is only part of the answer. Psychologic components may contribute to or cause overeating, leading to obesity. Self-therapy groups often help in treating the cause; use of pharmacologic agents tends to treat only the symptoms. In addition, caloric expenditure by physical activity can promote the maintenance of a nonobese state in the motivated individual. The rate of caloric expenditure of various physical activities is included in Table 2. When one considers that basal metabolism over a typical 24-hour period consumes approximately 1,000 cal per square meter of body surface area (average body surface area is 1.73 m^2), it is easy to see how significant exercise can be in accelerating weight loss. However, it must be emphasized that excessive eating (caloric intake) is the major cause of obesity and that caloric restriction should be the cornerstone of any weight control program.

Etiology of Obesity

The question of why individuals ingest more calories than they expend is complex. The answer may be related to physiologic, genetic, social, environmental, or psychologic factors or to an interrelationship of two or more of these factors. Endocrine disorders, such as hypothyroidism or

TABLE 2	Caloric expenditure rates
Activity (1 hr)	Calories expended
Bicycling (6 mph)	240
Bicycling (12 mph)	410
Cross country skiing	700
Jogging (5.5 mph)	740
Jogging (7 mph)	920
Jumping rope	720
Running in place	650
Swimming (50 yd/min)	500
Tennis (singles)	400
Walking (2 mph)	240
Walking (3 mph)	320
Walking (4.5 mph)	440

Cushing's syndrome, are apparently rarely involved in causing obesity per se. Obesity may result from an anatomical or biochemical lesion in the brain's feeding centers, although this hypothesis has not been proven in humans.

Some researchers believe that thin and obese people differ in the degree of thermogenesis that occurs after food ingestion. Overeating in nonobese subjects causes increased heat production, which tends to dissipate the excess calories. In obese subjects, the dissipation of thermal energy may be less pronounced, resulting in fat storage. Animal models of obesity have been shown to have a defective thermogenic component, but the evidence for this metabolic defect in human obesity is largely circumstantial. Additionally, some individuals gain fat more easily than others. A subnormal thermogenic response to food has been reported in the obese and the postobese. Although these studies may be criticized on the basis that reductions in diet-induced thermogenesis (DIT) may not be a cause but rather a result of the obesity and/or metabolic adaptation to a low caloric intake, the concept of a defective DIT in the etiology of obesity remains provocative.

The thermogenesis theory was expanded to include a specialized form of fat tissue (brown fat), which participates in thermogenesis. The exact role of brown fat is unclear, but it appears to favor increased triglyceride hydrolysis. Animal studies have indicated that sympathetic denervation of brown fat results in an increase in body fat in lean animals. Additionally, an increase in norepinephrine turnover in brown fat during elevated DIT, as well as the ability of norepinephrine to stimulate activity of brown adipose tissue, further implicates the sympathetic branch of the autonomic nervous system in obesity. Several reports present evidence that, in humans, the thermogenic response to food plays an important role in the relationship of the sympathetic nervous system to brown fat.

A biochemical basis for obesity involving sodium–potassium adenosine triphosphatase (ATPase) has been suggested. This enzyme facilitates the sodium–potassium pump process in body cells, which could result in caloric expenditure. Red blood cells in obese people were noted to have lower levels of sodium–potassium ATPase as compared with those in individuals of normal weight. In other words, individuals with reduced sodium–potassium ATPase activity are more likely to store fat than those with normal enzyme activity because they burn fewer calories.

The correlation of a primitive "hibernation response" with human obesity has been proposed. Adaptive reactions that prepare the body for an impending shortage may be predominant in the obese individual. Although humans do not hibernate, an "endomorphic system" representing a relic of the human evolutionary past may be present to initiate the overeating typical of most obese persons. It is suggested that this "hunger reaction" may be initiated by the beta endorphins.

The connection that exists between metabolism and sleep may be related to obesity. Obesity has been correlated with the frequency of an ultraradian brain rhythm (rapid eye movement and non-rapid eye movement sleep). This observation lends credence to the proposal that the amount of sleep decreases in obese people when they lose weight whereas sleep time has been observed to increase when anorectic patients gain weight.

Another hypothesis suggests that the presence of excess fat cells in infancy may predispose an individual to obesity later in life. Obese patients not only have larger than normal fat cells but also have an increased number of these cells. Apparently, as people lose weight on a low-calorie diet, the size of each fat cell decreases but their total number remains the same; when these people return to increased weight levels, their fat cells regain their original size. Obesity in children may result from the addition of new fat cells whereas "adult onset obesity" may represent an expansion of fat cells already present. Previous experiments suggest that the earlier the onset of obesity, the greater the number of fat cells. After the age of 20, obesity is caused almost exclusively by the expansion of existent cells. Accordingly, an overweight child or adolescent may be more susceptible to obesity as an adult.

A child who has one obese parent has a 40% chance of being obese; if both parents are obese, the child's chance of obesity increases to 80%. These data suggest a direct genetic component, and although it has not been absolutely proven in human obesity, it has been indicated in animal studies. In experimental animals, genetic transmission of obesity is associated with modified organ size and composition. Human data also suggest fundamental relationships between body build and obesity. Studies revealed that obese women differed from nonobese women in morphologic characteristics other than the degree of adiposity: obese women were more endomorphic than nonobese women; abdomen mass overshadowed thoracic bulk, all regions were notable for their softness and roundness, and the hands and feet were relatively small.

Obesity may result from environmental influences such as the widespread advertising of food products. Occupational, economic, and sociocultural factors also may be considered in the broad environmental sense. It now appears that socioeconomic status and related social factors are important in obesity development. Obesity is seven times more common among women of low socioeconomic groups than among those of higher status, a trend that is similar although less marked in men. The mental health indices of obese subjects in the low socioeconomic group reflected immaturity, rigidity, and suspiciousness in comparison with those of individuals in the same group with normal weight; a defect in impulse control may be suggested by the immaturity rating. The prevalence of obesity in lower socioeconomic classes is first noted in early adulthood. Suggestive relationships between ethnic and religious factors and obesity have been noted for both sexes.

Obesity has a psychogenic component in 90% of the cases. Although the psychologic aspect of caloric excess is usually exemplified by compulsive overeating replacing other gratifications, other factors are also involved. Decreased physical activity often coexists with mental depression and may play a role in the development and maintenance of obesity. This observation involves the aspect of caloric expenditure rather than caloric ingestion and stresses the function of caloric disequilibrium in obesity. Therefore, depression may not be an incidental occurrence in obese people but rather one of the main reasons for the obesity.

Appetite Control

The hypothalamus of the brain contains centers that are involved in the food ingestion process: studies of the rat hypothalamus show a "satiety center" and an "appetite center." Destroying the satiety center leads to marked overeating with subsequent obesity; obliterating the appetite center results in emaciation. These results indicate that impulses from the satiety center may inhibit feedback of the appetite center after food is ingested. The glucostatic hypothesis of appetite regulation states that hunger is related to the degree by which glucose is used by cells called glucostats. When glucose use by glucostats in the satiety center is low, the inhibitory effect on the appetite center is reduced, favoring eating behavior. Conversely, when glucose use is high, the appetite center is inhibited and the desire for food intake is reduced.

The hypothalamus contains a high concentration of noradrenergic terminals. A discrete fiber system that supplies the hypothalamus with most of its norepinephrine-secreting terminals is called the ventral noradrenergic bundle. Food-induced enhancement of sympathetic activity is modulated by the ventral noradrenergic bundle; in animals with lesions of this region, food intake increased significantly. It has been suggested that the ventral noradrenergic bundle normally mediates satiety and may serve as a substrate for amphetamine-induced appetite suppression. Destroying the noradrenergic terminals in the hypothalamus or damaging the ventral noradrenergic bundle results in obesity in animals.

Visual and chemical food-related stimuli are interpreted in the cerebral cortex, the area of the central nervous system (CNS) that is involved in accepting or rejecting the sight, aroma, or taste of food. An obese person may respond differently than a person of normal weight to the appearance, taste, or smell of food. Endogenous opioids increase food intake in animals, and naloxone (an opioid antagonist) decreases food intake in animals and in obese humans. Opiate receptors, which exist in the taste pathways, are believed to modulate human taste. Thus, an emerging hypothesis suggests that an endogenous opioid system is involved in human gustatory perceptions. Research involving the trigeminal nerve, a pathway relaying sensory input from the oral cavity to the hypothalamus, supports this system's possible role in food intake. The trigeminal circuit is a system of oral touch, and the excessive nibbling common to obese individuals may be caused by their greater sensitivity to this stimulus.

Role of Obesity in Other Conditions

Studies have shown a significant association between morbidity, early mortality, and obesity. Cardiovascular diseases (e.g., hypertension, myocardial infarct, heart failure, and coronary artery disease) and cerebrovascular diseases (e.g., stroke) are associated with obesity. There is evidence that sustained hypertension is more common in overweight people; therefore, persons at high risk for hypertension, such as those with a family history of youthful obesity, should consider controlling their weight and reducing their salt intake. The pharmacist should recommend salt-intake reduction to persons who cannot control their obesity by other reasonable means. However, although reduced sodium intake may reduce weight through water loss, thereby providing some psychologic benefits, it should be stressed that this type of weight loss has no effect on fat cells or on true weight loss.

The relationship between obesity and diabetes mellitus is well documented. (See Chapter 16, "Diabetes Care Products and Monitoring Devices.") An early study revealed that 85% of patients over 40 years of age who developed diabetes mellitus were overweight. Glucose intolerance commonly occurs with obesity, and relative insulin resistance is noted in obese subjects although insulin production may be normal or high. Obesity that persists over long periods of time is generally associated with partial exhaustion of the beta cells and a resultant hypoinsulinemia. The hyperinsulinemia that occurs in obesity of shorter duration is related to increased body fat. Weight reduction results in improved glucose tolerance in the obese person with diabetes and reduced hyperinsulinemia in obese persons both with and without diabetes. It may also decrease or eliminate the severity of diabetes mellitus and the need for insulin or oral sulfonylureas. Hyperostosis of the spine (formation of bony bridges between the vertebrae) has been associated with hyperglycemia and obesity, although these factors are at least partly independent of one other.

Certain skin disorders, including candidiasis, tinea infections, furunculosis, pruritus vulvae, and trophic ulcerations, occur more often in obese individuals. These conditions have also been associated with diabetes mellitus, which may explain their particularly high incidence in obese persons. Entrapment of moisture in skinfolds, which produces a better culture medium for some microorganisms, is certainly a contributing factor.

In postmenopausal women, obesity appears to be positively related to the risk of both breast and endometrial cancer. Obesity is also associated with increased estrogen production, which is proportionately more significant in postmenopausal women because the ovaries no longer contribute to production of estrogen. The peripheral aromatization of androstenedione (a major adrenal hormone) to estrone via the aromatase reaction in adipose tissue is the principal source of estrogen in postmenopausal women; an increased rate of this reaction has been reported in obese women.

In addition to the correlation of obesity with the above-named disease states, obese individuals have larger and more cellular organs (heart and liver). Obesity-associated hyperlipidemia may be related to cholesterol gallstone formation because the level of cholesterol is characteristically elevated in obesity.

Excessive obesity may contribute to respiratory distress, impaired gas exchange, and pulmonary embolism. Obesity alters pulmonary function resulting in reduced lung volume, hypercapnia, and pulmonary hypertension. Charles Dickens' description of Joe, the fat boy in *The Pickwick Papers*, as obese and somnolent may be the first account of this condition in literature; the "pickwickian syndrome" describes a person who is obese, exhibits narcoleptic behavior, and has an excessive appetite.

Although obesity is generally caused by overeating, it may mask malnutrition. Often the obese individual overconsumes carbohydrates while omitting other nutrients such as protein, vitamins, and minerals from the diet. Obesity may predispose individuals to the development of gout, may aggravate degenerative joint disease (osteoarthritis) in weight-bearing joints (e.g., knees and ankles), may produce or aggravate lower back pain, and may be associated with menstrual irregularities. In addition, obesity may create a psychologic burden and lead to low self-esteem. Dexterity, coordination, and mobility may be impaired, which can have serious implications in a job situation.

Symptoms of Obesity

The cardinal symptom of obesity is an increase in body weight and the obvious mass of fatty tissue. Common complaints regarding obesity are often cosmetic, involving a desire to look slim. However, remarks such as "I can't tie my shoes without getting out of breath" indicate dyspnea and actual physical discomfort. The obese individual may also complain of persistent backache, inflammation in weight-bearing joints, and low back pain.

Long-term (> 8–12 weeks) regular use of nonprescription products to correct obesity may indicate a more severe underlying problem, and persons who remain obese after weeks to months of intermittent or continuous self-medication with nonprescription anorexigenic products should be referred to a physician. A psychogenic component involving inactivity due to mental depression or a compulsive anxiety reaction related to repeated snacking may be involved in such cases. The pharmacist should emphasize that weight loss will not occur unless caloric imbalance is corrected.

Treatment

Drug treatment of obesity is of limited value because the only satisfactory means of long-term weight control is lifestyle change incorporating caloric reduction and increased physical activity. In 1992, the Food and Drug Administration (FDA) issued a final rule establishing that 111 active ingredients in over-the-counter (OTC) weight control products are not generally recognized as safe and effective.[1] These products are listed in Table 3. The final monograph on OTC weight control products includes only phenylpropanolamine (PPA) and benzocaine as Category I drugs.

Anorexiants of the amphetamine class suppress appetite and reduce body weight via activation of beta-adrenergic and/or dopaminergic receptors within the perifornical hypothalamus. Although PPA is often considered to be a member of the amphetamine class of anorexiants, this drug is an atypical adrenergic anorexiant.[2] Unlike amphetamine, PPA microinjected into the perifornical hypothalamus does not suppress feeding. Moreover, PPA-induced anorexia is not reversed by the dopamine antagonist haloperidol. Instead, the anorexic action of PPA may result, in part, from its interaction with $alpha_1$-adrenergic receptors within the paraventricular medial hypothalamus.

Another theory of appetite suppression is that anorexiants act primarily by lowering the body's metabolic set point and only secondarily by suppressing appetite.[3] This theory is supported largely by anecdotal reports of the rapid regaining of body weight after cessation of appetite suppressants in contrast to the relative stability of weight loss achieved without medication.

Phenylpropanolamine

PPA is a sympathomimetic agent related chemically and pharmacologically to ephedrine. PPA stimulates both alpha and beta receptors and also has an indirect effect by releasing norepinephrine from peripheral nerve endings. PPA exerts predominant peripheral adrenergic effects and weak central stimulant actions. In the past, controversy has existed as to PPA's effectiveness as an anorexigenic agent. Early animal studies indicated its usefulness in diminishing food intake in animals, and a qualitative difference between the anorexigenic activities of PPA and amphetamines was reported.[4] The weight-reducing action of PPA may reflect a combined effect on both food intake[5,6] and brown adipose tissue thermogenesis.[7]

In a physician-managed weight-reduction program that included behavior modification, mild caloric restriction, and exercise, subjects taking PPA lost significantly more weight (6.1 kg) than subjects taking placebo (4.3 kg).[8] And a 14-week study that evaluated the anorectic activity of 75-mg daily doses of PPA in 102 overweight subjects found PPA to be associated with significant weight loss as early as week 6 of the study and to be a superior anorexiant compared with placebo.[9] Studies evaluating

TABLE 3 Ingredients determined by the FDA to be not generally recognized as safe and effective

Alcohol	Ferric ammonium citrate	Papain
Alfalfa	Ferric pyrophosphate	Papaya enzymes
Alginic acid	Ferrous fumarate	Pepsin
Anise oil	Ferrous gluconate	Phenacetin
Arginine	Ferrous sulfate (iron)	Phenylalanine
Ascorbic acid	Flax seed	Phosphorous
Bearberry	Folic acid	Phytolacca
Biotin	Fructose	Pineapple enzymes
Bone marrow, red	Guar gum	Plantago seed
Buchu	Histidine	Potassium citrate
Buchu, potassium extract	Hydrastis canadensis	Pyridoxine hydrochloride (vitamin B_6)
Caffeine	Inositol	Riboflavin
Caffeine citrate	Iodine	Rice polishings
Calcium	Isoleucine	Saccharin
Calcium carbonate	Juniper, potassium extract	Sea minerals
Calcium caseinate	Karaya gum	Sesame seed
Calcium lactate	Kelp	Sodium
Calcium pantothenate	Lactose	Sodium bicarbonate
Carboxymethylcellulose sodium	Lecithin	Sodium caseinate
Carrageenan	Leucine	Sodium chloride (salt)
Cholecalciferol	Liver concentrate	Soybean protein
Choline	Lysine	Soy meal
Chondrus	Lysine hydrochloride	Sucrose
Citric acid	Magnesium	Thiamine hydrochloride (vitamin B_1)
Cnicus benedictus	Magnesium oxide	Thiamine mononitrate (vitamin B_1 mononitrate)
Copper	Malt	Threonine
Copper gluconate	Maltodextrin	Tricalcium phosphate
Corn oil	Manganese citrate	Tryptophan
Corn syrup	Mannitol	Tyrosine
Corn silk, potassium extract	Methionine	Uva ursi, potassium extract
Cupric sulfate	Methylcellulose	Valine
Cyanocobalamin (vitamin B_{12})	Mono- and diglycerides	Vegetable
Cystine	Niacinamide	Vitamin A
Dextrose	Organic vegetables	
Docusate sodium	Pancreatin	
Ergocalciferol	Pantothenic acid	

Source: *Federal Register*. 1991 Aug 8; 56 (153): 37797.

the safety and efficacy of nonprescription anorexiants beyond 12–14 weeks are lacking. Long-term maintenance of weight loss remains the ultimate goal.

In 1982, the FDA Advisory Review Panel on Over-the-Counter Miscellaneous Internal Drug Products found PPA to be generally safe and effective for short-term weight control.[10] The FDA permits a PPA dose of up to 37.5 mg in immediate-release products and of up to 75 mg in sustained-release products. The maximum daily dose is set at 75 mg.[10]

Side effects such as nervousness, restlessness, insomnia, dizziness, perspiration, anxiety, headache, nausea, and an excessive increase in blood pressure may occur with PPA, especially if the recommended dose is exceeded. Cardiovascular adverse reactions, including hypertensive episodes and stroke, have been reported following both excessive doses and recommended doses of products containing PPA alone or in combination with other drugs.[11] Hypertension has been cited as the most likely cause of PPA-associated intracranial hemorrhage.[12] Intracerebral hemorrhage and cerebral vasculitis have been associated with prolonged PPA use and with use at doses in excess of those recommended in package labeling.[13,14] Vascular etiology involving multiple focal areas of arterial narrowing and segmental vascular injury has been implicated in lobar subcortical and subarachnoid hemorrhages.[13] Various cardiac rhythm disturbances, myocardial infarct, and atrioventricular blockage have also been attributed to PPA.[15–19] Acute renal failure, sometimes associated with rhabdomyolysis, has been reported after PPA ingestion.[20–23]

Hypertensive reactions in previously normotensive individuals have been reported with exaggerated single oral doses of 85 mg of PPA in an immediate-release dose form.[24,25] A double-blind study in young normotensive adults revealed that significant elevations in blood pressure may occur after a single dose of PPA.[26] There is evidence that the immediate-release product in these studies was a different isomer, (+)norpseudoephedrine, than the racemic form, (±)norephedrine, which is available in the United States.[27] It has been suggested that hypertensive effects are more likely to occur when PPA is in the immediate-release form than when it is in a sustained-release preparation.[28]

However, a review of prospective clinical trials indicated that PPA was an appropriately marketed OTC drug with an acceptable margin of safety.[29] Controlled clinical studies have demonstrated an absence of significant side effects or hypertensive activity with PPA in either obese patients[30] or healthy nonobese subjects.[31,32] A recent study of obese normotensive patients[33] demonstrated the absence of significant pressor effects with a 75-mg sustained-release PPA dose form, even when combined with caffeine. Other reports[34–36] document the absence of significant pressor effects with PPA in recommended nonprescription doses. Finally, in a pilot study, the safety and efficacy of PPA at therapeutic doses was noted in a population of adult patients with stable, controlled hypertension.[37]

CNS stimulation as evidenced by PPA-associated convulsive seizures has been noted,[38] as have been psychiatric adverse effects attributed to PPA.[39] Mental disturbances have been described in considerable detail, and the possibility of PPA-associated psychotic episodes clearly exists.[40,41] Amphetamine-like reactions to PPA have been reported from emergency room records over a 6-month period. All adverse CNS effects, which included respiratory stimulation, tremor, restlessness, increased motor activity, agitation, and hallucinations,[42] occurred within 1 to 2 hours after ingestion of PPA in combination with caffeine. Pharmacists should advise patients of the possible CNS adverse effects of PPA. However, although some clinicians believe PPA poses a danger to the public and should be regarded as a drug with potential for abuse,[43] a recent study provides evidence that PPA administered at recommended doses does not produce the euphoriant or stimulant subjective effects that characterize drugs of abuse.[44]

Although the FDA Advisory Review Panel on Over-the-Counter Cold, Allergy, Bronchodilator, and Antiasthmatic Drug Products did not review anorexiants as such, it concluded that the incidence of side effects with oral PPA is low at recommended doses.[45] Additionally, an analysis of 70 cases of accidental or deliberate overdose with PPA or PPA with caffeine revealed that symptoms such as nausea or vomiting, nervousness, headache, tachycardia, or dizziness occurred in adults only if the dose ingested exceeded the manufacturer's recommended dosage.[46]

Because PPA is an adrenergic substance, it may elevate blood glucose levels and produce cardiac stimulation. For these and other reasons, the labels on products containing PPA warn that individuals with diabetes mellitus, heart disease, hypertension, or thyroid disease should seek medical advice before taking this drug.

A severe hypertensive episode was reported when indomethacin was taken with an 86-mg dose immediate-release form of PPA,[47,48] and psychotic reactions have been described with 50 mg of PPA consumed in combination with isopropamide and phenyltoloxamine.[49] PPA has also been implicated in drug–drug interactions with monoamine oxidase inhibitors,[50] and severe hypertensive episodes may be more likely when patients who are already taking monoamine oxidase inhibitors ingest preparations containing PPA in an immediate- rather than a sustained-release form.

Among other drug–drug interactions, PPA was found to cause various adverse effects when ingested concurrently with aspirin and acetaminophen (nausea, vomiting, headaches, weakness, malaise, and severe muscle tenderness; brown-colored urine; and acute interstitial nephritis);[51,52] with thioridazine (fatal ventricular arrhythmia);[53] with methyldopa or oxyprenolol (severe hypertension);[54] and with fluphenazine treatment in conjunction with PPA overdose (catatonia).[55]

Evidence exists that suggests a pharmacokinetic interaction of PPA with caffeine. Coadministration of a sustained-release preparation of PPA increased plasma caffeine concentration fourfold and the concentration–time curve approximately threefold after administration of sustained-release caffeine preparation in human volunteers.[56] A pharmacodynamic interaction also has been reported between caffeine and PPA in which an additive increase in blood pressure occurs.[57] In a study of the effects of five drug preparations (75 mg PPA, 150 mg PPA, 75 mg PPA plus 400 mg caffeine, 400 mg caffeine, and placebo) in 16 resting, normotensive subjects, significant blood pressure increases occurred over several hours following the 150-mg dose of PPA and the 75-mg dose of PPA plus 400 mg caffeine but occurred less frequently after ingestion of 75 mg PPA alone and the 400 mg caffeine alone.[58] PPA-induced hypertension has been treated with nifedipine[59] and propranolol.[60]

There is one report of a positive phentolamine test for pheochromocytoma in PPA-induced hypertension,[61] and a pseudopheochromocytoma syndrome has been described following PPA use.[62]

The reports of adverse reactions with PPA and PPA-containing combinations should be interpreted within the total context of use. Many of these reports involve only one case or report of multiple drug ingestion and are, in a sense, anecdotal in nature. Factors such as hypersensitivity, dose and dosage forms ingested, concurrent pathology, and the presence of other drugs should be established before use of PPA is discounted.[63]

Benzocaine

Benzocaine was first incorporated into a weight-control preparation in 1958.[64] A preparation containing benzocaine and methylcellulose in chewing gum wafers was tried for 10 weeks in 50 patients who were 5.5–46 kg overweight. Results showed that 90% of the subjects lost weight. However, the study did not use a placebo control group, and the weight loss could have been caused by benzocaine, methylcellulose, or the diet alone. The benzocaine dose was small, and any marked degree of numbness in the oral cavity was questionable. It is conceivable that subtle effects on taste sensitivity or taste modification may occur, and perceived analgesia or numbness is not necessary for possible appetite suppressant activity.

When the two nonprescription anorectic drugs, PPA and benzocaine and their combination, were compared in a 30-patient study, benzocaine produced less weight loss than PPA ($p < .05$). Weight loss with PPA was not enhanced by combination with benzocaine.

Constant snacking is characteristic of the "oral syndrome" in many obese persons. A nontraditional appetite-control plan using benzocaine, glucose, caffeine, and vitamins in a hard candy form was tried. The subjects ingested the candies when they wanted a snack and before and after meals; this approach kept the patients orally active while elevating their blood glucose levels. The influence of benzocaine was considered an essential component of the significant weight reduction in the study group.

Because capsules or tablets containing benzocaine are designed to be swallowed, the drug does not come into contact with the oral cavity. Thus, any appetite suppression would depend on an effect on the gastrointestinal mucosa. However, no conclusive clinical data support such an activity. The FDA Advisory Review Panel on Over-the-Counter Miscellaneous Internal Drug Products classified benzocaine as generally effective for short-term weight control. This panel also determined that a dose of 3–15 mg for use in gum, lozenges, or candy just prior to food consumption was generally safe and effective for weight control.

Although they are rare, cyanotic reactions such as methemoglobinemia have been reported following benzocaine administration. These reactions occur primarily among infants and are therefore not specifically relevant to the use of the drug in the noninfant obese population. It is important, however, to be aware of potential benzocaine toxicity because benzocaine-induced methemoglobinemia has been reported recently in an adult. In addition, a fatal anaphylactic reaction occurred in an adult a few minutes after ingesting a throat lozenge containing benzocaine. Obese individuals who take preparations containing benzocaine over long periods may predispose themselves to the consequences of drug-induced hypersensitivity.

Other Products

Vitamins and minerals are present in some nonprescription weight-control products. If a dieting patient is not receiving adequate quantities of vitamins and minerals in the diet regimen chosen, the administration of vitamins and minerals is warranted. However, recommended daily allowances for vitamins and minerals are present in any well-balanced, low-calorie diet. (See Chapter 17, "Nutritional Products.")

Low-Calorie Balanced Foods

The "canned diet" products are considered substitutes for the usual diet. One product typical of this group supplies 70 g of protein per day, an amount the manufacturer states "is the recommended daily dietary allowance of protein for normal adults." It also contains 20 g of fat and 110 g of carbohydrate in a daily ration for a total daily calorie intake of 900 cal. Powder, granule, and liquid forms are available; these products are also formulated as cookies and soups.

These dietary products are low in sodium. Weight loss in the first 2 weeks is probably caused, in part, by water loss from the tissues. It is questionable, however, whether a weight loss over a short period is significant with regard to the effective long-term treatment of obesity.

The pharmacist should be aware that products that substitute 900 cal per day for the usual diet are usually effective in reducing weight. Moreover, it appears that any diet of 900 cal that supplies adequate protein and lowers carbohydrate and fat intake should enable an obese patient to lose weight.

Artificial Sweeteners

Sucrose overuse is common. A sucrose substitute, saccharin, is about 400 times more potent than sucrose as a sweetener and provides no calories. Although it produces a bitter taste in some individuals, it is the most popular artificial sweetener, especially since the prohibition of nonregulated use of cyclamates. Saccharin may have considerable importance in reducing caloric intake in some individuals. For instance, if it is used instead of one heaping teaspoonful of sugar to sweeten a cup of coffee, 33 cal are removed from the diet.

In 1972, after bladder tumors were discovered in rats fed exaggerated doses of saccharin in utero and throughout life, the FDA removed saccharin from the list of food additives generally recognized as safe. Saccharin is currently permitted in products labeled specifically as diet foods or beverages. Human epidemiologic studies have not revealed a clear-cut relationship between saccharin consumption and urinary bladder carcinoma. However, saccharin may accumulate in fetal tissues and therefore should not be used during pregnancy.

Aspartame is a synthetic dipeptide that is about 180 times as sweet as sugar. The FDA has determined that it too is safe as a food additive. However, because phenylalanine is contained in aspartame, individuals with phenylketonuria or patients who should avoid protein foods must be alerted to this fact. Thus, products containing aspartame must carry the warning: "Phenylketonurics: Contains Phenylalanine." In addition, directions not to use aspartame in cooking or baking (because the compound loses its sweetness) are required on table products containing aspartame.

Acesulfam, a newly available artificial sweetener, is a chemical relative of saccharin. Approximately 200 times sweeter than sucrose, acesulfam has been approved by the FDA for use in certain food products, including chewing gum, dry beverage mixes, instant tea and coffee, puddings, gelatins, and nondairy creamers.

Fructose, sorbitol, and xylitol may be used as alternatives to saccharin, but these sweeteners contain calories and should not be viewed as being "sugar-free" diet items. Fructose and xylitol are sweeter than sucrose, and xylitol is less calorigenic and more expensive. Apparently, neither sorbitol nor xylitol causes tooth decay, and some products containing xylitol have a more pleasant taste. However, some evidence implicates xylitol in the development of urinary tract abnormalities, kidney stones, and tumors in laboratory animals. Further tests are under way to evaluate this possibility. The ingestion of sufficient amounts of dietetic candies containing sorbitol may result in an osmotic catharsis in small children.

Several naturally occurring compounds show promise as substitutes for sucrose. Monellin, thaumatin, and miraculin are proteins from plant sources and are currently being investigated as possible sucrose substitutes.

Fat Substitutes

These substitutes mimic the "mouth-feel" of fat but contain fewer calories. For example, Simplesse®, a blend of egg white and/or milk protein whipped to a creamlike consistency, is a frozen dessert that contains less than 1 g of fat per serving. Oatrim® is a cholesterol-free fat substance designed to replace the fat in meats, cheeses, baked goods, and frozen desserts. Olestra® looks and tastes like fat but is not absorbed by the body; because it is heat resistant, it can be used for cooking and frying.

Dosage Forms

Nonprescription products for obesity control are available as liquids, powders, granules, tablets, capsules, sustained-release capsules, wafers, cookies, soups, chewing gum, and candy preparations. If wafers, chewing gum, or candy cubes are substituted for high-calorie desserts or snacks, the candy-like nature of the dosage form may offer patients a psychologic aid that is not found when a standard tablet or capsule is used. Ingesting large quantities of diet candy would, of course, contribute significantly to caloric intake.

Adjunctive Therapy

The therapy for most cases of obesity is dietary restriction alone or in conjunction with other therapeutic measures such as exercise. Patients who are having difficulty losing weight may find reinforcement in self-help groups and behavior modification programs.

Diet

Total fasting or semistarvation is sometimes proposed as a means of weight reduction in severely obese persons. However, starvation, either total or partial, depletes the body of some lean tissue (protein) and essential electrolytes in addition to fat. The ketosis and ketoacidosis resulting from a fasting state represents a significant metabolic alteration. If total fasting is used to treat obesity, hospitalization and intensive medical supervision is recommended to deal effectively with the alteration of physiologic functions.

High-protein, low-carbohydrate diets of 800–1,000 cal (kcal) a day are often used in weight-reduction programs. Low-carbohydrate diets have been advocated on the premise that individuals may eat as much as they desire as long as no carbohydrates are ingested. However, fat from food may be deposited as fat in the body, and proteins may be converted to fat. The excess fat metabolized may result in an increased production of ketones to the degree that ketosis, acidosis, and dehydration may occur.

Some low-carbohydrate diets recommend inclusion of large quantities of fat in the diet. But although a high-fat diet may suppress fat synthesis, it does not prevent fat deposition. An additional problem encountered in high-fat diets is the elevation of serum lipids. And while a carbohydrate-free, high-fat diet does cause an immediate weight reduction due to water loss (dehydration), it does not significantly affect adiposity. The "drinking-man's diet" adds alcohol to this regimen, which tends to add more calories and the increased liability of fat deposition. A high-meat (protein and fat), no-carbohydrate diet presents an extra burden to the kidneys because of the resultant increase in urea load. In addition, an increase in the uric acid levels in this diet may precipitate gouty arthritis in susceptible persons.

A low-protein, low-fat rice diet that was advocated several years ago is unbalanced and could lead to ill health. A diet containing kelp, vinegar, lecithin, and vitamin B_6 has been proposed. Excess kelp, which contains high amounts of iodine, may decrease thyroid function by negative feedback mechanisms. The other ingredients in this diet do not have any established value in weight reduction. The weight loss in this diet is due to the low caloric intake rather than to the use of these specific additives.

The extent of injuries and deaths caused by the use of extremely low-calorie protein diets is unclear. The complaints reported to the FDA often include nausea, vomiting, diarrhea (liquid preparations), constipation (dry preparations), faintness, muscle cramps, weakness or fatigue, irritability, cold intolerance, decreased libido, amenorrhea, hair loss, dry skin, cardiac arrhythmias, recurrence of gout, dehydration, and hypokalemia. Studies oriented toward geographic incidence, concurrent pathology, age, and other factors need careful scrutiny. The possibility of drug–food interactions with these diets also exists. Patients taking prescription medicines such as diuretics, antihypertensives, hypoglycemic agents, insulin, adrenergics, high doses of corticosteroids, thyroid preparations other than those used in replacement therapy, and lithium should not use the liquid protein diet.

The patient's age should also be taken into consideration because elderly obese persons may be more susceptible to cardiovascular stress and gout. Thus, the pharmacist should warn the patient not to undertake this type of diet without proper medical supervision.

A low-calorie, balanced diet containing no less than 12–14% protein, no more than 30% fat (preferably unsaturated), and the remainder composed of complex carbohydrate (low sucrose) is recommended over potentially dangerous unbalanced diets of questionable value.

Group Therapy

Group therapy and behavior modification are effective in treating obesity. Groups such as Weight Watchers® have been successful in providing long-term treatment. The peer group dynamic is an effective deterrent to overeating for many persons. Behavior modification that considers eating as a "pure" activity (not combined with any other activity) and that focuses on eating more slowly may be beneficial. In addition, keeping a diet diary and using a unit-dose concept for food may prove helpful in a weight-reduction program. Psychotherapeutic approaches show promise in obesity control.

Surgical Intervention

In refractory cases of severe obesity that pose a serious health threat, intestinal bypass operations have been performed. This procedure is probably the most hazardous and debatable measure used to treat extreme obesity, and it has led to alternative, perhaps safer, procedures such as gastric partitioning.

Product Selection Guidelines

As a health care professional, the pharmacist should emphasize the importance of a rational, low-calorie, balanced diet and proper exercise to correct caloric imbalance, as well as of individual effort in maintaining a diet management program. The patient may be referred to a support group.

In recommending a nonprescription product for weight control, the pharmacist should stress that weight cannot be reduced without a concerted effort to change one's eating and exercise lifestyle and to maintain the new behavior long term. The patient should be made aware of the caloric value of various food types. The pharmacist should inquire about previous diet control regimens the patient has attempted so that other nonprescription diet management adjuncts may be considered. However, a nonprescription obesity control product should be considered only as an adjunct to a planned weight-reduction program. Vitamins sometimes are added to such products on the assumption that dieting individuals may not have an adequate vitamin intake. This practice may be justified in individual cases but should not be applied to all patients. The pharmacist may also participate in monitoring the patient's weight-reduction efforts.

Summary

A patient should recognize that a successful weight-reduction program includes physical activity, reduced caloric intake, and possibly a pharmacologic aid such as a nonprescription product, and that its effectiveness depends largely on the patient's motivation, education, and acceptance of a regimen necessary to achieve long-term weight control. The role of the pharmacist is to supply pertinent and accurate information regarding these matters.

References

1. *Federal Register.* 1991 Aug 8; 56: 37792–9.
2. Wellman PJ. Overview of adrenergic anorectic agents. *Am J Clin Nutr* 1992 Jan; 55 (1 suppl): 193S–8S.
3. Stunkard AJ. In: Garattini S, Somani R, eds. *Anorectic Agents: Mechanisms of Action and Tolerance.* New York: Raven Press; 1981: 191–210.
4. Wellman PJ. The pharmacology of the anorexic effect of phenylpropanolamine. *Drugs Exp Clin Res* 1990; 16 (9): 487–95.
5. Hoebel BG, Cooper J, Kamin M, et al. Appetite suppression by phenylpropanolamine in humans. *Obes Bariatr Med* 1975; 4: 192.
6. Hoebel BG, Krauss J, Cooper J, et al. Body weight decreased in humans by phenylpropanolamine taken before meals. *Obes Bariatr Med* 1975; 4: 200.
7. Wellman PJ. Weight loss induced by chronic phenylpropanolamine: anorexia and brown adipose tissue thermogenesis. *Pharmacol Biochem Behav* 1986 Mar; 24: 605–11.
8. Weintraub M, Ginsburg G, Stein C, et al. Phenylpropanolamine OROS (Acutrim) vs. placebo in combination with caloric restriction and physician-managed behavior modification. *Clin Pharmacol Ther* 1986 May; 39: 501–9.
9. Greenway F. A double-blind evaluation of the anorectic activity of phenylpropanolamine versus placebo. *Clin Ther* 1989 Sep–Oct; 11: 584–9.
10. *Federal Register.* 1982; 47: 8466.
11. Lake CR, Gattant S, Masson E, et al. Adverse drug effects attributed to phenylpropanolamine: a review of 142 case reports. *Am J Med* 1990; 89: 195–208.
12. Fallis RJ, Fisher M. Cerebral vasculitis and hemorrhage associated with phenylpropanolamine. *Neurology* 1985; 35: 405–7.
13. Maertens P, Lum G, Williams JP, et al. Intracranial hemorrhage and cerebral angiopathic changes in a suicidal phenylpropanolamine poisoning. *South Med J* 1987 Dec; 80: 1584–6.
14. Glick R, Hoying J, Cerullo L, et al. Phenylpropanolamine: an over-the-counter drug causing central nervous system vasculitis and intracerebral hemorrhage. Case report and review. *Neurosurgery* 1987; 20: 969–74.
15. Clark JE, Simon WA. Cardiac arrhythmias after phenylpropanolamine ingestion. *Drug Intell Clin Pharm* 1983; 17: 737–8.
16. Pentel P et al. Myocardial injury after phenylpropanolamine ingestion. *Br Heart J* 1982; 47: 51–4.
17. Weesner KM et al. Cardiac arrhythmias in an adolescent following ingestion of an over-the-counter stimulant. *Clin Pediatr* 1982; 21: 700–1.
18. Woo OF et al. Atrioventricular conduction block caused by phenylpropanolamine. *JAMA* 1985; 253: 2646–7.
19. Burton BT et al. Atrioventricular block following overdose of decongestant cold medication. *J Emerg Med* 1985; 2: 415–9.
20. Bennett W. Hazards of the appetite suppressant phenylpropanolamine [letter]. *Lancet* 1979; 2: 42–3.
21. Swenson RD et al. Acute renal failure and rhabdomyolysis after ingestion of phenylpropanolamine-containing diet pills. *JAMA* 1982; 248: 1216.
22. Rumpf KW et al. Rhabdomyolysis after ingestion of an appetite suppressant. *JAMA* 1983; 250: 2112.
23. Duffy WB et al. Acute renal failure due to phenylpropanolamine. *South Med J* 1981; 74: 1548.
24. Frewin DB, Leonello P, Frewin M. Hypertension after ingestion of Trimolets. *Med J Aust* 1978; 2: 497–8.
25. Horowitz JD, McNeil JJ, Sweet B, et al. Hypertension and postural hypotension induced by phenylpropanolamine (Trimolets). *Med J Aust* 1979; 1: 175–6.
26. Horowitz JD, Howes LG, Christophidis N, et al. Hypertensive responses induced by phenylpropanolamine in anorectic and decongestant preparations. *Lancet* 1980; 1: 8159, 60–1.
27. Morgan JP. In: Morgan JP, ed. *Phenylpropanolamine.* Fort Lee, NJ: Burgess; 1986: 13–25.
28. Cuthbert MF. Anorectic and decongestant preparations containing phenylpropanolamine. *Lancet* 1980; 1: 367.
29. Morgan JP, Funderburk FR. Phenylpropanolamine and blood pressure: a review of prospective studies. *Am J Clin Nutr* 1992 Jan; 55 (1 suppl): 206S–10S.
30. Noble RE. Phenylpropanolamine and blood pressure. *Lancet* 1980; 1: 1419.
31. Silverman HI et al. Lack of side effects from orally administered phenylpropanolamine and phenylpropanolamine with caffeine: a controlled three-phase study. *Curr Ther Res* 1980; 28: 185.
32. Saltzman MB, Dolan MM, Doyne N. Comparison of effects of two regimens of phenylpropanolamine on blood pressure and plasma levels in normal subjects under steady-state conditions. *Drug Intell Clin Pharm* 1983; 17: 746–50.
33. Noble R. A controlled clinical trial of the cardiovascular and psychological effects of phenylpropanolamine and caffeine. *Drug Intell Clin Pharm* 1988; 22: 296–9.
34. Goodman RP et al. The effect of phenylpropanolamine on ambulatory pressure. *Clin Pharmacol Ther* 1986; 40 (2): 144–7.
35. Liebson I, Bigelow G, Griffith RR, et al. Phenylpropanolamine: effects on subjective and cardiovascular variables at recommended over-the-counter dose levels. *J Clin Pharmacol* 1987; 27: 685–93.
36. Klesges RC, Klesges LM, Meyers AW, et al. The effects of phenylpropanolamine on dietary intake, physical activity, and body weight after smoking cessation. *Clin Pharmacol Ther* 1990 June; 47: 747–54.
37. Bradley MH, Raines J. The effects of phenylpropanolamine hydrochloride in overweight patients with controlled stable

hypertension. *Curr Ther Res* 1989 July; 46 (1): 74–84.
38. Deocampo PD. Convulsive seizures due to phenylpropanolamine. *Med Soc N J* 1979; 76: 591–2.
39. Lake CR, Masson EB, Quirk RS. Psychiatric side effects attributed to phenylpropanolamine. *Pharmacopsychiatry* 1988; 21 (4): 171–81.
40. Norvenius G et al. Phenylpropanolamine and mental disturbances. *Lancet* 1979; 2: 1367–8.
41. Scavullo BC, Dementi B. Psychotic reactions following the naive ingestion of an anorectic, phenylpropanolamine, in psychiatric patients. *J Am Coll Toxicol* 1986; 5: 577–81.
42. Dietz AJ. Amphetamine-like reactions to phenylpropanolamine. *JAMA* 1981; 245: 601–2.
43. Blum A. Phenylpropanolamine: an over-the-counter amphetamine? [editorial]. *JAMA* 1981; 245: 1346–7.
44. Morgan JP, Funderburk FR, Blackburn GL, et al. Subjective profile of phenylpropanolamine: absence of stimulant euphorigenic effects at recommended dose levels. *J Clin Psychopharmacol* 1989 Feb; 9: 33–8.
45. Summary minutes of the FDA OTC Panel on Cold, Cough, Allergy, Bronchodilator, and Antihistamine Drug Products. Washington, DC; 1973 June.
46. Ekins BR, Spoerke DG. An estimation of the toxicity of nonprescription diet aids from seventy exposure cases. *Vet Hum Toxicol* 1983; 25: 81–5.
47. Lee KY et al. Severe hypertension after ingestion of an appetite suppressant (phenylpropanolamine) with indomethacin. *Lancet* 1979; 1: 1110–1.
48. Lee KY et al. Severe hypertension after administration of phenylpropanolamine [letter]. *Med J Aust* 1979; 1: 525–6.
49. Kane FJ, Green BQ. Psychotic episodes associated with the use of common proprietary decongestants. *Am J Psychiatry* 1966; 123: 484–7.
50. Smookler S, Bermundez AJ. Hypertensive crisis resulting from an MAO inhibitor and an over-the-counter appetite suppressant. *Ann Emerg Med* 1982; 11: 482–4.
51. Yu PH. Inhibition of monoamine oxidase activity by phenylpropanolamine, an anorectic agent. *Res Commun Chem Pathol Pharmacol* 1986; 51: 163–71.
52. Bennett WM. Hazards of appetite suppressant phenyl propanolamine. *Lancet* 1979; 2: 8132.
53. Chouinard G et al. Death attributed to ventricular arrhythmia induced by thioridazine in combination with a single Contact C capsule. *Can Med Assoc J* 1978; 119: 729–30.
54. McLaren EH. Severe hypertension produced by interaction of phenylpropanolamine with methyldopa and oxyprenolol. *Br Med J* 1976; 2: 283–4.
55. Castellani S. Catatonia associated with phenylpropanolamine overdose and fluphenazine treatment: case report. *J Clin Psychiatry* 1985; 46 (7): 288.
56. Lake CR, Rosenberg D, Gallant S, et al. Phenylpropanolamine increases plasma caffeine levels. *Clin Pharmacol Ther* 1990; 47: 675–85.
57. Brown NJ, Ryder D, Branch RA. A pharmacodynamic interaction between caffeine and phenylpropanolamine. *Clin Pharmacol Ther* 1991; 50: 363–71.
58. Lake CR, Zaloga G, Bray J, et al. Transient hypertension after two phenylpropanolamine diet aids and the effects of caffeine: a placebo-controlled follow-up study. *Am J Med* 1989; 86: 427–32.
59. Gibson RG et al. Nifedipine therapy of phenylpropanolamine-induced hypertension. *Am Heart J* 1987; 113: 406–7.
60. Pentel PR, Asinger RW, Benowitz NL. Propranolol antagonism of phenylpropanolamine-induced hypertension. *Clin Pharmacol Ther* 1985 May; 37: 488–94.
61. Duvernoy EC. Positive phentolamine test in hypertension induced by a nasal decongestant. *N Engl J Med* 1969; 280: 877.
62. Hyans JS et al. Pseudopheochromocytoma and cardiac arrest associated with phenylpropanolamine. *JAMA* 1985; 253: 1609–10.
63. Appelt GD. The safety of phenylpropanolamine. *J Clin Psychopharmacol* 1983; 3: 322–3.
64. Plotz M. Obesity. *Med Times* 1958; 86: 860–3.

CHAPTER 20

Ophthalmic Products

Jimmy D. Bartlett and Mark W. Swanson

Questions to ask in patient assessment and counseling

- *Is your vision blurred?*
- *Do your eyes hurt? Is the pain sharp or dull? Is it constant or intermittent?*
- *Do your eyes itch or sting?*
- *How long have these symptoms been present? What were you doing when you noticed them? Have you had a similar problem before?*
- *Have you recently used a nonprescription eye product? Which one(s) did you use? For what symptoms?*
- *Have you recently been in an accident or injured your head in any way?*
- *What is the nature of your work?*
- *Have you been working outside or in an environment that would cause your eyes to water, itch, or burn?*
- *Have your eyes been exposed recently to irritants such as smog, chemicals, or sun glare? Have you recently applied any pesticides or fertilizers?*
- *Do you have any other eye problems (double vision, redness, scratchy feeling, discharge, or twitch)?*
- *Do you have a chronic disease such as diabetes, glaucoma, or hypertension?*
- *Have you recently had a head cold or sinus problem?*
- *Are you currently taking any prescription or nonprescription medications?*
- *Do you have any allergies? If so, to what are you allergic?*
- *Do you wear contact lenses? Are they hard or soft lenses?*
- *What contact lens products do you use?*
- *Do you use eye cosmetics? Have you changed brands of eye makeup or used a friend's eye makeup?*
- *Do you use hair spray or spray deodorants?*

Editor's Note: This chapter is based in part on the chapter with the same title that appeared in the 9th edition but was written by Dick R. Gourley.

Many common conditions causing ocular discomfort are minor and self-limiting. In some instances, however, relatively minor symptoms may be associated with severe, potentially blinding conditions. Pharmacists should be well versed in eye anatomy and physiology and in common ocular conditions to provide the best possible guidance to patients who seek assistance in choosing between self-treatment or professional medical care.

Eye Anatomy and Physiology

External Eye

The external location and exposure of the eye make it susceptible to environmental and microbiologic contamination. However, the eye has many natural defense mechanisms to protect it against such contamination. The eyelids are one of the major protective elements (Figure 1).

The eyelids are a multilayer tissue covered externally by the skin and internally by a thin mucocutaneous epithelial layer, the palpebral conjunctiva. The intermediate portion of the eyelid contains glandular tissue and muscles for lid closure and opening. There are five main types of glandular tissue found within the eyelid: the meibomian glands, the glands of Zeis and Moll, and the accessory lacrimal glands of Krause and Wolfring.[1] The meibomian, Zeis, and Moll glands are sebaceous in nature and are found near the cilia (eyelashes). The glands of Krause and Wolfring are lacrimal glands found deep within the palpebral conjunctiva near the junction of the eyelid and globe. Their secretion constitutes the bulk of nonstimulated tears.

The eyelids serve primarily to protect the front surface of the eye. Through neural reflex mechanisms, the lids are physically able to block many foreign contaminants from reaching the ocular surface. The cilia also collect debris before it encounters the eye. The second principal function of the eyelids is to spread the tears produced by the glandular tissue. The eyelids close in a zipper-like manner from the outer margin to the inner margin, thereby forcing the flow of tears toward the nose, where drainage canals are located in the upper and lower eyelids. The drainage canals converge, forming the lacrimal sac between the inner eyelid and nose. The lacrimal sac is drained by a canal opening just below the inferior turbinate of the nasal cavity. The lacrimal drainage system is lined by a highly vascularized epithelium, and absorption into the systemic circulation along this pathway gives rise to potential systemic effects of topically administered eye medications.[1]

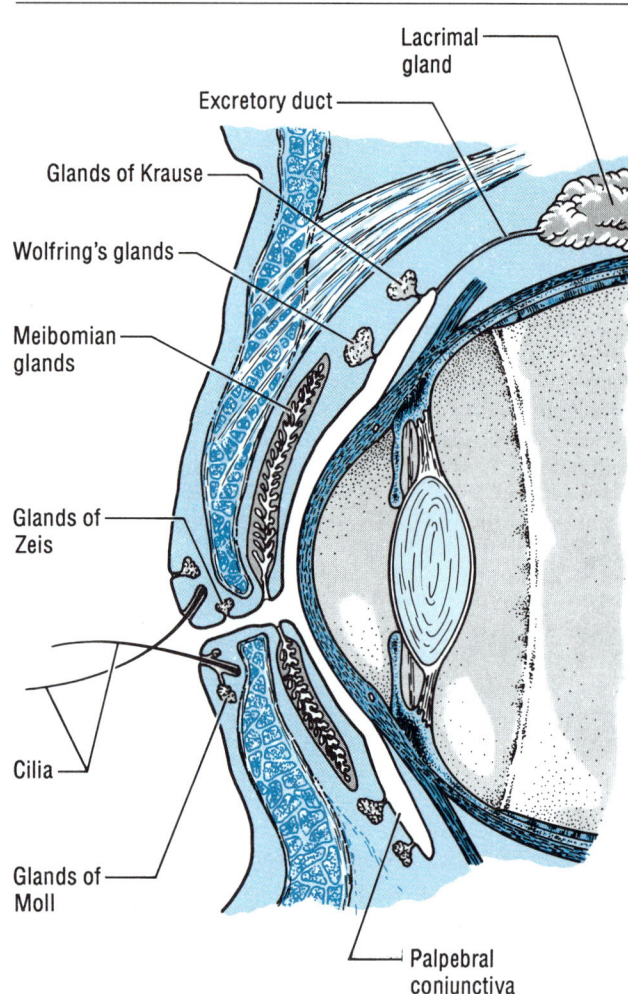

FIGURE 1 Cross-sectional anatomy of the eyelid.

The tear layer functions to keep the ocular surface lubricated, provides a mechanism for removing debris that touches the ocular surface, and has a potent antimicrobial action provided by specific enzymes and a number of immunoglobulins, notably IgA. The tear layer is a trilayer film. The outer surface is a thin lipid layer produced by the meibomian, Zeis, and Moll glands of the lids. The lipid layer complex prevents evaporation and maintains the optical properties of the tear layer. Even with the beneficial effect of the lipid layer, however, as much as 25% of total tear volume is lost to evaporation.[2] The middle, and largest, layer of the tear film is aqueous and is produced by the accessory lacrimal glands of Krause and Wolfring. This layer is largely responsible for the wetting properties of the tear film. The inner layer of the film is mucinous and is produced by goblet cells found within the conjunctiva. The mucinous layer allows the aqueous and lipid layers to maintain constant adhesion across the cornea and conjunctiva. Abnormalities within any one of these three layers can result in ocular discomfort.

The tears are produced at a rate of 1 to 2 mcL per minute with a turnover of approximately 16% total volume per minute.[2,3] An ambient tear volume of approximately 7–10 mcL is found on the ocular surface at any point in time.[2] During episodes of ocular irritation, reflex tearing is stimulated by the lacrimal gland found underneath the outer portion of the upper eyelid, and tear production increases to more than 300% of the nonstimulated production rate.[4]

The visible external portion of the eye is composed of the cornea and sclera (Figure 2). The sclera is a tough, collagenous layer that gives the eye rigidity and encases the internal eye structures. The visible sclera is covered by two epithelial layers, the episclera and the bulbar conjunctiva. The bulbar conjunctiva is contiguous with the palpebral conjunctiva at the junction between the eyelid and the ocular surface (the fornix). The episcleral and bulbar conjunctival layers contain the vascular and lymphatic systems of the anterior eye surface and are the source of visible eye redness during ocular irritation or inflammation. The sclera, episclera, and bulbar conjunctiva join the cornea in a transitional zone (the limbus).

The cornea is an aspherical, avascular tissue that is the principal refractive element of the eye. Approximately 12 mm wide and 0.5 mm thick,[1] it consists of five distinct layers: the epithelium, Bowman's layer, stroma, Descemet's membrane, and the endothelium. The epithelium and endothelium maintain corneal hydration, Bowman's and Descemet's layers serve barrier and protective functions, and the stroma provides the cornea with its clarity.

The unique anatomic structure of the cornea affects drug penetration. The corneal epithelium is lipophilic and allows the passage of fat-soluble drugs. The corneal stroma is hydrophilic and allows the passage of water-soluble drugs. The penetration of a drug into the eye through the cornea therefore depends on biphasic solubility. Damage to the corneal epithelium may markedly change drug absorption rates. Comparative studies with intact and compromised epithelium have shown that drug penetration into the aqueous layer may be increased by as much as threefold in corneas with compromised epithelium.[5]

Reflex tearing occurs immediately upon the instillation of a drug into the eye, diluting the drug's concentration. It has been shown that solutions as hypertonic as 2.5% sodium chloride are diluted to the concentration of tears (0.9–0.95%) within 1 to 2 minutes.[2] The difficulty for drugs to penetrate through the cornea, combined with their rapid removal through the tear system and their dilution by reflex tearing, can hinder efforts to maintain therapeutic drug concentrations in the eye. Studies have shown that as much as 90% of an instilled dose administered to the eye may be lost.[6]

Internal Eye

Directly behind the cornea is the anterior chamber, a cavity filled with aqueous humor (Figure 2). The aqueous functions to maintain the normal internal eye pressure and provides nutritional support for the cornea and crystalline lens. It is produced at a constant rate by the epithelium of the ciliary body and is drained from the anterior chamber via the trabecular meshwork found at the junction between the iris and back surface of the cornea. During episodes of internal eye inflammation, the aqueous becomes filled with white blood cells and protein released by the ciliary body. Large amounts of inflammatory cells may block the drainage system, causing the internal eye

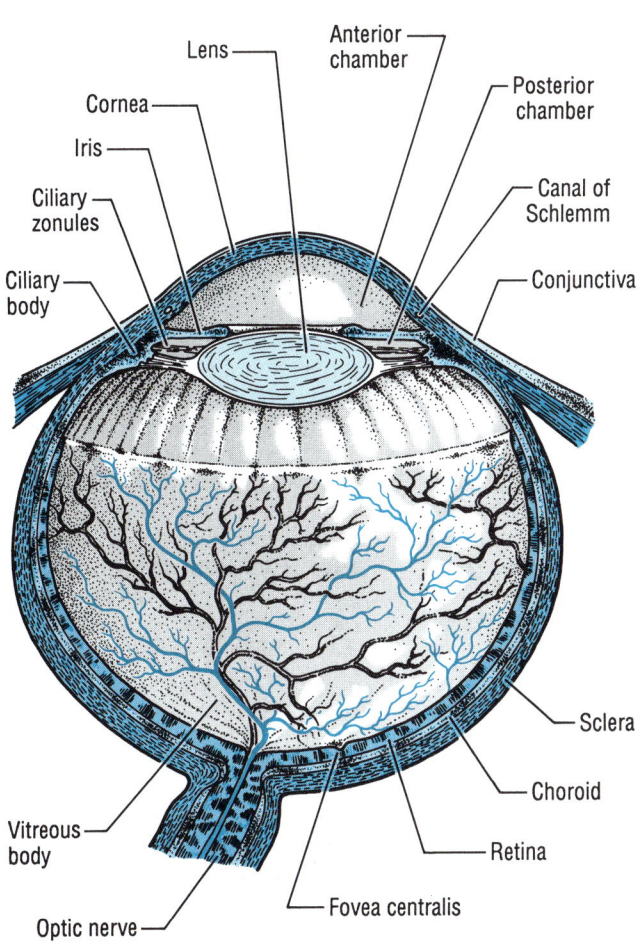

FIGURE 2 Major anatomic features of the eye.

able to focus light, and at some point the individual must rely on optical devices to focus near objects on the retina. Presbyopia, or lack of near focusing ability, commonly begins to manifest itself at around ages 40–45. Focusing of the lens is directly controlled by the ciliary body.

The ciliary body is bordered anteriorly by the iris and is continuous with the choroid posteriorly. The ciliary body is composed of the ciliary muscle and the ciliary epithelium. The lens is connected to the ciliary body by the ciliary zonules, threadlike protein fibrils attached to the lens surface. The ciliary muscle is largely controlled by the parasympathetic nervous system. During accommodation, the ciliary muscle constricts, releasing tension on the ciliary zonules and allowing the lens to change shape. During episodes of ocular inflammation, the ciliary muscle may begin to spasm, resulting in fluctuating vision and pain. For this reason, inhibition of the ciliary muscle (cycloplegia) using anticholinergic agents is a frequent treatment during internal ocular inflammation.

Behind the lens lies the vitreous body. It composes about 80% of the total eye volume and is filled with vitreous humor, a gellike, fluid collagen matrix that helps maintain eye volume. Posteriorly, the vitreous humor abuts the retina, a multilayer neural tissue that begins the visual pathway. Light is initially captured by the rods and cones of the retina in a complex photochemical process. Ultimately, the photic message is transmitted by the optic nerve and visual pathways to the posterior cerebral cortex, where the visual information is decoded. The retina adheres relatively loosely to the retinal pigment epithelium beneath it. Trauma may cause the retina to separate from the pigment epithelium, resulting in retinal detachment. A number of inflammatory conditions of the retina can occur, and most have prominent symptoms. Some, however, have relatively mild symptoms mimicking common irritative conditions.

pressure to rise. Similarly, during episodes of angle-closure glaucoma, the trabecular meshwork is physically blocked by the iris with a resultant increase in intraocular pressure.

The iris is the visible colored portion of the eye. It functions in much the same way as an aperture on a camera to regulate light striking the retina. The central opening in the iris is the pupil. The pupillary diameter is controlled by two opposing muscles within the iris, the sphincter and the dilator. As the names imply, the sphincter decreases the pupil diameter whereas the dilator increases it. The sphincter is controlled by the parasympathetic nervous system, and the dilator is controlled by the sympathetic nervous system. Both topical and systemic drugs may affect the tonus of these muscles, thereby altering the pupil diameter. Prostaglandins released by the iris during episodes of inflammation may also affect the sphincter muscle, resulting in constriction of the pupil. This constriction may help distinguish simple external irritation from more severe internal inflammation.

Directly behind the pupillary aperture is the crystalline lens, an avascular, biconvex structure that alters its shape to focus light on the retina. The focusing is a response to the viewing of a near object and is referred to as accommodation. With normal aging, the lens becomes less

Common Ocular Disorders

Ocular inflammation and irritation can be caused by many conditions. Nonprescription ophthalmic products are safe and effective in treating some of these conditions. Their primary use is in the relief of minor symptoms of burning, stinging, itching, and watering. The Food and Drug Administration (FDA) has suggested that self-medication may be indicated for tear insufficiency, corneal edema, and external inflammation or irritation.[7] Self-medication also may be effective in managing hordeolum (stye), blepharitis, and conjunctivitis.[8] Referral for medical care is mandatory for embedded foreign body, uveitis, flash burns, tear duct infection, and corneal ulcers.

The FDA has recommended that consumers not self-treat ophthalmic conditions for longer than 72 hours without consulting a doctor.[7] It refers specifically to self-treatment with ophthalmic lubricants and vasoconstrictor products. The pharmacist should advise patients of this general rule on duration of use when recommending nonprescription ophthalmic products. Care should be taken when counseling patients because many seemingly harmless ocular conditions can prove to be devastating. Figures 3 and 4 provide general algorithms that may be used in the decision-making process in managing eyelid irritation and red eye. It must be emphasized that if the etiology is not clearly

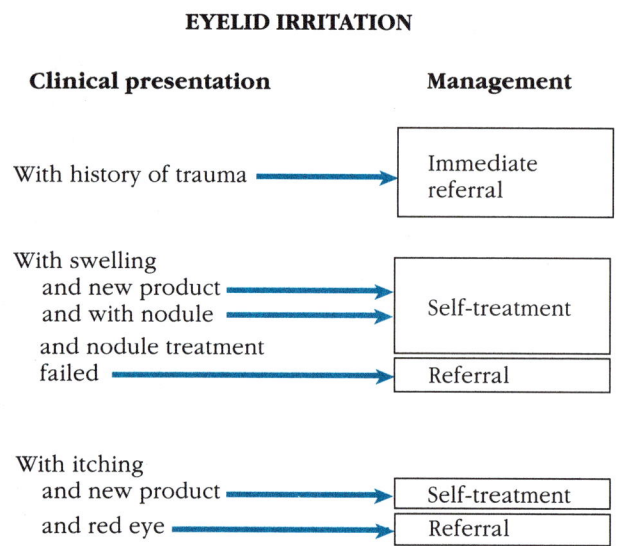

FIGURE 3 Decision-making algorithm for management of patients with eyelid irritation.

due to simple external irritation, referral to an optometrist or ophthalmologist is strongly encouraged.

Eyelid Conditions

Because the eyelids are a highly vascular tissue, blunt trauma can easily rupture blood vessels and cause bleeding into the eyelid tissue space, resulting in swelling and ocular discomfort. Under most circumstances, blunt trauma does not result in internal damage and treatment is largely supportive, entailing cold compresses and oral nonprescription analgesics as needed. However, all individuals with blunt trauma should be evaluated by an ophthalmologist or optometrist as soon as possible after the event. In addition to the visible external damage, blunt trauma can result in internal eye bleeding, secondary glaucoma, and retinal detachment.

Blepharitis is an inflammatory condition of the eyelid margins. It is almost always due to *Staphylococcus epidermidis,* *Staphylococcus aureus,* seborrheic dermatitis, or a mixture of these conditions.[9] Red, scaly, thickened eyelids, often with loss of the eyelashes, are typical of blepharitis. Itching, burning, and redness are the most common accompanying complaints. All forms of blepharitis tend to be chronic, and individuals are often aware of their diagnosis. Treatment may include topical antibiotics or nonprescription lid hygiene preparations. Lid scrubs with baby shampoo are also effective. Lid scrubs consist of cleansing along the eyelid margin with gauze pads or cotton applicators soaked with prepackaged solution, baby shampoo, or topical antibiotic ointment. The chronic nature of blepharitis makes the use of careful lid hygiene preferable to the long-term use of topical antibiotics.

Infestation of the eyelids with the organisms *Phthirius pubis* (crab louse) or *Pediculus humanus capitis* (head louse) may cause symptoms similar to blepharitis. These organisms are also responsible for sexually transmitted lice infestation. Children are rarely affected by the crab louse but are commonly affected by the head louse. Adults with eyelid infestation will often be aware of the involvement of other body areas. Pediculicides (e.g., RID®, Nix®, and A-200®) are useful for treating noneyelid areas but should not be used around the eye because they could cause severe hypersensitivity reactions. A 1% yellow mercuric oxide ointment used twice a day is effective for eyelid infestation. A bland ophthalmic ointment (e.g., petrolatum) used for 10 days is also effective because it suffocates the louse and deprives its eggs of adequate oxygen. A 0.25% physostigmine ointment is effective, but the side effects due to its powerful anticholinesterase activity are not well tolerated. Pharmacists should also carefully instruct patients about the need to take hygienic measures, including washing clothing and bedding, which may contain unhatched eggs.

Swelling, scaling, or redness of the eyelid along with profuse itching are common with contact dermatitis. A change in makeup or soap or exposure to some foreign substance is usually the cause. The equal involvement of each eyelid suggests allergy because both eyes are often exposed. Questioning the patient about new products used (e.g., eyeliner and eye shadow) quickly identifies the offending substance, removal of which is the best treatment. Swelling of the eyelid can be marked in some cases, and nonprescription oral antihistamines along with cold compresses will help reduce the inflammation and itching.

Hordeolum is an inflammation of either the meibomian gland (internal hordeolum) or the glands of Zeis and Moll (external hordeolum). A palpable, tender nodule is always present. Swelling of the eyelid, almost to the point of closure, can occur with a severe internal hordeolum. The cause is invariably one of the staphylococcal species associated with blepharitis. Hordeola typically respond well to hot compresses applied three to four times daily for 5–10 minutes at each session. Clearing usually occurs within 1 week. Although external hordeola may be treated with a topical antibiotic, internal hordeola do not respond well to such treatment and are best treated with a course of oral antibiotics. In recalcitrant cases, surgical drainage may be required. A chalazion is very similar to an internal hordeolum except that the former is a sterile, nontender condition. Hot compresses applied the same as for treatment of hordeola are usually sufficient to drain chalazia. Recalcitrant chalazia may require an intralesional steroid injection or surgical excision. Recurrences of chalazion and hordeolum may be reduced by the periodic use of lid scrubs.

Ocular Surface Conditions

Despite the protective effect of the lids, foreign substances often contact the ocular surface. The immediate response of the eye is watering. If reflex tearing does not remove the foreign substance, the eye may need to be flushed. Lint, dust, and similar materials can usually be removed by rinsing the eye with sterile saline or specific eyewash preparations (irrigants). Foreign particles trapped between the upper lid and the bulbar conjunctiva can be particularly difficult to flush and may need to be removed by an optometrist or ophthalmologist. Metallic foreign bodies are often not removed by self-irrigation and can cause abrasion, scarring, and chronic red eye if not removed.

Moreover, when such particles contact the eye as a result of high-speed grinding or activities that entail metal striking metal, intraocular penetration is possible. Thus, immediate medical referral is indicated.

Contact with foreign matter can also cause abrasions of the cornea and conjunctiva. These injuries result in partial or total loss of the epithelium and are especially painful if the cornea is involved. Scratches by fingernails and metallic foreign bodies are a common source of this type of injury. Self-treatment is not recommended owing to the risk of bacteria or fungi contaminating and infecting the eye.

Chemical exposure by splash injury, a solid chemical, or fumes can be a serious problem and should be considered a medical emergency. The initial treatment should include flushing the eye with sterile saline for at least 10 minutes. If saline is not available, water may be used. Because the lids and ocular surface are particularly sensitive to alkali damage, severe scarring can occur. This type of injury should be referred immediately to an emergency facility.

Thermal damage may range from minor to severe. One common form of thermal damage occurs from exposure to ultraviolet radiation during snow skiing without protective goggles. This form of irritation is typically minor and usually responds well to artificial tear solutions or ointments. If such treatment does not provide relief within 24 hours, medical referral is indicated. More severe forms of thermal injury, however, may occur from welder's arc. These injuries may require a visit to the optometrist or ophthalmologist to provide definitive care, including eye patching.

Conjunctivitis is the term given to inflammation of the bulbar conjunctiva. Four general types of conjunctivitis are commonly seen: viral, allergic, bacterial, and chlamydial. Viral conjunctivitis is probably the most common form. A recent cold, sore throat, or exposure to someone with pinkeye is a common precursor of this condition. Individuals with viral conjunctivitis will usually have a "pink eye" with a copious amount of watery discharge. Symptoms include nondescript ocular discomfort and mild to moderate foreign body sensation; vision may occasionally be blurred. Low-grade fever may be present, and swollen preauricular or submandibular lymph nodes may be found. Viral conjunctivitis is usually self-limiting, with symptoms resolving over 1–3 weeks. Treatment is aimed at relief of the major symptoms using artificial tear preparations and ocular decongestants. Because certain forms of viral conjunctivitis can be extremely contagious, counseling should include warnings about washing hands, sharing towels, and properly disposing of tissues used to blot the eye.

Allergic conjunctivitis is characterized by a red eye with watery discharge. The hallmark symptom accompanying ocular allergy is itching. Vision is usually not impaired but may be blurred due to excessive tearing. The list of antigens that can cause ocular allergy is virtually endless, but the most common allergens include pollen of various types, animal dander, and topical eye

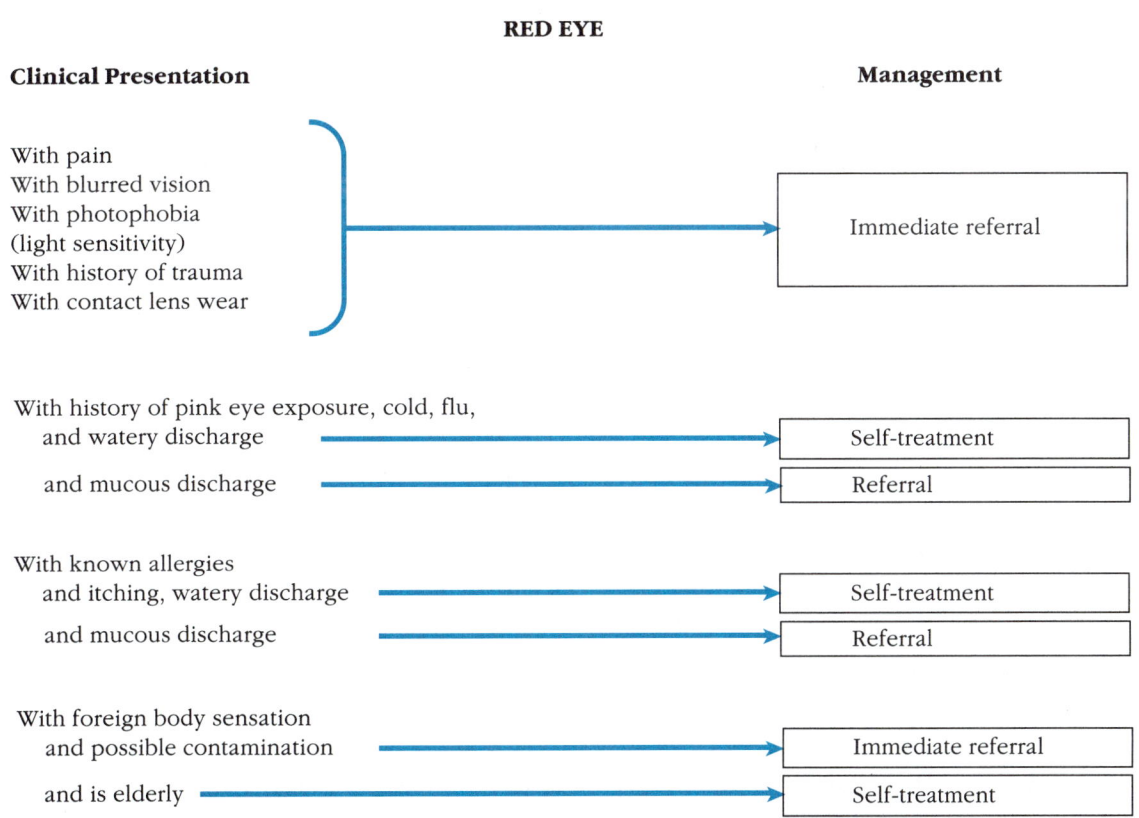

FIGURE 4 Decision-making algorithm for management of patients with red eye(s).

preparations. Persons with ocular allergy will often report seasonal allergic rhinitis as well. Questioning the patient about exposure to an allergen may help identify the offending substance. Removal or avoidance of the cause is the best treatment, but ocular decongestants, nonprescription oral antihistamines, and cold compresses will help relieve symptoms.

Bacterial conjunctivitis can be caused by a number of organisms, including *S. aureus, S. epidermidis, Streptococcus pneumoniae,* and *Haemophilus influenza.*[9] This condition is characterized by a red eye with purulent discharge. The most common complaint is of general eye discomfort along with the key symptom of the eyelids sticking together on awakening. Bacterial conjunctivitis is typically self-limiting within 2 weeks, but topical antibiotics can clear the infection more quickly.

A fourth type of conjunctivitis is caused by chlamydial infection. In the United States, this is a sexually transmitted disease and thus is often seen in the sexually active population. Chlamydial conjunctivitis may have many signs and symptoms in common with both viral and bacterial conjunctivitis and is often initially misdiagnosed. Misdiagnosis of chlamydial conjunctivitis can be a serious problem because afflicted individuals often harbor other sexually transmitted diseases. Women with chlamydial urethritis are at risk of pelvic inflammatory disease. Because of the pitfalls in separating chlamydial infection from self-limiting viral and bacterial conjunctivitis, self-treatment should be discouraged if symptoms and signs are vague.

Keratitis is the inflammation of the cornea. It may accompany any of the forms of conjunctivitis or exist as a separate entity. Individuals with keratitis, which is potentially a vision-threatening problem, will generally have signs of conjunctivitis accompanied by one or more additional symptoms, including blurred vision, photophobia, and pain. Individuals with red eye and signs of keratitis need to be evaluated as soon as possible by an optometrist or ophthalmologist. This is especially true for patients who wear contact lenses who are contemplating self-treatment of red eye. Corneal ulceration and loss of the eye are more likely among those who wear contact lenses than among those who do not. *Pseudomonas aeruginosa,* the most common cause of corneal ulcer among contact lens wearers, produces a collagenase that can destroy the cornea within 24 hours.[10]

Corneal edema may occur from a variety of conditions, including overwear of contact lenses, surgical damage to the cornea, and inherited corneal dystrophies. The edematous area of the cornea is often confined to the epithelium. Because fluid accumulation distorts the optical properties of the cornea, halos or starbursts around lights, with or without reduced vision, are a hallmark symptom of corneal edema. Once the initial diagnosis is established, hypertonic saline in solution or ointment form, usually in 2% and 5% concentrations, can be used to dehydrate the cornea. Pharmacists should forewarn individuals using a 5% solution that profound stinging may occur on instillation.

Dry eye is among the most common disorders affecting the anterior eye. This condition is characterized by a white or mildly red eye; a sandy, gritty feeling or complaint of something in the eye is common. Contrary to what the name suggests, dry eye is often accompanied by excess tearing. Abnormalities in the tear layer cause less than optimal lubrication of the ocular surface. This leads to the production of more inadequate tears, and a vicious cycle is set up. Dry eye is most often associated with the aging process, but it can also be caused by lid defects; loss of lid tissue turgor; Sjögren's syndrome; a variety of collagen diseases, including rheumatoid arthritis; and systemic medications. Antihistamines, anticholinergics or drugs with anticholinergic properties (e.g., antihistamines and antidepressants), diuretics, and beta blockers are some of the more common pharmacologic causes of dry eye.

Treatment of dry eye is the instillation of nonprescription artificial tears and lubricants. The products are similar, but the buffering agents, preservatives, pH, and other formulation factors may vary. Preparations without preservatives have been shown to have a greater beneficial effect on the ocular surface than do those with preservatives.[11] Both drop and ointment preparations are available. Because all ointments tend to blur vision for some time after instillation and have longer contact time with the eye, their preferred usage is at bedtime; drops are generally recommended for use during the day. Vitamin A preparations are also available for treatment of dry eye. Although these have generally been shown to be no more effective than artificial tear preparations in the treatment of routine dry eye, they may be of greatest benefit in treating severe dry eye associated with glandular tissue destruction.[12] The most severe cases of dry eye may be treated with ocular inserts or hyaluronidase, or by occlusion of the lacrimal drainage system to increase the available tear pool.

Internal Eye Conditions

Uveitis is the general term for inflammation of the uveal tract (iris, ciliary body, or choroid). This disorder is divided into anterior, posterior, and panuveal (affecting both anterior and posterior) types. Anterior uveitis is also known as iritis, whereas posterior uveitis is often associated with vitritis. In these conditions, white blood cells are found within the anterior chamber or vitreous body. Uveitis can be caused by a number of conditions, including trauma and systemic inflammatory disease, but in many individuals it is idiopathic. Persons with uveitis can have symptoms very similar to those of viral conjunctivitis or keratitis, with pain, blurred vision, and photophobia commonly reported. The eye is usually mildly to markedly red with reflex tearing. The absence of contact with infected individuals may help determine whether the cause is simple viral conjunctivitis. Untreated uveitis can cause secondary glaucoma, destruction of the iris, and in some cases blindness. Treatment involves topical, depot, or systemic oral steroids, depending on the underlying cause. Because of the severe consequences of untreated or improperly treated uveitis, care must be taken in recommending self-treatment.

Narrow-angle or angle-closure glaucoma may present as a red, painful eye. Symptoms associated with angle closure occur as a result of obstruction of the trabecular meshwork and the aqueous draining system. The angle-closure attack may be precipitated by dilation of the pupil with mydriatics; the attack often occurs as the pupil is returning to its normal state several hours after the mydriatic has been instilled. The most common symptoms are brow-ache or headache, often accompanied by nausea and vomiting; these symptoms are typically severe enough to cause the individual to visit an eye doctor. Individuals complaining about headache or eye pain after an eye examination should be referred immediately to their eye doctor.

Ophthalmic Drug Formulations

Ophthalmic medications available without a prescription are necessarily formulated to reduce the stinging and other side effects common with many prescribed ophthalmic drugs. The pH, buffers, tonicity adjusters, and preservative systems must be carefully controlled to produce a product that is comfortable to use and will therefore encourage compliance with the self-medication process. Ophthalmic products that sting, burn, or otherwise irritate ocular tissues will, of course, be poorly tolerated by the patient who self-treats. Among the inactive ingredients of nonprescription ophthalmic products, the drug vehicle and preservative systems are the most important, and the pharmacist must have adequate knowledge of these components to assist the patient in selecting the appropriate ophthalmic product. In addition, various other ingredients are often included as excipients.

Vehicles

An ophthalmic vehicle is an agent other than the active drug that is added to a formulation to enhance drug action by providing increased viscosity. Although aqueous solutions can be used, the vehicles listed in Table 1 are more viscous and thus retard drainage of the active ingredient from the eye; this increases the retention time of the active drug and enhances bioavailability at the external ocular tissues. These polymers are generally of high molecular weight, and some of the molecules can even bind at the corneal surface to increase drug retention and stabilize the tear film. Among the most commonly used vehicles for ophthalmic solutions are polyvinylpyrrolidone (PVP, povidone), polyvinyl alcohol (PVA), hydroxypropylmethylcellulose (HPMC), and poloxamer 407.

TABLE 1	Selected ophthalmic vehicles

Carboxymethylcellulose (CMC) sodium
Dextran 70
Gelatin
Glycerin
Hydroxyethylcellulose (HEC)
Hydroxypropylmethylcellulose (HPMC)
Methylcellulose
Poloxamer 407
Polyethylene glycol
Polyvinyl alcohol (PVA)
Polyvinylpyrrolidone (PVP, povidone)
Propylene glycol

TABLE 2	Preservatives commonly used in ophthalmic products

Benzalkonium chloride (BAK)
Benzethonium chloride
Cetylpyridinium chloride
Chlorhexidine
Chlorobutanol
Disodium ethylenediaminetetraacetic acid (EDTA)
Methylparaben
Phenylethyl alcohol
Phenylmercuric acetate
Phenylmercuric nitrate
Propylparaben
Sodium benzoate
Sodium propionate
Sorbic acid
Thimerosal

PVP is not bound to membrane surfaces and thus does not provide long-lasting viscosity enhancement beyond its normal residence time in the tears. The viscosity of PVP does not change until near pH 1.0, when it doubles. Thus, there is no appreciable ionic character to the PVP molecule at pharmaceutical or physiologic pH values. Consolute binding, however, can cause a change in the size of the polymer molecule, influencing the viscosity and other properties of the solution.

PVA is a water-soluble viscosity enhancer commonly used in a concentration of 1.4%.[13] This vehicle is generally nonirritating to the eye and documentation has shown that it actually facilitates healing of abraded corneal epithelium.[14]

Like PVA, the viscosity enhancer HPMC is available in several molecular weights and in formulations with different substitutions. These polymers are often called "substituted cellulose ethers." When used as ophthalmic lubricants, these vehicles enhance tear film stability. HPMC (0.5%) has been documented to exhibit twice the ocular retention time of 1.4% PVA.[15]

The first polyionic vehicle to be evaluated in the eye was poloxamer 407, a vehicle with a hydrophobic nucleus, hydrophilic end groups, and surfactant properties. Polyionic vehicles such as poloxamer 407 are unique in their ability to produce an artificial microenvironment in the tear film, which can greatly enhance the bioavailability of certain drugs used in the eye.[16]

Preservatives

Preservatives are incorporated into ophthalmic products designed for multidose use. These components are intended to destroy or limit multiplication of microorganisms inadvertently introduced into the product. Commonly used preservatives in commercial ophthalmic products are listed in Table 2.

Preservatives currently available for ophthalmic use are of two distinct types. One group, the surfactants, are molecules that disrupt the plasma membrane and are usually bactericidal. Other groups include the metals mercury and iodine, their derivatives, and alcohols. These compounds are considered bacteriostatic if they only inhibit growth, or bactericidal if they destroy the ability of bacteria to reproduce.

The quaternary surfactants, benzalkonium chloride (BAK) and benzethonium chloride, are preferred by many manufacturers because of their stability, excellent antimicrobial activity, and long shelf life. Unfortunately, these agents have toxic effects on both the tear film and the corneal epithelium.[17] A single drop of 0.01% BAK can break the superficial lipid layer of the tear film into numerous oil droplets. This preservative can reduce the tear film breakup time and thus may represent a poor choice for an antimicrobial preservative in artificial tear products.[18] The inclusion of BAK in artificial tear formulations does not provide protection to corneal epithelium or promote a stable oily tear surface.

Chlorhexidine is useful as an antimicrobial agent in the same range of concentrations as BAK, yet it is used at lower concentrations in commercial ophthalmic formulations. Because it does not alter corneal permeability to the same extent as does BAK, chlorhexidine is not as toxic to the eye.

Of the mercurial preservatives, thimerosal is less likely to degrade into toxic mercury than either phenylmercuric acetate or phenylmercuric nitrate. Compared with BAK, which undermines tear film stability, thimerosal has no known effects on the tear film. An important clinical point, however, is that some patients develop contact blepharitis or conjunctivitis after several weeks of exposure to thimerosal and must therefore discontinue use of products containing this preservative. Moreover, products containing thimerosal are rapidly disappearing from the commercial marketplace because this preservative induces contact allergy.

Chlorobutanol is less effective than BAK as an antimicrobial preservative and, indeed, tends to disappear from bottles during prolonged storage.[13] Compared with thimerosal, however, chlorobutanol does not appear to produce allergic reactions associated with prolonged use.

During the past decade, methylparaben and propylparaben have been introduced into some ophthalmic medications, especially artificial tears and nonmedicated ointments. However, these preservatives are unstable at high pH and can sometimes induce allergic reactions.

Ethylenediaminetetraacetic acid (EDTA) is a chelating agent that preferentially binds and sequesters divalent cations. The role of EDTA in preservative systems is to assist the action of thimerosal, BAK, and other agents. As with those other preservatives, EDTA can sometimes induce contact allergies.[19]

Useful excipients are antioxidants, wetting agents, buffers, and tonicity adjusters. Antioxidants prevent or delay deterioration of products exposed to oxygen in the air, and wetting agents reduce surface tension, allowing the drug solution to spread more easily over the ocular surface. Buffers help to maintain ophthalmic products in the range of pH 6.0–8.0, thus promoting ocular comfort upon instillation. Tonicity adjusters allow the medication to be isotonic with the physiologic tear film. Products in the sodium chloride equivalence range of 0.9% ± 0.2% are considered isotonic and will help reduce ocular irritation and tissue damage. Solutions in the range of 0.6–1.8% are usually comfortable when placed on the human eye.

Ointments

Ophthalmic ointments represent a special type of vehicle produced by mixing white petrolatum and mineral oil with or without a water-miscible agent such as lanolin. The mineral oil is added to the petrolatum to allow the vehicle to melt at body temperature, and the lanolin is added to absorb water. This allows for water and water-soluble drugs to be retained in the delivery system. Commercial ophthalmic ointments are generally derivatives of a hydrocarbon mixture of 60% petrolatum (USP) and 40% mineral oil (USP), which is a semisolid at room temperature but which melts at body temperature. In general, ointments are well tolerated by the ocular tissues.

The primary clinical purpose for an ophthalmic ointment is to increase the ocular contact time of the instilled product. The ocular contact time of the ointment vehicle is about twice as long in the blinking eye and four times as long in the nonblinking or patched eye as that of a saline vehicle. Nonmedicated ophthalmic ointments are often used for self-medication in treating dry eye syndromes. Patients should be informed, however, that their use may cause temporary blurred vision because ointments coat the eye.

Major Therapeutic Categories of Nonprescription Ophthalmic Products

Numerous nonprescription ophthalmic products for treating minor ocular irritations are commercially available for self-administration by the patient under minimal or no supervision. Such products are also adequate for treating certain clinical conditions that have been diagnosed by health practitioners. The pharmacist must actively assist patients in selecting the appropriate product that will enhance compliance, minimize or avoid side effects, and reduce the attendant costs of therapy. Nearly all ophthalmic conditions amenable to nonprescription therapy can be treated by using the appropriate product chosen from the following categories of medications.

Lubricants

Many advances have been made in understanding the mechanisms involved in tear film formation, but the role of tears in maintaining a normal conjunctival and corneal surface is still not completely understood. The availability of synthetic chemicals suitable for topical application to the eye has resulted in the development of various solutions to help alleviate dryness of the ocular surface. The use of water-soluble polymer solutions and bland, nonmedicated ointments remains the primary therapy for the dry eye. Because almost all these products are available without a prescription, the pharmacist has a primary responsibility to assist and counsel the patient regarding their selection and proper use. Although a benefit of ophthalmic lubricant therapy is to increase the viscosity of existing tears, it must be emphasized that high viscosity alone does not necessarily provide relief for all dry eye conditions. Consequently, other, less viscous hydrophilic substances are now included as the primary polymeric ingredients of many artificial tear formulations.

Artificial Tear Solutions (Demulcents)

Lubricants formulated as solutions consist of inorganic electrolytes to achieve tonicity and maintain pH, preservatives, and water-soluble polymeric systems. These solutions are usually administered three to four times daily (Table 3), but depending on the patient's clinical needs and response to therapy, they may be given as often as hourly or only occasionally.

The substituted cellulose ethers are commonly incorporated into many artificial tear solutions. These include HPMC, hydroxyethylcellulose (HEC), hydroxypropylcellulose (HPC), methylcellulose, and carboxymethylcellulose (CMC). These solutions are colorless and vary in viscosity.

Methylcellulose is usually used in a concentration of 0.25–1.0%. At a concentration above 2%, the methylcellulose solution becomes sufficiently viscous to be classified as an ointment. Most contemporary artificial tear solutions incorporate other substituted cellulose ethers, especially HEC and HPC. Solutions of these polymers are usually less viscous than, but have emollient properties equal or superior to, those of methylcellulose. These ethers can also be combined with other polymers for use as artificial tears. Perhaps the most important property of the cellulose ethers in artificial tear formulations is that they stabilize the tear film and prevent tear evaporation, both of which are beneficial effects for patients with dry eye.[20] These beneficial effects generally occur without irritation or toxicity to the ocular tissues. Thus, their relative lack of toxicity, their viscous properties, and their beneficial effects on the tear film have made cellulose ethers extremely useful components of artificial tear preparations.

PVA is another commonly used viscosity enhancer for artificial tear preparations. This polymer is usually used in a 1.4% concentration and is considerably less viscous than methylcellulose. Like the cellulose ethers, PVA also enhances stability of the tear film without causing ocular irritation or toxicity. Although PVA is compatible with many commonly used drugs and preservatives, certain compounds can thicken or gel solutions that contain it. Such compounds include sodium bicarbonate; sodium borate; and the sulfates of sodium, potassium, and zinc. For example, sodium borate, found in some extraocular irrigants, may react with contact lens wetting solutions containing PVA.[21] Thus, it is important to be cautious when clinically using solutions containing PVA with solutions containing any of these other agents.

PVP has surface-active properties similar to those of the cellulose ethers. This compound is thought to form a hydrophilic layer on the corneal surface, mimicking natural conjunctival mucin. This "mucomimetic" property has firmly established the role of PVP as an artificial tear formulation. Because PVP promotes wetting of the ocular surface, both mucin- and aqueous-deficient dry eyes seem to benefit.

Vitamin A deficiency can affect many epithelial-lined organs, including the eye; therefore, the topical administration of retinol, the alcohol form of vitamin A, has been advocated for treating various dry eye disorders. Unfortunately, few controlled clinical trials have been conducted to substantiate the usefulness of retinol solution in dry eye syndromes. Some preliminary studies claim possible benefits for patients with conjunctival hyperemia, superior limbic keratitis, superficial punctate keratitis, and giant papillary conjunctivitis. Many patients may respond favorably to solutions that contain vitamin A because of their emollient qualities. Until more definitive data become available, however, the specific benefits of topically applied vitamin A solution for treating dry eyes will remain speculative. Retinol is available in nonprescription formulations, usually containing 5,000 IU of vitamin A and polysorbate 80.

In recent years, artificial tear preparations have been introduced in preservative-free formulations. This is beneficial for patients who are sensitive to preservatives such as BAK and thimerosal. Nonpreserved artificial tear preparations are now available in a variety of unit-dose dispensers, and some of these products are formulated to provide electrolyte support to the damaged surface epithelium of the eye. For example, Cellufresh® and Celluvisc® are designed in lower (Cellufresh®) and higher (Celluvisc®) viscosity vehicles to provide nutritional support to the ocular surface of patients with moderate to severe dry eye syndromes.[22] In general, however, nonpreserved formulations have the disadvantage of increased cost compared with preserved artificial tear solutions, and they can become easily contaminated by the patient during use. Thus, strict hygienic procedures for self-administration must be followed, and any unused solution should be properly discarded.

Clinical results and patient acceptance remain the final criteria for determining efficacy in the treatment of patients with dry eyes. It must be emphasized that no single formulation has yet been identified that will universally improve clinical signs and symptoms while maintaining patient comfort and acceptance.[21]

TABLE 3 Procedure for self-administration of eyedrops

1. Wash hands thoroughly.
2. Tilt head backward.
3. Gently grasp lower outer eyelid below lashes and pull eyelid away from eye to create a pouch.
4. Place dropper over eye by looking directly at it.
5. Just before applying a single drop, look upward.
6. After applying the drop, look downward for several seconds.
7. Release the eyelid slowly.
8. Close eyes gently for 1 to 2 minutes. Minimize blinking or squeezing the eyelid.
9. With a finger, put gentle pressure over the opening of the tear duct at the inner corner of the eye.
10. Blot excessive solution from around eye.

Finally, a sterile, buffered isotonic solution containing 0.25% tyloxapol and 0.02% BAK is available specifically for cleaning and lubricating artificial eyes. Tyloxapol is a detergent surfactant that liquefies solid matter on the prosthesis, and BAK aids tyloxapol in wetting the artificial eye. This solution is used in the same manner as ordinary artificial tears. With the artificial eye in place, one or two drops of solution should be applied three or four times daily. In addition, the solution can be used as a cleaner to remove oily or mucous deposits; in this case, the artificial eye is then rubbed between the fingers and rinsed with tap water prior to insertion.

Bland (Nonmedicated) Ointments (Emollients)

The principal advantage of bland ointments is their enhanced retention time in the eye, which appears to enhance the integrity of the tear film. Thus, both mucin- and aqueous-deficient eyes can benefit from the application of lubricating ointments.

Ointment formulations are usually administered twice daily (Table 4), but depending on the patient's clinical needs and therapeutic response, they may be administered as often as every few hours or only occasionally as needed. Many patients prefer to instill the ointment at bedtime to keep the eyes moist during sleep and to improve morning symptoms of dry eye.

Because of the viscosity of the melted ointment base in the tear film, many patients complain of blurred vision during ointment therapy. This problem can usually be resolved by decreasing the amount of ointment instilled or by administering it at bedtime. Although ointment preparations are generally nonirritating, preservatives can be toxic to ocular tissues. Some patients develop hypersensitivity reactions, which prompt them to discontinue therapy. Alternatively, symptoms associated with preserved ointment products can often be eliminated by changing to nonpreserved formulations; this is especially true for patients who require long-term treatment for dry eye. As a rule, it is better to recommend nonpreserved bland ointments for the treatment of dry eye to overcome potential problems that might occur with the use of preserved products.

Decongestants

Phenylephrine

Phenylephrine, which acts primarily on alpha-adrenergic receptors of the ophthalmic vasculature, is commercially available in concentrations ranging from 0.12 to 10%. However, only the 0.12% or 0.125% concentration is available without a prescription. Higher concentrations are generally reserved for the short-term dilation needed for eye examinations. To prolong its shelf life, sodium bisulfite, an antioxidant, is often added to the phenylephrine vehicle. Expiration dates should be strictly enforced because loss of pharmacologic activity may occur without visible changes in solution color.

Nonprescription concentrations of phenylephrine are used as a topical decongestant (vasoconstrictor), but even at these low concentrations, the drug may dilate the pupil if enough of it penetrates the corneal epithelium. This is not uncommon in persons who wear contact lenses who may instill the medication following lens wear. Because a patient can use phenylephrine indiscriminately to quiet

TABLE 4 Procedure for self-administration of eye ointments

1. Wash hands thoroughly.
2. Tilt head backward.
3. Gently grasp lower outer eyelid below lashes and pull eyelid away from eye.
4. Place ointment tube over eye by looking directly at it.
5. With a sweeping motion, place 1/4- to 1/2-inch of ointment inside the lower eyelid by gently squeezing the tube.
6. Release the eyelid slowly.
7. Close eyes gently for 1 to 2 minutes.
8. Blot excessive ointment from around eye.
9. Vision may be temporarily blurred. Avoid activities requiring good visual ability until vision clears.

an irritated eye, the drug can induce pupillary dilation and precipitate angle-closure glaucoma in eyes predisposed with narrow anterior chamber angles. This adverse effect is more likely if the cornea is damaged or diseased, allowing increased corneal drug penetration. Thus, patients should be cautioned against instilling this and other ophthalmic decongestants too often and should be encouraged to seek professional eye care if offending ophthalmic signs or symptoms do not resolve within 72 hours.

The most important and common side effect following chronic use of phenylephrine for ocular decongestion is rebound congestion of the conjunctiva, in which the conjunctival vessels become progressively more dilated with continued use of the drug. This phenomenon can create a vicious cycle in which phenylephrine is instilled to quiet an inflamed conjunctiva, which becomes progressively more inflamed with repeated instillation of the medication. Patients with apparent rebound effect should be referred for professional eye care for differential diagnosis and management.

Systemic adverse effects are extremely rare following the topical instillation of nonprescription phenylephrine for ocular decongestion. Although not reported in the literature, certain drug–drug interactions involving low concentrations of phenylephrine are theoretically possible. The pressor effects of phenylephrine may be enhanced in patients taking atropine, tricyclic antidepressants and monoamine oxidase inhibitors, reserpine, guanethidine, or methyldopa. The drug should therefore be used cautiously by patients with cardiovascular disease or diabetes, or by patients taking the concomitant medications listed above. Because of these possible adverse reactions, phenylephrine and other ocular decongestants should not be used as ocular irrigants.

Imidazoles

Three additional decongestants are available in nonprescription strength for topical application to the eye: naphazoline, tetrahydrozoline, and oxymetazoline. Like phenylephrine, the imidazoles have greater alpha- than beta-receptor activity and are therefore clinically useful in constricting conjunctival vessels. Moreover, these drugs have only minimal effect on underlying vessels of the episclera and sclera.

Naphazoline has been documented to be effective in constricting conjunctival vessels as well as in reducing tearing and pain associated with superficial ocular inflammation.[23] However, patients with lightly pigmented irides (e.g., blue eyes or green eyes) appear to be more sensitive to the mydriatic effects of naphazoline.

Satisfactory results have similarly been obtained with tetrahydrozoline in most patients with allergic or chronic conjunctivitis, and the beneficial effects can last from 1 to 4 hours. Unlike phenylephrine or naphazoline, tetrahydrozoline does not appear to alter pupil size. However, certain patients may experience mild, transient stinging immediately following instillation of the drops.

Oxymetazoline has been evaluated as a topical agent for treatment of allergic and noninfectious conjunctivitis. Topical treatment will improve most symptoms associated with allergic or noninfectious conjunctivitis, including burning, itching, tearing, and foreign body sensation. The clinical effects of oxymetazoline can last up to 4–6 hours. Oxymetazoline (0.025%) appears to be relatively free of both ocular and systemic side effects.

It is difficult to reach definitive conclusions regarding clinical comparisons of the available nonprescription ocular decongestants. Although most of the tested preparations produce blanching of conjunctival vessels, 0.02% naphazoline seems to produce greater blanching when compared with other nonprescription decongestants containing 0.05% tetrahydrozoline or 0.12% phenylephrine.[24] Investigators have observed no significant differences in conjunctival blanching with preparations containing naphazoline in concentrations of 0.02%, 0.05%, or 0.1%.[24] Thus, 0.02% naphazoline is an excellent choice for nonprescription therapy of mild to moderate conjunctivitis that is of environmental or noninfectious origin.

The imidazoles generally do not induce ocular or systemic side effects. However, patients should be cautioned that their liberal or indiscriminate use can lead to excessive systemic absorption and the possibility of cardiovascular side effects. Moreover, some patients may experience epithelial xerosis (abnormal dryness) occurring with prolonged topical instillation of local vasoconstrictors. Because rebound congestion appears to be less likely following topical ocular use of naphazoline or tetrahydrozoline, these agents should generally be recommended over phenylephrine or oxymetazoline. And because it has superior documented efficacy and produces a relative lack of side effects, 0.02% naphazoline can be recommended with confidence as an ocular vasoconstrictor of choice.[25]

Irrigants

Extraocular irrigating solutions, or irrigants, are used to cleanse ocular tissues while maintaining their moisture; these solutions must be physiologically balanced with respect to pH and osmolality. Because the tissues with which they come in contact obtain nutrients elsewhere, the role of irrigants is primarily to clear away unwanted materials or debris from the ocular surface. Extraocular irrigants are used only on a short-term basis. All the ophthalmic irrigating solutions are available without a prescription and therefore can be used by patients and practitioners alike.

In the ophthalmic practitioner's office, these solutions come in handy after certain clinical procedures, and they are often used to wash away mucus or purulent exudates from the eye. They are also administered in the hospital to clean out eyes between changes of ocular dressings. When used for these routine purposes, ocular irrigants should not be applied with contact lenses in place because the solutions tend to cause contact lens irritation by reducing the mucin component of the tear film or, in the case of rigid gas permeable lenses, by reducing the hydrophilicity of the lens surface.[26] Furthermore, absorption of the preservatives BAK or phenylmercuric acetate by soft contact lenses can have a deleterious effect on the corneal epithelium. Although irrigating solutions may be used to wash out the eyes after contact lens wear, they have no particular value as contact lens wetting, cleansing, or cushioning solutions.

One of the most useful applications of extraocular irrigants is in ocular lavage following chemical injuries to the eye. Penetrating chemicals, such as alkalis, must be washed out immediately. Although the ideal irrigating solution for this purpose is physiologic saline, water may be the only available, practical substance, and it can be recommended when no commercial ocular irrigant is handy. In the particular case of alkali burns to the ocular surface, however, lavage with extraocular irrigants may be inadequate to prevent or minimize ocular damage. In emergency situations involving alkali or acid burns, prompt professional evaluation and treatment by an ophthalmologist or optometrist are strongly encouraged.

In cases in which the patient experiences continuous eye pain, changes in vision, or continued redness or irritation of the eye, or in which the ocular condition persists or worsens, evaluation by an eye care professional should similarly be strongly encouraged. Extraocular irrigants should not be used for open wounds in or near the eyes. As previously discussed, ocular irrigants should not be used in conjunction with contact lens wetting solutions or with other eye care products containing PVA. Commercial irrigating products that use an eyecup should generally be avoided because of difficulties in cleaning the eyecup, with the resultant risk of bacterial or fungal contamination.

Hyperosmotics

Topically applied hyperosmotic formulations are intended to increase the tonicity of the tear film, thereby promoting movement of fluid from the cornea. When applied to the eye, these agents withdraw water from the cornea to the more highly osmotic tear film, which, in turn, is eliminated through the normal tear flow mechanisms. Many patients with mild to moderate corneal epithelial edema may experience improved subjective comfort and vision following appropriate use of these medications. Of the topical ophthalmic hyperosmotic agents that are commercially available, only sodium chloride can be obtained without a prescription in both solution and ointment formulations.

For clinical use, sodium chloride is available in 2% and 5% solution as well as in 5% ointment. In general, the 5% concentration in ointment form is the most effective in reducing corneal edema and improving vision. However, application of 5% sodium chloride tends to produce symptoms of stinging and burning. Thus, patients often prefer the 2% concentration for long-term therapy. Usually one or two drops of the solution are instilled every 3 to 4 hours (Table 3). The ointment formulation, however, requires less frequent instillation and is usually reserved for use at bedtime to minimize symptoms of blurred vision (Table 4). Because vision associated with edematous corneas is often worse on arising, several instillations of the solution during the first few waking hours may be helpful. Hypertonic saline is nontoxic to the external ocular tissues, and allergic reactions are rare.

Perhaps the most important contraindication to topical hyperosmotic sodium chloride is its use to clear edematous corneas with traumatized epithelium. The intact corneal epithelium exhibits only limited permeability to inorganic ions; therefore, an absent or compromised corneal epithelium will promote increased corneal penetration of the hyperosmotic and thereby reduce the osmotic effect. Consequently, the management of corneal edema associated with traumatized epithelium requires the use of organic hyperosmotic agents that are available only on prescription.[27] Patients whose history or physical appearance suggests a damaged corneal epithelium should be referred for immediate professional eye care.

Antiseptics

Several nonprescription agents are commercially available to reduce the bacterial population on the ocular surface, including the eyelid margins. Although the efficacy of most of these agents is largely unsubstantiated, they may be recommended for patients with only minor conjunctival or eyelid inflammation that is possibly associated with an infectious organism. Of the commercially available agents, only yellow mercuric oxide has received adequate scientific attention to document its effectiveness for some minor ocular infections. The others (silver protein, boric acid, and zinc sulfate) have not been adequately studied clinically for use in most ocular surface infections.

Patients with staphylococcal blepharitis may benefit from the use of yellow mercuric oxide ointment applied to the eyelid margins as a lid scrub, especially when there is only minimal involvement or when the condition has already been brought under control with prescription antibacterial agents. Nightly application of this ointment may prevent exacerbation of the condition. Use of the 1% ointment has been shown to effectively reduce bacterial lid counts in almost 90% of patients with blepharitis who use the medication twice daily;[28] it has also proved useful for treating phthiriasis palpebrarum (lice infestation of the eyelids). In this condition, yellow mercuric oxide ointment is applied twice daily for 1 week. Frequent or prolonged use should be avoided because it can lead to mercury poisoning. If irritation or rash develops, or if the condition persists, the patient should be evaluated medically.

Silver protein is indicated for treatment of ocular infections and for preoperative use in ocular surgery. At low doses, this agent has antimicrobial activity against both Gram-positive and Gram-negative organisms. When instilled prior to surgery, silver protein stains and coagulates mucus; all stained material should then be removed before operating to reduce the incidence of postoperative infection. For preoperative use, two or three drops are instilled into the eye and then rinsed with sterile irrigating solution. For treatment of mild ocular infections, several drops of silver protein are generally instilled every 3 to 4 hours for several days. Frequent topical application to the eye for prolonged periods should be avoided, however, because it can result in permanent discoloration of the eyelid skin or conjunctiva, a condition known as argyria. Silver protein is incompatible with topically applied sodium sulfacetamide preparations.[29]

Boric acid is indicated for the treatment of irritated or inflamed eyelids. Available in 5% or 10% ointment formulations, boric acid should generally be applied in a small quantity to the inner surface of the lower eyelid once or twice daily. If ocular irritation persists or increases, the patient should receive medical attention.

Zinc sulfate is a mild astringent for temporary relief of minor ocular irritation. It is generally used in a dosage of one to two drops up to four times daily. Zinc salts have also been used for infections caused by *Moraxella*. But the application of 0.25% zinc sulfate solution, although effective against the bacteria, is not as effective as prescription antibacterial therapy.

Detergents/Abrasives (Eyelid Scrubs)

Although there are many forms of blepharitis, the mainstay of therapy is generally careful eyelid hygiene. The patient can easily accomplish this at home by using hot compresses for 15–20 minutes, two to four times daily. Each application should be followed by lid scrubs using a mild detergent cleanser compatible with ocular tissues (Table 5). These lid scrub procedures are usually effective and well tolerated.

Although baby shampoo is often used for this purpose, recent experience has shown other commercially available cleansers to be as effective with potentially less ocular stinging, burning, and toxicity.[30] Commercial lid scrub products are intended for use in the removal of oils, debris, or desquamated skin associated with the inflamed eyelid. The lid scrubs can also be used for hygienic eyelid cleansing in people who wear contact lenses. These products are designed to be used full strength on eyelid tissues and must not be instilled directly into the eyes. The most effective application technique is to close the eyes and gently scrub the eyelids and eyelashes using side-to-side strokes. The solution should be rinsed thoroughly, and the applications should generally be repeated twice daily. Some of the commercial products are packaged with gauze pads, which provide an abrasive action to augment the cleansing properties of the detergent solution. Eyelid scrubs using commercially available detergents are most effective in patients with noninfectious blepharitis. Thus, if the

TABLE 5	Procedure for eyelid scrubs

1. Wash hands thoroughly.
2. Apply three to four drops of baby shampoo or eyelid cleanser to cotton-tipped applicator or gauze pad.
3. Close one eye and clean the upper eyelid and eyelashes using side-to-side strokes, being careful not to touch eyeball with applicator or fingers.
4. Open eye, look up, and clean lower eyelid and eyelashes using side-to-side strokes.
5. Repeat the procedures on other eye using a clean applicator or gauze pad.
6. Rinse eyelids and eyelashes with clean, warm water.

patient's signs or symptoms fail to improve, the patient should be referred for professional ocular examinations and treatment with appropriate antibacterial agents.

Multivitamins

Deficiencies of vitamin A and zinc have been associated with certain adverse ocular effects. Beyond replacement of documented nutritional deficiencies, which occur rarely in the United States, treatment or prevention of ophthalmic diseases using vitamins and/or minerals is not clearly established.

In recent years, investigations have explored the prophylactic use of vitamins A, C, and E as well as zinc to guard against the degenerative ophthalmic changes that appear to be associated with the aging process. The primary mechanisms of action offered to explain the theoretical efficacy of such therapy include antioxidation and free radical scavenging. Several products are now commercially available for the prevention and treatment of macular degeneration, but considerably more data will be required before these products can be generally recommended.[31]

Guidelines for Ocular Pharmacotherapy

The pharmacist has an important responsibility in guiding patients to appropriate nonprescription ocular therapy. Both the safety and effectiveness of ophthalmic products can be enhanced by paying strict attention to drug selection, contraindications, and appropriate dosage schedules and administration technique. Careful consideration of the patient's medical history, including concomitant medication use, will often minimize the risk of adverse reactions. Appropriate dosing procedures are important to ensure maximum effectiveness of the self-administered medications.

History Taking

A careful history not only alerts the pharmacist to possible adverse drug reactions, but also may assist the pharmacist to select the best product for the patient's ocular condition. Among the most important issues to be investigated in the patient's history is concomitant medications. Drug interactions can play a significant role in potentiating or impairing drug effects and may even exacerbate any potential adverse reaction. For example, topically applied phenylephrine may heighten the pressor effects of certain prescription drugs.[25]

Inquiry regarding a history of drug allergies is essential. Hypersensitivity to thimerosal and other mercurial compounds is not uncommon among those who wear contact lenses, and topically applied ophthalmic medications containing mercurial preservatives, especially when used long term, can lead to allergic reactions.

Patients with systemic hypertension, arteriosclerosis, and other cardiovascular diseases may be at risk when topically applied ocular decongestants such as phenylephrine or the imidazoles are used. Adverse cardiovascular events are also possible when these agents are used in patients with hyperthyroidism.[25]

Although most topically administered drugs can be used safely during pregnancy, it is prudent to limit topical ophthalmic dosing in pregnant women. Artificial tears can be used without limit, but agents with ingredients that affect the autonomic nervous system, such as ocular decongestants, should be used sparingly during pregnancy.

The pharmacist should carefully consider the nature and extent of ocular involvement. Because a definitive ocular diagnosis requires professional examination by an ophthalmologist or optometrist, it is difficult to give precise guidelines on when the pharmacist should refer patients who are not responding to nonprescription therapy. As a general rule, however, patients who fail to respond within 72 hours should be referred for medical evaluation, especially if they are not currently under the care of an ophthalmic practitioner. It is important for patients with acute ocular disease to receive a prompt definitive diagnosis, including baseline visual acuity, before the appropriateness of nonprescription therapy is considered. Some acute conditions, presenting with or without ocular pain or blurred vision, can be appropriately treated with nonprescription agents, but a recent diagnosis from the ophthalmic practitioner can give the pharmacist additional reassurance and confidence in recommending such treatment.

On the other hand, many patients with chronic ocular conditions, especially dry eye, may fail to respond to initial nonprescription therapy with artificial tears or other lubricants. In many of these cases, the most appropriate strategy is to change to a different lubricant, especially one with a different polymer or preservative system. Then, if there is still no response, the patient should be strongly encouraged to seek professional assessment and care from an ophthalmic practitioner. Although the cost-effectiveness of ophthalmic care can be greatly improved through the use of nonprescription agents, severe visual impairment, including blindness, can be a serious clinical and medicolegal complication if referral for definitive diagnosis and treatment is delayed.

Self-Administration of Ophthalmic Medications

Proper drug instillation technique is critical if the target tissue (the eye) is to receive the maximum benefit from the medication. The following general guidelines should help promote the safe and effective use of nonprescription ophthalmic products, and should help the pharmacist decide whether the patient should be referred for professional ophthalmic care.[32,33]

- Nonprescription ophthalmic products should be used only in situations in which vision is not threatened, and they should generally not be used for longer than 72 hours without medical referral if the condition being treated persists or worsens.
- Nonprescription ocular medications should not be recommended to patients who have demonstrated an allergy to any of the active ingredients, preservatives, or other excipients in the product.
- Patients who are already using a prescription ophthalmic product should use nonprescription products only after consulting with an ophthalmic practitioner or pharmacist.
- Patients with a history of narrow anterior chamber angles or narrow-angle glaucoma should not use topical ocular decongestants because of the risk of angle-closure glaucoma.
- The lowest concentration and conservative dosage frequencies should be used, and overdosage should be avoided.
- Drug application should be conservative in patients with hyperemic conjunctiva because of the potential for increased systemic drug absorption and the risk of adverse effects.
- Patients should be reminded to use all medications only as directed. There is generally no additional benefit from receiving more than the intended amount of the drug.
- If multiple drop therapy is indicated, the best interval between drops is at least 5 minutes. This helps to ensure that the first drop is not flushed away by the second, or that the second drop is not diluted by the first.
- If both drop and ointment therapy are indicated, the drop should be applied at least 10 minutes before the ointment so that the ointment does not become a barrier to tear film or corneal penetration of the drop.
- Patients should wipe excessive solution or ointment from the eyelids and lashes after instillation.
- Because ointments may blur the patient's vision during the waking hours, they should be used with caution if visual acuity is critical; otherwise, bedtime instillation is most appropriate.
- Use of eyecups should be discouraged because of potential bacterial, fungal, or viral contamination.
- Ophthalmic medications should not be used beyond their expiration dates. Eyedrop bottles should be replaced or discarded 1 month (30 days) after the sterility safety seal is opened because the manufacturer's expiration date does not apply once the seal is broken.
- Patients should store all medications out of children's reach.
- The pharmacist should recognize adverse drug reactions, including the clinical signs of drug toxicity or allergy.
- Ophthalmic solutions and ointments, as well as eyelid scrubs, are often misused. The pharmacist should help to ensure maximum safety and effectiveness of these agents by carefully instructing patients in the proper self-administration procedures. Appropriate patient education and counseling must accompany dispensation of any ophthalmic product. Tables 3, 4, and 5 summarize the step-by-step procedures in using ophthalmic drops, ointments, and eyelid scrubs.

Summary

The pharmacist is strategically positioned in the community to treat patients with ophthalmic pathology or to recommend self-management with one or more nonprescription drugs. Several such pharmaceuticals are available to manage the symptoms of minor acute or chronic conditions of the eye and eyelid. By understanding the pathophysiology of certain ocular conditions and knowing how to assess patients who present with such conditions, a pharmacist should be able to optimize the safe, appropriate, effective, and economical use of nonprescription drugs in the management of various conditions of the eye and eyelid.

References

1. Warwick R. *Anatomy of the Eye and Orbit*. 7th ed. Philadelphia: W. B. Saunders; 1975: 195–219.
2. Milder B. The lacrimal apparatus. In: Moses RA, Hart WM, eds. *Adler's Physiology of the Eye*. 8th ed. St. Louis, Mo: CV Mosby; 1987: 15–35.
3. Mishima S, Gasset A, Klyce SD, et al. Determination of tear volume and tear flow. *Invest Ophthalmol* 1966; 3: 264–76.
4. Jordan A, Baum J. Basic tear flow. Does it exist? *Ophthalmology* 1980; 9:920–30.
5. Pfister RR, Burstein N. The effects of ophthalmic drugs, vehicles, and preservatives on corneal epithelium; a scanning electron microscope study. *Invest Ophthalmol* 1976; 15: 246–59.
6. Harris LS, Galin MA. Dose response analysis of pilocarpine-induced ocular hypotension. *Arch Ophthalmol* 1970; 1: 605–8.
7. Ophthalmic drug products for over-the-counter human use; final monograph. *Federal Register* 1988; 53 (43).
8. Ophthalmic drug products for over-the-counter human use; establishment of a monograph; proposed rulemaking. *Federal Register* 1980; 45 (89): 30002–50.
9. Jones DB, Liesegang TJ, Robinson NM. Laboratory diagnosis of ocular infections. Paper presented at Washington, DC: American Society for Microbiology; 1981.
10. Cohen EJ, Gonzalez C, Leavitt KG, et al. Corneal ulcers

associated with contact lenses including experience with disposable lenses. *CLAO J* 1991; 1: 173–6.
11. Lopez-Bernal D, Ubels JL. Quantitative evaluation of the corneal epithelial barrier effect: effect of artificial tears and preservatives. *Curr Eye Res* 1991; 7: 645–66.
12. Schilling H, Koch JM, Waubke TN, et al. Treatment of dry eye with vitamin A acid: an impression cytology controlled study. *Fortschr Ophthalmol* 1989; 5: 530–4.
13. Mullen W, Sheppard W, Leibowitz J. Ophthalmic preservatives and vehicles. *Surv Ophthalmol* 1973; 17: 469–83.
14. Sabiston DW. The dry eye. *Trans Ophthalmol Soc N Z* 1969; 21:96–100.
15. Linn ML, Jones LT. Rate of lacrimal excretion of ophthalmic vehicles. *Am J Ophthalmol* 1968; 65:76–8.
16. Burstein NL. Basic science of ocular pharmacology. In: Bartlett JD, Jaanus SD, eds. *Clinical Ocular Pharmacology*. Boston: Butterworth Publishers; 1989: 3–28.
17. Burstein NL. Preservative cytotoxic threshold for benzalkonium chloride and chlorhexidine digluconate in cat and rabbit corneas. *Invest Ophthalmol Vis Sci* 1980; 19: 308–13.
18. Wilson WS, Duncan AJ, Jay JL. Effect of benzalkonium chloride on the stability of the precorneal tear film in rabbit and man. *Br J Ophthalmol* 1975; 59: 667–9.
19. Mondino BJ, Salamon SM, Zaidman GW. Allergic and toxic reactions in soft contact lens wearers. *Surv Ophthalmol* 1982; 26: 337–44.
20. Norn MS. Desiccation of the precorneal film: I. corneal wetting time. *Acta Ophthalmol* 1969; 47:865–80.
21. Jaanus SD. Lubricants and other preparations for the dry eye. In: Bartlett JD, Jaanus SD, eds. *Clinical Ocular Pharmacology*. Boston: Butterworth Publishers; 1989: 301–12.
22. Grene B, Harrold M, Mordaunt J, et al. A clinical study comparing the efficacy of two ophthalmic lubricating solutions using impression cytology. *Invest Ophthalmol Vis Sci* 1990; 31 (suppl): 529.
23. Miller J, Wolf EM. Antazoline phosphate and naphazoline hydrochloride, singly and in combination for the treatment of allergic conjunctivitis—a controlled double-blind clinical trial. *Ann Allergy* 1975; 35: 81–6.
24. Abelson MB, Yamamoto GK, Allansmith MR. Effects of ocular decongestants. *Arch Ophthalmol* 1980; 98: 856–8.
25. Jaanus SD, Pagano VT, Bartlett JD. Drugs affecting the autonomic nervous system. In: Bartlett JD, Jaanus SD, eds. *Clinical Ocular Pharmacology*. Boston: Butterworth Publishers; 1989: 69–148.
26. Hales RH. Contact lenses: a clinical approach to fitting. Baltimore: Williams & Wilkins; 1978: 32–50.
27. Lamberts DW. Topical hyperosmotic agents and secretory stimulants. *Int Ophthalmol Clin* 1980; 20: 163–9.
28. Kastl PR, Ali Z, Mather F. Placebo-controlled, double-blind evaluation of the efficacy and safety of yellow mercuric oxide in suppression of eyelid infections. *Ann Ophthalmol* 1987; 19: 376–9.
29. Rowsey JJ. Anti-infective agents. In: Bartlett JD, Chormley NR, Jaanus SD, et al., eds. *Ophthalmic Drug Facts*. St. Louis, Mo: Facts and Comparisons; 1992: 77–135.
30. Polack FM, Goodman DF. Experience with a new detergent lid scrub in the management of chronic blepharitis. *Arch Ophthalmol* 1988; 106: 719–20.
31. Sperduto RD, Ferris FL, Kurinij N. Do we have a nutritional treatment for age-related cataract or macular degeneration? *Arch Ophthalmol* 1990; 108: 1403–5.
32. Bartlett JD, Cullen AP. Clinical administration of ocular drugs. In: Bartlett JD, Jaanus SD, eds. *Clinical Ocular Pharmacology*. Boston: Butterworth Publishers; 1989: 29–66.
33. Bartlett JD. Dosage forms and routes of administration. In: Bartlett JD, Ghormley NR, Jaanus SD, et al., eds. *Ophthalmic Drug Facts*. St. Louis, Mo: Facts and Comparisons; 1992: 1–7.

CHAPTER 21

Contact Lens Products

Janet P. Engle

> **Questions to ask in patient assessment and counseling**
>
> - What types of lenses do you wear? Hard, soft, or rigid gas-permeable (RGP)? Are your lenses for extended wear?
> - How long have you been wearing lenses? When did you start wearing this pair in particular?
> - What types of problems are you having with your lenses? Are they related to eye irritation or to changes in vision? When did the problems start?
> - How many hours per day do you wear your lenses before problems start? Do you remove your lenses during the day?
> - When did you last see your optometrist or ophthalmologist?
> - How do you take care of your lenses?
> - Have you recently changed brands of any of your solutions?
> - How often do you change your storage solutions?
> - How often do you clean your storage container? Does it need to be replaced?
> - Have you become pregnant or begun using oral contraceptives since you were fitted for lenses?
> - What nonprescription and prescription medications are you now taking?
> - Do you have any allergies?

Annual sales of contact lens care products exceed $400 million in pharmacies and $900 million overall, and are growing faster than any other category of nonprescription items. With the introduction of soft contact lenses in the 1970s, the greatly enhanced comfort of lenses has led to a significant expansion of the contact lens market. Similarly, developments with rigid gas-permeable (RGP) hard lenses provide the comfort of soft lenses and the enhanced optical qualities of hard lenses. Extended-wear lenses, toric lenses for astigmatism, tinted lenses, bifocal contact lenses, and disposable lenses have also greatly expanded the potential patient population. It is estimated that, by the year 2000, the number of persons wearing contact lenses (contacts) will be the same as the number using eyeglasses.

Of the 25 million Americans currently wearing contacts, nearly 90% use the lenses to correct the vision of an otherwise healthy eye. Figure 1 illustrates the demographic characteristics of contact lens wearers. Although much of the motivation to wear contacts may be cosmetic, properly fitted lenses can provide significant vision advantages over spectacles. Contact lenses reduce size distortion and prismatic effects and improve peripheral vision. Elimination of spectacle fogging, dirt accumulation, and frame distraction may also be a significant advantage to many users. Most soft contact lens wearers state that their lenses are more comfortable than eyeglasses.

However, it has been well established that corneal contact lenses, even when expertly fitted, somewhat alter ocular tissues and change the corneal metabolism. These effects make it imperative that both the user and the health professional understand the proper care, maintenance, and safe use of these products. Failure to do so can greatly increase the chance of corneal infection, corneal ulcers, and other ocular conditions that may result in permanent eye damage. Fortunately, however, most side effects of contact lens use are reversible if attended to promptly.

More than 200 nonprescription contact lens care products are available and consumers are likely to be overwhelmed by the variety. Except for the prescriber, pharmacists are the most qualified to counsel contact lens wearers as to which products to choose.[1] Product selection depends on the products' compatibility with each other as well as with the specific contact lens. These considerations place a direct responsibility on the pharmacist to understand this area of professional practice and provide effective, up-to-date information when consulting with the contact lens wearer.

Characteristics of Contact Lenses

Contact lenses are often broadly classified into three distinct groups based on their chemical makeup and physical properties (Table 1). Lenses that are relatively inflexible, do not appreciably absorb water, and retain their shape when removed from the eye are commonly called hard lenses. RGP lenses, which are also rigid in shape, are oxygen permeable. Lenses that are moderately to highly flexible, absorb a high percentage of water, and conform to the shape of a supporting surface are commonly called soft lenses. Subgroups of contact lenses are extended-wear lenses and disposable lenses. Extended-wear lenses can

---

This chapter is based in part on the chapter with a similar title that appeared in the 9th edition but was written by Thomas A. Gossel and J. Richard Wuest.

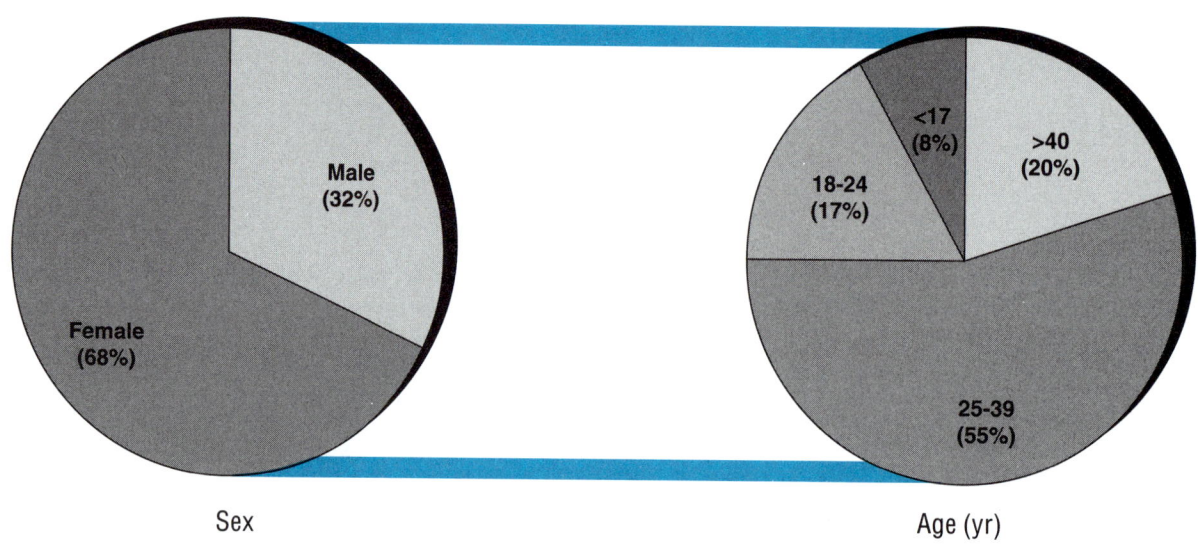

FIGURE 1 Demographics of lens wearers.

be either RGP hard lenses or soft lenses and are designed to be worn for an extended time before removal. Disposable lenses are designed to be worn for 1 week and then thrown away.

Contact lenses are manufactured from polymers that vary widely in their chemical and physical properties. Each material has physical and surface characteristics that correlate to the specific problems the patient may encounter.[2]

Physical characteristics of contact lenses include dimensional stability, physical breakage, and polymer stability. Generally, hard lenses are dimensionally stable and tend to hold their parameters with little change. Soft lenses, however, are much less stable physically; water content, to a large extent, will dictate their physical strength. RGP lenses generally have a high degree of dimensional stability. As the lens dehydrates, however, curvature of the plastic changes.

The characteristics of the different contact lenses account for most of the problems the patient will encounter. Unfortunately, most patients do not know which type of lens they are wearing. This underscores the importance of establishing an excellent relationship with contact lens practitioners in the area.

To maintain a healthy cornea, an adequate amount of oxygen is needed. The more oxygen that passes through the contact lens, the more adequately corneal metabolism can be maintained. Several terms are important when discussing oxygen transmission of a contact lens. *Oxygen permeability* describes the ability of a specific material to permit the passage of oxygen. Oxygen permeability is expressed as the Dk value of the material, where D is the diffusion coefficient and k is the solubility coefficient. The higher the Dk value is, the higher the oxygen permeability. The Dk/L value, in which the L value corresponds to the thickness of the material, is a measure of oxygen transmissibility (i.e., the amount of oxygen that can be transmitted through a contact lens of specific thickness) and is thus the value to which most practitioners and manufacturers refer. Because the lens thickness will vary depending on the power of the lens, many manufacturers will report the Dk/L value for a lens with a −3.00D prescription. For example, a lens that corrects a large myopia (minus lens) will be thinner in the center than a lens that corrects hyperopia (plus lens), which will be thicker in the center than on the periphery.

The minimal oxygen transmission values needed to prevent corneal edema in most patients have been extensively debated. For a daily wear lens, the Dk/L value ([cm mL O_2]/[sec mL mm Hg]) should be at least 24.1×10^{-9}; for extended-wear lenses, the Dk/L should be 34.3×10^{-9}. This limits overnight corneal swelling to approximately 8% and provides for adequate daytime deswelling to occur.[3]

Oxygen transmission also depends on the water content of the lens. The higher the water content, the more oxygen is transmitted through the lens. However, as water content increases, durability decreases, and the lens must be made thicker, which hinders oxygen permeability. Thus, a thick lens with a high water content may transmit the same amount of oxygen as a thin lens with a lower water content.[4] Another problem is that, as water content increases, the lenses tend to attract tear deposits such as lipids, proteins, and polysaccharides. Further, and especially if large pores or many pores are present, lenses with a high water content tend to be more susceptible to the growth of bacteria and fungi on the surface than lenses with a lower water content.[5]

Types of Contact Lenses

During 1990, the majority of contact lens–wearing patients (51%) were fitted with soft daily wear contact lenses. Daily wear RGP lenses were prescribed for 24% of patients. Approximately 12% of patients obtaining contact lenses were given disposable soft contact lenses. Extended-wear soft

TABLE 1	Comparisons of contact lens characteristics		
	Conventional hard lenses	Soft contact lenses	Rigid gas-permeable hard lenses
Lens characteristics			
Rigidity	+++	0	+++
Durability	+++	+	++
Oxygen transmission	0	+	+++
Adsorbs chemicals	0	+++	0
Optical quality			
Visual acuity	+++	+	+++
Corrects astigmatism	Yes	Toric	Yes
Photophobia	+++	+	++
Spectacle blur	+++	0	++
Convenience			
Comfort	+	+++	++
Adaptation period	Weeks	Days	Days
Extended wear	No	Yes	Yes
Intermittent wear	No	Yes	No

Key:
+ indicates the degree to which the characteristic is present.
0 means the characteristic is not present.

lenses were worn by 10% and extended-wear RGP lenses were worn by 2% of patients. Table 1 provides a comparative summary of the characteristics that differentiate conventional hard lenses, soft lenses, and RGP hard lenses.

Hard Lenses

Hard contact lenses were the first lenses to be used in the United States. Hard lenses are polymerized products of esters of acrylic acid or methacrylic acid. The most common plastic found in hard lenses is polymethylmethacrylate (PMMA), which is known commercially as Lucite® or Plexiglas®.

PMMA is not significantly permeable to oxygen; therefore, for the cornea to remain healthy, the lens must be able to slide and rock over the corneal surface in response to a blink so that oxygenation can occur. As the hard lens moves, a layer of tears forms under it and is continually recirculated by the sliding and rocking motion. This process provides oxygen-coated tears to the corneal surface and is commonly referred to as the tear pump phenomenon. To allow this movement over the eye, hard lenses are made relatively small in diameter and thus may pop out of the wearer's eye.

Another phenomenon associated primarily with hard lenses is "spectacle blur." A hard lens, while in place on the cornea, alters the surface topography of the eye. As a result, the patient may not see well with glasses immediately after removing the lens. Generally, spectacle blur abates in 20–30 minutes.

Contact lenses made of PMMA are hydrophobic. However, PMMA possesses many characteristics that make it ideal for an over-the-eye corrective lens:

- Lenses are very light because of a specific gravity of 1.18–1.20.
- The refractive index, 1.49–1.50, is similar to that of glass spectacle lenses.
- Lenses allow a light transmission of 90–92%.
- Lenses are not affected by weak alkalis or weak acids.
- The plastic does not cause sensitivity reactions when placed on the cornea.

The "hardness" of these hard contact lenses is less than that of glass but is more than that of RGP or soft lenses. Reasonable care must be exercised with hard lenses to avoid scratching or chipping them. PMMA is now rarely used for new contact lens fittings.

In hard lenses, a small colored dot marker or an etch mark on one lens identifies it as being for the left or right eye. This marker, located at the outer periphery of the lens, is not perceived by the wearer when the lens is on the cornea.

Inadequate care or neglect of hard lenses may lead to corneal problems or wearer discomfort, but the lens will still maintain its optical qualities.

Rigid Gas-Permeable Hard Lenses

The new generation of RGP lenses combines the optical qualities of PMMA and the oxygen permeability of soft lenses. Generally, RGP lenses can deliver two to three times more oxygen to the cornea than soft lenses of the same thickness. However, to maintain rigidity (important for the correction of astigmatism and the fit of the lenses), RGP lenses are generally much thicker than soft lenses. RGP lenses, unlike soft lenses, also exchange up to 20% of the postlens tear volume per blink.

RGP hard lenses have been investigated for extended-wear use, and some have been approved for 1–7 days of extended wear. However, RGP lenses have been implicated in causing corneal ulcers (eruptions on the corneal surface). In rare instances, these ulcers can lead to partial or complete blindness.

RGP hard lenses are available in several materials. One type of lens is composed of silicone acrylates that combine PMMA and silicone in varying amounts. This material is relatively stable and inflexible. A disadvantage of most silicone acrylates when compared with PMMA, however, is a decrease in surface wettability owing to the relatively higher hydrophobicity of silicone.

Another type of RGP hard lens is made of cellulose acetate butyrate (CAB). CAB lenses transmit more oxygen than PMMA lenses but much less than other RGP lenses. Like PMMA, CAB is very wettable on the eye and is now used for patients who require rigid lenses but who have wetting incompatibilities with newer RGP materials. However, CAB also has several disadvantages, including its relative ease of surface scratching and its tendency to warp. CAB lenses tend to flex when on the eye and must be made very thick on patients whose corneas are toric (bulging).

TABLE 2 Examples of rigid gas-permeable contact lenses

Brand name	Manufacturer	Composition
AIRlens	Wesley-Jessen	t-Butyl styrene
Boston Lens II	Polymer Technology	Silicone acrylate
Boston RXD	Polymer Technology	Fluorosilicone acrylate
Polycon II	Sola/Barnes Hind	Silicone acrylate
RX-56	Rynco Scientific	Cellulose acetate butyrate (CAB)
Sila Rx	Sola/Barnes Hind	Silicone
Silsoft	Bausch & Lomb	Silicone
Bifocal lenses		
Dura-sil Front Surface Bi-focal	Danker Labs	Silicone acrylate
Tangent Streak	Fused Kontacts	Fluorosilicate acrylic
Extended-wear (1–7 days) or daily wear RGP lenses		
Boston Equalens	Polymer Technology	Fluorosilicone acrylate
Fluoroperm 92	Paragon Optical	Fluorosilicone acrylate
Paraperm EW	Paragon Optical	Silicone acrylate

TABLE 3 Soft contact lens classification

Group I: low water, nonionic	Group III: low water, ionic
Polymacon	Bufilcon A (45%)
Hefilcon A and B	Etrafilcon
Tefilcon	Phemfilcon A (38%)
Tetrafilcon A	
Group II: high water, nonionic	**Group IV: high water, ionic**
Lidofilcon A and B	Bufilcon A (55%)
Surfilcon	Perfilcon
Vifilcon	Phemfilcon A (55%)

Fluorine may also be a component of RGP lenses. This may be in the form of fluorosilicone acrylate or fluoropolymer lenses. Fluorine increases oxygen permeability of the lens. Fluorinated lenses have the advantages of decreasing deposits, increasing oxygen transmissibility, and reducing problems with lipophilicity. Their disadvantages are that they tend to have greater mass, which may change the way they fit, and tend not to be highly wettable.

t-Butyl styrene, another type of RGP hard lens, is moderately oxygen permeable and lighter than other RGP lens materials. However, it is brittle, has poor wettability, and lacks surface stability.[6]

Pure silicone contact lenses have been available for many years but have experienced limited market success and consumer popularity. These lenses can be made in both a hard resin and a flexible, elastomeric variety. The elastomeric version is the most permeable to oxygen of all contact lenses. However, pure silicone lenses are uncomfortable because silicone is extremely hydrophobic. These lenses are also lipophilic, making their surfaces susceptible to lipid deposits.

Of the many materials available, the silicone acrylates (Boston Lenses®) and the fluorosilicone acrylates (i.e., Boston Equalens®) are the most commonly used.[7] Table 2 lists examples of RGP hard contact lenses currently available in the United States.

Soft Lenses

The main chemical difference between the hydrophobic, rigid hard lens and the hydrophilic soft lens is that the soft lens contains hydroxyl or hydroxyl and lactam groups, which allow it to absorb and hold water. Table 3 classifies the different types of soft contact lenses into four groups according to water content. Nearly all lenses are composed of 2-hydroxyethylmethacrylate (HEMA) with small amounts of cross-linking agents that form a hydrophilic gel (hydrogel) network. The degree of cross-linking determines lens hydrophilicity. Greater cross-linking means that fewer hydrophilic groups are available for interaction with water, which in turn produces a less flexible, less hydrated lens than those originally available.

Ionic lenses tend to attract more protein deposits than nonionic lenses; soaking ionic lenses in sorbate-preserved saline will yellow the lens prematurely. High water lenses, which tend to attract tear-film deposits into their matrix, usually cannot withstand daily heat disinfection. If soaked in enzymes for prolontged period to time, these lenses may also cause sensitivity reactions.

The water content of soft lenses has gradually decreased since they were introduced. The water content of a HEMA-type material can vary between 5 and 90%, but a theoretical "ideal" value might be 75–78%, which matches the hydration of the corneal stroma. Increasing the water content improves the oxygen permeability of a material. However, permeability also depends on lens thickness. Highly hydrated lenses are more comfortable but are also more fragile. Because lenses with a high water content must therefore be thicker to offset fragility, the two factors often cancel each other out regarding oxygen transmissibility. Lowering the water content produces a more durable and longer lasting lens. In addition, reducing the percentage of water in a soft HEMA lens also reduces the thickness of the hydrated lens, thereby improving the wearer's comfort.

Soft lenses in the nonhydrated (dry) state are rigid and extremely brittle and should not be handled by the wearer. When hydrated, the lenses expand as water is absorbed into the gel matrix. They are most comfortable when they are larger than the diameter of the cornea, have thin edges, and undergo just enough movement on the eye to ensure lubrication of the ocular surface under the lens. Many lens wearers find they cannot tolerate lenses with a thickness above 0.4 mm because of lid discomfort. For those who cannot tolerate regular soft lenses, several ultrathin soft lenses are available with a thickness as low as 0.04 mm.

Subgroups of Soft Lenses

Increased oxygen permeability of soft contact lenses enables certain lenses to be "broken in" more quickly and worn continuously. Table 4 lists examples of soft contact lenses approved for wear in the United States. Extended-wear lenses were originally intended to be worn for weeks. However, because of problems with contamination and infection, they should not be worn for more than 7 days.[8] Recent evidence strongly supports removing them overnight to reduce the risk of ulcerative keratitis.[9,10]

Some soft contact lenses are classified as "specialty" lenses. These include toric, bifocal, tinted, and disposable lenses. Toric soft lenses have been developed specifically to correct astigmatic visual conditions. Traditional soft lenses do not correct astigmatism because they conform to the corneal surface rather than retain their original shape, as do hard lenses. Toric soft lenses are fabricated with both spherical and cylindrical optical corrections and remain "on axis" because of design features such as weighting the bottom edge of the lens. Spherical soft lenses can be fitted to eyes with an upper limit of astigmatism of about 1.00 diopters, a figure highly dependent on the criticality and motivation of the patient. (A diopter is a unit of refracting power used as a quantitative measure of the abnormal refraction of light at surfaces such as the cornea.)

Bifocal lenses, which can be weighted in a fashion similar to that of toric lenses, are prescribed to correct presbyopia (ocular changes due to age). Table 4 lists examples of available toric soft lenses and bifocal lenses.

Tinted lenses are available for cosmetic purposes (to change eye color) as well as for corrective uses. Other types of lenses are tinted, not to change eye color but to facilitate the handling and increase the visibility of the lens. Prosthetic tinted lenses are also available; these may be used to mask corneal scarring, cover an amblyopic (lazy) eye, or help rectify color deficiency. Table 4 lists examples of available tinted lenses.

Disposable lenses, which are worn for 1 week and then discarded, are also available. Because the lenses are discarded after wear, the care regimen for disposable lenses is greatly simplified.

Advantages of Soft Lenses

Soft lenses are easier to insert and are considerably more comfortable than hard lenses. This effect is most apparent during the initial break-in period. Photophobia is not likely to occur with soft lenses, and glare is significantly reduced. As with hard lenses, however, flare around the periphery may be noticed at night, particularly in individuals who have large pupils. This flare is caused by refractive light entering the eye through the edge margin of the contact lens.

Soft lens wearers can change more easily from their lenses to eyeglasses after a period of wear. The typical soft lens wearer does not usually experience the spectacle blur common among hard lens wearers.

Soft lenses are less likely than hard lenses to trap dust particles, eyelashes, or other foreign material under the lens. Soft lenses are also less likely to dislodge or fall out than hard lenses. Therefore, soft lenses are often better suited for occasional wear and sports, including contact sports.

Disadvantages of Soft Lenses

Although many people prefer the comfort of soft lenses, not all soft lens wearers can achieve excellent visual acuity. The hydration of the lens may change either in or out of the eye, particularly with extreme temperatures and low relative humidity; this change can decrease the quality of the visual image. Because a soft lens conforms in large part to the corneal shape, it is difficult to project the degree of vision improvement before the lens is actually placed on the eye.

Because soft lenses cannot be as precisely tailored to the specific requirements of an individual cornea, the fitting process is less exact than it is with rigid lenses. As a result, the overall quality of vision with soft contact lenses does not usually equal that of a properly fitted pair of rigid lenses. Fortunately, these differences are small and should not concern the average wearer.

Unlike hard lenses, soft lenses can absorb chemical compounds from topically administered ophthalmic products.[11] As previously discussed, ocular irritation may result, and the lens may be damaged. With the exception of a few specially formulated rewetting solutions, no solutions should be placed into the eye with the soft lens in place. If a drug solution is placed into the eye prior to lens insertion, the wearer must wait until the solution has cleared from the precorneal (conjunctival) pocket—about 5 minutes. In some instances, the prescriber may prefer the lenses to be worn while a prescription medication is being instilled in the eye so that they may serve as a reservoir for the drug. If no instructions accompany an ophthalmic prescription for a soft lens wearer, the prescribing physician should be contacted. This is also true for a nonprescription ophthalmic product not specifically designed for use with contact lenses. When topical ophthalmic ointments are being used, the lenses should not be worn at all.

Unlike hard lenses, soft lenses cannot be easily marked to identify which is for the left and right eyes. A soft lens wearer who is uncertain of the identity of the lenses may have to see the vision specialist.

TABLE 4 Examples of soft contact lenses

Brand name	Manufacturer	% water/saline	Group[a]
Daily wear soft lenses			
AO Soft	CIBA Vision	42.5	I
Cibasoft	CIBA Vision	37.5	I
DuraSoft	Wesley-Jessen	38.0	III
Hydrocurve II	Sola/Barnes-Hind	55.0	III
Sof-Form 67	Salvatori Ophthalmics	67.0	II
Soflens	Bausch & Lomb	38.6	I
Softcon	CIBA Vision	55.0	IV
Extended-wear soft lenses			
Cibathin	CIBA Vision	37.5	I
DuraSoft 3	Wesley-Jessen	55.0	IV
Permaflex Natural	CooperVision	74.0	II
Permalens	CooperVision	71.0	IV
Softmate I	Sola/Barnes-Hind	45.0	III
Softmate II	Sola/Barnes-Hind	55.0	IV
Soft toric lenses			
Hydrocurve II Toric	Sola/Barnes-Hind	45.0	III
Optima Toric	Bausch & Lomb	45.0	I
Spectrum Toric	CIBA Vision	55.0	IV
Soft bifocal lenses			
Bi-Soft	CIBA Vision	37.5	I
Hydrocurve II	Sola/Barnes-Hind	45.0	III
PA1	Bausch & Lomb	38.6	I
Soft daily wear tinted lenses			
Cibasoft soft colors (blue, green, aqua, amber, royal blue)	CIBA Vision	37.5	I
Hydron Sero 4 Sof Blue (soft blue visibility tint)	Allergan Optical	38.0	I
Soft extended-wear tinted lenses			
Cibathin soft colors (blue, green, aqua, amber, royal blue)	CIBA Vision	37.5	I
Natural Tint 03/04 (aqua, jade, sable, crystal blue)	Bausch & Lomb	38.0	I

[a]Group I: low water, nonionic.
Group II: high water, nonionic.
Group III: low water, ionic.
Group IV: high water, ionic.

Soft lenses generally cost more than hard lenses. Although the initial cost of acquiring soft lenses has decreased, the overall cost is greater because they must be replaced more often owing to changes in the refractory requirements of the eye. Soft lenses are also more costly because they are less durable than hard ones and require more lens-cleaning and disinfecting products.

The care given to contact lenses varies considerably with each wearer. Soft lenses rapidly degenerate to useless pieces of plastic if they are neglected. When used with a fastidious care and cleaning program, daily wear soft lenses can be expected to have an average life of 12–18 months compared with 18–36 months for similarly used RGP lenses.

Indications for Contact Lenses

The decision to wear contact lenses rather than eyeglasses is sometimes based on therapeutic necessity. For example, with keratoconus, a gradual protrusion of the central cornea, satisfactory vision is usually unattainable with ordinary eyeglasses but can be obtained with rigid contact lenses.12 Other examples of therapeutic necessity are lenses used as collagen shields and soft contact lenses saturated with antibiotic agents.

Aphakia results when the crystalline lens of the eye is removed because of an opacified lens or cataract and an intraocular lens is not implanted. Aphakic individuals characteristically see better with cataract contact lenses than with cataract spectacles. Extended-wear contacts are particularly beneficial for such patients because their poor vision makes it difficult for them to insert and remove lenses.

Visual aberrations caused by corneal scarring are also often better corrected by rigid contact lenses. Whereas eyeglasses simply correct refractive error by changing the focus of light incident on the cornea, the proximity of the contact lens actually masks irregularities in the corneal topography. Prosthetic lenses may also make corneal scarring cosmetically unnoticeable.

Perhaps the main reason for choosing contact lenses is the perceived improvement in personal appearance. Other strongly influencing factors include no obstruction of vision from eyeglass frames, greater clarity in peripheral vision, no fogging of lenses caused by sudden temperature changes, and more freedom of motion during vigorous activity (e.g., sports).

Contraindications for Contact Lenses

Some individuals who require vision correction cannot or should not wear contact lenses. Contraindications are often based on lifestyle as well as on medical history. Occupational conditions that may prohibit the wearing of contacts include exposure to dust and particulate matter, wind, glare, molten metals, irritants, chemicals, tobacco smoke, and chemical fumes.13 Certain chemical fumes have been suggested as being particularly hazardous because of the potential concentration of irritants under a hard lens or inside a soft lens. The lens theoretically prolongs contact of such substances with the cornea and can lead to corneal toxicity. However, these theoretical occupational contraindications have not been proven.

The successful wearing of contact lenses depends on adequate tear production. Insufficient tear production, a deficiency or excess of mucin, excessive lipid production, or excessively dry environments may preclude successful contact lens use. So, too, may dry spots on the cornea, often found in postmenopausal women. These spots, possibly caused by the absence of the precorneal film, are often identified with lacrimal insufficiency.

Contact lenses should not be used for cosmetic reasons if a patient has active pathologic intraocular or corneal conditions. Medical reasons that contraindicate contact lens wear include chronic conjunctivitis; blepharitis; recurrent viral, bacterial, or fungal infections; poor blink rate or incomplete blink; and insufficient or abnormal tear production. Diabetic patients are often advised against extended-wear contact lenses because of retarded healing processes and the tendency toward prolonged corneal abrasion with such use. This precaution is probably unnecessary for daily wear of lenses unless problems occur. Chronic common colds or allergic conditions such as hay fever and asthma may also make lens wear extremely uncomfortable or impossible.

Contact lenses should be used with caution by patients with epilepsy, high blood pressure, heart disease, or severe arthritis. The corneal topography may be altered by pregnancy or use of oral contraceptives. The fluid-retaining properties of estrogen may lead to edema of the cornea and eyelids as well as to decreased tear production.

Contact lenses should also be used with caution by elderly persons, because of possible lacrimal insufficiency and loose lid tissues, which create a sagging conjunctival cul-de-sac and therefore make lens retention difficult. Individuals with arthritis may lack the dexterity needed to insert lenses. Lens wearers moving from a low to a high altitude may encounter hypoxia or metabolic deficiency, resulting in irritation and corneal abrasions.

During the period needed for adapting to rigid contact lenses, the eyelids may become hyperemic; this condition may lead to blepharitis, especially in the upper lid. Short pseudoblinks, by new wearers of hard lenses, may irritate the conjunctiva of the upper eyelid. Chin elevation and squinting may result from the patient's efforts to minimize the irritation.

Contact lenses generally can match or exceed the vision obtained with spectacles. However, depending on the type of lens, there are situations in which vision may become worse.14 Light may be scattered through soft lenses because of the water content. Some patients wearing lenses with high water content may experience hazy vision around the edges of objects. In some cases, patients wearing hard contact lenses experience nighttime "ghosting," which occurs when the patient's pupil dilates enough to see the edges of the hard lens. This can sometimes be corrected with larger diameter lenses. Other patients complain of "spiderweb" vision, usually at night; this can be due to crazing, the development of fine cracks, usually in RGP lenses.

Problems with Contact Lenses

AIDS/HIV/Herpes

The human immunodeficiency virus (HIV) has been isolated from the tears of infected individuals as well as from the contact lenses worn by infected individuals. This becomes an issue for a patient in the case of trial contact lenses. These lenses may be reused by different patients in the lens fitter's office. After the lens is used in any patient, it is disinfected. Generally, these lenses are not dispensed to a patient except as a "loaner" lens (i.e., patient waiting for new replacement lenses). Even in this scenario, the lenses are disinfected with heat or chemicals before being dispensed. Studies have shown that heat and the routinely available hydrogen peroxide products are effective in inactivating HIV viruses. The Food and Drug Administration (FDA) also requires that all contact lens regimens kill the herpes simplex virus, another enveloped virus. There have been no reported cases of HIV transmission via a contact lens fitting.15

Drugs

Many undesired effects have been reported when a patient who wears contact lenses ingests or topically applies certain drugs (Table 5). The pharmacist must understand the problems these medications may cause. In general, patients should be counseled not to place any ophthalmic solution or ointment into the eye when contact lenses are in place. The only exceptions to this rule are products specifically formulated to be used with contact lenses, such as rewetting drops, or those products that an eye care practitioner has specifically recommended for use with contact lenses.

Topical administration of ophthalmic drugs may have physiologic consequences or may modify pharmacologic responses to drugs. The use of solutions that may be considered benign, such as artificial tears, may reduce tear breakup time and alter the distribution of the mucoid, aqueous, and lipid components of tears, perhaps causing initial discomfort upon instillation of the drops.[11] The pharmacologic effect of a topically administered drug while soft lenses are in place may be exaggerated: the soft lens may absorb the drug and release it over time, thus creating a sustained-release dosage form; or the drug effect may be decreased as the lens may absorb the drug and bind it tightly so that none of it is released into the eye. Further, the contact time of the medication with the eye may be increased due to the presence of any type of contact lens. Finally, some increased drug absorption may occur secondary to a compromised corneal epithelium that is present during contact lens wear.[11]

Additionally, the preservatives, vehicles, tonicity factors, and pH of the solution to be instilled into the eye could alter the lenses. For instance, instillation of hypertonic solutions such as 10% sodium sulfacetamide or 8% pilocarpine may cause soft lens dehydration and lens disfigurement. Topical medications with an acidic pH promote lens dehydration and steepening; alkaline medications promote hydration and flattening.[16] Topical suspensions may lead to lens intolerance due to buildup of particulate matter and discomfort. Gel and oil formulations may alter the surface relationship between the contact lens and the cornea.[11] Finally, the active ingredient of certain topical products (e.g., epinephrine) may discolor lenses.

Some drugs that are present in indoor air may damage lenses. Two examples are ribavirin and nicotine. Some nurses who care for patients receiving ribavirin have reportedly experienced cloudy lenses after repeated exposure to the drug.[17,18] Similarly, contact lens wearers who are exposed to a large amount of cigarette smoke may discover a brown discoloration and nicotine deposits on the lenses. This is especially true for those who smoke and have nicotine-stained fingers.[19]

Some systemic medications are secreted into tears and may interact with (primarily soft) contact lenses through this mechanism. For example, rifampin will stain the lenses and tears orange. Drugs such as gold salts are secreted into the tears and may cause ocular irritation. Others drugs may affect tear production, the refractive properties of the eye, the shape of the cornea, or the actual lens (Table 5).[20]

Cosmetics

Patients who wear contact lenses should choose—and use—cosmetics with care.[21] Women should insert lenses before applying makeup and should avoid touching the lens with eyeliner or mascara. Cosmetics with an aqueous base should be used because oil-based products may cause blurred vision and irritation if they are deposited on the lens. Cream eye shadows are preferable to powder shadows. Mascara should be applied only to the very tips of the lashes. Eyeliners should never be applied inside the eyelid. Any aerosol products, in particular, must be used with caution. Irritation may occur if some of the spray particles are trapped in the tear layer beneath the lens, and some sprays may actually damage the lens. One way to avoid a problem is to insert the lenses, go to another room, cover the eyes with a cloth, use the spray, and then leave the area with the eyes still closed.

TABLE 5 Drug–contact lens interactions

Changes in tear film and/or production

Tear volume decreased
- Anticholinergic agents
- Antihistamines
- Diuretics
- Timolol (topical)
- Tricyclic antidepressants

Tear volume increased
- Cholinergic agents
- Reserpine

Color changes in lenses (primarily soft lenses)
- Diagnostic dyes (i.e., fluorescein)
- Epinephrine (topical)
- Fluorescein (topical)
- Nicotine
- Nitrofurantoin
- Phenazopyridine
- Phenothiazines
- Phenylephrine
- Rifampin
- Sulfasalazine
- Tetracycline
- Tetrahydrozaline (topical)

Tonicity changes
- Pilocarpine (8%)
- Sodium sulfacetamide (10%)

Lid/corneal edema
- Chlorthalidone
- Clomiphene
- Oral contraceptives
- Primidone

Ocular inflammation/irritation
- Gold salts
- Isotretinoin
- Salicylates

Refractive changes (i.e., induction of myopia)
- Acetazolamide
- Sulfadiazine
- Sulfamethizole
- Sulfamethoxazole
- Sulfisoxazole

Miscellaneous
- Digoxin (increased glare)
- Ribavirin (cloudy lenses)

Adapted with permission from Engle JP. Contact lens care. *Am Druggist* 1990 Jan: 54–65.

Nail polish, hand creams, and perfumes should be applied only after the lenses have been inserted. Nail polish and remover can destroy a lens. Men often contaminate their lenses with hair preparations; they should take special care to clean their hands thoroughly before handling contact lenses. Soaps containing cold cream or deodorants should be avoided because they can leave a film on the fingers after rinsing. This residue is readily transferred to a lens and can cause blurred vision. Moreover, if the lens comes in contact with residual petrolatum-based lotion on the patient's fingers, the lens' surface can be modified. This modification cannot be detected by inspection; it will be noted, however, once the lens is worn. Approximately 20–30 minutes after insertion of the lens, the surface-wetting properties of the lens are disrupted.[22]

Corneal Hypoxia and Edema

An adequate supply of oxygen exists only if the cornea is continuously bathed with oxygenated tears.[23] During blinking, metabolic byproducts from the surface epithelium are flushed from under the contact lenses and oxygen is brought in as the lenses move toward and away from the cornea. Even when properly fitted, however, both rigid and soft lenses can produce a progressive hypoxia of the cornea while the lenses are in place, especially in persons who have low blink frequency or incomplete blinks.

One major effect of this hypoxia is edema of the corneal tissues. It has been demonstrated that corneal thickness is increased to a greater extent by hard (PMMA) lenses. After approximately 16 hours of continuous wear, hard and, to a lesser extent, soft lenses cause the glycogen content of the cornea to fall to a level that is accompanied by significant edema. Symptoms associated with corneal edema include photophobia, rainbows around a light, sensations of hotness, grittiness and itchiness, fogging of vision, and blurred vision. A patient experiencing corneal edema from overuse of contact lenses can be treated with one to two drops of sodium chloride (2 or 5%) every 3 to 4 hours after the lenses have been removed. The patient should be counseled that transient stinging or burning may occur upon instillation of the drops. Further, the patient should be counseled not to overuse the lenses.

If lenses are removed for 6 hours, the glycogen levels return to approximately 93% of the normal value and to about 98% in 8 hours. To prevent edema from reaching this extent, lenses should be removed for a 1-hour rest period after 7–9 hours of wear. The lenses may then be reinserted for up to 8 hours if necessary. Wearing RGP or soft lenses uninterrupted for 14–18 hours once or twice a week will not usually cause problems; continuing such a practice on a daily basis should be discouraged. Tolerance to contact lens wear does occur.

Another effect of corneal hypoxia is neovascularization. The development of new vessels is potentially irreversible. Routine follow-up visits to the lens care specialist are important for monitoring for this effect of contact lens wear.

Corneal Abrasions

Corneal abrasions are surface defects in the epithelial layer of the cornea. Causes of these abrasions range from poorly fitted lenses or simple overwear to scratches caused by the entrapment of foreign bodies under the lens. The cornea is sensitive to abrasion, so reflex lid closure (blepharospasm), tearing, and rubbing the affected eye are immediate. However, rubbing the eye must be avoided because it can cause more extensive damage while the lens remains in the eye.

Fortunately, the pain associated with corneal abrasion is usually of greater magnitude than the damage. The epithelium regenerates quickly: most minor epithelial defects (i.e., those that are 22 mm in diameter or less) generally heal within 12–24 hours. The lens should be left out for 2 days to a week. The wearer may then proceed using a modified break-in schedule suggested by the vision specialist. More extensive abrasions require the attention of an eye care specialist.

Symptoms of Lens Problems

Lens wearers may initially encounter various problems in adapting to lenses, particularly RGP ones; even longtime wearers occasionally experience difficulty. Many of these problems arise from different causative factors, and identifying and solving a specific problem may require a trained vision specialist. The following list provides a perspective for counseling a lens wearer who seeks advice. Most of this information is particularly applicable to rigid lens wear.

- *Deep aching of eye:* This pain persists even after the lens is removed and may be caused by poorly fitted lenses. The lens care practitioner must be consulted.
- *Blurred vision:* This effect may be produced by improper refractive power, tear film buildup, cosmetic film buildup, switched lenses, corneal edema, or use of oral contraceptives.
- *Excessive tearing:* Tearing is normal when lenses are first worn; however, tearing may also be caused by poorly fitted lenses or chipped, rough edges on the lenses.
- *Fogging:* "Misty" or "smoky" vision can be caused by corneal edema, overwearing of contact lenses, coatings or deposits on lens surfaces, or poor wetting of the lens while on the eye.
- *Itching:* This may be caused by allergic conjunctivitis and may be treated with short-term use of topical steroids.
- *Lens falls out of eye:* Poorly fitted lenses are probably the cause. However, even properly fitted hard lenses may occasionally slide off the cornea or be blinked out of the eye.
- *Inability to wear lenses in morning:* This may be caused by corneal edema or mild conjunctivitis.
- *Pain after removal of lens:* This effect is usually caused by corneal abrasion. The presence of the lens anesthetizes the cornea owing to hypoxia; sensation returns after 4–6 hours and pain develops.
- *Sudden pain in the eye:* A foreign body or chipped lens may be the problem.
- *Squinting:* This effect is caused by excessive lens movement or a poorly fitted lens. The wearer squints to center the optical portion of the lens over the pupil.

Products for and Care of Contact Lenses

Contact Lens Solutions

Formulation Considerations

The manufacturing and marketing of contact lenses are regulated by the ophthalmic devices division of the FDA. Even though contact lens solutions are not considered drug products, formulation considerations still apply. Contact lens wearers should use only lens care products that have been approved by the FDA for use with their specific contact lens material.

The basic considerations for a well-formulated contact lens solution include pH, viscosity, isotonicity with tears, stability, sterility, and provision for maintenance of sterility (bactericidal action). The pH range of comfort is not well defined because tear pH varies among individuals; normal tear pH is 7.4. It is best to have a weakly buffered solution that can readily adjust to any tear pH because highly buffered solutions can cause significant discomfort, even ocular damage, when instilled. However, as with therapeutic ophthalmic solutions, stability of the solution components takes precedence over comfort. For this reason, many contact lens solutions are formulated with pH values above or below 7.4. However, these systems are weakly buffered and are usually well tolerated by the eye.

Routine daily use of any contact lens solution allows the potential for bacterial contamination. Depending on specific lens care procedures, a single container may last for a month or more. The solution must therefore contain a bactericidal agent that is both effective over the long term and nonirritating with daily use in the eye. Few preservatives fulfill these criteria. Commonly used agents are benzalkonium chloride, thimerosal, and sorbic acid products, all of which can cause irritation, depending on concentration and patient sensitivity.

Solutions from different manufacturers should not be mixed because a precipitate may result. For instance, a product containing alkaline borate buffers forms a gummy, gel-like precipitate on lenses if mixed with a wetting solution containing polyvinyl alcohol. Further, solutions containing cationic preservative, such as chlorhexidine, polyquaternium-1 (Polyquad), or polyaminopropyl biguanide (Dymed), should not be mixed with solutions containing an anionic preservative such as sorbic acid, because this, too, will cause a precipitate.[24]

Preservatives

Benzalkonium Chloride   Benzalkonium chloride is a surface-active agent and germicide that is effective against a variety of Gram-positive and Gram-negative bacteria. In sufficient concentration, it is also effective against perhaps the most worrisome ocular pathogen, *Pseudomonas aeruginosa*. Several properties of benzalkonium chloride require that care be exercised with respect to its concentration in a hard lens solution. It is incompatible and should not be used with soft contact lenses because it is adsorbed onto the matrix of the lens. Severe toxicity may occur due to sustained release of benzalkonium chloride from the lens.

High concentrations of benzalkonium chloride cause ocular damage, either directly by instillation into the eye or indirectly by adsorption onto the lens.[25] The maximum tolerable concentration is reportedly about 0.03% (1:3,000), with solutions of 0.02% having been shown to be tolerated up to several times a day. However, most solutions for direct instillation into the eye contain concentrations between 0.004 and 0.01%.[25]

Some persons using a solution preserved with benzalkonium chloride develop ocular irritation because the surfactant builds up on their lenses. Switching to a solution with a lower benzalkonium chloride concentration may alleviate this, but change to a solution with a completely different preservative or cleaning agent may be required.

Thimerosal   Thimerosal, or sodium ethylmercurithiosalicylate, was introduced as an alternative to benzalkonium chloride, with which it is incompatible. Like benzalkonium chloride, it acts by interfering with cell metabolism, glycolysis, and respiration. It is effective against *P. aeruginosa*, but it is slow to act because it depends on sustained release of mercurial ions that penetrate the bacterial cell. Like other mercurials, thimerosal may also cause sensitization in some individuals after repeated application. The reaction can be delayed and may take months to occur.

In general, thimerosal does not pose a significant problem except when used with soft contact lenses. Thimerosal may bind to debris in soft lenses and remain in contact with the eye for as long as the lens is in place. Moreover, the concentration of the preservative carried to the eye via soft lenses appears to cause a significant incidence of irritation. Thus, most practitioners have discouraged its use in soft lens care products because of the high incidence of sensitivity in the patient. On the other hand, thimerosal is rapidly cleared from the tear fluid when instilled with RGP lenses and therefore is less likely to be problematic for these patients.

Phenylmercuric Nitrate   Phenylmercuric nitrate is also a mercurial preservative, similar in action to thimerosal. It is usually used in dilute concentration and only in hard lens products. When used alone, however, it is not very effective against *P. aeruginosa*. Organic mercurials can be effective preservatives, but their usefulness in ophthalmic solutions is severely limited because of their slow action.

Sorbic Acid or Potassium Sorbate   Sorbic acid was, at one time, very popular as a preservative. Less irritating than mercurials, it is the preservative ingredient often included in products labeled "thimerosal-free" or "for sensitive eyes." However, it reportedly may increase age-associated yellowing of some lenses, particularly those containing a methacrylic acid.[26] In addition, sorbic acid's maximum antimicrobial activity is at a pH that is too low to be of optimum value for use on the eye.

Chlorhexidine   Chlorhexidine can irritate the eyes, and its degradation products may produce a yellow-to-green coloration.[27] It can be precipitated by borates, phosphates, and carbonates. At the concentration that chlorhexidine is used in soft lens solutions, it is less effective against several yeasts and fungi than is optimal. There are also problems associated with its use in RGP lens soaking or conditioning solutions, which generally contain high molecular weight wetting agents that may impair its disinfecting action. Solutions containing chlorhexidine that appear greenish should not be used because the color change indicates decomposition of the product.[27]

Sodium Salts of EDTA Sodium salts of ethylenediaminetetraacetic acid (EDTA) are often used in lens solutions because EDTA disrupts the integrity of bacterial cell walls. In so doing, it enhances the action of other preservatives. It also complexes with other substances, such as metallic ions, that might reduce benzalkonium chloride activity; by complexation, calcium deposits on lenses may be prevented. EDTA is often used in contact lens solutions that contain another chemical agent as their primary preservative. Solutions of EDTA cannot be claimed to be preservative-free, even if there is no other primary preservative. Addition of EDTA to nonpreserved saline solutions will increase their shelf life after opening.

Polyquaternium-1 Polyquaternium-1 (Polyquad) is a quaternary ammonium lens care preservative shown to be effective against certain bacteria, fungi, and yeast. Few toxicity or sensitivity problems have been noted with this preservative thus far. When first introduced to the market, formulations containing Polyquad were not compatible with lenses that had a high water content. The methacrylic acid component of the lens had the ability to adsorb the preservative in toxic levels. However, recent formulations do not seem to have this problem.

Polyaminopropyl Biguanide Polyaminopropyl biguanide (Dymed) is a cationic polymeric biguanide effective against certain bacteria, fungi, and yeast. Some solutions were formerly preserved with chlorhexidine, and there were reports of contamination of the solution with *Serratia marcescens*, which is able to feed on the high molecular weight wetting agents. However, no adverse effects to polyaminopropyl biguanide have been reported. One manufacturer of RGP solutions uses higher concentrations of this preservative than are found in soft lens solutions; this is necessary because the RGP solutions contain high molecular weight wetting agents, which decrease the effectiveness of the preservative. The higher concentrations do not seem to cause toxicity to the wearer because RGP lenses do not adsorb the preservatives to the degree that soft lenses do.

Hard Contact Lenses

Lens care products help to minimize the stress on the eye from hard contacts. These products aid the wearer, providing comfort and safety.

Hard lens care involves three important steps: cleaning, soaking, and wetting (Figure 2). For optimal lens care, all three steps should be performed each time the lenses are removed from the eye.

Cleaning Solutions

Normal tears are composed of secretions from many specialized glands lining the lacrimal apparatus, conjunctiva, and lids. Many components are somewhat hydrophobic and tend to adhere to the surface of a hard lens during normal daily wear. This residue, primarily proteinaceous

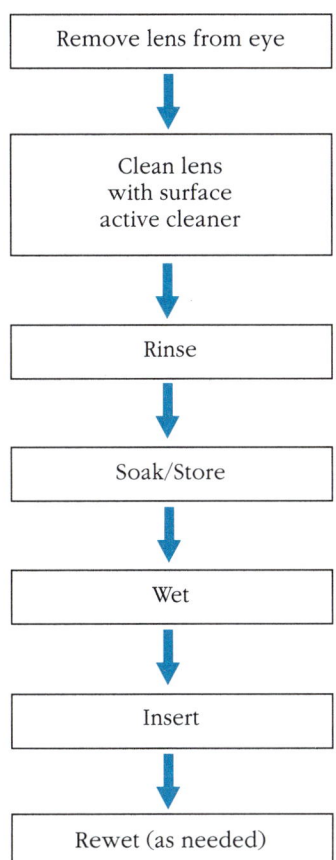

FIGURE 2 Hard contact lens care.

debris and oils, acts as a growth medium for bacteria. If it is not routinely removed by daily cleaning, it may harden to form coatings or tenacious deposits that create an irregular surface on the lens. This residue will eventually irritate the lids and corneal epithelium, and may progress to infection or other pathology. Decreased visual acuity and lens wear time are likely consequences of a cloudy lens or allergenic reactions.

Typical cleaning solutions contain nonionic or amphoteric surfactants that emulsify oils and aid in solubilizing other debris. Proteins and lipids are soluble in highly alkaline media, but a high pH can cause lens decomposition. Weak alkaline solutions may be helpful in dislodging deposits from the lens in conjunction with the surface tension–lowering properties of the surfactants.

Lenses should be thoroughly rinsed after cleaning because residual cleaning agents may lead to ocular irritation. Lenses should never be wiped dry with tissue because this can cause surface scratches. Also, homemade cleaning solutions, such as mixtures of baking soda with distilled water or cleaning solution, should not be used; they may scratch the lens and may not be easily rinsed off.[28] Similarly, dishwashing detergent, lighter fluid, toothpaste, or other cleaners not formulated for contact lens use may accumulate on the lens and cause damage or ocular irritation.

There are four basic techniques for cleaning hard lenses.

Friction Rubbing A contact lens cleaning solution or gel is applied to both surfaces of the lens. The lens is then rubbed between the thumb and forefinger or between the forefinger and palm of the opposite hand for about 20 seconds. Friction rubbing is the most common cleaning method and it is effective, but it may result in scratched and warped lenses if rubbing is too vigorous.

Spray Cleaning The lenses are placed into a perforated holder and held under a stream of running water from an ordinary faucet. The pressure of the water flow dislodges debris that has been loosened by overnight soaking in the storage case.

Hydraulic Cleaning The lenses are placed into separate baskets in a plastic container that has a rotating cap (e.g., Hydra-Mat II®). The cap, which is connected to the baskets, is rotated for 20–30 seconds to provide a high level of turbulence. The unit is filled with a special cleaning solution to assist in the removal of deposits.

Ultrasonic Cleaning The lenses are placed in a water bath through which ultrasound waves are passed. These specialized cleaning units have not been shown to be superior in cleaning contact lenses, and their cost is high.

Soaking Solutions

A soaking solution is used to store hard contact lenses whenever they are removed from the eyes. The solution maintains the lens in a constant state of hydration for maximum comfort and visual acuity. It also aids in removing deposits that accumulate on the lens during wear.

A rigid lens absorbs between 1 and 3% moisture by weight. Upon exposure to air, the lens dehydrates; it subsequently rehydrates when it comes in contact with a soaking solution or the lacrimal fluid. Placing a dehydrated lens into the eye causes discomfort as the lens absorbs tears from the precorneal area. In addition, a dehydrated lens is flatter than a hydrated lens; this factor causes problems with both comfort and visual acuity.

If lenses are allowed to dry out during overnight storage, accumulated deposits are more difficult to remove by normal cleaning. Storage in a soaking solution reduces the likelihood of deposits forming.

To maintain sterility, storage solutions use essentially the same preservatives as wetting solutions. The main difference is that the concentration can be somewhat higher in a soaking solution because the solution is rinsed from the lens before insertion. However, preservative levels are carefully selected because higher levels do not necessarily give increased effectiveness and may lead to impaired wetting or corneal irritation because of the adsorption of preservatives onto the lens.

Wetting Solutions

The functions of an ideal wetting solution are:

- To convert the hydrophobic lens surface to a hydrophilic surface by means of a uniform film that does not easily wash away;
- To increase comfort by providing cushioning and lubrication between the corneal surface and the inner surface of the lens, and between the lens and the inner surface of the eyelid;
- To place a viscous coating on the lens to protect it from oil on the fingers during insertion;
- To stabilize the lens on the fingertip to ease insertion, particularly for individuals with poor manual dexterity or unsteady hands.

If the lens is thoroughly cleaned before insertion, lacrimal fluid can adequately wet the lens. Indeed, the wetting action of popular wetting solutions is not significantly better than that of saline, and patients whose tears are capable of wetting a lens almost immediately upon insertion often do not use these solutions.

The basic wetting solution comprises components from four main categories:

- *Cushioning agents:* for example, viscosity-inducing additives (usually cellulose gum derivatives such as methylcellulose or hydroxypropyl methylcellulose);
- *Wetting agents:* for example, polyvinyl alcohol or other surfactants;
- *Preservatives:* for example, benzalkonium chloride, thimerosal, polyquaternium-1, sorbic acid, and polyaminopropyl biguanide;
- *Buffering agents and salts:* substances used to adjust pH and tonicity.

The cushioning effect of a wetting solution is achieved by hydrophilic polymers that lubricate the interface between the lens and the surfaces of the cornea and eyelid. Cellulose gum derivatives are often used. Although compounds such as methylcellulose possess a degree of surfactant activity, they do not promote uniform wetting of a rigid lens. For this reason, polyvinyl alcohol is also used often to decrease surface tension.

The concentration of the cushioning polymer in wetting solutions affects both eye comfort and the quality of vision immediately following insertion. In some individuals, a concentration that is too low causes discomfort after only a short time. In other wearers, a high polymer concentration results in blurred vision because the viscous solution mixes poorly with tears. Overspill of solution onto the lids and eyelashes causes crusting as the solution dries; this crusty residue can be a source of foreign material falling into the eye. Saliva should never be used to wet contact lenses because it can lead to infection by *Acanthamoeba*, *P. aeruginosa*, or other pathogens.

Multifunctional Products

Initially, manufacturers recommended three different solutions for the cleaning, soaking, and wetting of hard contact lenses. However, there has been a trend toward using combination solutions for these functions: single solutions claimed to be effective for all three procedures.

The major problem with an all-purpose solution is that ingredients required in its formulation perform different and somewhat incompatible functions. For example, high concentrations of benzalkonium chloride are necessary to kill bacteria in soaking solutions; however, these same concentrations can cause ocular irritation when placed directly on the eye with a contact lens. If lenses are stored overnight in a solution containing a high concentration of polymers for cushioning and wetting, the lenses may become gummy and cause discomfort. Similarly, if lenses are stored overnight in a cleaning solution containing an anionic surfactant, the detergent may eventually build up on the lens and cause irritation.

No single agent that will adequately perform all three basic functions currently exists. The present all-purpose solutions are compromises. They are marginally effective but cannot be expected to perform as well as separate solutions.

Rewetting Products

Rewetting solutions are intended to clean and rewet the contact lens while the lens is in the eye. They depend on the use of surfactants to loosen deposits; removal is assisted by the natural cleaning action of blinking. An agent used to promote this action is polyoxyl 40 stearate. Although these products function well to recondition the lens, the cornea benefits more if the lens is actually removed, cleaned, and rewetted. Removing the lens for even a brief time allows the cornea to recover some of its depleted glycogen levels.

Other Products

Other ophthalmic products are available to the hard lens wearer for occasional use. Some, such as artificial tears and ocular decongestants, are not recommended for use with the lenses in place. Because of their emollient and lubricating effect, artificial tears can be used to soothe the eye. Ocular decongestants reduce mild conjunctival hyperemia associated with prolonged lens wear. However, these topical decongestants can induce conjunctival hypoxia, which may harm the patient.[29] Routine use of these products should be avoided. If symptoms requiring their use persist, a visit to a vision specialist is advised.

Product Selection Guidelines

The variety of lens care solutions available to hard lens wearers poses a selection problem. The availability of single- and multiple-function products within the same product line can further frustrate and confuse some wearers. Thus, product selection is an area in which pharmacists can perform a much needed role as a consultant. Unfortunately, information is not always sufficient to provide a complete foundation for patient consultation. Product labeling is often incomplete or limited to general information. The specific agents and concentrations of preservatives are usually listed adequately, but concentrations of cushioning and lubricating polymers are often absent. Furthermore, other ingredients are often listed simply as "cleaning agents" or "buffers," making alternate selections a random process. One factor that could help determine which products to recommend is the adequacy of the labeling. A surfactant cleaner, a soaking solution, a wetting solution, and a rewetting solution should be recommended.

Insertion and Removal

Hard contact lens wearers should be instructed in the proper procedures for inserting and removing their lenses as follows: After washing hands, remove the lens from the lens storage case. Rinse the lens with fresh conditioning/soaking solution. Inspect the lens for cleanliness and signs of damage (cracks or chips). If you use a wetting or conditioning solution, place a few drops on the lens. Place the lens on the top of the index finger. Place the middle finger of the same hand on the lower lid and pull it down. With the other hand, use a finger to lift the upper lid and then place the lens on the eye. Release the lids and blink. Check vision immediately to ascertain that the lens is in the proper position. If the lens is not placed correctly after three to four blinks (blurry vision), it may be off center, on the wrong eye, or dirty. Instill one to three drops of rewetting or reconditioning drops into the eye. If there is no improvement, remove the lens, place several drops of wetting/conditioning solution onto both surfaces, and reinsert. Repeat this procedure with the other lens.

Before removing the lens, fill the storage cases with soaking/conditioning solution. Remove the top from the cleaning solution. Place your hand (or a towel) under your eye. Two methods are appropriate for removing the lens from the eye:

- *Two-finger method:* Place the tip of your forefinger of one hand on the middle of your eyelid by the lashes. Place the forefinger of the other hand on the middle lower lid margin. Push the lids inward and then together. The lens should pop out. If it only becomes decentered onto the white part of your eye, recenter and try again.
- *Temporal pull/blink method:* Place an index finger on the temporal edge of the lower and upper lids. Stretch the skin outward and slightly upward without allowing the lid to slide over the lens. Blink briskly. The lens will pop out because of the pressure of the eyelids at the top and bottom of the lens. Blinking facilitates removal after the lids have been tightened around the lens.

Rigid Gas-Permeable Lenses

The diversity and variation in materials used in RGP lenses preclude generalizations. Lens wearers should be advised by their eye care professionals about the products and regimens recommended for their particular lenses. The labeling for contact lens products also indicates the lenses for which they are approved.

The care of an RGP lens is similar to that of a hard contact lens (Figure 3). The first step, after removing the lens from the eye, is to clean the lens. After cleaning, the lens is soaked in a soaking or conditioning solution. The lens may be wetted and then inserted into the eye. Rewetting or reconditioning drops may be used while the lens is on the eye. With some lenses, once weekly enzymes are also recommended.

Some RGP lenses have a high silicone content. These lenses have decreased surface wettability. The lens surface tends to have a negative charge, which promotes the binding of positively charged tear constituents. Cleaners that are designed for conventional hard or RGP lenses may not be effective in removing the more tenacious deposits. Other cleaners that are formulated for this type of lens (i.e., Boston Daily Cleaner®) contain polymeric beads, which act to mechanically break the adhesive bonds that have formed between the lens and the deposits. However, these cleaners have also been associated with hairline scratches on the RGP lens.[30]

It is important to counsel the patient to rinse the lens carefully and not apply too much pressure when cleaning. RGP lenses tend to coat on the concave surface rather

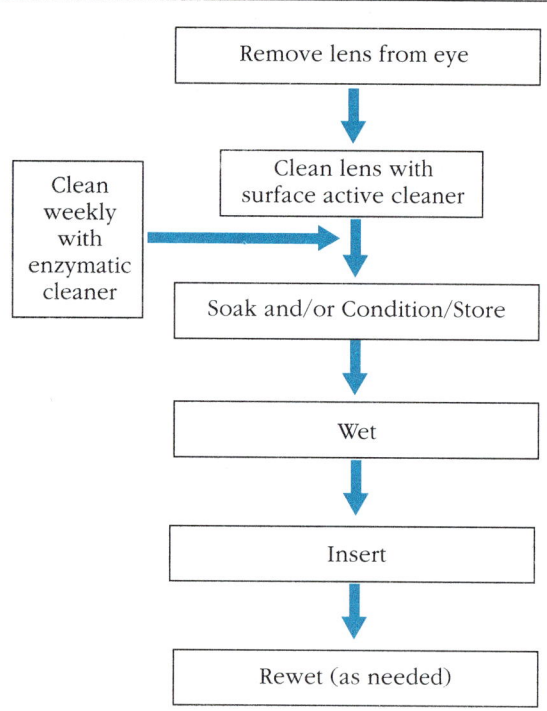

FIGURE 3 Gas-permeable lens care.

than on the convex surface, as is the case with hard lenses. Care should be taken to clean both surfaces of the lens thoroughly, even though the concave surface may be harder to reach. The lenses should be cleaned in the palm of the hand to decrease the risk of chipping an edge, which may occur when the lens is cleaned between the fingers.[30]

Because these high-silicone lenses have decreased surface wettability, conditioning solutions are used instead of soaking solutions to facilitate the formation of a cushioning tear layer. A conditioning solution is essentially a specially formulated wetting solution. The conditioner system enhances wettability of the lens, increases comfort, and disinfects the lens. It is important to counsel the patient that the Boston Advance Conditioning® solution must be discarded 90 days after opening the bottle. There is a space on the label to record the date that the product is opened.

Reconditioning/rewetting drops may also be used while the lens is on the eye to rewet the lens as necessary. Boston Reconditioning Drops® must also be discarded 90 days after opening. Heat disinfection cannot be used with RGP lenses.

As the silicone content of RGP lenses increases, so does the amount of protein adherence. Silicone acrylate lenses have an active surface that promotes the binding of tear constituents. Protein deposits on the lens will decrease the oxygen permeability, and the patient may experience discomfort.[31] Lenses of this type should be cleaned with an enzymatic product once weekly. Failure to comply with this cleaning step may result in the need for professional polishing or replacement of the lens.

Products containing chlorhexidine gluconate should not be used with silicone or styrene lenses because this agent will make the lens surface more difficult to wet and may also cause surface clouding. Fluorosilicone acrylate lenses should not be disinfected with hydrogen peroxide or cleaned more than one time with Miraflow®. Cracking, changes in parameters, and brittleness have been noted when this type of lens is cleaned repeatedly with Miraflow®.

Product Selection Guidelines

The appropriate lens care regimen for RGP lenses must be compatible with the particular lens. Lens wearers should be advised against substituting other products for those specifically recommended by their eye care professional. Patients wearing RGP lenses should be advised to purchase a surface-active cleaning product, an enzymatic product, and a conditioning or soaking solution, depending on the type of lens worn. A rewetting or reconditioning product should also be recommended.

Insertion and Removal

Wearers of RGP lenses should be counseled to follow the insertion and removal procedures for hard lenses.

Soft Contact Lenses

Conventional hard lens solutions should never be used with soft lenses because absorption of the ingredients can damage the lenses. Because soft lenses contain a high percentage of water, they are most prone to bacterial contamination. Good lens disinfection is crucial to prevent ocular infection and damage to the lens material by bacteria and fungi. Wearers of soft hydrophilic contact lenses should also be particularly cautious in exposing their lenses to chemicals. These chemicals, many of which penetrate and bind with the lens material, can come from cosmetics, environmental pollutants, and ophthalmic and systemic products.

The basic regimen of care for soft lenses is different from that for hard lenses (Figure 4). All steps must be completed to avoid ocular complications.

Cleaning Products

A troublesome aspect of soft lens wear is the accumulation of deposits on the lens.[32] The nature of these deposits varies, but generally they consist of proteins and lipids from the wearer's lacrimal secretions. Deposits are a greater problem with the more highly hydrated lenses, but the rate at which these deposits accumulate depends on the lens and the tears. Some wearers experience little difficulty and wear soft lenses for long periods without significant buildup; others may show deposits in as little as 2 or 3 days. Whatever the cause or accumulation rate, the result is an uncomfortable lens of poor optical quality.

Soft contact lenses require two cleaning steps to rid them of debris. Cleaning with a surface-active cleaner must be done daily or, in the case of extended-wear lenses, each time they are removed from the eye. Cleaning with an enzymatic cleaner should be done weekly.

Surface-Active Cleaners A common method of cleaning soft lenses uses surface-active materials and friction rubbing. Several drops of a cleaning product are placed onto the lens surface, and the lens is gently rubbed between the thumb and forefinger. Another method is to place the lens in the palm of the hand and rub gently with a fingertip. With both methods, care must be used to avoid cutting the soft lens with

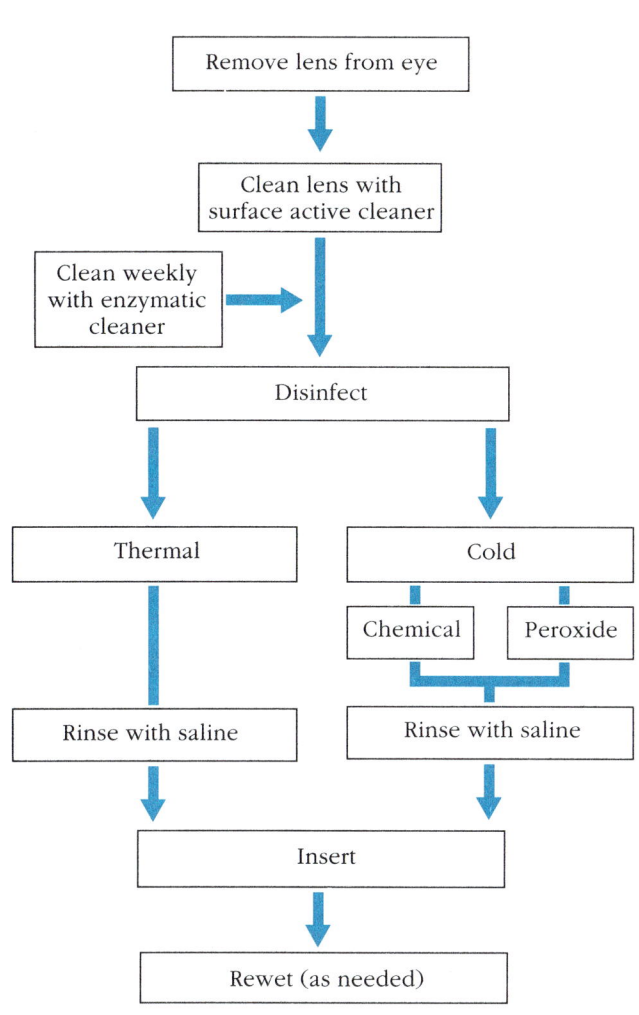

FIGURE 4 Soft contact lens care.

a fingernail or scratching the lens surfaces with grit or dirt on the hands. Soft lens cleaning solutions generally contain a nonionic detergent, a wetting agent, a chelating agent, buffers, preservatives, and, in some cases, polymeric cleaning beads. Friction cleaning usually takes about 20–30 seconds, and then the cleaner must be thoroughly rinsed from the lens. Rinsing is an essential part of soft lens care; it should be carried out using a sterile isotonic buffered solution. Tap water should *never* be used with soft contact lenses because it is not isotonic and it contains harmful pathogens.

Enzymatic Cleaners Although the surface-active cleaners generally are quite effective in removing lipid deposits, they are less successful in removing tenacious protein debris. Enzymatic cleaners are an additional cleaning aid that can help solve this problem. These enzymes hydrolyze polypeptide bonds of protein and dissolve the protein deposits. For the enzyme solution to work properly, however, the lens must be cleaned with a surface-active cleaner first; enzymes are ineffective in the presence of debris covering or mixed with protein.

Generally, enzymatic cleaners are used in the following manner. The enzyme tablet (papain, pancreatin, or subtilisin) is placed in a solution recommended by the manufacturer and the lens is allowed to soak from as briefly as 15 minutes (high-water lenses) to as long as overnight (low-water lenses). The enzymatic cleaner is then thoroughly rinsed from the lens to prevent eye irritation. With most enzymatic products (the exception being certain subtilisin products), the lens then must be disinfected to complete the cleaning procedure. It is usually sufficient to use enzyme cleaning as a once-a-week supplement to daily cleaning with surface-active chemicals. Some enzymatic regimens have been developed to be used simultaneously with thermal and chemical disinfection.

Table 6 shows some of the differences between various enzymatic products. Of particular note are the products that allow the patient to combine the enzymatic cleaning and disinfecting steps. These products are dissolved in

TABLE 6 Enzymatic cleaners

	Extenzyme	Optizyme	ReNu Effervescent	ReNu Thermal	Softlens	Ultrazyme
Odor	Yes	No	No	No	Yes	No
Disinfection necessary	Yes	Yes	Yes	No	Yes	No
Effective with short soak	Yes	Yes	Yes	Yes	Yes	Yes
Use concurrently with heat disinfection	No	No	No	Yes	No	No
Use concurrently with H_2O_2 disinfection	No	No	No	No	No	Yes

Adapted with permission from Engle JP. Contact lens care. *AM Druggist* 1990 Jan: 54-65.

the hydrogen peroxide used for disinfection or in the saline that will be heated in the disinfecting step. This decreases the number of steps necessary for lens care and may increase compliance.

Disinfecting Methods

The FDA recommends disinfection of soft contact lenses before each reinsertion. Disinfection occurs after cleaning the lens. Two methods of disinfection are currently approved: thermal and chemical. Studies have shown that microorganisms do not actually enter the matrix of soft lenses but that surface contamination could lead to ocular infection.[33] Both disinfecting methods are reliable for most ocular pathogens. Chemical disinfection with hydrogen peroxide has increased in popularity with certain types of lenses over thermal and earlier chemical disinfectants.

Thermal Disinfection The basic method of thermal disinfection involves placing the cleaned lenses into separate compartments of a storage case filled with saline. The case is then placed into a heating unit, and the temperature is increased to a specific level for a prescribed time. Originally, the lenses were disinfected by raising the temperature to the boiling point for about 20 minutes. Units that use a lower temperature (about 176°F [80°C]) for a longer time are now available. The FDA requirement is at least 176°F (80°C) for at least 10 minutes. This process is as effective as boiling for most organisms, and it prolongs lens life. The procedure is usually done at night.

For situations in which it is not possible to use a heat disinfecting unit, the patient may place the tightly closed lens case containing the lenses and saline in a pot of boiling water for at least 10 minutes (15 minutes if at an altitude above 7,000 feet). The water must not boil away. The pot with the water and lenses should then be removed from the heat and allowed to cool for 30 minutes. The patient should resume use of the heat disinfecting unit as soon as possible.

Thermal disinfection has several advantages. It can be done with a preservative-free solution and is therefore less likely to cause eye irritation. Additionally, it kills microbial contamination better than any other method. Thermal disinfection is the only contact lens disinfecting method known to be effective against cysts of *Acanthamoeba*, and it is generally more effective against chemically resistant microorganisms such as fungi and bacillus species. It also kills organisms on and surrounding the contact lens case, further preventing potential contaminants from entering the lenses.

Thermal disinfection also has several drawbacks. Lenses with a high water content cannot withstand daily heating. Some individuals find the method cumbersome and less convenient than chemical disinfection. There is also a high initial cost for equipment, although long-term costs of chemical disinfectant solutions may offset this. The user must take care to remove proteinaceous and other debris by cleaning lenses before thermal disinfection. Lens cases used with thermal units, and the units themselves, should be routinely inspected for damage, cracks, or leaks and replaced at the earliest sign of a problem.

Chemical Disinfection In chemical disinfection, the lenses are stored for a prescribed period of time in a solution containing bactericidal agents that are compatible with soft lens materials. There are two basic forms of chemical disinfecting systems available in the United States. The original chemical disinfecting solutions consisted of antimicrobial preservatives of sufficient concentration in storage solutions primarily composed of saline. These initial disinfecting solutions contained chlorhexidine and thimerosal, which induces sensitivity reactions in many soft lens wearers. These solutions no longer contain thimerosal, but several solutions still contain chlorhexidine. Patients are less sensitive to chlorhexidine and apparently can tolerate it better than thimerosal. To avoid sensitivity reactions, solutions with several new disinfecting preservatives are currently being marketed for soft contact lens solutions. These preservatives are sorbic acid, Polyquad, and Dymed, touted to be much less toxic or allergenic than their predecessors. However, these agents may also be less effective against fungi and protozoans.

Patients should soak their lenses in the disinfecting solution for a minimum of 4 hours. The lenses may be stored for longer periods in these solutions; however, if they are stored longer than 3 days, the patient should clean and disinfect the lenses with fresh solution for at least 4 hours prior to inserting the lenses.

The second chemical method uses hydrogen peroxide as the antimicrobial agent. Soft lenses are placed in purified hydrogen peroxide, and the liberation of oxygen from peroxide disinfects. Following disinfection, the peroxide is neutralized to trace levels by the catalytic action of platinum or peroxidase, by soaking lenses in sodium thiosulfite solution, or by dilution techniques.

Patients who use the platinum disk (i.e., AO Sept®) for neutralization should be counseled to replace the disk after 100 uses or 3 months, whichever comes first. Failure to comply with these instructions may result in disk failure, and the patient may sustain a peroxide burn on the cornea. Moreover, although the catalytic disk systems only require one step, that step takes 6 hours for disinfection and neutralization, which decreases the flexibility of the system. Another disadvantage to catalytic disks is that, depending on the design of the case, bacteria beneath the disk may be protected from the disinfecting action of the hydrogen peroxide.[34] Once the catalytic disk neutralizes the peroxide, a nonpreserved solution remains. If the lenses are left in the case for several days, bacterial contamination may occur. Patients should not store their lenses in neutralized AO Sept® for more than 24 hours unless they disinfect the lenses again prior to insertion.

Most hydrogen peroxide systems that require two steps for disinfection and neutralization require only 20–30 minutes to work. The patient may use these products in the morning just before insertion. For most patients, one of the products that use a neutralizing solution is appropriate. This product requires only 20–30 minutes to use; the neutralizing step is easy; and if there is a preservative in the neutralizing agent, there is less chance that the resultant solution will become contaminated. Table 7 outlines the differences among the various peroxide products.

One potential disadvantage of hydrogen peroxide disinfection is that patients may insert the lens directly from the peroxide solution without neutralization. A peroxide-soaked lens placed on the eye will cause great pain, photophobia, redness, and, perhaps, corneal epithelial damage. If this occurs, the patient should immediately remove

TABLE 7	Differences in peroxide products				
	Neutralizing dilution agent	Flexibility		Potential risks	
		Overnight	Morning		
AO Sept	Platinum disc	Yes	No	Disc failure[b]	
Consept	Chemical solution	Yes	Yes	None	
Lensept	Chemical solution	Yes	Yes	None	
Mirasept[a]	Chemical solution/tablets	Yes	Yes	None	
Oxysept	Chemical solution/tablets	Yes	Yes	None	
UltraCare	Chemical Tablets	Yes	No	None	
Pure-Sept	Saline (osmotic extraction)	Yes	Yes	Possible irritation from leftover peroxide	
Quik-Sept	Saline (osmotic extraction)	Yes	Yes	Possible irritation from leftover peroxide	

[a] Mirasept neutralizing solution (multiuse bottles) must be discarded 4 months after opening.
[b] Disc wears out and must be replaced every 3 months or after 100 uses.
Adapted with permission from Engle JP. Contact lens care. *Am Druggist* 1990 Jan: 54–65.

the lens from the eye and flush the eye with sterile saline solution. The pain should subside within a few hours. If it does not, the patient should consult a lens care specialist. If the patient has any doubt as to whether the peroxide was neutralized, the entire disinfecting cycle should be started over again to avoid the risk of inserting a peroxide-soaked lens without a neutralizing step.

Another potential problem for patients using hydrogen peroxide systems is soaking the lenses in the peroxide solution for longer than the manufacturer recommends. This is not a good practice because it may take longer to neutralize the peroxide.

One new product, UltraCare®, avoids the risk of peroxide burns in a convenient process. The neutralizing tablet is a delayed-release tablet that the user adds at the beginning of the disinfecting cycle. Disinfection and neutralization occur without any additional steps.

Household hydrogen peroxide solutions should not be used to disinfect soft lenses because contaminants and other chemicals within such solutions may discolor the lenses. Also, the pH of topical hydrogen peroxide may be too low for use with contact lenses.[35]

Saline Solutions

The hydrophilic soft contact lens must be maintained in a constant state of hydration. Furthermore, the hydrated lens must be isotonic with tears because changes in tonicity can alter the conformation and optical properties of the lens. Isotonic normal saline is the basic solution used for rinsing, thermally disinfecting, and storing soft contact lenses.

Prepared saline is available in either preserved or preservative-free forms. Because thimerosal and chlorhexidine can cause sensitivity reactions or irritation in a great many patients, sorbic acid–preserved products are commonly promoted for sensitive eyes and appear to be acceptable to most wearers. Salines preserved with Polyquad and Dymed are also available for patients who are sensitive to other preservatives.

Several preservative-free salines are also available. Preservative-free buffered saline is available in unit-of-use containers (which should be used and discarded once opened) and in several sizes of multiuse bottles (which must be discarded 14–30 days after opening, depending on the product formulation). Nonpreserved salines are also available as aerosol sprays.

Some nonpreserved saline products contain EDTA, which prevents deposits of calcium and other divalent ions on the surface of the lens. EDTA, although not a preservative, will inhibit the growth of certain bacteria, thus extending the shelf life of the product. Nonpreserved, nonaerosol saline generally has a shelf life of 15 days once opened. When EDTA is added to the product, that shelf life may be extended to 30 days.

Patients should avoid using other forms of saline such as intravenous normal saline or saline "squirts" because these products are usually too acidic for use with soft contact lenses.

Some persons prepare their own preservative-free saline using salt tablets and USP purified water. The use of salt tablets is inexpensive, but the clear superiority of commercial salines argues strongly against it. The use of homemade saline from salt tablets and the application of improper lens care are the greatest predisposing factors to acanthamoeba keratitis, a rare but vision-threatening eye disease, and to many anterior eye infections contracted by hydrophilic lens wearers.[36] The FDA no longer condones the use of salt tablets, and neither should a concerned pharmacist.

Acanthamoeba, of which there are 15 species, is an opportunistic protozoan. Usually nonpathogenic, *Acanthamoeba* has been isolated from airborne dust, soils, surface water, tap water, and even distilled water. In unfavorable environments, it forms a very resistant cyst that can survive many antimicrobial agents, even though its vegetative form (trophozoite) may be susceptible. Viable cysts have been found in swimming pools and hot tubs that are adequately chlorinated to kill trophozoites.

Most victims of acanthamoeba keratitis have used nonsterile saline solution made from salt tablets and distilled water or have used tap water in the maintenance of their soft contact lenses. Because they are very resistant, *Acanthamoeba* cysts often can survive attempts to eradicate them antimicrobially from the eye. Multiple antibiotic regimens have been applied with variable or poor therapeutic response. Many cases of acanthamoeba keratitis are severe enough to require keratoplasty, a partial or complete cornea transplant, in an attempt to save the eye. Unfortunately, the persistent presence of cysts gives this eye infection a poor prognosis which, in many cases, ultimately leads to enucleation—the partial or total removal of the affected eye. As a diagnosis of the keratitis has become more definitive and awareness of the disease has become more acute, the apparent incidence of acanthamoeba keratitis has risen from 11 cases reported between 1973 and 1983, to 24 cases between mid-1985 and February 1986. More than 200 cases were diagnosed through the first quarter of 1989.

Rewetting Products

Accessory solutions for use with soft lenses permit lubricating and rewetting (and, in some cases, cleaning) of the lens in the eye. These solutions typically contain a low concentration of a nonionic surfactant to promote cleaning and a polymer to lubricate the lens surface, along with buffering agents. These solutions are particularly useful to patients with highly hydrated lenses, such as the extended-wear type. Exposure of lenses to wind and high temperature causes some dehydration, even of the lens in the eye. The resulting discomfort can sometimes be relieved by one or two drops of rewetting solution. To minimize contaminations, the tip of the applicator bottle should not touch the eye, eyelid, or any other surface. The pharmacist should be aware of the preservative content of these products. Some are available without thimerosal and may be less sensitizing to patients with preservative allergies.

Product Selection Guidelines

Many problems associated with soft lens wear arise from the way people handle their lenses. Unsatisfactory results with soft lens products may stem from improper procedures rather than from inadequate products.[37] In one investigation, only 26% of contact lens wearers fully complied with care instructions. Noncompliance was directly correlated to the occurrence of signs and symptoms of potential wearing problems. Specific questions about the care and maintenance regimen used by a wearer can often bring these problems to light.

Surface-Active Cleaners Some surface-active cleaners have a lower viscosity and may be easier to rinse off the lens (e.g., Bausch & Lomb Sensitive Eyes Daily Cleaner®). These products are good choices for patients who have difficulty completely rinsing the cleaner off their lens.

In addition to surfactants, some products (e.g., Opti-Clean II®) contain mild abrasives, which aid in the removal of lens deposits. Patients who have difficulty removing deposits from their lenses will benefit from this type of cleaner. These products should be shaken before use. Some patients may have difficulty in rinsing these cleaners off their lens. Care should be taken to be sure that no residue from the cleaning solution remains on the lens prior to insertion.

Finally, one surfactant cleaner (i.e., Miraflow®) contains isopropyl alcohol. This product is useful for patients who discover heavy lipid deposits on their lenses.

Enzymatic Cleaners Enzymatic cleaners can be recommended based on the disinfecting system the patient uses. If the patient uses thermal disinfection, ReNu Thermal® is a good choice because it eliminates the need to perform the enzymatic cleaning and disinfecting step separately. An exception to this is a patient who wears crofilcon A soft lenses (e.g., CSI®, CSI-T®, or AZTECH®); the plastic in these lenses has been found to stiffen when used with ReNu Thermal® enzymatic cleaner. If the patient uses a hydrogen peroxide cleaning system, Ultrazyme® is a good choice. This product can be placed in the peroxide solution, thus cleaning and disinfecting at the same time. If the patient uses a chemical disinfecting system, the comparisons between products become very idiosyncratic unless the patient has an allergy to one of the components.

In some cases, manufacturers market the same enzymatic tablet under different trade names. For example, Allergan markets its line of papain products under three different trade names: Allergan Enzymatic®, Extenzyme®, and Pro-free/GP®. These three products are marketed for soft contact lenses, extended-wear soft contact lenses, and RGP lenses, respectively. Pharmacists should be aware that these three products are essentially the same and can be interchanged.

Disinfecting Methods When counseling a patient about the best disinfecting method to use, the pharmacist should ask what type of lenses the patient wears. If the patient wears low-water lenses, heat disinfection is best because it is the only method that eradicates *Acanthamoeba*. If a patient wears high-water lenses or is not sure what type of lenses he or she has, a hydrogen peroxide system or a second-generation chemical system (i.e., Opti-free® or ReNu®) can be recommended.

Soft lens wearers may freely switch from thermal to chemical disinfecting methods, but the switch from chemical to thermal may present problems. If lenses that have been chemically disinfected are not completely free from all traces of the chemicals, they can be damaged by heating. Prolonged soaking in several changes of saline is recommended to clean the lenses before using a heating unit.

Insertion of Soft Lenses

When inserting soft lenses, the wearer should carefully follow these steps:

- Wash the hands with noncosmetic soap and rinse thoroughly; dry the hands with a lint-free towel.
- Remove the lens for the right eye from its storage container. Rinse it with saline solution to dilute any preservatives left from disinfection.
- Place the lens on the top of a finger and examine it to be sure it is not inside out. This can be done by using the "taco test." Gently fold the lens at the apex (not the edges) between the thumb and forefinger. The edges should look like a taco shell with the edges pointed inward. If the edges roll out, the lens is inverted and must be reversed.
- Examine the lens for cleanliness. If necessary, clean it and rinse again with saline.
- Insert the lens on the right eye.
- Repeat the process for the left eye.

Formulation Considerations for Soft Lens Products

Several incompatibilities may occur when mixing soft lens products. Most manufacturers test for compatibility within their own product lines; however, compatibility with other manufacturers' products is usually not determined. Generally, cold disinfecting solutions should not be interchanged or used concurrently. If a patient mixes a disinfecting solution containing chlorhexidine and thimerosal (i.e., Flexcare®) with a product containing a quaternary ammonium compound (i.e., Allergan Hydrocare®), a toxic keratopathy known as mixed solution syndrome may occur. Patients should be counseled not to switch from a chemical disinfecting system containing chlorhexidine to a hydrogen peroxide system unless they procure new lenses. A fine black precipitate may form on the lenses if chlorhexidine is still present in the lens matrix. Other chemical disinfecting system residue on soft lenses may cause the lens to turn pink, yellow, brown, black, or purple if the lens is exposed to a hydrogen peroxide system. Barnes Hind Daily Cleaner® should not be mixed with a cleaner containing poloxamer 407 (i.e., Mirasoft®) because cloudy precipitates may form on the lens.[24]

Patient Assessment and Counseling

Although contact lenses are usually safe, lens wearers can experience a variety of problems. Most lens care–related problems are minor and can be easily solved by the knowledgeable pharmacist. Others require ocular inspection and should be referred to the prescriber. A few problems are serious and may be vision threatening. In these cases, the pharmacist must certainly refer the patient to an appropriate specialist.

The Contact Lens Case

As important as lens care is the proper care and cleaning of the contact lens storage case. A storage case should be able to hold at least 2.5 mL of the storage solution.[38] This minimizes the chance that the soaking solution will be overwhelmed by an inoculum of bacteria. The lens case should be cleaned thoroughly or replaced regularly. This entails air drying the case between periods of use and scrubbing it weekly. Some manufacturers recommend cleaning the case twice weekly using a few drops of lens cleaner and hot water.[39] If the case can withstand boiling (such as those made of polycarbonate or noryl plastic), it can be boiled in a pot of water for 10 minutes weekly.[40] It should be examined for cracks and replaced periodically. Lens cases can attract a biofilm that will attract pathogens. This may cause infections.

All Lens Wearers

Pharmacists should ask all patients wearing contact lenses the questions at the beginning of this chapter. The answers to these basic questions will give the pharmacist a sense of the urgency and a general sense of the etiology of the problem, and will help the pharmacist determine whether the problem is related to noncompliance with care regimens or to drug–lens interactions. The pharmacist should then ask specific questions related to the type of lens the patient is currently wearing. Only then can the pharmacist give appropriate counseling information.

The following are general instructions the pharmacist can give patients for successful contact lens wear.

- The hands should be washed with noncosmetic soap and thoroughly rinsed before contact lenses are touched.
- Oily cosmetics should be avoided while lenses are being worn. Bath oils or soaps with a bath oil or cream base may leave an oil film on the hands that will be transferred to the lenses.
- When lenses are being handled over a sink, the drain should be covered or closed to prevent loss of a lens.
- If the lenses are not comfortable after insertion or if vision is blurred, the patient should check to be sure that they are not on the wrong eye or on inside out.
- Lenses should be checked to be sure that they are not scratched, chipped, or torn; that there are no foreign particles on them; and that they are clean and thoroughly rinsed of cleaner. Lens warpage and discoloration may also cause discomfort.
- Contact lenses are individually fitted to correct the refractive error of each eye. To avoid mixing up the lenses, it is helpful always to work with the same lens first. Hard lenses may be marked or etched with a dot in the periphery to avoid confusion.
- Aerosol cosmetics damage the lens and should be applied either before lens insertion or with eyes closed until the air is clear of spray particles.
- Lenses should not be inserted in red or irritated eyes. If the eyes become irritated while lenses are being worn, the lenses should be removed until irritation subsides. Should irritation or redness not subside, a lens practitioner should be consulted.
- Except for extended-wear lenses, contact lenses must not be worn while sleeping.
- Lenses should not be worn while sitting under a hair dryer if excessive dryness of the eyes results. The same caution applies to overhead fans or air ducts.

- When cleaning the lens, the wearer should rub it in a back-and-forth rather than a circular direction.
- The eyes should be protected when lenses are worn outside on windy days because soot and other particles may become trapped under the lens and scratch the cornea.
- Contact lenses do not preclude the use of eye protection in industry, sports, or any other occupation or hobby that has the potential for eye damage.
- Contact lens solutions should never be reused.
- Contact lenses should always be stored in a proper lens case when not in use.
- Soaking solutions in lens cases should be replaced after each use. Lenses must never be stored in tap water.
- Contact lenses should be cleaned only with agents specifically made for that purpose.
- Each type of lens should be cared for only with commercially manufactured products made specifically for that type of lens.
- Contact lens care products from different manufacturers may not be chemically compatible with each other and should not be mixed unless they are identified as compatible by a lens care specialist.
- Care products should be discarded if the labeled expiration date has passed.
- Contact lenses should generally not be worn in swimming pools, hot tubs, ocean waters, or other natural bodies of water unless there is external eye protection such as goggles.
- To prevent contamination, dropper tips or the tips of lens care product containers should not be touched.
- Contact lenses and contact lens care products should be kept out of the reach of children.
- Saliva should never be used to wet contact lenses. This practice can result in eye infections.
- If an eye infection is suspected, medical attention should be sought immediately.
- Only ophthalmic solutions specifically formulated for contact lens use should be used in the eye while wearing lenses.
- All instructions for care should be carefully followed.

Hard Lens Wearers

Pharmacists should ask hard lens wearers the following additional questions:

- Do you soak your lenses when they are not in use? Lenses should not be stored dry.
- How often do you clean your lenses? Patients should clean their lenses every time they remove them from their eyes.
- What lens care products do you use? Do you use a combination-type solution, which may not provide optimal lens care?
- Do you inspect your lenses regularly for chips and scratches?

The following special instructions will help ensure successful hard contact lens wear.

- The eyes should not be rubbed while lenses are in place.
- Contact lenses should not be rinsed with very hot or very cold water because temperature extremes may warp the lenses.
- Lenses should be cleaned before storage.
- Wearers should not get oils or lanolin on the lens.

Rigid Gas-Permeable (RGP) Lens Wearers

Pharmacists should ask RGP lens wearers the following additional questions:

- What brand of RGP lenses do you wear?
- Do you routinely use enzymatic cleaners? How often? How do you dilute the enzymatic tablet?
- Do you clean your lenses immediately upon removal from the eye?
- Do you routinely use a soaking/conditioning solution formulated for your type of RGP lenses?

The following special instructions will help ensure successful RGP lens wear:

- Patients should be sure to apply cleaner to and clean both sides of the lens.
- When cleaning the lens, patients should not apply too much pressure.
- If tap water is used to rinse the cleaner off the lens (not recommended), the lens must be disinfected before being placed in the eye.[41]
- Heat disinfection should not be used with RGP lenses.

Soft Lens Wearers

Pharmacists should ask soft lens wearers the following additional questions:

- What type of soft lenses do you wear (i.e., brand, high-water or low-water content, ionic or nonionic)?
- Do you clean your lenses before disinfection?
- What method of disinfection do you use?
- How often do you disinfect your lenses?
- Do you use commercial saline solutions or do you mix your own? How often do you replace your solution?
- Do you use any cosmetics that are applied to the eye area? How do you apply these products?
- Do you routinely use enzymatic cleaners? How often? How do you dilute the enzymatic tablet?
- Are your lenses extended-wear lenses? How long do you wear them?

The following special instructions will help ensure successful soft contact lens wear:

- Soft contact lenses must be thoroughly cleaned before chemical or especially thermal disinfection.
- Chemical disinfectants must be completely rinsed off before the lens is placed in the eye.
- Hydrogen peroxide disinfectants must be completely neutralized before the lens is placed in the eye.
- Enzyme cleaner tablets should be discarded if any discoloration has appeared.
- Soft lenses must be handled with care because they are very fragile and can easily be torn.
- Soft contact lenses should be removed before instillation of any ophthalmic preparation that is not specifically intended for concurrent use with soft contact lenses. The wearer should wait at least 20–30 minutes before reinserting the lenses unless directed otherwise

by an eye care specialist. Lenses should not be worn at all when a topical ophthalmic ointment is being used.
- Soft contact lenses should not be worn in the presence of irritating fumes or chemicals.
- Extended-wear soft lenses should not be worn continuously for more than 7 days without complete cleaning and disinfection.
- Disposable soft contact lenses should be used strictly in accordance with manufacturer's guidelines and under supervision of a lens specialist.

Extended-Wear Lens Wearers

Extended-wear lenses can be either RGP or soft. The following instructions should be given to patients wearing extended-wear lenses:[13]

- Each morning, look carefully at your eyes. Is there unusual, persistent redness? (Some redness is normal upon wakening; it should abate within 45 minutes.) Is there any unusual discharge? Pain? If any of the above are present, remove the lens and call your lens care practitioner.
- Can you see well with your lenses? (Some hazy vision is normal upon awakening because of corneal hypoxia, which develop overnight.) Application of a few drops of rewetting agent may improve the hydration of the lens and help resolve the hypoxia. If it does not, remove the lenses, clean them, and reinsert. If your vision still has not improved within an hour, remove your lenses and call your lens care practitioner.
- If your lenses appear to be lost upon awakening, check your eyes to see if the lenses were displaced. Soft lenses can fold over on themselves and get lodged underneath the top or bottom eyelid.

References

1. MacKeen DL. Contact lens solutions. *Am Pharm* 1986 Oct; NS26: 691–6.
2. Feldman GL. Contact lens materials. *Int Ophthalmol Clin* 1981 Summer; 21 (2): 155–62.
3. Holden BA, Mertz GW. Critical oxygen levels to avoid corneal edema for daily and extended wear contact lenses. *Invest Ophthalmol Vis Sci* 1984; 25: 1161–7.
4. Hayworth NA, Asbell PA. Therapeutic contact lenses. *CLAO J* 1990 Apr; 16 (2): 137–42.
5. Yamaguchi T, Hubbard A, Fukushima A, et al. Fungus growth on soft contact lenses with different water contents. *CLAO J* 1984; 10: 166–71.
6. Lembach RG. Rigid gas permeable contact lenses. *CLAO J* 1990 Apr; 16 (2): 129–34.
7. Callender MG. Contact lenses and care systems. *Pharm Pract* 1990 Mar; 6 (2): 26–45.
8. Weinstock FJ, Zucker JL. Extended-wear cosmetic contact lenses. *Int Ophthalmol Clin* 1991 Spring; 31 (2): 25–33.
9. Schein OD, Glynn RJ, Poggio EC, et al. The relative risk of ulcerative keratitis among users of daily-wear and extended wear soft contact lenses. *N Engl J Med* 1989 Sep 21; 321 (12): 773–8.
10. Kershner RM. Infectious corneal ulcerations with over-extended wear of disposable contact lenses. *JAMA* 1989 Jun 23-30; 261 (24): 3549–50.
11. Krezanoski JZ. Topical medications. *Int Ophthalmol Clin* 1981 Summer; 21 (2): 173–6.
12. Lembach RG. Keratoconus. *Int Ophthalmol Clin* 1991 Spring; 31 (2): 71–82.
13. Freeman MI. Patient selection. *Int Ophthalmol Clin* 1991 Spring; 31 (2): 1–12.
14. Kastl PR. Is the quality of vision with contact lenses adequate? Not in all instances. *Cornea* 1990; 9 (suppl 1): S20–2.
15. Pepose JS. Contact lens disinfection to prevent transmission of viral disease. *CLAO J* 1988 Jul; 14 (3): 165–8.
16. Plotnik RD, Mannis MJ, Schwab IR. Therapeutic contact lenses. *Int Ophthalmol Clin* 1991 Spring; 31 (2): 35–52.
17. Diamond SA, Dupuis LL. Contact lens damage due to ribavirin exposure. *DICP, Ann Pharmacother* 1989 May; 23: 428–9.
18. Rodriguez WJ, Dang BR, Connor JD, et al. Environmental exposure of primary care personnel to ribavirin aerosol when supervising treatment of infants with respiratory syncytial virus infections. *Antimicrob Agents Chemother* 1987 Jul; 31: 1143–6.
19. Broich J, Weiss L, Rapp J. Isolation and identification of biologically active contaminants from soft contact lenses. *Invest Ophthalmol Vis Sci* 1980; 19: 1328–35.
20. Miller D. Systemic medications. *Int Ophthalmol Clin* 1981 Summer; 21 (2): 177–83.
21. Koetting RA. Cosmetics. *Int Ophthalmol Clin* 1981 Summer; 21 (2): 185–93.
22. Mandell RB, Respicio SG. Efficacy of contaminant removal by RGP lens cleaners. *Contact Lens Spectrum* 1988 Jun; 3 (6): 57–60.
23. White PF, Miller D. Corneal edema. *Int Ophthalmol Clin* 1981 Summer; 21 (2): 3–12.
24. Rakow PL. Mixing contact lens solutions. *J Ophthalmic Nurs Technol* 1989; 8 (2): 67–8.
25. Eriksen S, Dabezies OH. Preservatives. In: Dabezies OH, ed. *Contact Lenses, The CLAO Guide to Basic Science and Clinical Practice*. 2nd ed. Boston: Little, Brown; 1992: 28.1–.8.
26. Lowther G, Shannon BJ, Weisbarth R, eds. Contact lens care products and their use. In: *The Pharmacist's Guide to Contact Lenses and Lens Care*. Atlanta: CIBA Vision; 1988: 27–36.
27. Tripathi RC, Tripathi BJ. Lens spoilage. In: Dabezies OH, ed. *Contact Lenses, The CLAO Guide to Basic Science and Clinical Practice*. 2nd ed. Boston: Little, Brown; 1992: 45.1–.33.
28. Diefenbach CB, Seibert CK, Davis LJ. Analysis of two "home remedy" contact lens cleaners. *J Am Optom Assoc* 1988; 59 (7): 518–21.
29. Butrus SI, Abelson MB. Contact lenses and the allergic patient. *Int Ophthalmol Clin* 1986 Spring; 26 (1): 73–81.
30. Terry R, Schnider C, Holden BA. Rigid gas permeable lenses and patient management. *CLAO J* 1989 Oct; 14 (4): 305–9.
31. Mobley CL. Letter. *Contact Lens Forum* 1989 Apr; 14 (suppl 4): 13–14.
32. Stenson S. Soft contact lens deposits. *JAMA* 1987 May 22/29; 257 (20): 2823.
33. Tripathi BJ, Tripathi RC, Rhee JM. Adherence of bacteria to soft contact lenses. In: Dabezies OH, ed. *Contact Lenses, The CLAO Guide to Basic Science and Clinical Practice*. 2nd ed. Boston: Little, Brown; 1992: 42.1–.17.
34. Morgan JP. Problems associated with current care systems for contact lenses. Paper presented at Las Vegas: CLAO annual meeting; January 1990.
35. Harris MG. Practical considerations in the use of hydrogen peroxide disinfection systems. *CLAO J* 1990 Jan; 16 (suppl 1): S53–60.
36. Fiscella RG. New eye infection: difficult to detect, easier to prevent. *US Pharm* 1989 Apr; 14: 75–81.
37. Lowther G, Shannon BJ, Weisbarth R, eds. The importance of compliance. In: *The Pharmacist's Guide to Contact Lenses and Lens Care*. Atlanta: CIBA Vision; 1988: 23–5.

38. Krezanoski JZ, Dabezies OH. Hard lens hygiene. In: Dabezies OH, ed. *Contact Lenses, The CLAO Guide to Basic Science and Clinical Practice*. 2nd ed. Boston: Little, Brown; 1992: 31.1–.7.
39. Boston Equalens Patient Care Guide. Polymer Technology Corporation; 1987.
40. Callender MG. Contact lens care systems. Part 1. Hard and gas permeable lenses. *Pharm Pract* 1990 Mar; 6 (2): 26–31.
41. Campbell RC, Caroline PJ. RGPs and tap water. *Contact Lens Forum* 1990 Jul; 15: 64.

CHAPTER 22

Otic Products

Keith O. Miller

Questions to ask in patient assessment and counseling

Earache

- *Do you have an earache? How long have you had it?*
- *Is the pain sharp and localized or dull and generalized?*
- *Is the pain constant or made worse by pulling on the ears or chewing?*
- *Do you have or have you recently had a cold or the flu?*
- *Do you have a fever?*
- *Have you been swimming during the past few days?*
- *Have you attempted to clear your ears recently to remove earwax? If so, what method did you use?*
- *Are your ear canals dry and flaky or wet and sticky?*
- *Have you had similar symptoms in the past?*
- *What, if anything, have you already done to treat your earache?*
- *Do you wear dentures or have any dental problems?*
- *What is your occupation?*

Hearing Loss

- *When did you notice that your hearing is not as good as it used to be?*
- *Do you have a cold or the flu?*
- *Have you been swimming during the past few days?*
- *Are your eardrums damaged from a prior illness or injury?*
- *Have you been traveling in an airplane recently or been in any places where the air pressure has changed suddenly (e.g., fast elevators)?*
- *Does anyone else in your family have a hearing loss?*
- *Do any of your relatives wear a hearing aid?*
- *Would you be interested in taking a 5-minute hearing test for your own information only?*
- *Are you taking any prescription medications, even for other medical problems?*

- *Have you been hospitalized recently? If so, why?*

Tinnitus

- *Are the abnormal sounds you are sensing continuous or intermittent?*
- *Are you taking aspirin or any prescription or nonprescription medications? If so, what doses are you consuming?*

Discharge

- *Could you describe the appearance and the amount of discharge from your ear(s)?*
- *Was your ear itchy before the discharge appeared?*
- *Did you have any ear pain after the discharge appeared? Before the discharge started?*
- *Have you taken aspirin or pain-relieving eardrops, or have you tried to rinse out the ear?*
- *Do you have diabetes or any other medical condition?*
- *Do you have a problem with dandruff?*

Disorders of the ear are very common and usually cause discomfort. Patients often complain of earache, impacted ear, running ear, cold in the ear, itching in the ear, or a combination of these symptoms. Ear disorders may be caused by a disease of the auricle (most external portion of the ear), external ear canal (external auditory meatus), or middle ear, or by a disease in another area of the head and neck. A traumatic or pathologic condition of the tongue, mandibles, oropharynx, tonsils, or paranasal sinuses may cause referred pain to the ear and may appear to the patient as an earache. These conditions are often caused by an underlying disease process that requires accurate diagnosis and treatment by a physician. In such cases, self-treatment may be unwise.

Home remedies and nonprescription drugs are usually restricted to self-limited disorders that are related only to the external ear. Self-treatment should be reserved for minor conditions. In addition, self-treatment may be used effectively to prevent certain ear disorders, to aid the normal body defenses, and to improve the integrity of the skin that lines the auricle and external auditory canal.

Before recommending any nonprescription product to persons with ear disorders, the pharmacist should recognize the symptoms of the various disorders and their corresponding pathophysiology. This information will permit an accurate evaluation of the problem and assist the pharmacist in recommending treatment plans.

Anatomy and Physiology of the Ear

The external ear is composed of the auricle (pinna) and the external auditory canal (Figure 1). The auricle is the external appendage of cartilage (elastic type); it is covered by a thin layer of normal skin that is highly vascularized except for the lobule, which is composed primarily of fatty tissue. The auricle, which is oval, flattened, and irregular, is considered an extension of the cartilaginous ear canal. The cartilaginous projection anterior to the external opening of the ear (not shown in Figure 1) is called the tragus. A thin tissue layer called the perichondrium covers both the cartilaginous auricle and the outer cartilaginous half of the external auditory canal.[1] The periosteum, a specialized connective tissue, covers the inner bony half of the external auditory canal.[1] The skin covering the ear is thinner than skin elsewhere in the body because it lacks a protective layer of fat. The absence of this subcutaneous tissue makes this auricular skin subject to frostbite despite a rich supply of superficial blood vessels.[1,2]

The external auditory canal is tubular, forming a channel that permits sound waves to pass to the tympanic membrane (eardrum) and that protects the tympanic membrane from injury. In adults, the external auditory canal is typically 20–25 mm long.[2,3] Both the auricle and the external auditory canal show much individual variation in size and shape. The ear canal is the only epidermal-lined cul-de-sac in the body.

Excess water and fluids in the external auditory canal may cause a feeling of fullness in the ear. Fluid can be removed by having the patient tilt the head to one side with the affected ear down. This position allows the excess fluid to drain out of the ear by gravity. To permit direct visual examination of the tympanic membrane, it may be necessary to straighten the canal by applying traction to the auricle in an upward and backward direction.

The auricular skin is continuous and lines the entire ear canal and the outer covering of the tympanic membrane.[1] The skin covering the cartilaginous portion of the canal, which is thicker than the skin covering the bony portion, contains hair follicles, large sebaceous glands that open either to the skin surface or into the hair follicle lumen, and ceruminous glands.[3] There are 1,000–2,000 ceruminous glands in the average ear, although older individuals may have fewer.[3] Hair appears to serve a protective function, with its ability to trap foreign bodies in a waxy network. No hair follicles or glands (sebaceous and ceruminous) are found in the bony inner half of the external auditory canal.

Cerumen (earwax) is derived from the watery secretions of the apocrine glands (which mature and become functional at puberty) and the oily secretions of the sebaceous glands.[1] Collectively, these glands are referred to as ceruminous glands. The colorless, watery, fluid secretion is composed of polypeptides, lipids, fatty acids, amino acids, and electrolytes.[3,4] Cerumen turns brown when it mixes with desquamated epithelial cells and dust particles. The cerumen lubricates the skin and traps foreign material entering the external auditory canal, thus providing a protective barrier.[2,5] Semisolid cerumen is expelled unnoticed by epithelial migration. This migration involves movement

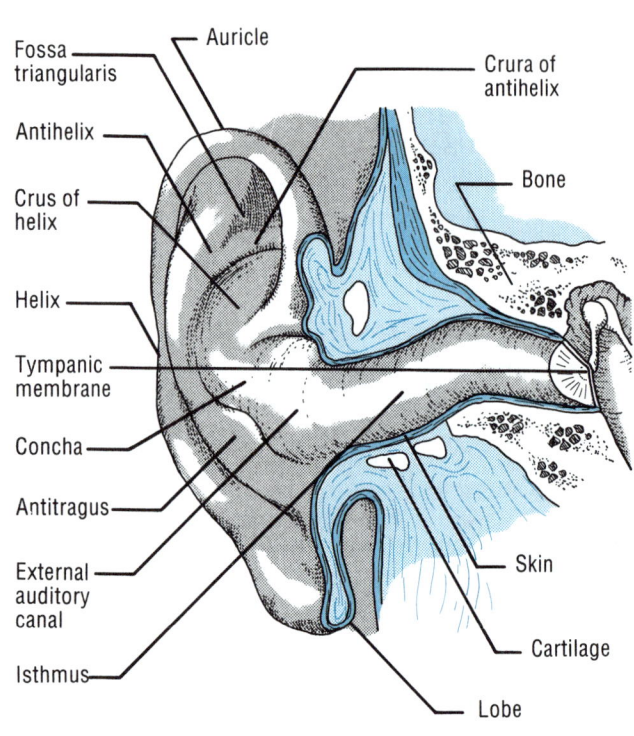

FIGURE 1 Anatomy of the auricle and external ear.

of epithelial cells across the surface of the tympanic membrane and the epithelial lining of the external auditory canal to the outside during the processes of chewing and talking.[2,6] The skin of the normal external auditory canal is water-resistant with a pH between 5.0 and 7.2, which helps prevent pathologic bacterial growth.[1,6,7]

The tympanic membrane is pearly gray, egg shaped, semitransparent, and about 0.1 mm thick and 8 to 9 mm wide.[3] The outer epithelial layer is continuous with the epidermis of the external auditory canal; the middle layer is tough, fibrous tissue; and the innermost layer is a mucous membrane continuous with the tympanic cavity lining.[6] In adults, the membrane forms approximately a 45° angle with the external canal floor; it is almost horizontal in infants.[3] It protects the middle ear from foreign material and also functions in transmitting airborne sound waves into the middle ear. Anatomically, the tympanic membrane is part of the external auditory canal (Figure 1); functionally, however, it is considered part of the middle ear (tympanic cavity).[3]

Etiology of Ear Conditions

Hairs in the outer half of the canal, the size of the ear canal and its isthmus, and cerumen act as natural defensive barriers of the normal ear canal, collectively preventing the introduction of foreign material that may cause

TABLE 1 Symptoms of selected otic disorders

	Boil	Otomycosis	Bacterial external otitis	Nonsuppurative otitis media	Impacted cerumen	Suppurative otitis media
Pain[a]	Often	Possibly	Often	Rarely	Rarely	Usually
Hearing deficit	Rarely	Possibly	Possibly	Possibly	Often	Usually
Purulent discharge	Rarely	Rarely	Often	Rarely	Rarely	Occasionally and indicative of perforation
Bilateral symptoms	Rarely	Rarely	Possibly	Often	Rarely	Occasionally
Appropriateness of self-medication	Auricle only	Never	Never	Never	Never	Never

[a] Pain is increased with chewing, traction on the auricle, and pressure on the tragus except in otitis media, where pain may be knifelike and steady.

---

injury or infection. The integrity of the skin layers and the acid pH of the canal also provide natural protection against infection.

Predisposing factors often lead to the breakdown of these natural defense barriers. An inherited narrowed ear canal, a malformation of the mandible, or excess hair growth in the canal may impair the normal cleansing process and decrease the efficiency of epithelial migration. In addition, hyperactive ceruminous glands may cause excessive wax to accumulate and become impacted. African Americans tend to have shorter and straighter ear canals, and thus they develop external otitis less often than non-African Americans.[8]

Certain conditions and activities contribute to the breakdown of natural defensive barriers of the normal ear canal. Intensely warm, humid climates, along with sweating and exposure to water (swimming and bathing during the summer months), have been implicated. The increased exposure to moisture may result in tissue maceration that breaks down the protective barrier of the skin and alters skin pH. These factors collectively predispose the ear canal to infection.[1,7] A positive correlation exists between the amount of water exposure in the ear canal and the incidence of external otitis.[8]

Ear disorders may also be due to various trauma-induced causes. Improperly cleaned or poorly fitted earplugs may cause trauma or maceration of the skin in the ear canal. Poorly fitted hearing aids or ear molds of hearing aids may be another source of trauma-induced injury.[7]

The removal of cerumen or the lack of natural protection provided by its presence may increase the predisposition for bacterial or fungal infection in the ear canal. Using an instrument, a cotton-tipped applicator, or other device to clean ears is likely to push the earwax deeper into the ear canal, causing it to become tightly impacted, increasing the difficulty of subsequent removal. This cleaning process also often causes trauma to the skin covering the ear canal, further predisposing the ear to infection. And because the normal healthy ear cleans itself, thus negating the need for cleaning with mechanical devices or instruments, mechanical cleaning of the ear decreases the ear's natural cleaning process.

After the protective layer of the skin of the ear canal has been compromised, a preinflammatory stage occurs in which the patient tends to scratch the ear involuntarily or rub the auricle in response to an itch.[9] These actions further abrade the skin, causing deep fissures in the epidermis of the cartilaginous portion of the ear canal. An inflammatory reaction follows this fissure formation, as evidenced by edema, pain, swelling, and redness of the affected area. This large area thus becomes a good culture site for bacteria or fungi, making subsequent infection likely.

Neurodermatitis is a condition that is presumably caused by chronic rubbing, scratching, or cleaning the ear in response to a vague itch or feeling of fullness that sometimes occurs. The itch sensation may also be characteristic of superficial fungal infection, contact dermatitis, or eczema.[1,10] Some individuals produce a scant amount of cerumen and may be subject to itching, maceration, and subsequent infection.[6]

Common Problems of the Ear

Many disorders of the external ear are minor and easily resolved. However, the pharmacist should keep in mind that pain associated with even minor disorders can be significant. Some untreated ear problems can result in hearing loss. The pharmacist can assist the patient by helping to evaluate and differentiate symptoms (Table 1), by discussing the proper course of action (self-treatment or referral to a physician), and by recommending an efficacious nonprescription product, if appropriate.

Disorders of the Auricle

Disorders associated with the auricle, the external part of the ear not within the head, are generally minor and

TABLE 2 Interpretation of physical findings associated with disorders of the external ear

Physical findings	Probable appearance	Physiologic basis	Example
Enlarged lymph node	Swollen, tender to touch, pre- and postauricular	Inflammation of lymph node; spread of infection outside the ear	Mastoiditis, otitis media
Tophus	Hard, pale node on helix, chalklike dust upon rupture	Urate crystals	Gout
Sebaceous cyst	Swollen, erythematous postauricle lesion in the skin of the ear	Inflammation of sweat gland	Skin infection
Cerumen	Red-orange pastelike discharge	Normal secretion of wax	Normal finding
Blood	Red-blue discharge	Ruptured blood vessel	External otitis
Serous fluid	Clear discharge	Blocked eustachian tube	Chronic (purulent) otitis media
Pus	Yellowish discharge	Acute inflammation	Acute suppurative otitis media

Adapted with permission from Longe RL, Calvert JC. *Drug Intell Clin Pharm* 1977; 11: 660.

involve lacerations, boils, and dermatitis. These conditions are also generally self-limiting. Table 2 provides examples of some common physical findings related to disorders of the external ear.

Trauma

Lacerations, including scrapes and cuts and involving only the skin of the auricle, usually heal spontaneously. Wounds that do not heal normally should be checked by a physician, as should deep wounds that may involve injury to the cartilage. Injury to the auricle that does not perforate the subperichondrium may cause subcutaneous bleeding and produce a hematoma. A hematoma may require aspiration or incision by a physician because it may obliterate normal auricular contours and often results in inflammation and perichondritis (cauliflower ear). The swelling can also cause local pruritus and pain upon touch.

Boils

Boils (furuncles) are usually localized infections of the hair follicles. In a high percentage of cases in young adults, no specific causative or predisposing factor can be established. Poor body hygiene may contribute to the development of boils. The etiologic organism of a boil is usually *Staphylococcus aureus*.[2,9]

A boil often involves the anterior external auditory canal. It usually begins as a red papule and develops into a round or conical superficial pustule with a core of pus and erythema around the base. The lesion gradually enlarges, becomes firm, and then generally softens and opens within 2 weeks, discharging the purulent contents. Because the skin is very taut, even minimal swelling may cause severe pain.

Boils are usually self-limiting; however, they may be severe, autoinoculable, and multiple. Deeper lesions may lead to perichondritis.

Small boils may be treated by good hygiene combined with topical compresses. Hot compresses of saline solution may be applied to the auricle and the side of the face. Boils that do not respond rapidly to topical therapy should be examined by a physician. In addition, patients with recurring boils should be referred to a physician for evaluation and possible systemic antibiotic therapy.

Perichondritis

Perichondritis is an inflammation involving the perichondrium (the fibrous connective tissue surrounding the auricular cartilage) usually following a poorly treated or untreated burn, injury, hematoma, or local infection. Its onset is characterized by a sensation of heat and stiffness of the auricle with pronounced pain. As the condition worsens, an exudate forms and the auricle becomes dark red, swollen, and shiny, with uniform thickening caused by edema and inflammation. Although the lesions are usually confined to the cartilaginous tissue of the auricle and external canal, some patients may experience generalized fever and malaise.

Perichondritis often results in severe auricular deformity, and atresia (a pathologic closure) of the external auditory canal may occur. A patient suspected of having perichondritis should be seen by a physician.

Dermatitis of the Ear

Inflammation of the skin may result from an abrasion of the auricle; if untreated, a dermal infection may develop. Inflammatory conditions such as seborrhea, psoriasis, and contact dermatitis (e.g., poison ivy and poison oak) may also affect the skin of the auricle and the external ear canal. Contact dermatitis may be caused by an allergic response to jewelry, cosmetics, detergents, or topical drug applications of antihistamines or antibiotics (dermatitis medicamentosa).[6,11,12] Lesions may spread to the ear canal, neck, and facial areas.[9]

Dry, scaly skin associated with an itchy ear canal suggests the presence of seborrheic dermatitis, especially in the presence of severe dandruff and other signs of seborrhea.[1] Symptoms of dermatitis of the ear usually include itching and local redness followed by vesication, weeping, and erythema. The lesions, which form scales and yellow crusts on the skin,[6,10] may spread to adjacent unaffected areas. Excessive scratching may cause the lesions to become infected. Topical drugs should be used cautiously in treating dermatitis because their potential allergenicity could exacerbate the condition. Because seborrheic dermatitis of the ear is usually associated with dandruff, treatment with dandruff-control shampoos is recommended.[9] Cases that are difficult to control should be referred to a physician.

Itching or Pruritus of the Ear

An itchy ear canal is a common symptom that may mask the preinflammatory stages of acute external otitis. Itching is usually related to dryness but may be a complaint when no abnormalities or lesions actually exist.[7] Abnormal cerumen content may be annoying to the patient and may be associated with dermatologic disorders such as seborrheic dermatitis. Symptoms include scaling, itching, and cracking of the ear canal.[2] For patients with chronic external otitis, itching rather than pain is the chief complaint.[2] In this case, the itching is caused by dry ears that may lack sufficient cerumen. Itching may also be caused by infections, allergic seborrheic dermatitis, eczema of the skin around the ears, psoriasis, contact dermatitis, superficial fungal infection, or neurodermatitis.[1]

Itching commonly begins as an annoying itch-scratch cycle that results in trauma, infection, epidermal barrier destruction, and inflammation of the affected areas following repeated scratching. Ear scratching may be a compulsive nervous habit.[9] Careful observation to determine the cause of itching is often helpful before any attempt is made to provide symptomatic relief.

Aural Drainage

Any patient with a discharge or drainage from the ear should be referred to a physician for proper diagnosis and treatment. The drainage or discharge may be blood, watery fluid (serum), or purulent or mucoid material. Head trauma may cause leakage of cerebrospinal fluid into the ear. Infection of the external ear canal may produce a watery discharge. A ruptured tympanic membrane usually produces a serosanguineous fluid. Any trauma of the ear canal may cause bleeding; and, if infected, the ear may exude a purulent fluid from which the causative organisms may be cultured and appropriate antibiotics chosen.

Self-treatment of ear disorders is inappropriate whenever drainage, pain, or dizziness is present; whenever an infection is suspected; whenever there is known injury in or perforation of the eardrum; or within 6 weeks following otic surgery.[13,14]

Disorders of the External Auditory Canal

Boils

Boils of the external auditory canal are pathologically similar to those of the auricle and external auditory canal. Symptoms include pain at the infected site, which is usually exacerbated by chewing. The ear canal may be partially occluded by swelling, but hearing is impaired only if the opening is completely occluded. Edema and pain over the mastoid bone directly behind the auricle may occur. Traction of the auricle or the tragus is very painful. Patients with boils in the external auditory canal should be referred to a physician because unresolved conditions may lead to more generalized infections.

Otomycosis

Otomycosis, an external fungal infection of the ear, is more common in warmer, tropical, or semitropical climates than in mild, temperate zones. Species of *Aspergillus* and *Candida* are the most common causative agents.[1,9] *Aspergillus niger* forms characteristic grayish membranes along the canal.[1] Antibiotic treatment of a bacterial ear infection, with resultant suppression of normal bacterial flora, and diabetes mellitus may predispose an individual to a fungal external ear infection.

A superficial mycotic infection of the external auditory canal is characterized by pruritus with a feeling of fullness and pressure in the ear. Intense itching is the primary complaint of patients with otomycosis.[2] Pain, if present, may increase with chewing and with traction on the pinna and tragus. The fungus leads to an accumulation of epithelial debris, exudate, and cerumen. In the acute state, the fungal infection may obstruct the external auditory canal, and hearing may be impaired.

Depending on the nature of the fungus, the color of the accumulated mass may vary. The skin that lines the external auditory canal and the tympanic membrane may become beefy-red and scaly. It may be eroded or ulcerated.[3] A scant, colorless mucoid discharge is common.

Otomycosis is particularly serious in diabetic patients because of the microangiopathy and associated cutaneous manifestations common to diabetes mellitus. Mycotic ear infections in diabetic patients should be treated promptly.

Keratosis Obturans

Keratosis obturans is a rare condition with an unclear etiology.[1] Wax accumulates in the deeper parts of the external auditory canal and, with adjacent epithelial cells, leads to an obstruction that exerts pressure on the surrounding tissue. The condition is probably related to faulty migration of squamous epithelial cells from the surface of the tympanic membrane. Pain may be present owing to erosion of the epithelial tissue surrounding the tympanic membrane.[1] The infection may form abscesses in the subcutaneous tissue or mastoid bone.

Pain in the ear and decreased hearing are common symptoms. A discharge and tinnitus may also occur. Mechanical removal of the obstruction is necessary but often difficult and should be performed by a physician, preferably an ear, nose, and throat specialist. Patients should not attempt to remove the obstruction themselves.

Foreign Objects in the Ear

Young children often insert small items into the ear canal; such items include candy, pretzel sticks, pencil erasers, toy stuffing, beans, peas, marbles, pebbles, beads, or metal nuts unscrewed from toys.[15] An object lodged in the ear canal will usually cause a hearing deficiency, pain, or pressure in the ear during chewing. An exudate may form because of secondary bacterial infection. Vegetable seeds, such as dried beans or dried peas, lodged in the external auditory canal swell when moistened during bathing or swimming and become wedged in the bony portion of the canal, causing severe pain. Furthermore, if an obstruction of the external auditory canal is not removed promptly, acute bacterial otitis may result. Insects enter the canal and cause stress by beating their wings and crawling. In such a case, olive oil (sweet oil) drops or mineral oil may be used to suffocate the insect and stop the movement.

Foreign objects lodged in the ear canal may not always cause symptoms and may be found only during a routine physical examination. Mechanical removal should be performed only by a physician because unskilled attempts at removal often damage the skin surrounding the external auditory canal or lodge the objects deeper into the ear canal.

Impacted Cerumen

The accumulation of cerumen in the external auditory canal may be caused by (1) overactive ceruminous glands; (2) a tortuous or small canal or abnormal narrowing of the canal, which may not permit normal migration of the cerumen to the outside; or (3) the secretion of abnormal cerumen, which may be drier or softer than normal cerumen and may interfere with the normal epithelial migration process. Individuals who get water in their ears while swimming or showering sometimes will experience a sudden loss of hearing in one ear. This may be caused by the increased bulk of the earwax or by water trapped behind the wax.[2] Cerumen is often packed deeper into the external auditory canal by repeated attempts to remove it with cotton-tipped devices and other instruments; ordinarily there is no pain unless the ear is secondarily infected.[2] There is usually no cerumen in the inner half of the canal unless it has been pushed there. In elderly persons, cerumen is often admixed with long hairs in the canal, preventing normal expulsion and forming a matted obstruction in the canal.

External Otitis

External otitis (inflammation of the skin lining the external auditory canal, often due to infection) is one of the most common diseases of the ear. It is also very painful and annoying. The external auditory canal is considered a blind cul-de-sac lined with skin. It is dark, warm, and well suited for collecting moisture. Prolonged exposure to moisture tends to disrupt the continuity of the epithelial cells, causing skin maceration and fissures that provide a fertile environment for bacterial growth. Additionally, this prolonged exposure to moisture tends to raise the pH above the normal range of 5–7,[15] which improves the growth environment for bacteria and fungi. Factors contributing to susceptibility to external otitis are race, age, climate, and occupation.[9] The most common causative organisms of external otitis include species of *Pseudomonas, Staphylococcus, Bacillus,* and *Proteus.* Fungi may be the causative organisms in some cases.[9]

There is very little subcutaneous tissue between the skin that is tightly bound to the perichondrium on the cartilaginous portion and the periosteum on the bony portion of the external auditory canal. When there is swelling, the lack of space available for expansion increases skin tension. Thus, the inflammation that causes edema provokes severe pain that is disproportionate to any visible swelling. As the inflammation increases, pain may increase significantly during chewing.

Symptoms often develop following attempts to clean the ear with cotton swabs, hairpins, matchsticks, pencils, fingers, or other objects. Symptoms may also be caused by foreign debris or scratching of the ear to relieve itching. This may traumatize and damage the horny skin layer, forming an opening that allows invasion by microorganisms. Because a normal, healthy, external auditory canal is impervious to potentially pathologic organisms, skin integrity generally must be interrupted before an organism can produce an infection.

Another type of trauma-induced external otitis is called swimmer's ear, or desquamative external otitis.[9] Excessive moisture in the external auditory canal may cause water to accumulate in the tympanic recess, resulting in tissue maceration and possibly predisposing the ear canal to infection. Attempts to clear the canal of water with objects that can abrade or lacerate the skin lining may result in infection. Also, cerumen accumulated in the external auditory canal absorbs water and expands, and the trapped water provides a medium for microbial growth.[3] Within a few hours to 1 day following exposure to excess water, symptoms of itching, pain, and possible draining from the ear with partial occlusion may occur.

Often the patient first complains of an itching feeling in the ear. Then, within a few hours up to 24 hours later, the complaints are followed by a feeling of wetness in the ear canal and discomfort leading to pain. The amount of wetness may vary from minimal to frank otorrhea (discharge). The discharge is usually cream colored or yellow. Any secondary hearing loss may be caused by epithelial debris mixed with a purulent discharge, which thus causes blockage.

A bacterial infection of the external auditory canal leads to inflammation and epidermal destruction of the tympanic membrane. The infection may progress through the fibrous layer of the tympanic membrane, causing perforation of the membrane and spreading the infection into the middle ear; this results in intense pain and discomfort. External otitis caused by bacterial infection, like otomycosis, is particularly difficult to control in individuals who have diabetes.[1,16]

Symptoms of acute external otitis are related to the severity of the pathologic conditions. There is usually mild or moderate pain, which becomes more pronounced by pulling upward on the auricle or pressing on the tragus. A discharge may be present. Hearing loss may occur if the ear canal is obstructed by swelling and edema, debris, or a cerumen plug.

Chronic external otitis is usually caused by the persistence of predisposing factors. The most common symptom

TABLE 3	Physical findings associated with selected conditions of the middle ear	
Physical findings	**Probable appearance**	**Interpretation**
Perforation	Dark, thin, oval discoloration	Rupture of the eardrum
Acute purulent otitis media	Yellowish pus behind eardrum; bulging, hyperemic membrane; light reflex absent	Acute infection of the middle ear
Chronic serous otitis media	Amber-like fluid behind eardrum; observable fluid level with air bubbles; retraction of handle of malleus	Blockage of eustachian tube

Reprinted with permission from Longe RL, Calvert JC. *Drug Intell Clin Pharm* 1977; 11: 661.

is itching, which prompts patients to attempt to scratch the ear canal to reduce or relieve the itching. This scratching can break the skin,[10] thereby allowing the entry of the pathogen(s).

In allergic external otitis and dermatitis of the external auditory canal caused by seborrhea, a common symptom is itching, burning, or stinging of the lesions. Often the complaints seem excessive compared with the visible signs.

Chronic cases and those with symptoms of severe pain, lymphadenopathy, discharge, possible hearing loss, and fever should be referred to a physician.[3] Tender lymph nodes may be felt anterior to the tragus, behind the ear, or in the upper neck just below the pinna. Minor cases of chronic and allergic external otitis, especially swimmer's ear, may be treated adequately with nonprescription drug products. However, all progressive symptoms of disease processes involving the external ear canal or auricle should be treated by a physician.

Malignant external otitis is the most progressive form of otitis. It occurs most often in elderly patients and in patients with chronic lymphocytic leukemia, granulocytopenia, or poorly controlled diabetes mellitus.[17,18] In these patients, the ear becomes inflamed and may involve the temporal bone area. The most common complaints are severe, persistent pain and swelling. Clinical findings include persistent aural drainage, severe tenderness, and swelling in the region of the ear and mastoid bone. The tragus is always tender to touch and the auricle is tender to traction.

Disorders of the Middle Ear

Disorders of the middle ear should not be treated with nonprescription otic products. A brief review of the common conditions involving the middle ear will aid the pharmacist in evaluating symptoms. Although some symptoms of middle ear disorders are the same as those of external ear disorders, others are not (Table 3). All bacterial infections of the middle ear should be promptly evaluated and treated by a physician. The usual treatment is systemic antibiotics therapy.

Otitis Media

Otitis media is an inflammatory condition of the middle ear that occurs most often during childhood. Conditions that interfere with eustachian tube function, such as upper respiratory tract infection, allergy, adenoid lymphadenopathy, and cleft palate, predispose individuals to otitis media.[1] Blockage of the eustachian tube allows oxygen in the middle ear cleft to be absorbed. This produces a relative negative pressure or vacuum that results in a transudation (movement) of fluid into the middle ear cleft. Generally, symptoms of eustachian tube blockage are mild intermittent pain, mild hearing loss, and fullness in the ear. If infection is absent, the color of the tympanic membrane, when retracted, is pearly gray. Inflation of the eustachian tube by Valsalva's maneuver (blowing against pressure) or by swallowing may help send air up the eustachian tube. The tube should not be inflated when the nasopharynx is infected because of the danger of spreading the infection into the middle ear.

Children often experience repeated episodes of eustachian tube obstruction caused by masses of adenoids that become edematous and block the eustachian tube opening, resulting in otitis media. Adenoidectomy usually prevents future occurrence. In adults, recurrent otitis media may be caused by nasopharyngeal tumors.

Chronic middle ear infections are often treated with myringotomy and placement of drainage tubes to relieve the pain and equalize the air pressure.[2] Nose blowing and sneezing against occluded nostrils may worsen the condition and therefore should be avoided.[19,20] If the serous fluid in the middle ear cavity remains sterile, the condition is called serous otitis media and is most often of viral origin; if the fluid is infected by bacteria, the condition is generally called purulent otitis media.

Symptoms of serous otitis media include a sensation of fullness in the ear accompanied by hearing loss.[7,21] The condition worsens as fluid accumulates and fills the middle ear cleft. The sensation of fullness is associated with voice resonance, a congested feeling in the ears, a hollow sound, or a popping or cracking noise in the ears during swallowing or yawning. These symptoms are usually not present in external otitis.

The most common symptoms in the acute phase of purulent otitis media are pain, hearing loss, fever as high as 104°F (40°C), and malaise.[21] As noted by one author, "the strategic location of middle cleft and mastoid cells separated from the sigmoid sinus and meninges by a mere thin shell makes every infection of the middle ear capable of intracranial infection."[1] The severity of symptoms increases as the condition worsens. Pain arises from the pressure of fluids in the middle ear. This causes an outward tension on the tympanic membrane, which is innervated by sensory nerves. The rapid production of fluid and tension in a short period of time is responsible for the acute pain, which is described as sharp, knifelike, and steady. The pain usually does not worsen with mastication or with traction applied to the auricle or tragus. Excessive nose blowing, especially against occluded nostril(s), may force additional purulent mucus into the eustachian tube and worsen the condition.

If patients are not treated promptly, pressure inside the middle ear may increase, leading to distension and bulging of the tympanic membrane. As bulging increases, so does necrosis, leading to perforation of the middle ear and the escape of the purulent material, which may cause a secondary bacterial external otitis infection. The appearance of a discharge is usually accompanied by a lessening of the pain because of the decreased tension on the tympanic membrane. The initial discharge may be blood stained, followed by foul-smelling, purulent, serous fluid.[6] The tympanic membrane usually loses the normal pearlish-gray luster and appears yellow to orange–pink to rusty–purple, representing a spectrum of increasing severity. Nonprescription eardrops or prescription antibiotic drops do not help to resolve acute otitis media while the tympanic membrane is intact. The use of nonprescription otic drugs to treat any form of otitis media is not recommended.

Chronic Otitis Media
In chronic serous otitis media, the fluid in the middle ear may be thin and serous or thick and viscous (glue ear).[6] Chronic serous otitis media occurs most often in small children. It may be caused by inadequate treatment of previous episodes of otitis media or by recurrent upper respiratory tract infections associated with eustachian tube dysfunction.[6]

The most common symptom is impaired hearing, but the onset is insidious. Children may have no acute symptoms,[6] and pain is usually absent. Frequently, parents may note that the child has become inattentive and disobedient. The child's school performance may decline. Diagnosis requires visual inspection of the tympanic membrane, which appears yellow or orange, lusterless, and less flexible. It is not perforated but often appears to be retracted. Often, long-standing fluid becomes more and more viscous, which accounts for the term *glue ear*.

Treatment may involve evacuation of the fluid by aspiration through an incision in the tympanic membrane (myringotomy) and implantation of temporary, pressure-equalizing tubes.[6] This procedure is usually performed bilaterally and is useful in patients who do not have hypertrophied adenoids and for whom an adenoidectomy is not indicated. The tubes allow equalization of pressure between the middle ear space and the atmosphere, thereby compensating for eustachian tube dysfunction.[2] It is common for children under 10 years of age to wear the tubes for 6–12 months. During this time, the tubes are typically extruded spontaneously, and it is generally unnecessary to implant them again.

The tubes are especially helpful during acute or persistent and frequent episodes of eustachian tube obstruction, a common complication of acute serous otitis media. They permit normal atmospheric environmental changes in the middle ear cavity and also allow for changes in air pressure that are independent of the eustachian tube. The mucosal and epithelial linings then return to normal function.

Chronic purulent otitis media is usually secondary to a persistent tympanic membrane perforation. With exacerbation of the condition, the patient may exhibit symptoms of acute purulent otitis media with mucopurulent discharge.

Tympanic Membrane Perforation
The most common causes of traumatic perforation of the tympanic membrane are water sports, such as diving or water-skiing.[6] Any corrosive agent introduced into the ear canal may also perforate the tympanic membrane. Other causes of perforation include blows to the head with a cupped hand, foreign objects entering the ear canal with excessive force, and forceful irrigation of the ear canal. At the moment of injury the pain is severe, but it decreases rapidly. Hearing acuity usually diminishes quickly, and if the condition is untreated, it may lead to otitis media. Other complications may include tinnitus, nausea, and vertigo (disequilibrium). Any patient suspected of having an acute perforated tympanic membrane should be referred to a physician for examination.

Barotrauma (Acute Aero-Otitis Media)
Barotrauma occurs during quick descent from high altitude.[10,22] The middle ear pressure fails to ventilate, resulting in a negative pressure in the middle ear. This negative pressure causes a suction and forces the tympanic membrane to retract, causing pain. Barotrauma may occur in individuals who fly with an upper respiratory tract infection or with any condition associated with impaired eustachian tube ventilation. For such patients, pretreatment with antihistamines or decongestants may help to avoid serious symptoms during air travel. Treatment of acute episodes consists of oral decongestants, antihistamines, and autoinflation of the eustachian tube (Valsalva's maneuver).[1,22] Swallowing or blowing against pressure may assist in sending air up the eustachian tube, thereby helping to equalize the pressure on both sides of the tympanic membrane.

Hearing Disorders
Obstructive Hearing Loss
Accumulated cerumen is a common cause of hearing loss, especially in persons with overactive cerumen glands. The accumulated cerumen causes an obstruction and produces a feeling of fullness or diminished hearing. Hearing impairment may occur when cerumen occludes the canal, impairing the transmission of sound waves to the tympanic membrane. After the patient swims or bathes, water can be trapped in the ear canal behind the cerumen. The trapped water is absorbed by the cerumen, causing expansion of the cerumen to worsen occlusion and thus

causing an acute hearing deficit. As discussed previously, temporary hearing impairment may also result from excessive edema, which, in combination with accumulated cerumen and debris, may occlude the canal. Impacted cerumen can be removed only by direct manipulation; the procedure should not be attempted by the patient or untrained persons.

Tinnitus

Tinnitus is defined as alien noise in the ear, which is subjective and audible only to the patient. It is described as sounding like steam escaping from a small pipe, ringing, roaring, pulsating, chirping (crickets), or humming. Tinnitus can be very annoying and may be constant or intermittent. The intensity of the disturbance varies from patient to patient, and patients' reactions may vary from minor distraction to severe mental depression.

Tinnitus can arise from a variety of causes involving the inner ear. It may be the result of blockage of the ear canal or of the eustachian tube and middle ear cavity, which is easily corrected following proper diagnosis. Tinnitus, which may be the first and only sign of a hearing disorder,[2] may be associated with hearing loss, exposure to high noise level, or acoustic trauma, or it may be a symptom of drug toxicity or systemic disease.[20] (Vertigo also may be of toxic origin, the result of intracranial or neurologic diseases, infection, hyperventilation, or severe ceruminal impaction.[23])

External otitis, serous otitis media, acute otitis media, and chronic otitis media seldom produce tinnitus as the sole or predominate complaint. Most patients with tinnitus have experienced a prior sensory insult from loud noise exposure, ototoxicity, head trauma, infection, Meniere's disease, or acoustic neuroma.[22]

Patients with tinnitus caused by such drugs as salicylates (arthritis patients), quinidine (heart patients), and quinine (malaria patients or patients using quinine to relieve leg cramps) usually will notice a decrease in the intensity of the tinnitus following discontinuation of the offending medication. Any patient who experiences tinnitus should receive a medical examination and evaluation. Nonprescription eardrops are not effective and are not recommended for the treatment of tinnitus.

Assessment

To choose appropriately between recommending patient self-treatment and physician referral, the pharmacist must be able to assess the nature and severity of the patient's otic condition by evaluating overt signs and symptoms (Table 1). The most common complaints may include one or more of the following: localized pain, itchiness in the ear canal, a feeling of fullness, hearing loss, lymphadenopathy, fever, and malaise.

Ear Pain

Pain in the ear, commonly identified by the patient as an earache, may be caused by various disorders. Careful inspection by trained personnel with proper instrumentation is often necessary to determine the etiology of the pain. External otitis, foreign material or cerumen packed against the tympanic membrane, and acute otitis media with its possible complications (e.g., mastoiditis or abscesses) are all common causes of ear pain. Pain may be referred to the ear from the sinuses, nasopharynx, tongue, hypopharynx, larynx, or temporomandibular joint. Loose-fitting dentures may also induce frank ear pain. In all such cases, the source of the pain should be determined and proper medical diagnosis should be made.

Pressure on the pinna or the tragus increases pain in external otitis.[7] Patients with otitis media rarely report increased pain with pressure on the pinna or tragus. Chewing may cause increased pain in patients with either external otitis or otitis media.

Boils

The signs and symptoms of a boil in the ear canal include localized, burning pain that increases when the patient chews, when traction is applied to the auricle, and when the tragus is pressed medially. A red, inflamed, raised lesion can be seen in the ear canal. The skin around the affected area is intact, provided the patient has not attempted to scratch the boil. The patient's subjective hearing is also usually intact. If lymphadenopathy, fever, malaise, or severe pain is present, the patient should be referred to a physician for treatment.

Foreign Objects

The signs and symptoms typically produced by a foreign object in the external ear usually include a feeling of fullness with hearing loss from the affected ear. Pain may be present and may increase with chewing, traction on the auricle, and pressure applied to the tragus. Lymphadenopathy, fever, or malaise do not occur acutely but may develop later, and there may be a foul-smelling discharge from the affected ear. Collectively, these characteristics indicate a secondary ear infection that is typically of bacterial or fungal origin. All patients with foreign objects in the ear, with or without secondary infection, should be evaluated and treated by a physician as promptly as possible.

External Otitis

The only means by which bacterial or fungal external otitis may be confirmed is by microbiologic culture. However, a culture is not always practical or necessary. Pain and swelling localized in the ear canal are usually the motivating symptoms that cause the patient to seek professional help (Table 4). A bacterial infection may be characterized by increased pain with chewing, traction applied to the auricle, and pressure applied medially on the tragus, as well as by a foul-smelling, mucopurulent discharge. Lymphadenopathy, a feeling of fullness, and fever and associated malaise may be additional characteristics of infection. Otoscopic examination may reveal a swollen, inflamed ear canal and an inflamed tympanic membrane. Patients with external otitis should be referred to a physician for thorough evaluation and treatment of the ear canal.

TABLE 4 Differential assessment of acute external otitis and acute otitis media		
	Acute external otitis	**Acute otitis media**
Season	Summer	Winter
Movement of tragus painful	Yes	No
Ear canal	Swollen	Normal
Eardrum	Normal (or red)	Perforated or bulging
Discharge	Yes	Yes, but through a perforation
Nodes	Frequent	Less frequent
Fever	Yes	Yes
Hearing	Normal or decreased	Always decreased

Adapted with permission from DeWeese D et al. *Otolaryngology—Head and Neck Surgery*. 7th ed. St. Louis: C. V. Mosby; 1988: 398.

Hearing Loss

Hearing loss is a complaint that should be evaluated and diagnosed by a physician or audiologist. Acute hearing loss without pain may be experienced and identified during an examination of the ear canal. Impacted cerumen in the ear canal obstructs the tympanic membrane and prevents its visualization.

Patients with impacted cerumen without secondary complications may be treated safely with nonprescription cerumen-softening agents. Patients with hearing loss without pain, and whose tympanic membrane is visible and not obstructed, should be evaluated and treated by a physician. Such decreased hearing may be due to a perforated tympanic membrane. Usually the patient with a perforated tympanic membrane has experienced a sharp pain of short duration at the time of injury. Treatment of a perforated tympanic membrane may include repair and medical therapy to prevent infection in the middle ear.

Otomycosis

Patients with otomycosis usually complain of itching and a feeling of fullness in the affected ear. The most common initial symptom of fungal external otitis is pruritus as opposed to the deep-seated pain and tenderness typically seen with predominately bacterial infections. Initially, the ear canal may reveal mild erythema and edema only. An established infection shows tender, red, and edematous tissue.[1] A colorless discharge may or may not be present. Pain is usually not present but may occur in severe cases. The pain increases with chewing, traction on the auricle, and pressure applied medially on the tragus. Systemic disturbances usually occur only in severe cases, which are often due to secondary bacterial infections with obstruction of the ear canal.

Otitis Media

The only conclusive means of diagnosing otitis media is via a complete patient history and physical examination using a pneumatic otoscope. Otitis media, which is most often caused by eustachian tube dysfunction, is found most commonly in children. Patients may be asymptomatic or may complain of occasional fullness and a cracking or hollow sound in the ears. The effect is usually bilateral. Otoscopic findings are specific and may demonstrate typical changes in tympanic membrane mobility consistent with the symptoms and degree of severity of the disorder.

A complication of prolonged serous otitis media is caused by bacteria and viruses extending along the eustachian tube and causing suppurative otitis media. Pneumatic otoscopic findings are specific and demonstrate a bulging, poorly resilient tympanic membrane resulting from the pus and exudate that accumulate behind the tympanic membrane. The patient usually experiences pain that is dull and throbbing at first and then rapidly becomes sharp, knifelike, and agonizing. The symptoms usually follow an upper respiratory tract infection. Systemic symptoms include chills, fever, and malaise. A bloody, purulent, foul-smelling discharge flows from the infected ear only after tympanic membrane perforation, at which time the patient experiences sudden relief from pain.

Patients with symptoms of either fever, malaise, or lymphadenopathy associated with any ear disorder should be thoroughly evaluated by a physician.

Treatment

Normally, the skin that lines the external auditory canal provides adequate protection against bacterial or fungal infection. Cerumen provides a continual, self-cleaning process that removes particulate matter and debris from the external auditory canal. An infection of the auricle or external auditory canal is a skin infection and should be treated as such.

Progressive symptoms of otic disease should be evaluated and treated only under a physician's supervision. Cerumen-softening and cerumenolytic agents only soften and loosen the cerumen to enable its easy removal by a physician. These agents do not readily remove cerumen. Effective mechanical removal by irrigation or instrumentation should be reserved for the physician. Surgical intervention may be necessary for deep cuts, bruises, or abrasions of the ear. Severe infections often require both systemic and local antibiotics. Self-treatment of boils may be instituted by applying heat followed by a bland antibiotic ointment to the affected area. A soft cotton applicator is useful for applying a topical drug over and around the boil. An antibiotic ointment may be used in the absence of known or suspected sensitivity. The lesion usually is self-limiting and clears after several days of frequent applications of heat and ointment. Resistant lesions require incision and drainage by a physician.

External Ear Disorders

Treatment of external otitis typically includes antibiotic and hydrocortisone drops applied in the ear canal. When cellulitis and lymphadenopathy are present, oral antibiotics are effective. Trauma to the ear should be avoided. The ear canals should be kept clean and dry at all times. After the patient swims or bathes, the ear canals may be filled for 1 to 2 minutes with two to four drops of acidified (acetic acid) solutions of alcohol, glycerin, propylene glycol, or water to a pH of 4 to 5 to help restore the normal acidic pH to the ear canal. A 1:1 mixture of warm water and 3% hydrogen peroxide can be used following swimming or bathing to enhance the removal of cerumen, but it will not contribute to the natural acidic environment of the ear canal.[1] Patients who have repeated episodes of external ear infections should be advised to use an acidifying agent or alcoholic solution when exposed to moisture.

A 5% aluminum acetate solution (Burow's solution) may be used as an astringent to obtain rapid resolution of eczematous or weeping skin.[1,2] Soaking with warm water, saline, or aluminum acetate solution is often useful in the treatment of crusting and edema involving the auricle and surrounding tissue.[18]

Cleansing the ear with a soft rubber bulb ear syringe may be uncomfortable but should never be painful. Severe, knifelike pain occurs if the tympanic membrane is ruptured, and it may be followed by intense vertigo. If frank pain does occur, irrigation must be stopped at once.

Cleansing repeatedly with saline or water at body temperature helps to clear debris from the ear canal. The irrigation solution should always be at body temperature; if it is too cold, the patient may experience vertigo.[7] Either a Water Pik® or a bulb ear syringe may be appropriate for cleansing purposes. Whichever instrument is chosen, proper technique is very important. The water column should be superior against the canal wall so that the returning stream may push the debris (cerumen) from behind.[6] External otitis should always be treated promptly to prevent spread to the mastoid bone or middle ear cavity. Severe cases may result in permanent hearing loss.

Nonprescription Pharmacologic Agents

Minor symptoms of external ear disorders may be treated prophylactically with alcohol, propylene glycol, glycerin, or water that has been acidified. Aluminum acetate solution also may be used for its astringent effects. These ingredients have been demonstrated to be safe and effective for maintaining a clean, dry ear canal and promoting aural hygiene.[1] The choice of the product depends on availability. Patients with otomycosis and those with impacted mycotic debris should have their ears cleaned and treated by a physician.

Nonprescription drug products used for palliative treatment of ear disorders should include selective products useful for treating skin disorders. For example, when applied to the skin, salicylic acid acts as an irritant; continuous application may cause dermatitis.[24] Thus, the use of salicylic acid in topical preparations applied to the ear is considered inadvisable unless recommended by a physician.

Topical antibiotic ointments, either with single or multiple antibiotics, are adequate for treating minor lesions of the auricle. They should be used only in the absence of known or suspected hypersensitivity. Antibiotics do not readily penetrate boils or abscesses; therefore, incision and drainage may be required.

Acetic Acid Solutions

Acetic acid solution in the form of household vinegar has been used successfully for many years to treat mild forms of external otitis.[1,25] Its application reduces redness, inflammation, and edema, thereby relieving the signs and symptoms of external otitis. It is also often recommended for treatment and prophylaxis of swimmer's ear. Acetic acid is well tolerated and nonsensitizing, and it does not produce resistant organisms. However, it does have an unpleasant vinegar-like odor, and it can be very painful if applied to the middle ear through a tympanoplasty tube or a perforation. If it does irritate or if sensitivity develops, use should be discontinued.[26]

Acetic acid has bactericidal and fungicidal properties when used properly, particularly against *Pseudomonas* sp., *Candida* sp., and *Aspergillus* sp. An environmental pH of 7.2–7.6 appears to be optimal for bacterial growth in the ear. This was confirmed in a study of 42 otitis cases in which pus cells and bacteria were observed in a pH range of 6.5–7.2.[27] Concentrations of 2 to 3% acetic acid provide effective and dependable treatment for mild forms of otitis by lowering the pH of the ear canal; however, solutions of less than 1% lack bactericidal properties.[28] The recommended treatment is four drops of dilute acetic acid (e.g., household vinegar) placed into the ear canal four times daily. This will provide an environmental pH of less than 3.[27] Recommended prophylaxis is four drops placed into the ear canal after swimming, showering, bathing, or hair washing.

A suitable concentration of acetic acid can be made easily and inexpensively in the pharmacy from white distilled household vinegar, which is usually 5% acetic acid. A 50:50 mixture of distilled household vinegar with either water, propylene glycol, glycerin, or rubbing alcohol (70% isopropyl or 70% ethyl alcohol) will provide a 2.5% acetic acid solution.[26] Because propylene glycol is viscous, mixing it with vinegar will increase the contact time of acetic acid on the epithelium. Anhydrous glycerin, alone or mixed with vinegar, will help to remove water from the ear. Alcohol alone or mixed with vinegar has anti-infective properties and provides a drying effect.[6,29] Decreasing the alcohol concentration may lessen the burning sensation and also decrease the drying effect, whereas increasing the alcohol concentration will increase the drying effect. Keeping the ear dry and instilling acidified alcohol into the ear canal at least three times a week as well as after swimming, showering, bathing, or hair washing has been shown to prevent the growth of bacteria, including *Pseudomonas* species.[5,6,30]

Patients can be treated at home with a dilute acetic acid solution (eight drops of white vinegar diluted to 10 mL with 10% isopropyl alcohol or aluminum acetate solution). The solution should be applied as two to four drops into the ear using proper technique.[1]

Aluminum Acetate Solution (Burow's Solution)

External otitis or local itching of the external ear caused by external ear dermatitis may be treated with an astringent such as 1:10 or 1:40 aluminum acetate solution.[3,28,31] One tablet or one packet dissolved in 500 mL of water yields a concentration of 1:40. Aluminum acetate solution is used widely for conditions involving the external ear. Its major value is its acidity, which restores the normal antibacterial pH of the ear canal.

Applied locally as protein precipitants, astringents dry the affected area by reducing the secretory function of the skin glands.[31] Contraction and wrinkling of the affected tissue may be seen; astringents also toughen the skin to help prevent reinfection. When applied properly, aluminum acetate may be used to treat bacterial infections as well as otomycosis.

When the ear canal is swollen, weeping, and inflamed, an aluminum acetate solution is helpful, given its anti-inflammatory, antipruritic, astringent, and limited antibacterial properties.[31] Aluminum acetate solution may also be used to treat the edema and crusting associated with acute moist ear canals, for which the abundant desquamative debris that forms requires special cleansing.[6]

A wet compress may be used with a gauze dressing on the auricle.[3,18] Drops may be instilled into the canal. The usual dosage of aluminum acetate solution is four to six drops every 4–6 hours until itching or burning subsides. The drops may also be used prophylactically against swimmer's ear to help clean and dry the ear canal after swimming or bathing. Aluminum acetate solution is suitable for children and adults. Used properly, it is nonsensitizing and well tolerated.[24] Adverse reactions are rare.

Antipyrine

The Food and Drug Administration (FDA) has concluded that antipyrine is neither safe nor effective for nonprescription use as a topical otic analgesic and anesthetic and that it should be used only under the advice and supervision of a physician.[30]

Benzocaine

The utility of benzocaine or other local anesthetics for local analgesia in the ear is not clear. The FDA has concluded that evidence is lacking to classify benzocaine as either safe or effective for nonprescription use as a topical analgesic, and it has suggested that benzocaine is ineffective topically as an analgesic and/or anesthetic on the tissue of the tympanic membrane and ear canal.[13,30] Hypersensitivity to benzocaine is considered a general contraindication to its topical use in the ear or elsewhere on the skin.

Reactions or complications caused by application of benzocaine are usually avoided or minimized by applying the minimal effective dose. Special caution should be exercised in patients with known drug hypersensitivities and in those with severe trauma or sepsis of the areas of application.

Boric Acid

Boric acid is an ingredient in some ear preparations. It is a weak, local anti-infective and is nonirritating to intact skin in a dilute solution of 1–5%. Alcohol–boric acid solutions show improved bactericidal action over alcohol alone (either 99% isopropyl or 70% ethyl alcohol) because the addition of boric acid increases the acidity of the preparation, which, when applied topically, increases the acidity of the skin.[5,28] Because of its toxicity, boric acid should be used with caution, particularly in children and on open wounds where the potential for systemic absorption is high.[31]

Camphor

The safety and effectiveness of camphor as an ingredient in nonprescription eardrops has not been substantiated.

Carbamide Peroxide

The antibacterial properties of carbamide peroxide (urea hydrogen peroxide) are due to release of the nascent oxygen, the primary value of which is in cleansing wounds. The effervescence caused by oxygen release mechanically removes debris from inaccessible regions. In otic preparations, the effervescence assists in disintegrating wax accumulations. Carbamide (urea) helps debride the tissue. These actions soften residue in the ear. Removal of the softened cerumen may be assisted by warm water irrigation.

The FDA has determined that 6.5% carbamide peroxide formulated in an anhydrous glycerin vehicle is safe and effective for occasional nonprescription use as an aid to soften, loosen, and remove excessive earwax.[14] The FDA recommends usage twice each day for up to 4 days if needed, or as directed by a physician. Five drops of the solution should be instilled into the affected ear and allowed to remain at least 15 minutes; this is done by either tilting the head (affected ear up) or inserting a small amount of cotton into the canal opening. The applicator tip should not enter the ear canal. Wax remaining after treatment may be removed by gently flushing the ear with warm water, using a soft rubber ear syringe. The process may be repeated a second time if necessary. Failure to obtain relief after 4 days of treatment could indicate a more serious condition, and a physician should be consulted. This process is not recommended for children under 12 years of age.

Unless it is under physician supervision, carbamide peroxide should not be used if there is ear drainage, pain, or dizziness; if there is known injury or perforation of the eardrum; or if ear surgery has been performed within the past 6 weeks. This treatment should be discontinued whenever irritation or rash appears. It is not recommended for treating pain of raw inflamed tissue, swimmer's ear, or itching of the ear canal.

Chloroform
The safety and effectiveness of chloroform as an ingredient in nonprescription topical ear products has not been established.

Glycerin
Glycerin may be used as a solvent or an emollient; it may also be used as a humectant because of its hygroscopic properties. Glycerin is widely used as a vehicle in many otic preparations (prescriptions and nonprescription). It is safe and nonsensitizing when applied to open wounds or abraded skin.

Dehydrated glycerin contains no less than 98.5% glycerin; glycerin (USP) contains no less than 95% glycerin (it may contain a maximum of 5% water).[31,32] Anhydrous glycerin may be prepared by heating glycerin (USP) at 302°F (150°C) for 2 hours to drive off moisture.[14] Because of glycerin's hygroscopic properties, patients should be advised not to rinse the applicator because this will dilute the glycerin and reduce its effectiveness.

Ichthammol
Ichthammol is a weak antiseptic and irritant with emollient properties. Its primary activity is as an emollient rather than an antiseptic. Ichthammol ointment (10%) is used for treating local inflammation associated with minor boils or abscesses. The safety and effectiveness of ichthammol in treating disorders of the ear is undefined at this time.

Menthol
The safety and effectiveness of menthol as a nonprescription ingredient in eardrops has not been substantiated.

Olive Oil (Sweet Oil)
Olive oil is used as an emollient and topical lubricant.[31] It may be instilled into the ear canal to alleviate itching and burning. It is also helpful for softening earwax.[16] If an insect becomes trapped in the ear canal, olive oil can be instilled to smother the insect.

Phenol in Glycerin
Phenol (5–10%) in glycerin has been used to treat pain caused by ear disorders. Its use is no longer recommended, however, because it poses inherent dangers of necrosis and perforation of the tympanic membrane.

Propylene Glycol
Propylene glycol is a solvent that has preservative and humectant properties. Used in both prescription and nonprescription otic preparations, propylene glycol is a clear, colorless, nonirritating, viscous liquid. It is useful as a vehicle because it is hygroscopic and its viscosity increases contact time with tissues of the external auditory canal.[6] Adding acetic acid to propylene glycol increases the solution's acidity, enhancing its anti-infective properties.[6] If used over a long period of time, propylene glycol may cause allergic dermatitis in susceptible individuals.[2,12]

Thymol
Thymol, a phenolic compound obtained from thyme oil, has a more agreeable odor than phenol. It has been used traditionally in topical preparations for its aromatic properties. It has antibacterial and antifungal properties in a concentration of 1%;[25] in the presence of large amounts of proteins, however, its antibacterial activity is greatly reduced. The clinical effectiveness of thymol for treating ear disorders has not been well studied and objectively determined. The value of thymol in managing any disorder of the external ear is unsubstantiated.

Other Cerumen-Softening Products
Direct visualization of the ear canal is important. Individuals having difficulty with hard, impacted cerumen can occasionally instill olive oil, mineral oil, glycerin, carbamide peroxide, diluted hydrogen peroxide solution, or propylene glycol in the ear to soften the cerumen and promote the normal process of removal.

The patient may irrigate the ear canal every few days with warm water, normal saline, a mixture of 20–30% alcohol and water, carbamide peroxide, or aluminum acetate solution to help prevent cerumen buildup. If the tympanic membrane is perforated or is not known to be intact, these cerumen-softening products should be used only under a physician's supervision. If perforation of the tympanic membrane is not suspected, a 1:1 solution of warm water and hydrogen peroxide can be used to flush the ear canal.[1] The overuse of undiluted 3% hydrogen peroxide and the indiscriminate or chronic use of aqueous hydrogen peroxide (1:1) instilled into the ear canal are unwise because maceration of the skin may predispose to infection.[9]

Cerumen-softening agents only soften the hardened, impacted cerumen. They do not and should not also be expected to remove cerumen. Patients can be instructed to use cerumen-softening agents for 3 to 4 days, at which time the cerumen should be softened enough to be easily removed by a physician.[2]

Removal of cerumen, desquamated debris, and dried secretions is often best accomplished by suction or use of a small cotton-tipped applicator and should only be performed by trained personnel. Gentle irrigation with an ear syringe or a forced water spray (Water Pik®) may be performed but only if the tympanic membrane is known to be intact. Tap water should be avoided because of potential contamination.[33] Sterile water may be used, but it must be at body temperature when instilled or the resultant vestibular stimulation will cause vertigo.[2]

Because most bacteria or fungi do not thrive in acidic environments, an important feature of any otic solution is that the pH is acidic.[2] In mild cases of external otitis, topical treatment is all that is necessary.[2] Following careful cleansing, an acidified soothing liquid suitable (i.e., dilute acetic acid in alcohol) placed in the ear canal is suitable. This treatment is preferred except in diabetic patients and in unusually severe cases of external otitis. In severe cases, these solutions may be used to flush debris from the ear canal to improve the effectiveness of topical antibacterial otic drops.¹ As inflammation diminishes, 30–70% acidified alcohol may be used to keep the ear canal clean and dry.

Patients may be advised to use an alcohol solution in the ear any time water enters the ear canal.⁶ Patients should also be advised that future episodes of external otitis may be avoided by keeping the ears dry with routine use of dilute acidified alcohol at least three times weekly, and especially after swimming.⁷ Patients should be cautioned against scratching their ear canal with cotton-tipped applicators.⁶ Patients with a known tympanic membrane perforation should not use any otic preparation without their physician's consent.

All nonprescription otic preparations may be contraindicated in individuals susceptible to local irritation and hypersensitivity. Patients should be advised to discontinue using the medication if rash, local redness, or other adverse symptoms occur.

Patient Evaluation

Evaluation of the patient's present health status must be based on information in the medical and drug history records, including current symptoms. The pharmacist should have the patient describe the symptoms, and should ask whether the patient has experienced similar symptoms previously and, if so, when and how they were treated. The pharmacist should also obtain information concerning the presence of chronic diseases that may impair healing, such as diabetes mellitus, or predisposing factors or conditions that may influence the patient's response to self-treatment, such as allergies.

Before suggesting self-treatment of an external ear disorder, the pharmacist should rule out an earache caused by otitis media secondary to an upper respiratory tract infection. A history of pressure in, or referred pain to, the ear may be caused by a pathologic condition in the area around the ear. Recent injury or trauma to the head or neck regions may also cause referred pain to the ear. Trauma to the ear canal is to be avoided at all times. Adults with recurrent otitis who respond poorly to treatment should be examined by a physician; recurrent otitis infections can be prevented by strict attention to predisposing causes such as seborrheic dermatitis, psoriasis, and eczema. Contact dermatitis must always be considered. Prophylaxis following swimming by adding two to four drops of acidified alcohol to both ears is encouraged.

Management of ear disorders may often be difficult because of underlying diseases or predisposing factors. The skin of patients with diabetes mellitus is more prone to infection (bacterial and fungal), especially when the diabetes is poorly controlled. Infections in diabetic patients tend to resolve more slowly and to recur more often. The increased predisposition to infection of the ear canal may be related to impairment of the skin's integrity and abnormalities in immunologic responses. Ear infections, especially external otitis, are difficult to treat in diabetic patients. Rigid control of diabetes cannot be overemphasized.

The pharmacist may assess the severity of the otic disorder and either provide appropriate nonprescription medication with instructions for proper use or refer the patient to a physician. Health professionals (pharmacists, physicians, and nurses) properly trained to visualize the tympanic membrane and ear canal with a suitable otoscope and properly instructed in aural hygiene may, in most cases, perform irrigation safely with an ear syringe or a forced water spray. Appropriately selected nonprescription drug products can be relied upon to provide a suitable therapeutic or prophylactic response in certain conditions. Proper product selection and patient instruction by the pharmacist requires a clear knowledge of the symptoms and pathophysiology of the condition being treated. Referral for medical evaluation and treatment requires an ability to recognize the severity of the illness and the potential or actual complications associated with the condition. The patient should always be referred to a physician if any of the following symptoms exist: severe pain, lymphadenopathy, discharge from ear, possible hearing deficit, or fever.

Patient Consultation

Cleansing procedures and self-treatment for treating ear disorders should not be delegated to patients unless they understand proper techniques in drug administration and use. Patients must be evaluated for their ability to understand the hazards of inappropriate self-treatment. The pharmacist with proper skill in aural visualization and irrigation procedures can usually make these judgments.

Patients should be instructed on the use of nonprescription drugs for the ear consistent with any other drug product dispensed by the pharmacist. They should also fully understand the proper use of medicine droppers for administering eardrops into the ear and of ear syringes for irrigating the ear. Water to irrigate the ear canal should be sterile or sterilized by boiling to prevent contamination.³³ Eardrops should be warmed to body temperature by holding the medication container in the palm of the hand or placing it into a vessel of warm water for a few minutes before administration. Heated eardrops should never be applied to the ear canal because they are likely to damage the ear. Also, excessive heat may damage the ingredients in the eardrop. Eardrops may be applied as often as four times daily. The involved ear should be tilted up for at least 2 minutes following the placement of two to four eardrops to permit effective contact of the medication.²

A cotton wick may be inserted gently into the ear canal to help the medication maintain contact with the affected area in the ear canal. Gently pulling the auricle backward may allow medication to reach a greater depth in the ear canal. Cotton wicks, however, usually require insertion with appropriate instruments and should be used only by trained personnel. If irrigation of the ear is necessary, it too should be performed only by trained personnel using either an ear syringe or a forced water spray, such as a Water Pik®; the direction of the water column should be superior against the canal wall so that the returning stream may push the debris from behind.² Although Water Pik® or ear syringe irrigations are generally safe, tympanic membrane perforations can occur. Therefore, the lowest possible effective pressure should be used to prevent mechanical trauma.⁷ Gentle irrigation, which assists in removing cerumen or debris, is most successful if the cerumen is not packed tightly.

TABLE 5	Five-minute hearing test

	Almost always	Half the time	Occasionally	Never
1. I have a problem hearing over the telephone.				
2. I have trouble following the conversation when two or more people are talking at the same time.				
3. People complain that I turn the television volume too high.				
4. I have to strain to understand conversations.				
5. I miss hearing some common sounds like the phone or doorbell ringing.				
6. I have trouble hearing conversations in a noisy background such as a party.				
7. I get confused about where sounds come from.				
8. I misunderstand some words in a sentence and need to ask people to repeat themselves.				
9. I especially have trouble understanding the speech of women and children.				
10. I have worked in noisy environments (on assembly lines, with jackhammers, around jet engines, etc.).				
11. Many people I talk to seem to mumble (or do not speak clearly).				
12. People get annoyed because I misunderstand what they say.				
13. I misunderstand what others are saying and make inappropriate responses.				
14. I avoid social activities because I cannot hear well and feel I will reply improperly.				
To be answered by a family member or friend: 15. Do you think this person has a hearing loss?				

Mark the column that best describes the frequency with which you experience each situation or feeling. To calculate your score, give yourself 3 points for every time you checked "almost always," 2 for every "half the time," 1 for every "occasionally," and 0 for every "never." If you have a blood relative who has a hearing loss, add another 3 points. Total your points.

0 to 5: Your hearing is fine. No action required.

6 to 9: Suggest you see an ear, nose, and throat (ENT) physician.

10 and above: Strongly recommend you see an ENT physician.

Reprinted with permission from the American Academy of Otolaryngology—Head and Neck Surgery, Inc., Alexandria, Va.

Patients should be advised that symptoms usually begin to subside within 1 to 2 days if self-treatment is appropriate. If symptoms persist or if an adverse reaction to the medication occurs, the patient should consult a physician immediately.

Prophylactic measures directed against the development of swimmer's ear, as recommended by the American Academy of Otolaryngology, should be instituted at the first sign of trapped water in the ear. The pharmacist should instruct the patient as follows:[34]

- Tilt head downward, affected ear up.
- If there is *no* possibility that there is a hole in the eardrum, carefully squeeze a medicine dropper full of rubbing (isopropyl) alcohol into the ear canal. (Alcohol dries the skin inside the ear, killing any bacteria or fungi.)
- With one hand, move the ear back and forth to move the solution all the way into the ear.
- Tilt the head to the other, affected side to let the alcohol out, gently tapping the unaffected side.
- Repeat the procedure in the opposite ear.

Some physicians add equal parts of white vinegar to the alcohol eardrops. However, anyone with a punctured eardrum should avoid swimming and avoid using any kind of eardrops without a physician's advice.

A 5-minute hearing test is sometimes useful to assess some patients with a suspected hearing deficit. It is not intended to be a test in sound discrimination (Table 5).

Summary

Otic disorders affect both young and old people, and visible signs are not always proportional to the degree of pain suffered. Nonprescription products are available to treat disorders of both the auricle and the external auditory canal. Disorders involving the middle ear should not be treated with nonprescription drug products.

By assessing the complaint and reviewing the patient's history, the pharmacist should be able to judge whether symptoms may be self-treated or referral to a physician is indicated. Health professionals trained in otic procedures may examine the tympanic membrane with an otoscope and irrigate the ear canal gently with a syringe or a forced water spray. This procedure should be performed only if the tympanic membrane is known to be intact and there are no underlying disorders as determined by a recent physician examination.

Objects such as hairpins, pencils, matchsticks, cotton swabs, or other sharp instruments should never touch the external auditory canal, and objects smaller than a finger draped with a clean washcloth should never enter the external auditory canal. Patients should be advised never to place objects in the ear canal. Good personal hygiene, especially of facial and neck areas, should be maintained at all times. Dandruff and dirty hair can be controlled with appropriate shampoos and washing. A skin infection must not be neglected because it may be transferred very easily to uninfected areas.

Many nonprescription otic products have been shown to be safe and effective. The pharmacist should advise the patient to consult a physician if symptoms do not subside within 1 or 2 days after treatment is initiated or if adverse reactions occur.

References

1. Paparella MM, Shumick DA. *Otolaryngology*. 3rd ed. Philadelphia: W. B. Saunders; 1991: 23, 26, 595, 1077, 1228–30, 1246, 1259, 1293.
2. DeWeese D et al. *Otolaryngology—Head and Neck Surgery*. 7th ed. St. Louis: C. V. Mosby; 1988: 347, 349, 351, 395–7, 399, 401–2, 409, 413, 423, 479, 1229, 1260.
3. Friedman I. *Pathology of the Ear*. London: Blackwell Scientific; 1974: 10, 14–5, 27.
4. Riegelman S, Sorby DL. *Dispensing of Medication*. 7th ed. Easton, Pa: Mack; 1971: 908.
5. Adams GL et al. *Fundamentals of Otolaryngology*. 5th ed. Philadelphia: W. B. Saunders; 1978: 181, 184.
6. Austin DF. Diseases of the external ear. In: Ballenger JJ et al., eds. *Diseases of Nose, Throat, Ear, Head, and Neck*. 14th ed. Philadelphia: Lea & Febiger; 1991: 925, 1069, 1075–6, 1106, 1117, 1179, 1229.
7. Meyerhoff WL, Rice DH. *Otolaryngology and Head and Neck Surgery*. Philadelphia: W. B. Saunders; 1992: 16, 18–9, 48, 157, 293, 353–4, 356, 1072, 1077, 1106, 1109–11.
8. *Federal Register* 1977; 42: 63559.
9. Mawson SR, Ludman H. *Diseases of the Ear*. 4th ed. Chicago: Yearbook Medical; 1979: 252, 257, 261, 267.
10. Senturia BH et al. *Diseases of the External Ear, An Otologic–Dermatology Manual*. 2nd ed. New York: Grune and Stratton; 1980: 79–80.
11. Rutka J, Alberti P. *Toxic and Drug Induced Disorders in Otolaryngology*. The Otolaryngology Clinics of North America; 1984: 761–74.
12. Booth J. In: Kerr A, ed. *Scott-Brown's Otolaryngology*. 5th ed. London: Butterworth's & Co Ltd; 1987: 55–6, 164.
13. *Federal Register* 1982; 47: 30014, 30018.
14. *Federal Register* 1986; 51: 28656–61.
15. Bordely J et al. *Ear, Nose, and Throat Disorders in Children*. New York: Raven Press; 1986: 56–7, 61, 89.
16. Cohn A. *Arch Otolaryngol* 1974; 99: 138.
17. Corcoran JG, Atline SG. Infectious diseases in the geriatric patient: symposium on geriatric otolaryngology. *Otolaryngol Clin North Am* 1983; 425.
18. Lucente FE. In: English GM, ed. *Otolaryngology—Diseases of the Ear and Hearing*. Vol 1. Philadelphia: Harper & Row; 1983: 1–2.
19. Bossi J, Jackman J. *Drug Intell Clin Pharm* 1977; 11: 665.
20. Smyth GDL. In: English GM, ed. *Chronic Otitis in Otolaryngology*. Philadelphia: Harper & Row; 1976: 2.
21. Elliott D et al. *Patient Care* 1971; 5: 20.
22. Lee KJ. *Differential Diagnosis, Otolaryngology*. New York: Arco; 1978: 91, 94, 115.
23. Wood RP, Northern FL. *Manual of Otolaryngology*. Baltimore: Williams & Wilkins; 1979: 39, 42.
24. Wade A, Reynolds JE. *Martindale, The Extra Pharmacopoeia*. 27th ed. London: Pharmaceutical Press; 1979: 212, 272.
25. Ochs I. *Arch Otolaryngol* 1950; 52: 935–7.
26. *AMA Drug Evaluations Annual*. Chicago: American Medical Association; 1992: 1128, 1480.
27. Goffin F. *N Engl J Med* 1963; 268: 287–9.
28. Jones E, McIain P. *Laryngoscope* 1961; 71: 928–35.

29. Wright D, Dinen M. *Arch Otolaryngol* 1972; 95: 245.
30. *Federal Register* 1977; 42: 63564.
31. *Remington's Pharmaceutical Sciences*. 18th ed. Easton, Pa: Mack; 1990: 761, 1310, 1316, 1318.
32. *USP DI*. 21st ed. Rockville, Md: U.S. Pharmacopoeial Convention; 1992: 158, 768.
33. Rubin J, Kamerer DB et al. Aural irrigation with water: a potential pathogenic mechanism for introducing malignant external otitis. *Ann Otol Rhino Laryngol* 1990: 99; 117–9.
34. Goldstein JC. What to advise patients on swimmer's ear. *Wellcome Trends Phar* 1989 Aug; 9.

American Pharmaceutical Association

2215 Constitution Avenue, NW
Washington, DC 20037-2985
(202) 628-4410 Fax (202) 783-2351

The National Professional Society of Pharmacists

Dear *Handbook* Purchaser:

As a result of a printer's error, several entries were omitted from page 884 of the general index in the *Handbook of Nonprescription Drugs*, 10th Edition.

Please cut out the information at the bottom of this page and tape it to the top of page 884.

We regret the inconvenience this error has caused our readers.

Special Projects Department
American Pharmaceutical Association

----

884 General Index

Afrin 12-Hour Pediatric, 704	*Alka-Seltzer Original*, 644, 716	*Almacone*, 716	*Amphogel*, 258
Afrin Tablets, 670	*Alka-Seltzer Plus Cold and Cough Medicine*, 670	*Almacone II*, 716	**Amphotericin B**, 547
Aftate, 879		*Almora*, 716	**Ampicillin**, 205

CHAPTER 23

Oral Health Products

Arlene A. Flynn

Questions to ask in patient assessment and counseling

General Assessment

- *What are your symptoms?*
- *How long have you had this dental problem?*
- *Have you seen a dentist about the problem? When?*
- *What remedies have you tried? How did you use them? How long did you use them? Did they work?*
- *Have you had this problem before?*

Mouth Pain

- *Where is the pain?*
- *Is the pain severe? Is there swelling in the area?*
- *Is the pain continuous and throbbing, or does it come and go?*
- *Is the pain triggered or made worse by hot or cold substances or by chewing?*
- *Do you feel ill?*
- *Do you have a cold, sinus infection, or ear infection?*
- *Do you have a fever?*
- *Are there any prior events such as trauma associated with the pain?*
- *Are there any other symptoms associated with the pain?*

Mouth Irritation or Discomfort

- *Where is the area of irritation or lesion? Is it visible? What color is it?*
- *Is the discomfort continuous?*
- *Is the discomfort aggravated by eating or drinking?*
- *Is there a discharge from the lesion?*
- *Do your gums bleed when you brush your teeth?*
- *Do you have a bad taste in your mouth?*
- *Do you have bad breath continuously?*
- *Are any of your teeth loose?*

- *Do you wear dentures? Are they loose?*
- *Do your dentures cause sore spots?*

General State of Oral Health

- *How do you brush your teeth or clean your dentures? How often?*
- *Do you use dental floss? How often?*
- *How often do you see your dentist for checkups?*
- *Do you use supplemental fluoride in any form (e.g., rinse or tablet)?*

Additional Patient-Specific Factors

- *Do you suffer from any chronic medical illness (e.g., diabetes mellitus, rheumatic heart disease, asthma, seizure disorder, or high blood pressure)?*
- *What prescription and nonprescription medications are you currently taking?*
- *Do you have a pacemaker?*
- *Have you had joint replacement surgery?*
- *Do you smoke or use any tobacco product (including smokeless tobacco products)?*
- *Do you have any food or drug allergies? If so, what are they?*

Dental diseases account for some of the most prevalent chronic diseases in our society. Pertinent statistics include the following:

- Fifty percent of the population needs dental treatment.
- Only 55% of the adult population visits a dentist during a year.
- Of all 17-year-olds, 84% have experienced tooth decay.
- The average adult has 23 decayed or filled tooth surfaces.
- Each year, dental diseases cause 6.73 million days of disability that results in confinement to bed.
- Nearly 80% of all Americans have some degree of periodontal disease.
- Forty-one percent of older Americans have lost all their natural teeth.
- Oral cancer accounts for 4% of all cancers.[1]

Since the 1970s, dental caries has declined significantly in school-age children in this country. The National Institute of Dental Research reports that 49.9% of all U.S. children aged 5–17 in 1990 had no episodes of dental caries in their permanent teeth, as compared with 36.6%

Editor's Note: This chapter is based in part on the chapter with the same title that appeared in the 9th edition but was written by Karen A. Baker.

in 1980 and 28% in 1970.[2] But although the incidence of dental caries is declining, it remains a public health problem, and the importance of prevention should not be ignored. In addition, root caries, an age-related problem that affects the root surfaces of adult teeth exposed by gingival recession, is becoming increasingly important as adults retain greater numbers of teeth later in life and the number of older people increases. And periodontal disease, the prevalence and severity of which is related primarily to oral health care, remains the principal cause of tooth loss in adults over 35 years of age.[3] Yet this common and significant public health problem can be prevented or controlled.

Retail sales of oral hygiene products were estimated at $2.9 billion in 1991—a 30% increase in pharmacy sales since 1986.[4] The oral health care market has grown an average of 6.1% per year since 1986, and nonprescription products are widely available in the pharmacy for both the prevention and treatment of oral disease or discomfort. Therefore, a pharmacist may be the first health care professional to evaluate and counsel a patient with oral health care needs. On the basis of thorough patient assessment, the pharmacist can inform and advise the patient regarding self-care or the need for professional referral.

Patient Assessment and Counseling

Questions to ask the patient presenting with a dental problem relate to:

- The clinical manifestation of the particular problem (e.g., pain);
- The patient's general state of oral health;
- Possible etiology;
- Patient-specific factors (e.g., history of chronic disease, prescription medications, allergies, and previous dental care);
- Lifestyle risks;
- Product selection.

It is important for the pharmacist to assess each complaint to determine whether the problem (1) is a recurring one, (2) is likely to resolve with self-treatment using nonprescription products, (3) presents progressive and potentially serious consequences, or (4) presents a dental emergency requiring immediate professional care.

General Assessment Considerations

It is important for the pharmacist to determine if the patient is currently under a dentist's care and is experiencing a problem related to a recent dental procedure. Previous self-treatment with nonprescription oral products needs to be evaluated for possible misuse, abuse, or inappropriate response. A recurrent problem may signal a condition that warrants referral to a dentist.

Counseling a patient about nonprescription medication should include more than merely explaining that a product is preventive, curative, or palliative. The patient should be informed about how to use the product properly, how long to use it, what to expect from it, what precautions to take with its use, and what to do if it is ineffective. It is equally important for the pharmacist to tell the patient which nonprescription medications should not be used and why. The patient should realize that nonprescription drugs should improve the condition being treated. If their use results in no change, worsens the condition, or causes another problem, they should be discontinued and the patient should see a dentist or other physician.

Assessment of Clinical Manifestations

Pain

Pain can accompany many common oral problems. Different features of pain indicate different underlying problems. Tooth pain triggered or worsened by stimuli such as heat, cold, or pressure upon biting often indicates a pulpal response to deep carious lesions or a cracked or broken tooth. Continuous tooth pain may indicate pulpal infection and necrosis, an abscess, or serious periodontal disease. Fever, malaise, and swelling may indicate an oral abscess. A patient who feels ill, has a fever, or exhibits swelling should be referred to a dentist for immediate professional care.

Mouth Irritation or Discomfort

Continuous irritation, soreness, or pain that is associated with the soft tissues of the mouth and is more severe upon eating or drinking is a common symptom of canker sores and acute atrophic candidiasis. Pain along the gingival ridge under a denture prosthesis suggests ill-fitting dentures, denture stomatitis, or possible candidiasis. The color, shape, and location of various oral anomalies help in assessment. Recurrent oral sores on nonkeratinized oral mucosa (e.g., canker sores), recurrent vesicular sores on the skin bordering the lip (e.g., cold sores and fever blisters), and inflammation under seldom-cleaned dentures (e.g., denture stomatitis) are examples of location-specific lesions that can help define oral problems. Some examples of pathologic color changes include the white plaques of candidiasis, the erythema (redness) associated with the margins of canker and cold sores, and the gingival erythema associated with periodontitis. Halitosis may result from poor oral hygiene, trench mouth, or dentopyogenic infections, and it merits inquiry and possible referral.

Assessment of Patient-Specific Factors

If available, the patient's medication profile should be reviewed. This history, which should include prescription and nonprescription drug use, may suggest to the pharmacist potentially serious dental or medical complications, such as endocarditis secondary to an oral abscess in a patient with rheumatic heart disease. Patients who have undergone surgery for placement of a pacemaker or prosthetic joint may be at high risk for bacterial endocarditis. Use of oral irrigating devices may be contraindicated in these groups because of the possibility of bacteremia.[5] The pharmacist should also be alert to predisposing factors or conditions that might result in oral pathology. Examples include signs and symptoms of oral candidiasis in patients taking an antihistamine that dries the mouth owing to high anticholinergic activity, an orally inhaled steroid that decreases the immune response in the mouth, use of a broad-spectrum antibiotic that results in overgrowth of nonsusceptible organisms, and presence of a disease (e.g., leukemia, autoimmunodeficiency syndrome, or cancer) or use of a drug (e.g., cancer chemotherapy) that produces an immune deficiency disorder.

Assessment of General Oral Health

Poor oral hygiene or infrequent dental care can greatly increase the likelihood of dental caries, infection, periodontal disease, misfitting or broken dentures, and other oral health problems. Patients sometimes notice bleeding gingiva, the presence of plaque and calculus on teeth, and loose teeth during brushing and flossing. Such symptoms should prompt the pharmacist to refer the patient to a dentist for evaluation.

Assessment of Lifestyle Risks

Alcohol Consumption

Adverse effects of alcohol consumption on oral health include xerostomia (dry mouth) and increased risk for development of oral cancer.

Use of Tobacco Products

Use of tobacco products, both smoked and smokeless, has been associated with oral cancer, sinusitis, discoloration of the teeth, halitosis, xerostomia, periodontal disease, dental calculus, and other hard and soft tissue damage in the oral region.[6] Smoking accounts for about 30% of all cancer deaths, and about 390,000 premature, smoking-related deaths in the United States occur annually. If diagnosed early enough, however, many precancerous changes in the oral cavity can be reversed with the cessation of smoking or tobacco use.[6]

It is estimated that at least 10 million Americans, about 30% of whom are under 21 years of age, use smokeless tobacco. Use among teenage boys continues to increase. Epidemiologic and clinical case studies provide evidence of an increased risk of oral cancer among smokeless tobacco users, particularly those who regularly use snuff. Although the adverse effects associated with snuff use have been more fully documented than those associated with the use of other such products, the carcinogenic potential of all smokeless tobacco products is recognized.[7]

Evidence also supports an association of smokeless tobacco use with gingival inflammation and recession; increased dental caries (because these products contain sugar, which is kept in contact with the teeth); cervical erosion of the teeth; and oral leukoplakia, a precancerous oral lesion in 3–6% of squamous cell carcinomas.[8]

Any patient who complains of persistent mouth irritation and who uses tobacco products of any type should be advised to visit a dentist for evaluation and to seek help in stopping tobacco use. A National Cancer Institute program promotes the use of the "four A's," which pharmacists can adopt in counseling their patients:

- *Ask* patients about their smoking behaviors.
- *Advise* all smokers to quit.
- *Assist* patients in stopping.
- *Arrange* for supportive follow-up.[6]

Pharmacists might also seriously consider providing a smoke-free environment and eliminating the sale of tobacco products in the pharmacy.

Chewing Ice Cubes

Chewing ice cubes can cause tooth enamel to develop cracks because of pressure, shearing force, and the expansion and contraction caused by temperature changes. These tiny cracks provide surfaces for plaque and stain to accumulate.

Dental Anatomy and Physiology

The teeth and supporting structures are necessary for normal mastication and articulation and for aesthetic appearance. The primary dentition first appears at approximately 6 months of age with the eruption of the mandibular (lower jaw) central incisors; it is usually complete with the eruption of the upper second molars at approximately 24 months. There are 20 deciduous teeth, 10 in each arch. Generally, the permanent dentition first appears with the eruption of the mandibular first molar behind the deciduous second molar at approximately 6 years, and it continues in a regular pattern, replacing shedding deciduous teeth. The last permanent teeth to erupt are the third molars (wisdom teeth), which may appear between 17 and 21 years of age.

Anatomically, the teeth are grossly viewed as having two parts, the roots and the crown (Figure 1). The roots are normally below the gingival (gum) line or margin and are essential for support and attachment of the tooth to the surrounding tissues. The crown is above the gingival margin and is responsible for mastication. The teeth comprise four basic components: enamel, dentin, cementum, and pulp.

Enamel is composed of very hard, crystalline calcium salts (hydroxyapatite). It protects the underlying tooth structure and covers the crown of the tooth to the cementoenamel junction, enabling the crown to withstand the wear of mastication. Dentin, which is softer, lies beneath the enamel and makes up the largest part of the tooth structure. Its tubules enable transport of nutrients from the dental pulp. Dentin protects the dental pulp from mechanical, thermal, and chemical irritation.

The pulp occupies the pulp chamber and is continuous with the tissues surrounding the tooth by means of the apical foramen, an opening at the apex of the root. The pulp consists primarily of vascular and neural tissues. The only type of nerve endings in the pulp are free nerve endings; any type of stimulus to the pulp is interpreted as pain.

The periodontium comprises the tissues that support the teeth, including the cementum, the periodontal ligament, the encompassing alveolar bone, and the gingiva. The bonelike cementum is softer than dentin and covers the root of the tooth, extending apically from the cementoenamel junction. Its major function is to attach the tooth to the periodontal ligament via periodontal fibers. The periodontal ligament is connective tissue that attaches the tooth to the surrounding alveolar bone and gingival tissue. The four functions of

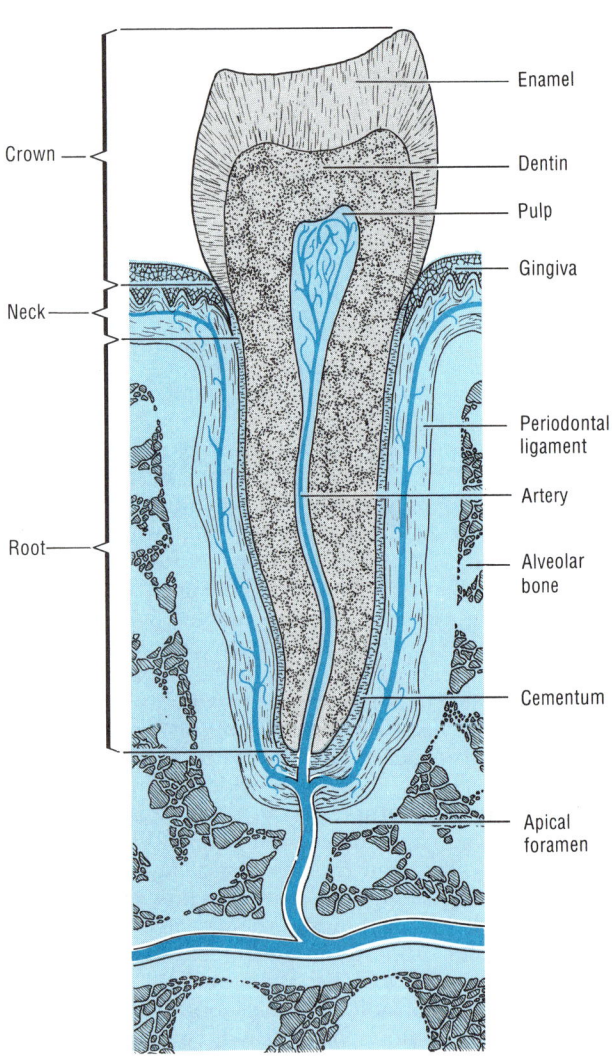

FIGURE 1 Anatomy of the tooth.

the periodontal ligament are supportive, formative, sensory, and nutritive. The alveolar bone forms the sockets of the teeth. Alveolar bone is thin and spongy, and it attaches to the principal fibers of the periodontal ligament as well as to the gingiva. And the gingiva is the soft tissue surrounding the teeth. It is normally pink and is keratinized. The gingiva is attached to the cementum by the gingival group of periodontal ligament fibers.

The mucosa covering the pharyngeal region, soft palate, floor of the mouth, vestibule (between the alveolar ridge and cheek), and cheeks is normally more pinkish-red than the gingiva. The outer surface of the mucosa is stratified squamous epithelium, but it does not have a keratinized stratum corneum outer layer as do the gingiva and hard palate, which accounts for the difference in color.

The tongue functions in mastication, swallowing, taste, and speech. Its dorsal or upper surface is usually irregular and rough in appearance. Taste buds are usually small, oval-shaped organs of flat epithelial cells surrounding a small opening (taste pore).

The major salivary glands are the parotid, submandibular, and sublingual salivary glands. They are responsible for secreting saliva, which is an alkaline, slightly viscous, clear secretion containing enzymes (lysozymes and ptyalin), albumin, epithelial mucin (a mucopolysaccharide), immune globulin, leukocytes, and minerals. Normal salivary gland function promotes good oral health in several ways. Saliva components clear carbohydrates and microorganisms from the oral cavity. Saliva also reduces the amount of acid formed by carbohydrate fermentation, and it buffers the pH fall caused by acid production. Its mineral components have a protective role in the demineralization and remineralization process of tooth enamel.

Common Oral Problems

The following sections discuss common oral problems, disease, and health concerns that pharmacists may encounter. Each section is organized to present etiology and pathophysiology; suggestions for preventive care; and guidelines for treatment, product selection, and patient counseling as appropriate.

Plaque and Calculus

Etiology and Pathophysiology

Plaque is commonly recognized as the source of microbes that cause caries and periodontal disease; thus, plaque buildup is related to the incidence of oral disease.[9] Plaque is thought to start with the formation of acquired pellicle on a clean tooth surface. Pellicle appears to be a thin, acellular, glycoprotein–mucoprotein coating that adheres to the enamel within minutes after a tooth is cleaned. Its source is thought to be saliva. The pellicle seems to serve as an attachment for cariogenic bacteria that produce, along with acids, long-chain polymers such as dextrans and levans that adhere to the pellicle and tooth surface. The resulting sticky adherent mass is called dental plaque. It is soft and readily disrupted by toothbrushing or flossing.

After meals, food residue may be incorporated into plaque by bacterial degradation. Left undisturbed, plaque thickens and bacteria proliferate. Plaque growth begins in protected cracks and fissures and along the gingival margin.[10] If not removed within 24 hours, dental plaque begins to calcify by calcium salt precipitation from the saliva and forms calculus, or tartar. This hardened, adherent deposit is removable only by professional dental cleaning.[10]

Calculus is generally considered to be a substrate on which additional plaque can develop, and it is not regarded as the primary causative oral accumulation in periodontal disease.[10] However, most periodontists agree that supra- (above) and subgingival (below the gingival margin) calculus can promote the progression of periodontal disease in several ways. Both can promote the retention of new bacterial plaque accumulation in contact with sensitive tissue sites, and both can interfere with local self-cleaning processes and patient plaque removal. Subgingival calculus also may intensify the inflammatory process. Thorough removal of subgingival calculus in periodontal therapy is an important step in delaying the reestablishment of periodontal pathogens and the resolution of inflammation.[11,12]

Plaque Removal

The best way to ensure healthy teeth and gingival tissues is to remove plaque buildup by brushing and flossing at least once a day. Toothbrushing removes plaque from the lingual (tongue) side, buccal (cheek) side, and occlusal (biting) surfaces of the teeth. Plaque found between the teeth (interproximal surfaces) can be removed efficiently only with dental floss and other aids (e.g., interproximal brush, dental tape, or rubber tip stimulator). Effective plaque removal will help prevent both dental caries and periodontal disease by removing disease-causing bacteria and preventing their growth. Eating fibrous foods such as celery, apples, or carrots does not prevent plaque accumulation or aid in its removal.[13]

Chemical management of plaque and calculus can enhance mechanical removal either by acting directly on the plaque bacteria or by disrupting components of plaque to facilitate its removal during routine oral hygiene. The use of chemical agents in plaque removal may be particularly appropriate for selected patients who may be either unable to brush and floss effectively or inhibited from doing so. Physically or mentally handicapped individuals (who may not be able to master the manual techniques necessary) and orthodontia patients or those with fixed prostheses may benefit from the addition of antiplaque agents to their oral hygiene regimen.

Products for Plaque Removal

Products for plaque removal may have cosmetic and/or therapeutic activity. Those that contain therapeutic ingredients specific to caries prevention (e.g., fluoride) or hypersensitivity are included below.

Toothbrushes and Similar Devices The toothbrush is the most universally accepted device available for removing dental plaque and maintaining good oral hygiene. Manual toothbrushes vary in size, shape, texture, and design. There are no specific recommendations as to which toothbrush is the best to use. Dentists recommend toothbrushes based on the individual patient's manual dexterity, oral anatomy, and periodontal health. The toothbrush should be of a size and shape to allow the patient to reach every tooth in the mouth. Many dentists and dental hygienists prefer soft, rounded, multitufted nylon bristle brushes. This is because nylon bristles are more durable and easier to clean than natural bristles and because soft, rounded bristle tips are more effective in removing plaque below the gingival margin and on proximal tooth surfaces. One study has shown that toothbrushes with greater bristle density are more effective at removing dental plaque.[14] Unfortunately, toothbrush firmness is not standardized; toothbrushes designated as soft, medium, or hard may not be comparable across manufacturers

Desirable characteristics to consider in selecting a toothbrush include:

- Flat head, sized to reach all parts of the mouth;
- Dense brushing surface;
- Slender, resilient nylon filaments with rounded ends.[15]

Most toothbrushes marketed in the United States have a flat handle design. There are many modifications, such as angle bends or flexible areas in the handle, that may allow contact between the bristles and some less accessible tooth surfaces. The handle should allow the patient to grasp and maneuver the brush easily.

The proper frequency and method of brushing will vary from patient to patient, depending on individual factors. After a clinical evaluation, the dentist or dental hygienist will recommend a method, time, and frequency for toothbrushing. Thoroughness of plaque removal without gingival trauma is more important than method. Patients should brush thoroughly at least once a day, preferably twice daily, taking time to clean all tooth surfaces systematically. A gentle scrubbing motion is indicated because the tips of the brush do the cleaning. Excessive force should be avoided because it may result in bristle damage, cervical abrasion, irritation of delicate gingival tissue, and gingival recession with associated hypersensitivity. Gentle brushing of the upper surface of the tongue is recommended to reduce debris, plaque, and bacteria.

How often should the patient buy a new toothbrush? There is no definite answer although 3 months has been suggested as a guide for toothbrush life expectancy. There are two major reasons for replacing toothbrushes frequently: wear and bacterial accumulation. Different methods of brushing cause bristles to wear differently. Worn, bent, or matted bristles do not remove plaque effectively. Thus, patients should replace toothbrushes at the first sign of bristle wear rather than after a set period of use, and ideally they should rotate two or three toothbrushes to allow each to dry completely between use, thereby decreasing bristle wear and matting. An innovation in the toothbrush product line is the Oral-B Indicator® (Oral-B Laboratories). This brush has a band of center bristles colored with a dye that fades with wear as a visual reminder to replace the brush.

Toothbrushes have been found to be a receptacle for bacteria. One study has reported that it takes just 17–35 days to accumulate a heavy buildup of bacteria on a toothbrush.[16] Patients with gingival or periodontal disease or with other infectious diseases of the oral tissues should change brushes every 2 weeks, and it is advisable to replace a toothbrush following a respiratory infection to prevent reinfection.[16] Patients should be advised to rinse their toothbrush thoroughly after each use to dislodge food debris and dilute sugar residue, both of which may serve as media for bacterial growth.

The American Dental Association (ADA) Council on Dental Materials, Instruments, and Equipment (CDMIE) has established a recognition program for products not currently covered by a formal acceptance program or certification. The council evaluates these products based on data regarding their safety and effectiveness for their intended use. Currently, more than 80 brands of manual toothbrushes representing more than 50 manufacturers may use the ADA logo on their packaging and advertisements, along with the statement that they are professionally recognized as being safe and effective.[17]

Standard electric toothbrushes mimic the motion of hand brushing. Although they have not proven superior to properly manipulated manual toothbrushes, electric toothbrushes may benefit patients who are mentally or physically handicapped, who lack manual dexterity, or who require someone else to clean their teeth, as well as some patients with orthodontic appliances. These devices may also be useful for young children when parents do the brushing and for patients who may be motivated by the novelty of a powered toothbrush to increase the frequency and efficiency of their oral hygiene.[18,19]

Electric toothbrushes, which are available from numerous manufacturers, use essentially three brush-head motions to clean (i.e., back and forth, up and down, and a combination pattern). Best results can be expected if a patient uses a brush carrying the ADA seal of acceptance and follows the specific directions of a dental professional. ADA criteria for acceptance are based primarily on safety concerns. Advertising may mention plaque reduction but may not claim improvement of any existing oral disease.[20] Selected ADA-accepted electric toothbrushes include the Braun/Oral-B Plaque Remover® (Braun, Inc), Epident® (Epi Products), Power Toothbrush® (Braun), Panasonic Power Floss and Brush® (Panasonic Personal Care, Inc), Plak Trac® (Windmere Corporation), Sunbeam Automatic Toothbrush® (Sunbeam Home Comfort), and Water Pik Powered Toothbrush® (Teledyne Water Pik).[21] Models such as the Water Pik® may offer an advantage for some handicapped individuals because the brushing action can be started by either depressing a button or simply applying pressure to the toothbrush bristles.

Other types of powered rotary devices for plaque removal have been marketed and evaluated. Because conventional dentifrices may clog these devices, a dentifrice specifically formulated for use with the device (e.g., Interplak® toothpaste by Bausch & Lomb) and/or a fluoride rinse is advised. The Rota-dent® (Pro-Dentec) comes with three interchangeable brush heads or tips shaped like interproximal brushes, and it rotates in a fashion similar to instruments used during a professional cleaning.[20] Clinical trials comparing the Rota-dent® with conventional manual plaque-removal devices show the Rota-dent® to be well accepted by users, generally superior to manual toothbrushes alone in removing plaque, and equivalent to manual toothbrushing when combined with a comprehensive oral hygiene program that includes instruction in the use of dental floss, toothpicks, interspace brushes, and disclosing agents.[22,23]

The Interplak Home Plaque Removal Instrument® (Bausch & Lomb Oral Care Division) has a brush head with 10 tufts of bristles arranged in two rows positioned to follow the gumline. Each tuft spins independently in the opposite direction of adjacent tufts at the rate of 4,200 rpm. If used properly, the Interplak® is more effective than manual brushing in eliminating plaque for most patients.[24] In addition, patients with orthodontic bands may find this device beneficial.

Both Rota-dent® and Interplak® have been accepted by the ADA.[21]

Oral Irrigating Devices Oral irrigators work by directing a high-pressure, steady or pulsating stream of water through a nozzle to the tooth surfaces. Studies have shown that these devices can remove only a minimal amount of plaque from tooth surfaces.[25,26] Thus, oral irrigators cannot be viewed as substitutes for a toothbrush, dental floss, or other plaque-removal devices but should be considered adjuncts in maintaining oral hygiene.[25] The ADA views these devices as potentially useful for "removing loose debris from those areas that cannot be cleaned with the toothbrush such as around orthodontic bands and fixed bridges."[25] Oral irrigators have also been valuable as vehicles for administering chemotherapeutic agents that inhibit microbial growth in inaccessible regions of the mouth.[27] Yet the ADA cautions that patients with advanced periodontal disease should use these devices only under professional supervision.[25] Oral irrigation devices should also be considered contraindicated in patients predisposed to bacterial endocarditis. Some periodontal groups have even concluded that "there is no scientific justification for recommending" the use of these devices as an aid in oral hygiene because the risks they pose for bacteremia and traumatic gingival damage may outweigh their value.[26]

Two types of oral irrigation devices are available: pulsating (intermittent low- and high-water pressure) and steady stream (constant water pressure). In general, steady-stream types are less expensive than pulsating models; however, neither type has shown superior ability to remove debris or plaque. Oral irrigators should be operated with warm or tepid water within recommended water pressure levels. Operating these devices parallel to the long axis of the teeth may traumatize soft tissue or impact food within a periodontal pocket.

The ADA has evaluated and given its seal of acceptance to several brands of irrigating devices, including Dento Spray® (Texell Products), Hydro Pik® (Gum Machine Company), Sunpak Aqua Floss Oral Irrigator® (Tocad Marketing Company), and Water Pik Oral Irrigator® (Teledyne Water Pik).[21]

Dental Floss Proximal caries and periodontal pocketing are related to plaque accumulation in the interdental areas. Interdental plaque removal has been reported to reduce gingival inflammation and prevent periodontal disease and dental caries.[25] Dental flossing is the most widely recommended method of removing dental plaque from proximal tooth surfaces not adequately cleaned by toothbrushing alone.[25] Besides removing plaque and debris interproximally, proper flossing also polishes the tooth surfaces, massages interdental papillae, and reduces gingival inflammation.

Floss is a multifilament nylon yarn that is available in waxed or unwaxed form and in varying widths, from thin thread to thick tape. Because no particular product has proven superior, patient factors such as tightness of tooth contacts, tooth roughness, and manual dexterity should be considered in product selection.[28] Clinical studies show no difference between waxed and unwaxed floss in terms of plaque removal and prevention of gingivitis,[29,30] and concern about a residual wax film deposited on tooth surfaces when using waxed floss is unfounded.[31]

Proper flossing technique requires some finger dexterity and practice. If done improperly, flossing can injure gingival tissue and cause cervical wear on proximal root surfaces.[32] Patients should be instructed to use approximately 18 in. of floss and wrap most of it around a middle finger. The remaining floss should be wound around the same finger of the opposite hand. About an inch of floss should be held between the thumbs and forefingers. The patient should not snap the floss between the teeth but should use a gentle, sawing motion to guide the floss to the gumline. When the gumline is reached, the floss should be curved into a C-shape against one tooth and gently slid into the space between the gum and tooth until there is resistance. The patient should hold the floss tightly against the tooth and gently scrape the side of the tooth while moving the floss away from the gums. Next, the patient should curve the floss around the adjoining tooth and repeat the procedure.

Waxed floss may pass interproximally between tight-fitting teeth without shredding easier than unwaxed floss. If contacts at the crowns of teeth are too tight to force floss interdentally, floss threaders can be used to pass floss between the teeth and around fixed bridges. Floss threaders, which are usually thin plastic loops or soft plastic, needle-like appliances, should be used cautiously so as not to physically traumatize the gingiva. One manufacturer offers special precut floss with a stiff "floss threader" at the end (Oral-B Super Floss®). Floss holders are recommended for patients lacking manual dexterity and for caregivers assisting handicapped or hospitalized patients. A floss holder should have one or two forks rigid enough to keep floss taut and a mounting mechanism that allows quick rethreading of floss.[28]

The ADA has recognized nearly 100 brands of dental floss and tape as safe and effective.[17]

Specialty Aids Cleaning devices that adapt to irregular tooth surfaces better than dental floss does are recommended for interproximal cleaning of teeth with large interdental spaces, such as is found in patients with periodontal disease.[28] Specialty brushes and aids are available to remove plaque from hard-to-clean areas (e.g., spaces around a fixed bridge or orthodontic bands) and dentures. The most common aids are tapered wooden toothpicks that are triangular (Stim-U-Dent®), holders for round toothpicks (Perio-aid®), miniature bottle brushes (Py-Co-Prox® or Proxabrush®), rubber stimulator tips, denture brushes, and denture clasp brushes.

Conflicting findings are reported for plaque-removal efficacy among these interproximal cleaning devices. Differences in methodology and patient populations prevent generalizations. Moreover, individual patient motivation and dexterity may influence results.[33] One study reported no difference in plaque-removal efficacy when comparing dental floss, an interdental brush, and a rubber tip stimulator used in addition to a toothbrush.[34] All three devices improved plaque removal in patients who brushed normally. Another study, which used a group of patients previously treated for periodontal disease, found the interdental brush superior to dental floss in removing plaque from large, open, interproximal spaces.[33] Patient oral anatomy, the presence of periodontal disease, the size of the interproximal spaces, and patient dexterity should all be considered when choosing an interdental cleaning aid.

Disclosing Agents Disclosing agents contain a vegetable dye (e.g., erythrosine or FD&C Red No. 3), which stains dental plaque so that the patient can easily see it. Disclosing agents are used at home by the patient for self-evaluation of plaque removal and in the dental office when the dentist is instructing the patient in proper cleaning technique. By staining the dental plaque and making it more visible, patients can evaluate their oral hygiene efforts and detect areas they missed, where more thorough brushing and flossing is indicated. The dye stains plaque but not tooth enamel, gingiva, or restorations, and it is easily rinsed away because it is soluble in water. (See color plates, photograph 2.)

Disclosing agents are available for home use as either a solution or a chewable tablet. These agents are not intended for daily or continuous long-term use; they should be used intermittently as a plaque indicator to monitor cleaning technique. Chewable tablets may be preferred for normal home use because they are individually wrapped in unit-of-use doses, thereby eliminating any problems with spilling that might occur with the liquids. The tablets are chewed, swished around the mouth, and then expectorated. Because they are sweet, usually containing mannitol or sorbitol, and brightly colored, the tablets may be mistaken for candy.[35] Thus, these products should be kept out of the reach of children, and use by children should be supervised. Solutions may be preferred in some cases because they can be applied with a cotton-tipped applicator to a handicapped patient's or child's dentition by another person, and they can be diluted with water. Disclosing products should be expectorated completely and not swallowed; the mouth should be rinsed with water and the water should also be expectorated.

Dentifrices Dentifrices are used with a toothbrush for cleaning accessible tooth surfaces. Use of a dentifrice enhances removal of dental plaque and stain, resulting in a decreased incidence of dental caries and gum disease, reduced mouth odors, and enhanced personal appearance.[36]

Dentifrices are available as powders, pastes, or gels. The powder forms commonly contain abrasive and flavoring agents and sometimes a surfactant (foaming agent). Dentifrice powders are either moistened to form a slurry and applied with a dry brush or used dry with a brush moistened with water. The powder is more abrasive when used dry. Powders have also been found to be imperfect as vehicles for therapeutic agents (i.e., fluoride).[37] The gels and pastes commonly contain an abrasive, a surfactant, a humectant (moistening agent), a binder/thickener, flavoring agents, a sweetener, and sometimes a therapeutic agent, such as fluoride for anticaries activity or potassium nitrate for treating hypersensitivity.

Dentifrice abrasives are pharmacologically inactive and insoluble compounds. Although dentifrices vary in their degree of abrasiveness, abrasiveness is an essential property for removal of stained pellicle from teeth.[36,38] Common abrasives include silicates, dicalcium phosphate, alumina trihydrate, calcium pyrophosphate, calcium carbonate, and sodium metaphosphate.[36] The ideal abrasive would maximally aid in cleaning and minimally cause damage to tooth surfaces. Unfortunately, because of the variance in patient brushing techniques and oral conditions, the ideal dentifrice abrasive does not exist. Although dentifrice abrasives do not pose a risk to dental enamel, the softer material of exposed root surfaces (cementum) and dentin can be damaged by toothbrushing action and excessive abrasiveness, which may lead to tooth hypersensitivity.[36] A radioactive dentin abrasion assay is used to determine relative dentifrice abrasivity. However, the lowest value of abrasivity required to remove stained pellicle has not been definitively established.[36]

Unless advised otherwise by their dentist, patients—especially those with periodontal disease, significant gum recession, and exposed root surfaces—should choose the least abrasive dentifrice that provides effective removal of stained pellicle. Low-abrasive dentifrices, which make up the great majority of dentifrice formulations currently marketed in the United States,[36] usually have a low concentration (10–25%) of silica abrasives, whereas high-abrasive dentifrices typically have higher concentrations (40–50%) of the inorganic calcium or aluminum salts listed above. Baking soda, a mild abrasive, has been added to some dentifrices (e.g., Colgate Baking Soda® and Arm & Hammer Dental Care®).

Surfactants are incorporated into most dentifrices because their detergent action aids in removing debris. The most frequently used surfactants are sodium lauryl sulfate and sodium dodecyl benzenesulfonate.[39] There is no evidence that surfactants in dentifrices possess anticaries activity or reduce periodontal disease, and they are considered inactive ingredients by the Food and Drug Administration (FDA).[40]

Humectants and binding agents are used in paste and gel dentifrices. The humectant (most commonly sorbitol or glycerin) provides a vehicle for other dentifrice components, prevents the preparation from drying out, and provides microbial resistance. The binder/thickener system, which commonly uses gums and silicas,[39] determines dentifrice texture, dispersibility, and appearance. Selection of the binder/thickener is determined by its compatibility with other components of the dentifrice formulation in producing the desired qualities.

Flavoring and sweetening agents are added to these preparations to make them more appealing. Sweeteners include sorbitol, glycerin, xylitol, saccharin, sodium saccharin, and aspartame. Flavoring agents, which are selected to provide a refreshing aftertaste, include essential oils and other flavorings (e.g., spearmint, wintergreen, and cinnamon).[39]

The most common therapeutic agent added to dentifrices is fluoride for its anticaries activity. Therapeutic agents are also added to treat hypersensitive dentin.

Chemical agents to control plaque and help prevent or reduce calculus formation have received much attention recently as additives to dentifrices and mouthrinses. Desirable characteristics for antiplaque agents include:

- Selective antibacterial activity and/or interference with the rate of accumulation or metabolism of supragingival plaque;
- Substantivity (sustained retention of the agent in the mouth);
- Compatibility with dentifrice ingredients;
- Lack of undesirable side effects for the user;
- Noninterference with the natural ecology of the normal oral microflora.[41,42]

Several dentifrice manufacturers make claims of antiplaque or tartar control effectiveness. Agents with antiplaque potential for inclusion in dentifrices include plant extracts (sanguinarine), metal salts (zinc and stannous), phenolic compounds (triclosan), and essential oils (thymol and eucalyptol).[41-43] The antibacterial triclosan is used in toothpastes marketed abroad. In a review of clinical studies on sanguinarine-containing dentifrices, however, only one in five trials reported a significant antiplaque effect.[44] There is little clinical data to support inclusion of enzymes (e.g., dextranases and oxidases) for antiplaque purposes, and quaternary ammonium compounds are incompatible with most conventional toothpaste ingredients.[43] Combinations of ingredients (e.g., triclosan and zinc citrate) have been shown to reduce plaque accumulation significantly and to be more effective at lower concentrations than either agent alone at higher concentrations.[41,43]

However, no dentifrice is currently accepted by the ADA as efficacious in the antiplaque/antigingivitis therapeutic category. Manufacturers of dentifrices with therapeutic potential for gingivitis and supragingival dental plaque control may voluntarily submit data to the ADA for evaluation. To gain the ADA seal for this therapeutic effect, the product must fulfill very stringent ADA guidelines.[45] Certain fluoride dentifrices for which antiplaque claims are made bear the ADA seal of approval for their anticaries effect only. Patients should not forgo the benefits of fluoride in favor of chemical antiplaque ingredients.

On the regulatory side, the FDA issued a call for data on oral health care products that make antiplaque and related claims.[46] The call for data was the initial step in developing the final segment of the rule making for over-the-counter (OTC) oral health care drug products, which will address antiplaque and related claims. Because plaque reduction or removal is intended to prevent disease (i.e., caries and periodontal disease), the FDA considers plaque removal and reduction claims to be drug claims.[46]

Two classes of oral health care products have made antiplaque claims. These classes include those products that rely on the mechanical action of abrasives to remove plaque, and those products that claim to reduce or remove plaque by chemical or antimicrobial activity. These products are available in multiple dosage forms (e.g., dentifrices, gargles, and mouthwashes). Manufacturers of products bearing antiplaque and related claims (e.g., for the "reduction or prevention" of plaque, tartar, calculus, or gingivitis) and containing active ingredients that have been marketed for such indications—and that meet conditions of FDA rules governing eligibility for review—may submit supporting safety and effectiveness data to the OTC drug review for consideration.[46]

A number of fluoride dentifrices containing anticalculus or tartar-control compounds are currently being marketed. Although plaque, not supragingival calculus, is the primary etiologic factor in marginal periodontal disease, the reduction of calculus formation is still a goal of oral hygiene.[10,47] The ingredients incorporated to prevent or retard new calculus formation are zinc chloride, zinc citrate, and soluble pyrophosphates, which act to inhibit crystal growth. A fluoride–pyrophosphate combination and a fluoride–zinc chloride dentifrice separately have yielded a range of 30–50% calculus reduction by occurrence and severity in placebo-controlled clinical trials.[47,48] Patients who form heavy calculus between dental visits may consider using a fluoride dentifrice with added tartar-control ingredients instead of a plain fluoride dentifrice. A patient's appearance may benefit from a lessening of visible supragingival calculus buildup, and reports indicate that professional dental cleaning may be easier because the calculus that does form is less adherent.[49]

The ADA regards inhibition of supragingival calculus as a nontherapeutic use and therefore does not evaluate anticalculus claims. However, all advertising claims made for accepted products are reviewed for accuracy. The ADA has directed that the following additional statement appear on all package and container labeling for accepted fluoride dentifrice products with calculus-control activity: "[Product name] has been shown to reduce the formation of tartar above the gumline, but has not been shown to have a therapeutic effect on periodontal diseases."[49]

Use of tartar-control toothpastes has been related to a type of contact dermatitis in the perioral region.[50] The addition of pyrophosphate compounds to these products increases alkalinity and requires increased concentrations of other components, such as flavorings and surfactants for solubilizing. It is hypothesized that the pyrophosphates, either alone or in combination with the higher concentrations of inactive ingredients, are implicated as the cause of an irritant contact dermatitis. Patients experiencing such a reaction should be advised to discontinue the tartar-control dentifrice and switch to a non–tartar-control fluoride product. The skin eruption has been shown to resolve by decreasing or eliminating exposure.[50]

Cosmetic dentifrices make no therapeutic claims and are usually chosen by patients because of taste, "whitening" ability, or antistain properties. Dentifrices claiming to remove stubborn coffee or tobacco stains are sometimes more abrasive than other formulations and should not be used by patients with exposed root surfaces. Baking soda or toothpastes containing baking soda will have a polishing effect. Other products may contain a pigment (e.g., titanium dioxide) that produces a temporary brightening effect. Rembrandt Whitening Toothpaste® (Den-Mat) contains a chemical complex of aluminum oxide, a citrate salt, and papain. Whitening dentifrices containing oxygenating agents are now considered drugs by the FDA and are discussed in the section on tooth whiteners.

Popular gel dentifrices are flavored and disperse rapidly in the mouth. Manufacturers of gel dentifrices have advertised that children brush longer and more thoroughly because of the gel's consistency, translucence, dispersibility, and flavor. This claim has not been substantiated, but many dentifrices marketed for children are of the gel type. The children's products usually have fruit flavors rather than the breath-freshening minty or cinnamon flavors that adults prefer.

Mouthrinses (Mouthwashes) Mouthrinse and dentifrice formulations are very similar. Like dentifrices, mouthrinses may be cosmetic or therapeutic. Both may contain surfactant(s), humectant(s), flavor, coloring, water, and therapeutic ingredient(s). A mouthrinse approximates a diluted liquid dentifrice containing ethanol and no abrasive. Alcohol adds bite and freshness, enhances flavor, solubilizes other ingredients, and contributes to the cleansing action and antibacterial activity. Flavor contributes to pleasant taste and breath freshening. Surfactants are foaming agents which aid in removal of debris. Other ingredients may include astringents, demulcents (soothing agents), antibacterial agents, and fluoride.[51] New additions to the mouthrinse category include dry formulations that contain ingestible surfactants rather than alcohol (Spritz® by Spectrum Consumer Products).

Mouthrinses can be classified by appearance, alcohol content, and active ingredients. In general, mouthrinses are minty (green or blue) or spicy (red), medicinal or alcoholic, and they contain various miscellaneous ingredients. Aromatic oils include thymol, eucalyptol, menthol, and methyl salicylate; these oils are antibacterial and have some local anesthetic activity. Benzoic acid is an antimicrobial agent, and cetylpyridinium chloride is a cationic surfactant capable of bactericidal activity although it does not penetrate plaque well. Domiphen bromide is a bactericidal agent similar to cetylpyridinium. Glycerin is a topical protectant that tastes sweet and is soothing to oral mucosa. Zinc chloride/citrate is an astringent that neutralizes odoriferous sulfur compounds produced in the oral cavity. Phenol is a local anesthetic, antiseptic, and bactericidal agent that penetrates plaque better than either cetylpyridinium or domiphen.

The alcohol content in mouthrinses ranges from 14 to 27% and constitutes a danger for young children who may be attracted by bright colors and pleasant flavors. Acute alcoholic intoxication and death resulting from high-dose ingestion is possible. Therefore, these products should be kept out of the reach of children.[52]

Cosmetic mouthrinses freshen the breath and clean some debris. The most popular cosmetic mouthrinses are phenolic (medicinal) and minty. To have some degree of oral malodor (e.g., morning breath) is normal in a healthy individual. This is because reduced activity of tongue, cheeks, and salivary flow enhance bacterial activity and production of odoriferous sulfur compounds.[51] Thus, products that are intended to eliminate or suppress mouth odor of local origin in healthy persons with healthy mouths are considered by the FDA Advisory Review Panel on Over-the-Counter Oral Health Care Products to be cosmetics unless they contain antimicrobial or other therapeutic agents,[53] and the ADA acceptance program does not evaluate mouthrinses labeled and advertised only as cosmetic agents. An important consideration is the potential for breath-freshening mouthrinses to disguise and delay treatment of pathologic conditions that may contribute to lingering oral malodor (e.g., periodontal disease, purulent oral infections, and respiratory infections). The ADA suggests that "if marked breath odor persists after proper toothbrushing, the cause should be investigated" and not masked with mouthwash.[54]

Over the last decade there has been a proliferation of nonprescription mouthrinses promoted for antiplaque or tartar-control activity. Ingredients added to mouthrinses for plaque control include agents with antimicrobial activity such as quaternary ammonium compounds (cetylpyridinium and domiphen), plant extracts (sanguinarine), and aromatic oils (thymol, eucalyptol, menthol, and methyl salicylate). Another approach uses a detergent system based on sodium benzoate to loosen plaque for easier removal.

Regarding products for chemotherapeutic control of plaque and gingivitis, the ADA acceptance program invites manufacturers to submit data voluntarily.[45] Listerine® (Warner-Lambert) was the first mouthrinse to be accepted by the ADA as a nonprescription antiplaque/antigingivitis mouthrinse. The ADA has authorized use of the following label statement:

> Listerine has been shown to help prevent and reduce supragingival plaque accumulation and gingivitis when used in a conscientiously applied program of oral hygiene and regular professional care. It has not been shown to have a therapeutic effect on periodontitis.[55]

The ADA has since accepted Cool Mint Listerine® and an increasing number of private-label antiseptic mouthrinses in the antiplaque/antigingivitis category of accepted therapeutic products.[56]

Viadent® (Vipont) rinse contains sanguinaria extract in combination with zinc chloride. Although sanguinarine has shown effectiveness against plaque-forming bacteria in vitro, results from controlled clinical trials using the rinse alone or in conjunction with Viadent® dentifrice have been mixed. Widely divergent findings ranging from significant reduction of plaque and gingivitis to negligible or no effect have been reported in numerous short-term and several long-term clinical studies.[44]

Clinical trials with mouthrinses containing cetylpyridinium chloride alone or in combination with domiphen bromide have reported reductions in plaque accumulation.[57] Based on available data, the potential for oral toxicity with these agents is low, and the potential for a gingival health benefit exists.[42,58,59] However, studies consistent with ADA guidelines have not been evaluated, and further study is needed to substantiate antigingivitis efficacy. At least one study has reported no difference in plaque control and gingival health between a cetylpyridinium rinse and placebo when the former was used as a prebrushing rinse.[59] It was suggested that the order of rinsing and brushing may be relevant: reduced activity may have been influenced by the interaction of the cationic surfactant with anionic detergents in the toothpaste. Rinsing after brushing or at a time separate from brushing may be indicated. Because cetylpyridinium is chemically related to chlorhexidine, it too may stain teeth, but to a much lesser degree.[59] Staining is usually associated with overuse.

Another approach to plaque control does not rely on antimicrobial activity but is based on principles of detergent action to loosen plaque. Plax® (Pfizer Oral Care Division) is intended for use as a prebrushing rinse. The detergent system includes sodium lauryl sulfate and sodium benzoate. However, findings reported in clinical trials are contradictory. Early reports of efficacy for plaque removal based on short-term clinical trials have not been consistently supported,[60,61] and a number of studies report that the use of Plax® yielded results comparable to those of placebo.[62–64]

Mouthrinses claiming anticalculus or tartar-control activity contain the same active ingredients as anticalculus dentifrices. The ADA regards inhibition of supragingival calculus as a nontherapeutic use and does not evaluate mouthrinse anticalculus claims. However, the mouthrinses are included with dentifrices in the FDA call for data and will be reviewed in evaluating antiplaque and related claims.

Patients should be cautioned that use of a mouthrinse with plaque or calculus control properties does not substitute for normal oral hygiene. These products are adjunctive to proper toothbrushing and flossing, and, in most cases, further research is necessary to determine how efficacious their antiplaque activity is. The benefits of fluoride should not be overlooked in favor of a plaque-control formula without fluoride. The rinses are intended for use twice daily after brushing, with the exception of Plax®, which should be used prior to brushing. In general, an amount equal to 1 to 2 tbsp of rinse should be swished vigorously in the mouth and between the teeth for about 30 seconds and then expectorated. The rinses should not be swallowed. Patients should be advised to refrain from smoking, eating, or drinking for 30 minutes following use. These products are generally safe when used as directed, but occasional adverse reactions have been reported. Overuse should be discouraged. Consultation with a health professional is indicated if irritation occurs and persists after use of the product is discontinued. Unsupervised use is contraindicated in patients with mouth irritation or ulceration. These products should be kept out of the reach of children.[57]

Tooth Whiteners Tooth whiteners containing oxidizing agents were previously marketed as cosmetics but are now considered drugs by the FDA. The drug classification makes the products subject to rigorous new drug application requirements to document their safety and effectiveness. Safety concerns relate to the long-term exposure of oral tissue to oxidizing agents. These concerns include (1) the possibility of soft tissue damage or delayed wound healing, (2) the potential for damage to tooth pulp, and (3) the potential for mutating or enhancing the carcinogenic effects of other agents (e.g., tobacco). The ADA accepts none of the available products for use as tooth-whitening agents, pending submission of sufficient safety and efficacy data.[65]

Tooth whiteners, which claim to bleach teeth, contain oxidizing ingredients such as hydrogen peroxide, carbamide peroxide, or perhydrol urea in gel or liquid form. Some kits marketed directly to consumers for unsupervised home use include a mouth tray for directly applying the bleaching agent to the teeth.

Early reports of dentist-supervised home bleaching of natural teeth began with the use of nonprescription products containing 10% topical carbamide peroxide (Gly-Oxide® and Proxigel®) that were intended for oral wound cleansing.[66] Products specifically marketed to dentists for home tooth bleaching also contain 10% carbamide peroxide as the active oxidizing agent (Omni White & Brite® by Omni International and Rembrandt Lighten Gel® by Den-Mat). Patients were instructed to expose extrinsically stained teeth to the peroxide gel by using custom-made mouth trays coated with a thin gel film. Anecdotal reports of successful tooth bleaching emerged. One double-blind study reported effective whitening with minimal and reversible adverse effects during treatment.[65] Further research is needed, however, to determine the long-term effects of oral tissue exposure to 10% carbamide peroxide and the degree of tooth whitening retained over time. Patients should be strongly discouraged from attempting tooth bleaching without a dentist's direct supervision because serious adverse effects from misuse or overuse of such products have been reported.[67]

Periodontal Disease

Periodontal disease is associated with oral hygiene status, not age. As life spans increase and people retain more teeth later in life, both the number of teeth at risk and the time for risk of periodontal disease increases.[68]

Etiology and Pathophysiology

The primary etiologic cause of periodontal disease is accumulated bacterial plaque.[69] The basic pathologic process is inflammatory. The more common forms of periodontal disease are gingivitis (an inflammation of the gingiva), which is the mildest form, is reversible, and affects nearly everyone; acute necrotizing ulcerative gingivitis (ANUG); and periodontitis, which, when severe, can cause significant, irreversible alveolar bone loss.

Gingivitis The etiology of gingivitis is thought to be associated with the accumulation of supragingival plaque. The marginal gingiva (the border of the gingiva surrounding the neck of the tooth) is held firmly to the tooth by a network of collagen fibers. Microorganisms present in the plaque in the gingival sulcus (the space between the gingiva and the tooth) are capable of producing harmful products such as acids, toxins, and enzymes that damage cellular and intercellular tissue. Dilatation and proliferation of gingival capillaries, increased flow of gingival fluid, and increased blood flow with resultant erythema of the gingiva are found in early stages. The gingiva may also enlarge, change contour, and appear puffy or swollen as a result of the inflammation. (See color plates, photograph 3.) The inflamed gingiva generally bleeds readily when probed or during toothbrushing; pink-tinted toothbrush bristles should be a sign to patients of possible gingivitis. In the early stage of gingivitis, it is possible to reverse the inflammatory process with effective oral hygiene.

In time and with neglect, the condition becomes chronic as capillaries become engorged, venous return is slowed, and localized anoxemia gives a bluish hue to areas of the reddened gingiva. The flat knife-edge appearance of healthy gingiva is replaced by a ragged or rounded edge. The presence of red cells in extravascular tissue and the breakdown of hemoglobin also deepen the color of gingival tissue. Progression of these conditions is usually slow, insidious, and often painless.

Chronic gingivitis may be localized to the area around one or several teeth, or it may be generalized, involving the gingiva around all the teeth. The inflammation may involve just the marginal gingiva, or it may be more diffuse and involve all the gingival tissue surrounding the tooth. Changes in gingival color, size, and shape, and ease of gingival bleeding, are common indications of chronic gingivitis that the patient as well as the pharmacist can recognize.

Left untreated, chronic gingivitis is a common precursor to the more advanced inflammatory condition of chronic destructive periodontal disease, or periodontitis. Bacterial species that predominate in periodontitis but are not present in healthy periodontium have been found in low proportions in gingivitis. Progression of pathophysiology in gingivitis may favor the growth of species implicated in periodontitis.

Acute Necrotizing Ulcerative Gingivitis ANUG, also referred to as Vincent's stomatitis and trench mouth, is an acute bacterial infection characterized by necrosis and ulceration of the gingival surface with underlying inflammation. The disease most commonly starts in the gingiva between teeth and displays "punched-out" papillae (the raised interproximal gingiva). The interdental and marginal gingiva exhibit a necrotic and grayish slough, while the adjacent gingiva usually exhibits marked erythema. The disease may involve a single tooth, a group of teeth, or the entire oral cavity. Accompanying symptoms often include severe pain, bleeding gingival tissue, halitosis, foul taste, and increased salivation. Lymphadenopathy, fever, and malaise may accompany the localized symptoms.

ANUG is seen most frequently in the United States in teenagers and young adults. Predisposing factors include anxiety, emotional stress, smoking, malnutrition, and poor oral hygiene. Factors resulting in decreased host resistance that alter the host–bacteria relationship have been implicated.[70] Treatment consists of local debridement and elimination of predisposing factors coupled with systemic drug therapy.

Periodontitis Periodontitis and gingivitis, the two most common periodontal diseases, can be distinguished in the following way. As previously discussed, gingivitis is the inflammation of the gingiva without loss or migration of epithelial attachment to the tooth. Periodontitis occurs when the periodontal ligament attachment and alveolar bone support of the tooth have been compromised or lost.[71] This process involves apical migration of the epithelial attachment from the enamel to the root surface. (See color plates, photograph 4.)

The American Academy of Periodontology (AAP) has classified periodontal disease in adults as follows:[71]

- *AAP classification*: Type I, Type II, Type III, and Type IV;
- *Epidemiologic*: moderately and rapidly progressing;
- *Clinical (based on response to treatment)*: refractory and recurrent.

The AAP describes Type I adult periodontitis as gingivitis characterized by changes in color, form, position, and surface appearance, and by the presence of bleeding or exudate. Type II is slight periodontitis characterized by the progression of gingival inflammation into deeper tissues and the alveolar bony crest. The periodontal pocket is 3 to 4 mm deep, and there is slight loss of connective attachment and alveolar bone. Type III is moderate periodontitis characterized by a noticeable loss of bone support and possible increased tooth mobility. Type IV is advanced periodontitis characterized by a major loss of alveolar bone support usually accompanied by increased tooth mobility.[71,72]

Adult periodontitis, especially slight or moderate, is very common. Most adults with periodontitis have moderately progressing disease, and perhaps 10% have rapidly progressing disease. As shown in the AAP classification system, diagnosis of adult periodontal disease can be based on the response to therapy.[71] Recurrent periodontitis is the destruction of the attachment apparatus occurring in a patient who has been successfully treated in the past. It often results from inadequate maintenance therapy and is relatively common. It appears to occur in localized areas but may be generalized in immunodeficient patients. Refractory, progressive periodontitis displays a continuous progression that is resistant to therapy.[71]

AAP has classified periodontal disease in juveniles as either localized or generalized. However, periodontitis in juveniles is relatively rare. Localized juvenile periodontitis (LJP) affects less than 1% of teenagers and young adults. Children in the 10- to 15-year age range are at greatest risk.[47] LJP is characterized by pocket formation, attachment loss, and alveolar bone loss primarily affecting the first molars and incisors. Occasionally, premolars and second molars are involved. These patients rarely display gingivitis and have little or no plaque or calculus. LJP displays a marked familial tendency and is associated with a particular type of bacteria. Generalized juvenile periodontitis (GJP) affects a slightly older age group and is much less prevalent than LJP. Severe gingival inflammation with extensive plaque and calculus deposits distinguishes GJP from LJP.

A dental periodontal examination includes an assessment of the gingiva and attachment apparatus and an examination of the entire periodontium with charting of all teeth in the dental record. The gingiva is assessed visually and by gingival bleeding measures. Periodontal probing measures pocket depth and attachment levels. Tooth mobility measurements and a radiographic survey of alveolar bone levels should also be included.[72] Patients have a good prognosis if an initial comprehensive course of therapy is successful. Unfortunately, alveolar bone loss is irreversible. Prospects for disease control are not good if plaque and calculus control is poor or if resolution of inflammation is inadequate despite comprehensive treatment.[72]

Prevention of Periodontal Disease

Adequate removal and control of supragingival plaque is the single most important factor in preventing and controlling periodontal disease. Accumulation of supragingival plaque over time can result in gingivitis. Removal of plaque can reverse gingivitis and reduce accumulation of calculus. If supragingival plaque accumulation is not controlled, it proliferates and invades subgingival spaces. At the same time, the composition of the bacterial flora changes to a more complex mix of organisms; specific types of bacteria are associated with plaque at different stages of accumulation.[73] The transition to subgingival plaque accumulation is significant because the patient cannot remove subgingival plaque adequately by mechanical means. Although not all periodontitis is preceded by gingivitis, the progression from supragingival plaque to gingivitis to periodontitis is relatively common, and an approach to limiting periodontitis is thus to control gingivitis.[45]

Dental Caries

Etiology and Pathophysiology

Dental caries is a destructive microbial disease that affects the calcified tissues of the teeth. Certain plaque bacteria generate acid from dietary carbohydrates; the acid demineralizes tooth enamel, leading to the formation of carious lesions that will eventually destroy the tooth if left untreated. Dental caries formation requires growth and implantation of cariogenic microorganisms (e.g., *Streptococcus mutans*, *Lactobacillus casei*, and *Actinomyces viscosus*) on exposed surfaces. If oral hygiene is neglected, dental plaque containing these organisms remains on the tooth surfaces, allowing the carious process to proceed.

Low molecular weight carbohydrates (sugars) readily diffuse into plaque and are quickly metabolized by the bacteria, resulting in a lowered plaque pH. The pH is reduced to a level which can cause demineralization of dental enamel. Repeated and frequent sugar intake will keep plaque pH depressed and thus support demineralization of enamel. Although sucrose is the most cariogenic sugar, other types of fermentable carbohydrates, such as fructose and lactose, also are cariogenic.[13]

Saccharin, a potent noncariogenic sugar substitute, is still widely used. Oral hygiene products such as mouthwashes and dentifrices contain low concentrations of saccharin that appear to present no hazard.[74] The FDA limit on saccharin is 1.0 g per day for adults; ingestion from normal use of both mouthwash and dentifrice would result in total saccharin expose of only about 20–40 mg per day.[74] Other sugar substitutes such as sorbitol, aspartame, and xylitol are currently used to sweeten a wide variety of products. Claims for the noncariogenicity of sorbitol need substantiation through further clinical trials.[75] Xylitol has been shown to be noncariogenic and aspartame appears to be so. Moreover, some clinical trials have reported that xylitol-containing chewing gum is cariostatic.[76] Gum chewing is associated with increased salivary flow, which apparently produces a beneficial buffering effect against acids in the oral cavity.[77]

The carious process is characterized by alternating periods of destruction and repair. Demineralization is caused by organic acids, such as lactic acid, produced (usually anaerobically) by microorganisms present in dental plaque. This demineralization is chronic in nature. A carious lesion starts slowly on the enamel surface and initially produces no clinical symptoms. Once the demineralization progresses through the enamel to the softer dentin, the destruction is much more rapid and becomes clinically evident as a carious lesion. At this point, the patient can become aware of the process by visualization or by symptoms of sensitivity to stimuli such as heat, cold, or percussion (chewing). If untreated, the carious lesion can result in damage to the dental pulp itself (with continuous pain as a common symptom) and, eventually, necrosis of vital pulp tissue. Because an opening exists between the pulp and surrounding supporting tissues via the apical foramen, the infectious process can progress apically and result in bone loss, abscesses, cellulitis, or osteomyelitis. Saliva, rich in calcium and phosphate ions, has a role in remineralizing early carious lesions. Fluoride ion in the mouth also promotes remineralization and thus retards enamel dissolution.

Prevention

Because a combination of diet (carbohydrate substrate), oral bacteria, and host resistance is involved in the process, intervention to prevent dental caries should be aimed at modifying these factors.[78] Frequency of refined carbohydrate intake should be reduced; plaque, which supports cariogenic bacterial growth, should be removed as discussed previously; and host resistance should be increased through appropriate exposure to fluoride ion. The declining prevalence of dental caries in children may be attributed to a combination of these interventions (e.g., increased exposure to fluoride in drinking water, dentifrices, and mouthrinses; changed patterns of diet; and improved oral hygiene).[13]

The Role of Fluoride   Fluoride is thought to help prevent dental caries owing to a combination of effects. Incorporated into developing teeth, fluoride systemically reduces the solubility of dental enamel by enhancing the development of a fluoridated hydroxyapatite (which is more resistant to demineralizing acids) at the enamel surface. The topical effect may aid in remineralizing early carious lesions during repeated cycles of demineralization and remineralization. There is some evidence that fluoride interferes with the bacterial cariogenic process. Fluoride that is chemically bound to organic constituents of plaque may interfere with plaque adherence and may inhibit glycolysis, the process by which sugar is metabolized to produce acid. Another possible mechanism proposes that fluoride may have specific bactericidal action on cariogenic bacteria in the plaque.[79]

Fluoridation of the public water supply is an effective and economically sound public health measure that has played a major role in decreasing the incidence of caries. More than half of the U.S. population resides in communities whose public water supply contains either naturally occurring or added fluoride at optimal levels for decay prevention (e.g., 1 ppm or 1 mg/L).[80] Besides the reduction of dental caries in children, benefits of fluoridation extend through adulthood, resulting in fewer decayed, missing, or filled teeth; greater tooth retention; and a lower incidence of root caries. Any decision to supplement fluoride intake depends on the concentration of fluoride present in the drinking water.[81,82] Systemic fluoride supplementation in children is based on the preventive mechanism of fluoride when incorporated into developing enamel. Current concepts of the action of fluoride relative to its presence in saliva and plaque provide a rationale for its topical application to prevent caries in all age groups.

Nonprescription topical fluoride-containing products such as dentifrices, mouthrinses, and self-applied gels provide a means of increasing contact of fluoride with the tooth surfaces.[83] Using a combination of fluoride-containing dental products results in additive anticaries activity. Fluoride exerts its greatest protection on the smooth surfaces of the teeth, but although brushing with a fluoride dentifrice provides anticaries protection, the fluoride does not reach the surfaces between teeth adequately. Patient groups with high caries activity or risk (e.g., orthodontic or medically compromised patients, patients with a nonfluoridated water supply, and patients with exposed root surfaces) may especially benefit from multiple sources of fluoride application. Fluoride-containing dental products are thought to be of greatest benefit when used in areas with a nonfluoridated public water supply; however, they can help reduce the caries incidence even in patients residing in communities with a fluoridated water supply.[84] The FDA has proposed that the following statement be applied to fluoride-containing dental care products: "The combined daily use of a fluoride treatment ('rinse' or 'gel') and a fluoride toothpaste can aid in reducing the incidence of dental cavities."[85]

Fluoride Dentifrices Use of fluoride-containing dentifrice is the one method of caries prevention common to all countries that show a reduction in caries.[86] Fluoride-containing toothpaste and gel dentifrice formulations with abrasive systems compatible with delivery of the fluoride compound, are accepted by the ADA as being safe and effective in caries prevention. Powder dentifrices have been found to be imperfect as vehicles for fluoride delivery because the amount of fluoride ion delivered to the teeth may vary significantly with patient application. The FDA has proposed classifying powdered fluoride-containing dentifrices in Category III.[37]

Sodium monofluorophosphate (0.76% or 0.80%) has been the most widely used fluoride compound because of its compatibility with a variety of abrasive systems. The number of accepted sodium fluoride dentifrices has increased with the development of compatible abrasive systems; most dentifrices contain 0.24% sodium fluoride.[84] Inadequate evidence exists to support differences in clinical effectiveness among different fluoride agents at the same 1,000-ppm fluoride ion concentration in toothpastes properly formulated with compatible components. The FDA has classified as Category I and equated the efficacy of 0.22% sodium fluoride, 0.76% sodium monofluorophosphate, and 0.4% stannous fluoride dentifrices containing 1,000 ppm fluoride ion in a compatible base.[87] No major differences were found in a review of approximately 51 studies comparing a fluoride toothpaste (either sodium fluoride or sodium monofluorophosphate) with placebo, and both agents produced an overall average caries reduction rate of 21 to 22%.[88]

Included among the ADA-accepted dentifrices are the standard 1,000-ppm and 1,100-ppm fluoride ion concentrations as well as a more recent 1,500-ppm fluoride ion product. This extra-strength monofluorophosphate product is clinically and statistically superior to its regular-strength monofluorophosphate counterpart.[89] However, because of concerns about excessive fluoride ingestion in children, the current ADA limit of 260 mg of fluoride per dentifrice container has been retained, and the ADA has required that the following directions appear on the Extra-Strength Aim® carton:

- Not for use by children under 2 years of age;
- To prevent swallowing, children 6 years of age or younger should be supervised while using the dentifrice;
- Brush teeth thoroughly, at least once daily.[89]

Conclusions from a recent review of clinical studies comparing high-potency fluoride dentifrices with conventional concentrations are reported in Table 1.[90]

Fluoride Mouthrinses and Gels ADA-accepted nonprescription fluoride mouthrinse products for topical home use include ACT®, ACT for Kids®, and Reach Fluoride Dental Rinse® (Johnson & Johnson); Fluorigard® (Colgate-Palmolive); and Ghostbusters Anti-Cavity Dental Rinse® (Perio Products).[91] These mouthrinses are therapeutic in that their common ingredient, 0.05% sodium fluoride, is a consistently effective anticaries agent. A number of fluoride gels are accepted by the ADA as well. Active ingredients of the gel formulations intended for home use are neutral or acidulated 1.1% sodium fluoride or 0.4% stannous fluoride.

Fluoride mouthrinsing enables patients to apply fluoride interproximally. Studies of fluoride mouthrinsing have given consistently positive results. Studies in which subjects used 0.05% sodium fluoride rinse once daily have demonstrated a significant reduction in caries incidence (17–47%), especially among children living in areas with nonfluoridated water.[92] Orthodontic patients may benefit because they are at risk of developing decalcified areas while under treatment and their ability to clean interdental spaces thoroughly may be inhibited.[92]

When recommending a nonprescription sodium fluoride mouthrinse, the pharmacist should stress that:

- The fluoride rinse should be used after cleaning the teeth and should be expectorated;
- Nothing should be taken by mouth for 30 minutes after use;
- The mouthrinse can benefit the patient for as long as the patient has natural dentition;
- The fluoride is preventive in action and will not cure already-carious teeth.[93]

TABLE 1 Review of clinical studies of high-potency fluoride dentifrices

Fluoride ion concentration (ppm) of compared dentifrices	Fluoride compound[a]	Cariostatic activity
1,500 versus 1,100	NaMFP	Higher concentration superior
2,000–2,500 versus 1,000	NaMFP	Higher concentration superior
2,800 versus 1,100	NaF	Higher concentration superior
2,000–2,500 versus 1,500	NaMFP	Insufficient evidence to support that higher concentration is superior
Combination versus either compound alone at equal total fluoride concentrations	NaF & NaMFP	No evidence to support that combination products are superior
High-potency combination (1,450–2,500) versus either mixed or single compound at conventional concentration (1,000–1,100)	NaF & NaMFP	Additional evidence needed to support trend that high-potency mixed products are superior

[a]NaMFP = Sodium monofluorophosphate; NaF = Sodium fluoride.
Adapted from Ripa LW. Clinical studies of high-potency fluoride dentifrices: a review. *J Am Dent Assoc* 1989; 118: 85–91.

Fluoride rinses provide a therapeutic fluoride treatment; they should not be confused with a mouthrinse, and package directions should be followed closely.

The self-applied fluoride gels are used once daily after the teeth are brushed with a fluoride dentifrice. The gel is a fluoride treatment and should not be confused with a gel form of fluoride dentifrice. The gel is brushed on the teeth, left for 1 minute, and then expectorated, not swallowed. Some concern has been raised about whether unsupervised home use of the fluoride gels is justified.[92]

Orofacial Pain

Toothache

Toothache usually indicates dental pathology involving tooth substance, dental pulp, or the supporting periodontium. Pain may also be referred to the teeth from the sinuses, eyes, or ears. Untreated dental caries will progress to destroy the barrier of enamel and dentin, allowing bacteria to reach the pulp. The inflammatory response to bacteria in the pulp will stimulate free nerve endings, resulting in pulpalgia or common toothache. The nociceptors in dental pulp are capable of only one perception in response to any stimulus strong enough to elicit a response.[94] That perception is pain. Pain may be intermittent, often indicating viable pulp with reversible damage. If pain is continuous and throbbing, this usually indicates irreversible pulp damage.

The patient with toothache should be advised to seek professional dental assistance. If swelling or fever is present, this usually indicates the need for antibiotic therapy. If the patient wears a removable prosthesis that attaches to the painful tooth, removing the appliance may help temporarily. Nonprescription analgesics such as ibuprofen, aspirin, or acetaminophen may be taken internally for short-term pain relief; however, none of these products, and particularly not aspirin, should ever be placed locally on gingival tissue or in a cavity; doing so can result in chemical burns of sensitive tissue. (See color plates, photograph 5.) Even if aspirin, ibuprofen, or acetaminophen is effective in relieving pain due to toothache, the patient should seek professional dental help as soon as possible.

The FDA has limited the definition of an agent for the relief of toothache to "ingredients placed in a tooth cavity to relieve throbbing, persistent pain resulting from an open cavity in the tooth."[95] Currently, there are no Category I agents for this purpose. Topical oral mucosal anesthetics/analgesics classified as Category I for relief of pain associated with minor irritation or injury to soft tissue are not considered effective for relieving toothache from a cavity and therefore have been classified as Category III for this purpose. Also, the FDA has reclassified eugenol from Category I to Category III, citing the need for controlled clinical investigations that demonstrate its effectiveness in relieving toothache.[95] The ADA accepts eugenol and clove oil for professional use by the dentist; however, although 85% eugenol has historically been used as a nonprescription toothache remedy, the ADA has not accepted eugenol or clove oil as safe and effective nonprescription drugs for toothache. These drugs are generally ineffective in the hands of the patient and can cause damage to viable pulp and soft tissue.

The FDA advisory review panel has recommended that beeswax not be included as an inactive ingredient in products intended for use in an open tooth cavity.[95] Such occlusive inactive ingredients are discouraged because they form a physical barrier and may prevent the escape of fluids and gases from a degenerating pulp. Of equal concern is the potential for patients to use the product as a temporary filling and to delay seeking professional treatment.

Hypersensitive Teeth
Tooth hypersensitivity affects approximately 40 million adults at some time, and about one-fourth of these adults experience a chronic condition.[38] Hypersensitive teeth result from exposed areas of the root at the cementoenamel junction. Exposed dentin allows stimuli to reach the nerve fibers within the pulp. Causes of dentinal hypersensitivity may relate to braces, postsurgical condition, gum recession, trauma, or excessive brushing with an abrasive dentifrice or hard bristle brush. Pain may be intense and may condition patients to limit oral hygiene, which in turn will contribute to plaque accumulation and progression of oral plaque diseases.[96] A patient who has self-diagnosed sensitive teeth should be referred to a dentist for consultation because there may be an underlying cause for pain that requires immediate treatment. However, once the dentist diagnoses it as dentinal hypersensitivity, this condition can be treated with a desensitizing dentifrice.

A tooth desensitizer acts on the dentin to block the perception of stimuli that are not usually perceived by subjects with normal teeth. Because the most common cause of tooth sensitivity is exposed dentin, a desensitizing dentifrice must inhibit sensitization while being nonabrasive. Two well-controlled clinical studies and three supportive studies provided sufficient data to the FDA to establish the effectiveness of 5% potassium nitrate for protection against painful sensitivity of the teeth due to cold, heat, acids, sweets, or contact. As a tooth desensitizer, 5% potassium nitrate remains the only Category I agent at this time.[95] Dibasic sodium citrate in pluronic gel and 10% strontium chloride were classified as Category III pending further evidence of effectiveness. ADA-accepted desensitizing dentifrices containing 5% potassium nitrate as the active ingredient include Denquel® (Proctor & Gamble), Mint Sensodyne®, and Promise® (Block Drug).[97]

Patients should be advised to apply at least a 1-in. strip of dentifrice to a soft bristle brush and to use the product twice daily for optimum effectiveness. Brushing thoroughly for at least 1 minute will apply the desensitizing agent to all sensitive surfaces. Onset of effect is not immediate and may take several days to 2 weeks. These dentifrices should be used until the sensitivity subsides or as long as recommended by a dentist. The patient should then switch to a low-abrasion dentifrice. Patients with hypersensitive teeth should avoid any toothpaste that is highly abrasive or promoted for whitening effect. The FDA has proposed a Category I classification for the combination of a Category I fluoride ingredient with 5% potassium nitrate for use in relieving dentinal hypersensitivity and preventing dental caries.[98] Such a product would be a good recommendation. However, dentifrices containing 5% potassium nitrate are not recommended for children under 12 years of age.

Fractured Dentition and Restorations
Fractures of the natural dentition should be treated by a dentist without delay. Besides being aesthetically unappealing (especially if it involves an anterior tooth), fractured teeth can result in pulp exposure, pain, irritation to adjacent soft tissues, malocclusion, rapid carious breakdown, compromised mastication, and infection. Minor chips in the tooth's crown may be adequately repaired with restorative materials and techniques. However, a large fracture may require endodontic treatment (root canal therapy), extensive restorative procedures, or extraction of the tooth.

Loose, displaced, or broken dental restorations (fillings) and nonremovable prostheses (crowns and bridges) may result in loss of normal function, tooth breakdown, or malocclusion. Only a dentist can evaluate and treat these conditions adequately.

Oral Mucosal Lesions

Oral Malignancies
Approximately 30,000 people are diagnosed with oral cancer each year in the United States. This presents approximately 4% of all cancers. Because of the serious consequences, oral cancer must always be considered in the differential diagnosis of persistent oral lesions. The most common form of oral cancer is squamous cell carcinoma, accounting for 90% of oral malignancies. Most oropharyngeal squamous cell carcinomas occur in persons over 50 years of age.[6] Clinically, oral carcinomas can appear as red or white lesions, ulcerations, or tumors.

As with other carcinomas, the cause of oral and perioral carcinomas is unknown; however, certain lifestyle behaviors have been identified as risk factors. Smoking, the use of smokeless tobacco products, and the excessive consumption of alcoholic beverages contribute to a higher risk for intraoral cancer. Snuff use, in particular, if started at an early age, seems to be associated with a higher incidence of oral cancer.[7] Unprotected sun exposure contributes to the increasing incidence of cancers of the face and lips. It is very important that the pharmacist question patients who seek product recommendations for treatment of persistent oral lesions and refer such individuals to a physician or dentist for evaluation.

Canker Sores and Cold Sores
Two of the most common oral problems for which patients will seek advice and nonprescription treatment are canker sores and cold sores (fever blisters). Both conditions yield to symptomatic self-treatment, and the conditions should be self-limiting unless a secondary infectious process occurs. Patients frequently and actively seek a pharmacist's recommendations for nonprescription products to relieve symptoms of canker sores and cold sores. This provides an excellent opportunity for the pharmacist to intervene on behalf of the patient. However, although many nonprescription products are available for symptomatic treatment of cold sores and canker sores, none has been shown conclusively to decrease the recurrence rate of lesions or to be curative.

Canker Sores Canker sores, also referred to as recurrent aphthous ulcers or recurrent aphthous stomatitis, affect approximately 20% of Americans, with the greater incidence in stressed populations and a slightly higher incidence in women than in men.[99] The cause of aphthous ulcers is unknown; however, evidence suggests that they may result from a hypersensitivity to bacteria found in the mouth. Precipitating or contributing factors may be food allergy, genetic predisposition, stress, hormonal changes, nutritional deficiency (possibly related to iron, B_{12}, or folic acid deficiency), systemic disease, or trauma (e.g., chemical irritation, biting the inside of cheeks or lips, or injury caused by toothbrushing or braces).[100] Evidence also suggests that cell-mediated immunity may play a role. Recent studies suggest that aphthous ulcers are caused by a dysfunction of the immune system and may be initiated by a trigger event such as a minor trauma.[100]

Aphthous lesions appear as an epithelial ulceration on nonkeratinized mucosal surfaces of movable mouth parts, such as the tongue, the floor of the mouth, the soft palate, or the inside lining of the lips and cheeks. Rarely, lesions affect keratinized tissue such as gingiva. Some patients may experience a painful sensation before the lesion actually appears. Patients may develop single or multiple lesions. Most aphthous lesions persist for 7–14 days and heal spontaneously without scarring.[100] Canker sores are neither viral in origin nor contagious.

Canker sores usually range from 0.5 to 3.0 cm in diameter; however, larger lesions can develop in clusters. Individual aphthous lesions are usually round or oval in shape and are either flat or crater-like in appearance. (See color plates, photograph 6.) The color is usually gray to grayish-yellow with an erythematous halo of inflamed tissue surrounding the ulcer. The lesions can be very painful and may inhibit normal eating, drinking, swallowing, and talking, as well as routine oral hygiene. Although many patients have recurrent episodes of oral lesions with periods of remission, some patients may chronically experience one or more lesions in the mouth for very long periods. There is usually no fever or lymphadenopathy accompanying aphthous lesions; however, these symptoms may arise if a secondary bacterial infection is present.

The main goal in treating canker sores is to control discomfort and protect the sores from irritating stimuli so that the patient can eat, drink, and perform routine oral hygiene. If predisposing factors can be identified, they should be eliminated if possible. Coating the ulcers with topical oral protectants such as Orabase® (Colgate-Hoyt), denture adhesives, or benzoin tincture can be effective in protecting lesions, decreasing friction, and affording temporary symptomatic relief.[101] These products can be applied as needed. The ADA accepts both Orabase Plain® and benzoin tincture as topical oral mucosal protectants.

Topical application of local anesthetic/analgesic pastes or gels also affords temporary pain relief. Benzocaine and butacaine are the most commonly used local anesthetics in nonprescription products. However, benzocaine is a known sensitizer (allergen) and should not be used by patients with a history of hypersensitivity to other benzocaine-containing products. The FDA has classified topical oral anesthetic/analgesic products containing 5–20% benzocaine, 0.05–0.1% benzyl alcohol, 0.05–0.1% butacaine sulfate, 0.05–0.1% dyclonine, 0.05–0.1% hexylresorcinol, 0.04–2.0% menthol, 0.5–1.5% phenol, 0.5–1.5% phenolate sodium, and 1–6% salicyl alcohol as safe and effective for temporary relief of pain associated with canker sores.[102]

Pharmacists should discourage the sustained use of potentially inflammatory products containing substantial amounts of menthol, phenol, camphor, and eugenol as anesthetic, counterirritant, or antiseptic treatments for canker sores. These agents may cause tissue irritation and damage or systemic toxicity, especially if overused.[103] None of these ingredients has been accepted as safe and effective by the ADA for treating canker sores.

Products that release nascent oxygen (e.g., 10–15% carbamide peroxide, 3% hydrogen peroxide, and perborates) can be used as debriding and cleansing agents to exert temporary relief of canker sore discomfort. These types of products can be used up to four times daily (after meals) but should be used for no more than 7 days. Depending on the dosage form, they are suitable either for direct application or as an oral rinse. It is important that the patient follow specific package directions. The solution should be expectorated and never swallowed. Safety of long-term use is not established, and if no improvement is seen in a week or if the condition worsens, professional consultation is indicated. Reports of tissue irritation, decalcification of enamel, and black hairy tongue are associated with chronic use.[104]

Systemic nonprescription analgesics (e.g., aspirin, ibuprofen, and acetaminophen) afford additional relief of discomfort. Aspirin should not be retained in the mouth before swallowing or placed in the area of the oral lesions because of the high risk for chemical burn with necrosis. (See color plates, photograph 5.)

Saline rinses (one to three teaspoons of table salt in four to eight ounces of warm tap water) may be soothing and can be used prior to topical application of a medication. If a nutritional deficiency is suspected as a contributing factor, nutritional supplements may be used. Zinc in astringent mouthwashes is of equivocal value in promoting healing. Silver nitrate should not be used to "cauterize" lesions because it lacks value and may stain teeth and damage healthy tissue.

Cold Sores Cold sores or fever blisters are lesions that are caused by the herpes simplex type 1 virus (HSV-1). They are referred to as herpes simplex labialis because they commonly occur on the lip or on areas bordering the lips; the usual site is at the junction of mucous membrane and skin of the lips or nose. The lesions are recurrent, often arising in the same location repeatedly. They are also painful and cosmetically objectionable. Patients who suffer from recurrent herpes labialis have sustained a primary (initial) infection with the herpes virus, which is reported most often in childhood. Patients may relate a history of primary herpetic stomatitis, which usually manifests itself by vesicles (blisters) in the mouth. Most primary oral infections of herpes seem to be subclinical, and most patients are unaware of their previous primary exposure. After the primary infection, the virus apparently remains in host cells. About half of all patients suffering a primary HSV-1 infection will experience recurrent local lesions after some unpredictable latent interval.

Cold sores are often preceded by a prodrome in which the patient notices burning, itching, tingling, or numbness in the area of the forthcoming lesion. The lesion first becomes visible as small, red papules of fluid-containing vesicles 1–3 mm in diameter. Often, many lesions coalesce to form a larger area of involvement. An erythematous, inflamed border around the fluid-filled vesicles may be present. A mature lesion often has a crust over the top of many coalesced, burst vesicles; its base is erythematous. The presence of pustules or pus under the crust of a cold sore may indicate a secondary bacterial infection and should be evaluated promptly and treated with an appropriate antibiotic.

Cold sores are self-limiting and heal without scarring, usually within 10–14 days. The recurrence rate and extent of lesions vary greatly from patient to patient. Some patients may experience several large lesions every few weeks; other patients may have only a single small lesion at infrequent intervals. Patients will often associate predisposing factors such as sun or wind exposure, fever, systemic infectious diseases (colds and flu), menstruation, extreme physical stress and fatigue, or local trauma with the onset of cold sores. Those who identify sun exposure as a precipitating event should be advised to use a lip sunscreen product routinely.

HSV-1 is contagious and thought to be transmittable by direct contact. Fluid from herpes vesicles contains live virus and may serve to transmit the virus from patient to patient.[105] Herpes simplex type 2 virus (HSV-2), which causes genital lesions, is sexually transmitted. However, it has been demonstrated in herpes lesions of the lip and can be caused by oral–genital contact or hand-to-mouth transfer.

The primary goals in treating cold sores are the same as for canker sores: to control discomfort, allow healing, and prevent complications. The cold sore should be kept moist to prevent drying and fissuring. Cracking of the lesions may render them more susceptible to secondary bacterial infection, may delay healing, and usually increases discomfort. Skin protectant ingredients (e.g., allantoin, petrolatum, and cocoa butter) can relieve dryness and keep lesions soft. Topical local anesthetics (e.g., benzocaine and dibucaine) in bland, emollient vehicles aid in relieving the discomfort of itching and pain. If there is evidence of secondary bacterial infection, topical application of a thin layer of triple antibiotic ointment (e.g., Mycitracin® or Neosporin®) three to four times daily is recommended, along with systemic antibiotics if indicated. Systemic nonprescription analgesics may provide additional pain relief.

The FDA review of OTC products for fever blisters and cold sores classified external analgesics, alcohols, ketones, and amine and "caine-type" local anesthetics as Category I.[106] These ingredients, which suppress cutaneous sensory receptors, offer analgesic, anesthetic, and antipruritic effects in relieving the pain and itching of fever blisters and cold sores. Counterirritant ingredients (e.g., menthol, phenol, and camphor), which stimulate cutaneous sensory receptors, are contraindicated.[106] Fever blisters and cold sores are not considered steroid-responsive dermatoses, and the use of topical steroids is also contraindicated.[105] The FDA has proposed the use of topically applied nonprescription skin protectants or externally applied analgesic/anesthetic drug products as the only currently effective nonprescription treatment for relieving the discomfort of fever blisters.[107]

Products that are highly astringent should be avoided. Tannic acid and zinc sulfate have been classified as Category III in the topical management of fever blisters and cold sores. Any combination product containing tannic acid as an active ingredient is also considered Category III. Because frequent applications of tannic acid to the lip and oral cavity could cause a patient to ingest it when eating or drinking, the FDA was concerned about the drug's potential for oral mucosal absorption and toxicity. This concern prompted the FDA to require further clinical data to support the safety and effectiveness of astringents in the symptomatic treatment of cold sores and fever blisters.[106]

Numerous orally administered products (e.g., preparations containing *Lactobacillus acidophilus*, *Lactobacillus bulgaricus*, the essential amino acid L-lysine, citrus bioflavinoids, or pyridoxine) have been proposed in the treatment of cold sores. However, evidence conclusively demonstrating efficacy is lacking. The FDA determined in a final ruling that "no orally administered active ingredient has been found to be generally recognized as safe and effective for OTC use to treat or relieve the symptoms or discomfort of fever blisters and cold sores."[107]

Lesions should be kept clean by gently washing with mild soap solutions. Hand washing is important in preventing lesion contamination and minimizing autoinoculation of HSV. Factors that delay healing (e.g., stress, local trauma, wind, sunlight, and fatigue) should be avoided.

Minor Oral Mucosal Injury or Irritation

Minor wounds or inflammation resulting from dentures, orthodontic appliances, minor dental procedures, accidental injury (e.g., biting the cheek or suffering abrasion from sharp, crisp foods), or other irritations of the mouth or gums may be treated with various drugs. Combination preparations to treat minor oral mucosal injury may contain (1) a single anesthetic/analgesic with either a single astringent, an oral mucosal protectant, or a denture adhesive; or (2) benzocaine combined with menthol or phenol preparations. Topical analgesic/anesthetics are applied for pain relief. Astringents cause tissues to contract, or arrest secretions by causing proteins to coagulate on a cell surface.[102] Oral mucosal protectants are pharmacologically inert substances that coat and protect the area. Debriding agents/oral wound cleansers may be used to (1) aid in the removal of debris or phlegm, mucus, or other secretions associated with sore mouth; (2) cleanse minor wounds or minor gum inflammation; and (3) cleanse canker sores.[108] Labeling of these products includes the following warning:

> Do not use this product more than 7 days unless directed by a dentist or doctor. If sore mouth symptoms do not improve in 7 days; if irritation, pain, or redness persists or worsens; or if swelling, rash or fever develops, see your doctor or dentist promptly.[102]

The FDA has determined that no ingredient is generally recognized as safe and effective for use as a nonprescription oral wound-healing agent.[109] The ingredients reviewed by the OTC panel include allantoin, carbamide peroxide in anhydrous glycerin, water soluble chlorophyllins, and hydrogen peroxide in aqueous solution. However, the nonmonograph status of these ingredients applies to their use as oral wound-healing agents only. After a thorough review process, the FDA has determined that four active ingredients are generally recognized as safe and effective for use as nonprescription oral health care debriding agents/oral wound cleansers. This proposed ruling applies to carbamide peroxide in anhydrous glycerin, hydrogen peroxide, sodium perborate monohydrate (1.2 g), and sodium bicarbonate.[108] Furthermore, allantoin is recognized as a safe and effective skin protectant.

Dentists may suggest that their patients use oxidizing mouthrinses or drops as an adjunctive treatment of specific conditions or as a postoperative aid to cleaning and to relieving discomfort. Peroxides and perborates release molecular oxygen. Hydrogen peroxide and carbamide peroxide do so immediately upon contact with tissue enzymes (catalase and peroxidase); however, tissue and bacterial exposure to the oxygen is very brief.[110] The foaming of the liberated oxygen exerts a mechanical action, which loosens particulate matter and cleanses debris from wounds. The efficacy of oxidizing products in killing anaerobic bacteria in the treatment of infections and periodontitis is equivocal and has not been established.[110]

For direct application, drops of the liquid (carbamide peroxide in anhydrous glycerin or hydrogen peroxide as a 3% aqueous solution) are placed on the affected area and allowed to remain in place for 1 minute. As a rinse, carbamide peroxide drops are placed on the tongue, mixed with saliva, and swished in the mouth for 1 minute. A 3% aqueous solution of hydrogen peroxide should be mixed with an equal amount of water before rinsing the mouth. Some products (e.g., Peroxyl Rinse® and Perimed®) are a 1.5% solution of hydrogen peroxide and should be used full strength. Sodium perborate monohydrate powder (1.2 g) should be dissolved in one ounce of water and used immediately. In all cases, it is important to follow package directions carefully. The solution should be spit out, not swallowed.

Prolonged rinsing with oxidizing products could lead to soft tissue irritation, decalcified tooth surfaces, and black hairy tongue.[110] Alternatives are a sodium bicarbonate rinse (one-half to one teaspoon in four ounces of water) or a salt water rinse (one to three teaspoons of salt in four to eight ounces of warm tap water). Mucolytic action is related to the alkalinity of the sodium bicarbonate solution. As a debriding agent/oral wound cleanser, the solution is swished in the mouth over the affected area for at least 1 minute and then spit out. A saline rinse can be used safely for cleansing and soothing.

Oral Infections

Dentopyogenic Infections
Dentopyogenic infections are pus-producing infections that are associated with a tooth or its supporting structures. The symptoms of these infections vary greatly, from minor generalized pain, throbbing, and sensitivity to fever, malaise, swelling, localized pain, erythema, warmth at the infection site, and septic shock. Symptoms and severity are determined by factors such as the anatomic features of the infection site, local and systemic host resistance, virulence of the causative organisms, and time between onset of infection and treatment. Dentopyogenic infections range in severity from small, well-localized abscesses with no systemic signs of infection to a diffuse, rapidly spreading cellulitis or osteomyelitis with high morbidity. Patients with severe symptoms associated with dentopyogenic infections usually seek dental attention as soon as possible; however, persons with minimal symptoms may unwisely delay dental treatment and attempt self-treatment. Dentopyogenic abscesses, even if well-localized and seemingly not serious, may progress to more severe acute or chronic infections, requiring dental surgical intervention with or without systemic antibiotic therapy.

The four common dental abscesses are periapical, periodontal, pericoronal, and subperiosteal. A periapical abscess, located around the apex of a tooth root, originates from a necrotic, infected dental pulp and gains access to the periapical area via the apical foramen. The two most common causes of dental pulp infection and necrosis with subsequent periapical abscess are dental caries that expose the pulp to oral bacteria and trauma that causes a decrease or stoppage of blood flow to and from the pulp.

A periodontal abscess is usually a result of periodontitis. Periodontitis leads to destruction of supporting tooth structures and the subsequent formation of deep periodontal pockets. The bacteria associated with periodontitis move toward the apex of the tooth within the deepening pocket. The accumulated bacteria within this pocket form an abscess in surrounding tissue if host resistance decreases or if the bacteria are forced into the surrounding tissue by trauma or occlusion of the pocket.

Pericoronal abscesses are most often associated with mandibular third molars (lower wisdom teeth). Mandibular third molars in the process of erupting or those that do not fully erupt often have gingiva covering a portion of the crown. This gingival tissue can be traumatized by the opposing upper third molar when the patient bites down. An abscess in the tissue surrounding the lower molar may also be caused by food, bacteria, and debris collecting beneath this flap of gingiva. Patients with healthy wisdom teeth may need a child-size toothbrush in addition to their regular toothbrush to reach that area effectively for thorough cleaning.

A subperiosteal abscess is a bone abscess located beneath the thin connective tissue (periosteum) covering the bone that surrounds or underlies a tooth socket. These infections are most common after a tooth extraction.

Candidiasis
Candidiasis is often called "the disease of the diseased" because it appears in debilitated patients, immunocompromised patients, and patients taking a variety of drugs. Predisposing factors include physiologic factors (early infancy, pregnancy, and old age); endocrine disorders (diabetes mellitus, hypothyroidism, hypoparathyroidism, and hypoadrenalism); malnutrition and malabsorption syndromes (iron deficiency anemia, pernicious anemia, postgastrectomy, and alcoholism); malignant diseases (leukemias and granulocytopenia); drugs causing depression of defense mechanisms (immunosuppressives, corticosteroids, cytotoxics, and radiation therapy); drugs causing xerostomia (anticholinergics, antidepressants, antipsychotics, antihypertensives, and antihistamines with anticholinergic activity contributing to a dry mouth); and other changes in the host environment (trauma, chemical damage, postoperative states, and chronic use of broad-spectrum antibiotics).

Candida albicans, a fungus commonly found in normal oral flora, is by far the most common opportunistic pathogen associated with oral infections. The acute pseudomembranous form of candidiasis is often referred to as "thrush," and it is characterized by white plaques with a "milk curd" appearance. These plaques, which are attached to the oral mucosa, can usually be detached easily, displaying erythematous, bleeding, sore areas beneath. (See color plates, photograph 7.) Thrush is most common in infants and debilitated patients.

Acute atrophic candidiasis, sometimes referred to as antibiotic tongue or antibiotic sore mouth, is characterized by erythematous, painful, sometimes bleeding areas of the mouth. The entire upper surface of the tongue or the entire oral cavity may be involved. This form is thought to be similar to thrush but lacks the white plaques. Broad-spectrum antibiotic therapy of long duration is the most common predisposing factor.

Chronic atrophic candidiasis, sometimes referred to as denture stomatitis or denture sore mouth, is commonly found in patients with full or partial dentures. Symptomatically, this form is characterized by generalized inflammation of the denture-bearing area. The tissue may be granular in appearance, or erythematous and edematous with soreness or a burning sensation.[111] Inflammation secondary to the trauma of ill-fitting dentures is usually localized to the specific area of the trauma; inflammation secondary to *Candida* is generalized to the entire denture-bearing tissue area. It appears that the candidal organisms adhere to the denture material or reside in pores of the denture material.[112] Failure to remove the denture at bedtime and to clean it regularly worsens this condition. Angular cheilitis (inflammation of the corners of the mouth) is commonly associated with chronic atrophic candidiasis and other forms of oral candidiasis.[111]

Candidiasis requires prompt treatment with local or systemic antifungal therapy. Patients with suspected candidiasis should be referred for medical or dental evaluation.

Halitosis

Halitosis, an offensive odor emanating from the oral cavity, may be symptomatic of oral pathology. Odor results from bacterial action of food debris. Some degree of oral malodor is normal in a healthy individual (e.g., morning breath). Foul breath can be a useful diagnostic aid, however, as in the case of trench mouth. The source of halitosis may be either oral or nonoral. Common oral causes include odoriferous decaying food particles, cellular and nutritional debris, plaque-coated tongue, periodontal disease, xerostomia, and stomatitis. Poor oral or denture hygiene, trench mouth, caries, postsurgical states, extraction wounds, purulent infections, chronic periodontitis, side effects of medication, and smoking can contribute to it. Common nonoral causes of halitosis include pulmonary disease such as purulent lung infections, tuberculosis, bronchiectasis, sinusitis, tonsillitis, and rhinitis. Other nonoral causes include the elimination of chemical substances from the blood through the lungs upon exhalation. Examples include alcoholic breath or acetone breath in severely hyperglycemic diabetics.

Any patient who complains of severe or lingering halitosis without a readily identifiable cause (e.g., smoking) should be advised to see a dentist for a thorough evaluation of possible pathology. Masking foul taste and odor with cosmetic mouthwashes may delay necessary dental or medical assessment and needed treatment.

Considerations in Special Populations

Geriatric Patients

The percent of the population aged 65 and older is increasing in the United States, and this increase is predicted to continue well into the twenty-first century. Projections for the year 2030 suggest that 20% of the population will be over age 65 and that 3%, or about 8.8 million people, will be over age 85.[113] Edentulism (toothlessness) is decreasing; more than half of older Americans have retained natural dentition. This has many dental implications. Topical fluoride application in the form of dentifrice, rinse, or gel is indicated for the prevention of coronal and root caries as long as there is natural dentition. Pharmacists should continue to recommend fluoride anticaries products to their older patients.

In counseling geriatric patients on oral health care, it becomes very important to consider medication profiles. Because the elderly are more likely to be taking multiple medications, the likelihood of drug-induced or disease-related changes in oral physiology increases.

Xerostomia

About 20% of the elderly are affected with xerostomia, a condition in which salivary flow is limited or completely arrested. Xerostomia was thought to be an age-related, degenerative process. However, it has been shown that healthy, nonmedicated geriatrics may experience a change in saliva composition but not necessarily a decreased flow.[114] The usual causes of xerostomia are disease (e.g., Sjögren's syndrome, diabetes, and depression), drugs (e.g., antihypertensives, antidepressants, and diuretics), or functional activity (e.g., breathing through the mouth or smoking). Radiation therapy of the head and neck can cause atrophy of the salivary glands. Drugs with anticholinergic activity or drugs that cause depletion of salivary flow volume have been implicated. Older persons are more likely to be taking multiple medications for chronic diseases; however, if xerostomia is drug induced and the medication can be changed, the condition may be reversed. Pharmacists should review medication profiles (prescription and nonprescription) for patients complaining of dry mouth to determine if the condition is drug induced.

Xerostomia can produce difficulty in talking and swallowing, stomatitis and burning tongue, increased caries, periodontal disease, or reduced denture-wearing time, depending on the status of dentition. Treatment should be directed toward the control of dental decay and the relief of soft tissue distress. The commercially available artificial salivas relieve soft tissue discomfort and are more effective and longer lasting than simple rinses and lozenges.

Artificial saliva preparations are designed to mimic natural saliva both chemically and physically. Because they do not stimulate natural salivary gland production, they must be considered as replacement therapy, not as a cure for xerostomia. Artificial saliva closely resembles natural saliva and is formulated with the following properties:

- *Viscosity*: Carboxymethylcellulose and glycerine are used to mimic natural saliva viscosity.
- *Mineral content:* All products contain calcium and phosphate ions, and some also contain fluoride. With normal use, no product has demonstrated the ability to remineralize enamel. Therefore, the ADA does not recognize any such claims made by the manufacturers.
- *Preservatives*: Salivart® (Westport Pharmaceuticals) does not contain preservatives because it is packaged as a sterile aerosol. Other products do contain preservatives, such as methyl- or propylparaben, which may cause hypersensitivity reactions in certain patients.
- *Palatability*: Flavorings such as mint or lemon and/or sweeteners such as sorbitol and xylitol are commonly used.

Artificial salivas can be used on an as-needed basis. The xerostomic patient with a history of caries susceptibility should use a professionally designed topical fluoride program in addition to artificial saliva products. These patients should also use a very soft toothbrush and avoid mouthrinses with high alcoholic content, given that alcohol contributes to xerostomia.

Among the ADA-accepted artificial salivas are Salivart®, Glandosane Synthetic Saliva® (Tsumura Medical), Moi-Stir Mouth Moistener® and Moi-Stir Oral Swabsticks® (Kingswood Laboratories), Orex Saliva Substitute® (Young Dental Manufacturing Company), Saliva Substitute® (Roxane Laboratories), and Xero-Lube® (Gel-Kam Division of Colgate-Palmolive).[97]

Denture Problems

Conditions such as denture stomatitis (an inflammation of the oral tissue in contact with a removable denture), inflammatory papillary hyperplasia, and chronic candidiasis can be caused by ill-fitting dentures, trauma, and poor denture hygiene. Denture stomatitis, a distressing and common finding in denture wearers, may also be attributed to infection with *C. albicans*, which can be found resident on the denture base.[112] Dentures accumulate plaque, stain, and calculus by a process very similar to that which occurs with natural teeth.[115] The denture plaque mass in contact with oral tissues produces predictable toxic results. Poor denture hygiene contributes to fungal and bacterial growth and so not only affects the patient aesthetically (unpleasant odors and staining), but also seriously affects the patient's oral health (inflammation and mucosal disease) and ability to wear the dentures successfully.[111]

Loose, misfitting, or broken removable dental prostheses (partial or full dentures) can also contribute to accelerated bone loss, ulceration, irritation, tumorous growths, and compromised oral function. Refitting, relining, or repairing dentures to ensure proper functioning requires professional dental treatment.

Denture Cleansers Patients should be instructed to clean dentures thoroughly at least once daily to remove unsightly stain, debris, and potentially harmful plaque. Only products specifically formulated for denture cleansing should be used; household cleansers (used for soaking) are not appropriate and may either be ineffective or damage denture material. The use of whitening toothpastes meant for use on natural dentition should be discouraged because their abrasivity is too high for them to be used safely on denture material.

A combination regimen of brushing and soaking is recommended.[116] Brushing with a denture brush, adapted to the denture's contour, and low-abrasion denture paste or powder will mechanically remove plaque and debris. These abrasive products should be used with care, and excessive force or pressure that could damage acrylic resin should be avoided. The brushing routine can be followed by soaking the denture in an alkaline peroxide cleansing solution to help remove remaining plaque and bacteria. Plaque removal is then enhanced by brushing the denture after it soaks in cleansers; instructions for doing so are included on some products.[117] The denture should be thoroughly rinsed before reinsertion in the mouth.

Denture cleansers are either chemical or abrasive in their cleaning action. The three types of chemical cleansers are alkaline peroxides, alkaline hypochlorites, and dilute acids. The abrasive cleaners are available as pastes, gels, or powders. The ideal denture cleansing product would:

- Remove both organic and inorganic denture deposits effectively;
- Possess bactericidal and fungicidal activity;
- Be nontoxic;
- Do no harm to denture materials.[112]

Because the ideal product does not yet exist, it is necessary to assess product characteristics in conjunction with patient circumstances. More than one product may be required to meet patient needs adequately.

Alkaline peroxide cleaners are the most commonly used chemical denture cleansers. These powders or tablets become alkaline solutions of hydrogen peroxide when dissolved. The ingredients are alkaline detergents and perborates, the latter of which cause oxygen release for a mechanical cleaning effect. Geriatric or handicapped patients may prefer an alkaline peroxide soak solution for daily, overnight cleaning. These products are most effective on new plaque and stains that are soaked for 4–8 hours. The alkaline peroxides have few serious disadvantages and do not damage the surface of acrylic resins.[117]

Alkaline hypochlorites (bleach) remove stains, dissolve mucin, and are both bactericidal and fungicidal. Denture plaque consists of cells embedded in a matrix that serves as a surface on which calculus may develop. Hypochlorite cleansers act directly on the organic plaque matrix to dissolve its structure, but they cannot dissolve calculus once formed.[117] The most serious disadvantage of hypochlorite is that it corrodes metal denture components such as the framework and clasps of removable partial dentures, solder joints, and possibly the pins holding the teeth.[112] The addition of anticorrosive phosphate compounds has greatly reduced this effect, but it is recommended that these products be used for 15-minute soaks to limit exposure[117] and not be used more often than once a week.

Dilute acids, often 3–5% hydrochloric acid, dissolve the inorganic (calcium) phosphate and are effective against calculus and stain on dentures. However, they corrode metal components and are harmful to fabrics, eyes, and skin if spilled during handling.[117] Therefore, these products are used in the dental office for professional cleaning but are not deemed suitable for routine patient home use.

Although many studies have been conducted on denture-cleansing products, only a few comparative trials have been published, and differences in methodology make direct comparisons of results very difficult. Published findings report that plaque accumulation of less than 24 hours is easier to remove but is not necessarily removed effectively by all products, even within the same class of cleaners. The relative ineffectiveness of all products tested during a short soaking time is often contrary to advertising claims.

The following denture cleansers are among those currently accepted by the ADA as safe and effective: Complete® (Vicks), Efferdent®, Efferdent paste®, and Fresh N' Brite® (Warner-Lambert).[118]

All denture-cleansing products should be completely rinsed off the denture before insertion. Contact with oral or other mucous membranes may result in serious tissue irritation or possibly severe chemical burns from the alkaline or acid product.[117] All denture cleansers should be kept out of the reach of children because of the potential for eye or skin irritation or toxicity from accidental ingestion.[117] Patients should not soak or clean dentures in hot water or hot soaking solutions because distortion or warping may occur. Stains that are resistant to proper denture brushing and soaking in available solutions should be evaluated by a dentist.[117]

Denture Adherents Denture adhesives may be the most overused dental products purchased by patients. Chronic bone resorption of the mandibular and maxillary ridges that support a denture occurs with even the best fitting denture. Furthermore, pathologic changes in soft tissue under the denture, such as ulcers and fibrous lesions, and accelerated bone resorption have been reported with the inappropriate use of denture adhesives and ill-fitting dentures.[119] Periodic dental examinations are necessary to evaluate bone resorption and ensure proper denture fit. Although denture adhesives may increase denture retention in some persons, the need for adhesives increases as the quality of the denture adaptation to underlying soft tissue deteriorates.[119] Excessive application of adherents could also cause denture repositioning with resultant malocclusion. The adhesive can actually interfere with correct positioning in relation to supporting bone. Patients who believe that daily use of denture adherents is necessary to attain denture security and comfort should be referred to their dentist for evaluation.

Denture adherents are usually composed of materials that swell, gel, and become viscous (e.g., karaya, pectin, or methylcellulose); materials that are antibacterial (e.g., sodium borate or hexachlorophene); and materials that serve as preservatives, fillers, or wetting or flavoring agents (e.g., propylparaben, magnesium oxide, sodium lauryl sulfate, or petroleum derivatives). Adherent powders either have a vegetable gum base or are composed of synthetic polymers. Adherent pastes usually contain karaya gum, petroleum jelly, colorings, and flavorings.

The ADA has accepted some denture adhesive products provided that the labeling indicates that they are to be used only temporarily or upon the recommendation of a dentist. All accepted denture adhesives contain the following warning label:

[Product name] is acceptable as a temporary measure to provide increased retention of dentures. However, an ill-fitting denture may impair your health—consult your dentist for periodic examination.

The ADA has accepted the following denture adherents as safe and effective: Co-Re-Ga®, Wernet's Denture Adhesive Cream®, Wernet's Powder®, and Super Wernet's Powder® (Block Drug); Extra Strength Effergrip® (Warner-Lambert); Firmdent® (Moyco); Perma-Grip® (Lactona); Rigident Cream® (Carter Products); and Secure® (Johnson & Johnson).[118]

Denture Reliners and Cushions Extended use of reliners or cushions for dentures invariably harms the patient and damages the denture. These products change the positioning of the denture, creating high-pressure points that can result in denture distortion, malocclusion, temporomandibular joint problems, decreased mastication function, and altered aesthetics.[119] Denture reliners and cushions have also been associated with bone resorption, traumatic ulcers, and gingival inflammation of the denture-bearing tissues.

The ADA does not accept any of these products as safe and effective, and it discourages their use. The FDA Bureau of Medical Devices requires the following warning label on these products:

WARNING For temporary use only. Long-term use of this product may lead to faster bone loss, continuing irritation, sores, and tumors. For use only until a dentist can be seen.

Patients with dentures need periodic professional dental evaluations. As time passes, it is normal to expect the original fit to need adjustment. This is accomplished effectively only by a dentist. Patients who feel their dentures are loose or otherwise uncomfortable should be referred to their dentist for evaluation. Any patients who are considering purchasing a denture reliner or cushion because of actual or perceived denture problems should be encouraged to see their dentist as soon as possible.

Denture Repair Kit

Broken dentures can be evaluated and repaired only by a dentist. Initial fitting and periodic refitting of dentures require extensive dental knowledge and skill. Patients should not attempt to glue or otherwise repair cracked, broken, or distorted dentures. Pharmacists should discourage the use of denture repair kits and advise patients to (1) save all pieces of the denture or appliance to take to the dentist, and (2) seek professional treatment without delay. Prolonged periods without wearing a partial denture can result in position changes among the remaining teeth and a loss of fit.[120]

Denture repair kits may contain methacrylate or other types of glue or acrylic materials. The FDA requires the following label on these products:

WARNING For emergency repairs only. Long-term use of home-repaired dentures may cause faster bone loss, continuing irritation, sores, and tumors. This kit is for emergency use only. See Dentist Without Delay.

Pediatric Patients

The 20 primary teeth that will erupt are present, but not visible, in the baby's jaws at birth. It is important to start oral hygiene early in life. A wet gauze pad may be used to wipe the baby's gums after each feeding to remove plaque and milk residue. The deciduous teeth will usually start to erupt around 6 months of age. Decay is a possibility at any time. "Baby bottle caries" results when an infant is allowed to nurse continuously from a bottle of juice, milk, or sugar water when put to bed. The prolonged time that teeth are in contact with the cariogenic liquid promotes caries. When the teeth have erupted, a soft child-size toothbrush can be used for cleaning. Parents must do the brushing and should take care to use only a very small amount of fluoride toothpaste or none at all. Children at this age will swallow the toothpaste, which will contribute to overall systemic fluoride ingestion.

Products for Teething

Teething is the eruption of the deciduous teeth through the gingival tissues. Usually this process is uneventful. However, when teething causes sleep disturbances or irritability, symptomatic treatment may be considered. Topical local anesthetics such as benzocaine and frozen teething rings may provide symptomatic relief. Systemic nonprescription analgesics (e.g., acetaminophen) may be used at appropriate doses. When teething is accompanied by fever, nasal congestion, or malaise, a dentist or physician should be contacted to rule out an infectious process.

The FDA review of nonprescription drug products for relief of oral discomfort has included benzocaine and phenol preparations as Category I topical anesthetic/analgesics for teething pain. Labeling reads: "For the temporary relief of sore gums due to teething in infants and children 4 months of age and older."[95] Products containing 5 to 20% benzocaine in solution or suspension that are intended to be used as teething preparations should be applied to the affected area not more than four times daily. Teething preparations containing phenol or phenolate sodium equivalent to 0.5% phenol in aqueous solution or suspension may be applied to the affected area up to six times daily. These preparations are not indicated for children under 4 months of age.[95] Moreover, products for teething must carry a warning that states that fever and nasal congestion are not symptoms of teething and may indicate the presence of an infection. ADA-accepted products include Baby Orajel Teething Pain Medicine® (Del Laboratories); Baby Anbesol Gel® (Whitehall); and Orabase Baby Analgesic Teething Gel® (Colgate). These products are alcohol free and contain 7.5% benzocaine.

Pediatric Toothbrushes

As with adult toothbrushes, soft bristles are recommended for children's toothbrushes. A child's toothbrush is generally smaller than an adult's and is available in a baby (for children up to age 6 or 7) and junior (age 7 to teens) size. Toothbrush size and shape should be individualized according to the size of the child's mouth. Children can usually remove plaque more easily with a brush having short and narrow bristles. No matter what type of toothbrush is used, however, children are usually unable to brush by themselves until they are 4 or 5 years old, and they may require supervision until 8 or 9 years of age to clean effectively.

Fluoride Cautions for Children

Fluoride dentifrices contribute to the total amount of fluoride ingested by children. Other sources are dietary, recommended systemic supplements, and any other topical fluoride preparations. When chronic fluoride ingestion from all sources is considered, children who live in a community with an optimally fluoridated water supply may exceed optimal daily amounts. This places them at risk for mild forms of dental fluorosis, a mottled appearance of surface enamel. Although a mild degree of fluorosis is an aesthetic concern, more severe cases can result in pitting and surface defects.[121] (See color plates, photograph 8.)

Studies of dentifrice ingestion by children show great variation in the amount of dentifrice retained and consistently show that younger children are more likely to swallow some dentifrice.[92] Limiting ingestion of fluoride dentifrice is advised. Parents should apply the toothpaste (only a pea-sized amount) to a child-size toothbrush and should brush the teeth of preschool children until the children can manage it properly. Children should be taught to rinse thoroughly and expectorate after brushing.[92] Only regular-strength fluoride toothpaste is recommended for use by children under 6 years of age.

A similar problem lies with fluoride rinsing in that children 3–5 years of age may swallow significant amounts of rinse each time they swish. A usual dose of 0.05% rinse contains 2 mg of fluoride ion and may contribute to mild fluorosis in the presence of a fluoridated public water supply. Ethanol content of nonprescription fluoride rinses ranges from 6 to 8% and may pose a hazard for very young children. Fluoride rinses should be used only by children over 5 years of age who have mastered the swallowing reflex. These products should be kept out of the reach of children, and children under 12 years of age should be supervised when rinsing. High-dose ingestion requires prompt medical assistance. Toxicity is related to fluoride content and ethanol content. Parents should be able to identify the product and estimate the amount ingested.[83]

Finally, fluoride gels are not recommended for children under 6, and children under 12 should use these products only under supervision.

Orthodontia

Fixed orthodontic appliances require very careful attention to oral hygiene to prevent gingivitis and caries. Patients with these appliances need a combination of toothbrush types to clean all surfaces effectively. Use of powered toothbrushes or oral irrigating devices may help to remove plaque and debris around orthodontic bands. It may be advisable for orthodontic patients to use a nonprescription fluoride mouthrinse while undergoing treatment.

Patients with removable orthodontic appliances should consult their orthodontist about using a denture cleanser. Some dental practitioners have recommended a denture cleanser in addition to brushing to remove plaque, tartar, odor-causing bacteria, and stain that accumulates on orthodontic appliances.[122]

Pregnant Patients

Pregnant patients are more susceptible to both dental caries and periodontal disease. Caries generally can be related to changes in eating habits, such as frequent snacking and "treats." Careful attention to frequent brushing and flossing is indicated to clear plaque and acid.[123]

Physiologic changes during pregnancy may contribute to changes in the soft oral tissues and result in an increased incidence and severity of gingivitis. An inflammatory condition so common that it is called pregnancy gingivitis is characterized by red, swollen gingival tissue that bleeds easily. This gingivitis is caused by local factors, as it is in any patient. Pregnancy causes modifications in the host's response, however, making gingival tissue more sensitive to bacterial dental plaque. Hormone levels or increased production of prostaglandins have been implicated in the heightened inflammatory response.[124] Pregnancy gingivitis can be prevented or resolved with thorough plaque control. The severity of the inflammatory response and resulting gingivitis will decrease postpartum, returning to prepregnancy levels after approximately 1 year.

The pharmacist will quite often be alerted very early in the pregnancy owing to counseling on prescription prenatal vitamins. Besides monitoring the pregnant patient's medications for safety, the pharmacist has an opportunity to advise a dental checkup and careful attention to brushing and flossing to avoid oral health complications.

Value-Added Pharmacy Services

Pharmacists can offer patients good oral health services in several other ways. As an initial step, pharmacists can contact local community dental practitioners and indicate a willingness to work together for optimal patient oral health care. The pharmacist may also want to consider one or more of the activities listed below:

- Contact the local public health agency to determine the level of community water fluoridation to assist dental and medical practitioners in prescribing supplements and patients in selecting fluoride-containing dentifrices, mouthrinses, and gels.[121]
- Monitor total fluoride ingestion in children, noting the use of fluoride prescription supplementation and family use of nonprescription fluoride products. Systemic supplements may be prescribed by both dentist and pediatrician. The pharmacist is in a unique position to coordinate children's fluoride supplementation.[121]
- Stock the oral health care section to highlight products accepted or recognized by the ADA. Advise patients of the significance of the ADA acceptance program.
- Make available, as an informational/educational addition to the oral health care section, the many types of brochures and patient information leaflets that the ADA provides on various oral health concerns.
- Take the initiative in counseling patients on the proper selection and use of nonprescription oral health care products. Because of the tremendous amount of advertising in this area, patients need knowledgeable and objective advice and assistance to be able to distinguish among product claims.
- Remember that older patients may be vision impaired and that lighting in the nonprescription product area becomes important for reading label directions and warnings.
- Include records of pertinent dental health information on patient profiles (e.g., dentures, orthodontics, and fluorosis).

Summary

Because dental disease is the most frequently encountered health problem in the United States, and because pharmacists see more people with dental problems than dentists do, today's pharmacist needs a well-developed knowledge of oral health care products and their use. The pharmacist–dentist team can improve oral health in the community. With useful references such as the *Journal of the American Dental Association*, *Clinical Products in Dentistry*, and the special dental issue of *Pharmacy Times* every July; awareness of ongoing FDA and ADA evaluation of nonprescription dental products; and open lines of communication with dental practitioners, pharmacists can better serve their patients as oral health consultants and members of the dental health care team.

References

1. Harris NO, Christen AG, *Primary Preventive Dentistry*. 3rd ed. Norwalk, Conn: Appleton & Lange; 1991: 399, 406.
2. Harris NO, Christen AG. *Primary Preventive Dentistry*. 3rd ed. Norwalk, Conn: Appleton & Lange; 1991: 419.
3. Striffler DF, Young WO, Burt BA. *Dentistry, Dental Practice, and the Community*. 3rd ed. Philadelphia: W. B. Saunders Co; 1983: 123, 140, 236.
4. Anon. Latest Nielsen data. *Drug Topics* 1992 Apr 20; 136 (8): 71.
5. Harris NO, Christen AG. *Primary Preventive Dentistry*. 3rd ed. Norwalk, Conn: Appleton & Lange; 1991: 156–7.
6. Harris NO, Christen AG. *Primary Preventive Dentistry*. 3rd ed. Norwalk, Conn: Appleton & Lange; 1991: 406, 470–1.
7. Anon. NIH consensus development conference: health implications of smokeless tobacco use. *Am Pharm* 1986 Apr; NS26 (4): 18–20.
8. Glover ED, Edmundson EW, Edwards SW, et al. Implications of smokeless tobacco use among athletes. *The Physician and Sportsmedicine* 1986; 14 (12): 95–104.
9. McHugh WD. Role of supragingival plaque in oral disease initiation and progression. In: Loe H, Kleinman DV, eds. *Dental Plaque Control Measures and Oral Hygiene Practices*. Oxford, England: IRL Press; 1986: 1–12.
10. Pader M. *Oral Hygiene Products and Practice*. New York: Marcel Dekker, Inc; 1988: 45–59.
11. Greenwell H, Bissada NF, Wittwer JW. Periodontics in general practice: professional plaque control. *J Am Dent Assoc* 1990: 642–6.
12. Low SB, Ciancio SG. Reviewing nonsurgical periodontal therapy. *J Am Dent Assoc* 1990: 467–70.
13. Kidd EAM, Joyston-Bechal S. *Essentials of Dental Caries*. Bristol, England: IOP Publishing Ltd; 1987: 3–15, 82.
14. Pretara-Spanedda P, Grossman E, Curro FA, et al. Toothbrush bristle density: relationship to plaque removal. *Am J Dent* 1989; 2 (6): 345–8.

15. Nathan A, Anderson C. Oral health: part 2. oral hygiene. *Pharm J* 1991 May 25; 246: 657–8.
16. Anon. Toothbrush may be link to sore throat, infections. *Med World News* 1986 Mar 10; 27 (5): 68.
17. Council on Dental Materials, Instruments, and Equipment, Council on Dental Therapeutics. *Clinical Products in Dentistry: A Desktop Reference*. Chicago: American Dental Association; 1992 Jan: 27–9.
18. Bratel J, Berggren U, Hirsch J-M. Electric or manual toothbrush? *Clin Prev Dent* 1988; 10 (3): 23–6.
19. Council on Dental Therapeutics. *Accepted Dental Therapeutics*. 40th ed. Chicago: American Dental Association; 1984: 386–7.
20. Harris NO, Christen AG. *Primary Preventive Dentistry*. 3rd ed. Norwalk, Conn: Appleton & Lange; 1991: 91–3.
21. Council on Dental Materials, Instruments, and Equipment, Council on Dental Therapeutics. *Clinical Products in Dentistry, A Desktop Reference*. Chicago: American Dental Association; 1992 Jan: 9–10.
22. Glavind L, Zeuner E. The effectiveness of a rotary electric toothbrush on oral cleanliness in adults. *J Clin Periodontol* 1986; 13: 135–8.
23. Mueller LJ, Darby ML, Allen DS, et al. Rotary electric toothbrushing: clinical effects on the presence of gingivitis and supragingival dental plaque. *Dent Hyg* 1987; 546–50.
24. Coontz EJ. The effectiveness of a new home plaque-removal instrument on plaque removal. *Compend Cont Educ Dent* 1985; 6 (suppl): 117–22.
25. Council on Dental Therapeutics. *Accepted Dental Therapeutics*. 40th ed. Chicago: American Dental Association; 1984: 388.
26. Frandsen A. Mechanical oral hygiene practices. In: Loe H, Kleinman DV, eds. *Dental Plaque Control Measures and Oral Hygiene Practices*. Oxford, England: IRL Press; 1986: 100.
27. Greenstein G. Effects of subgingival irrigation on periodontal status. *J Periodontol* 1987 Dec; 58: 827–36.
28. Carranza FA Jr. *Glickman's Clinical Periodontology*. 7th ed. Philadelphia: W. B. Saunders; 1990: 706.
29. Lamberts DM, Wunderlich RC, Caffesse RG. The effect of waxed and unwaxed dental floss on gingival health: part I. plaque removal and gingival response. *J Periodontol* 1982; 53: 393–9.
30. Hill HC, Levi PA, Glickman I. The effects of waxed and unwaxed dental floss on interdental plaque accumulation and interdental gingival health. *J Periodontol* 1973; 44: 411–3.
31. Perry DA, Pattison G. An investigation of wax residue on tooth surfaces after the use of waxed dental floss. *Dent Hyg* 1986; 60: 16–9.
32. Harris NO, Christen AG. *Primary Preventive Dentistry*. 3rd ed. Norwalk, Conn: Appleton & Lange; 1991: 115–21.
33. Kiger RD, Nylund K, Feller RP. A comparison of proximal plaque removal using floss and interdental brushes. *J Clin Periodontol* 1991; 18: 681–4.
34. Mauriello S, Bader J, George M, et al. Effectiveness of three interproximal cleaning devices. *Clin Prev Dent* 1987; 9: 18–22.
35. Anon. Controlling plaque limits periodontal disease. *US Pharm* 1987 Aug; 12: 70–6.
36. Pader M. *Oral Hygiene Products and Practice*. New York: Marcel Dekker, Inc; 1988: 426–39.
37. *Federal Register* 1988; June 15; 53: 22443–6.
38. Kanapka JA. Over-the-counter dentifrices in the treatment of tooth hypersensitivity. *Dent Clin North Am* 1990 Jul; 34 (3): 545–60.
39. Pader M. *Oral Hygiene Products and Practice*. New York: Marcel Dekker, Inc; 1988: 439–53.
40. *Federal Register* 1980; Mar 28; 45: 20670.
41. Marsh PD. Dentifrices containing new agents for the control of plaque and gingivitis: microbiological aspects. *J Clin Periodontol* 1991; 18: 462–7.
42. Hogg SD. Chemical control of plaque. *Dent Update* 1990 Oct; 17: 330, 332–4.
43. van der Ouderaa F, Cummins D. Anti-plaque dentifrices: current status and prospects. *Int Dent J* 1991; 41 (2): 117–23.
44. Balanyk TE. Sanguinarine: comparisons of antiplaque/antigingivitis reports. *Clin Prev Dent* 1990; 12 (3): 18–25.
45. Council on Dental Therapeutics. Guidelines for acceptance of chemotherapeutic products for the control of supragingival dental plaque and gingivitis. *J Am Dent Assoc* 1986; 112: 529–32.
46. *Federal Register* 1990; Sep 19; 55: 38560–2.
47. Lobene RR. Reduced formation of supragingival calculus with the use of zinc chloride dentifrice. *J Am Dent Assoc* 1987; 114: 350.
48. Zacherl WA, Pfeiffer HJ, Swancar JR. The effect of soluble pyrophosphates on dental calculus in adults. *J Am Dent Assoc* 1985; 110: 737–8.
49. Naleway CA, Whall CW Jr. What benefits do tartar control dentifrices provide your patrons? *Pharm Times* 1987 Jul; 53: 32–7.
50. Beacham BE, Kurgansky D, Gould WM. Circumoral dermatitis and cheilitis caused by tartar control dentifrices. *J Am Acad Dermatol* 1990 Jun; 22: 1029–32.
51. Pader M. *Oral Hygiene Products and Practice*. New York: Marcel Dekker, Inc; 1988: 489–504.
52. Harris NO, Christen AG. *Primary Preventive Dentistry*. 3rd ed. Norwalk, Conn: Appleton & Lange; 1991: 148.
53. *Federal Register* 1982; May 25; 47: 22842–4.
54. Council on Dental Therapeutics. *Accepted Dental Therapeutics*. 40th ed. Chicago: American Dental Association; 1984: 324.
55. American Dental Association. Council on Dental Therapeutics accepts Listerine. *J Am Dent Assoc* 1988; 117: 515–7.
56. Council on Dental Materials, Instruments, and Equipment, Council on Dental Therapeutics. *Clinical Products in Dentistry: A Desktop Reference*. Chicago: American Dental Association; 1992 Jan: 35–6.
57. Gossel TA. Counseling the consumer on antiplaque mouthrinses. *US Pharm* 1988 Dec; 13: 46–8, 51.
58. Pader M. *Oral Hygiene Products and Practice*. New York: Marcel Dekker, Inc; 1988: 333–8.
59. Moran J, Addy M. The effects of a cetylpyridinium chloride prebrushing rinse as an adjunct to oral hygiene and gingival health. *J Periodontol* 1991; 62: 562–4.
60. Bailey L. The effect of a detergent-based pre-brushing dental rinse on plaque accumulation. *J Clin Dent* 1990; II (1): 6–10.
61. Emling RC, Yankell SL. An analysis of the clinical plaque removal efficacy of a pre-brushing dental rinse in a three center study design. *J Clin Dent* 1990; II (1): 11–6.
62. Grossman E. Effectiveness of a prebrushing mouthrinse under single-trial and home-use conditions. *Clin Prev Dent* 1988; 10: 3–6.
63. Beiswanger BB, Mallatt EM, Mau SM, et al. The relative plaque removal effect of a prebrushing mouthrinse. *J Am Dent Assoc* 1990; 120: 190–2.
64. Freitas BL, Collaert B, Attstrom R. Effect of the pre-brushing rinse, Plax, on dental plaque formation. *J Clin Periodontol* 1991; 18: 713–5.
65. Howard WR. Patient-applied tooth whiteners: are they safe, effective with supervision? *J Am Dent Assoc* 1992; 123: 57–60.
66. Haywood VB, Heymann HO. Nightguard vital bleaching. *Quintessence Int* 1989; 20: 173–6.
67. Cubbon T, Ore D. Hard tissue and home tooth whiteners. *CDS Rev* 1991 Jun; 84 (5): 32–5.
68. Harris NO, Christen AG. *Primary Preventive Dentistry*. 3rd ed. Norwalk, Conn: Appleton & Lange; 1991: 66–78.
69. Barrington EP, Nevins M. Diagnosing periodontal diseases. *J Am Dent Assoc* 1990 Oct; 121: 460–4.
70. Pinkham JR. *Pediatric Dentistry: Infancy Through Adoles-*

cence. Philadelphia: W. B. Saunders; 1988: 507–8.
71. Genco RJ, Goldman HM, Cohen DW, eds. *Contemporary Periodontics*. St. Louis: Mosby; 1990: 63–81.
72. Genco RJ, Goldman HM, Cohen DW, eds. *Contemporary Periodontics*. St. Louis: Mosby; 1990: 348–59.
73. Loe H. The specific etiology of periodontal disease and its application to prevention. In: Carranza FA, Kenney EB, eds. *Prevention of Periodontal Disease*. Chicago: Quintessence Publishing Co, Inc; 1981: 15–22.
74. Pader M. *Oral Hygiene Products and Practice*. New York: Marcel Dekker, Inc; 1988: 226–8.
75. Harris NO, Christen AG. *Primary Preventive Dentistry*. 3rd ed. Norwalk, Conn: Appleton & Lange; 1991: 338–43.
76. Bar A. Caries prevention with xylitol. *World Rev Nutr Diet* 1988; 55: 1–27.
77. Anon. Consensus: oral health effects of products that increase salivary flow rate. *J Am Dent Assoc* 1988; 116: 757.
78. Pader M. *Oral Hygiene Products and Practice*. New York: Marcel Dekker, Inc; 1988: 89, 101.
79. Striffler DF, Young WO, Burt BA. *Dentistry, Dental Practice, and the Community*. 3rd ed. Philadelphia: W. B. Saunders Co; 1983: 204–5.
80. Anon. Fluoride: still a good public health value. *Pharm Times* 1990 Jul; 56: 105–7, 111.
81. Pray WS. Fluoridation: the battle continues. *US Pharm* 1990 Oct; 15 (10): 20–4.
82. Council on Dental Therapeutics. *Accepted Dental Therapeutics*. 40th ed. Chicago: American Dental Association; 1984: 395–420.
83. Adair SM. Risks and benefits of fluoride mouthrinsing. *Pediatrician* 1989; 16: 161–9.
84. Council on Dental Therapeutics. *Accepted Dental Therapeutics*. 40th ed. Chicago: American Dental Association; 1984: 402–11.
85. *Federal Register* 1985; Sep 30; 50: 39859.
86. Glass RL. Fluoride dentifrices: the basis for the decline in caries prevalence. *J R Soc Med* 1986; 79 (suppl) 14: 15–7.
87. *Federal Register* 1985; Sep 30; 50: 39872.
88. Mellberg JR. Fluoride dentifrices: current status and prospects. *Int Dent J* 1991 Feb; 41 (1): 9–16.
89. Council on Dental Therapeutics. *J Am Dent Assoc* 1988; 117: 785.
90. Ripa LW. Clinical studies of high-potency fluoride dentifrices: a review. *J Am Dent Assoc* 1989; 118: 85–91.
91. Council on Dental Materials, Instruments, and Equipment, Council on Dental Therapeutics. *Clinical Products in Dentistry: A Desktop Reference*. Chicago: American Dental Association; 1992 Jan: 39.
92. Ripa LW. A critique of topical fluoride methods (dentifrices, mouthrinses, operator-, and self-applied gels) in an era of decreased caries and increased fluorosis prevalence. *J Public Health Dent* 1991 Winter; 51 (1): 23–41.
93. Gossel TA. The role of fluorides in preventing cavities. *US Pharm* 1986 Mar; 11: 28–32, 34.
94. Maher WP. Anatomy of a toothache. *Pharm Times* 1992 Mar; 58: 43–9.
95. *Federal Register* 1991; Sep 24; 56: 48308–10, 48315–6, 48325, 48335–46.
96. Gossel TA. Hypersensitive teeth: OTCs take the pain away. *US Pharm* 1991 May; 16 (5): 23–32.
97. Council on Dental Materials, Instruments, and Equipment, Council on Dental Therapeutics. *Clinical Products in Dentistry: A Desktop Reference*. Chicago: American Dental Association; 1992 Jan: 37.
98. *Federal Register* 1992; May 11; 57: 20115.
99. Pray WS. Oral mucosal lesions. *US Pharm* 1990 Feb; 15 (2): 21–2, 24–5, 66.
100. Antoon JW, Miller RL. Aphthous ulcers—a review of the literature on etiology, pathogenesis, diagnosis, and treatment. *J Am Dent Assoc* 1980 Nov; 101: 603–8.
101. Council on Dental Therapeutics. *Accepted Dental Therapeutics*. 40th ed. Chicago: American Dental Association; 1984: 79.
102. *Federal Register* 1991; Sep 24; 56: 48342–3.
103. *Federal Register* 1982; May 25; 47: 22809.
104. Gossel TA. Debriding agents and oral wound cleansers. *US Pharm* 1990 Feb; 15 (2): 28–36.
105. Council on Dental Therapeutics. *Accepted Dental Therapeutics*. 40th ed. Chicago: American Dental Association; 1984: 64–5.
106. *Federal Register* 1990; Jan 31; 55: 3372, 3379.
107. *Federal Register* 1992; Jun 30; 57: 29173.
108. *Federal Register* 1988; Jan 27; 53: 2453, 2456.
109. *Federal Register* 1986; Jul 18; 51: 26113.
110. Council on Dental Therapeutics. *Accepted Dental Therapeutics*. 40th ed. Chicago: American Dental Association; 1984: 321–2.
111. Budtz-Jorgensen E, Bertraum U. Denture stomatitis: I. the etiology in relation to trauma and infection. *Acta Odont Scand* 1970; 28: 71–92.
112. Abelson DC. Denture plaque and denture cleansers: review of the literature. *Gerodontics* 1985; 1: 202–6.
113. Niessen LC, Williams GC. Aging in America: implications for dentistry. *Pharm Times* 1988 Jul; 54: 36–40.
114. Baum BJ. Changes in salivary function in older subjects. In: Ferguson DB, ed. *The Aging Mouth*, Vol 6 of *Frontiers of oral physiology*. Basel, Switzerland: Karger; 1987: 126–34.
115. Gossel TA. Counseling patients on denture cleansing products. *US Pharm* 1988 Jun; 13: 56–8, 61–2, 76.
116. Zacharczenko N. Dentures and denture care. *Pharm Times* 1991 Jul; 57: 42.
117. Council on Dental Materials, Instruments, and Equipment. Denture cleansers. *J Am Dent Assoc* 1983; 106: 77–9.
118. Council on Dental Materials, Instruments, and Equipment, Council on Dental Therapeutics. *Clinical Products in Dentistry: A Desktop Reference*. Chicago: American Dental Association; 1992 Jan: 8.
119. Gossel TA. The proper use of denture adhesives and reliners. *US Pharm* 1987 Sep; 12: 42, 46, 48, 51.
120. Klatell J, Kaplan A, Williams G Jr. *Family Guide to Dental Health*. New York: Macmillan; 1991: 37.
121. Baker KA, Levy SM. Review of systemic fluoride supplementation and consideration of the pharmacist's role. *Drug Intell Clin Pharm* 1986; 20: 935–42.
122. Wilson M. Fighting plaque. *Am Drug* 1988 Sep; 198: 102–4.
123. Klatell J, Kaplan A, Williams G Jr. *Family Guide to Dental Health*. New York: Macmillan; 1991: 83.
124. Harris NO, Christen AG. *Primary Preventive Dentistry*. 3rd ed. Norwalk, Conn: Appleton & Lange; 1991: 487.

CHAPTER 24

Ostomy and Wound Care Products

Michael L. Kleinberg and Moya J. Vazquez

> **Questions to ask in patient assessment and counseling**
>
> **Ostomies**
>
> - *What type of ostomy do you have? Where is it located?*
> - *How long have you had the ostomy?*
> - *Do you irrigate and/or use a pouch?*
> - *What type of appliance are you using?*
> - *What is the stoma size?*
> - *Do you have problems with the skin surrounding the stoma?*
> - *Have you noticed any change in the contents of your fecal discharge or urinary output?*
> - *Are you experiencing any problems related to your ostomy, such as diarrhea or gas?*
> - *Are you having any problems with odor or gas control?*
> - *Are you taking any prescription or nonprescription medications?*
>
> **Wounds**
>
> - *What type of wound do you have?*
> - *How long has the wound been present?*
> - *Is there redness or swelling around the wound?*
> - *Does the wound emit any odor?*

Ostomy Care

An ostomy is the surgical formation of an opening, or outlet, through the abdominal wall for the purpose of eliminating waste. It is usually made by passing the colon, small intestine, or ureters through the abdominal wall. The opening of the ostomy is called the stoma.

An understanding of the digestive process is important because ostomy surgery interrupts this process. The particular problems associated with each type of ostomy are directly related to the phase of digestion that is interrupted. Major functions of the digestive system include the digestion and absorption of foodstuffs and the absorption of water. Digestion begins in the mouth and continues in the stomach and small intestine; water absorption takes place in the large intestine. (The anatomy of the lower digestive tract and the urinary tract is shown in Figure 1.) (See Chapter 11, "Antacid Products," and Chapter 13, "Antidiarrheal Products.")

Ostomy surgery necessitates the use of an appliance designed to collect the waste material normally eliminated through the bowel or bladder. Approximately 90,000 ostomies are created annually in the United States, and more than 1 million patients have established stomas.[1]

The idea of cutting into the abdominal cavity and creating an artificial opening is not new. This type of surgery was first suggested in 1710 by a French physician, Alexis Littre.[2] Since that time, the technique of ostomy surgery has been refined greatly. The surgical creation of a stoma is only the first step in the rehabilitation of an ostomate (a person with an ostomy). Complete recovery depends on how well ostomy patients understand and adjust to their changed medical and physical circumstances.

Because each ostomy patient is different, one patient may benefit from a particular type of appliance, whereas another may develop problems with it. The ostomy patient should know how to apply and fit an appliance that affords maximum benefit.

Pharmacists who are involved in ostomy care must be familiar with the various types of ostomies and with the use and maintenance of the appliances for each type of surgery. They should also be prepared to provide patients with information on special needs related to ostomy care, such as skin care, diet, fluid intake, and drug therapy.

Pharmacy involvement in ostomy care is important. The American Pharmaceutical Association identifies ostomy care as an area in which the pharmacist plays a clinical role in direct patient care. The American Society of Hospital Pharmacists specifies experience in ostomy care in its accreditation standards for residency training. Procurement and distribution of ostomy supplies and patient counseling are necessary services that can be provided by the pharmacist.

Types of Ostomies

Several types of ostomies are performed regularly. They include ileostomy, in which the entire colon and possibly part of the ileum are removed; colostomy (ascending, transverse, descending, and sigmoid), in which the colon is partially removed; and urostomy, or urinary diversion, in which the bladder may be removed. A discussion of each type follows. Special problems affecting patients often depend on the location of the ostomy. Skin irritation and

---

This chapter is based in part on the chapter with a similar title that appeared in the 9th edition but was written by Michael L. Kleinberg and Melba C. Connors.

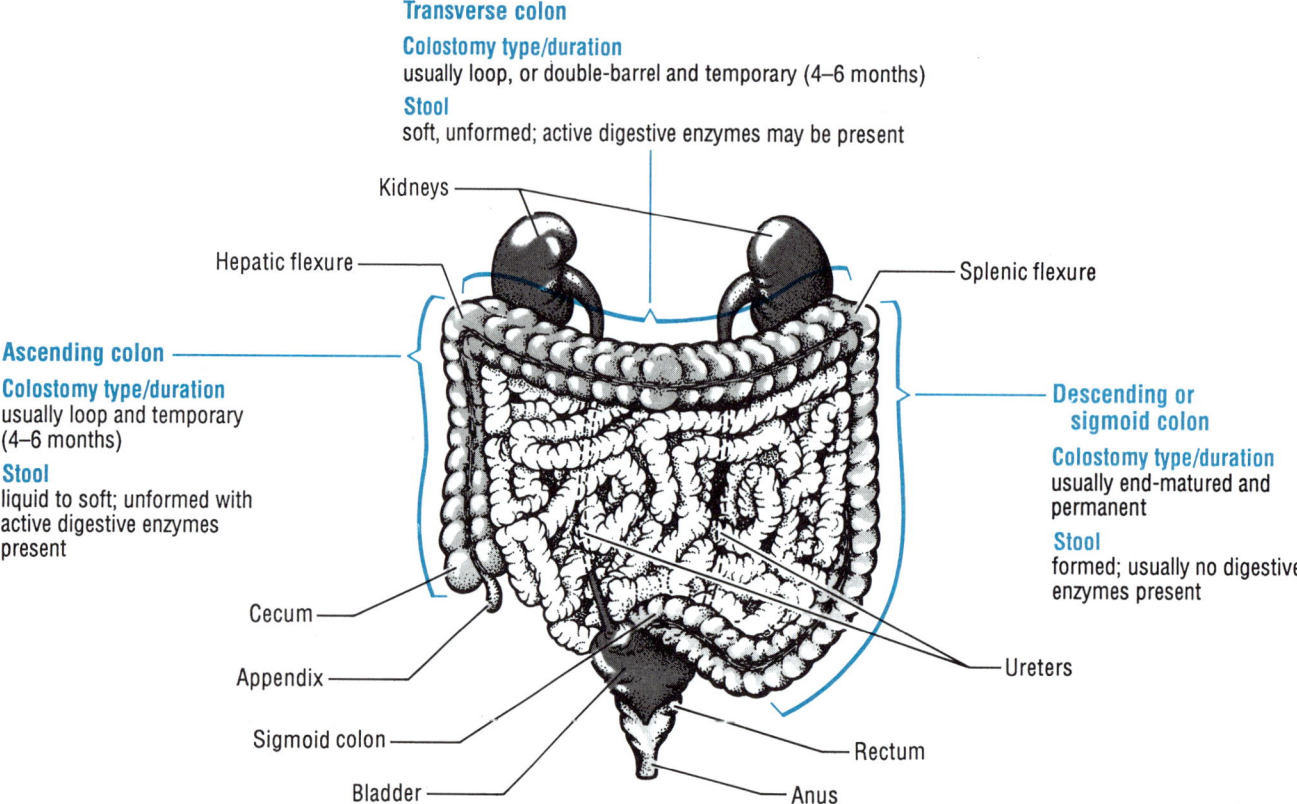

FIGURE 1 Anatomic drawing of the lower digestive and urinary tracts, which depicts the location and permanence of colostomies. Adapted with permission from *Am J Nurs* 1977; 77 (3): 443.

electrolyte and fluid imbalance cause more problems in ostomates with a fluid or semisoft stoma discharge. This is a factor for ileostomates, for ascending and transverse colostomates, and for urostomates. Urostomates and ileostomates may also experience an increased incidence of kidney and gallbladder stone formation. Constipation may be a problem in patients with descending and sigmoid colostomies.

Ileostomy

An ileostomy is a surgically created opening between the ileum and the abdominal wall. Reasons to have ileostomy surgery include ulcerative colitis, Crohn's disease, trauma, familial polyposis, and necrotizing enterocolitis. The two most common disorders requiring ileostomy surgery, ulcerative colitis and Crohn's disease, are inflammatory conditions affecting the intestines. Ulcerative colitis affects the large intestine and rectum. Its clinical course is often prolonged, with the patient experiencing remissions and exacerbations. Crohn's disease may involve any part of the gastrointestinal tract. As the disease progresses, the bowel wall thickens, causing the lumen to narrow. Obstruction may result, requiring surgery. Patients with these diseases may develop debilitating extraintestinal manifestations. In an acute episode, toxic megacolon and perforation are possible. These conditions require surgery. The entire colon is surgically removed, and the ileum is brought to the surface of the abdomen (Figure 2A).

It should be mentioned that a total proctocolectomy, which results in an ileostomy, is considered a cure for the ulcerative colitis patient. Because of the possibility of the disease's recurrence, coupled with the total loss of large bowel function, the same surgical procedure is used less often in patients with Crohn's disease. Mortality for elective surgery for ulcerative colitis is in the range of 0–2%; for emergency surgery mortality is about 4 to 5%, and for toxic megacolon it increases to 17%. A major complication of any surgical procedure is sepsis, either in the wound or in the intra-abdominal cavity. The most common late complication of ileostomy surgery is intestinal obstruction, which occurs in about 10% of ileostomy patients.

The discharge from an ileostomy ranges from liquid to semisoft because it contains fluid that normally would be absorbed from the large bowel. When the colon is removed, the body loses the capacity to reabsorb water. Therefore, ileostomates must maintain adequate fluid intake to compensate for this water loss.

Excoriation of the skin is a common problem for ileostomates. The continuous flow of liquid or semisoft discharge contains active pancreatic enzymes that irritate and digest unprotected skin. Diligent hygiene and special protective measures can help prevent these problems. Patients with standard ileostomies are never continent. The flow is continuous, and an appliance must be worn at all times.

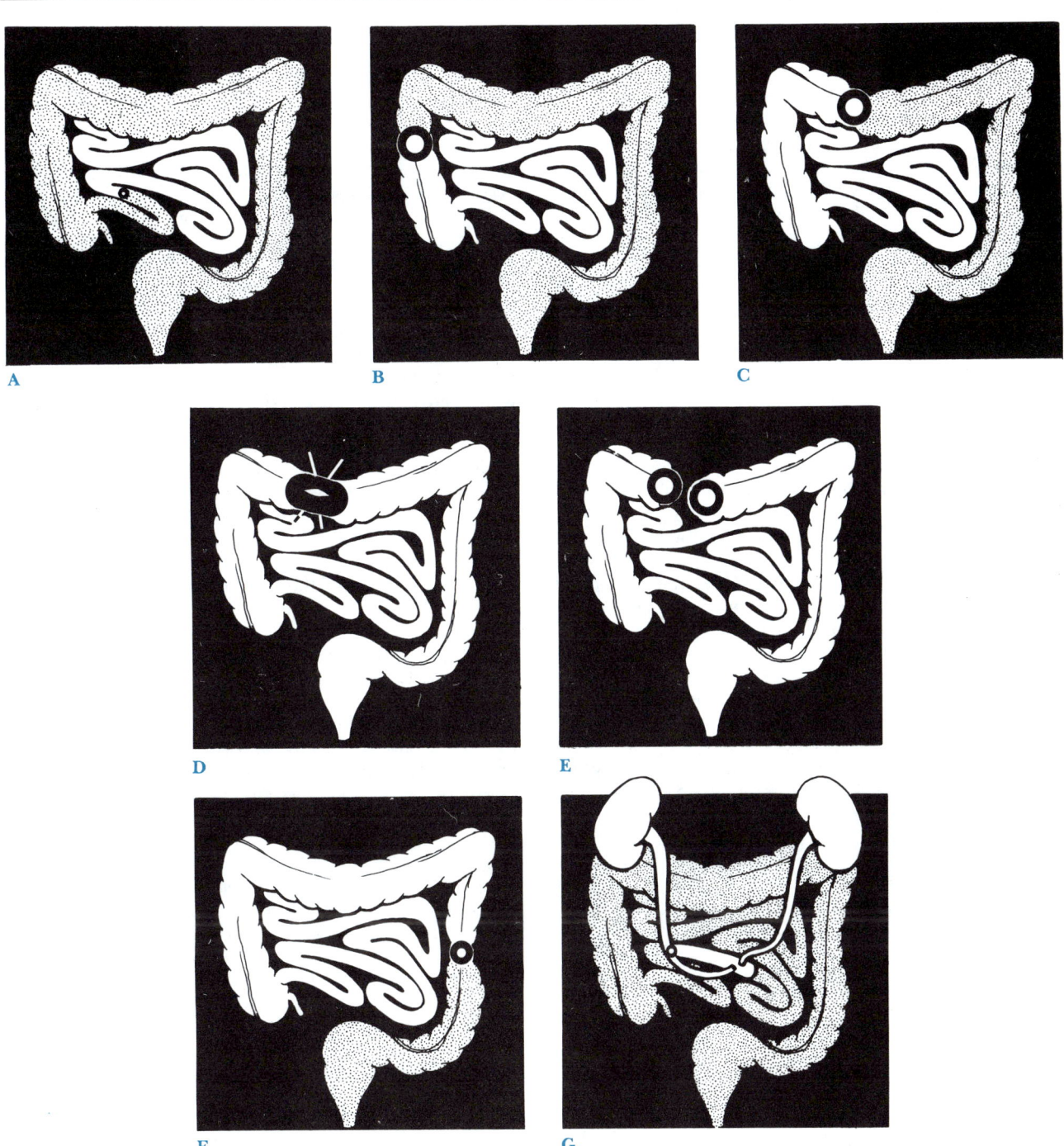

FIGURE 2A–G Types of ostomies: A, ileostomy; B, ascending colostomy; C, transverse colostomy; D, loop ostomy; E, double-barrel colostomy; F, descending or sigmoid colostomy; G, ileal conduit. Adapted from the Hollister Ostomy Reference Chart, Copyright© 1978, 1979, 1980, Hollister, Incorporated (all rights reserved) and from Wuest JR. *J Am Pharm Assoc* 1975; NS15: 626.

Researchers are continually working on ways to render the ileostomate continent. One procedure, developed by Dr. Nils Kock of Sweden, may be an alternative for those who meet certain criteria.[3] The surgeon creates a pouch internally, made from 35–50 cm of ileum. An intussusception of the bowel is used to create a "nipple" that renders the patient continent for stool and flatus. The distal limb of the ileum is brought to the abdomen. A flush stoma is made just above the hairline. The pouch is emptied by inserting a catheter through the nipple into the pouch. At first, the pouch holds approximately 75 mL. It stretches with use so that 6 months postoperatively it can hold 600–800 mL without discomfort or danger. At this time, the pouch needs to be drained only three or four times a day.

Restorative Proctocolectomy

A newer operation, restorative proctocolectomy, involves sparing the rectum of those with ulcerative colitis or familial polyposis. The mucosa is stripped from the rectum, rendering it free of disease. An internal pouch is created from the small bowel, but without a nipple valve. The distal end of the ileum is then pulled through the rectum and attached. Thus the sphincter is preserved and no ostomy is necessary. Because of the different ways the internal pouch can be constructed, one may hear this operation described as an S or J pouch. Recipients of this procedure have more frequent bowel movements and may experience some perianal skin irritation.

Because the diseases and conditions requiring ileostomy surgery are found primarily in persons 15–25 years of age, the advantages of this operation are obvious. For those in the prime of their athletic, social, and sexual lives, the absence of an external pouch allows a speedy adjustment and rehabilitation. Not everyone is a candidate for this surgery, however. Among the factors taken into consideration are the patient's age (between 15 and 50 is believed to be ideal), intelligence, absence of Crohn's disease, motivation, other handicaps, and general health.

Colostomy

A colostomy is the creation of an artificial opening using part of the large intestine or colon. Major indications for performing a colostomy include obstruction of the colon or rectum, cancer of the colon or rectum, genetic malformation, diverticular disease, trauma, and loss of anal muscular control. The three types of colostomies (Figure 1) are named for the portion of the bowel that is brought to the outside of the body to form the stoma: ascending colostomies, transverse colostomies (further subdivided into temporary loop ostomies, double-barrel colostomies, and permanent stoma colostomies), and descending or sigmoid colostomies.

When certain conditions are present in the lower bowel, it may be necessary to perform a temporary colostomy so that the lower bowel can heal. Healing of the diseased bowel may take several weeks, months, or years. Eventually the colon and rectum are reconnected and bowel continuity is restored. A permanent colostomy is formed when the rectum is removed. A colostomy, permanent or temporary, may be made in any part of the colon.

The type of colostomy the surgeon will perform depends on the condition being treated. If the disease entity is cancer, the section of bowel may be resected without a colostomy. If the lesion is in the lower rectum, however, the entire rectum is removed, resulting in a permanent colostomy. The most common disease that may result in a colostomy is diverticulitis. It presents as small balloon-like areas in the lining of the large intestine. Sometimes these areas become irritated and rupture, resulting in peritonitis, which usually requires emergency surgery. To protect the perforated section and the suture line when this area is surgically removed, a temporary colostomy may be performed. The opening can be made at any point in the bowel above the lesion. The more proximal the colostomy, the more watery and frequent the output will be. When the disease process is resolved and the suture line is healed, a comparatively minor operation is performed to restore the continuity of the large intestine.

Ascending Colostomy

In an ascending colostomy, the ascending colon is retained but the rest of the large bowel is removed or bypassed. This ostomy appears on the right side of the abdomen (Figure 2B). Its discharge is semiliquid because the fluid has not been reabsorbed. The patient must wear an appliance continuously.

Transverse Colostomy

In a transverse colostomy, an opening is usually created on the right side of the transverse colon (Figure 2C) in one of two ways. One method entails lifting a loop of the transverse colon through the abdominal incision. A rod or bridge is then placed under the loop to give additional support (Figure 2D) and is removed after a few days. Another method is to divide the bowel completely and have two openings (double-barrel colostomy) (Figure 2E). In this case, the proximal stoma discharges fecal material and the distal stoma secretes small amounts of mucus. Although the remaining colon increases its hydrating function with time, the discharge generally stays semisoft. Generally, irrigation does not produce control in patients who have transverse colostomies; therefore, an appliance must be worn continuously.

Descending and Sigmoid Colostomies

Descending and sigmoid colostomies are on the left side of the abdomen (Figure 2F). They can be made as double-barrel or single-barrel openings. Because the fecal discharge is firm and often can be regulated by irrigation, an appliance may not be needed. However, many patients prefer appliances to irrigation. Several factors should be considered in connection with the decision to irrigate, including the following:[4]

- The capability of the patient to manage the irrigation procedure;
- The prognosis of the patient;
- The presence of either stomal stenosis or peristomal hernia;
- The presence of radiation enteritis.

Urinary Diversions (Urostomies)

Urinary diversions are performed as a result of bladder loss or dysfunction usually caused by cancer, neurogenic bladder, or genetic malformation. An ileal or colon conduit is created by implanting the ureters into an isolated loop of bowel, the distal end of which is brought to the surface of the abdomen (Figure 2G). An appliance must be worn continuously. In another procedure, a ureterostomy, the ureters are detached from the bladder and brought to the outside of the abdominal wall. This procedure is performed less frequently because the ureters tend to narrow unless they have been dilated permanently by previous disease.

Continent Urostomy

Dr. Kock has developed an operation to render urinary diversion patients continent. It is very much like the continent ileostomy previously described, except that the ureters are inserted into the proximal limb of the ileum leading into the isolated internal ileal pouch and an additional nipple valve is created at the proximal opening of the pouch. This keeps the urine from refluxing into the kidneys, thus lessening the chance of infection. Other continent urinary operations, such as the Indiana pouch, are being devised, but they are all similar in that the pouch is drained by a catheter.

Appliances and Accessories

The appliance is an extremely important aspect of the ostomate's well-being. The ostomate has lost a normal body function; the appliance takes over that lost function and almost becomes a part of the body. The type of appliance depends on the type of surgery performed. Patients with regulated colostomies (who irrigate routinely with no output from the stoma between irrigations) may wear closed-end appliances or a gauze square. Those with unregulated colostomies and ileostomies usually wear open-end appliances to allow frequent emptying. The ideal appliance would be leak-proof, comfortable, easily manipulated, odor-proof, inconspicuous, inexpensive, and safe.[5] Unfortunately, no one appliance meets all of these criteria. (Major manufacturers of ostomy products and accessories are listed in the appendix to this chapter.)

Appliances

In the past, most ostomy appliances were reusable. The advantages of reusable appliances are their durability, availability in many complexities, and relatively low cost. Their disadvantages are that they require cleaning before each use and that they are heavy, tend to retain odor, and often require a separate skin barrier. Reusable appliances may still be the best choice for some patients because of the many modalities available for treatment.

Most ostomates are now fitted with disposable appliances. Most of these appliances incorporate a skin barrier in each flange, eliminating the need for a separate skin barrier. The disposable equipment is available in one- and two-piece systems. The two-piece system allows the patient to center the flange easily and to change the pouch, if desired, without removing the flange from the skin. The one-piece system is very flat; it has no ring that might be noticeable through clothes. The one-piece system is also easy to apply because it does not require the dexterity needed for the two-piece system. Some manufacturers offer different depths of convexity, which make the two-piece system available to more people. Reusable and disposable appliances are available in both transparent and opaque styles.

Belts

Special belts attached to various appliances give additional support. Belts are made for specific appliances and generally are not interchangeable. Not all ostomates need to wear belts. Indications for use are a deeply convex faceplate, poor wearing time, activity (especially in children), heavy perspiration, and personal preference. Belts may cause ulcers if worn too tight. To be effective, the belt must be kept even with the belt hooks. If the belt slips up around the waist, it may cause poor adherence and possibly a cut of the stoma.

Skin Barriers

Skin barriers are intended to protect the skin immediately adjacent to the stoma and to provide a barrier between the skin and the stoma discharge. They also correct imperfections in the skin surface, allowing the appliance to fit securely. Except in patients with urinary diversions, a skin barrier should always be used with appliances. Skin barriers (e.g., Stomahesive® wafers, HolliHesive® wafers, and Colly-Seels®), powders, and pastes are available for special skin problems. The powder is used on weeping skin. The paste (which is not a glue but has a pasty consistency) is used to seal around the stoma and to fill in creases in the skin. These products produce a flat surface for application of other skin barriers.

Skin Protective Dressings

A waterproof dressing can be applied to the skin in a thin film, which might be described as a chemical bandage. After application, the product leaves a thin protective layer on the skin that aids in the removal of adhesive tape and absorbs the stress normally applied to the top layers of the skin when the ostomy appliance is removed. Although these dressings promote skin protection, they do not replace skin barriers such as Stomahesive®. When the skin is reddened but unbroken, these preparations briefly protect the skin from the contact agent causing the redness. They also can help to waterproof tape around a draining wound. These dressings come in varying forms: gel, bottle (with brush), spray can, roll-on, and wipe-on packets.

Transparent, semipermeable dressings come in many sizes, from one used for intravenous sites to a complete body wrap. These dressings are transparent, sterile materials that are sticky on one side; they can be used as a dressing, as a second skin to which appliances are affixed, or as a prophylactic for preventing skin irritation. They take some dexterity to apply, however, and two persons may be needed to apply larger pieces. Op Site®, Tegaderm®, and Bioclusive® are examples of these dressings.

Special Skin Care

Several companies manufacture products especially for the incontinent patient or others at high risk of excoriation.

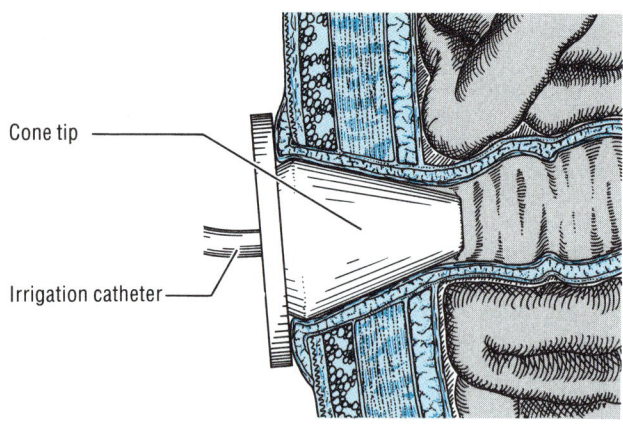

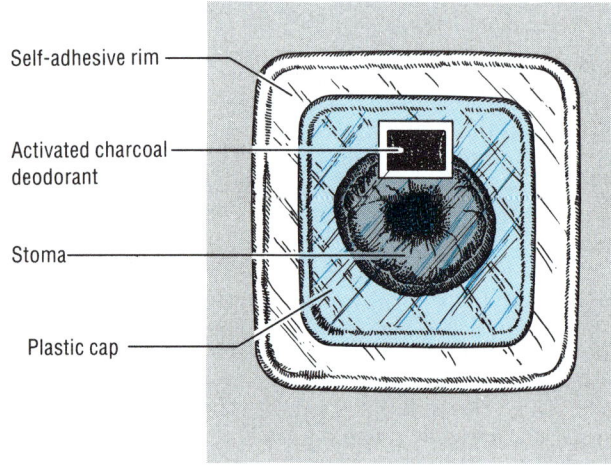

FIGURE 3 Colostomy irrigation set. A cone-tipped irrigator is preferred to a plain catheter to avoid possibility of false passage and bowel perforation. Adapted with permission from *Clinical Symposia*, illustrated by John A. Craig, M.D. Copyright© 1978 CIBA-GEIGY Corporation (all rights reserved.

The products include a gentle liquid cleaner that renders output odorless, a cream that can be rubbed into the skin and to which the appliance will adhere, and an ointment that is not water soluble and gives high-grade protection to vulnerable areas where pouching is not appropriate.

Tape
Hypoallergenic tape supports appliances. A strip may be applied across the top, bottom, and sides of the faceplate, with half on the faceplate and half on the skin.

Irrigating Sets
A patient with a colostomy distal to the splenic flexure who gives no history of an irritable bowel, who is not a child, who does not have a disabling handicap, and who wants to maintain control without a pouch is a candidate for irrigation. To be safe and effective, a colostomy irrigation set, rather than a standard enema set, should be used. This set consists of a reservoir for the irrigating fluid, a tube, a graduated clamp, a soft catheter, and a dam or cone (Figure 3). Perforation of the bowel is a serious complication of irrigation, but it has almost been eliminated by use of a cone, which is inserted 1/2 to 1 in. into the colostomy. In patients who are not able to use a cone, the catheter should not be inserted more than 2 in. past the dam. Although introducing water into the bowel stimulates peristalsis, control (meaning at least 24 hours without any output) is rarely achieved unless the colostomate instills and holds in a prescribed amount of water. Therefore, the dam, takes the place of the absent sphincter, allowing the patient to hold in the water.

The irrigating set also includes a sleeve that attaches to a faceplate that is held on the patient by a belt. The distal end of the sleeve is inserted into the toilet. Thus the returns go into the toilet, leaving no waste material to be cleaned up after this procedure. Frequency of irrigation depends somewhat on the colostomate's normal bowel habits. After control is achieved, the patient may wear a piece of gauze over the stoma or wear a security pouch. The irrigation is not necessary for health; it is merely one method of management.

Deodorizers
Odor control is either local or systemic. Some agents are placed directly in the appliance to mask the odor of the fecal discharge. Liquid concentrates are available as companion products of most ostomy devices; they can be placed directly into the pouch to neutralize odor. Specially formulated bathroom sprays are also available. Ostomates sometimes place aspirin tablets in the pouch to control odor, but this practice should be discouraged because aspirin may irritate the stoma.

In addition to local methods of odor control, devices are available that fit directly on the pouch to filter and control gas and odors. One such commercial device is a charcoal filter, which is placed on the pouch. Newer pouches are formulated with an odor-barrier film.

Fitting and Application
Measuring the stoma to determine the proper fit of an appliance is an important part of ostomy care. An appliance with an opening smaller than the stoma may cause abrasion of the stoma and poor wearing time. An appliance with an opening larger than necessary, even with a snug-fitting skin barrier, may allow skin excoriation and hyperplasia formation. Considerations in fitting the appliance include body contour, stoma location, skin creases and scars, and type of ostomy. The lack of uniformity in types of ostomies and ostomy equipment makes it difficult to give standard instructions for application. Some procedures for applying different types of appliances and their accessories (Figure 4) are discussed in greater detail in readily available patient-oriented pamphlets.[6,7] An enterostomal therapy (ET) nurse is an excellent source of assistance in the custom fitting of these appliances.

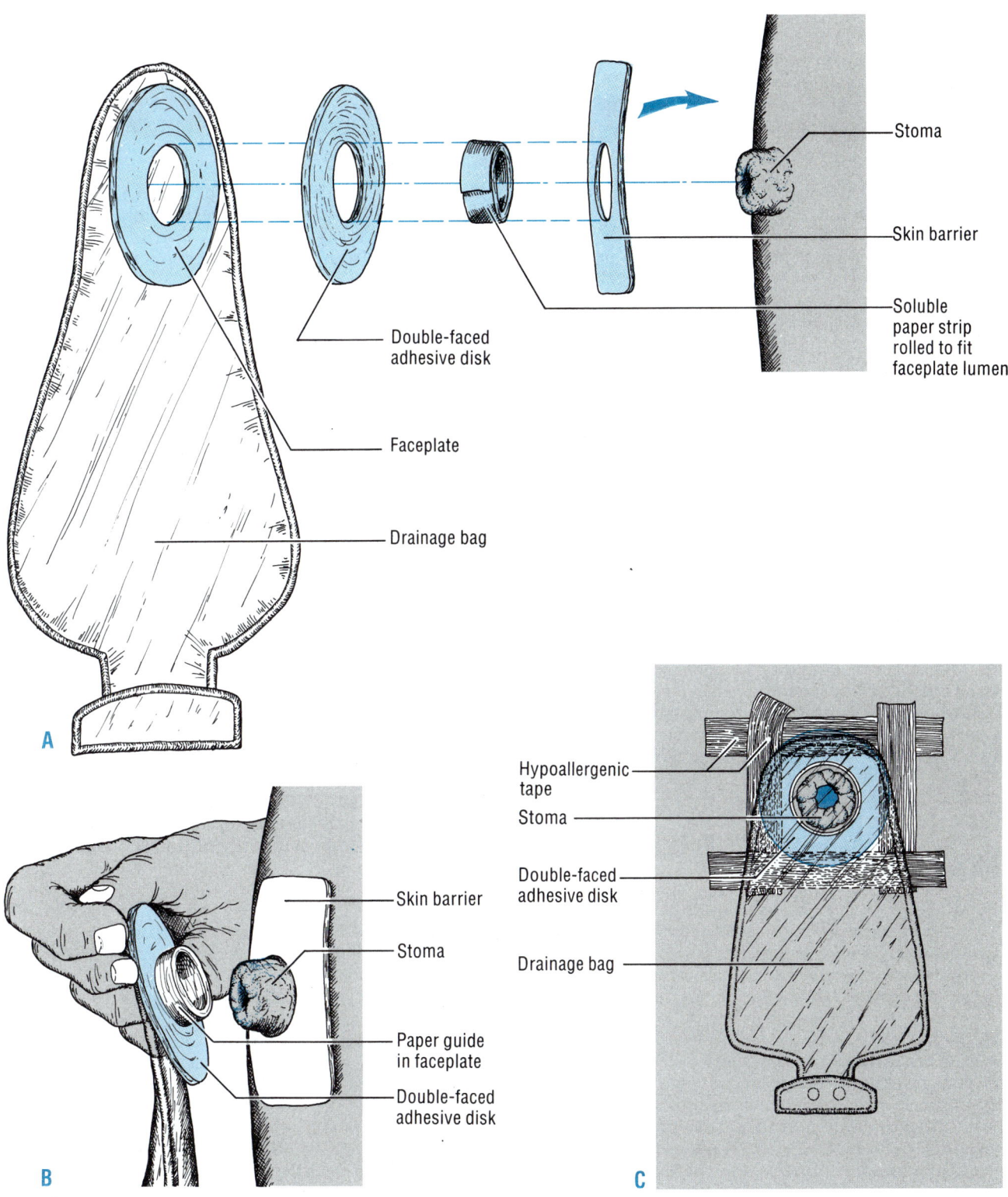

FIGURE 4A–C Components of an ileostomy appliance: A, drainable bag and skin barrier; B, after skin barrier is affixed to skin, the appliance is placed, using paper strip guide to align faceplate lumen over stoma; C, hypoallergenic tape placed around faceplate in "picture frame" fashion.

Potential Complications

Ostomates may experience both psychologic and physical complications. The pharmacist should be prepared to handle these complications or to refer patients to an ET nurse. A thorough explanation before surgery of the type of surgery to be performed, what to expect during the postsurgical recovery period, and the appliances and supplies the patient will use often alleviates the patient's anxiety.

Psychologic Complications

After ostomy surgery, depending on previous mental status and self-confidence, the patient may be psychologically depressed. There may also be fears of not being able to engage in former work, participate in sports, perform sexually, or have children. The pharmacist should reassure the patient that the ability to carry out these activities or functions generally remains unchanged. However, the pharmacist should be aware that most men who have a radical resection of the rectum or bladder are rendered organically impotent. Penile implants or other erection aids could enable a man to regain part or all of this function. If the patient is concerned about impotence, a referral to his urologist would be appropriate.

The United Ostomy Association, formed in 1962, comprises various ostomy organizations in the United States whose main purpose is to help ostomy patients by giving moral support and supplying information. The United Ostomy Association (36 Executive Park #120, Irvine, CA 92714, [714-660-8624]) sponsors national, regional, and local meetings and publishes a quarterly journal and other literature.

ET is a comparatively new nursing specialty. Registered nurses with postgraduate education from an accredited school for ET may specialize in ostomy care. A representative listing of ET nurses may be obtained from the Executive Secretary, International Association of Enterostomal Therapy, 2081 Business Center Drive #290, Irvine, CA 92715 (714-476-0268).

Physical Complications

Physical complications of ostomies include stenosis of the stoma, fistula formation, prolapse, retraction, and skin irritation. A continuing series of articles concerning physical problems, their assessment, and care have been published in the medical literature.[8]

Stenosis

Stenosis (narrowing) of the stoma is caused by the formation of scar tissue. Excessive scar tissue usually is caused by improper surgical construction, postoperative ischemia, active disease, or alkaline stomatitis or dermatitis. Although dilation of the stoma is often advocated to prevent or palliate this problem, the only cure is revision of the stoma.

Fistula

The formation of an opening, or fistula tract, from inside the body to the skin most often is a manifestation of inflammatory bowel disease. Other causes of this complication are cancer, abscess formation, foreign body retention, radiation, tuberculosis, and trauma. Treatment is with hyperalimentation, surgery, or both.

Prolapse

Prolapse, the abnormal extension of the bowel beyond the abdominal wall, frequently results when the opening in the abdominal wall is too large. The danger of prolapse is the resultant decrease in blood supply to the bowel outside the abdominal cavity. Treatment is surgical correction.

Retraction

Retraction is the recession of the stoma to a subnormal length. It may be caused by several factors, including active Crohn's disease. It also may lead to damage of the skin surface. Treatment is surgical correction.

Skin Irritation

Skin irritation can occur from a number of causes, most commonly excoriation from the output, sensitivity to a product, monilial infection, epithelial hyperplasia, alkaline dermatitis, infection, or Crohn's disease.

Output Excoriation   Excoriation, an abrasion of the epidermis by digestive enzymes from output, occurs when an improper pouch is worn, the lumen in the faceplate is too big, or the pouch has leaked and has not been promptly replaced. This allows fecal or urinary output to come in contact with the skin. Fecal output may contain active pancreatic enzymes (especially in the case of an ileostomy) that digest the skin protein. The alkaline nature of the fecal output also is irritating to unprotected skin. Alkaline urine is similarly irritating and causes excoriation. These two conditions are treated differently. After diagnosis and treatment, a skin barrier and pouch may be applied. The pouch should be changed as infrequently as possible to lessen irritation and treatment should be continued until the skin is clear.

Sensitivity   Preoperative patch testing of patients with a history of allergy, adhesive tape reaction, eczema, or psoriasis and those with very fair skin can help prevent skin irritation caused by sensitivity to a product. Patch testing can easily be done by the physician or ET nurse and checked by the patient at home.

Monilial Infection   Monilial infection may be a problem in patients who wear appliances continuously. A dark, warm, moist environment provides an area for growth of species of Candida. The primary symptom is itching. If the condition is diagnosed early, an application of nystatin powder is useful. If the infection is allowed to continue unchecked, the skin will become denuded, the faceplate will not stick, and additional skin irritation will result from the output. The nystatin preparation should be used every other day and for 1 week after the skin has become clear.

In treating monilial infections, it is also important to ascertain whether the ostomate is taking antibiotics. Any antibiotic, but especially a broad-spectrum agent, changes the flora of the skin, and the entrenched monilia become difficult to eradicate. For ostomy patients taking antibiotics, nystatin powder should be continued for 1 month after the yeast is gone.

Hyperplasia   Hyperplasia, the overgrowth of hyperplastic skin, occurs when the faceplate opening is too large. In the early stages there is no pain, but later the affected skin cells multiply and cause agonizing pain. The condition resembles a mucosal malignancy. To treat the condition, a Colly-Seel® is placed over the skin, fitting closely around the stoma. A convex faceplate that is just 1/16 in. larger than the stoma is applied, and a snug belt is added. A mild case of hyperplasia generally resolves in 1 week. Severe cases, although treated the same, may take from 1 month to 6 weeks to heal. Other treatment methods are cauterization and surgical removal.

Alkaline Dermatitis Many patients with urinary diversions have problems with alkaline urine. Although normal urine is not particularly irritating on intact skin, urine that is alkaline may have gross effects on the stoma and skin. It is a major cause of frank blood in the pouch because it renders the stoma extremely friable.

The treatment is to acidify the urine. The patient should avoid alkaline ash foods, especially citrus fruits and juices, which, although originally acidic, are excreted in alkaline form. Ascorbic acid or cranberry juice acidifies the urine.

The stoma and skin may be soaked with a 50% solution of white vinegar and water. The saturated cloth is renewed with new solution as often as necessary. This treatment must be repeated every 4 hours while the patient is awake. The appliance can then be applied. If the manifestation is mild, this procedure should be performed once every other day until the skin is clear. Most of the new urinary appliances have an antireflux feature, which keeps the urine from resting on the stoma or exposed skin.

Infection With the possible exception of patients with Crohn's disease, ostomates do not have more frequent infections of the peristomal skin, or other skin, than do nonostomates. However, an infection under the faceplate can be a problem. If the skin is indurated, swollen, and red, it may need incision and draining. At that time, a culture is taken and sent to the lab for culture and sensitivity testing. The appropriate antibiotic can be prescribed topically, systemically, or both. It may be a challenge to devise a way of containing the discharge while leaving the affected area accessible for treatment.

Excessive Sweating Sweating under the faceplate can decrease wearing time and cause monilial infection. Cement and a belt may be necessary to hold the appliance in place. Discomfort from perspiration underneath the collection pouch can be alleviated by purchasing or making a cover or bib to keep the pouch material from touching the skin.

Diet

Diet does not play an important role in management of the ostomy patient. Most patients can eat a liberal diet, including all of the foods eaten before surgery, if the foods are chewed well. However, it is wise to remain on a diet low in fiber for the first 6 weeks after surgery to allow the intestine to heal and swelling to resolve. After that time, a regular diet can be resumed. Urostomates may want to avoid asparagus or other foods that cause odor. Irrigating colostomates should avoid any food that causes them to have loose stools. (This varies with each individual.) Patients with ileostomies are more prone to obstruction from high-roughage foods eaten in large quantities or exclusive of other food. These patients should chew certain foods well and eat them in small amounts and with other food; these foods include popcorn, nuts, corn on the cob, mushrooms, bran products, citrus fruits, coconut, Chinese vegetables, raw celery, and raw carrots.

Because they have no control over gas passage, fecal ostomates may prefer to cut down on gas-forming foods such as beans, vegetables of the cabbage family, onions, beer, and carbonated drinks.

Osteomates may also want to avoid odor-producing foods such as cheese, eggs, fish, beans, onions, vegetables of the cabbage family, some vitamins or medications, and asparagus.

Patients with a urostomy, ileostomy, or ascending colostomy must include an adequate amount of fluid in their diets to prevent the precipitation of crystals or kidney stones in the urine. Absence of the large bowel may not allow normal absorption of water needed to maintain urinary volume.

Use of Medications

Because part or all of the colon is removed and intestinal transit time may be altered, the ostomate may experience adverse affects from taking prescription or nonprescription medications, or the medications may be ineffective (Table 1).

Coated or sustained-release preparations may pass through the intestinal tract without being absorbed, and the patient may receive a subtherapeutic dose. The ostomate should look for any undissolved drug particles in the pouch. Liquid preparations or preparations that are crushed or chewed before swallowing are best.

The ostomate also must be careful in taking antibiotics, diuretics, and laxatives. Antibiotics may alter the normal flora of the intestinal tract, causing diarrhea or fungal infection of the skin surrounding the stoma. If diarrhea occurs, fluid and electrolyte intake should be increased. Antidiarrheal and antimotility drugs may affect ileal excreta.[9] The physician may prescribe nystatin powder to treat fungal overgrowth.

Sulfa drugs should be used with caution. Crystallization in the kidney may occur more often in patients having difficulty with fluid balance. To minimize this problem, fluid intake should be increased and the urine should not be acidified. In ileostomy patients, whose fluid and electrolyte balance is more difficult to maintain, diuretics should be given with care because additional loss of fluid may cause dehydration and electrolyte imbalance.[10] The ileostomate should be monitored for signs of hyponatremia if salt substitutes are prescribed.

Laxatives may be used by colostomy patients, but only under close supervision. Ostomates tend to become obstructed, and the laxative's particular action may cause perforation. If the colostomate is constipated, a stool softener may be recommended. Antacids may cause problems and should be taken with caution. Products containing calcium may cause calcium stones in the urostomate; products containing magnesium may cause diarrhea in the ileostomate; and aluminum products may cause constipation in the colostomate. To alleviate any anxiety, the

TABLE 1 Effects of certain medications on the ostomate

	Colostomate	Ileostomate	Urostomate
Dosage Forms			
Chewable tablets	1	1	1
Enteric-coated tablets	1	3	1
Sustained-release medication	1	3	1
Liquid medication	1	1	1
Gelatin capsules	1	1	1
Compounds			
Alcohol	1	1	1
Antibiotics (poorly absorbed)	1	2,3	1,2
Antidiarrheal agents	1,2	1	1
Calcium-containing antacids	2	2	2
Corticosteroids	1	2	1
Diuretics	1	2	2
Magnesium-containing antacids	2	2	1
Opiates	1,2	1	1
Salicylates	1	1	1
Salt substitutes	1	2	1
Stool softeners	1	2	1
Sulfa drugs	1	1	2
Vitamins	1	2	1

Key:
1. means medication probably has no adverse effects.
2. means medication may cause an increase in adverse effects; patient should be monitored.
3. means medication may be ineffective; patient should be monitored.

patient should be counseled about medications that may discolor the feces (Table 2).

Summary: Ostomy Care

With proper instructions and equipment, ostomates can lead normal, healthy lives. Pharmacists can help by giving patients information about treatment and ostomy supply services and by referring patients to an ET nurse when appropriate.

Wound Care Overview

The approach to wound care has dramatically changed over the last decade. In the past, problems related to wound healing were approached empirically and solutions were usually based on anecdotal experience. Popular opinion dictated that wounds be left exposed to air to encourage dryness and scab formation. Occlusive dressings were expressly avoided because it was thought that the moist, warm environment they created would promote bacterial colonization. Winter and colleagues first showed in the

TABLE 2 Medications that may discolor feces

Medication (brand name)	Effect
Aluminum antacids	Whitish color or speckling
Antibiotics (oral)	Greenish gray
Anticoagulants (excess)	Pink to red to black (bleeding)
Bismuth salts	Black
Charcoal	Black
Ferrous salts	Black
Heaprin	Pink to red to black (bleeding)
Indomethacin (Indocin)	Green
Oxyphenbutazone (Tandearil)	Pink to red to black (bleeding)
Phenazopyridine (Pyridium)	Orange red
Phenophtalein	Red
Phenylbutazone (Butazolidin)	Pink to red to black (bleeding)
Pyrvinium pamoate (Povan)	Red
Salicylates	Pink to red to black (bleeding)
Senna (and other anthraquinone derivatives)	Yellow-green to brown

Reprinted from Strauss S. *Your Prescription and You—A Pharmacy Handbook for Consumers*. 3rd ed. Ambler, Pa: Medical Business Services; 1978.

TABLE 3 Growth factors influencing wound healing

Factor	Source	Target Receptor
TGF-ß[a]	Platelets Macrophage Lymphocyte Bone Most tissues	All cells
PDGF[b]	Platelets Macrophage Endothelial cell Smooth muscle cell	Fibroblast Smooth muscle cell Glial cell
aFGF[c] and bFGF/HBGF[d]	Macrophage Cartilage (CGDF)[e] Brain (ECGF)[f]	Endothelial cell Fibroblast Chondrocyte Glial cell, etc.
EGF[g]	Saliva Urine	Epithelial cell Fibroblast
TGF-α[h]	Platelets Keratinocyte Macrophage	Epithelial cell Fibroblast Endothelial cell
EDF[i]	Epithelial cell	Epithelial cell Fibroblast
MDGF[j]	Macrophage	Fibroblast Smooth muscle cell
IGF-I/Sm-C[k]	Plasma Liver Fibroblast	Fibroblast Endothelial cell Fetal tissues
IL-1, IL-2[l]	Macrophage (IL-1) T-lymphocyte (IL-2)	Fibroblast Synovial cell ?

[a]Transforming growth factor beta.
[b]Platelet-derived growth factor.
[c]Acidic fibroblast growth factor.
[d]Basic fibroblast growth factor/heparin-binding growth factors.
[e]Cartilage-derived growth factor.
[f]Endothelial cell growth factor.
[g]Epidermal growth factor.
[h]Transforming growth factor alpha.
[i]Epidermal cell-derived growth factor.
[j]Monocyte/macrophage-derived growth factor.
[k]Insulin-like growth factor-I/somatomedin-C.
[l]Interleukin-1, interleukin 2.
Reprinted from McGrath MH. *Wound Healing* 1990; 17 (3): 423.

early 1960s that superficial wounds heal faster when they are kept moist than when they are allowed to scab over.[11] Winter's research showed that epidermal cells are better able to migrate to the surface of a moist wound. The formation of a scab forces the epidermal cells to detour underneath the scab to get to their destination, delaying healing. Subsequent clinical research confirmed Winter's findings.[12]

Despite clear evidence to support the benefits of a moist wound healing environment, clinical practice lagged behind. Traditional gauze dressings continued to predominate over the newer synthetic products that provided a moist environment. Although it is true that the moist environment that promotes healing can also support bacterial growth, a wound need not be completely sterile under a dressing and the presence of some bacteria is not necessarily deleterious, especially in individuals with intact immune systems.[13]

Wound healing is a complex cascade of biochemical and cellular events regulated by the cellular immune system, specifically the macrophages and the T-lymphocytes.[14–16] Polypeptide growth factors regulate the immune system and play distinct roles in the various phases of wound healing. These growth factors, found naturally in a wound site, are being manufactured through recombinant DNA technology and tested for their ability to accelerate healing when applied to a wound. Clinical trials involving recombinant growth factors as wound healing agents are in progress. Eventually, recombinant growth factors may be used sequentially or in combination to speed healing, especially in chronic wounds. One day they may even be incorporated into nonprescription wound care products.

Growth Factors

Polypeptide growth factors are agents of the immune system that promote cell proliferation. They interact with an external receptor on a target cell and this interaction leads to intracellular changes that prepare the cell for DNA synthesis and division. These proteins also have chemoattractant properties, meaning they induce a unidirectional migration of cells (i.e., into the wound site).[17,18]

The nomenclature for growth factors is confusing because some are named for their tissue of origin, others for their target cells, and still others for their activity in tumor cell cultures. Table 3 lists growth factors that are known to play a role in the regulation of wound healing.[16–18] As the list illustrates, many growth factors are closely related and some are actually identical.

The Wound Healing Process

Mechanisms of Healing

Healing involves the mechanisms of contraction, epithelialization, and connective tissue deposition. Contraction is the process of myofibroblasts pulling the margins of the wound inward. Excessive wound contraction is a pathologic process that results in contracture. Epithelialization is the process of residual epithelial cells migrating across the surface of the wound and proliferating to provide new surface epithelial cells. Connective tissue deposition is the process whereby fibroblasts move into the wound site, proliferate, and produce collagen and proteoglycans ("ground substance") which form the scar tissue.[19]

Classifications of Wounds

Wounds can be classified as either partial thickness or full thickness. Partial-thickness wounds have a base containing living epithelial elements such as hair shafts and sweat ducts that provide epidermal cells to the wound site and enable the skin to regenerate. Partial-thickness wounds usually heal completely in less than a month and scarring is rare. These wounds contract less than full-thickness wounds and they contract in direct proportion to their depth. Superficial wounds may not contract at all. Full-thickness wounds have no source of new epithelium in the wound site other than from tissue at the edges of the wound. Reepithelialization, contraction, and connective tissue deposition are all part of the healing process for these wounds. Full-thickness wounds larger than 15 cm in diameter are slow to heal and often require skin grafts. Contraction of scar tissue in large wounds can be a serious complication requiring treatment to minimize pain, disfigurement, and disability.[19]

Phases of Healing

The chronologic steps of healing overlap significantly, but for simplicity's sake they can be broken down into three stages: inflammation, proliferation, and remodeling.[20]

Acute Inflammation

The inflammatory stage lasts 3 to 4 days and begins with hemostasis or clotting, which protects the individual from excessive blood loss and the wound from exposure to bacterial contaminants. Blood flows into the wound site and the clotting cascade is triggered, leading to the accumulation of platelets and the formation of a clot to halt bleeding. Platelets release the initial growth factors that help to attract inflammatory cells and fibroblasts. Mast cells react to tissue damage by releasing histamine. Histamine stimulates nerve endings and activates chemical mediators that cause redness, pain, swelling, and heat. Inflammatory exudate containing antibodies, neutrophils, and macrophages leaks into damaged tissues. Initially, neutrophils effectively clear the wound of contamination if bacteria are not excessive (i.e., if there are fewer than 10^5 per gram of tissue).[21] Approximately 24 hours after wounding, the macrophage takes over as the key cell in wound healing. Macrophages clear dead bacteria and tissue through phagocytosis; secrete enzymes for necrotic tissue debridement; and, when signaled by prostaglandins, endotoxins, and lymphokines, activate oxygen metabolism and secrete a host of enzymes and growth factors. During the inflammatory phase, the matrix filling the wound site changes in composition from primarily fibrin (a major component of blood clots) to proteoglycan (a glycoprotein that facilitates cellular interactions).[16–18]

Proliferation

During the proliferative stage of healing, which lasts approximately from day 3 to day 21, new tissue is formed. The key cell during this phase is the fibroblast. The dermis starts to be repaired by growth factor–mediated proliferation of fibroblasts that synthesize collagen (the major component of repaired dermal tissue). The epidermis begins to repair itself through growth factor–mediated proliferation and migration of cells from the borders of the wound. Keratinocytes migrate most easily across the moist surface of the wound; if the surface becomes dry, they are forced to migrate through the underlying matrix, a detour that slows the healing process.[11]

New blood vessels form within the wound matrix through a process known as angiogenesis. Angiogenesis growth factor is the stimulus for the formation of endothelial buds at the end of injured blood vessels, a very important part of wound healing because these new blood vessels supply the wound with essential nutrients and oxygen. During this stage, the matrix is changed from proteoglycan to collagen, its final and permanent structure. Between days 5 and 15, the tensile strength of the wound increases significantly because of collagen deposition. During this stage of healing, growth factors such as transforming growth factor beta (TGF-ß, fibroblast growth factor (FGF), and platelet-derived growth factor (PDGF) play important roles.[18]

Collagen Remodeling

Remodeling is the final phase of healing, during which granulation tissue is formed and collagen is remodeled. This phase starts on approximately day 21 and may last for a year or two. Synthesis and deposition of collagen slow down, but connective tissue strength increases. The scar may continue to mature for months or years but will never reach more than 80% of the strength of the skin before injury. Normally, in uninjured tissue, collagen fibers lie parallel and the tissue can withstand great stress. Injury alters this symmetry and new collagen is laid down in random fashion, which decreases its strength. Eventually, enzymes lyse some of the newly formed collagen, making it more flexible and streamlined. At the same time, the collagen fibers cross-link and become more organized and therefore stronger.[22] TGF-ß, PDGF, and FGF continue to play important roles during this remodeling phase of healing.[18]

Deficient Wound Healing

Healing can be compromised by any of three mechanisms: (1) inadequate blood circulation to the wound, (2) an inadequate inflammatory response by the host, or (3) an altered repair process that results in the formation of fibrous adhesions.[22] The factors that most often lead to compromised healing are pharmacologic agents such as steroids or cytotoxic drugs; extrinsic factors such as infection, foreign bodies, or desiccation; and intrinsic factors such as diabetes, peripheral vascular disease, poor nutrition, aging, or an immunocompromised host.[23] Wounds that typically heal slowly and are considered chronic include diabetic ulcers, venous stasis ulcers, pressure ulcers, and severe burns. In each case, there is at least one underlying defect in healing.[22] Recombinant growth factors are expected to have their greatest impact in the treatment of these chronic wounds.[24]

Management of Wounds

The management of a wound is dictated by its etiology, location, and severity, along with the nutritional and medical status of the patient. The choice of dressing may be affected by several factors, including vascular status; the risk or presence of infection; the environment and the depth of the wound; the volume of wound exudate; the location of the wound; patient comfort and preferences; the availability of particular dressings; the cost–benefit equation; durability and adaptability; odor control requirements; and the capabilities of the patient and the patient's caregivers. In addition to care of the local wound site, management of a wound may involve systemic interventions. For instance, all patients need attention to their nutritional status; patients with pressure ulcers require pressure relief; and patients with venous stasis ulcers require compression of the involved extremity.[22,25]

Thousands of wound care products are available in the United States today. An understanding of the wound healing process can help the pharmacist to assist clinicians and patients in selecting effective products that are known to support healing.

Until recombinant growth factors become commercially available, wound management will be limited to optimizing the wound healing environment. This means keeping the wound clean, moist, and free from physical trauma. The key to faster, painless healing is to occlude or partially occlude the wound to create a moist environment.[13] As discussed earlier, the idea that exposure to air is best has been disproven. The primary goal in wound healing is to minimize scarring, and scarring is closely related to the type of dressing used—occlusive dressings result in less scarring than gauze dressings.[13] The timing of dressing placement is also important—immediate occlusion leads to resurfacing of epithelium faster than delayed occlusion.[13] In some individuals, occlusive dressings may produce irritation, maceration, and dermatitis on the surrounding skin.

Bacterial infections slow the healing process but some topical antibacterial agents may be toxic to cells and can actually retard healing.[21] Cleansing of the wound should be accomplished with a physiologic solution such as isotonic saline. If a superficial wound is contaminated with dirt, mild soap and tap water can be used to clean it gently. If antimicrobial solutions such as povodine are used, they should be extremely dilute to avoid destroying delicate tissue.[20]

For wounds with high bacterial counts, topical preparations containing antimicrobials such as silver sulfadiazine may be prescribed. To be successful, topical preparations must be in continual contact with the surface and must penetrate the wound effectively; they can be used in conjunction with dressings such as hydrogels. The goal of topical antimicrobial therapy is to convert the wound's bacterial count to fewer than 10^5 per gram of tissue. The bacterial colony count, and not the type of bacteria contaminating a wound surface, is the crucial factor. Systemic antibiotics are of limited use in the treatment of an infected wound because they do not penetrate the fibrous bed of a granulating wound; they are useful only when the infection has spread beyond the wound site.

Wound Dressings

Turner has developed a set of criteria for the optimal dressing.[26] According to Turner, the ideal dressing (1) removes excess exudate, (2) maintains a moist environment, (3) is permeable to oxygen, (4) thermally insulates the wound, (5) protects the wound from infection, (6) is free of particulate or toxic contaminants, and (7) can be removed without disrupting delicate new tissue.[26] A plethora of solutions and coverings for wounds are available today, and the range of choices may be overwhelming to an individual trying to choose an appropriate dressing.

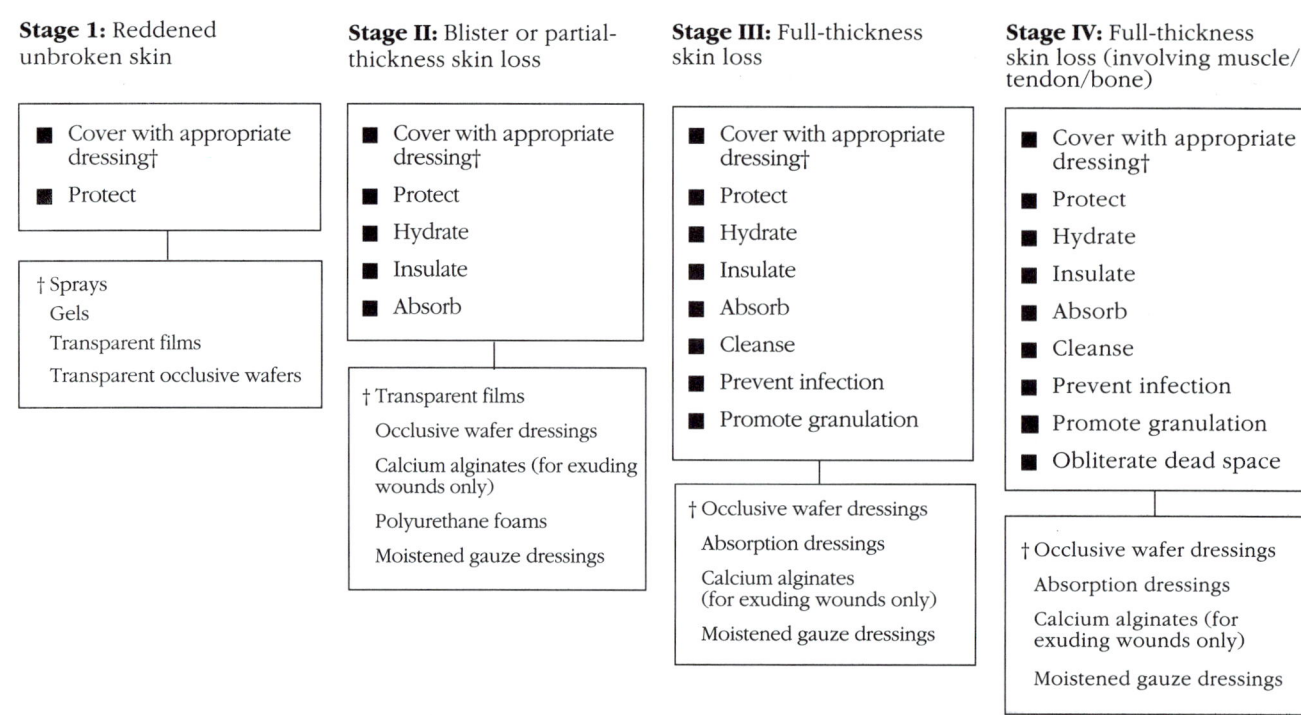

FIGURE 5 Algorithm guidelines for product selection based on wound severity. Adapted with permission from Jeter KF, Tintle TE. *Clin Podiatr Med Surg* 1991; 8 (4): 805.

Jeter and Tintle have developed a schema to assist clinicians in choosing the most appropriate dressing for their patients' wounds (Figure 5).[27] In addition to wound dressings, several pharmacologic agents classified as antimicrobial soaps, antiseptics, skin wound cleansers, and skin wound protectants are available. (See Chapter 28, "Topical Anti-Infective Products.")

Product Selection Guidelines For Pharmacists

Table 4 describes the major categories of wound care products available today and provides an overview of their indications, advantages, and disadvantages. Although none of these products meets all of Turner's criteria, many do approach his description of the optimal dressing.

Basic Instructions for Treating Acute Wounds

Patients who have acute wounds should do the following:

- Position the wound above the level of the heart to slow bleeding and relieve throbbing pain.
- If it is dirty, clean the wound with mild soap and water or a mild wound cleanser that is not toxic to cells. Avoid antiseptic solutions unless they are extremely dilute.
- Occlude the wound with a dressing that will keep the wound site moist and is an appropriate size and contour for the affected body part.
- Avoid disrupting the dressing unnecessarily; change it only if it is dirty or not intact (frequent changes may remove resurfacing layers of epithelium and slow the healing process).
- Use a mild analgesic to control pain.
- Observe the wound for signs of infection (redness, swelling, and exudate are a normal part of healing; foul odor is not).
- Consult a physician if infection is suspected.
- Consult a physician if the wound occurred in dirty conditions and the patient is unsure about his or her tetanus immunization status.

Basic Instructions for Treating Chronic Wounds

The basic instructions for treating acute wounds may not apply to chronic wounds. For that reason, patients who have chronic wounds should be advised to seek medical advice concerning wound care. These patients should also:

- Consult a physician about any slow-healing wound because the underlying defect in healing probably requires systemic treatment as well as local wound care;
- Prevent pressure ulcers by repositioning the body regularly and frequently and by using pressure-relieving devices;
- Watch for early signs of skin redness over bony prominences (prompt intervention can prevent skin breakdown.)

TABLE 4 Options in wound management

Description (brand name)[a]	Use indications	Advantages	Disadvantages
Transparent adhesive films			
Semiocclusive translucent dressings with partial or continuous adhesive composed of polyurethane or copolyester thin film (e.g., ACU-derm, Op-Site, Uniflex)	Stages I, II, shallow stage III Clean, granular wounds Minimally exuding wounds Autolysis Can use with absorption products and alginates Can be used in conjunction with some enzymatic debriders	Semiocclusive Gas permeable Easy inspection Autolysis Protection Impermeable to fluids/bacteria Conformable Self-adherent Reduce pain Moist environment Resist shear	For uninfected wounds only Not absorptive May cause periwound trauma on removal With continuous adhesive, may reinjure wound on removal With large amounts of exudate, maceration may occur
Nonadherents/nonimpregnated dressings			
Nonadherent, porous dressings. Lightly coated dressings allow easy flow-through of exudate (e.g., Adaptic, Telfa)	Skin donor sites Stage II, shallow stage III Staple/suture lines Abrasions Lacerations	Readily available Less adherent than plain gauze	Need secondary dressing May have traumatic/painful dressing removal Some impregnated dressings may delay healing May require frequent dressing changes Some may cause exudate pooling
Alginates			
Hydrophilic, nonwoven dressings of calcium–sodium (percentages vary between products) alginate fibers. Alginates are processed from brown seaweed into pad or twisted fiber form. Exudate transforms fibers to gel at wound interface (e.g., Kaltostat, Sorbsan)	Light to heavy exuding wounds Stages II, III, IV Moist wound environment Autolysis Skin donor sites	Absorptive Reduce pain Nonocclusive Moist wound environment Conformable Easy, trauma-free removal Can use on infected wounds Accelerate healing time Less frequent dressing changes Potential to aid in control of minor bleeding	Require secondary dressing Characteristic odor May need wound irrigation May desiccate May promote hypergranulation
Absorptive wound fillers			
Hydrophilic dressings that absorb exudate dead cells and bacteria (e.g., Debrisan Beads, Hydragran)	Stages II, III Exuding wounds Nontunneling deep wounds Infected wounds	Absorb exudate Moist environment Nonocclusive Reduce odor Conformable Inert Clean debris Many distributed in unit dose packs	Contraindicated with tunneling May be difficult to remove May increase wound pH May sting on application Need secondary dressing Application techniques vary

continued

TABLE 4 Options in wound management

Description (brand name)	Use indications	Advantages	Disadvantages
Enzymatic debriders			
Debriders digest necrotic tissue by differing methods (e.g., Elase, Santy)	Stages II, III, some stage IV Dermal ulcers Second- and third-degree burns	Nonsurgical method of debridement Some will not damage healthy tissue	May require frequent dressing changes Require secondary dressing May require cross-hatching of eschar Some may damage healthy tissue Application techniques vary significantly Need moist wound environment Some require refrigeration
Gauze			
Nonocclusive fiber dressing with loose, open weave	Stages II–IV Minimal to heavy exuding wounds/topicals Infected wounds Debridement Wound rehydration	Readily available Deep wound packing May use with infected wounds/topicals Mechanical debridement Nonocclusive Conformable	Wound bed may desiccate if dressing dry Nonselective debridement May cause bleeding/pain on removal Need secondary dressing Frequent dressing changes Some dressings may "shed"
Hydrogels/gels			
Nonadherent, nonocclusive dressings with high moisture content that come in the form of sheets and gels (e.g., Elasto-Gel, Vigilon)	Stages II, III, some approved for stage IV Granular or necrotic wound beds Autolysis Some used on partial- and full-thickness burns	Nonadherent Most are nonocclusive Trauma-free removal Varying absorption capabilities Conformable Some can be used in conjunction with topicals Thermal insulation Reduce pain Moist environment	Most require secondary dressings May macerate periwound skin Some products may dehydrate Slow to minimal absorption rate in most Most require frequent/daily dressing change
Island dressings			
Nonadherent absorptive center barrier with adhesive at perimeter (e.g., Airstrip, Viasorb)	Stages II, III Moderate to heavy exuding wounds Autolysis Suture/staple lines	Nonadherent over wound Semiocclusive No secondary dressing required Impermeable to fluids/bacteria Protective Reduce pain	May cause periwound trauma on removal

continued

TABLE 4 *continued*

Description (brand name)	Use indications	Advantages	Disadvantages
Foams			
Semipermeable, absorptive, nonwoven, inert polyurethane foam dressings (e.g., EPIGARD, LYOfoam)	Stage II, shallow stage III Minimal to moderate drainage Autolysis Donor sites First- and second-degree burns Contraindicated for third-degree burns	Most are nonadhesive Some can be used with infected wounds/topicals Thermal insulation Reduce pain Nonocclusive Moist environment Conformable Less frequent dressing changes Trauma-free removal Absorbent	Most require secondary dressing May require cutting May cause wound desiccation May be difficult to determine wound contact surface
Hydrocolloids			
Wafer dressings composed of hydrophilic particles in an adhesive form covered by a water-resistant film or foam (e.g., Comfeel, ULTEC)	Stages I, II, and shallow stage III Clean, granular wounds Autolysis Minimal to moderate exuding wounds Can use with absorption products and alginates	Occlusive Manage exudate by particle swelling Autolysis Long wear time Self-adherent Impermeable to fluids/bacteria Conformable Protective Thermal insulation Reduce pain Moist environment	For uninfected wounds only May cause periwound trauma on removal Difficult wound assessment Characteristic odor Impermeable to gases Some may leave residue on skin or in wound
Carbon-impregnated dressings			
Dressings with an outer layer of carbon for odor control (e.g., LYOfoam "C" Odor Absorbent Dressing)	Malodorous wounds	Control odor	Require appropriate seal or odor may escape Carbon is inactivated when it becomes wet
Biosynthetics			
Semipermeable dressings that are designed to adhere to a clean or debrided wound and remain in place without removal throughout the course of reepithelialization (e.g., BioBrane II)	Partial-thickness burns Donor sites Meshed autografts	Gas permeable Adherent to wound May be used in conjunction with topical antibacterial agents Reduce pain Wound visible	Permeable to fluids/bacteria May require secondary dressing or skin staples May adhere to skin at removal Not for use on necrotic tissue

[a]The brand names listed for each type of wound dressing are given as examples of available products; however, these brand names do not constitute an all-inclusive list of available wound-dressing products.

Adapted with permission from an unpublished document prepared by McIntosh A, Raher E. Silver Cross Hospital, Joliet, Ill, 1991.

References

1. Benfield BR et al. *Arch Surg* 1973; 107: 62.
2. Cromar CD. *Dis Colon Rectum* 1968; 7: 256.
3. Cohen Z and Stone R. *Ostomy Manage* 1980; 2: 4.
4. Watt R. *Am J Nurs* 1977; 77: 442.
5. Sparberg M. *Ileostomy Care*. Springfield, Ill: Charles C. Thomas; 1971: 18.
6. Gross L. *Ileostomy: A Guide*. Los Angeles, Calif: United Ostomy Association, Inc; 1974: 28.
7. Gill NN et al. *Instructions for the Care of the Ileostomy Stoma*. Cleveland, Ohio: Cleveland Clinic Foundation; 3.
8. Travers C. *J Enterostomy Ther* 1980; 7: 8.
9. Kramer P. *Dig Dis* 1977; 22: 327.
10. Gallagher ND et al. *Gut* 1962; 3: 219.
11. Winter GD. Formation of scab and rate of epithelialization on superficial wounds in the skin of the domestic pig. *Nature* 1962; 193: 293–4.
12. Hinman CC, Maibach HI, Winter GD. Effect of air exposure and occlusion on experimental skin wound. *Nature* 1963; 200: 377.
13. Epstein WL, ed. *Dermatol Focus* 1988 Nov; 7 (3).
14. Hunt TK. Basic principles of wound healing. *J Trauma* 1990; 30 (suppl 12): 122–8.
15. Barbul A. Immune aspects of wound repair. *Clin Plast Surg* 1990; 17 (3): 433–42.
16. Epstein WL, ed. *Dermatol Focus* 1989 Jan; 7 (4): 7–16.
17. Servold SA. Growth factor impact on wound healing. *Clin Podiatr Med Surg* 1991; 8 (4): 937–96.
18. McGrath MH. Peptide growth factors and wound healing. *Clin Plast Surg* 1990; 17 (3): 421–32.
19. Cohen IK, Diegelmann RF, Lindblad WJ. *Wound Healing: Biochemical and clinical aspects*. Philadelphia: W. B. Saunders; 1992.
20. Cooper DM. Optimizing wound healing: A practice within nursing's domain. *Nurs Clin North Am* 1990; 25 (1): 165–80.
21. Cuzzell JZ, Stotts NA. Wound care. Trial and error yields to knowledge. *Am J Nurs* 1990; 90 (10): 53–60.
22. Albritton JS. Complications of wound repair. *Clin Podiatr Med Surg* 1991; 8 (4): 773–85.
23. Tepelidis NT. Wound healing in the elderly. *Clin Podiatr Med Surg* 1991; 8 (4): 817–26.
24. Servold SA. Growth factor impact on wound healing. *Clin Podiatr Med Surg* 1991; 8 (4): 937–96.
25. Bryant RA, ed. *Acute and Chronic Wounds: Nursing Management*. St. Louis: Mosby-Year Book; 1992.
26. Turner TD. Recent advances in wound management products. In: Advances in Wound Management. London: John Wiley & Sons, Ltd; 1986.
27. Jeter KF, Tintle TE. Wound dressings of the nineties: indications and contraindications. *Clin Podiatr Med Surg* 1991; 8 (4): 799–816.

Appendix: Major Manufacturers of Ostomy Products and Accessories

- Atlantic Surgical Company, Inc.
  1834 Landsdowne Avenue
  Merrick, Long Island, NY 11566
  516-868-4545
  Full line of appliances and auxiliary products.

- Bard International Division
  730 Central Avenue
  Murray Hill, NJ 07974
  201-277-8000
  Full line of appliances and auxiliary products.

- Blanchard Ostomy Products
  2216 Chevy Oaks Circle
  Glendale, CA 91206
  213-242-6789
  Reversible appliances and karaya wafers.

- Convatec
  (A Squibb Company)
  CN5254
  Princeton, NJ 08543-5254
  201-359-9200
  Appliances and supplies.

- Coloplast, Inc.
  5610 West Sligh Avenue
  Suite 100
  Tampa, FL 33634
  813-886-5634
  800-237-4555
  Full line of supplies and auxiliary products.

- Cymed, Inc.
  3447 Investment Boulevard Suite #2
  Hayward, CA 94545
  415-782-7550
  Appliances and supplies.

- Foxy Enterprises
  Plaza 16-E Lancaster Avenue
  Ardmore, PA 19003
  215-642-6207
  Custom-made pouch covers.

- Hy Tape Surgical Products Corporation
  772 McLean Avenue
  Yonkers, NY 10704
  914-237-1234
  Type L closed-end pouches, tape.

- Hollister, Inc.
  2000 Hollister Drive
  P.O. Box 250
  Libertyville, IL 60048
  312-642-2001
  Pouches and auxiliary products.

- Johnson & Johnson Company
  501 George Street
  New Brunswick, NJ 08903
  201-524-0400
  Paper tape; transparent, semipermeable dressing.

- Marlen Manufacturing and Development Company
  5150 Richmond Road
  Bedford, OH 44146
  216-292-7060
  Full line of appliances and auxiliary products.

- Mason Laboratories
  119 Horsham Road
  Horsham, PA 19044
  215-675-6044
  Colly-Seel and Colly-Seel appliances.

- 3M Medical Products Division
  3M Center 225-52-01
  St. Paul, MN 55144-1000
  612-733-1100
  Micropore paper tape: transparent, semipermeable dressing.

- Nu-Hope Labs, Inc.
  P.O. Box 39348
  Los Angeles, CA 90039
  213-666-5249
  Appliances and supplies.

- Palex Medical, Inc.
  8807 Northwest 23rd Street
  Miami, FL 33172
  305-592-1830
  800-446-6786
  One-piece appliances and skin barriers.

- The Perma-Type Company, Inc.
  P.O. Box 175
  Farmington, CT 06032
  203-677-7388
  Appliances and supplies.

- Perry Products
  3803 East Lake Street
  Minneapolis, MN 55406
  612-722-4783
  Nonadhesive appliances.

- Robinson Surgical Appliance Company
  21 East Main Street
  Auburn, WA 98002
  206-833-3161
  Appliances.

- H. W. Rutzen and Son
  345 West Irving Park Road
  Chicago, IL 60618
  Appliances.

- Torbot Company
  1185 Jefferson Boulevard
  Warwick, RI 02886
  401-739-2241
  Appliances and auxiliary supplies.

- Smith & Nephew Limited, Inc.
  11775 Starkey Road
  Largo, FL 34643
  813-392-1261
  Auxiliary products.

- VPI
  P.O. Box 266
  Spencer, IN 47460
  800-843-4851
  One-piece nonadhesive nondisposable appliances.

COLOR PLATES

Plate 1

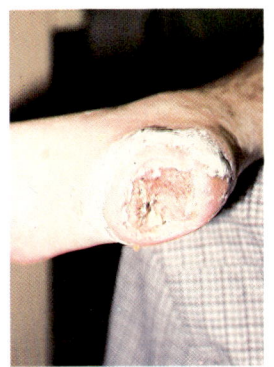

1 Gangrene of the foot is a serious and common complication of diabetes caused by trauma that has gone unrecognized because of neuropathy (loss of sensation) or vascular lesions. Eventually, the trauma may lead to gangrene when the necrotic (dead) skin is removed and ulceration results (as shown). (See Chapter 16, "Diabetes Care Products and Monitoring Devices.")

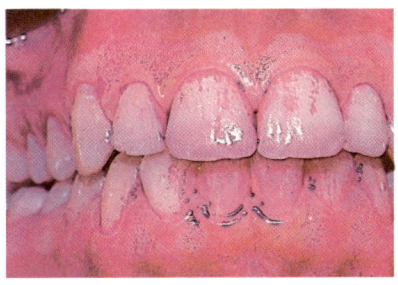

2 Disclosing agents, such as erythrosin (FD&C Red No. 3), aid patients in evaluating the effectiveness of their brushing and flossing by staining mucinous film and plaque on teeth. These agents reveal the presence and extent of deposits on teeth that otherwise appear clean. (See Chapter 23, "Oral Health Products.")

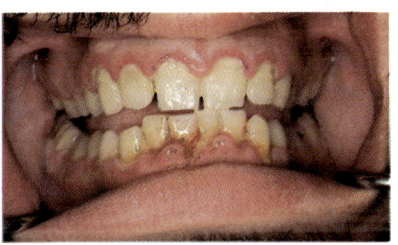

3 Chronic gingivitis, an asymptomatic inflammation of the gingivae (gums) at the necks of the teeth, is an early stage of periodontitis and is usually caused by poor oral hygiene. The gingivae are erythematous (red) and may have areas that appear swollen and glossy. In addition, mild hemorrhage may occur during teeth brushing. (See Chapter 23, "Oral Health Products.")

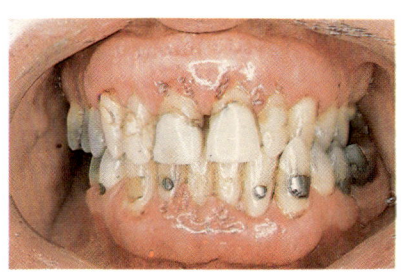

4 Chronic periodontitis (pyorrhea), an inflammation of the tissues surrounding the teeth, including the gingivae, periodontal ligaments, alveolar bone, and the cementum (bony material covering the root of a tooth), is caused by plaque accumulation resulting from poor oral hygiene. The gingivae may be erythematous and swollen and may recede from the necks of the teeth. The condition is not painful and usually is accompanied by halitosis, loosening of the teeth, and mild hemorrhage during teeth brushing. (See Chapter 23, "Oral Health Products.")

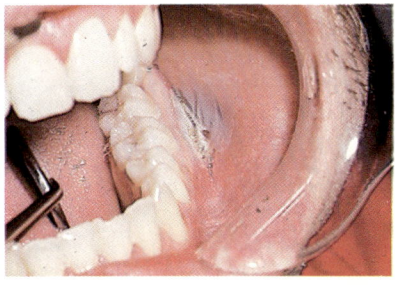

5 Aspirin burn results from the topical use of aspirin to relieve toothache. An aspirin tablet is placed against the tooth where it is held in place by pressure from the buccal (cheek) mucosa. The mucosa becomes necrotic and is characterized by a white slough that rubs away, revealing a painful ulceration. (See Chapter 23, "Oral Health Products.")

Plate 2

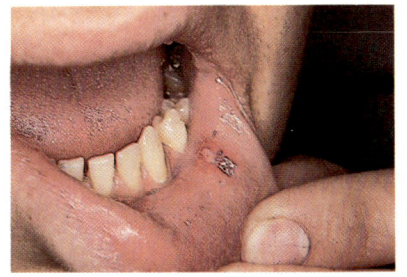
6

6 Aphthous ulcers (canker sores) are recurrent, painful, single or multiple ulcerations of bacterial origin. The central ulceration is sharply demarcated, often has a yellow to white surface of necrotic debris, and is surrounded by an erythematous margin. (See Chapter 23, "Oral Health Products.")

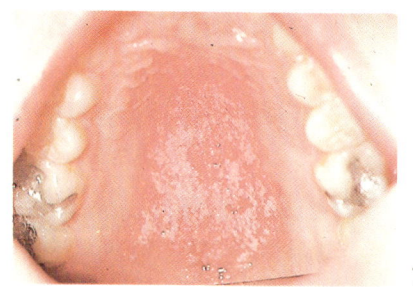
7

7 Candidiasis (candidosis, moniliasis, thrush), an infection caused by overgrowth of *Candida albicans*, tends to occur in people with debilitating or chronic systemic disease or those on long-term antibiotic therapy. Candidiasis commonly presents as a whitish-gray to yellowish, soft, slightly elevated pseudomembrane-like plaque on the oral mucosa; the plaque is often described as having a "curdled-milk" appearance. If the membrane is stripped away, a raw bleeding surface remains. A dull burning pain is often present. (See Chapter 23, "Oral Health Products.")

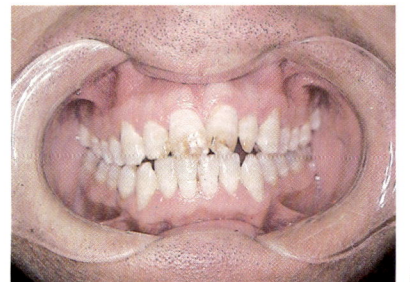
8

8 Dental fluorosis (mottled enamel) occurs during the time of tooth formation and is caused by the long-term ingestion of drinking water containing fluoride at concentrations greater than 1 ppm. Discoloration of the teeth varies, depending upon the level of fluoride in the water, and ranges from white flecks or spots to brownish stains, small pits, or deep irregular pits that are dark brown in color. (See Chapter 23, "Oral Health Products.")

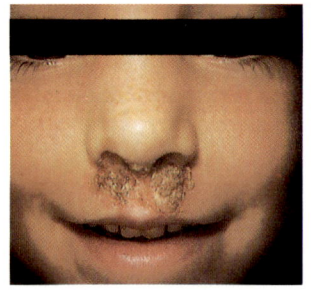
9

9 Impetigo is a bacterial infection characterized by honeycomb crusts on erythematous bases. A bullous (blistering) form can also occur. (See Chapter 28, "Topical Anti-Infective Products.")

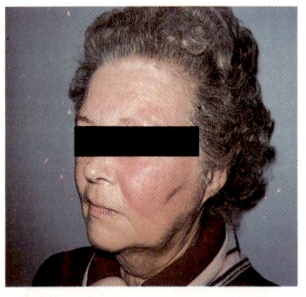
10

10 Erysipelas is a streptococcal infection that often involves the face or extremities. The infected area is red and raised with local warmth and edema. The margins of the infected area change rapidly, often forming serpiginous (irregular) patterns. (See Chapter 28, "Topical Anti-Infective Products.")

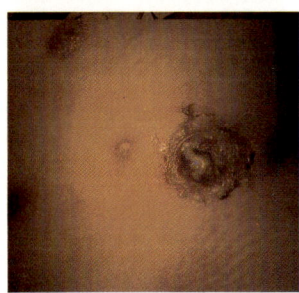
11

11 Infections of the hair follicles are usually caused by staphylococcal or streptococcal organisms. Superficial infections (folliculitis) can occur; deeper infections are called furuncles (small boils). Carbuncles form when adjacent hair follicles are involved. (See Chapter 28, "Topical Anti-Infective Products.")

Plate 3

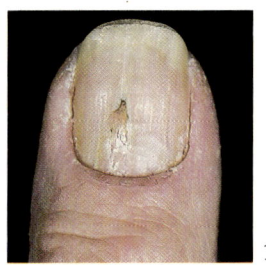

12 Paronychia is caused by overexposure of the nails to water, causing cuticle loss and inflammation around the nail folds. About 50% of cases involve candidal infection. (See Chapter 28, "Anti-Infective Products.")

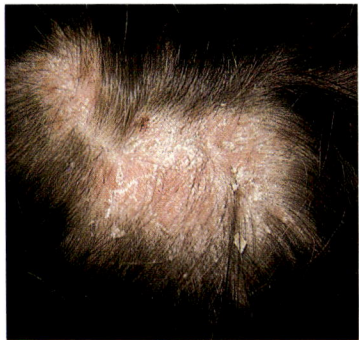

13 Tinea capitis, a fungal infection of the scalp, is marked by scale on the scalp with local breaking or loss of hair; erythema (redness) is usually not observed. (See Chapter 28, "Topical Anti-Infective Products.")

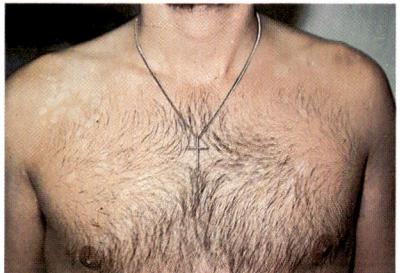

14A and B Tinea versicolor is caused by a yeast organism that overgrows locally, resulting in hyperpigmentation or hypopigmentation (**A**). These mildly scaling eruptions characteristically occur on the chest, upper back, and arms (**B**). (See Chapter 28, "Topical Anti-Infective Products.")

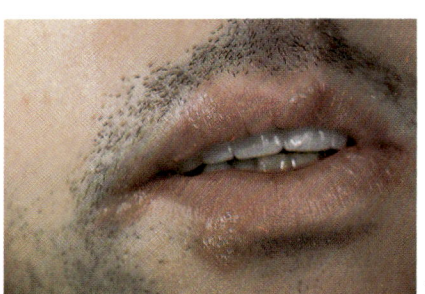

15 Herpes simplex lesions of the mouth and the eye usually start as a small cluster of vesicles (tiny blisters) that subsequently heal over with a serosanguinous (blood-tinged) crust. Local stinging, burning, and pain often herald the onset of lesions. Eye involvement should always be referred to an ophthalmologist. (See Chapter 28, "Topical Anti-Infective Products.")

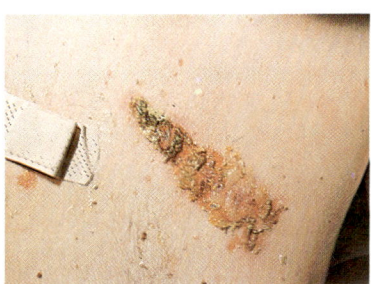

16A and B Herpes zoster is a reactivation of previous chickenpox virus that has remained latent in the nerve roots. Pain precedes small clusters of vesicles (blisters) on an erythematous base that are distributed along the cutaneous (skin) area supplied by the infected nerve (**A**). The inflammation characteristically stops in the midline of the body (**B**). (See Chapter 28, "Topical Anti-Infective Products.")

Plate 4

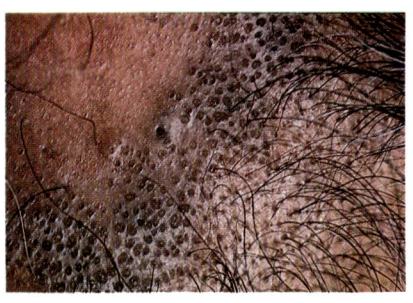

17 Comedonic acne (noninflammatory) occurs when follicles become plugged with sebum, forming a comedone on the surface. The black color is caused by oxidation of lipid and melanin, not dirt as is commonly believed. (See Chapter 29, "Acne Products.")

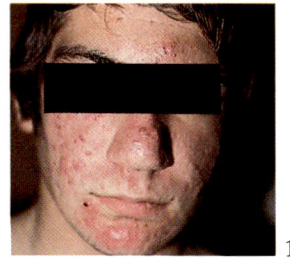

18 Pustular acne (inflammatory) presents as inflamed papules that are formed when superficial hair follicles become plugged and rupture at a deeper level. Superficial inflammation results in pustules; deep lesions cause large cysts to form with possible resultant scarring. (See Chapter 29, "Acne Products.")

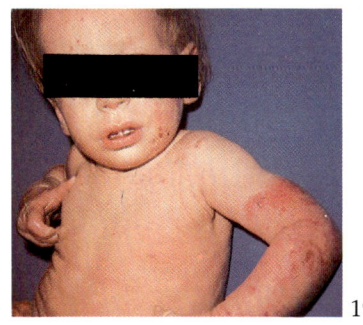

19A, B, and C Atopic dermatitis (eczema) is an inflammatory condition that occurs on the outer aspect (extensor) surface of the elbows and knees (**A**) during the first year of life and then involves predominantly the flexors (**B**). The hands, feet, and face are often involved as well (**C**). The dermatitis is characterized by erythema, scale, increased skin surface markings, small blisters, and crusting; secondary infection is common. (See Chapter 30, "Dermatologic Products.")

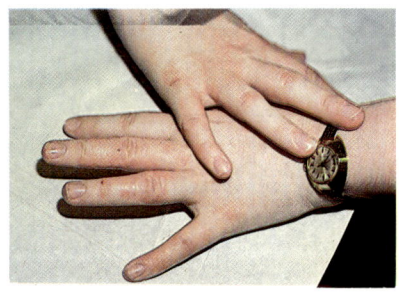

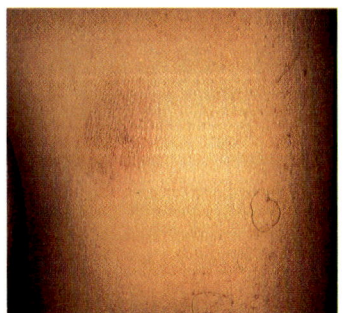

20 Fixed drug reaction is an adverse reaction that can appear as erythematous oval patches, which recur in the same site upon reexposure to the causative drug. The patches resolve with characteristic tan-brown pigmentation. (See Chapter 30, "Dermatologic Products.")

Plate 5

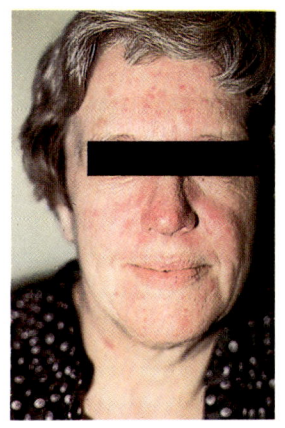

21 Seborrhea (seborrheic dermatitis) is a red scaling condition of the scalp, midface, and upper midchest of adults. Characteristic greasy, yellow scale is shown here in the eyebrows and around the folds of the nose. (See Chapter 30, "Dermatologic Products.")

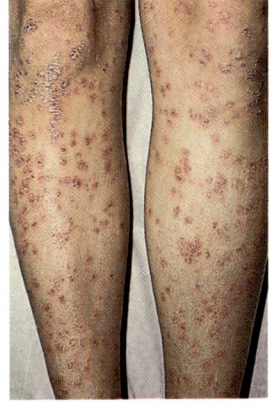

22A, B, and C **Psoriasis** is a scaling condition in which erythematous plaques (red raised areas) are covered by a thick adherent scale. The borders of the lesions are well developed and vary from guttate (very small plaques) to large plaque types: (**A**) guttate; (**B**) medium-sized plaques; (**C**) large plaques. (See Chapter 30, "Dermatologic Products.")

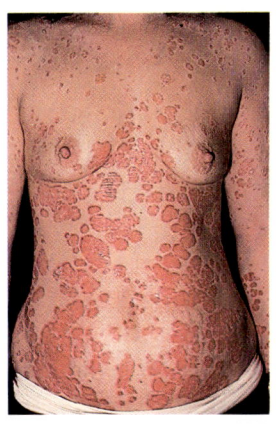 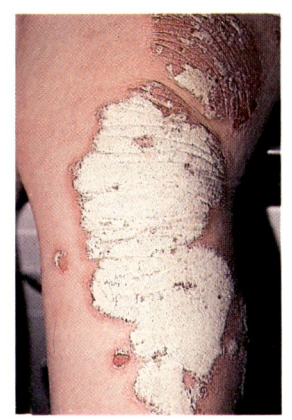

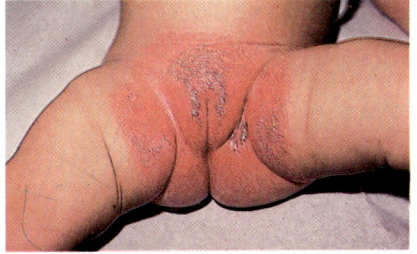

23 Diaper dermatitis presents as erythema of the groin (crease area around the genitals) and is common in infants. The case shown here was caused by a contact allergen. Contact irritants, such as urine and feces, and secondary bacterial and yeast infections may also cause problems in this area. (See Chapter 31, "Diaper Rash and Prickly Heat Products.")

Plate 6

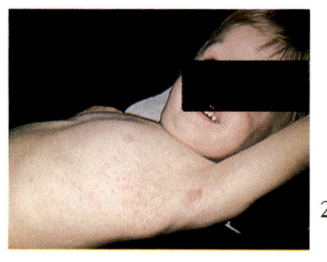

24 Miliaria rubra (heat rash) is an obstruction of sweat glands. Superficial involvement results in only tiny vesicles (blisters) appearing on the skin surface (miliaria crystallina). When deeper inflammation is present, the surrounding erythema is characteristic of miliaria rubra. (See Chapter 31, "Diaper Rash and Prickly Heat Products.")

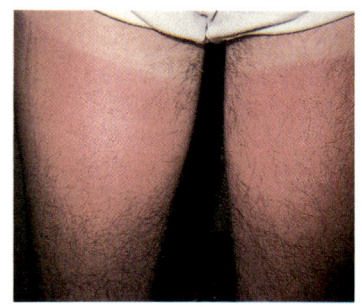

25 Sunburn presents as an erythema that occurs after excessive sun exposure; severe burns can result in large blister formation. Proper sunscreen application can provide photoprotection for susceptible patients. (See Chapter 33, "Burn and Sunburn Products.")

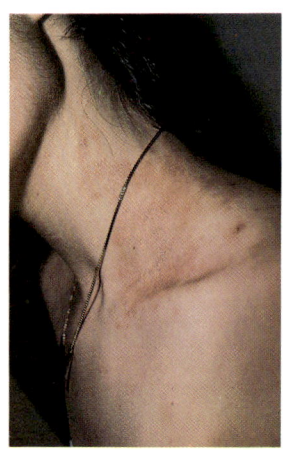

26 Cosmetic-induced photosensitivity can be caused by ingredients in certain topical colognes and perfumes. This immunologic reaction produces a local erythema that leaves characteristic postinflammatory pigmentation. (See Chapter 33, "Burn and Sunburn Products.")

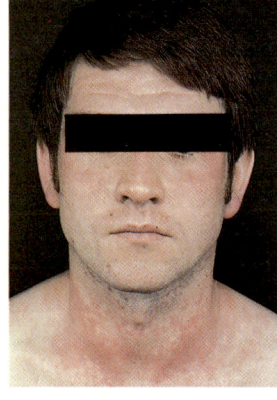

27 Drug-induced photosensitivity is a reaction that occurs on sun-exposed surfaces of the head, neck, and dorsum (back) of the hands. The erythema does not occur on photoprotected areas (under the nose and chin, behind the ears, and between the fingers). (See Chapter 33, "Burn and Sunburn Products.")

Plate 7

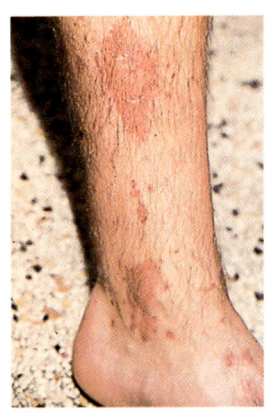 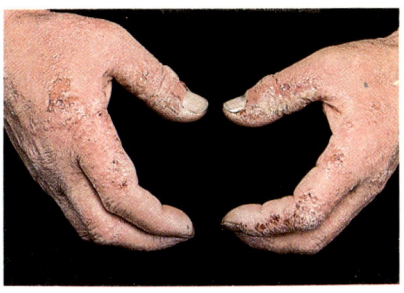

28A and B **Poison ivy** causes a linear erythema that can develop into large blisters (**A**, **B**). Similar reactions can also be caused by poison oak and poison sumac. (See Chapter 35, "Poison Ivy and Poison Oak Products.")

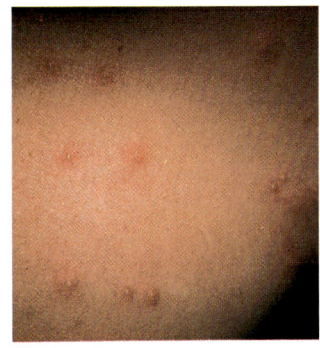

29 **Insect bites** are often characterized as small clusters of itchy red papules. A small overlying superficial vesicle may be present. (Chapter 36, "Insect Sting and Bite Products.")

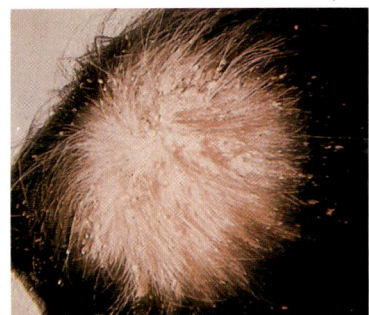 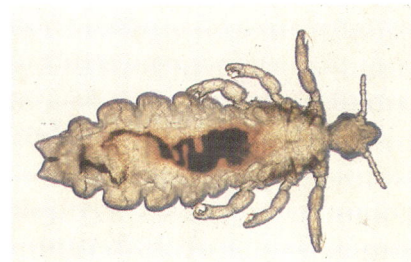

30A and B **Pediculosis capitis** is a louse infestation of the scalp. Examination of the scalp hair in this infestation shows tiny nits (eggs) attached to the hair shaft (**A**). The organism shown is only occasionally seen (**B**). (See Chapter 36, "Insect Sting and Bite Products.")

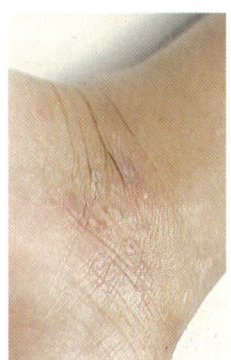

31 **Scabies** is caused by a small mite that burrows under the superficial skin layers. Small linear blisters that cause intense itching can be seen between the finger webs, on the inner wrists, in the axilla, around the areola (nipple) of the breast, and on the genitalia. (See Chapter 36, "Insect Sting and Bite Products.")

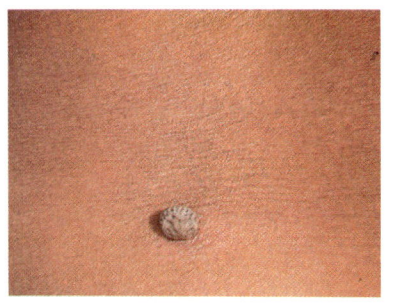

32 Ticks can attach to human skin and burrow into superficial skin layers. With careful examination, the back of the organism is usually visible on the skin surface. Ticks are vectors of several systemic diseases. (See Chapter 36, "Insect Sting and Bite Products.")

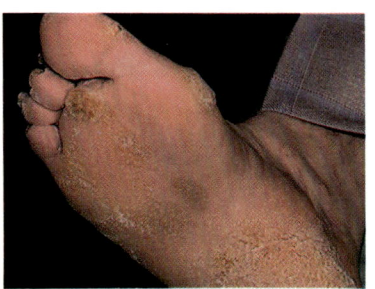

33 **Calluses** are thickened scales that often form on joints and weight-bearing areas. A callus on the plantar surface of the foot is shown here. (See Chapter 37, "Foot Care Products.")

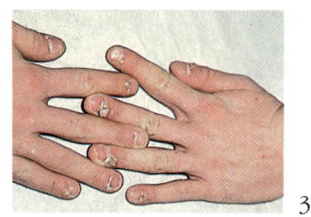

34 **Common warts** are viral-induced lesions that present as localized rough accumulations of keratin (hyperkeratosis) containing many tiny furrows. If the wart's surface is pared, small bleeding points can be seen. (See Chapter 37, "Foot Care Products.")

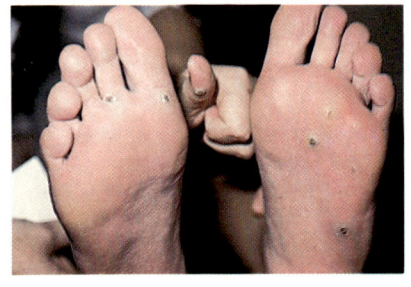

35 **Plantar warts**, caused by a viral infection, are often found on the plantar surface of the foot and present with hard localized accumulations of keratin. The punctate bleeding points seen when the lesions are pared distinguish plantar warts from calluses. (See Chapter 37, "Foot Care Products.")

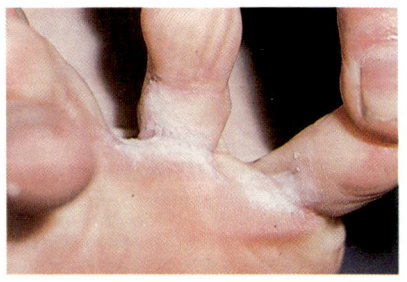

36 **Tinea pedis** infection of the toes characteristically starts between the fourth and fifth web space and spreads proximally. Scaling can progress to maceration with resultant small fissures. (See Chapter 37, "Foot Care Products.")

CHAPTER 25

Contraceptive Methods and Products

Louise Parent-Stevens and Roberta S. Carrier

> **Questions to ask in patient assessment and counseling**
>
> - *What type of contraceptive method are you now using?*
> - *What contraceptive products have you used before?*
> - *What did you like or dislike about your current or previous contraceptive method?*
> - *Are you in a stable relationship now?*
> - *What does your partner like or dislike about your current or previous contraceptive method?*
> - *Have you discussed contraception and sexual health matters with your physician or another health care provider?*
> - *Do you belong to a religious faith that has specific guidelines concerning family planning?*
> - *Do you have children already? Do you want additional children?*
> - *Do you know what your risks are for being infected with the virus that causes acquired immunodeficiency syndrome (AIDS) or with other sexually transmitted diseases?*
> - *How do you protect yourself from sexually transmitted diseases, including AIDS?*

Throughout history people have sought ways to control their fertility in order to choose the number and timing of pregnancies. As knowledge of reproductive physiology has evolved, a wider variety of safe and reliable methods of contraception has been developed.

The earliest recorded methods of contraception include coitus interruptus, mentioned in the Book of Genesis of the Bible; barrier methods, such as the vaginal pessaries made of crocodile dung used in ancient Egypt; and early cervical caps made from lemon halves, a method said to have been used by Casanova.[1]

According to the 1991 Ortho Birth Control Study of 15- to 50-year-old U.S. women at risk for unintended pregnancy, sterilization of either the female or the male continues to be the most widely used method of conception control. The next most prevalent method of contraception is the birth control pill; 28% of all women ages 15 to 44 use an oral contraceptive as their primary method of birth control. Three percent of the women surveyed use the diaphragm, and 1% of the women surveyed rely on the intrauterine device (IUD). IUD use in 1991 was considerably lower than the 1982 figure of 7%, most likely because of the adverse publicity the IUD has received. With 76% of women aged 15 to 44 years using some form of birth control, the 24% who do not use any consistent method of contraception represent an at-risk population.[2]

In the United States and worldwide, reliance on nonprescription methods of contraception is widespread. The fact that nonprescription contraceptive products are accessible and relatively inexpensive makes them very important for those who do not have access to family planning services or who, for personal reasons, choose not to use physicians or clinics. Even if a prescription product is chosen as the primary contraceptive method, low-cost and low-risk nonprescription methods may be appropriate at different times in a person's reproductive life. Some people use nonprescription contraceptive methods as their primary method because they are unable to use or prefer not to use a prescription contraceptive method.

Consistent and proper use of a contraceptive, whether prescription or nonprescription, will significantly reduce the incidence of unwanted pregnancies. Moreover, a recent survey of women undergoing counseling for unplanned pregnancies found that inconsistent or improper use of contraceptives was responsible for 74% of unwanted pregnancies.[3] Given that an estimated 40% of pregnancies in the United States are unplanned,[4] it is apparent that much more attention needs to be paid to family planning and contraceptive counseling.

Of particular concern is the high risk of pregnancy in the adolescent population. The 1988 National Survey of Family Growth found that 38% of 15- to 17-year-old women and 74% of 18- to 19-year-old women had experienced sexual intercourse. Of the teenagers who were sexually active, only 65% used a contraceptive method during their first sexual encounter. The most popular choice of contraceptive in this age group was condoms (47%). Withdrawal (8%) was used as frequently as birth control pills (8%). Thirty-five percent of the sexually active adolescents used no contraceptive method.[4] The comparatively high teenage pregnancy rate in the United States (10% of 15- to 19-year-olds) compared with other developed countries may have much to do with the fact that the average teenager is exposed to unprotected intercourse for an average of 1 year before seeking contraceptive advice. In this age group, fully 73% of pregnancies are unintended.[4] Only one in three sexually active teenagers consistently uses contraception. Efforts to disseminate accurate reproductive information as well as to provide access to contraceptive products are vital to addressing this serious public health problem. Often contraceptives are not used until after the young woman becomes pregnant.

This chapter is based in part on the chapter with the same title that appeared in the 9th edition but was written by Roberta S. Carrier.

TABLE 1 Lowest expected, typical, and lowest reported failure rates during the first year of use of a method and first-year continuation rates

Method (1)	% of women experiencing an accidental pregnancy in the first year of use			% of women continuing use at one year[d]	
	Lowest expected[a] (2)	Typical[b] (3)	Lowest reported[c] (4)	Exc. preg. (5)	Inc. preg. (6)
Chance[e]	85	85	43.1		
Spermicides[f]	3	21	0.0	55	43
Periodic abstinence		20		84	67
Calendar	9		14.8[g]		
Ovulation method	3		10.5[g]		
Symptothermal[h]	2		12.6		
Postovulation	1		2.0[g]		
Withdrawal	4	18	6.7[g]		
Cap[i]	6	18	8.0	77	63
Sponge					
Parous women	9	28	27.7	73	53
Nulliparous women	6	18	13.9	73	60
Diaphragm[i]	6	18	2.1	69	57
Condom[j]	2	12	4.2	73	64
IUD		3		75	73
Progestasert®	2.0		1.9		
Copper T 380A	0.8		0.5		
Pill		3		75	73
Combined	0.1		0.0		
Progestogen only	0.5		1.1		
Injectable progestogen				70	70
DMPA	0.3	0.3	0.0		
NET	0.4	0.4	0.0		
Implants				90	90
NORPLANT® (6 capsules)	0.04	0.04	0.0		
NORPLANT®-2 (2 rods)	0.03	0.03	0.0		
Female sterilization	0.2	0.4	0.0		
Male sterilization	0.1	0.15	0.0		

[a]Among couples who initiate use of a method (not necessarily for the first time) and who use it *perfectly* (both consistently and correctly); the authors' best guess of the percentage expected to experience an accidental pregnancy during the first year if they do not stop use for any other reason.

[b]Among *typical* couples who initiate use of a method (not necessarily for the first time), the percentage who experience an accidental pregnancy during the first year if they do not stop use for any other reason.

[c]In the literature on contraceptive failure, the *lowest reported* percentage who experienced an accidental pregnancy during the first year following initiation of use (not necessarily for the first time) if they did not stop use for any other reason. However, see Note h.

[d]Among couples attempting to avoid pregnancy, the percentage who continue to use a method for 1 year, under the alternative assumptions that no one becomes pregnant (col. 5) and that the proportion becoming pregnant is given by col. 2 (col. 6).

[e]The lowest expected and typical percents are based on data from populations where contraception is not used and from women who cease using contraception in order to become pregnant. These represent our best guess of the percent who would conceive among women now relying on reversible methods of contraception if they abandoned contraception altogether. The lowest reported percent is based on U.S. women who use no contraception even though they do not wish to become pregnant. This group is selected for low fecundity or low coital frequency, and some fraction may use an unreported variant of periodic abstinence.

[f]Foams and vaginal suppositories.

[g]Too low, because rate is based on more than 1 year of exposure.

[h]Cervical mucus (ovulation) method supplemented by calendar in the preovulatory and basal body temperature in the postovulatory phases.

[i]With spermicidal cream or jelly.

[j]Without spermicides.

Reprinted with permission from Hatcher RA et al. *Contraceptive Technology 1990–1992*. 15th ed. New York: Irvington Publishers Inc; 1990: 134.

Choice of Contraceptive

There is no perfect method of birth control. Throughout life a woman's reproductive priorities change; her contraceptive choice may change as well. The method selected should be well thought out by the couple involved. The major points to be considered should include safety, effectiveness, accessibility, and acceptability of each method to each sexual partner.

Safety factors to consider in choosing a method of contraception include the risk of side effects as well as protection against sexually transmitted infectious diseases, including human immunodeficiency virus (HIV), the AIDS virus. It is important that sexually active individuals who are infertile, through either surgical or natural causes, be aware that they are still at risk for contracting and transmitting sexually transmitted diseases (STDs). Other safety considerations are the potential for method-associated effects on future fertility and possible method-associated adverse effects on the fetus, should unintended conception occur.

The effectiveness of a contraceptive method (Table 1) is reported in two ways: the *lowest expected* accidental pregnancy rate in the first year of use (method-related failure rate) and the *typical* accidental pregnancy rate (use-related failure rate). The lowest expected rate is very difficult to measure and indicates the method's theoretical effectiveness, assuming accurate and consistent use of the method every time intercourse occurs. The more realistic typical rate includes pregnancies that may have occurred because of inconsistent or improper use of the method. Reported use-related failure rates may vary, depending on the population studied. Effectiveness increases with increasing length of use of a particular method. Declining fertility in an older user population may contribute to increased effectiveness rates. In addition, couples who use contraception to prevent pregnancy have fewer failures than those who use contraceptives to space the births of their children.[5]

The percentage of people who continue with a given contraceptive method after a year of use is an indication of the method's acceptability (Table 1). Important factors in determining a method's acceptability include religious beliefs, future reproductive plans, complexity of method use, degree of interruption of spontaneity, "messiness," partner supportiveness, and cost. Pharmacists should be aware of the safety, effectiveness, accessibility, acceptability, and relative cost of the different contraceptive methods to help their patients make informed decisions.

Natural Family Planning

Natural family planning methods, also called periodic abstinence, rhythm, or fertility awareness methods, make use of various techniques to determine a woman's period of fertility. The information provided by these techniques is helpful in pinpointing the time of ovulation and optimal time for conception. Natural family planning is the only method of contraception approved by the Roman Catholic Church and is widely used around the world. Natural family planning can be divided into four methods: calendar, basal body temperature, cervical mucus, and symptothermal, each of which requires keeping detailed records of the woman's menstrual cycles and other symptoms associated with cyclical hormonal levels.

The data acquired, such as basal body temperature or the character and quantity of cervical mucus (Figure 1), are recorded on detailed monthly charts. After a period of instruction and with the information provided by charts from several months, a woman is usually able to predict her most fertile time. With this information, the couple can choose to abstain from sexual intercourse during this period if they want to avoid pregnancy.[6] (See Chapter 7, "Menstrual Products," for a review of menstrual physiology and biochemistry.)

Calendar Method

The calendar method (also known as the rhythm method) is based on records of monthly menstrual cycle lengths. The estimated day of ovulation, considered to be 14 ± 2 days before the onset of menstruation, is used to determine the woman's fertile period. The fertile period is calculated on the basis of estimates of the viable life of ova and sperm.[7] The fertilizable life of the ovum (egg) is estimated to be from 6 to 24 hours following ovulation, as measured by peaks in estrogen and luteinizing hormone (LH). Sperm is considered to be viable for 48 to 72 hours. The fertile period for a woman with records of her last 12 months of cycles is found by subtracting 18 days from the shortest cycle to determine the first fertile day and subtracting 11 days from the longest cycle to determine the last fertile day. For example, if a woman's shortest cycle in the last year was 25 days and her longest was 30 days, her fertile period would be from day 7 to day 19 of her cycle (Table 2). The calendar method is considered the least

TABLE 2	How to calculate the interval of fertility using the calendar or rhythm method		
If the shortest cycle has been (no. of days)	The first fertile (unsafe) day is	If the longest cycle has been (no. of days)	The last fertile (unsafe) day is
21[a]	3rd day	21	10th day
22	4th	22	11th
23	5th	23	12th
24	6th	24	13th
25	7th	25	14th
26	8th	26	15th
27	9th	27	16th
28	10th	28	17th
29	11th	29	18th
30	12th	30	19th
31	13th	31	20th
32	14th	32	21st
33	15th	33	22nd
34	16th	34	23rd
35	17th	35	24th

[a]Day 1, first day of menstrual bleeding.

Reprinted with permission from Hatcher RA et al. *Contraceptive Technology 1990–1992*. 15th ed. New York: Irvington Publishers Inc; 1990: 341.

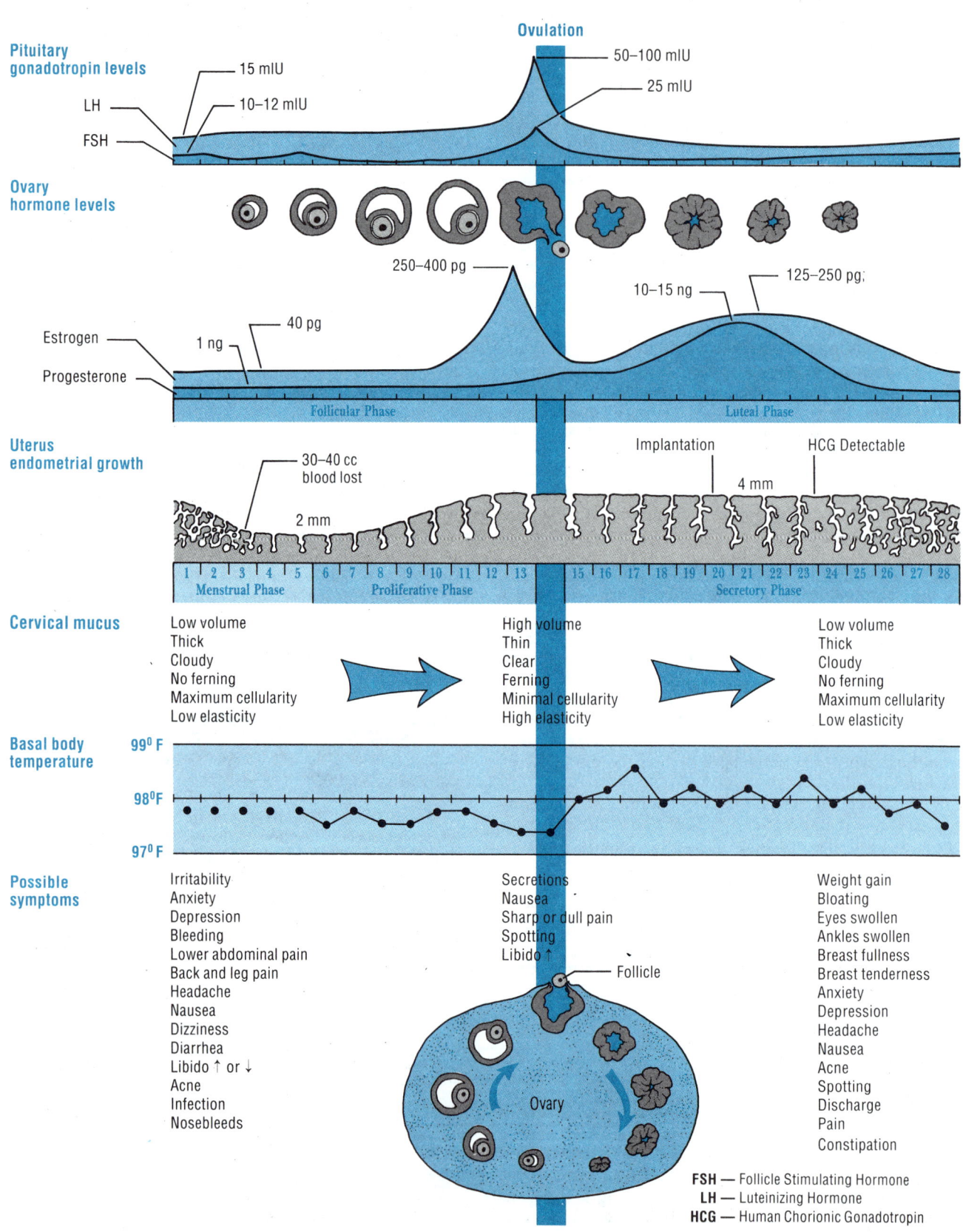

FIGURE 1 Primary menstrual cycle events: hormone levels, ovarian and endometrial patterns, cyclical temperature, and cervical mucus changes. Reprinted with permission from Hatcher RA et al. *Contraceptive Technology 1990–1992*. 15th ed. New York: Irvington Publishers Inc; 1990: 42.

effective of natural family planning methods, primarily because of natural variations in the length of a woman's normal menstrual cycle. Family planners do not currently recommend using the calendar method as the sole method of contraception, but it may be used in conjunction with other natural family planning methods described below. The calendar method is still widely employed as the sole contraceptive method; however, such reliance results in many unintended pregnancies (Table 1).[6,7]

Basal Body Temperature Method

In the basal body temperature (BBT) method, the woman measures her body temperature every day before arising and charts this temperature. The temperature should be taken with a mercury or electronic digital thermometer that is calibrated in increments of 0.1°F (0.5°C). Such a thermometer allows the detection of small changes in body temperature. It is very important to obtain the temperature before any physical activity and to obtain it at the same time every day. Oral or rectal temperature may be used, but any given individual should use one method (site) consistently.

These charts can be used to estimate the time of ovulation because there is usually a characteristic drop in BBT 12–24 hours before ovulation. The BBT then usually rises sharply over a 24–48-hour period to about 0.4–0.8°F (0.2–0.4°C) above the lowest point (the *nadir*) (Figure 2).[6–8] This sharp rise, called the *thermal shift*, is due to high progesterone levels. The *safe* (infertile) *period* is considered to begin after 3 days of postnadir temperature elevation and lasts until the start of the next cycle (menstruation). Because this method is not absolutely accurate in predicting when ovulation occurs, the postmenstrual or preovulatory safe period is difficult to determine, and those who engage in unprotected intercourse during this period have a higher pregnancy rate.

Electronic digital thermometers are more accurate than mercury thermometers and have a shorter recording time (45–90 seconds). Because the activity of shaking down a thermometer may cause the woman's body temperature to change, mercury thermometers must be shaken down each night rather than immediately before use in the morning.

Poor correlation of the thermal shift with ovulation reduces the accuracy of the BBT method. Furthermore, some women have monophasic menstrual cycles and do not have a definite or significant temperature dip or rise. Stress, fever, lactation, and use of an electric blanket may affect BBT, and temperature changes are difficult to interpret just before and during menopause.[8] At such times it is best for the couple to use one or more alternative methods of contraception.

Cervical Mucus Method

The cervical mucus method is based on the rather consistent changes in cervical mucus that take place during a normal menstrual cycle. Every day, the woman observes the mucus at the vulva (vaginal orifice) and charts its character and the amount produced (Figure 1). After menstruation, there are days when most women notice a sensation of dryness at the vaginal orifice. As estrogen levels rise, the cervical mucus increases in quantity and elasticity and becomes clear, resembling raw egg white.[6-8] The peak symptom, the last day of the clear, stretchy, estrogenic mucus, has been shown to be within a day of ovulation for most women. With the postovulatory rise in progesterone, the mucus becomes thick and sticky or is absent. The

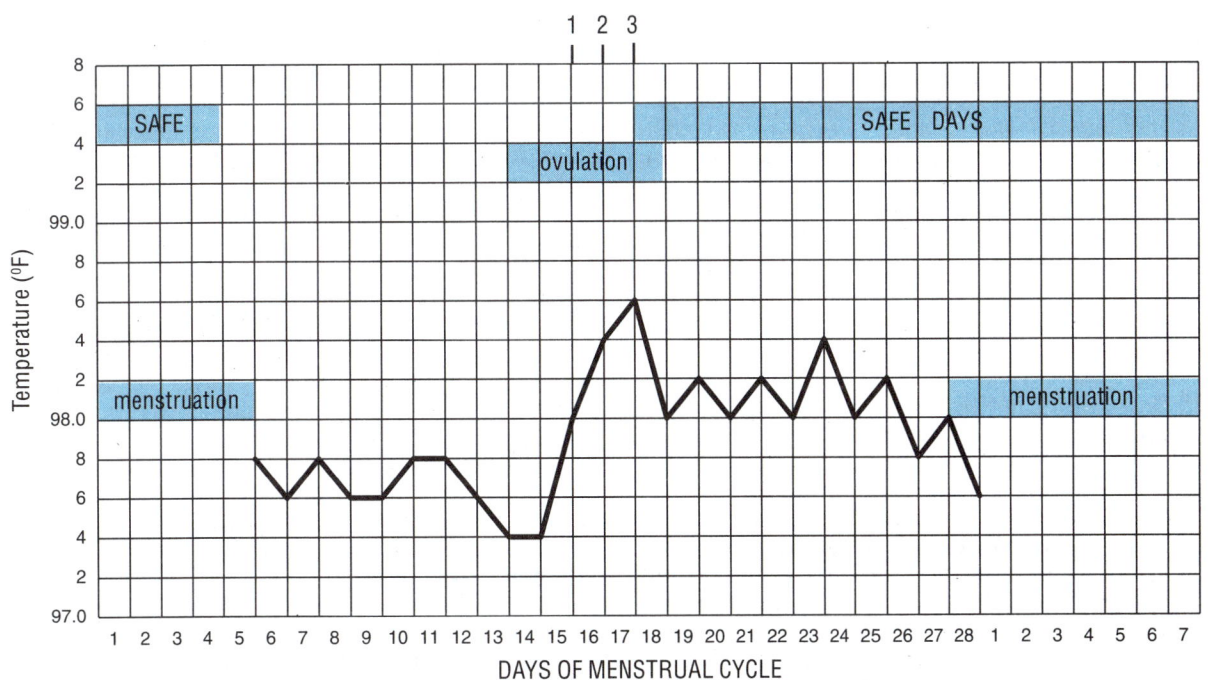

FIGURE 2 Basal body temperature variations during a model menstrual cycle. Reprinted with permission from Hatcher RA et al. *Contraceptive Technology 1990–1992*. 15th ed. New York: Irvington Publishers Inc; 1990: 343.

TABLE 3 Characteristics of cervical mucus throughout the normal menstrual cycle with the corresponding rules for intercourse

Phase	No. days in 28-day cycle	Characteristics of mucus	Rules for intercourse
Menses	3–5	Present but obscured by menstrual flow	Abstain
Thick mucus or dry days	2–4	No mucus or present in small amounts	Intercourse permitted on alternate days
Wet mucus days	2	Cloudy, yellow or white, and of sticky consistency	Abstain
Ovulation	3–5	Clear, slippery, wet, and stretchy, with the consistency of raw egg white—last day of this phase is known as the "peak symptom"	Abstain
Thick mucus or dry days	0–3	Small amount of cloudy, sticky mucus or no mucus	Intercourse beginning 4th day after last days of wet, stretchy mucus
Dry days	7–12	Usually no mucus, dry	Intercourse permitted
Wet mucus days	0–3	Clear and watery	Intercourse permitted

Reprinted with permission from Hatcher RA et al. *Contraceptive Technology 1990–1992*. 15th ed. New York: Irvington Publishers Inc; 1990: 345.

woman is considered fertile from the first day after menstruation on which mucus is detected until 72 hours after the appearance of the peak symptom (Table 3). With experience, a woman learns to differentiate other vaginal secretions, such as an infectious discharge or seminal fluid, from normal mucus. Most women can learn this method after three cycles. The average number of days of abstinence required per cycle is 17.[6] This method of natural family planning is preferred over the BBT method for postpartum lactating women and those nearing menopause. Women who use this method are also apt to detect abnormalities in their normal mucus patterns that may be due to infections, and thus are able to seek early treatment.

Symptothermal Method
The symptothermal method combines BBT charting with notations of other cyclical signs of ovulation (Figure 1). These signs might include breast tenderness, intermenstrual pain (mittelschmerz), labial edema, peak symptom cervical mucus, and changes in the character and position of the cervix. Most studies on the effectiveness of this method use the thermal shift (the temperature rise after the nadir) of the BBT method to determine the postovulatory safe period and use the cervical mucus or calendar method to determine the end of the preovulatory or postmenstrual infertile period.[8] Combinations of these methods have good predicted effectiveness; the lowest reported annual failure rate is 12.6% (Table 1).

Withdrawal
Coitus interruptus (withdrawal), although used intentionally by only a small percentage of couples in the United States, is more commonly practiced in some European countries[9] and in undeveloped countries around the world. The practice involves coital activity until ejaculation is imminent, then withdrawal of the stimulated penis and ejaculation away from the vagina or vulva. Accidental pregnancy rates with this method are in the range of 18 pregnancies per 100 couples in the first year of use.[9] Method failures (pregnancy even when the method is used correctly and consistently) are due in part to the fact that involuntary preejaculation secretions may contain millions of sperm. Disadvantages of this method include a higher pregnancy rate, a lack of protection against STDs, the requirement for considerable self-control by the man, and the potential for diminished pleasure for the couple due to interrupted lovemaking. Although this method should not be recommended, it is better than no contraceptive method.

Lactational Infertility
In many developing countries, breast-feeding is used as a contraceptive method for spacing the birth of children. When the infant receives only breast milk and the mother has not menstruated, protection against conception may persist for up to 6 months.[10] However, if breast feedings are supplemented with bottle feedings, lactational amenorrhea may not be a reliable form of contraception.

Although menstrual periods in lactating women may be anovulatory, ovulation may also occur before the return of menses. In general, if a breast-feeding woman is sexually active, other contraceptive measures should be employed no later than 5 weeks postpartum.[7]

In-Home Ovulation Prediction Tests

Ovulation prediction test kits, which are designed to aid couples in conceiving, detect the surge in LH that occurs shortly before ovulation. (See Chapter 4, "In-Home Testing and Monitoring Products.") These kits detect an increase in urinary excretion of LH, usually 8–40 hours before actual ovulation. Because the life expectancy of sperm may be as long as 72 hours, these ovulation predictors do not give warning of impending ovulation with enough accuracy to be effective contraceptive agents when used alone.

Home urine assays for estrogen and pregnanediol have been developed to detect the beginning and end, respectively, of the fertile phase.[6,11] These tests can warn of impending ovulation at least 3 days before its occurrence and can also detect the rise in progesterone that signals the end of the fertile period. In one group of women using these assays, there were only four unplanned pregnancies over 55 woman-years. (This figure can be extrapolated to 7.3 pregnancies per 100 woman-years).[11] These urine assays, when commercially available, may be used as a nonprescription method of fertility prediction for contraceptive purposes.

Advantages of Natural Family Planning

Natural family planning methods have the positive effect of encouraging communication within a relationship and may be the only truly shared contraceptive method. The cost of monitoring symptoms is minimal. Many couples like the fact that no chemicals are used in preventing conception, producing no chemical risk to the fertility or health of the couple (or to the fetus, if pregnancy should occur).

Risks of Natural Family Planning

The risks of natural family planning methods fall into three areas. First is the risk of pregnancy: these techniques have higher pregnancy rates than most other contraceptive methods. Second is the risk of STDs, because these methods involve no barriers to such infections, such as condoms or spermicides. The risk for STDs may be relatively low overall because these methods are most often practiced by couples in stable, long-term, monogamous relationships. The third and most controversial risk is that of abnormal pregnancy outcomes, such as birth defects or fetal wastage, should a couple conceive unintentionally. This risk is related to the possible association of such a conception with aged gametes (either sperm or ovum). Comparative studies have found a relative risk of 1.0 to 5.2 for birth defects or spontaneous abortion among those practicing natural family planning at the time of conception. At this time, however, the evidence for an increased risk of abnormal pregnancy outcomes is not conclusive. This controversial issue may become clearer as surveillance continues.[12]

The Pharmacist's Role in Natural Family Planning

Natural family planning methods, especially the BBT and cervical mucus methods, require extensive training and support from those who have experience and training with these methods. The pharmacist may supply BBT thermometers and monitoring charts. The pharmacist should be supportive and available to answer questions or to refer individuals to certified trainers in natural family planning. Couples should be reminded of medications that may interfere with physical signs and symptoms. For instance, phenothiazines, aspirin, and other medications may alter body temperature,[13] and vaginal foams, gels, creams, and douches will interfere with cervical mucus. A pharmacist with the proper training might consider counseling in natural family planning as a unique practice possibility.

Vaginal Contraceptives

Vaginal contraceptives (spermicides) use surface active agents to immobilize (kill) sperm. The effective spermicides include nonoxynol-9, octoxynol-9, and menfegol. Nearly all currently available products use nonoxynol-9. No products containing menfegol are currently marketed in the United States; however, several are available in Asia.

Spermicides come in a variety of dosage forms: jelly, cream, foam, suppository, film, and sponge. Spermicides used alone have a relatively high failure rate among typical first-year users (Table 1).[14] Of these products, vaginal foam appears to be most effective when it is used consistently. Use-effectiveness improves greatly if spermicides are used in conjunction with barrier methods such as diaphragms, cervical caps, or condoms. If the woman wants to douche, she should wait at least 8 hours after intercourse before doing so.

Spermicides are easy to use and readily available without prescription, and most forms are relatively inexpensive. Unit-dose containers of foam and suppositories can be carried in a purse quite discreetly. Spermicides are very useful as a backup method to other contraceptive products such as condoms and can also serve as a backup method if a birth control pill has been missed. If vaginal lubrication is desired, spermicidal creams or jellies are very good choices. There is also a growing body of literature suggesting that spermicides are possibly somewhat protective in vivo against many STDs, including chlamydia and gonorrhea.[15–17] Although studies have shown that nonoxynol-9 inactivates HIV in vitro and can apparently decrease transmission of simian immunodeficiency virus in monkeys, data on its efficacy in preventing the transmission of HIV between humans are lacking and efficacy should not be assumed.[18,19]

The relatively low use-effectiveness rate of spermicides used alone is their major disadvantage. Each product has very specific directions for use, dosage, and timing of administration with respect to coital activity. Users must be reminded to pay strict attention to the directions for use for each product. Some people are hypersensitive (allergic) to the components and others find spermicidal products excessively messy. Very frequent use may lead to irritation or damage of the vaginal and cervical epithelium.[20] There has been concern about a possible association between spermicide use and birth defects or miscarriage. After two very large population studies,[21,22] however, the Food and Drug Administration (FDA) has concluded that no increased risk of birth defects can be attributed to spermicides.[23]

Vaginal Creams and Jellies

When using a vaginal cream or jelly without a diaphragm or cervical cap, the user should be careful to choose a cream or jelly with a higher concentration of spermicide, not one with a lower concentration designed for use in conjunction with barrier methods. Creams have better lubricating and spreading qualities, whereas gels may be less messy. A full applicator of spermicide should be deposited high in the vagina, near the cervix. These agents are effective immediately and may be inserted up to 30–60 minutes in advance of intercourse. The product should be reapplied if intercourse is repeated or if intercourse is more than 60 minutes after initial application. In addition, douching should be delayed until at least 8 hours after the last act of intercourse. Allergic reactions, although rare, may be experienced by either partner. Couples having oral–genital sex may find the taste of some of these products unpleasant.[14]

Vaginal jellies and creams that are designed for use with diaphragms and cervical caps have lower concentrations of spermicide. Because of the lower concentration of spermicide, these products should not be used alone. Products designed for use alone, which contain higher concentrations of spermicide, may also be used with a diaphragm or cervical cap. The diaphragm or cervical cap is filled one-third full with spermicide and positioned over the cervix with placement checked as instructed by the health care practitioner. The diaphragm or cervical cap with the spermicide may be inserted up to an hour before intercourse.

The diaphragm is to be left in place for at least 6 hours after intercourse; if coitus is repeated before 6 hours have elapsed, additional cream or jelly should be inserted intravaginally without removing the diaphragm. If 6 hours have elapsed since intercourse, the diaphragm should be removed and washed and new spermicide should be applied before it is used again.[24] A study by Leitch found that contraceptive jelly retained its spermicidal activity for up to 12 hours and cream was effective for up to 24 hours after application.[25] If this finding is confirmed by other research, the time restrictions on insertion before intercourse and on reapplication of spermicide for repeated intercourse may be liberalized.

The cervical cap need not be removed if intercourse is repeated and it may be left in place for up to 48 hours. To ensure full protection in the event of repeated intercourse, it is advisable to apply another dose of spermicide intravaginally without removing the cervical cap.[24]

Vaginal Foams

When used alone, contraceptive foams appear to have better efficacy rates than do other vaginal contraceptives, possibly because they are more evenly distributed and adhere better to the cervical area and vaginal walls. Their availability and ease of use also make vaginal contraceptive foams an excellent product to use in combination with condoms, a good backup contraceptive method for women who use oral contraceptives, and useful for women with newly inserted IUDs. Women experiencing vaginal dryness may find vaginal contraceptive foams to be inadequate lubrication compared with creams and jellies. Strict attention must be paid to the directions for use for each product; some require two full applicators, whereas others require only one for an effective dose. For convenience, applicators may be prefilled before use. Prefilled unit-dose applicators are also commercially available. Vaginal foam is effective immediately on insertion and, like the other vaginal preparations, should be applied as close to the cervix as possible. Contraceptive foam, like creams and jellies, may be inserted up to an hour before coitus. Douching should be delayed until at least 8 hours after the last act of intercourse to allow adequate time for the spermicide to act.

Vaginal Suppositories

Vaginal suppositories are solid or semisolid dosage forms that are activated by the moisture in the woman's vaginal tract. They must be inserted high up in the vagina at least 10–15 minutes before intercourse. There may be some occasions when the suppository will not completely dissolve, resulting in an unpleasant, gritty sensation. As with other medicated suppositories, there is a risk that the woman may forget to unwrap the product or choose the wrong orifice for insertion, so the pharmacist should make certain the user understands the directions. Efficacy of vaginal suppositories is low. They are generally not recommended because more efficacious vaginal products are available. Vaginal suppositories do not require refrigeration.

Contraceptive Film

Vaginal contraceptive film, available in the United States since 1987, is made in England and has been used in Europe for 12 years. The active ingredient is nonoxynol-9, and the film is available in packets of 3, 6, or 12 paper-thin 2-inch square sheets. The film is activated by vaginal secretions. It is inserted on the tip of a finger and placed at the cervix, where it should be allowed to dissolve for at least 5 minutes before intercourse. Patients should be advised not to place the film over the penis for insertion. This method does not ensure proper placement and does not allow adequate time for dissolution. The film is effective for 2 hours. It is unknown how widely marketed or used this product is, or how the film compares in effectiveness with other vaginal contraceptive products.[14]

Contraceptive Sponge

The contraceptive sponge was approved by the FDA in 1983. It is a small, circular, disposable sponge, 2.5 cm thick and 5.5 cm in diameter, made of polyurethane permeated with 1 g of nonoxynol-9. The sponge must be moistened with about 2 tbsp (1.0 oz) of water to activate the spermicide. It is then inserted into the vagina so that the concave side covers the cervix. The sponge is believed to act as a contraceptive in three ways: (1) by serving as a mechanical barrier, (2) by the direct action of the spermicide, and (3) by absorbing semen. The sponge is considered active for 24 hours, regardless of the number of times intercourse is repeated. Like the diaphragm, the sponge should be kept in place for 6–8 hours after coital activity. Removal of the sponge is facilitated by a woven polyester loop attached to the convex side.

Typical failure rates for the contraceptive sponge range from 13.4 to 28.3 pregnancies per 100 women in the first year of use.[26,27] When data from a United States multicenter study were analyzed, it was found that whether women had previously given birth was a major factor in predicting effectiveness. Women who had not given birth (nulliparous women) who used the vaginal contraceptive sponge experienced an accidental pregnancy rate of 13.9%, which was not statistically different from the rate of diaphragm users studied. Women who had given birth (parous women) who used the sponge had a 28.3% risk of accidental pregnancy.[27] Theories for this variance include the possibility of poor fit in women who had delivered vaginally and the possibility that parous women had different contraceptive objectives—that is, that they were spacing their children rather than preventing births. At this time, it may be prudent not to routinely recommend the contraceptive sponge to parous women because of its poor efficacy.

The contraceptive sponge is convenient, safe, portable, and widely available without prescription. Populations at risk for STDs who use the contraceptive sponge may experience a decreased risk of infection caused by gonorrhea and chlamydia.[28–30]

The vaginal contraceptive sponge may be dislodged during intercourse. A woman must be able to locate her cervix and be comfortable in doing so to place the sponge correctly. Some women have difficulty removing the sponge, and the product has been known to fragment on removal. Contraindications to use include spermicide sensitivity, anatomic abnormalities of the vagina, and a history of toxic shock syndrome. Although the toxin-producing bacteria responsible for toxic shock syndrome are apparently inhibited in vitro by the contraceptive sponge,[31] an increased risk of about the same magnitude as that for tampon users has been identified by the Centers for Disease Control and Prevention.[32] The relative risk of toxic shock syndrome for tampon users has been estimated at 8 to 30 times baseline; the risk for sponge users is estimated to be 7.8 to 40 times baseline. Women should take special care to wash their hands before inserting the sponge, should not use the sponge during menstruation or postpartum, and should not exceed the 24-hour maximum recommended retention time. Users should also be advised to make sure that the entire sponge is removed, as fragments left in the vagina may serve as a focus for infection. There have also been reports of a small increase in the incidence of vaginal fungal infection among sponge users.[30]

In-vitro research has found that the nonoxynol-9 in the contraceptive sponge inactivates HIV at concentrations of nonoxynol-9 that are much lower than are attainable in vaginal fluid. However, one study showed that the sponge provided no more protection against HIV infection than did a placebo vaginal insert. Sponge users in that study did have a significantly decreased rate of infection with gonorrhea.[33] Sponge use was associated with a significant increase in vaginal and genital ulcers. Such lesions may enhance transmission of HIV and other STDs. Until it is proven otherwise, one must assume that the vaginal contraceptive sponge is not an effective method of preventing the transmission of HIV and subsequent infection.

Condoms

Condoms—also known as rubbers, sheaths, prophylactics, safes, skins, or pros—are the most important barrier contraceptive device in an era of sexually transmitted infectious diseases. The condom was originally described in the 16th century by Fallopius as a means of protecting the wearer from syphilis.[1] Apart from its role as a contraceptive, its importance in disease prevention is second only to that of abstinence.

The sheath described by Fallopius was made of linen. Current-day materials are much more comfortable for users and their partners. Latex condoms come in a variety of colors, styles, shapes, and thicknesses (ranging from 0.02 mm to approximately 0.1 mm). Other available features include reservoir tips, ribs, studs, lubrication, and spermicidal lubrication.[34] Condom sales increased by 20% from 1986 to 1988, and the sale of latex condoms treated with spermicide increased by 116%. This increase was attributed to an extensive public health campaign following the release of the U.S. Surgeon General's report on AIDS, which recommended the regular use of condoms by persons at risk in order to assist in the prevention of HIV transmission.[35] Condoms made from lamb cecum (skins) provide less protection from STDs than do latex condoms because of their higher porosity. They are also more expensive. Skins should be recommended only for those who have a latex allergy[36] or for those who are not at risk for STDs, such as those in a long-term, mutually monogamous relationship with an uninfected person.

Since 1976 condom quality has been under the purview of the FDA. The Center for Devices and Radiological Health is responsible for monitoring the quality of domestically produced condoms as well as imported condoms.[37,38] In 1987 the testing program was expanded because of concerns about protection from the AIDS virus. The United States uses a water-leak test as the standard. The failure rate per batch is not to exceed 4 condoms per 1000. Of batches that met the quality guidelines, the average failure rate was 2.3 per 1000 tested.[38] A newer test method being evaluated uses a fluorescent microsphere that approximates the size of the human immunodeficiency virus.[39]

The typical use-failure rate for condoms is 10–13 pregnancies per 100 women during the first year of use.[14,34] The most common cause of use-failure with condoms, as with all other contraceptive methods, is the lack of consistent, proper use. An important part of being able to use a product effectively is understanding the directions for use. A recent review of the reading level required to understand the printed instructions included in condom packaging found that although many Americans do not have the reading skills of a high school graduate, condom instructions are written at or above a high school reading level.[40] Because condoms are frequently purchased in drug stores, pharmacists are the obvious primary source of verbal information on the correct use of condoms. Unfortunately, in one recent survey of 31 pharmacies, only 31% of the pharmacists were able to appropriately educate a patient on the proper selection and use of a condom.[41] It is imperative that pharmacists maintain and continually update their contraceptive knowledge base.

If the condom user wants a lubricant, the pharmacist must stress the importance of using lubricants that do not harm or weaken the strength and integrity of the condom. Condom users should definitely avoid any oil-based lubricants, including Vaseline®, Vaseline Intensive Care® lotion, baby oil, and corn oil.[42,43] These products cause rapid deterioration of the latex and may lead to breaks in the condom. Appropriate water-based lubricants to use with latex condoms include products such as K-Y Jelly®, Ortho Personal Lubricant®, or any of the spermicidal creams or jellies. Several manufacturers now offer lubricants specifically designed for use with condoms, such as CondomMate®.

TABLE 4 Guidelines for proper condom use

1. Use only condoms that are fresh (not previously opened) and that have been stored in a dry, cool place (not a wallet or car glove compartment).
2. *Always* use latex condoms unless you are in a monogamous relationship with someone you *know* is not infected with HIV.
3. Do *not* attempt to test the condom for leaks before using; this only increases the risk of tearing.
4. Condoms occasionally break. You should always have a vaginal spermicidal product (foam, cream, or jelly) available and insert it as soon as possible if a condom break or spill occurs.
5. Be aware that long fingernails or jewelry may easily tear condoms.
6. Unroll the condom onto the erect penis before the penis comes into *any* contact with the vagina. *This is very important for preventing both pregnancy and disease*. If you start to put the condom on backward, discard that condom and use a fresh one.
7. If you are not using a reservoir-tipped condom, leave 1/2 inch of space between the end of the condom and the tip of the penis by pinching the top of the condom as you unroll it. This leaves space for the ejaculate and decreases the risk of breakage.
8. If your partner has vaginal dryness, you may want to use additional lubrication. This will help decrease the risk of tears and breakage. Only *water-based lubricants* such as K-Y Jelly®, Lubrin®, and CondomMate® are safe for use with condoms. Oil-based lubricants, such as Vaseline® and Crisco®, weaken condoms and increase the chance of breakage. Spermicidal agents may be used as lubricants with condoms and may increase the effectiveness of the condom as well.
9. After ejaculation, withdraw the penis immediately. Hold on to the rim of the condom as you withdraw to prevent the condom from slipping off, especially if you have used additional lubrication.
10. Check the condom for tears and then discard.
11. If a tear has occurred, *immediately* insert spermicidal foam, cream, or jelly containing a high concentration of spermicide into the vagina. *Do not* use *suppositories* or a vaginal *film* in these cases, as the delay time for dissolution may decrease the product's efficacy.

Excessive heat or overexposure to ozone at levels found in some metropolitan areas will significantly decrease the integrity of the latex within 6 hours; consequently, proper storage of condoms is very important. Pharmacists should emphasize that condoms must be protected from light and excessive heat.[44] The shelf life of condoms under optimal conditions, as packaged by the manufacturers, is 3–5 years; the user should always check for discoloration, brittleness, or stickiness, and condoms displaying any of these characteristics should be discarded.[38]

Condoms should be placed on the erect penis before any genital contact, because precoital involuntary urethral secretions of the male may contain semen or viable sperm. Rather than interrupting foreplay, many couples find it very pleasurable to incorporate condom use into foreplay by having the woman put it on her partner.[34] If the condom does not have a reservoir tip, one should be improvised by leaving a half-inch space at the tip. Air should be squeezed from this reservoir by pinching it as the condom is unrolled to its full length. To minimize tears, care should be taken with rings and fingernails, and adequate lubrication should be ensured before vaginal or anal entry. If the condom should break while it is being put on, it must be replaced immediately. If breakage or leakage occurs after ejaculation, a spermicidal product (cream, jelly, or foam) should be inserted immediately, although the protective value of this procedure is uncertain. Once ejaculation has occurred, the man should withdraw his penis while it is still erect, holding on to the base of the condom to prevent it from slipping off and spilling semen. Spermicidal condoms or the combined use of a vaginal spermicide and a condom may minimize the risk of pregnancy should leakage occur. Specific guidelines for proper condom use are given in Table 4.

The incidence of condom breakage is unknown. Breakage rates from studies vary widely: 1 break per 164 acts of intercourse (a rate of 0.6%) was reported in a general population of health care workers;[34] rates of 0.5% for anal acts and 0.8% for vaginal acts were reported in a study conducted in brothels in Australia;[45] a rate of 5% was reported in a Danish study using both female prostitutes and hospital personnel;[46] and an 8% incidence of tearing or slippage during anal intercourse was reported in a study of Dutch homosexuals.[47] In one report of three study sites, breakage rates ranged from 6.7 to 12.9%. Some individuals in this study had multiple incidences of breakage, indicating that breakage may be related as much to the individual user as it is to manufacturing defects.[48] One study found that the use of additional lubrication with lubricated condoms increased the likelihood of condom slippage, leading to possible spillage of semen.[49]

For the vast majority of people, condoms are an effective, acceptable, inexpensive, safe and nontoxic method of birth control. The most frequent complaint is decreased sensitivity of the glans penis and decreased sexual pleasure for the male. Strategies for countering this problem might include the use of very thin condoms, ridged condoms, or—in a monogamous relationship with an HIV-negative individual—lamb cecum condoms.

It is estimated that 1 to 2% of the population may be sensitized to latex.[50] These patients may develop condom contact dermatitis. Patients should be asked if they can wear rubber gloves or blow up a balloon without developing itching. The sensitizers are usually antioxidants or accelerators used in processing the rubber.[36] Because different manufacturers use different processes, changing brands may alleviate the problem. In one study, the range of reactions in patients allergic to latex ranged from 0 to 76%, depending on the brand used.[51] If switching brands does not eliminate the irritation, lamb cecum condoms may be used if their limitations are recognized. Also, patients may be sensitized to components of the lubricant. Again, changing brands may resolve the problem.

Female Condom

Because of concerns over the lack of means for women to protect themselves against pregnancy and STDs (especially HIV), several types of vaginal barrier pouches are under development.[52] Some of these are in the final stages of testing necessary for marketing in the United States.

Reality®, a female condom made by Wisconsin Pharmacal, is made of polyurethane rather than latex. It is thinner than the male condom and is resistant to degradation by oil-based lubricants. It is prelubricated and is designed for one-time use. It is secured by a circular ring that fits like a diaphragm over the cervix. An outer ring, which dangles outside the vagina, is designed to protect the external genitalia.

The Bikini Condom®, which is produced by International Prophylactics Inc, resembles a G-string panty. It is made of latex twice as thick as that used in the average male condom. The pouch contains a water-based lubricant, and it is unrolled as the penis is inserted into the vagina.

A third type of vaginal pouch, called Women's Choice®, more closely resembles the male condom but is wider. The open end has a ring that stays outside the vagina; the closed end consists of a thicker dome-shaped patch of latex. This product is inserted with an applicator, like a tampon, and is lubricated with a silicone lubricant.

Advantages of these devices include a reduced chance of breakage, less mess than spermicides, no known significant adverse effects, and easy access without prescription. They offer a means of control and protection for women and by women. Some women have reported heightened clitoral stimulation with the Women's Choice® product. The female condom has been shown to be impermeable to HIV in vitro.[53]

Some disadvantages noted include the expense (female condoms cost significantly more than male condoms), a cumbersome and unattractive appearance, vaginal irritation, decreased sensation for some women, and some difficulty with insertion for those not experienced in using tampons. Most of these disadvantages are considered minor and should not significantly affect proper use of the female condom.

Douching

Vaginal douches should never be considered a method of contraception. Under favorable conditions in the female reproductive tract, active sperm have been found in the cervical crypts and oviducts within 5 minutes after ejaculation.[7] Postcoital douching would have no effect in removing sperm from the upper reproductive tract and might, in fact, force or propel sperm higher in the reproductive tract. Because consistent users of douches have a higher incidence of pelvic infections and ectopic pregnancies,[54] it is questionable whether the practice of douching, even for personal hygiene, is of any benefit to a woman's vaginal health. (See Chapter 27, "Personal Care Products.")

Sexually Transmitted Diseases

Acquired Immunodeficiency Syndrome

The incidence of AIDS is increasing almost exponentially. The first 100,000 cases of the full-blown disease were reported over a 99-month period (June 1981–August 1989); the next 100,000 cases were reported over a period of just 27 months (September 1989–November 1991).[55] Given these facts and the fact that well over 1 million Americans are HIV-positive, the prevention of STDs must be a priority. As health care practitioners in a position to offer much-needed health information, pharmacists must keep current in their knowledge of all aspects of prevention and treatment of STDs, especially with respect to AIDS.

In the United States, at least 65% of HIV infections are transmitted via heterosexual or homosexual intercourse.[56] Between 1990 and 1991 the rate of heterosexual transmission of AIDS increased by 21% and the number of AIDS cases reported in women increased by 15%.[56] The known routes of transmission are (1) blood and blood products (via transfusions, sharing contaminated needles and syringes, and accidental contaminated needle sticks); (2) mucous membrane exposures (saliva, seminal fluid, and vaginal fluids, including menstrual blood); and (3) perinatal and peripartum transmission to infants. Table 5 provides a list of safer sex options as well as high-risk sexual activities. The only sure way to guard against infection with the AIDS virus through sexual contact is to abstain from sex or to remain in a mutually monogamous relationship with an uninfected individual. If neither of these is feasible, the next option is to use latex (not natural membrane) condoms for any oral, anal, or vaginal intercourse.[57] In populations at risk, individuals who have consistently used condoms have a rate of seroconversion (an indicator of infection with the AIDS virus) that is significantly lower than the seroconversion rate seen in those who do not use condoms or who use condoms inconsistently.[58-60] It is very important to emphasize that condom use does not guarantee safety because of the possibility of condom breakage.[46,47] Laboratory data are being accumulated that suggest that the spermicide nonoxynol-9 in proper concentrations may be somewhat effective in killing the AIDS virus and might offer additional protection when used with condoms.[38,59,61]

Because compliance with safer sex practices, especially with regard to condom use, is poor even among those at risk, other behavioral factors aimed at lowering risk should be stressed.[62] These changes include changes in lifestyle and sexual practices.

Other Sexually Transmitted Diseases

There are over 20 STDs, both bacterial and viral, that may have severe longstanding consequences on the health and reproductive capabilities of those infected. A thorough discussion of these diseases is beyond the scope of this chapter. The presence of some other STDs may increase a person's susceptibility to and risk of acquiring HIV infection.[63] Chlamydia, now the most commonly occurring STD in the United States, causes pelvic inflammatory disease, cervicitis, and infertility in women; urethritis and epididymitis in men; and conjunctivitis and pneumonia in neonates.[64] Gonorrhea is

TABLE 5 Safer sex practices

Safe activities
Massage
Hugging
Body rubbing
Kissing (dry)
Masturbation
Hand-to-genital touching (hand job) or mutual masturbation
Erotic books and movies

Possibly safe activities
Kissing (wet)
Vaginal/rectal intercourse using latex condom (use spermicide for extra safety)
Oral sex on a man using a latex condom
Oral sex on a woman who does not have her period or a vaginal infection with discharge (use latex barrier such as dental dam for extra safety)

Unsafe activities
Any intercourse without a latex condom
Oral sex on a man without a latex condom
Oral sex on a woman during her period or a vaginal infection with discharge without a latex barrier such as a dental dam
Semen in the mouth
Oral–anal contact
Sharing sex toys or douching equipment
Blood contact of *any* kind, including menstrual blood, sharing needles, and any sex that causes tissue damage or bleeding

Reprinted with permission from Hatcher RA et al. *Contraceptive Technology 1990-1992*. 15th ed. New York: Irvington Publishers Inc; 1990: 76.

---

still a major problem, as are herpes simplex, venereal warts, and syphilis.[65] Tactics to prevent transmission by using barrier contraceptives such as latex condoms and vaginal contraceptive spermicides, along with changes in sexual practices as previously described for AIDS prevention (Table 5), are strongly recommended and can have a major positive effect on the prevalence of STDs.[15]

As previously mentioned, spermicidal contraceptive sponges appear to offer some protection against chlamydia and gonorrhea (but not HIV and other sexually transmitted infections)[16,29,33,65] and may add to the protective effects of condom use. It is also important to keep in mind that some STDs, such as syphilis and herpes, may be spread via external skin lesions. Condoms and spermicides may not be effective in preventing these types of infection.

all options to be presented in a clear and nonjudgmental manner. All sexually active individuals who are not in a mutually monogamous relationship should be aware that they must protect themselves and their partners from AIDS and other STDs and should choose a contraceptive method accordingly.

Pharmacists should thoroughly familiarize themselves with the proper use of currently available nonprescription contraceptive products and should provide opportunities for consultation with patients by removing barriers that may prevent dialogue. Contraceptive products and information should be available in an area where the patient can browse and where the pharmacist can easily interact with the patient, such as next to or directly in front of the prescription counter. A private area for education and counseling is important if adequate discussion is to take place.

Special efforts should be made to offer contraceptive information and services to adolescents. This population group is especially likely to be uninformed or misinformed about reproductive matters. Many pharmacists are uncomfortable discussing reproductive health with young people. Such a pharmacist should refer adolescents to a clinic that specializes in services to young people, if one is available. Adolescents need clear, accurate information on all aspects of reproductive health. The pharmacist should keep in mind that printed instructions are often written above the reading level of most adolescents (as well as many adults); therefore, verbal instructions are very important. Nonprescription methods particularly useful for the impulsive adolescent might include condoms and contraceptive foam in prefilled applicators.

Condom use should be stressed as a method of disease prevention for all, including those who currently use prescription methods of birth control (e.g., oral contraceptives or the IUD). Reservoir-tip and spermicidally lubricated latex condoms add additional protection against STDs and the risk of condom rupture.

The diaphragm, cervical cap, or natural family planning methods may be an acceptable approach to contraception for a couple in a stable relationship. These methods require either special fitting or training. In addition to stocking spermicidal products and BBT thermometers, pharmacists may serve as referral centers for those desiring to use these methods of family planning.

Further information on reproductive health and AIDS may be found by contacting the organizations listed in Appendices 1 and 2.

Pharmacists, as the most accessible health care professionals, can be invaluable in contributing to the reproductive health and knowledge of people in their communities. Reproductive health and contraceptive information may well be one of the most challenging areas of a pharmacist's practice, and one that has a profound impact on the public health and individual well-being of those we serve.

Summary

Not many decisions in life are more personal or more important than the choice of a contraceptive method. Optimally, the decision should be made by both sexual partners. Because no single method is likely to be suitable throughout a person's reproductive life, it is important for

References

1. Eichhorst BC. Contraception. *Prim Care* 1988 Sep; 15 (3): 437–9.
2. *Ortho 1991 Birth Control Survey*. Raritan, NJ: Ortho Pharmaceutical Corp; 1991.
3. Sophocles AM Jr, Brozovich EM. Birth control failure among patients with unwanted pregnancies: 1982–1984. *J Fam Pract* 1986 Jan; 22 (1): 45–8.

4. Forrest JD, Singh S. The sexual and reproductive behavior of American women, 1982–1988. *Fam Plann Perspect* 1990 Sep/Oct; 22 (5): 206–14.
5. Schirm AL, Trussell J, Menken J, et al. Contraceptive failure in the United States: the impact of social, economic and demographic factors. *Fam Plann Perspect* 1982 Mar/Apr; 14 (2): 68–94.
6. Brown JB, Blackwell LF, Billings JJ, et al. Natural family planning. *Am J Obstet Gynecol* 1987 Oct; 157 (4 pt 2): 1082–9.
7. Klaus H. Natural family planning: a review. *Obstet Gynecol Survey* 1982 Feb; 37 (2): 128–50.
8. Gross BA. Natural family planning indicators of ovulation. *Clin Reprod Fertil* 1987 5: 91. Invited review.
9. Hatcher RA, Stewart F, Trussell J, et al. *Contraceptive Technology 1990–1992.* 15th ed. New York: Irvington Publishers Inc; 1990: 351–54.
10. Kennedy KI, Rivers R, McNeilly AS. Consensus statement on the use of breastfeeding as a family planning method. *Contraception* 1989 May; 39 (5): 477–91.
11. Brown JB, Holmes J, Barker G. Use of the home ovarian monitor in pregnancy avoidance. *Am J Obstet Gynecol* 1991 Dec; 165 (6 pt 2): 2008–11.
12. Gray RH, Kambic RT. Epidemiological studies of natural family planning. *Hum Reprod* 1988 3: 693.
13. Frazier JL, Schumock GT. Drug-induced alterations in body temperature. *P&T* 1991 Mar; 16 (3): 164, 271–5.
14. Hatcher RA, Stewart F, Trussell J, et al. *Contraceptive Technology 1990–1992.* 15th ed. New York: Irvington Publishers Inc; 1990: 134.
15. Stone KM, Grimes DA, Mageder LS. *Am J Obstet Gynecol* 1986 Jul; 155 (1): 180–8.
16. Louv WC, Austin H, Alexander WJ, et al. A clinical trial of nonoxynol-9 for preventing gonococcal and chlamydial infections. *J Infect Dis* 1988 Sep; 158 (3): 518–23.
17. Niruthisard S, Roddy RE, Chutivongse S. Use of nonoxynol-9 and reduction in rate of gonococcal and chlamydial cervical infections. *Lancet* 1992 Jun 6; 339: 1371–5.
18. Voeller B. Nonoxynol-9 and HTLV-III. *Lancet* 1986 May 17; 1 (8490): 1153. Letter.
19. Miller CJ, Hendrickx AG, Alexander NJ, Marx, PA, Gettie A. The effect of contraceptives containing nonoxynol-9 on the genital transmission of simian immunodeficiency virus in rhesus macaques. *Fertil Steril* 1992 May; 57 (5): 1126–8.
20. Niruthisard S, Roddy RE, Chutivongse S. The effects of frequent nonoxynol-9 use on the vaginal and cervical mucosa. *Sex Transm Dis* 1991 Jul/Sep; 18 (3): 176–9.
21. Mills JL, Reed GF, Nugent RP, et al. Are there adverse effects of periconceptional spermicide use? *Fertil Steril* 1985 Mar; 43 (3): 442–6.
22. Harlap S, Shiono PH, Ramchara S, et al. Chromosomal abnormalities in the Kaiser-Permanente Birth Defects Study, with special reference to contraceptive use around the time of conception. *Teratology* 1985 Jun; 31 (3): 381–7.
23. Data do not support association between spermicides, birth defects. *FDA Drug Bull* 1986 16: 21.
24. Hatcher RA, Stewart F, Trussell J, et al. *Contraceptive Technology 1990–1992.* 15th ed. New York: Irvington Publishers Inc; 1990: 218–221.
25. Leitch WS. Longevity of Ortho Creme® and Gynol II® in the contraceptive diaphragm. *Contraception* 1986 Oct; 34 (4): 381–93.
26. Edelman DA, North BB. Updated pregnancy rates for the Today contraceptive sponge. *Am J Obstet Gynecol* 1987 Nov; 157 (5): 1164–5.
27. McIntyre SL, Higgins JE. Parity and use-effectiveness with the contraceptive sponge. *Am J Obstet Gynecol* 1986 Oct; 155 (4): 796–801.
28. Polsky B, Baron PA, Gold JWM, et al. In vitro inactivation of HIV-1 by contraceptive sponge containing nonoxynol-9. *Lancet* 1988 Jun 24; 1 (8600): 1456.
29. Rosenberg MJ, Feldblum PJ, Rojanapithayakorn W. The contraceptive sponge's protection against chlamydia trachomatis and Neisseria gonorrhoeae. *Sex Transm Dis* 1987 Jul/Sep; 14(3): 147–52.
30. Rosenberg MJ, Rojanapithayakorn W, Feldblum PJ, et al. Effect of the contraceptive sponge on chlamydial infection, gonorrhea, and candidiasis: a comparative clinical trial. *JAMA* 1987 May 1; 257 (17): 2308–12.
31. Remington KM, Buller RS, Kelly JR. Effect of the Today contraceptive sponge on growth and toxic shock syndrome toxin-1 production by *Staphylococcus aureus*. *Obstet Gynecol* 1987 Apr; 69 (4): 563–9.
32. Faich G, Pearson K, Fleming D, et al. Toxic shock syndrome and the vaginal contraceptive sponge. *JAMA* 1986 Jan 10; 255 (2): 216–8.
33. Kreiss J, Ngugi E, Holmes K, et al. Efficacy of nonoxynol-9 contraceptive sponge use in preventing heterosexual acquisition of HIV in Nairobi prostitutes. *JAMA* 1992 Jul 22; 268 (4): 477–82.
34. Hatcher RA, Stewart F, Trussell J, et al. *Contraceptive Technology 1990–1992.* 15th ed. New York: Irvington Publishers Inc; 1990: 161–3.
35. Moran JS, Janes HR, Peterman TA, et al. Increase in condom sales following AIDS education and publicity, United States. *Am J Public Health* 1990 May; 80 (5): 607–8.
36. Fisher AA. Condom dermatitis in either partner. *Cutis* 1987 Apr; 39 (4): 281, 284–5.
37. Provencher GC, Miller PJ. Who's responsible for condom quality? *Am J Nurs* 1988 May; 88 (5): 640, 643. Letter.
38. Centers for Disease Control. Condoms for prevention of sexually transmitted diseases. *MMWR* 1988 Mar 11; 37 (9): 133–7.
39. FDA develops latex condom permeability test method. *The Gray Sheet* 1990 16:22.
40. Richwald GA, Wamsley MA, Coulson AH, et al. Are condom instructions readable? Results of a readability study. *Public Health Rep* 1988 Jul–Aug; 103 (4): 355–9.
41. Gebhart F. Pharmacists fail condom quiz, other AIDS prevention questions. *Drug Topics* 1992 Mar 9; 136 (5): 14–5.
42. Voeller B, Coulson AH, Bernstein GS, et al. Mineral oil lubricants cause rapid deterioration of latex condoms. *Contraception* 1989 Jan; 39 (1): 95–102.
43. White N, Taylor K, Lyszkowski A, et al. Dangers of lubricants used with condoms. *Nature* 1988 Sep 1; 335 (6185): 19.
44. Clark LJ, Sherwin RP, Baker RF. Latex condom deterioration accelerated by environmental factors: I. ozone. *Contraception* 1989 Mar; 39 (3): 245–51.
45. Richters J, Donovan B, Gerofi J, et al. Low condom breakage rate in commercial sex. *Lancet* 1988 Dec 24/31; 2 (8626–7): 1487–8.
46. Gotzsche PC, Hording M. Condoms to prevent HIV transmission do not imply truly safe sex. *Scand J Infect Dis* 1988 20 (2): 233–4.
47. Van Griensven GJP, De Vroome EMM, Tielman RAP, et al. Failure rate of condoms during anogenital intercourse in homosexual men. *Genitourin Med* 1988 Oct; 64 (5): 344–6.
48. Russel-Brown P, Piedrahita C, Foldsey R, Steiner M, Townsend J. Comparison of condom breakage during human use with performance in laboratory testing. *Contraception* 1992 May; 45 (5): 429–37.
49. Trussell J, Warner DL, Hatcher RA. Condom slippage and breakage rates. *Fam Plann Perspect* 1992 Jan/Feb; 24 (1): 20–3.
50. Fisher AA. Condom conundrums: part 1. *Cutis* 1991 Nov; 48 (5): 359–60.
51. Turjanmaa K, Reunala T. Condoms as a source of latex allergen and cause of contact urticaria. *Contact Dermatitis* 1989 May; 20 (5): 360–4.
52. Female condoms scheduled to reach U.S. market this year. *Contraceptive Technology Update* 1991 12(8): 117–22, 127.

53. Drew WL, Blair M, Miner RC, Conant M. Evaluation of the virus permeability of a new condom for women. *Sex Transm Dis* 1990 Apr/Jun; 17 (2): 110–2.
54. Hatcher RA, Stewart F, Trussell J, et al. *Contraceptive Technology 1990–1992*. 15th ed. New York: Irvington Publishers Inc; 1990: 63, 186.
55. Centers for Disease Control. The second 100,000 cases of acquired immunodeficiency syndrome—United States, June 1981–December 1991. *MMWR* 1992 Jan 17; 41 (2): 28–9.
56. Centers for Disease Control. Update: acquired immunodeficiency syndrome—United States, 1991. *MMWR* 1992 Jul 3; 41 (26): 463–8.
57. Food and Drug Administration. Counseling patients about the prevention of AIDS. *NY State J Med* 1988 May; 88 (5): 264–5.
58. Ngugi EN, Plummer FA, Simonsen JN, et al. Prevention of transmission of human immunodeficiency virus in Africa: effectiveness of condom promotion and health education among prostitutes. *Lancet* 1988 Oct 15; 2 (8616): 887–90.
59. Feldblum PJ, Fortney JA. Condoms, spermicides, and the transmission of human immunodeficiency virus: a review of the literature. *Am J Public Health* 1988 Jan; 78 (1): 52–4.
60. Darrow WW. Condom use and use-effectiveness in high-risk populations. *Sex Transm Dis* 1989 Jul–Sep; 16 (3): 157–9.
61. Rietmeijer CAM, Krebs JW, Feorino PM, et al. Condoms as physical and chemical barriers against human immunodeficiency virus. *JAMA* 1988 Mar 25; 259 (12): 1851–3.
62. Henry K, Osterholm MT. Reduction of HIV transmission by use of condoms. *Am J Public Health* 1988 Sep; 78 (9): 1244. Letter.
63. Wasserheit JN. Epidemiological synergy. interrelationships between human immunodeficiency virus infection and other sexually transmitted diseases. *Sex Transm Dis* 1992 Mar–Apr; 19 (2): 61–77.
64. Sanders LL, Harrison HR, Washington AE. Treatment of sexually transmitted chlamydial infections. *JAMA* 1986 Apr 4; 255 (13): 1750–6.
65. North BB. Vaginal contraceptives: effective protection from sexually transmitted diseases for women? *J Reprod Med* 1988 Mar; 33 (3): 307–11.

Appendix 1: Family Planning Information

In addition to the resources listed below, many states and counties have their own chapters of family planning organizations such as Planned Parenthood. Check with your local board of health or look in your local telephone directory.

- The Alan Guttmacher Institute
  111 Fifth Avenue
  New York, NY 10003
  212-254-5656

- Planned Parenthood Federation of America, Inc.
  810 Seventh Avenue
  New York, NY 10019
  212-541-7800

- The Population Council
  Office of Communications
  1 Dag Hammarskjold Plaza
  New York, NY 10017
  212-644-1300

- Population Information Program
  The Johns Hopkins University
  624 North Broadway
  Baltimore, MD 21205
  410-659-6300

- Special Programme of Research, Development and Research Training in Human Reproduction
  World Health Organization
  Avenue Appia
  CH 1211, Geneva 27
  Switzerland

Appendix 2: AIDS Information Resources

The 15 AIDS Education and Training Centers are listed in alphabetical order by state. Each center serves a geographic area and provides information and ongoing education for health care providers.

- AIDS Education & Training Center
  University of California at Davis
  5110 East Clinton Way, Suite 115
  Fresno, CA 93727
  209-252-2851

- AIDS Education & Training Center
  University of Southern California
  1420 San Pablo Street, B207
  Los Angeles, CA 90033
  213-224-7711

- Mountain Plains Regional AIDS
    Education & Training Center
  University of Colorado
  4200 East 9th Avenue, Box A-906
  Denver, CO 80262
  303-270-5885

- Comprehensive AIDS Program
  University of Miami
  P.O. Box 016960 (D-90)
  Miami, FL 33101
  305-549-6003

- Emory AIDS Training Network
  Emory University
  735 Gatewood Road, NE
  Atlanta, GA 30322
  404-727-2929

- Midwest AIDS Training & Education Center (MATEC)
  University of Illinois
  808 South Wood Street M/C779
  P.O. Box 6998
  Chicago, IL 60612
  312-996-1373 or 312-996-1426

- Delta Region AIDS Education and Training Center
  Louisiana State University
  1542 Tulane Avenue
  New Orleans, LA 70112
  504-568-3855

- Mid-Atlantic AIDS ETC
  University of Maryland at Baltimore
  East Hall
  520 West Lombard Street
  Baltimore, MD 21201
  410-328-8334

- New England AIDS Education and Training Center
  University of Massachusetts
  55 Lake Avenue North
  Worcester, MA 01655
  508-856-3255

- Center for AIDS Education
  University of Medicine and Dentistry of New Jersey
  30 Bergen Street
  Newark, NJ 07107
  201-456-6640

- AIDS Education & Training Center
  New York University
  429 Shimkin Hall
  Washington Square
  New York, NY 10003
  212-998-5332

- East Central AIDS Education and Training Center
  Ohio State University
  B0902 UHC, 456 West 10th Avenue
  Columbus, OH 43210
  614-293-8188

- Pennsylvania/New York Regional AIDS
    Education and Training Center
  University of Pittsburgh
  200 Meyran Avenue
  Pittsburgh, PA 15213
  412-624-1023

- AIDS Education & Training Center
  The University of Texas
  P.O. Box 20186
  Houston, TX 77225
  713-792-4471

- WAMI AIDS Education & Training Center
  University of Washington
  820 NE 45th Street, Suite 1 XD-20
  Seattle, WA 98105
  206-543-9750

CHAPTER 26

Hemorrhoidal Products

Benjamin Hodes

Questions to ask in patient assessment and counseling

- *What are your symptoms?*
- *How long have your symptoms been present? Do they recur?*
- *Are your symptoms associated with straining at a bowel movement?*
- *Have you noticed any bleeding? Describe it.*
- *What improves or worsens your symptoms?*
- *Have you treated your symptoms without the use of medication? What nondrug measures have you used?*
- *Have you previously used any nonprescription or prescription drugs for these symptoms?*
- *Do you take laxatives regularly? If so, which ones and how often?*
- *What other medications do you take?*
- *Have you recently changed your diet or amount of fluid intake?*
- *Are you now or have you recently been pregnant?*
- *Do you often experience constipation or diarrhea?*
- *Do you have any other medical conditions such as heart failure, liver disease, inflammatory disease of the intestine, or varicose veins?*

Anorectal diseases, including hemorrhoids, are annoying, discomforting, and potentially serious. Several of these diseases are not amenable to self-treatment and require medical attention; however, many of their symptoms can be self-treated, as can other anorectal disorders that are relatively minor. The pharmacist should carefully evaluate any symptoms reported by the patient. Numerous nonprescription products are available for the symptomatic relief of the burning, pain, itching, inflammation, irritation, swelling, and general discomfort of hemorrhoids.

Anatomy and Physiology

With respect to anorectal diseases, three parts of the body are of concern: the perianal area, the anal canal, and the lower portion of the rectum (Figure 1).

The perianal area (about 7 cm in diameter) is the portion of the skin and buttocks immediately surrounding the anus. The presence of sensory nerve endings makes this area very sensitive to pain. Perianal tissue differs from most other skin tissue in that it is constantly moist and occluded.

The anal canal (about 4 cm long) is the channel connecting the end of the gastrointestinal (GI) tract (rectum) with the outside of the body. The lower two-thirds of the canal is covered by modified anal skin, which is structurally similar to the skin covering other parts of the body. The canal contains sensory nerve endings as well as pressure receptors that allow the perception of distention pain.

The point in the mid-upper anal canal at which the skin lining changes to mucous membrane is the dentate or pectinate line, also known as the anorectal line.

Two powerful sphincter muscles that encircle the anal canal control the passage of fecal material. The external sphincter, located at the bottom of the anal canal, is a voluntary muscle. The internal sphincter, which allows passage into the anal canal, is an involuntary muscle. Both sphincters lie under the tissues of the anal canal and extend downward. Under normal conditions, the external sphincter is closed and prevents the involuntary passage of feces or discharges.

In healthy individuals, the skin covering the anal canal serves as a barrier against absorption of substances into the body. Therefore, treatment applied to this area can be expected to manifest only local effects. If disease is present, the loss of protective oils or breaks in the surface may alter the character of the skin covering the canal, thereby diminishing the skin's protective capabilities.

The most prominent parts of the vasculature in the region above and below the anorectal line are the three hemorrhoidal arteries and the accompanying veins. Veins and arteries above the anorectal line are referred to as internal; those below, as external.

Anal crypts are normal pocket-like formations located on the internal side of the anorectal line. They face upward and, because of their position, sometimes retain small amounts of fecal material that may cause irritation. This irritation may lead to infection and foster the development of anorectal disease.

Investigators commonly distinguish between rectal mucosa and anal mucosa and consider the anorectal line to be the end of the anal canal. For purposes of this chapter, the appearance of the mucosal region will be considered the beginning of the rectal area.

The rectum (about 12–15 cm long) is the lower end of the GI tract and extends from the anorectal line up to the sigmoid colon. It is lined with semipermeable mucous membranes, is highly vascularized, and contains no sensory pain fibers. Like the anal canal, however, it does contain pressure receptors. And like the skin of the anal canal, the mucous membranes in the rectum protect the body from invasion by the bacteria present in feces.

Because of the plexus of hemorrhoidal vessels beneath the rectal mucosa and the paths followed by the blood returning to the heart through the hemorrhoidal veins, substances absorbed through the rectal mucous membranes may enter the systemic circulation without passing through the liver. This possibility is important in evaluating the potential systemic toxicity of locally applied drugs. The rectal pH, which ranges from neutral to basic, is important in determining the extent to which substances in the rectum are absorbed.

Anorectal Disorders

Miscellaneous Anorectal Disorders

Some potentially serious anorectal disorders, including fissures, fistulas, inflammatory bowel diseases, and tumors, may present hemorrhoidal-like symptoms and should not be self-treated. Patients should be promptly referred to a physician if any of the following conditions are suspected:

- *Abscess:* a painful swelling in the perianal or anal canal area caused by a bacterial (primarily staphylococcal) infection and resulting in the formation of a localized area of pus;
- *Anal fistula:* a channel-like lesion near the anus, associated with swelling, pain, constraint or intermittent discharge, and pruritus, and usually resulting from an anorectal abscess;
- *Anal fissure:* a slitlike ulcer in the anal canal lining, which may be painful, may exist alone or in conjunction with hemorrhoids, and often causes bleeding (as evidenced by bright red blood on toilet tissue);
- *Condyloma latumi:* a firm, wartlike, usually painless lesion, and one of the secondary lesions of syphilis;
- *Condyloma acuminata:* venereal warts, usually sexually transmitted, that appear as multiple, polymorphic, painless lesions in the genital or perianal region;
- *Cryptitis:* inflammation and hypertrophy of the anal crypts, a condition that probably originates in an anal gland and is primarily symptomized by pain aggravated by defecation;
- *Malignant neoplasm:* a serious disease, often characterized by constipation, in which bleeding and pain may be associated with malignant anal tumors (the

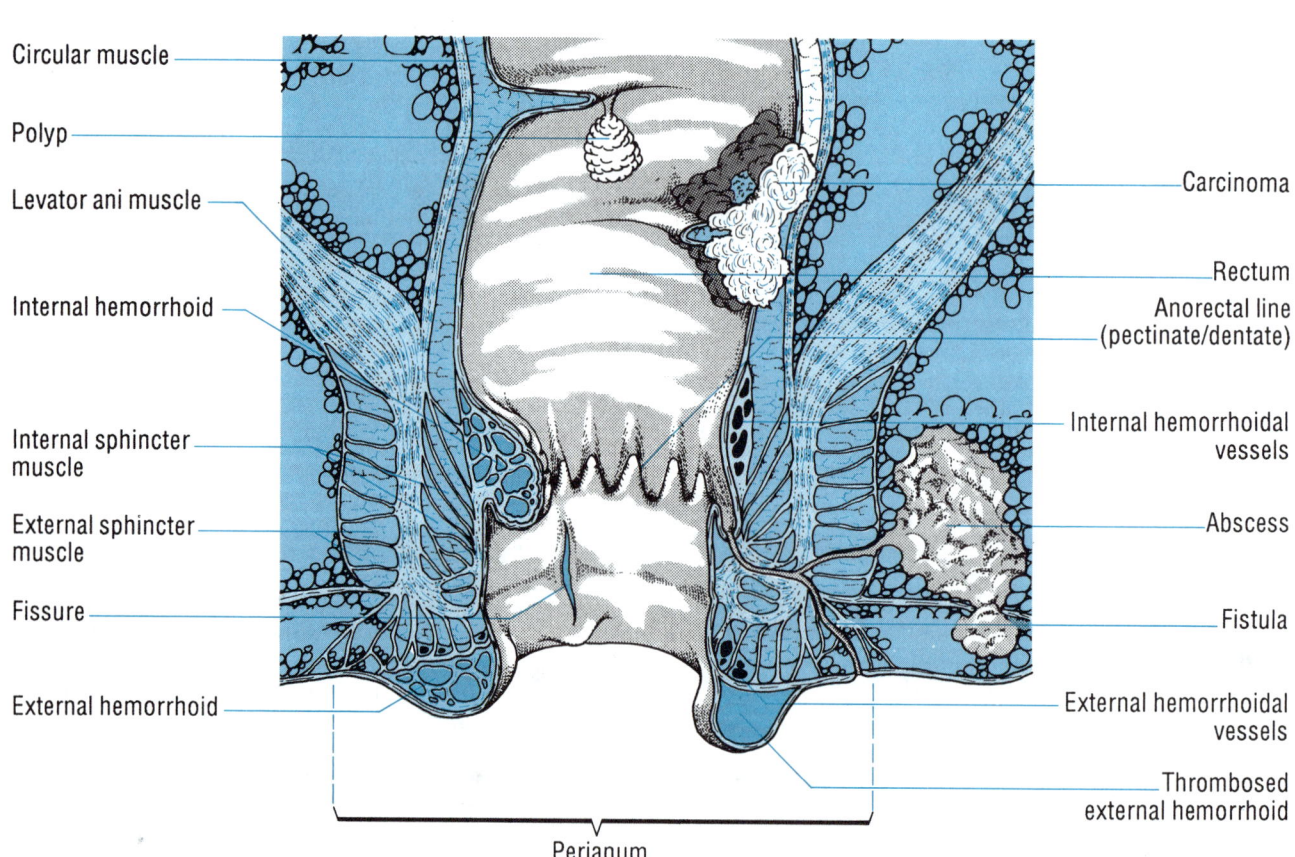

FIGURE 1 Selected disease states in anorectal region.

most common of which is squamous cell carcinoma), which are usually unnoticeable and located in the rectum;
- *Polyps:* benign or malignant rectal tumors that are characterized by bleeding and, rarely, by a mass protruding through the anus or a feeling of fullness or pressure in the rectum.

Hemorrhoids

Hemorrhoids (also known as piles) are abnormally large, bulging, symptomatic conglomerates of veins, supporting tissues, and overlying mucous membranes or skin of the anorectal area. They may be classified according to either their degree of severity or their location[1] (Figure 1).

Classification

External The two types of external hemorrhoids, thrombosed and cutaneous, occur below the anorectal line. A thrombosed hemorrhoid is a hemorrhoidal vein either in the anal canal or adjacent to the anus that contains a blood clot or thrombus. Such hemorrhoids may be quite painful. The clot may vary in size from that of a pea to that of a walnut. Cutaneous hemorrhoids, which consist of fibrous connective tissue covered by anal skin, are located outside the anal sphincter at any point on the circumference of the anus. They may result either from a previously thrombosed external hemorrhoid in which the clot has become organized and been replaced by connective tissue[2] or from uneven skin healing after a hemorrhoidectomy.

Internal Internal hemorrhoids occur above the anorectal line and are further classified according to location (e.g., left lateral, right posterior, or right anterior). Occasionally, because of its size and distention, an internal hemorrhoid descends below the anorectal line and outside the anal sphincter. It is then referred to as a prolapsed hemorrhoid.

Internal–External Internal and external hemorrhoids sometimes occur together. Also known as mixed hemorrhoids, they appear as baggy swellings. The following types occur:

- *Prolapsed.* A prolapsed hemorrhoid is characterized by pain until the prolapse is reduced; blood, which is bright red, may or may not be present.
- *Without prolapse.* A hemorrhoid without prolapse may be characterized by bleeding but not by pain.
- *Strangulated.* A strangulated hemorrhoid is one that has prolapsed to such a degree and for so long that its blood supply is occluded by the anal sphincter's constricting action; it is very painful and usually becomes thrombosed.

Etiology

Hemorrhoidal disease appears most often in persons 20–50 years of age.[1] It has been estimated that, in the United States, 58% of individuals over 40 years of age have hemorrhoids to some extent.[3] Many factors have been implicated in the etiology of hemorrhoidal disease;[4] these factors include heredity, erect posture, pregnancy, prolonged standing, lack of dietary bulk, heavy lifting, constipation, sneezing, portal hypertension, diarrhea, pelvic tumors, and anal infection.[5] Common denominators are physiologic vulnerability and pressure on hemorrhoidal veins that results in excessive venous engorgement. Symptomatic hemorrhoids develop only in susceptible individuals; socioeconomic and cultural factors (e.g., diet or lifestyle) may be precipitating factors.[6]

Although controversial, heredity appears to be a factor in hemorrhoidal formation.[7] Dietary and cultural patterns may also predispose persons to hemorrhoids.[8] Low-fiber diets and inadequate fluid intake contribute to hard stools and constipation. Constipation leads to straining at defecation, which in turn leads to increased pressure within the hemorrhoidal vessels, thereby precipitating the formation of hemorrhoids. Certain bowel habits, such as prolonged sitting on the toilet during bowel movements, may also precipitate hemorrhoids because of increased strain on the hemorrhoidal veins.[9]

Hemorrhoids may also be brought on by chronic diarrhea, cardiac failure, obesity, coughing, sneezing, vomiting, physical exertion, and portal hypertension.[10]

Pregnancy is by far the most common cause of hemorrhoids in young women. The gravid uterus produces increased pressure in the middle and interior hemorrhoidal vessels. Labor may also intensify the hemorrhoidal condition and produce intense symptoms after delivery. Pelvic tumors may give rise to hemorrhoids by a similar process. Another possible cause of anorectal disorders is an infection that may occur initially in the anal crypts and spread to the nearby tissue, causing inflammation that may result in a fistula or abscess.

Internal Hemorrhoids Internal hemorrhoids occur when three "cushions" that are considered normal anatomic structures[11] become engorged and protrude into the anal canal. Aging and other factors cause deterioration of connective tissue; therefore, these cushions become loosened from their submucosal anchoring, gradually become elongated, and descend toward the anus.[12] Because of this weakening, the veins also become distended. As the loose anal lining descends, the hemorrhoids and weakened cushions become increasingly exposed and susceptible to increased pressure from straining or trauma resulting from constipation. Engorgement of the blood vessels may eventually result in clot formation, swelling, and the erosion of the lining and vessel wall with bleeding.[12] In support of this etiology, microscopic analysis of hemorrhoidectomy specimens has revealed fragmented supportive connective tissue.[13] After repeated episodes of straining with a relaxed sphincter, the hemorrhoids dilate and ultimately prolapse out of the anus. Eventually, this protrusion leads to hemorrhoids that are permanently prolapsed and enlarged.

External Hemorrhoids External hemorrhoids are recognized as a swelling of the skin and associated blood vessels around the rim of the anus.[14] External hemorrhoids are covered by highly innervated skin, and when this skin is stretched by a thrombosis, sudden and severe pain can result.

Symptoms of Anorectal Disease

Itching, burning, inflammation, pain, irritation, swelling, and discomfort are symptoms of anorectal disease. If these symptoms are caused by hemorrhoids rather than by a more serious anorectal disease, they may be relieved by self-treatment.

Itching, or pruritus, occurs as a manifestation of mild inflammation associated with many anorectal disorders. *Pruritus ani* refers to persistent itching in the anal and perianal area that even occurs in the presence of good hygiene. Itching is one of the most common symptoms of anorectal disease and may be secondary to swelling, irritation caused by dietary factors, or moisture in the anal area.

Itching is typically associated with hemorrhoidal disease when there is mucous discharge from prolapsing internal hemorrhoids. Sensitivity to fabrics, dyes and perfumes in toilet tissue, detergents, local treatment, and fecal contents are common causes of itching. Fungal infections, parasites, allergies, and associated anorectal pathologic lesions may also cause itching. Broad-spectrum antibiotic therapy may trigger itching as a result of infection secondary to the overgrowth of nonsusceptible organisms, particularly fungi. Chronic use of mineral oil can lead to pruritus ani. Itching may also be attributed to a psychologic cause on rare occasions.

Burning, a common symptom of anorectal disease, suggests a somewhat greater degree of irritation of the anorectal sensory nerves than that associated with itching. The burning sensation may range from a feeling of warmth to a feeling of intense heat and may be constant or associated with defecation.

Inflammation, a tissue reaction distinguished by heat, redness, pain, and swelling, is often caused by trauma, allergy, or infection. The inflammation itself, but not the underlying cause, may be relieved by self-treatment.

Acute inflammation of the anal tissue may cause pain. Hemorrhoidal pain, which is steady and aching, is usually worsened by standing or defecating. Pain is experienced consistently and predictably with acute external hemorrhoids. Chronic external hemorrhoids often exhibit no pain. Because of the absence of sensory nerve endings above the anorectal line, uncomplicated internal hemorrhoids rarely cause pain. However, when strangulation, thrombosis, or ulceration occurs, pain may be severe.[2] Patients with severe, persistent pain should be referred to a physician.

Irritation is a response to stimulation of the nerve endings and is characterized by burning, itching, pain, or swelling. Swelling is caused by an accumulation of excess fluid associated with engorged hemorrhoids or hemorrhoidal tissue. Discomfort, a vague and generalized uneasiness, may result from any or all of these symptoms.

Bleeding, seepage, protrusion, prolapse, and thrombosis should not be self-treated, both because a more serious disorder may be masked and because no appropriate nonprescription therapy is available.

Bleeding is almost always associated with internal hemorrhoids and may occur before, during, or after defecation. Painless bleeding during defecation is the most common symptom of hemorrhoids.[15] The amount of bleeding experienced often varies and is not necessarily related to the amount of hemorrhoidal tissue present. When bleeding occurs from an external hemorrhoid, it is typically due to an acute thrombosis accompanied by rupture. Pain often accompanies such bleeding, although a patient may experience some relief of the pain with the onset of the bleeding. Blood from hemorrhoids is usually bright red and covers the fecal matter. Bleeding is stimulated by defecation but may occur as an "oozing," which will soil underclothes.

The chronic blood loss associated with bleeding hemorrhoids infrequently produces severe anemias. Bleeding may indicate the presence of serious anorectal disease (e.g., abscess, fistula, cancer, colitis, or diverticulitis) and should not be self-treated.

Seepage, the involuntary passing of fecal material or mucus, is caused by an anal sphincter that does not close completely because of pain, swelling, or inflammation. This symptom cannot be self-treated, and the patient should be referred to a physician.

Protrusion, a frequent sign or symptom of uncomplicated internal and external hemorrhoids, is defined as the projection of hemorrhoidal or rectal tissue outside the anal canal. The rectal protrusion may vary in size and usually appears after defecation, prolonged standing, or unusual physical exertion. It is painless except when thrombosis, infection, or ulceration is present. Strangulation of a protruding hemorrhoid by the sphincter may lead to thrombosis. Self-treatment is not appropriate and should not be encouraged.

A painful lump may develop when contraction of the anal sphincter interferes with blood flow from a prolapsed internal or mixed hemorrhoid, resulting in thrombosis. If this prolapsed hemorrhoid is returned to an area above the anal sphincter before thrombosis occurs, the pain and lump usually disappear. However, when defecation occurs, both pain and lump are likely to recur. Permanently prolapsing internal hemorrhoids cause a mucoid discharge, which in turn may lead to perianal irritation, itching, pain, and swelling.

Thrombosis within a hemorrhoid is a common complication. Abrupt onset of severe, constant pain in the anal area, accompanied, for example, by a grape-sized lump, is a sign that thrombosis of a mixed or external hemorrhoid may have occurred. If untreated, the burning pain persists for about 5–7 days, diminishing in intensity after the first day. A hard, tender lump at the site of the pain typically appears; after the second day this lump slowly dissipates and eventually leaves a skin tag.

If a thrombosed hemorrhoid persists, gangrene and ulcers may develop on its surface. This condition may lead to an oozing of blood as well as to hemorrhaging, particularly when the patient is defecating or standing. If the clot remains exposed, infection may occur, and an abscess or fistula may result.

If the thrombosed hemorrhoid resides entirely above the anorectal line (a pure internal hemorrhoid), there may be minimal pain because of the lack of sensory nerve supply. Patients are likely to be unaware that such a hemorrhoid is present unless there are sudden changes in bowel habits.

Assessment

By questioning the patient, the pharmacist should be able to determine whether self-treatment is desirable and, if so, which nonprescription drug product is suitable.

The first step in the assessment process is to determine the nature of the symptoms. Bleeding, pain, itching, and prolapse are most common. Abdominal symptoms, seepage, prolapse, blood in the stool, or severe and persistent pain could indicate another potentially serious medical problem that cannot be self-treated, in which case the patient should be advised to see a physician promptly. If the patient has not used any medication previously, the pharmacist should determine if there are any contributing factors such as diarrhea or constipation, obesity, cardiovascular disease, hepatic disease, pregnancy, and chronic cough. The pharmacist should also determine causative or precipitating factors such as bowel habits, physical exertion, prolonged sitting or standing at work, insufficient fiber or liquids in the diet, and laxative abuse. Based on information received in the assessment process, the pharmacist may either recommend an appropriate nonprescription product for the temporary relief of minor anorectal symptoms (itching, burning, pain, swelling, or discomfort) or refer the patient to a physician for further medical evaluation.

Treatment

Pharmacologic Agents

The nonprescription pharmacologic agents recommended to relieve symptoms of anorectal disease include local anesthetics; vasoconstrictors; protectants; counterirritants; astringents; analgesics, anesthetics, and antipruritics; and keratolytics. Products containing an excessive number of agents may not be optimally effective because of potential interaction among ingredients.

Local Anesthetics

Local, topical anesthetics temporarily relieve pain, burning, itching, discomfort, and irritation by preventing the transmission of nerve impulses. These products should be used in the perianal region or the lower anal canal; symptoms within the rectum generally are not relieved by topical anesthetics because of the lack of rectal sensory nerve fibers.[16] Further, their application should be limited to the area below the rectum because local anesthetics may be rapidly absorbed through the rectal mucosa and cause potentially toxic systemic effects. Absorption through the perianal skin, even if abraded, would not be particularly rapid.

Local anesthetics may produce allergic reactions, both locally and systemically. Such reactions may cause burning and itching that are indistinguishable from symptoms of the anorectal disease being treated. If symptoms return after cessation of therapy, a physician should be contacted.

The following local anesthetics are recommended for use in hemorrhoidal preparations for application to the perianal or lower anal canal regions:

- Benzocaine, when used externally in the base form, is safe and effective in concentrations of 5–20% applied up to six times a day.[17] The most common adverse reaction to topical benzocaine is sensitization.
- Benzyl alcohol is effective in concentrations of 5–20%[17] and may be applied up to six times a day.
- Dibucaine and dibucaine hydrochloride are considered pharmacologically equivalent[16] for external use as local anesthetics in concentrations of 0.25–1% applied up to three or four times a day.
- Dyclonine hydrochloride is effective in concentrations of 0.5–1% and may be applied up to six times a day.[17]
- Lidocaine is effective for external use in concentrations of 2–5% and may be applied up to six times a day.[17]
- Pramoxine hydrochloride may be used externally as a topical aerosol foam, ointment, cream, or jelly in a water-miscible base. The concentration typically used as a local anesthetic is 1%.[17] Adverse effects are rare, and pramoxine hydrochloride exhibits less cross-sensitivity than do other local anesthetics because of its distinct chemical structure. Pramoxine-containing anorectal products may be applied up to five times a day.
- Tetracaine and tetracaine hydrochloride are effective when used externally in concentrations of 0.5–1% and may be applied up to six times a day.[17]

Other local anesthetics used in hemorrhoidal preparations are not recommended because they have not met Food and Drug Administration (FDA) safety and efficacy standards. Additional evidence is required to demonstrate the effectiveness of diperodon used externally or intrarectally.

Vasoconstrictors

Vasoconstrictors are chemical agents structurally related to the naturally occurring catecholamines, epinephrine and norepinephrine. Applied locally in the anorectal area, vasoconstrictors stimulate the alpha-adrenergic receptors in the vascular beds, causing constriction of the arterioles. Although it has been demonstrated that locally applied vasoconstrictors promptly alter the blood supply to the mucosa, the FDA does not recognize or approve the use of these products to control minor bleeding.[18] Because rectal bleeding may be a sign of a more serious disease, a physician should be consulted.

Vasoconstrictors, in addition to shrinking swollen hemorrhoidal tissue a small amount, also relieve itching somewhat because they produce a slight anesthetic effect by an unknown mechanism. The reduction of swelling associated with irritated hemorrhoidal tissue is transient.

The FDA has concluded that potentially serious side effects, including the elevation of blood pressure, the risk of producing cardiac arrhythmia, nervousness, tremor, sleeplessness, and aggravation of symptoms of hyperthyroidism, are less likely to occur when vasoconstrictors are used locally in recommended dosages.[18] Because of the slight possibility of systemic adverse reactions from topically applied vasoconstrictors, these products should be avoided in patients who have diabetes, hyperthyroidism, hypertension, difficulty in urination due to prostate enlargement, and cardiovascular diseases, and in those patients who are taking monoamine oxidase inhibitors. Some topical anorectal products containing ephedrine sulphate may cause nervousness, tremor, sleeplessness, nausea, and loss of appetite.

Four vasoconstrictors are recommended for external use: aqueous solutions of ephedrine sulfate, epinephrine hydrochloride, phenylephrine hydrochloride solutions, and epinephrine base. Ephedrine sulfate and phenylephrine hydrochloride solutions are also recommended for internal (intrarectal) use.[17] These agents are not commercially available for anorectal use in a solution dosage form. Additional data are needed to establish the safety and effectiveness of epinephrine base for intrarectal use and of epinephrine undecylenate for external use. Selected facts about the vasoconstrictors used to manage the symptoms of uncomplicated hemorrhoids are included below:

- Ephedrine sulfate (aqueous solution), which is readily absorbed through mucous membranes in the rectum, has a more prolonged effect than epinephrine and acts on both alpha- and beta-adrenergic receptors. The hypertensive effects of ephedrine are potentiated by monoamine oxidase inhibitors as well as by tricyclic antidepressants. When ephedrine is applied topically, its onset of action ranges from a few seconds to 1 minute, its duration of action is 2 to 3 hours, and it effectively relieves itching and swelling. The recommended concentration is 0.1–1.25% applied up to four times a day.[17]
- Epinephrine hydrochloride (aqueous solution) and epinephrine base are effective in the relief of itching and swelling only when they are used externally because epinephrine is inactivated at the pH of the rectum. Epinephrine is absorbed from the mucous membranes and acts on both alpha- and beta-adrenergic receptors. The recommended concentration is 0.005–0.01% applied up to four times a day.[17]
- Phenylephrine hydrochloride (aqueous solution) is believed to relieve itching caused by histamine release and reduces congestion in the anorectal area. It acts primarily on the alpha-adrenergic receptors and produces vasoconstriction by a direct effect on receptors rather than by norepinephrine displacement. The recommended dosage is 0.25% applied up to four times a day.[17]

Protectants

Protectants prevent irritation of the anorectal area and water loss from the stratum corneum by forming a physical barrier on the skin. Protection of the perianal area from irritants such as fecal matter leads to a reduction in irritation and concomitant itching. Little or no absorption of protectants occurs.

Absorbents, adsorbents, demulcents, and emollients are included in the protectant classification. Many substances classified as protectants are also used as vehicles, bases, and carriers of pharmacologically active substances (e.g., vasoconstrictors and local anesthetics).

Adverse reactions to protectants as a class are minimal. Wool (lanolin) alcohols may cause allergies and are probably responsible for most cases of lanolin allergy.[19]

The protectants recommended for use are aluminum hydroxide gel (in moist conditions only), cocoa butter, glycerin in aqueous solution, hard fat (cocoa butter substitutes, hydrogenated cocoglycerides, and hydrogenated palm kernel glycerides), kaolin, lanolin, mineral oil, white petrolatum, petrolatum, and topical starch. All these protectants are recommended for external and internal (intrarectal) use, with the exception of glycerin, which is recommended for external use only. Protectants recommended only when used in combination with one, two, or three other protectants and subject to limitations are calamine, cod liver oil, shark liver oil, and zinc oxide.[17] Calamine (based on the zinc oxide content of calamine) and zinc oxide must not exceed 25% (weight per weight) per dosage unit. Cod liver oil or shark liver oil may be used if the product containing either protectant is labeled so that the amount of oil used in 24 hours represents a quantity that provides 10,000 USP units of vitamin A and 400 USP units of cholecalciferol.[17] Protectants may be applied up to six times a day or after each bowel movement.

If a protectant is used in a nonprescription preparation, it should make up at least 50% of the dosage unit; if two to four protectants are used, their total concentration should represent at least 50% of the whole. Adequate thickness to prevent water loss from the epidermis determines the amount of protectant required. With the exception of cod liver oil and shark liver oil, any protectant ingredient used in combination should contribute at least 12.5% by weight. Glycerin is approved in a 20–45% (weight per weight) aqueous solution so that the final product contains not less than 10% and not more than 45% glycerin (weight per weight). Any combination product containing glycerin must contain at least this minimum amount of glycerin.[17] Hard fat is defined according to the official *National Formulary* monograph and, according to the FDA, includes Witepsol ingredients (cocoa butter substitutes, hydrogenated cocoglycerides, and hydrogenated palm kernel glycerides) under the designation of "hard fat" in the over-the-counter anorectal drug product monograph.[20,21]

The bismuth salts that are found in some hemorrhoidal products are not recommended as protectants. Bismuth subnitrate is not considered safe because it may be absorbed, producing toxic symptoms from the bismuth ion as well as from the nitrate ion. The effectiveness of bismuth oxide, bismuth subcarbonate, wool alcohols, and bismuth subgallate as protectants in the anorectal area has not been established.

Counterirritants

Counterirritants (e.g., camphor, menthol, or juniper tar) distract from the perception of pain and itching by stimulating cutaneous receptors to evoke a feeling of comfort, warmth, cooling, or tingling. Because the rectal mucosa contains no sensory nerve endings, counterirritants exert no effect in this area and are recommended for external use only.

Effective August 1991, the FDA allowed the inclusion of menthol, camphor, and juniper tar in hemorrhoidal products. (See Chapter 32, "External Analgesic Products.") Camphor (greater than 3%), turpentine oil (rectified) (6–50%), and menthol (1.25–16%) are not considered to be safe and effective for this purpose.[22]

Astringents

Applied to the skin or mucous membranes for a local and limited effect, astringents coagulate the protein in skin cells, thereby protecting the underlying tissue and decreasing cell volume. When appropriately used, astringents contribute to drying by lessening mucus and other secretions. This drying effect helps relieve local anorectal irritation and inflammation.

Calamine and zinc oxide in concentrations of 5–25% are recommended as astringents for both external and internal use when applied up to six times a day or after each bowel movement.[17] Zinc, a heavy metal, acts as a protein precipitant and provides an astringent effect. Witch hazel (hamamelis water) in a concentration of 10–50% is recommended as an astringent for external use in anorectal disorders; its effectiveness is due primarily to its alcohol content (14%). The FDA concluded that witch hazel provides temporary relief of itching and burning,[17] and is safe and effective for external use when applied up to six times a day or after each bowel movement. Witch hazel is incorporated in several commercially available rectal pads or wipes that are advertised as being useful for hemorrhoids. Recommended products should be limited to those containing the appropriate concentration of an astringent ingredient.

Wound-Healing Agents

Several ingredients in nonprescription hemorrhoidal products are claimed to be effective in promoting wound healing or tissue repair in anorectal disease. In particular, skin respiratory factor (SRF), a water-soluble extract of brewer's yeast, also referred to as live yeast cell derivative (LYCD), is the subject of considerable controversy. Although some clinical trials have supported the manufacturer's claims, insufficient evidence currently exists to confirm that SRF/LYCD is effective in promoting the healing of diseased anorectal tissue.[23] Commercial preparations containing SRF/LYCD as primary ingredients remain on the market pending review of additional clinical trials. Reformulation of products such as Preparation H® and Wyanoids® will be necessary if data from clinical trials do not support the manufacturer's indications or claims of efficacy. Peruvian balsam, vitamin A, and vitamin D lack demonstrated effectiveness as wound healers.[22] The value of cod liver oil and shark liver oil as hemorrhoidal wound healers remains equivocal;[22] their value as protectants in hemorrhoidal products is somewhat less equivocal.

Antiseptics

Antiseptics generally inhibit the growth of microorganisms. Some nonprescription anorectal products contain compounds intended for use as antiseptics. However, because of the large numbers of microorganisms in feces, it is unlikely that applying antiseptics to the anorectal area provides a degree of antisepsis greater than that achieved by washing the area with mild soap and water. There is no compelling evidence that antiseptic use prevents anorectal infection.

Compounds claimed to have antiseptic properties include boric acid, boric acid glycerite, hydrastis, phenol, resorcinol, and sodium salicylic acid phenolate. Serious questions remain about the safety and effectiveness of these compounds as antiseptics in products designed to relieve the symptoms of hemorrhoids.

Keratolytics

Keratolytics cause desquamation and debridement or sloughing of epidermal surface cells. By fostering cell turnover and loosening surface cells, keratolytics may help to expose underlying tissue to therapeutic agents. Used externally, they are somewhat useful in reducing itching, although their exact mechanism of action is not known. Because mucous membranes contain no keratin layer, the intrarectal use of keratolytics is not justified and may cause harm.

The two keratolytics recommended for external use in hemorrhoidal products are aluminum chlorhydroxy allantoinate (alcloxa) and resorcinol. The dosage ranges established by the FDA are up to six 2-g applications per day of a 0.2–2.0% ointment for alcloxa and of a 1–3% ointment for resorcinol.[17] Precipitated and sublimed sulfur do not meet safety or efficacy conditions for either internal or external use in anorectal preparations.[22]

Anticholinergics

Anticholinergics inhibit or prevent the action of acetylcholine, the transmitter of cholinergic nerve impulses. Because anticholinergics act systemically, they are not effective in ameliorating the local symptoms of anorectal disease.

Although atropine and belladonna extract were used in anorectal preparations, they are not considered safe and effective for this purpose.

Analgesics, Anesthetics, and Antipruritics

To promote consistency in the rule-making process, the FDA has redesignated as "analgesic, anesthetic, and antipruritic" several ingredients that were formerly classified as "counterirritants."[24] This nomenclature was adopted to conform with the FDA pharmacologic designations of the active ingredients despite the inherent redundancy of the terms *anesthetic* and *antipruritic* as defined in this section.

In the anorectal area, a topically applied drug that relieves pain by depressing cutaneous sensory receptors is defined as an analgesic, anesthetic drug. Similarly, a topically applied drug that relieves itching by depressing cutaneous sensory receptors is defined as an antipruritic drug.[24]

Menthol (0.1–1%), juniper tar (1–5%), and camphor (0.1–3%) are safe and effective for external use in the anorectal area and may be applied up to six times a day.[17]

Hydrocortisone

Topically applied hydrocortisone-containing products have the potential to reduce itching, inflammation, and discomfort by producing vasoconstriction, lysosomal membrane stabilization, and antimitotic activity.[25] The combination of hydrocortisone with other appropriate ingredients in nonprescription products is currently available to manage selected hemorrhoidal symptoms (see product information tables). Nonprescription topical hydrocortisone-containing products are indicated for temporary relief of minor external anal itching due to minor irritation or rash.

Bulk-Forming Laxatives

Because constipation is a precipitating factor in hemorrhoidal disease, patients may be advised to consider using bulk-forming laxatives. (See Chapter 15, "Laxative Products.") Ingredients commonly found in these products include barley malt extract, methylcellulose, and psyllium hydrocolloid. Patients must strictly follow directions for proper use to prevent adverse effects and increase efficacy. Adequate fluid intake should also be encouraged.

Miscellaneous

Collinsonia (stoneroot), *Escherichia coli* vaccines, lappa (burdock), leptandra (culver's root), and mullein are ingredients that have been included in nonprescription hemorrhoidal products and do not fall within the previously discussed pharmacologic classifications. With the exception of *E. coli* vaccines, these compounds are antiquated remnants of herbal medicine. There is no evidence that

TABLE 1	Indications for the use of nonprescription anorectal pharmacologic agents					
Symptom	Analgesic, anesthetic, antipruritic	Vaso-constrictor	Protectant	Astringent	Local anesthetic	Keratolytic
Discomfort	yes	yes	yes	yes	yes	yes
Irritation	no	yes	yes	yes	no	no
Itching	yes	yes	yes	yes	yes	yes
Pain	yes	no	no	no	yes	no
Soreness	yes	no	no	no	yes	no
Swelling	no	yes	no	no	no	no
Burning	yes	no	yes	yes	yes	no

they are effective in treating symptoms of anorectal disease. The safety and effectiveness of *E. coli* vaccines are also unproven.[26]

A summary of the indications for nonprescription anorectal pharmacologic agents is presented in Table 1.

Dosage Forms

Drugs for the treatment of anorectal symptoms are available in many dosage forms. For intrarectal use, suppositories, creams, ointments, gels, and foams are available. Applicators, fingers, and pile pipes are used to facilitate their application. Creams, ointments, gels, pastes, wipes, pads, liquids, and foam are used externally.

Although there are considerable pharmaceutical differences among ointments, creams, pastes, and gels, the therapeutic differences are not significant. The term *ointment* is thus used here to refer to all semisolid preparations designed for external or intrarectal use in the anorectal area. Although a suppository is defined as a solid dosage form, it differs very little from semisolids in its vehicle formulation.

Ointments are vehicles for drugs used in treating anorectal disease symptoms; moreover, they also possess inherent protectant and emollient properties. The primary function of an ointment base is the efficient delivery of the active ingredients.

When used externally, ointments should be applied as a thin covering to the perianal area and the anal canal. For intrarectal use, pile pipes and fingers can be used to apply ointments. Pile pipes have the advantage over fingers in that the drug product may be introduced into the rectal mucosa where a finger cannot reach. For most efficient use, the pile pipe should have lateral openings, as well as a hole in the end, to allow the drug product to cover the greatest area of rectal mucosa. The pile pipe should be lubricated before insertion by spreading the ointment around the pipe tip. The potential for systemic absorption is greatest from the rectal mucosa.

The lubricating effect of a suppository may ease straining at defecation. However, because of disadvantages, suppositories are not generally recommended as a dosage form in treating anorectal disease symptoms. In prone patients, suppositories may leave the affected region and ascend into the rectum and lower colon. If the patient remains prone after inserting a suppository or an ointment, the active ingredients may not be evenly distributed over the rectal mucosa. Suppositories and ointments are relatively slow acting because they must melt to release the active ingredient.

Foam products present no proven advantage over ointments; however, theoretically, they provide more rapid release of active ingredients. Their disadvantages include the difficulty in establishing that the foam remains in the affected area and the fact that the size of the foam bubbles determines the concentration of active ingredient available.

Anal Hygiene

Cleansing the anorectal area with mild, unscented soap and water regularly and after each bowel movement helps to relieve hemorrhoidal symptoms and may prevent recurrence of perianal itching. Practical means of cleansing after a bowel movement include the use of commercially available hygienic and lubricated wipes or pads. Patients should be advised to blot or pat rather than rub the irritated perianal area with these wipes. This advice also applies to the use of toilet tissue, which should be unscented, uncolored, and soft.

Sitz baths are often useful in relieving hemorrhoidal symptoms and in promoting good hygiene. Patients should sit in warm water (110–115°F [43.3–46.1°C]) two to three times a day for 15 minutes. Plastic sitz baths, which fit over the toilet rim for convenient patient use, are easily cleaned and are available at pharmacies.

Surgical Treatments

Modern surgical treatments for hemorrhoids include injection of sclerosing agents, rubber band ligation, dilation of the anal canal and lower rectum, cryosurgery, hemorrhoidectomy, and laser coagulation.

Product Selection Guidelines

Patient Considerations

Knowledge of a patient's present medical condition, medical history, and medication profile is necessary to determine how an individual may respond to self-treatment. First, the pharmacist must determine whether the patient has symptoms amenable to self-treatment. Then the pharmacist should determine a suitable anorectal product, if any, taking into account what other diseases the patient may have, what medications the patient may be taking, and any other factors that may affect treatment.

Pregnant and nursing women should only use products recommended for external use except for the recommended protectants, which may be used internally. Children with hemorrhoids or other anorectal disease should be referred to a physician.

Product Considerations

Nonprescription anorectal preparations are intended to provide temporary symptomatic relief of the burning, itching, pain, swelling, irritation, and discomfort of anorectal disorders. A wider range of products is available by prescription for use in treating other anorectal diseases.

In recommending an appropriate nonprescription product, the pharmacist should consider the type and amount of ingredients and the dosage form. A product containing recommended ingredients in appropriate combination at effective dosage levels should be offered. For intrarectal use, the only approved ingredients are vasoconstrictors, protectants, and astringents. A pile pipe of appropriate length (2 in.), with a well-lubricated and flexible tip and with holes on the sides, may be used to apply an ointment-type product. Suppositories are not generally recommended for use as a dosage form for the self-treatment of anorectal conditions.

As a general rule, products containing the least number of recommended ingredients should be suggested. Those with one or a few specific ingredients are most likely to minimize undesirable interactions and maximize effectiveness. In general, scented and tinted products should be avoided. Symptoms should be managed as specifically as possible. Shotgun therapy is generally best avoided.

In evaluating nonprescription anorectal products, the pharmacist should attempt to ensure that the vehicle is appropriate for anorectal use and that the active ingredient(s) will be properly released from the formulation. The FDA has not demanded final formulation testing to assess the appropriateness of specific vehicles for anorectal preparations.

Biopharmaceutical Considerations

The bioavailability of drugs from anorectal dosage forms is a result of a complex activity involving physicochemical, physiologic, manufacturing, dosage form, dosage, and application variables. The precise relationship between theoretical bioavailability considerations and therapeutic effectiveness of anorectal dosage forms remains to be established. Absorption from anorectal dosage forms involves release from the vehicle, dissolution into the surrounding medium, diffusion to a membrane, and penetration of the membrane. For oleaginous bases, diffusion from the base is the rate-limiting step in the release of a drug from its vehicle. The rate at which a drug diffuses from its base depends on a number of factors, including the vehicle pH, the drug concentration, the dissociation constant of the drug, the presence of surfactants, and the drug's particle size. Most drugs used in hemorrhoidal products are basic amines (local anesthetics and vasoconstrictors). The un-ionized base is soluble in lipid ointment bases; the salt form is not. Salt forms from weak bases are converted to the un-ionized base at tissue pH. The un-ionized form penetrates the lipid tissue barriers such as nerve membranes. The solubility of the drug and its partitioning in a vehicle largely determine the drug's release rate from the vehicle.

If a drug has a greater affinity for the vehicle than for the surrounding medium, a relatively slow release rate is expected. Conversely, if a drug has a greater affinity for the surrounding medium than for the vehicle, a relatively rapid release rate occurs. Ephedrine sulfate dissolved in an oleaginous base such as cocoa butter is released relatively rapidly into a surrounding aqueous medium.

In the case of oleaginous bases, the rate-limiting step in absorption seems to be the rate at which the drug leaves the vehicle and dissolves in the surrounding fluid. For a water-soluble or water-miscible base (polyethylene glycol), a water-soluble drug form is preferred to facilitate absorption. The water soluble drug form is preferred because the absorption rate appears to be controlled by the transfer of the drug through the mucosa.

In ointments, creams, and suppositories, additives such as viscosity-increasing agents or surfactants are often required to achieve a high-quality product. Surfactants may increase or decrease drug absorption.

The drug absorption rate of an anorectal product may be affected by the manufacturing process. For example, the release rates associated with cocoa butter may vary according to the temperature at which the cocoa butter is melted. This effect may be explained by the polymorphic nature of cocoa butter.

Patient Consultation

The pharmacist should emphasize the importance of good care and hygiene in helping to prevent and alleviate symptoms of anorectal disease. Specific advice should include the following guidelines:

- For maximum effect, nonprescription anorectal products should be used after, rather than before, bowel movements.
- If seepage, bleeding, protrusion, or severe pain occurs, a physician should be contacted as soon as possible.
- Products designed for external use only should not be inserted into the rectum.
- Products to be used externally should be applied sparingly.

- Patients should be warned that certain people may develop allergic or hypersensitivity reactions to external-use products that contain any approved concentration of local anesthetic, menthol, or resorcinol. Should redness, irritation, swelling, pain, or other symptoms develop or worsen, use of the product should be discontinued and a physician consulted.
- If insertion of a product in the rectum causes pain, use of the product should be discontinued and a physician consulted promptly.
- Patients with cardiovascular disease, diabetes, hypertension, or hyperthyroidism, or patients experiencing difficulty in urination, should not generally use a topical anorectal product containing a vasoconstrictor.
- Patients taking prescription drugs to treat hypertension or depression should not use an anorectal product containing a vasoconstrictor without consulting a physician.
- Patients should be warned that products containing ephedrine sulfate may cause nervousness, tremor, sleeplessness, nausea, and loss of appetite.
- Patients using an anorectal product containing aluminum hydroxide gel or kaolin should be informed that, for these products to come in contact with the skin, any previously used petrolatum-containing or greasy ointment should be removed.
- Patients should be advised that products containing resorcinol should not be used on any open wound anywhere.
- If possible, before any nonprescription anorectal product is applied, the anorectal area should be washed with mild soap and warm water, rinsed thoroughly, and gently dried by patting or blotting with toilet tissue or a soft cloth.
- If bleeding occurs or if symptoms worsen or do not improve after 7 days of self-treatment, a physician should be consulted promptly.

Cleansing the anorectal area with moistened, unscented, and uncolored toilet tissue or a wipe after defecation is recommended. Sitz baths are an alternative nondrug approach for managing mild symptoms of uncomplicated anorectal disease. The importance of maintaining normal bowel function by eating properly, drinking adequate amounts of fluid, and avoiding excessive laxative use should be emphasized as a means of preventing anorectal disease. A diet high in fiber and fluid will promote the formation of easily passed stools, thereby preventing constipation and the accompanying straining. Patients with symptomatic hemorrhoids may experience a significant reduction in bleeding and pain within a few weeks after beginning the regular use of a bulk laxative. Stool softeners such as docusate may also be useful in preventing straining that may lead to or aggravate hemorrhoids. (See Chapter 15, "Laxative Products.")

Summary

For external use, an ideal hemorrhoidal formulation would contain a vasoconstrictor, a local anesthetic, and one to four recommended protectants totaling at least 50% of the formulation. Another appropriate formulation might contain a protectant, an analgesic, a local anesthetic, an antipruritic, and a vasoconstrictor. Either of these combinations should be effective in relieving the itching, irritation, burning, swelling, discomfort, and pain associated with hemorrhoids.

For internal use, a model product would contain an appropriate astringent (e.g., calamine or zinc oxide), a vasoconstrictor (e.g., ephedrine sulfate or phenylephrine hydrochloride), and from one to four recommended protectants totaling at least 50% of the formulation. An ointment-type dosage form applied with a suitable pile pipe is recommended. This product should relieve the itching, swelling, discomfort, and irritation associated with hemorrhoids.

When used externally, products containing benzocaine (5–20%) in a polyethylene glycol base would be expected to be effective in relieving itching, burning, discomfort, soreness, and pain associated with hemorrhoids. For intrarectal use, a product consisting of 100% petrolatum is appropriate to recommend and is safe for use by pregnant women.

The pharmacist should make clear to the patient that if symptoms worsen or do not improve after 7 days of self-treatment, or if bleeding, protrusion, or seepage occurs, a physician should be consulted as soon as possible.

References

1. Bubrick MP, Benjamin RB. *Postgrad Med* 1985; 77: 165.
2. Shackelford RT. In: Turrell R, ed. *Diseases of the Colon and Anorectum*. Philadelphia: W. B. Saunders; 1969: 896.
3. Cohen Z. *Can J Surg* 1985; 28: 230–1.
4. Smith LE. *Gastroenterol Clin North Am* 1987; 16: 81.
5. Driscoll D et al. *U.S. Pharm* 1981; 5 (50): 43–4.
6. Hyams L, Philpot J. *Am J Proctol* 1970; 21: 177.
7. Granet E. *Manual of Proctology*. Chicago: Year Book Medical Publishers, Inc; 1954: 115.
8. Holt RL. *A Cure and Preventative: Hemorrhoids*. Laguna Beach, Calif: California Health; 1977: 50–69.
9. Smith LE. *Consultant*. July 1985: 95.
10. Jacobs DM et al. *Dis Colon Rectum* 1980; 23: 567–9.
11. Thompson WHF. *Br J Surg* 1975; 62: 542–52.
12. Dennison AR et al. *Surg Clin North Am* 1988; 68 (6): 1403.
13. Smith LE. *Gastroenterol Clin North Am* 1987; 16: 83.
14. Dennison AR et al. *Surg Clin North Am* 1988; 68 (6): 1402.
15. Cochran JL. *Postgrad Med* 1991; 89 (1): 149.
16. *Federal Register* 1988; 53: 30759.
17. *Federal Register* 1990; 55: 31780.
18. *Federal Register* 1980; 45: 35621.
19. *Federal Register* 1980; 45: 35635.
20. *The United States Pharmacopoeia XXII and the National Formulary XVII*. Rockville, Md: United States Pharmacopeial Convention, Inc; 1989: 1931.
21. *Federal Register* 1990; 55: 31778.
22. *Federal Register* 1988; 53: 30777.
23. *Federal Register* 1988; 53: 30765.
24. *Federal Register* 1988; 53: 30779.
25. *AMA Drug Evaluations*. 4th ed. New York: John Wiley and Sons; 1980: 1009–1052.
26. *Federal Register* 1990; 55: 31777.

CHAPTER 27

Personal Care Products

Donald R. Miller and Mary Kuzel

> ### Questions to ask in patient assessment and counseling
>
> #### Feminine Cleansing and Deodorant Products
>
> - *Have you noticed any difference in your vaginal discharge? Are you having pain or itching?*
> - *Are there any sores in the vaginal area?*
> - *How long has the condition been present?*
> - *Have you had this condition before?*
> - *Have you ever seen a physician for this condition or treated it yourself?*
> - *Do you douche? If so, how frequently? What product do you use?*
> - *Are you taking any prescription drugs?*
> - *Are you using any nonprescription feminine cleansing or deodorant products?*
> - *Do you currently use an intrauterine device (IUD)? Have you ever used one?*
> - *Are you pregnant?*
> - *Do you have any medical problems such as diabetes?*
>
> #### Antiperspirants and Underarm Deodorants
>
> - *Do you want to purchase an antiperspirant, a deodorant, or a combination of both types?*
> - *Do you perspire heavily even in cool temperatures? When you are nervous and excited?*
> - *Do you feel that you need an extra-strength product? Why?*
> - *Do the palms of your hands and the soles of your feet perspire heavily?*
> - *Has the amount of perspiration changed recently?*
> - *Have you ever had an allergic reaction to any antiperspirant or deodorant product?*
>
> #### Skin-Bleaching Products
>
> - *Have you been using a skin-bleaching product? If so, for how long?*
> - *For what type of freckle or "skin spot" do you use it?*
> - *How long have you had that freckle?*
> - *Has the freckle changed color or increased in size?*
> - *Do you have any medical problems?*
> - *Is there any possibility that you are pregnant?*
> - *Are you taking any medications, including birth control pills?*
>
> #### Depilatories
>
> - *Why do you want to use a depilatory?*
> - *Have you used a depilatory before?*
> - *Have you discussed use of a depilatory with your physician?*
> - *Are you currently taking any medications?*
> - *Is your skin very sensitive?*
>
> #### Nonmedicated Shampoos
>
> - *What special problems do you have with your hair (oily, dry, easily tangled)?*
> - *In what age group is the primary user? (Young children need a decreased irritant; teens may need shampoos for oily hair.)*

American society is probably unsurpassed in its concern for cleanliness, personal hygiene, and elimination of body odors. The many available products are intended to keep us clean and odor-free from head to toe. Included among these are feminine cleansing and deodorant products, antiperspirants and underarm deodorants, skin-bleaching products, depilatories, and nonmedicated shampoos. Many of these products are intended to affect normal physiologic processes. Therefore, the pharmacist must consider the use of such products from the cosmetic, medical, and therapeutic points of view.

Feminine Cleansing and Deodorant Products

A multitude of feminine vaginal products are commercially available. These products claim and advertise many benefits to use, including:

- General cleansing of the vaginal and perineal areas;
- Relief of vaginal itching and burning;
- Removal of vaginal discharge and secretions;
- Treatment of minor irritations;
- Reduction or coverup of vaginal odor;
- Production of a soothing and refreshed feeling in the vaginal area.

With today's prevalence of sexually transmitted disease, it should be stressed that self-treatment with nonprescription personal hygiene and anti-infective products may be dangerous. The actions and benefits of most of these products are purely cosmetic or limited to the treatment of recurrent vaginal *Candida* (fungal) infections. Feminine deodorant sprays and douche preparations should not be recommended for self-treatment of any disease.

Physiology of the Vaginal Tract

The healthy vagina cleanses itself daily by producing secretions that lubricate the vaginal tract. The external genitalia may be further cleansed and deodorized effectively by washing with mild soap and water. Factors important for vaginal health include good external hygiene, proper pH balance, normal hormonal concentrations, and the presence of normal vaginal bacterial flora.

Estrogens play a major role in determining the vaginal environment. Vaginal surfaces are lined with squamous epithelium. Estrogens control the thickness of this lining and the epithelial cell glycogen content. Glycogen breakdown produces lactic acid, which is necessary for maintaining the normal acidic pH of the adult vagina. Epithelial cell thickness and glycogen content increase as menstruation begins (menarche) and decrease at menopause. In menstruating women, this thicker vaginal epithelium provides some protection against bacterial, fungal, and protozoal infections. Conversely, such infections constitute the most common vaginal disorder in prepubertal girls and postmenopausal women.

Normal vaginal bacteria and their ecologic balance have become better understood in recent years. The indigenous microflora are a complex mixture of aerobic and anaerobic organisms including *Staphylococcus*, *Gardnerella*, *Bacteroides*, and *Streptococcus* species, and a strain of *Lactobacillus* known as Döderlein's bacillus, which metabolizes epithelial glycogen to lactic acid.[1] Vaginal pH is normally acidic during the childbearing years and alkaline in prepubertal girls and postmenopausal women. During the reproductive years, vaginal pH ranges from 3.0 to 5.5. An acidic vaginal pH and the presence of normal bacterial flora usually preclude pathogenic growth of microorganisms; a shift in pH toward alkalinity may render the patient more susceptible to vaginal infection. Pregnancy and the pseudopregnancy induced with oral contraceptive therapy markedly increase the vaginal glycogen content and may predispose these women to microbial infection. *Candida albicans* is the most common causative agent of vaginal infections in the pregnant population.[2]

Normal vaginal secretion is composed of endocervical mucus, bacteria, and desquamated vaginal epithelium. The quantity and composition of this secretion varies with age, phase of menstrual cycle, sexual arousal and sexual activity, use of oral contraceptives, pregnancy, frequency of douching, changes in estrogen and progesterone levels (e.g., menopause), or emotional state.

A normal vaginal discharge is a natural cleansing process. In the absence of personal cleanliness or during times of excessive vaginal discharge, accumulated secretions may produce an odor. Additional causes of vaginal odor are associated with the presence of semen, old blood, infection, intrauterine devices (IUDs), and forgotten foreign objects (e.g., a tampon or contraceptive sponge fragments).

Selected Pathology of the Vaginal Area

Symptoms of vaginitis are responsible for a large percentage of outpatient physician visits by female adults.[2] Symptoms described typically include abnormal vaginal discharge or spotting, odor, pain, burning, and itching. One cause of these symptoms is an inflammation of vulvar and vaginal epithelium due to disturbances in the balance of the normal flora or to the presence of pathogenic organisms. The inside of the vagina does not have nerve endings to perceive pain and itching, so the patient is asymptomatic until the external genitalia become involved in the infection. Vaginitis varies by infection type, organism, and age group affected. There are three major types of vaginal infections: bacterial vaginosis, trichomonal vaginitis, and *Candida* vulvovaginitis. These are presented in more detail in Chapter 28, "Topical Anti-Infective Products."

Bacterial vaginosis is the most prevalent vaginal infection and is the leading cause of abnormal vaginal discharge in women of reproductive age.[3] Bacterial vaginosis is the preferred name for what was formerly referred to as *Haemophilus* vaginitis, nonspecific vaginitis, and, most recently, *Gardnerella* vaginitis. *Gardnerella vaginalis*, once believed to be the causative pathogen, is probably one of several endogenous organisms that may overgrow in bacterial vaginosis. Risk factors for development of this infection include previous or current *Trichomonas* (protozoal) infection, increased sexual activity, or use of an IUD.[4] In fact, vaginitis in patients using Norplant®, a levonorgestrel-releasing subdermal implant, is reported to be half as prevalent as it is in IUD users.[5]

Bacterial vaginosis may be linked with adverse pregnancy outcomes. A recent study showed a significant association between preterm rupture of membranes and onset of preterm labor in women with this infection.[6] Diagnosis and treatment of bacterial vaginosis must be made by a physician. Metronidazole (Flaygl®), 500 mg twice daily for 7 days, remains the treatment of choice.[3] Douche products will not effectively cure a bacterial infection and may only mask symptoms. Douches should never be recommended to treat a vaginal infection of any kind.

Candida vaginitis is common in women of childbearing age. Factors predisposing to this fungal infection include antimicrobial therapy, corticosteroid therapy, cancer chemotherapy, pregnancy, diabetes mellitus, oral contraceptive use, IUD use, or tight-fitting underclothing made from synthetic fabrics.

Vaginal candidiasis is often incorrectly called a yeast infection; a more correct term would be *yeast-like* fungal infection. Vulvar and vaginal pruritus are common symptoms of *Candida* infection. This itching is often associated with a thick, white, odorless discharge that resembles cottage cheese.[7] *Candida* infection may also be sexually transmitted. Male partners may harbor the organism, remain asymptomatic, and transmit it through sexual contact.

Initial diagnosis and treatment of *Candida* infection must be made by a physician. A recent development is the nonprescription status of former prescription agents for the effective treatment of *Candida* vaginitis. If the fungal infection is recurrent and symptoms are recognizable, the nonprescription products, if properly used, should afford cure of vaginal infection in most patients. Sporadic use may lead to the development of resistance or may mask underlying disorders. Pharmacists must actively counsel patients on the proper selection and use of vaginal antifungal products because more products are expected to achieve nonprescription status in the future. Proper selection, use, and counseling advice is included in Chapter 28, "Topical Anti-Infective Products." Referral to a physician should be made when the following situations are present:

- Purulent vaginal discharge;
- A thin watery discharge with pruritis in postmenopausal women;
- Pruritis with or without an odorous vaginal discharge;
- Self-treatment failure;
- Persistent, severe, or recurrent symptoms.

Trichomonas infection is due to a flagellated protozoa. The prevalence of trichomoniasis correlates with sexual activity and is highest among women with multiple sexual partners.[1] This infection is sexually transmissible; all sexual partners should be treated to prevent treatment failure.[2] Antibiotic therapy for trichomonal infection includes metronidazole, 2 g as a one-time dose, 1 g taken twice in the same day, or 250 mg three times daily for 1 week.[1] The dose in children is 5 mg/kg three times daily for 7 days. *Trichomonas* infection also occurs in older women. *Candida* and trichomonal infections may occur simultaneously, and both organisms may be present in the healthy vagina.

Another common condition is atrophic vaginitis. In this syndrome, which occurs after menopause, estrogen deficiency leads to thinning of the vaginal wall, reduced normal vaginal secretions, and a shift toward an alkaline pH. These changes bring an increased risk of traumatic irritation and infection.[1] Local and/or systemic estrogen therapy may be prescribed for this condition because estrogen both stimulates vaginal epithelium, increasing its thickness, and improves resistance to infection. Various products, including convenient vaginal gels and inserts, are available for the symptomatic relief of vaginal atrophy and dryness.

Vaginal Douche Products

Because vaginal douches mechanically irrigate the vagina, thus clearing away mucus and other accumulated debris, they may be used as cosmetic cleansing agents. A recent study confirmed that douching remains a relatively common practice, given that more than half of all women douche regularly or intermittently.[8] The most frequent reason stated for douching was to achieve good vaginal hygiene.

It is not known how often women douche for nontherapeutic purposes. Some nonprescription douche products recommend douching no more often than twice a week.[9] An alternative cleansing method for vaginal and perineal areas involves gently washing the vulvar, perineal, and anal regions, and the vagina with the fingers using lukewarm water and mild soap.[10]

Douche products are available as liquids, liquid concentrates to be diluted with water, powders to be dissolved in water, and powders (insufflations) to be instilled as powders. Premixed douche products in disposable applicators are widely available and convenient to use, as they eliminate the care and cleansing requirements of nondisposable equipment.

Ingredients

Antimicrobial Agents Most antimicrobial agents in douche products are present in concentrations that provide preservative properties but no antimicrobial therapeutic activity. These agents include benzethonium and benzalkonium chloride, chlorothymol, hexachlorophene, and parabens.[11] Other compounds such as boric acid, cetylpyridinium chloride, oxyquinoline, and sodium perborate may be included for their supposed antiseptic or germicidal activity; however, their value as antimicrobials is also highly questionable in the concentration employed. Because many manufacturers do not list concentrations of ingredients when the products are considered cosmetics, it is impossible to assess the efficacy of those ingredients for their intended purpose.

The possibility of local irritation, sensitization, and contact dermatitis exists with many antimicrobial agents found in douches. If these effects are encountered, the patient should discontinue using the product and consult a physician.

Counterirritants Counterirritant compounds such as eucalyptol, menthol, phenol, and thymol are included in douche products for their local anesthetic or antipruritic effects; however, the efficacy of these agents has not been substantiated. Aromatic agents may be added to mask odors and to produce a soothing and refreshing feeling in general.

Astringents Astringent substances such as ammonium and potassium alums and zinc sulfate are included in some douches to reduce local edema, inflammation, and exudation. The astringent concentration is important because many astringents are irritants in moderate or high concentrations but are ineffective if too dilute.

Proteolytics At least one proteolytic agent, papain, is included in a douche product to "break down" the excess vaginal discharge. Papain is an enzyme that attacks proteinaceous material and may elicit inflammatory and allergic reactions.

Surfactants Docusate sodium, nonoxynol 4, and sodium lauryl sulfate are used to facilitate the douche's spread over vaginal mucosa and its penetration of mucosal folds. This surfactant or detergent effect lowers surface tension and increases wettability; its cosmetic or clinical value, however, is not readily apparent. Cetylpyridinium chloride, benzalkonium chloride, and benzethonium chloride also have mild surfactant properties.

Substances Affecting pH Many vaginal douche products are buffered or contain substances that purposely render them either acidic or alkaline. For example, sodium perborate and sodium bicarbonate provide alkalinity, and lactic acid and citric acid provide acidity. However, even daily use of douches will not significantly alter vaginal pH. A douche solution itself may actually wash out glycogen, lactic acid, and other acids and render the pH alkaline for a short time.

Povidone–Iodine Povidone–iodine (e.g., Betadine®) has been claimed to relieve minor irritation. Although few allergic reactions have been reported with povidone–iodine, it may be systemically absorbed and should not be used by individuals allergic to iodine-containing products. Absorption poses a particular hazard to pregnant women, in whom repeated vaginal applications may result in iodine-induced goiter and hypothyroidism in the fetus.

Douche Equipment
Several types of syringes are available for douching purposes. The douche bag (fountain syringe or folding feminine syringe) should be held at hip level and instilled via gentle gravity pressure. This system holds one to two quarts of fluid and comes with tubing and a shut-off valve. Two types of tips are supplied, one for enema use (the shorter rectal nozzle) and one for douching. The two tips are not interchangeable: vaginal infections may occur if the rectal tip is also used for douching. Bulb douche syringes hold 8–16 oz of fluid; the disposable units contain 3–9 oz. The flow rate is regulated by the amount of hand pressure exerted when the bulb is squeezed. Gentle pressure is recommended because excess force may introduce fluid into the cervix and cause inflammation.

Administration Guidelines for Douching
To use douches safely, appropriately, and effectively, patients should be instructed to:

- Not use these products if they are pregnant;
- Not use these products for birth control;
- Discontinue product use if irritation develops;
- Keep all douche equipment clean and dry;
- Use all products strictly according to manufacturer instructions;
- Never instill a douche with forceful pressure;
- Use lukewarm water to dilute products;
- Not douche until at least 8 hours after intercourse if a diaphragm, cervical cap, contraceptive jelly, cream, foam, or contraceptive sponge is used;
- Not douche 24–48 hours before any gynecologic examination.

Adverse Effects from Douching
An association between douching and acute pelvic inflammatory disease (PID) has been proposed.[12] PID has been found to be related to frequency of douching. Because of variables that cannot be controlled, it is difficult to draw any conclusion from this information. There also may exist an association between douching and the risk of tubal pregnancy.[13] Additional problems include irritation or sensitization from douche ingredients and disruption of normal vaginal flora and vaginal pH.

Feminine Deodorant Sprays

Feminine deodorant sprays, mists, or powders are intended for use on the external genital area to mask or reduce objectionable odor. These products are intended for cosmetic use only; they do not possess any therapeutic effect. Ingredients may include an antimicrobial agent, an emollient carrier, a perfume, and a propellant.

Ingredients

Perfumes Fragrances or perfumes, the primary ingredients of feminine deodorant sprays, are responsible for deodorant activity. Fragrances are characterized as mild or strong, short or long lasting, sweet, medicinal, and floral, among other categories. Some products contain encapsulated perfumes that are released slowly on contact with vaginal moisture. The sprays should be selected with care because some may be irritating to perineal and vaginal mucosa.

Antimicrobials Antimicrobial compounds in sprays are preservatives rather than therapeutic agents. Properly used, they do not alter normal vulvovaginal flora.

Emollients A number of emollient substances are included in these formulations, both as vehicles and for their soothing effect on the skin. The most commonly used are fatty alcohols, esters such as isopropyl myristate, and polyoxyethylene derivatives of fatty esters. Unfortunately, some of these substances also may be sensitizers.

Propellants With proper application, propellants are not likely to be irritants. However, if the spray is held too close to the body and the propellant reaches the skin, the chilling effects or even tissue freezing induced by evaporation of the spray may cause vaginal irritation and edema. The fluorinated hydrocarbon propellants that were previously used have been largely replaced by aliphatic hydrocarbons such as propane and isobutane that appear to be less hazardous to the environment.

Guidelines for Proper Usage
Patients should be instructed to observe the following guidelines for the proper application and use of feminine deodorant sprays:

- Hold the product at least 20 cm (8 in.) from the body when spraying;
- Discontinue use if irritation occurs;
- Do not use to mask an odor that may be one symptom of a more serious condition that requires medical attention;
- Do not use frequently;
- Do not use on inflamed vaginal areas.

Miscellaneous Products

Premoistened towelettes are used for their vaginal deodorant, cleansing, or cosmetic properties. Women who are sensitive to aerosol propellants might be informed of the towelette formulations because, except for the propellants in sprays, the ingredients in these towelettes are similar to those of deodorant aerosols. However, direct irritation or sensitization from other towelette ingredients may occur.

Products claiming to relieve vaginal pain and itching are available. However, if symptoms indicate some type of infectious vaginitis, the pharmacist should not recommend a vaginal cream or similar local anesthetic vaginal product without a concurrent recommendation by a physician. Vaginal products that claim to treat vaginal pain and itching may simply mask the underlying cause of symptoms and delay an accurate diagnosis and proper treatment.

Nonprescription hydrocortisone products are also available. Patients should be instructed to use vaginal hydrocortisone products with caution because they may mask symptoms of vaginitis. Also, vaginal mucosal absorption of hydrocortisone may occur. These products should not be used intravaginally.

Antiperspirants and Underarm Deodorants

Commercial products to prevent or alleviate body odor have been sold since the late 1800s. Nearly every adult in North America uses one of the many antiperspirants (antiwetness), deodorants (antiodor), or deodorant soaps available. However, many consumers are unaware of the difference between antiperspirants and deodorants, and they may buy one product expecting the other's effect. Pharmacist input into the selection of an underarm product is desirable.

Anatomy and Physiology of Sweat Glands

Commercial products may be aimed at affecting the products of two types of sweat glands: eccrine and apocrine. Eccrine glands (true sweat glands) are distributed over most of the skin surface but particularly on the palms, soles, face, and axillae (armpits). They consist of a secretory coil in the lower dermis and subcutaneous tissue, and a duct that travels in a helical manner to the skin surface (see Figure 1 in Chapter 29, "Acne Products"). The duct contains an intraepidermal unit that modifies the composition of the sweat. Constituents of eccrine secretion are water, sodium, potassium, chloride, urea, lactate, and very small amounts of glucose. The secretion is hypotonic and has a pH of 4–6.8.

Adequate eccrine gland function is vital to the maintenance of normal body temperature. Heat can be dispelled by the evaporation of moisture on the skin surface. However, the cooling function of sweat is provided by glands all over the body, so the inhibition of sweating in just one area, such as the axillae, is not harmful.[14] Although perspiration contains "waste products" such as urea and lactate, perspiring is not important in purification of the blood. People who live in cool environments do not suffer from a lack of perspiration.[14]

The eccrine glands are unusual because they are cholinergic in function but are supplied with sympathetic nerves. Intact innervation is necessary for function. Three stimuli activate glandular response: thermal stimulation produces sweating mainly on the face and upper trunk; emotional stimulation causes perspiration primarily on the palms, soles, and axillae; and sensory stimulation can produce local perspiration (e.g., hot spicy food causes sweating around the face). Thermal stimulation has a latent period before sweating starts, but emotional and sensory stimulation produce an immediate response. Eccrine glands in the axillae are unique in being responsive to both thermal and emotional stimulation.[15] In the normal adult, the quantity of eccrine perspiration varies from negligible under basal conditions to 12 L in 24 hours at maximal stimulation.[14]

The average production is about a liter a day, but this varies with race, age, sex, conditioning, and acclimatization to heat. Eccrine sweat is normally odorless although food and drug substances may be excreted with it.

Apocrine glands consist of a coiled secretory tubule and a duct that normally opens into the neck of the hair follicle above the sebaceous gland. These glands, which are confined mainly to the axillae, areola, groin, and perineum, produce a scanty, milky substance that is odorless upon secretion but becomes odoriferous upon bacterial decomposition. Apocrine glands are poorly developed in children and begin to enlarge at puberty. The secretion serves no known useful purpose but may have evolved as a mechanism for sexual attraction.[14] There are differences in apocrine activity among races. Apocrine secretion is intermittent and produced at a very slow rate. The secretion rate is indifferent to thermal stimulation but responds to emotional stress and mechanical stimulation. However, apocrine secretion in the axillae may be unique in its responsiveness to heat or to the combination of heat and emotional stimulation.

Disorders of Sweat Glands

Although some underarm moisture (hidrosis) or odor (bromhidrosis) is normal, our culture considers it offensive. Excess wetness may be embarrassing as well as damaging to clothes. Wetness and odor are related but distinct problems. Wetness is caused by eccrine glands whereas odor is primarily caused by bacterial decomposition of apocrine secretion. It is hard to determine which causes more concern because most people consider the problems to be inseparable.

Wetness

Wetness is caused by water being secreted faster than it evaporates. The axillae normally retain moisture because evaporation is retarded there. Transient hyperhidrosis is a physiologic response to heat or emotion. Severe axillary hyperhidrosis may be familial, may or may not be associated with palmar and plantar hyperhidrosis, and is usually not associated with odor problems.[16] Generalized pathologic hyperhidrosis may be caused by certain medical disorders such as thyrotoxicosis, lymphomas, diabetes mellitus, tuberculosis, anxiety, fever, and abnormalities of the autonomic system.[15,17] Primary idiopathic hyperhidrosis usually presents as a symmetrical problem involving the axillae, soles, or palms. Women are more likely to seek treatment for hyperhidrosis than are men.[16]

In contrast to hyperhidrosis, anhidrosis may be caused by hypothermia, local lesions in the autonomic nervous system, diabetic neuropathy, or malfunction of the sweat gland itself. Compensatory hyperhidrosis occurs in the remaining normal sweat glands.[17]

Prickly heat (miliaria rubra) involves closure of the pores of the eccrine sweat glands and blockage of sweat delivery. This causes sweat to enter the surrounding epidermis with consequent irritation. (See Chapter 31, "Diaper Rash and Prickly Heat Products.")

Body Odor

Both eccrine and apocrine secretions are sterile and initially odorless. When left to stand, however, perspiration undergoes considerable change, mainly because of bacterial degradation of apocrine secretions. The odor of freshly collected perspiration may be mild but not generally objectionable. The odor varies with the individual, activity, emotional state, and diet.[18] Body odor arises with the growth of bacteria in the secretion of apocrine sweat glands. Which apocrine component actually produces the odor is unclear, but degradation of apocrine secretions produces short-chain fatty acids such as isovaleric acid (which causes a typical acidic "sweaty" odor),[19] mercaptans, indoles, ammonia, amines, and hydrogen sulfide. The presence of hair increases axillary odor because hair acts as a collecting site for oily secretions, cellular debris, dirt, and bacteria. Wetness from eccrine secretion promotes bacterial growth and dispersion of apocrine secretion. Oddly enough, however, excessive watery eccrine sweat may wash away apocrine sweat so that no odor is present.[15,20] Conversely, patients with axillary odor may have no problem with wetness.[20]

Because bacterial decomposition of apocrine secretion is required for odor, differences in flora between subjects have been examined. Data suggest that subjects with pungent body odor are relatively few in number and have a much higher number of lipophilic diphtheroids in their microflora than subjects without strong body odor.[19] In most cases, the body odor is not caused by biologic dysfunction but is simply a matter of personal hygiene. The presence of sebum, perspiration, and other debris greatly increases axillary odor. Regular removal of debris by bathing will reduce odor, but washing alone does not remove all products of degraded perspiration and cannot remove many of the resident bacteria on the skin. Shaving the axillae may help by removing hair that serves to retain moisture, which acts as a substrate for bacteria.

Treatment

Disorders of perspiration can be approached in multiple ways. In assessing the most appropriate method of dealing with perspiration problems, the pharmacist must first determine whether the person is more concerned about wetness or odor. A substance can be applied to reduce the amount of eccrine perspiration secreted. (No product can effectively reduce apocrine secretion.) Such substances are labeled antiperspirants and are classified as drugs by the Food and Drug Administration (FDA) because they are intended to influence a physiologic body process. Another substance may prevent, mask, or change perspiration odor without attempting to block its flow. These preparations are termed deodorants and are regarded as cosmetics. Deodorants may contain perfumes to mask odor, germicides to inhibit bacterial growth, or powders to absorb moisture. Many commercial products are combinations of antiperspirants and deodorants; however, any product labeled as a deodorant cannot make antiperspirant claims. The fact that numerous products are marketed for these purposes speaks for their popularity. Antiperspirants alone tend to be the least acceptable because their action is relatively hard to perceive immediately, whereas the failure of a deodorant product is much more obvious.

The second thing the pharmacist should determine is whether the problem is pathologic. In pathologic hyperhidrosis, patients will complain of constant heavy perspiration inappropriate to the climate and situation, and may complain more often of palmar or plantar sweating than of axillary sweating. Nonprescription antiperspirants are not adequate to relieve pathologic hyperhidrosis. Patients with such a problem should be referred to a physician for diagnosis and treatment.

Wetness problems that do not respond to nonprescription products may be treated in several other ways. Stronger concentrations of aluminum chloride in absolute ethanol (e.g., Drysol®, or Xerac-AC®) are available by prescription. These preparations are applied to the hyperhidrotic areas at bedtime; the area may be covered with a plastic wrap, and the residue is washed off in the morning.[20,21] Systemic anticholinergics or phenoxybenzamine, an alpha-adrenergic antagonist,[22] may also be prescribed to reduce perspiration flow.

The technique of iontophoresis (passing an electrical current through the area of the sweat glands) has been used.[16,21] This technique, which may work by producing keratotic plugs within sweat glands that temporarily block the flow of sweat,[23] is recommended especially for local hyperhidrosis of the palms or soles.[15,16] A battery-run device called the Drionic® (General Medical Co., Los Angeles, Calif.) is available for home use. However, some authorities believe the Drionic® is no more effective than topical antiperspirants,[21,23] On rare occasions, in refractory cases of hyperhidrosis, various operative procedures—including sympathectomy, liposuction, and excision or curettage of eccrine glands—may be attempted.[16,21]

Ingredients

The FDA has determined that aluminum chloride, aluminum chlorohydrates, aluminum zirconium chlorohydrates, and buffered aluminum sulfate are safe and effective as topical antiperspirants in the appropriate concentration. However, only aluminum chlorohydrates have sufficient safety data to permit their use in an aerosolized dosage form.[24]

Currently used ingredients have evolved from the empirical use of astringent metal salts, many of which were tried and discarded because of undesirable properties such as staining or irritation. Although the action of antiperspirants in reducing the flow of eccrine perspiration can be measured objectively, the mechanism of action has been a subject of intense debate that is still unresolved. The oldest theory focused on a simple astringent action, which causes shrinkage of the pore: it was speculated that an antiperspirant might act on a sweat gland to produce inflammation and swelling around the duct, thereby contracting its orifice. However, a number of chemicals that are strong astringents have minimal antiperspirant activity. Another theory is that an antiperspirant increases the permeability of the sweat duct, causing reabsorption of sweat (the "leaky hose" theory).

Studies have indicated that a physically demonstrable obstruction of the duct accounts for anhidrosis.[25,26] However, after the stratum corneum is stripped from the skin, antiperspirant activity still remains; thus, obstruction is more than superficial. A plug may be caused by keratin precipitated by the antiperspirant. However, the keratin plug is probably a late, nonspecific reaction to injury, whereas the initial plug is caused by an amorphous, aluminum-containing cast that extends down the length of the duct. There is no inflammation.[25] The individual sweat duct remains physically occluded until it is replaced by normal cell renewal in several days. Thus, antiperspirants have prolonged action.[14] The degree to which antiperspirants decrease wetness is relatively slight and could not be enough to cause an appreciable decrease in odor.[14] However, antiperspirants are also strong antibacterials and therefore may be effective deodorants.[27]

The most common adverse effect of nonprescription antiperspirants is skin irritation (e.g., tingling, stinging, or burning), which is caused by the formation of hydrochloric acid; sensitization is very rare.[14] Normally, irritation can be reduced by decreasing the frequency or amount of antiperspirant used. Antiperspirants should not be applied to freshly shaved skin. If erythema or papules develop, use of the product should be discontinued for a few days, during which period a deodorant can be applied instead. The patient can usually return to the same antiperspirant later, using it in lesser amounts. The contents of all antiperspirant products are fully labeled, so a user who is sensitive to a specific ingredient can choose a different formulation.

No evidence exists to suggest that antiperspirants cause permanent harm to sweat glands. Normal sweating resumes within a week after discontinuation of use. Also, no evidence of systemic toxicity caused by topical application of antiperspirants has been reported. However, antiperspirants should not be applied to broken or irritated skin because axillary granulomas have been reported.[28]

Because acidity is irritating to the skin and damaging to clothing, nonprescription antiperspirant formulations may be buffered by adding urea or glycine in 5–10% concentrations. These buffers do not appreciably increase the pH of a preparation or act as alkalis to precipitate aluminum hydroxide, which would reduce antiperspirant activity. However, at ironing temperatures, they decompose to ammonia and neutralize acidity to protect clothing.[18]

Aluminum Chloride Aluminum chloride ($AlCl_3$) hydrolyzes in water to aluminum hydroxide and hydrochloric acid, forming strongly acidic solutions. This high acidity tends to damage fabrics in contact with treated skin and is very irritating to the skin at higher concentrations. Therefore, the FDA has recommended that only concentrations of 15% or less (in aqueous solution) should be considered both effective and safe. Solutions of aluminum chloride show significantly greater efficacy than less irritating antiperspirant compounds.[14] Although alcoholic solutions of aluminum chloride are available by prescription, there are no data on the safety of this formulation for unsupervised use.

Ideally, aluminum chloride should be applied at night when sweat glands are inactive, and the affected area should be occluded for 2–8 hours. The high degree of acidity may be desirable to help deposit the aluminum salts deep in the epidermis. Dry skin enhances penetration and reduces irritation from formation of hydrochloric acid.[29]

Aluminum Chlorohydrates Aluminum chlorohydrates are available commercially in several products that differ in the ratio of aluminum to chlorine. The empirical formulas of the most widely used ingredients are $Al_2(OH)_4Cl_2$ and $Al_2(OH)_5Cl$, which are known as two-thirds basic and five-sixths basic aluminum chloride, respectively. Aluminum chlorohydrates are also available as polyethylene glycol or propylene glycol complexes. These complexes are formulated to provide greater alcohol solubility and do not affect the safety or efficacy of the salts from which they are prepared.[14] The advantage of chlorohydrate salts over aluminum chloride is their lower acidity. The greater the aluminum-to-chloride ratio in the salt, the less acidic is the solution.

The panel found that aluminum chlorohydrates are safe and effective when applied topically to the underarms in concentrations of 25% (anhydrous) or less. These concentrations have produced very little skin irritation in patch testing or market experience.

Aluminum Zirconium Salts Aerosol products containing zirconium have been banned because they may cause lung granulomas if inhaled.[30] Skin changes have been found in rabbits injected with aluminum zirconium glycine complex. However, the efficacy of aluminum zirconium glycine complex is good, and the combination is effective in concentrations of not more than 20% anhydrous weight.

Buffered Aluminum Sulfate Aluminum sulfate itself produces a high degree of irritation. However, it is available as an 8% solution buffered with 8% sodium aluminum lactate. This preparation is effective and virtually nonirritating.[14]

Glutaraldehyde and Tannic Acid Both glutaraldehyde 2% in buffered solution and tannic acid are available without prescription. Used to treat hyperhidrosis of the palms and soles but not of the axillae, these ingredients are thought to act by occluding the sweat ducts. A drawback is that they stain the skin brown.[21,22]

Antimicrobials Deodorants may contain perfumes and colognes to mask body odor, or they may contain substances that inhibit bacterial action. Among the latter group, the phenolic compounds are long lasting and compatible with soaps. Triclosan and trichlorocarbanilide are often found in deodorants and deodorant soaps such as Dial® and Coast®. The astringent aluminum salts also have antiseptic properties. Compounds of metals other than aluminum are used as deodorants. Zinc phenolsulfonate is used in liquid products; zinc oxide, peroxide, or stearate is used in powders.[18] Sodium bicarbonate, a time-honored deodorant, absorbs moisture, and its alkalinity may inhibit bacteria.

Internal Deodorants Chlorophyll and its salts have been reported anecdotally to have deodorant properties. There is no objective evidence that chlorophyll taken orally is effective as a systemic deodorant for reducing normal body or urinary odors.[31,32] However, the FDA has found chlorophyllin copper complex (e.g., Pals®) 100–200 mg per day and bismuth subgallate 200–400 mg four times daily to be safe and effective for reducing odor from a colostomy or ileostomy.[32] Chlorophyllin copper complex may cause some cramping or diarrhea.

Dosage Forms

The ideal antiperspirant or deodorant should apply conveniently, dry quickly, not stain clothing, be nonirritating, and last all day after a single application. However, available products are far from ideal. Creams were the first available delivery system for antiperspirants but were largely abandoned for more convenient dosage forms. Aerosols became immensely popular in the 1960s, capturing up to 85% of the market, but their use has plummeted because of publicity about adverse effects on the lungs and the environment. Furthermore, their effectiveness is low. Powders are generally deodorants that absorb moisture. To be active, antiperspirant ingredients must be in solution.[18]

Not all dosage forms are equally effective. The FDA believes that a 20% reduction in wetness is the minimum required to be noticeable by the user. Therefore, it has suggested, but not required, that an average sweat reduction of 20% be ensured for each antiperspirant formulation.[24] In recommending products, the pharmacist should note the following points:

- No nonprescription product inhibits wetness completely in the axillae; during normal use, only a 20–40% sweat reduction can be expected.[14]
- Minor variations in formulation may have a critical effect on a product's activity;[33] thus, two similar products may be quite different in effectiveness.
- There is extreme individual variability in response to antiperspirants; some subjects actually perspire more after some applications.

Labeling Claims

The FDA determined that there were insufficient data on nonprescription antiperspirants for certain label claims to be allowed. Unless appropriate data are submitted for each product, the FDA prohibits claims of "long-lasting" or "all-day" effectiveness and of being effective for "emotional" or "troublesome" perspiration. Claims about "extra strength" are disallowed entirely because concentration does not necessarily correlate with effectiveness. The only claim allowed is a statement to the effect that the product reduces underarm wetness.[24]

Guidelines for Proper Use

The pharmacist should be sure that the consumer understands the difference between deodorants and antiperspirants. Deodorants are not a substitute for cleanliness; their use should follow bathing. Antiperspirants reduce but do not stop wetness, especially during thermal or emotional stress. Antiperspirants are not effective immediately after application. Repeated applications over time are needed to achieve the maximal effect.[14]

Before applying antiperspirants, the user should let the underarm dry. This reduces discomfort from moisture-induced hydrolysis of aluminum salts to hydrochloric acid. In addition, the antiperspirant effect is completely abolished if the subject is perspiring during application. Antiperspirants should not be applied to open, broken, abraded, or freshly shaved skin.

Finally, the patient should be advised of the marked variation in response to antiperspirants from person to person and product to product. If one product does not perform satisfactorily, it is quite appropriate to try others.

Skin-Bleaching Products

Hyperpigmentation of the skin may result from various causes. It is usually asymptomatic and of no medical consequence although it may occasionally signify systemic illness. Hyperpigmentation, particularly on the face, can be a source of cosmetic disability and mental distress. Thus, agents that can bleach away excess pigment when applied topically enjoy a large market among racial and ethnic groups around the world. Although these products serve a cosmetic function, it is important to emphasize that they are drugs and have potential toxicity.

Physiology of Skin Pigmentation

Normal skin color is contributed by melanocytes in the basal layer of epidermis, which produce pigment granules called melanosomes. These granules contain a complex protein called melanin, a brown-black pigment. Melanocytes can be viewed as tiny one-celled glands with long projections to pass pigment particles into the keratinocytes, which synthesize skin keratin. As keratinocytes migrate upward, they carry the pigment with them and deposit it on the surface of the skin as they die. Melanocytes are also present in the hair bulb cells, and they pass pigment granules on to the hair.

Melanin is the most efficient sunscreen known. It prevents damaging ultraviolet (UV) rays from the sun from entering deeper parts of the skin and causing sunburn. Solar radiation stimulates melanocytes to provide more melanin resulting in gradual skin darkening or a "tan." The various human races have roughly the same number of melanocytes, but dark-skinned people have more active cells.[34]

Hyperpigmentation Syndromes

Certain systemic and skin diseases cause pigment cells to become overactive, resulting in a darkening of the skin, or to become underactive, with a resultant lightening of the skin. Endocrine imbalances caused by Addison's disease, Cushing's disease, hyperthyroidism, pregnancy, estrogen therapy (including oral contraceptives), and skin cancer (melanoma) will affect skin pigmentation. Metabolic alterations affecting the liver and certain nutritional deficiencies can be associated with diffuse melanosis.[35] Physical trauma or inflammatory dermatoses may cause a postinflammatory pigmentation. Also, certain drugs such as chlorpromazine and hydroxychloroquine have an affinity for melanin and may cause hyperpigmentation. Thus, the pharmacist must inquire about concurrent drug therapy and systemic illnesses before recommending a nonprescription product. Diffuse pigmentation disorders and those caused by systemic factors should never be self-treated without prior evaluation by a physician. Similarly, lesions that are changing in size, shape, or color may be cancerous and should never be self-treated. Prompt referral to a physician is indicated in all such cases.

Several types of hyperpigmentation, including freckles, melasma, and lentigines, are amenable to self-treatment.[35,36] Freckles are simple spots of uneven pigmentation that are exacerbated by the sun. Melasma (also called chloasma) is a condition in which blotchy patches appear on the face or neck, usually because of a hormonal imbalance. Melasma is often caused by pregnancy ("the mask of pregnancy") or oral contraceptives, and sun exposure is necessary for its development. Lentigines, hyperpigmented spots that may appear at any age anywhere on the skin or mucous membranes, are caused by an increased deposition of melanin and an increased number of melanocytes. They are darker than freckles and not induced by UV radiation. However, solar or "senile" lentigines, commonly but incorrectly known as liver spots, appear on the exposed surfaces of fair-skinned people and are induced by UV radiation.

Treatment

The intensity of localized hyperpigmentation in producing freckles, melasma, lentigines, or postinflammatory pigmentation may be decreased by topical nonprescription skin-bleaching agents. Nonprescription products are directed at suppressing melanin formation within the skin. The pharmacist must emphasize to patients the importance of avoiding excessive exposure to sunlight and of using sunscreen agents or protective clothing.

Specific systemic therapy is required for diffuse systemic pigmentation disorders. Physician-directed management of hyperpigmentation may include more effective prescription agents such as ointments formulated with 0.1% tretinoin (retinoic acid), 5% hydroquinone, and 0.1% dexamethasone. Monobenzone should not be used because it produces irreversible depigmentation of normal as well as darkened skin. Light cryosurgical freezing with liquid nitrogen may also be used.

Ingredients

Historically, a number of topical agents have been used in skin-bleaching preparations. These agents have included hydroquinone, the monobenzyl and monomethyl ethers of hydroquinone, ammoniated mercury, ascorbic acid, and peroxides.[37] Only preparations containing hydroquinone were submitted to the FDA Advisory Review Panel on Over-the-Counter Miscellaneous External Drug Products.[35]

Hydroquinone The FDA has recommended that only hydroquinone (*p*-dihydroxybenzene) in concentrations of 1.5–2.0% be available for nonprescription use.[36] Hydroquinone produces reversible depigmentation of the skin and hair of mice, guinea pigs, and humans by a complex mechanism of action. Hydroquinone and its derivatives are oxidized by tyrosinase to form highly toxic free radicals that cause selective damage to the lipoprotein membranes of the melanocyte, thereby reducing conversion of tyrosine to dopa and subsequently to melanin.[38] However, experiments on guinea pigs also indicate that hydroquinone has toxic effects at the subcellular level in both follicular and nonfollicular melanocytes in that it disrupts membranous cytoplasmic organelles and affects the formation, melanization, and degradation of melanosomes.

Several studies demonstrate that topical preparations of 2–5% hydroquinone are effective in producing cutaneous depigmentation.[35] The 2% concentration is safer and has produced results equal to those of higher concentrations.[39] Side effects of topical hydroquinone are mild when used in low concentrations. Tingling or burning on application and subsequent erythema and inflammation were observed in 8% of patients using a 2% concentration and in 32% of patients using a 5% concentration of hydroquinone.[39] Higher concentrations frequently irritate the skin and, if used for prolonged periods, may cause disfiguring effects including epidermal thickening, pitch-black pigmentation, and colloid milium (yellowish papules associated with colloid degeneration).[35,40]

The effectiveness of hydroquinone varies among patients. The results are best on lighter skin and lighter lesions. In African Americans, the response to hydroquinone depends on the amount of pigment present. Additionally, the earlier that hydroquinone is used to treat minor skin blemishes, the more likely that results will be satisfactory. When depigmentation does occur, melanin production is generally reduced by about 50%.[35] Hyperpigmented areas fade more rapidly and completely than surrounding normal skin. Although treatment may not lead to complete disappearance of hypermelanosis, the results are often satisfactory enough to reduce self-consciousness about hyperpigmentation.

When treatment is begun, melanin excretion may transiently increase. A decrease in skin color usually becomes noticeable in about 4 weeks; however, the time of onset varies from 3 weeks to 3 months. Depigmentation lasts for 2–6 months but is reversible. Darker lesions repigment faster than lighter lesions. Because the ability of the sun to darken lesions is much greater than that of hydroquinone to lighten them, strict avoidance of sunlight is imperative. Although sunscreens may help, even visible light may cause some darkening, and sun protection should preferably be opaque.[39] Some hydroquinone products are available in an opaque base (Eldopaque®) or together with a sunscreen (Selaquin®).

In some cases, lesions become slightly darker before fading. A transient inflammatory reaction may develop after the first few weeks of treatment. Occurrence of inflammation makes subsequent lightening more likely, although inflammation can occur without the development of depigmentation. The appearance of mild inflammation need not be considered an indication to stop therapy except in the patient whose reaction increases in intensity. In such situations, sensitization should be considered. Topical hydrocortisone may be used temporarily to alleviate the inflammatory reaction. Contact with the eyes should be avoided. A patch test can be done to test for allergy to hydroquinone; however, most reactions are irritant rather than allergic in nature.

If hydroquinone is accidentally ingested, it seldom produces serious systemic toxicity. However, oral ingestion of 5–15 g has produced tremor, convulsions, and hemolytic anemia.[41]

Reversible brown discoloration of nails has been reported occasionally following the application of 2% hydroquinone to the back of the hand.[42] The discoloration is probably caused by formation of oxidation products of hydroquinone. Hydroquinone is readily oxidized in the presence of light and air. Any discoloration or darkening of the cream is an indication of deterioration and a possible decline in the strength of available hydroquinone.[35] Thus, the preferable method of packaging is in small squeeze tubes.

The dosage of hydroquinone is a thin topical application of a 2% concentration rubbed into affected areas twice daily. If no improvement is seen within 3 months, its use should be discontinued and the advice of a physician sought.[36] Once the desired benefit is achieved, hydroquinone can be applied as often as needed in a once- or twice-daily regimen to maintain depigmentation of the skin. Because of the lack of safety data, hydroquinone is not recommended for children under age 12 except under the supervision of a physician.

Hydroquinone Adjuvants and Combinations Because hydroquinone is oxidized by contact with air, antioxidants such as sodium bisulfite may be added to the formulation. Hydroquinone is incompatible with alkali or ferric salts.[41] Iodochlorhydroxyquin or oxyquinolone sulfate may be added as antimicrobial preservatives.[35] The inclusion of a sunscreen agent is rational and appropriate, provided that combination products are advertised not primarily as sunscreens but as skin-bleaching agents with added sunscreen.

Monobenzone Monobenzone, the monobenzyl ether of hydroquinone, is restricted to prescription-only use. Its action and onset time are similar to that of hydroquinone except that depigmentation may be permanent. Its use is restricted to depigmenting residual areas of normal skin in patients with extensive vitiligo (a condition resulting in patches of depigmentation, often with hyperpigmented borders).

Ammoniated Mercury Ammoniated mercury was in common use as a skin-bleaching agent before monobenzone became available. However, chronic application of ammoniated mercury can cause systemic mercury intoxication, and sensitization is common. There also is a lack of efficacy data. Therefore, ammoniated mercury is not approved by the FDA for nonprescription use as a skin-bleaching agent.[43]

Guidelines for Proper Use

Before selecting a nonprescription skin-bleaching product, the pharmacist should be sure that a physician has confirmed the patient's need for using it. These products are intended to lighten only limited areas of hyperpigmented skin and should be used only in areas of brownish discoloration; reddish or bluish areas, such as diffuse port wine discolorations, are not amenable to treatment. These products should not be used on areas that are changing in size, shape, or color. If the product is effective, the results should be noticeable within 2 to 3 months. These products will not permanently injure the skin. Hydroquinone may be applied to a small area of unbroken skin and should be assessed for 24 hours to observe for irritation or allergic reactions. It should never be applied near the eyes or to cut, abraded, or sunburned skin.

Depilatories

Although the biologic significance of human hair is minute, its cosmetic importance is considerable. Any discrepancy between cosmetic standards and normal biologic range may be embarrassing. Excessive growth of facial or body hair has been a common complaint among women for centuries.

Physiology of Hair Growth

Racial and cultural factors affect both the type of normal hair growth and people's attitude about it. In North American culture, any hair except that on the scalp is considered a masculine trait. However, the growth of upper lip and preauricular hair soon after puberty is a normal racial characteristic among females of some ethnic groups. This is attributed to sensitivity of the skin to androgens.[44] Excessive hair growth of essentially normal distribution is termed hypertrichosis; a change in hair growth distribution inconsistent with sex and racial background is called hirsutism.[44] Either condition may be caused by a change in one of two distinct features of hair growth: cycle or pattern.

The hair growth cycle comprises successive stages of growth (anogen) and rest (telogen). During the rest period, fully developed hair is retained in the follicle for a while and then shed. If the rest phase is long and hair is shed well before the next growth phase for that follicle, the skin appears relatively hairless. If the rest phase is short and the succeeding hair appears in the follicle shortly after or even before the earlier hair is gone, the skin appears hairy. Androgens influence the growth cycle by increasing the length of the growth phase and decreasing the length of the rest phase.

The hair growth pattern refers to the type of hair made by the follicle, either vellus or terminal. Follicles over most of the body produce only fine, fuzzlike vellus hair; however, follicles can be transformed to produce longer, coarser, pigmented terminal hair. In both sexes, androgens cause terminal hair to replace vellus hair in the pubic area and axillae. Additional androgen stimulation causes transformation of follicles on the face, chest, and abdomen.

Hirsutism can usually be traced to an endocrine origin.[44] It may be caused by the virilizing effects of excessive androgen or progestin production or by excessive adrenal corticosteroids. Hypertrichosis may be caused by drugs such as acetazolamide, phenothiazines, diazoxide, cyclosporine, minoxidil, penicillamine, psoralens, or phenytoin.[45] The central issue in determining whether self-treatment is advisable is separating the infrequent instances of endocrine or drug-induced disease from the vast majority of cases in which excess hair is purely a cosmetic problem. Whenever the signs of virilization are present or the pattern of hair growth has changed markedly, the patient should be referred to a physician for diagnosis. The patient's menstrual history can also be valuable; if menstruation is completely normal, the patient is unlikely to have serious endocrinopathy.

Methods of Hair Removal

Medical demands for hair removal are rare. Occasionally, ingrown beard hairs need to be removed and surgeons still remove hair from operative sites.[46] Pseudofolliculitis barbae is a frequent condition in African Americans in which the sharp tips of shaven beard hairs curve in a 180° arc toward the epidermis and penetrate the skin causing papules and pustules. Chemical depilatories can be useful in this condition because hair is cleanly removed at the skin surface to produce a blunt tip, which is less likely than a shaved hair to penetrate skin.[47]

There is no method to increase or decrease the number of hair follicles in the skin; these are fixed at birth. However, a hair can be removed at either the surface (depilation) or the roots (epilation). Because epilation removes the hair at a deeper point, it has to be repeated less often. All practical methods except electrolysis are temporary (Table 1). Women often shave hair from their legs and trunk but generally find shaving the face unacceptable.

TABLE 1	Methods of hair removal
Method	**Implement or process**
Depilation (action on the hair shaft)	
Shaving	Razor or electric shaver
Abrasion	Pumice or fiber
Dissolving	Chemicals, enzymes
Bleaching	Peroxides, organic acids
Epilation (action on the hair root)	
Extraction	Tweezers, wax, adhesives, powered devices for home use (e.g., Epilady®)
Toxins	Metabolic: endocrine or nutritional disorders
	Disease: infection, immune deficiency
	Poison: metals, drugs
Destruction	Electrolysis: galvanic
	Cautery: short-wave
	Chemical: phenol, acid
	Ionization: X-rays or gamma rays

Adapted with permission from Spoor HB. *Cutis* 1978; 21: 283.

Little evidence exists that shaving makes hair grow faster or coarser.[48,49]

Epilation

Local epilation by plucking may be a reasonable method of removing a few strong hairs. If removal of the hair is complete and includes the hair bulb, hair is not noticeable again for 3–6 weeks. However, damage to the follicles may sometimes cause infection or scarring.[48]

Wax epilation is essentially a form of mass plucking. A wax of low melting point (or adhesive semisolid on a backing material) applied to the skin rapidly solidifies and enmeshes hair. It is then quickly pulled off the skin, against the direction of hair growth, along with embedded hairs. If not done skillfully, this technique can be painful and allergic reactions to the adhesives can occur. It should not be used by diabetics or those with poor circulation because they are at greater risk for infection. The patient should be cautioned to make sure the wax is not too hot prior to use. Moreover, hair must be at least 1 mm long to be grasped by the wax. More recently, battery-powered devices such as Epilady® have become available. These devices catch hairs and pluck them as the device is moved across the skin.

Electrolysis

Permanent removal of hair by electrolysis (galvanic or shortwave diathermy) can be very tedious and expensive, even on facial hair, because only a few nonadjacent hairs should be treated at one time. Thus, it is useful for women with a few coarse hairs. Galvanic electrolysis is less traumatic but slower than wax epilation.[46] Even with good technique, the 15–25% of hairs in the telogen phase regrow, and the operation has to be done again. Although electrolysis is somewhat painful (the needle must be inserted into the bulb of the hair shaft), some dermatology experts feel that competent operators can produce excellent results. Self-operated electrolysis is not advisable because significant scarring may occur if the hair follicle is not destroyed correctly.

Depilation

Depilatory creams and lotions represent a logical and convenient alternative for hair removal. Most chemical depilatories are substituted mercaptans used in the presence of alkaline-reacting materials (e.g., calcium thioglycolate with calcium hydroxide). This combination has generally supplemented the sulfides of barium, strontium, and calcium, which are faster acting but are poisonous and have strong odors.

Chemical depilatories act by reducing disulfide bonds between cystine molecules in hair keratin. Increasing osmotic pressure within the hair fiber results in swelling and deterioration of the hair to a soft mass, which is easily wiped off the skin in 5–15 minutes. To some extent, skin is subject to the same degradation as hair because cystine makes up 15% of keratin in hair and 2% of keratin in skin.[50] Also, thioglycolate is a known contact allergen.[50] However, its presence seldom causes skin reactions, and when reactions do occur, they are usually irritant rather than allergic. Irritation is more likely to be a problem on the face.[48] Hair that regrows is less bristly than it is after shaving, so there is less itching during regrowth. Coarse, highly pigmented hair is harder to remove than vellus hair.

Thioglycolates Thioglycolates are present in the large majority of commercial preparations and are available as pastes, lotions, and creams. A 2–4% concentration is sufficient; higher concentrations do not work appreciably faster or better.[51] Increasing the concentration of alkali increases the depilation rate but also increases skin irritation. Thioglycolates are safe when applied topically and, at appropriate concentrations, have little systemic toxicity if absorbed.[51] They have only a mild odor. These preparations are oxidized by air; they should not be kept too long and they should be stored in a tightly covered container

Alkaline Sulfides Barium, calcium, or strontium sulfides act two to three times faster than thioglycolate[51] but are more irritating. They have a strong odor caused by hydrolysis of hydrogen sulfide and are poisonous if ingested. Sulfides are indicated for men with thick beard hair because thioglycolates act too slowly in such cases.[50]

Guidelines for Proper Use

The depilatory may be tested by applying it to a small patch of normal skin for 15 minutes and then washing it off. If no reaction occurs within 24 hours, a thick layer of depilatory may be applied with the enclosed plastic glove or applicator against the direction of hair growth. The depilatory is left on for 5–15 minutes, depending on the formulation; package directions should be followed carefully. The depilatory is then removed with a spatula or tissue (avoiding contact with water to minimize odor), and the skin is washed with mild soap and water. Some manufacturers provide an emollient lotion to soothe the skin and prevent dryness after treatment. If necessary, 1% hydrocortisone cream can be applied to treat irritation. The treatment may be repeated as needed, normally every 2–4 weeks.

Nonmedicated Shampoos

In contrast to body hair, scalp hair has long been a source of beauty and social distinction. Interestingly, it has only been in this century that much attention has been paid to cleansing it.

Originally, shampoos were made of relatively harsh soaps; today, synthetic detergents are used almost exclusively in commercial products. The success of modern shampoos is based not only on their cleansing properties, but also on their cosmetic properties—that is, ability to impart luster, beauty, and manageability to hair. A good shampoo makes hair feel clean, provides it with a gloss or sheen, and does not leave it "frizzy" or unmanageable or otherwise adversely affect its physical properties. Shampoos are often formulated to emphasize special properties, such as conditioning, adding body, having an appealing fragrance, or minimizing eye sting.

Physiology of Hair

Hair has three layers: the medulla, which receives nourishment from the root; the cortex, which contains pigment; and the cuticle, which is a thin, translucent layer that lets color shine through to the outside. An undamaged cuticle reflects light to give hair a healthy, shiny look. Damage to the cuticle reduces shine, allows split ends to occur, and makes hair susceptible to static electricity.[52] Normal hair varies in thickness (texture) from coarse to fine. Because hair is dead tissue, no product can "feed" hair to make it healthier.

Hair soil includes natural skin secretions, skin debris, dirt from the environment, and residue of hair grooming products. The scalp normally secretes enough oil to keep the hair glossy and the scalp comfortable. However, a buildup of oil between shampooing makes the hair limp and stringy, whereas too little oil makes hair dull, lifeless, "flyaway," and easily breakable.

Specialty Shampoos

Today's shampoos may promote any number of special components or properties. However, their primary benefit is still cleansing. Manufacturers must be cautious regarding therapeutic claims because such products would then be considered drugs by the FDA.

A conditioner is a product applied to the hair to restore oils, sheen, elasticity, and manageability. It is useful on dry, damaged, or overprocessed hair. Many shampoos include conditioners in the formulation, but conditioners are best applied after the shampoo. A cream rinse is a product used after a shampoo to smooth the cuticle, eliminate tangles, and make the hair manageable.

Protein shampoos may be used on fine, limp, or damaged hair. They may increase hair bulk because amino acids and small polypeptide fragments of hydrolyzed protein can become linked to the keratin of damaged hair shafts.[52,53] Most of the protein does not become a permanent part of the hair; it is only adsorbed temporarily and washed off again at the next shampoo.

Herbal shampoos may simply include a herbal fragrance or one of many botanical extracts that are present in small amounts and add nothing to the efficacy of the product. Although saponins are also a source of natural detergents, they are toxic and not included in current formulations.[54]

Baby shampoos contain nonirritating amphoteric detergents and few, if any, additives such as perfumes that could irritate eyes. Their mild cleansing action is desirable for fine or chemically treated hair.

Consumers should be wary of marketing claims for specialty shampoos because there is little real difference among them. In blinded tests, Ivory Dishwashing Liquid® performed as well as expensive specialty brands.[55]

Primary Ingredients

Soaps are sodium or potassium salts of fatty acids. Unfortunately, they tend to form insoluble mineral salts, which leave a dulling scum on the hair, especially in geographic areas with a hard public water supply. No major soap-based shampoos are currently on the market.[53]

With synthetic detergents, the carboxyl group of the fatty acid is replaced by another hydrophilic group, thus avoiding the negative properties of soaps. Detergents tend to be classified by their hydrophilic groups (e.g., anionic, cationic, amphoteric, or nonionic). Adult shampoos are usually anionic whereas those for children are more likely to be amphoteric or nonionic in composition. Cationic materials are more likely to be found in hair rinses and conditioners to neutralize static electricity imparted by anions. The most widely used detergent in shampoos is the anionic agent, sodium lauryl sulfate (a sulfated derivative of lauryl alcohol). It and other alkyl sulfates are completely effective in hard water, provide excellent foam, and leave hair feeling smooth and soft. They are also easily perfumed and easily rinsed out, and they do not become rancid. Sodium salts were used originally, but now ammonium or tri- and diethanolamine salts are often used because they are less drying to hair.

Nonionic and amphoteric detergents are also popular. They have low foaming properties but are especially mild to the eyes. Many shampoos contain a combination of detergents to balance their desirable characteristics.

Additives

Many secondary ingredients are routinely added to shampoos. Because most surfactants cleanse hair so well that it becomes unmanageable, conditioning agents are added to coat the hair with a very small amount of lubricating material to restore defects in the cuticle. These agents are emollients such as lanolin and its derivatives, glycerol, propylene glycol, and lauryl or octyl sarcosines. Cationic materials (e.g., fatty amines and quaternary ammonium compounds) are added to reduce the electrostatic charge on hair, but they are irritating to the eyes and are also adsorbed onto hair and retained after rinsing.

Foam builders and stabilizers (e.g., fatty acid alkanolamides) make the product more pleasing to use although a lot of foam is not a prerequisite to good cleansing. Thickeners, which may be simple salts (e.g., sodium chloride) or methylcellulose derivatives, also make the product more aesthetically acceptable by creating a rich feel. Sequestering agents, which include ethylenediaminetetraacetic acid (EDTA), citric acid, and pyrophosphates, prevent formation of calcium, magnesium, and iron soaps. Short-chain alcohols act as clarifying agents and make it easier to rinse the shampoo out. In creams and lotions, stearate and palmitate salts are added as opacifying agents. Finally, the formulation may include preservatives, antioxidants, buffering agents, perfumes, and dyes.

Shampoo Formulations

Shampoos are available in clear liquids, lotions, pastes, and gels, allowing for great latitude in physical and performance capabilities. Dry shampoos are mixtures of absorbent powders and mild alkalis that pick up soil from hair and scalp; they are valuable for ill or incapacitated persons who cannot wet their hair. Dry shampoos are left in the hair for a specified period and then are brushed or combed out.

Adverse Effects from Shampoos

Detergents can damage the stratum corneum skin barrier by removing natural skin oils, and can produce redness and cracking. Dermatologic conditions, and even vulvovaginitis in females, are more likely to occur when a child's hair is shampooed while the child is seated in the bathtub.[56] Most complaints about shampoos concern skin or eye irritation, but occasionally users may have an allergic skin reaction to a specific ingredient or additive, especially perfumes. Accidental oral ingestion of nonmedicated shampoo is unlikely to cause toxicity other than mild gastrointestinal irritation.[57]

Guidelines for Proper Use

All modern shampoos work very well with little to distinguish among them with regard to consumer acceptability.[55] The more effective a shampoo is in cleansing, the harsher it will be on hair. Those who shampoo more often (e.g., daily) should choose a gentle shampoo such as baby shampoo or one labeled for dry hair. Teenagers tend to have oily hair and should avoid conditioning shampoos, although a cream rinse will aid in combing and provide manageability. Structural differences in the hair of African Americans make their hair more inclined to dryness and fragility. Thus, African Americans should use milder shampoos or apply conditioner after shampooing.[34] Shampoos for dry or oily hair vary in the amount of detergent and conditioners in the formulation.

One sudsing and rinse is enough for frequent shampooing. Hair should be rinsed very well to remove all traces of shampoo. For best results, hair should be gently dried with a towel or blow dryer set at low temperatures.

Summary

The psychologic and cosmetic benefits of using personal care products are unquestionable. However, such products may be misused in terms of selection, frequency of use, or technique of application. Many products can cause direct contact irritation or allergic sensitivity, but perhaps the greatest hazards lie not with the product but with inadequate counseling regarding proper selection and use.

The available literature is not compelling about the value of vaginal deodorant and cleansing products used routinely. Antiperspirants and underarm deodorants, skin-bleaching agents, depilatories, and nonmedicated shampoos are appropriate for routine use if the user understands what can be reasonably expected from the product. The pharmacist's advice and counsel in product selection and use can be of great value.

References

1. McCue JD. Evaluation and management of vaginitis. *Arch Intern Med* 1989; 149: 565–8.
2. Foreman A, Smith CB. Vaginitis. *Postgrad Med* 1990; 88 (5): 123–33.
3. Thomason JL, Gelbart MD, Scagliane NJ. Bacterial vaginosis: current review with indications for asymptomatic therapy. *Am J Obstet Gynecol* 1991; 165: 1210–7.
4. Weaver CT, Mengel MB. Bacterial vaginosis. *J Fam Pract* 1988; 27 (2); 207–15.
5. Roy S. Nonbarrier contraceptives and vaginitis and vaginosis. *Am J Obstet Gynecol* 1991; 165: 1240–4.
6. Gravelt MG. Independent associations of bacterial vaginosis and chlamydia trachomatis with adverse pregnancy outcome. *JAMA* 1986; 256: 1899–1903.
7. Biffee JM. Vaginal candidiasis. *US Pharm* 1992; 17 (Feb suppl): 41–7.
8. Rosenberg MJ et al. Vaginal douching. *J Reprod Med* 1991; 36 (10): 753–8.
9. Gossel TA. Feminine hygiene products. *US Pharm* 1992; 17 (5): 24–32.
10. McGowan L. Peritonitis following the vaginal douche and a proposed alternative. *Am J Obstet Gynecol* 1965; 90 (4): 506–9.
11. Gossel TA. Feminine hygiene products: why your advice is needed. *US Pharm* 1986; 11 (5): 20–7.
12. Wolner-Hanssen P, Eschenbach DA, Paavonen J, et al. Association between vaginal douching and acute pelvic inflammatory disease. *JAMA* 1990; 263: 1936–41.
13. Dalin JR et al. Vaginal douching and the risk of tubal pregnancy. *Epidemiol* 1991; 2: 40–8.
14. *Federal Register* 1978; 43: 46694–732.
15. Sato K, Kang WH, Saga K, et al. Biology of sweat glands and their disorders: II. Disorders of sweat gland function. *J Am Acad Dermatol* 1989; 20: 713–26.
16. Lillis PJ, Coleman WP. Liposuction for treatment of axillary hyperhidrosis. *Dermatol Clin* 1990; 8 (3): 479–82.
17. Sato K. Hyperhidrosis. *JAMA* 1991; 265: 651.
18. Plechner S. Antiperspirants and deodorants. In: Balsam MS,

Sagarian E, eds. *Cosmetics: Science and Technology.* 2nd ed. New York: Wiley-Interscience; 1972, 2: 373–416.
19. Labows JN, McGinley KJ, Kligman AM. Axillary odor: current status. In: Frost P, and Horwitz SN, eds. *Principles of Cosmetics for the Dermatologist.* St. Louis, Mo: C.V. Mosby; 1982: 89–97.
20. Hurley HJ. Combined axillary hyperhidrosis and bromhidrosis. *JAMA* 1983; 250: 419.
21. White JW. Treatment of primary hyperhidrosis. *Mayo Clin Proc* 1986; 61: 951–6.
22. Manusov EG, Nadeau MT. Hyperhidrosis: a management dilemma. *J Fam Pract* 1989; 28: 412–5.
23. Electrical current for excessive sweating. *Med Lett Drugs Ther* 1986; 28: 109.
24. *Federal Register* 1982; 47:36492–505.
25. Holzle E, Kligman AM. Mechanism of antiperspirant action of aluminum salts. *J Soc Cosmetic Chem* 1979; 30: 279–95.
26. McWilliams SA, Montgomery I, Jenkinson DM, et al. Effects of topically-applied antiperspirant on sweat gland function. *Br J Dermatol* 1987; 117: 617–26.
27. Shelley WB, Hurley HJ. Anhydrous formulation of aluminum chloride for chronic folliculitis. *JAMA* 1980; 244: 1956–7.
28. Williams S, Freemont AJ. Aerosal antiperspirants and axillary granulomata. *Br Med J* 1984; 288: 1651.
29. Holzle E, Kligman AM. Factors influencing the antiperspirant action of aluminum salts. *J Soc Cosmetic Chem* 1979; 30: 357–67.
30. *Federal Register* 1977; 42: 41374–6.
31. Blake R. Determination of extent of deodorizing properties of chlorophyl. *J Am Podiatr Med Assoc* 1968; 58: 109–12.
32. *Federal Register* 1990; 55: 19862–8.
33. Majors PA, Wild JE. The evaluation of antiperspirant efficacy-influence of certain variables. *J Soc Cosmetic Chem* 1974; 25: 139–52.
34. Grimes PE, Davis LT. Cosmetics in Blacks. *Dermatol Clin* 1991; 9: 53–68.
35. *Federal Register* 1978; 43: 51546–55.
36. *Federal Register* 1982; 47: 39108–17.
37. Bleehan SS. Skin bleaching preparations. *J Soc Cosmetic Chem* 1977; 28: 407–12.
38. Jimbow K, Obeta H, Pathak M, et al. Mechanism of depigmentation by hydroquinone. *J Invest Dermatol* 1974; 62: 436–49.
39. Arndt KA, Fitzpatrick TB. Topical use of hydroquinone as a depigmenting agent. *JAMA* 1965; 194: 965–7.
40. Hoshaw RA, Zimmerman KG, Menter A. Ochronosis-like pigmentation from hydroquinone bleaching creams in American Blacks. *Arch Dermatol* 1985; 121: 105–8.
41. "AHFS Drug Information 92." Bethesda, Md: American Society of Hospital Pharmacists; 1992: 2187.
42. Mann RJ, Harman RM. Nail staining due to hydroquinone skin lightening creams. *Br J Dermatol* 1983; 108: 363–5.
43. *Federal Register* 1990; 55: 46914–21.
44. Casey JH. Hirsutism: pathogenesis and treatment. *Aust N Z J Med* 1980; 10: 240–5.
45. Miwa LJ, Shaefer MS, Stratta RJ, et al. Drug-induced hypertrichosis: case report and review of the literature. *DICP: Ann Pharmacother* 1990; 24: 365–8.
46. Spoor HB. Depilation and epilation. *Cutis* 1978; 21: 283–7.
47. Dunn JF. Pseudofolliculitis barbae. *Am Fam Physician* 1988; 38 (3); 169–74.
48. Richards RN, Uy M, Meharg G. Temporary hair removal in patients with hirsutism: a clinical study. *Cutis* 1990; 45: 199–202.
49. Wagner RF. Physical methods for the management of hirsutism. *Cutis* 1990; 45: 319–26.
50. Natow AJ. Chemical removal of hair. *Cutis* 1986; 38 (2): 91–2.
51. Barry RH. Depilatories. In: Balsam MS, Sagarian E, eds. *Cosmetics: Science and Technology.* 2nd ed. New York: Wiley-Interscience; 1972; 2: 39–72.
52. Draelos ZK. Hair cosmetics. *Dermatol Clin* 1991; 9: 19–27.
53. Goldenberg RL. Shampoo formulations and their effects on the scalp and hair. In: Frost P, Horwitz SN, eds. *Principles of Cosmetics for the Dermatologist.* St. Louis, Mo: C.V. Mosby; 1982: 13–5.
54. Hunting ALL. *Encyclopedia of Shampoo Ingredients.* Cranford, NJ: Micelle Press; 1983: 245.
55. Shampoos. *Consumer Rep* 1989; 54: 95–9.
56. Brown JL. Hair shampooing technique and pediatric vulvovaginitis. *Pediatrics* 1989; 83: 146.
57. Tyre DJ, Paloucak F. Personal shampoos and safety considerations. *Am J Hosp Pharm* 1991; 48: 937–8.

CHAPTER 28

Topical Anti-Infective Products

Dennis P. West and Susan V. Maddux

> **Questions to ask in patient assessment and counseling**
>
> - *What area of the skin is affected? How extensive is the area involved?*
> - *Is the skin broken? Is there pus? Is it painful?*
> - *How long have you had this condition? Have you ever had it before? Are any other members of your family affected?*
> - *Has the condition developed as the result of a previous rash or skin problem?*
> - *Has the condition worsened?*
> - *Do you have a fever or any flulike symptoms?*
> - *Do you have diabetes? Do you have any other medical conditions?*
> - *Do you have any allergies to topical medications?*
> - *What treatments have you tried for this condition? Were they effective?*
> - *What oral or topical medications are you presently using? Have they been effective?*

Topical anti-infectives are used to treat and prevent infection of various tissues (skin, hair, nails, and mucous membranes). The active ingredients of the products are antimicrobials; most are antibacterial or antifungal agents. Because this product classification is so broad, this chapter's content is limited to antimicrobial products for use in prevention and self-treatment of skin and vaginal infections.

Skin Assessment

Before recommending a topical product for self-medication of cutaneous infections, the pharmacist should assess the nature of the patient's complaint. Noninfectious processes, including drug-induced eruptions, should be considered.[1] Antimicrobial agents should generally be considered in cases of infectious etiology and in cases where secondary infection may occur.

Referral to a physician should be considered, especially if:

- There is doubt as to the causative factor or organism.
- Initial treatment has not been successful or the condition is getting worse.
- Applications of topical drug products have been used for prolonged periods over large areas, especially on denuded skin (potential for systemic toxicity).
- Exudate is excessive and continuous.
- Widespread infection has occurred.
- There is a predisposing illness, such as diabetes, systemic infection, or an immune deficiency.
- Fever, malaise, or both occur.
- A primary dermatitis (allergic dermatitis, psoriasis, or seborrhea) exists and becomes secondarily infected.
- Lesions are deep and extensive.
- Lancing is needed to aid drainage of exudate or provide pain relief.

The Normal Skin

The skin is the largest organ of the body and is involved in numerous physical and biochemical processes.[2] Normal skin thickness is 3–5 mm; it is thickest on the palms of the hand and soles of the feet and thinnest on eyelid and scrotal tissue. Human skin is composed of three functionally distinct regions (Figure 1). The outermost region (epidermis) is compact and nonvascular and consists of stratified squamous epithelial cells. The middle region (dermis) is vascular and contains connective tissue. These two regions are not similar in composition but they interconnect. The hypodermis, or subcutaneous tissue, is the innermost area; it is actually loose connective tissue and adipose tissue firmly anchored to the dermis.

The epidermis is composed of several distinct sublayers. The innermost, in close association with the dermis, is the stratum germinativum (basal cell layer), which consists of columnar/cuboidal epithelial cells. Above this layer is the prickle cell unit (stratum spinosum), composed of polygonal epithelial cells, which is thicker in the palms and soles than in other anatomic skin sites. These two epidermal sublayers are involved in mitotic processes of epidermal regeneration and repair. Prickle cells are produced by cellular division and contain keratinocytes, the pigment-forming melanocytes that contain melanin precursors, and melanin granules. As keratinocytes migrate to the skin surface, they change from living cells to dead, thick-walled, flat nonnucleated cells containing keratin, a fibrous protein.

Above the prickle cells is the granular sublayer (stratum granulosum), which is actually several thicknesses of

---

This chapter is based in part on the chapter with the same title that appeared in the 9th edition but was written by Michael R. Jacobs and Paul Zanowiak.

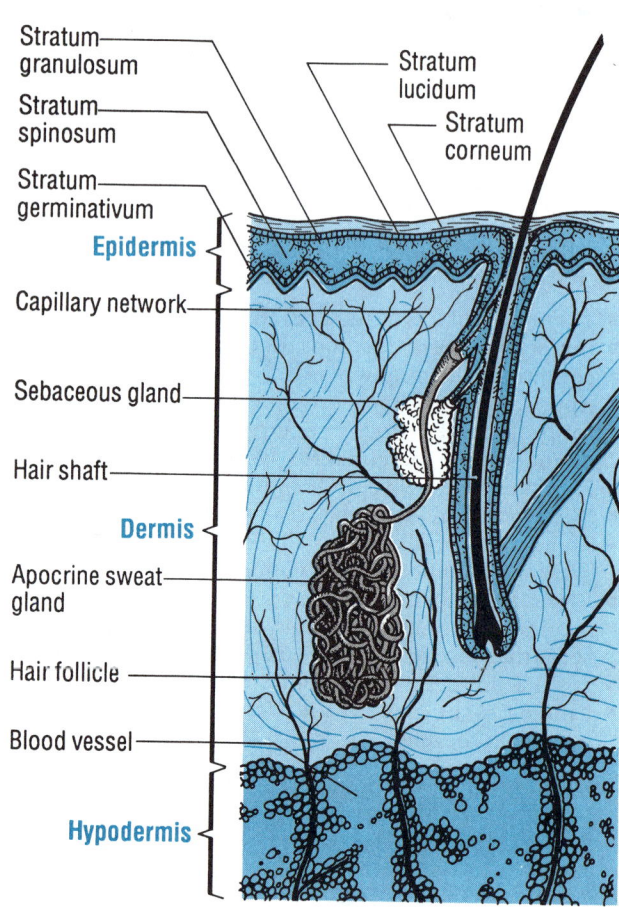

FIGURE 1 Cross section of human skin.

flattened polygonal cells. These cells contain granules of keratohyalin, which are changed to keratin in the outermost portion (the stratum corneum or horny outer layer) of the epidermis. A translucent, thin area (stratum lucidum), present in the palms and soles, lies between the stratum granulosum and the stratum corneum. The stratum lucidum is a narrow band of flattened, closely packed cells believed to be derived from keratohyalin. The stratum corneum is composed of flat, scaly, dead (keratinized) tissue. Its outermost cells are flat (squamous) plates that are constantly shed (desquamated).

Desquamated cells lost from the outer surface of the epidermis are replaced by new cells generated by the mitotic processes of the stratum spinosum and stratum germinativum. The newer cells push older ones closer to the surface. In the process they become flattened, decrease their water content, become more compact, and gradually lose their nuclei, taking their place on the skin surface.

The dermis, which supports the epidermis and separates it from the lower fatty layer, consists mainly of collagen and elastin embedded in a mucopolysaccharide substance. Fibroblasts and mast cells are found throughout. A network of nerves and capillaries is found in the dermis; this network comprises the neurovascular supply to dermal appendages (hair follicles, sebaceous glands, and sweat glands). Main regions of the dermis are known as papillary or reticular layers. The papillary sublayer, adjacent to the epidermis, is rich in blood vessels, and the papillae probably act as conduits to bring nutrients near the avascular epidermis. Below the papillae, the reticular layer contains coarser tissue that connects the dermis with the hypodermis.

Subcutaneous tissue, composed of relatively loose connective tissue of varying thickness, provides necessary pliability for human skin. This layer also includes a fatty component that facilitates thermal control and food reserve and provides cushioning or padding.

Skin Components

Hair Follicles

A hair shaft is generated by a hair papilla at the base of a follicle. A follicle is basically an inward tubular folding of the epidermis into the dermis. Within the follicle is a fiber (hair shaft) of keratinized epithelial cells that grows as a result of multiplication of cells in the papilla. Capillaries are also present in the follicle to provide nutrients to the hair.

Sebaceous Glands

Most sebaceous (sebum-producing) glands are located in the same anatomic area as the hair because they are usually adjacent to follicles. Sebaceous glands not associated with hair follicles may be found in genital areas, around the nipples, and on the border of the lips. Ducts of these glands are lined with epithelial cells that are continuous with basal cell layers of the epidermis. Sebum, which covers the hair and skin surface, is a mixture of free fatty acids (mainly palmitic and oleic), triglycerides, waxes, cholesterol, squalene, other hydrocarbons, and traces of fat-soluble vitamins. With sweat, sebum forms an emulsion that includes surface waste products of cutaneous cells.

Sweat Glands

Two types of sweat glands are identified in association with dermal anatomy: the eccrine and apocrine glands. Both are considered exocrine because their secretions (sweat) reach the skin surface.

Eccrine glands are independent of hair follicles and develop from the epithelium of the skin surface, extending in a coil to the dermis. Secretory epithelia are located in the hypodermis, and the ducts ascend through the epidermis. They are present over most of the body surface, except for genital areas and legs, and are especially numerous on palms and soles.

Eccrine sweat production is controlled by a heat regulatory center of the hypothalamus. Emotional stress and cholin-

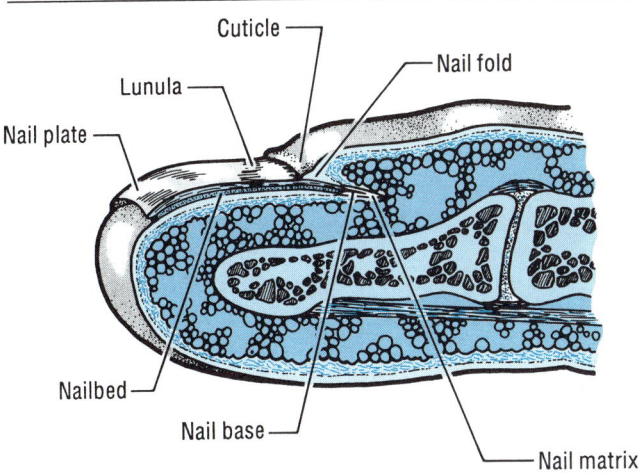

FIGURE 2 Anatomic features of the nail. Adapted with permission from *Integumentary Systems*. Roanoke, Va: CMRI; 1992: 22.

ergic drugs can also trigger eccrine sweating. The volume of eccrine sweat produced (several liters per day) is much greater than that of apocrine sweat.

An apocrine sweat gland is generally attached to a hair follicle by a duct, leading down into a coiled, secretory glandular tubule. These tubules are covered with myoepithelium, allowing contraction to adrenergic stimulation. Such stimulation, as in stress, releases a milky secretion that contains proteins, sugars, and lipids. This secretion is odorless until skin bacteria act on its contents, producing the characteristic pungent odor. Apocrine glands are present around the nipples, in axillae, and in the anogenital region. The glands do not function in body temperature regulation but are responsive to hormone secretion. Consequently, the onset of action of these glands is associated with puberty.

Nails

Nails are modifications of the keratinized region of epidermal tissue. The nail bed, on which the nail plate lies, derives from basal epidermis. At its periphery, the body of the plate is surrounded by the nail matrix. This matrix is derived from the nail groove, which is a process of the basal cell layer of the epidermis. At the base of the nail is the white area called the lunula (Figure 2).

Skin Surface

Secretions that accumulate on the skin surface are weakly acidic, with a pH of 4.5 to 5.5 (the acid mantle).[2] This pH varies slightly from individual to individual and from one area of the body to another; it is somewhat higher in areas where perspiration evaporates slowly.[3]

Various microorganisms live on the surface of intact skin. Individual species that make up the flora exist in a normal ecologic balance. Skin flora is diverse, including aerobic and anaerobic bacterial species. The species and number of organisms found on the skin may change over one's lifetime. Some individuals have a constantly high microbial population.

Percutaneous Absorption

The skin acts as a barrier between the environment and the body, partially protecting the body from harmful external agents such as pathogenic organisms and chemicals.[4] Its ability to carry out this function depends on a variety of factors, including the age of the individual, underlying disease states, use of certain oral or topical medications, and preservation of an intact stratum corneum.[5] The skin also contributes to sensory experiences and is involved in temperature control, development of pigment, and synthesis of some vitamins. It is important in hydroregulation because it controls moisture loss from the body and moisture penetration into the body.

Except for the stratum corneum, the cells of all layers use nutrients and oxygen and excrete water and carbon dioxide. Most oxygen is supplied from the blood, although a small amount is supplied from the external environment. Similarly, carbon dioxide is removed from the tissues mainly by the blood, but small amounts are discharged directly to the atmosphere.

Skin hydration is important to the health and normal function of the skin. If the corneal layer becomes dehydrated, it loses elasticity and its permeation characteristics become altered. The stratum corneum can be hydrated by water transfer from lower regions of the skin and by water accumulation (perspiration) induced by occlusive coverings, such as tight, impervious bandages or oleaginous pharmaceutical vehicles (e.g., petrolatum). Generally, such moisture accumulation seems to "open" the compactness of the stratum corneum for renewed suppleness and more effective penetration by some drug molecules. (See Chapter 30, "Dermatologic Products.")

The acid mantle has been postulated to be a protective mechanism because microbes tend to grow better at a pH of 6–7.5. Infected areas have higher pH values than those of normal skin. Several fatty acids (propionic, caproic, and caprylic) found in sweat and sebum inhibit microbial and fungal growth. Therefore, the importance of the acid mantle concept lies not solely in the inherent pH of the acid mantle, but also in the specific compounds responsible for the acidity.

Another protective mechanism is the buffer capacity of skin surface secretion. When pH is raised or lowered, the skin readjusts to a normal pH. Moreover, normal skin flora acts as a defense mechanism by controlling the growth of potential pathogenic organisms and their possible invasion of the skin and body.

A drug must be released from its vehicle if it is to exert an effect at the desired site of activity (the skin surface, the epidermis, or the dermis). Release of the drug from its vehicle occurs at the interface between the skin surface and the applied layer of product. The physical–chemical relationship between the drug and the base determines the rate and amount of drug released. Considerations such as the solubility of the drug in the vehicle, its diffusion coefficient in the vehicle, and its partition coefficient into sebum and stratum corneum are significant to its efficacy.6 A drug with a strong affinity for the vehicle has a lower rate and extent of percutaneous absorption than does a drug with weaker affinity to its vehicle. Thus, a drug with a proper balance of polar and hydrocarbon moieties (a partition coefficient approaching 1) penetrates the stratum corneum more readily than do drugs that are either highly polar or highly lipoidal, because that portion of the skin possesses both hydrated proteins and lipids.

Other factors influencing drug release include degree of hydration of the stratum corneum, pKa of the drug, pH of the drug vehicle and the skin surface, drug concentration, thickness of the applied layer, and temperature. Blood flow is altered dramatically by the temperature at the anatomic site of application. As temperature increases, blood flow in the area also increases, as does the rate of percutaneous absorption. These factors apply to drug release from all topical forms (e.g., powders, ointments, pastes, emulsified creams or lotions, gels, suspensions, and solutions).

Oily hydrocarbon bases such as petrolatum are transiently occlusive, promote hydration, and generally increase molecular transport. Hydrous emulsion bases are less occlusive; water-soluble bases (polyethylene glycols) are minimally occlusive. The latter, in fact, may attract water from the stratum corneum, thereby decreasing drug transport. Powders with hydrophilic ingredients presumably decrease hydration because they promote evaporation from the skin by absorbing available water.

Substances are transported from the skin surface to the general circulation through percutaneous absorption. The routes of such transport have not been proved, but it is presumed that they involve passage between the keratinized units of the stratum corneum and through skin appendages (hair follicles, sweat glands, and sebaceous glands). The major route of drug absorption is by passive diffusion through the stratum corneum, followed successively by transport through deeper epidermal regions and the dermis.

After application of a topical drug product, transport of the drug cannot begin until the surface of the stratum corneum is in contact with the applied drug. A lag time occurs while a drug is transferring from its vehicle into the sebum and stratum corneum.

Depending on the physical–chemical properties of a drug, the sebum, and various skin regions, drug movement into and through the skin meets with varying degrees of enhancement or inhibition. The stratum corneum provides the greatest resistance and is often a rate-limiting barrier to percutaneous absorption. Because it is nonliving tissue, the stratum corneum may be viewed as having the general characteristics of an artificial and semipermeable membrane, and molecular passage through it is mostly passive diffusion. Once a molecule has crossed the stratum corneum, there is much less resistance to its transport through the rest of the epidermis and into the dermis.

When the stratum corneum is hydrated, drug diffusion is generally accelerated. Because occlusion increases hydration of the stratum corneum, it enhances the transfer of most drugs; hydration swells the stratum corneum, loosening its normally tight, densely packed arrangement and making diffusion easier. The increased amount of water present in the skin under such conditions probably further enhances the transfer of polar molecules.

Wounds, burns, chafed areas, and extensive lesions of various dermatoses alter the integrity of the stratum corneum and result in artificial shunts of the percutaneous absorption process. Scarring and inflammation can also alter absorption. Such enhanced drug absorption could lead to potentially dangerous systemic drug levels by percutaneous absorption. Caution should be used in applying topical medication to damaged skin, especially if large surface areas are involved.

Causes of Skin Infection

Cutaneous infections may be caused by bacteria, fungi, viruses, or parasites. Many bacterial and fungal infections are amenable to topical therapy. The condition should be carefully assessed before a treatment is selected or the patient counseled.

Bacterial Skin Infections

Bacterial skin infections are commonly classified as pyodermas because exudate is often present. They are caused principally by species of beta-hemolytic *Streptococcus* and *Staphylococcus*.[5] The lesions result from external infection or reinfection and may be superficial or may involve deeper tissue. These pyodermic infections may be either primary (in which case no previous dermatoses exist) or secondary (in which case a predisposing problem preceded the infection). Other organisms may be present in secondary pyodermas, including Gram-negative bacteria (e.g., *Pseudomonas aeruginosa*), which are especially prevalent on warm moist skin such as axillae, ear canals, and interdigital spaces.

Infections by pathogenic organisms are related to the breakdown of the skin's "disinfecting" protective mechanisms or to the development of an abundance of colonies of pathogenic organisms.[5] A breakdown of the normal ecological balance may be enhanced by alterations in the skin's defense mechanisms.

Normally, the stratum corneum has only about 10% water content, which ensures elasticity but is generally below that needed to support luxuriant microbial growth.[5] An increase in moisture content may allow microbial growth, leading to infection. A break in the intact skin surface has a deleterious effect on the skin's defensive properties, allowing large numbers of pathogenic organisms to be introduced into the inner layers.

In addition, the risk of infection may be increased by excessive scrubbing and irritation of the skin (especially with strong detergents), excessive exposure to water, prolonged occlusion, excessively elevated skin temperature, or local injury.[5,7–9] Therefore, the presence and severity of microbial skin infection is generally dependent on the condition of the skin's defense mechanisms, the number of pathogenic organisms present, and the supportive nutrient environment for those organisms.

The main pyodermic infections are impetigo, ecthyma, erysipelas, folliculitis, furuncles (boils), carbuncles, and paronychia.

Impetigo

Impetigo, typically caused by species of *Staphylococcus*, *Streptococcus*, or both, is a relatively superficial infection. Direct contact with the infected exudate may result in transmission of organisms. Lesions first appear as small red spots that may evolve into characteristic vesicles (tiny sacs or blisters) filled with amber fluid.[10] Exudate accumulates and forms yellow or brown crusts (scabs) on the skin surface, often surrounded by erythematous skin. Eruptions may be annular (circular) with clear central areas or may be clustered or grouped. The exposed parts of the body are most easily affected, but no area of the skin is immune if autogenous reinfection is not controlled. (See color plates, photograph 9.) Impetigo is most common in children and is considered contagious. Generally, in primary impetigo (impetigo vulgaris) the responsible bacteria cause the infection directly.

Ecthyma

Ecthyma, like impetigo, may involve species of *Staphylococcus*, *Streptococcus*, or both, but the lesions extend much deeper into the dermis. The legs are most commonly affected, and the lesions often occur singularly and tend to be localized. The lesion usually begins as an erythematous pustule that rapidly erodes and becomes crusted. This condition often occurs as a secondary infection after mild trauma or injury to the skin. In humid tropical environments, the lesions may become quite destructive.

Erysipelas

Erysipelas, caused by species of Group A beta-hemolytic *Streptococcus*, is characterized by a rapidly spreading, red, edematous plaque. This superficial infection has sharply established borders and a glistening surface.[10] It occurs most often on the scalp and face, and the organisms enter through a break in the skin. (See color plates, photograph 10.) Erysipelas is usually accompanied by fever, chills, and malaise.

Folliculitis

Follicular pustules are usually superficial but may be deep, depending on the pathogen or the site involved. They involve only the hair shafts; surrounding tissue is usually minimally affected. Skin areas regularly exposed to water, grease, oils, tars, and other contaminants seem most susceptible to folliculitis.

Furuncles and Carbuncles

Furuncles and carbuncles are generally staphylococcal infections located in or around hair follicles. In these pyodermas, the lesion may start as superficial folliculitis but may develop into a deep nodule. (See color plates, photograph 11.) The fully established furuncle has elevated swelling, is erythematous, and is often painful. Furuncles are more common in males. Hairy areas and areas subject to maceration and friction (collar, waist, buttocks, and thighs) seem most vulnerable. The initial erythema and swelling stage is followed by thinning of the skin around the primary follicle, centralized pustulation, destruction of the pilosebaceous structure, discharge of the core (plug), and central ulceration. Scarring may occur.

Although furuncles are usually primary infections, they may occasionally be secondary infections related to other dermatoses or diseases. Diabetes mellitus or agammaglobulinemia may predispose an individual to furuncles or carbuncles. Chronic cases of these pyodermas should be referred to a physician for evaluation of a possible underlying disease.

Carbuncles begin in a manner similar to furuncles and may have similar etiologies. Carbuncles involve clusters of follicles, with deeper and broader penetration over a larger area than furuncles. Furuncles may develop into carbuncles by infiltration or infection of adjacent follicles.

Paronychia

Paronychia is a pyogenic infection of the nails, accompanied by swelling and tenderness of the surrounding tissue. Paronychia is caused primarily by beta-hemolytic species of *Streptococcus* or *Staphylococcus*. Moderate pressure may force a pus exudate, and the nail may develop with irregularities. (See color plates, photograph 12.) It is important that this condition be differentiated from candidal or other fungal infections of the nails.

Fungal Skin Infections

Fungal skin infections, often called dermatomycoses, are among the most common cutaneous disorders.[11] Characteristically, they exhibit single or multiple lesions that may produce mild scaling or deep granulomas (inflamed nodular-sized lesions). Superficial infections affect the hair, nails, and skin and are generally caused by three genera of fungi: *Trichophyton*, *Microsporum*, and *Epidermophyton*. Species of *Candida* may also be involved.[12] Fungal infections of hairless skin are generally superficial and the organisms are found in or on the uppermost skin layers.

Tinea Pedis

Tinea pedis, also known as athlete's foot or ringworm of the feet, is caused by several species of fungi. (See Chapter 37, "Foot Care Products.")

Tinea Capitis

Transmitted by direct contact with infected persons or animals, ringworm of the scalp is caused by species of *Microsporum* or *Trichophyton*. Most cases occur in children. Depending on the causative organism, the clinical presentation varies from noninflamed areas of hair loss to deep, crusted lesions, which may lead to scarring and permanent hair loss. (See color plates, photograph 13.) These large lesions, similar to carbuncles in appearance, are called kerions.

Tinea Cruris

Tinea cruris (also called jock itch) is caused by *Epidermophyton floccosum*, *Trichophyton rubrum*, or *Trichophyton mentagrophytes*. It occurs on the medial and upper parts of the thighs and the pubic area and is more common in males. The lesions have specific margins that are elevated slightly and are more inflamed than the central parts; small vesicles are found at the margins. Acute lesions are bright red and turn brown in chronic cases; they may scale. This condition is generally bilateral with severe pruritus.

Tinea Corporis

Species of *Trichophyton* or *Microsporum* are the causative organisms of ringworm of the skin. There is a higher incidence of tinea corporis among persons living in humid climates. The lesions involve glabrous (smooth and bare) skin and begin as small, circular, erythematous, scaly, pruritic areas. They spread peripherally and the borders may contain vesicles or pustules. Tinea corporis should be differentiated from noninfectious dermatitis; the lesions may be similar in appearance.

Moniliasis (Candidiasis)

Moniliasis or candidiasis, caused mainly by *Candida albicans*, usually occurs in intertriginous areas such as the groin, axillae, interdigital spaces, under the breasts, and at the corners of the mouth. Involvement of the mucous membranes may be known as thrush, vaginal candidiasis, or pruritus ani, depending on the area affected. Candidal paronychia is most common in people whose activities involve routine immersion of the hands in water. Infection, malignancy, and systemic diseases such as diabetes may lower general resistance and allow candidal infections to flourish. Certain drugs, including oral antibiotics and steroids, may also contribute to candidal infection when used over prolonged periods of time.

Tinea Versicolor

Tinea versicolor is a common superficial fungal infection of the stratum corneum caused by *Pityrosorum orbiculare*. This organism is part of the normal flora in most individuals but is capable of becoming pathogenic under certain conditions. The most distinctive clinical feature is the change in pigmentation on the affected sites, ranging from white to medium brown. The shade of the macular lesions depends on the pigmentation of the individual; lesions usually occur on seborrheic areas of the body in a confetti-like configuration (See color plates, photographs 14A and B). Because mild scaling and pruritus are the only other sequelae, tinea versicolor is generally considered a disease of cosmetic disfigurement.

Viral Skin Infections

Viral infections may occur directly in or on the skin and may present as warts, molluscum contagiosum, herpes simplex,[13,14] or varicella-zoster infections (shingles, [herpes zoster] usually in adults, and varicella [chickenpox], usually in children).

Herpes Simplex

Herpes simplex virus may infect the skin and mucous membranes. The causative agent is a large virus, *Herpesvirus hominis*. (See color plates, photograph 15.) There are two types: type 1 (HSV-1), which causes fever blisters or cold sores and is most commonly found in the perioral area, and type 2 (HSV-2), which is most commonly seen as genital lesions.

Varicella-Zoster Infections

Chickenpox, which is highly contagious and generalized, usually develops in the nonimmune host; shingles, which is localized and painful, tends to develop in the partially immune host. Immunosuppressed patients are quite vulnerable to the varicella-zoster virus.

Shingles probably results after reactivation of a latent virus, which resides in the dorsal root or cranial nerve ganglion cells. Patients with shingles usually have a past history of chickenpox. Lesions usually occur along a single dermatome unilateral to the midline of the body; they appear as clustered vesicles on an erythematous base. The involved area may coalesce to form plaques that may be very painful. Peripheral neuropathy (nerve pain) may develop and persist over weeks or months. Regional lymph nodes are generally tender. (See color plates, photographs 16A and B.)

Molluscum Contagiosum

Molluscum contagiosum is a viral tumor caused by a poxvirus containing deoxyribonucleic acid. The disease is contracted by direct contact with an infected person, by contact with a fomite, or by autoinoculation.

The virus is manifested by one or more small (3–5 mm), pink, slightly raised lesions usually found on the abdomen, inner thigh, or perianal area. The mature lesion has a slight depression on the top and a soft core that can be expressed easily.

Patient Information

For bacterial and fungal infections, intermittent applications are considered poor therapy; regular applications are preferable. If increased irritation occurs, the patient should be instructed to contact a physician. Proper application technique should be described to the patient to prevent overmedication or undermedication. In addition to information about nonprescription drug usage, the pharmacist may also provide information that will help eradicate the infection and minimize the likelihood of future infections. Such information would address proper cleaning of the infected area, avoiding the use of tight-fitting or occlusive clothing, and avoiding situations that could lead to recurring infections.

Moreover, the patient should be told the expected duration of therapy and what conditions would indicate a need for physician-directed care (e.g., the development of a secondary bacterial infection). In general, the patient should see substantial improvement in 1 week; if this does not occur, the patient should be referred to a physician. Recurring skin infections may be a sign of undiagnosed diabetes or other organic problems. Patients with recurring infections should be referred to a physician.

Treatment and Prevention of Bacterial Skin Infections

The therapeutic and prophylactic use of nonprescription topical antimicrobial products should be limited to superficial conditions that involve small areas of the body surface. Self-administered topical products should be viewed as extensions of supportive treatment (proper cleaning, proper hygiene, and clean bandaging). Inappropriate self-treatment may cause scarring and spread the infection.

Topical self-medication with anti-infective products should be reserved for superficial first-aid uses or uncomplicated infections. More serious or deeper tissue infections usually require systemic therapy. Although many anti-infective nonprescription products are available, few have been studied under controlled conditions. Comparative studies are also limited in number.

For the treatment of impetigo, systemic or topical prescription antibiotics are preferred. Topical nonprescription agents seem to be most effective when lesions are superficial and are not extensive.[15] Cleaning the area with mild soap and water and gently removing loose crusts should improve response to topical therapy. Streptococcal infection can occur in other tissues (renal, heart valve, etc.) concurrent with impetigo. Most physicians, therefore, treat impetigo infections with systemic as well as topical products.

Although less objective information is available for other bacterial skin infections (e.g., erysipelas, ecthyma, and folliculitis), treatment with the medications listed above may be effective as long as the infection is not extensive. Furuncles and carbuncles may require lancing, which should be done by or under the direction of a physician. Bacterial infection of the nails is rare and may require drainage as well as treatment with systemic antibiotics.

The use of first-aid antibiotics helps to prevent infection in minor cuts, scrapes, and burns. Cleaning the wound with mild soap and water or with hydrogen peroxide and covering it with an appropriate dressing may be the only treatment necessary. A physician should be consulted if the area becomes inflamed or painful or if pus develops

First-Aid Antibiotics

Topical nonprescription antibiotics (e.g., bacitracin, chlortetracycline hydrochloride, neomycin sulfate, and polymyxin B sulfate in combination with neomycin, bacitracin, or both) are indicated to help prevent infection in minor cuts, scrapes, and burns.[16] Oxytetracycline, in combination with polymyxin B sulfate, is also indicated. Polymyxin B sulfate, neomycin, and bacitracin may also be used in combination with local-anesthetic active ingredients for this purpose.

Bacitracin

Bacitracin, including its zinc salt, is a polypeptide antibiotic that is generally bactericidal. Bacitracin acts to inhibit cell-wall synthesis. Topically, the drug is minimally absorbed. However, hypersensitivity reactions ranging from localized pruritus and edema to anaphylactic reactions may occur. The drug is active against several Gram-positive organisms. The development of resistance in previously sensitive organisms is rare. Topical nonprescription preparations usually contain 400–500 units per gram of ointment and are applied one to three times a day.[17]

Neomycin

Neomycin, an aminoglycoside antibiotic, is effective against many Gram-negative organisms and some species of *Staphylococcus*. Resistant organisms may develop. Neomycin appears to inhibit protein synthesis by irreversibly binding to the 30S ribosomal subunit. Neomycin is considered to be bactericidal. Neomycin applied topically produces a relatively high rate of hypersensitivity; reactions occur in 5–8% of patients.[18] Although it is not absorbed when applied to intact skin, application to large areas of denuded skin has been known to cause systemic toxicity (ototoxicity and nephrotoxicity).[18]

Neomycin is available in cream and ointment forms, alone or in combinations. The concentration commonly used in nonprescription products is 3.5 mg/g (equivalent to 5 mg/g of neomycin sulfate). Applications are made one to three times a day. Neomycin is most frequently used in combination with polymyxin and bacitracin to prevent the development of neomycin-resistant organisms. Because neomycin is a relatively common cause of allergic contact dermatitis and because it is not essential to topical antibacterial coverage of skin infections, it is rarely recommended by the dermatologic community. The combination of bacitracin and polymyxin B sulfate is more widely accepted for clinical use in dermatology than the combination of bacitracin, polymyxin B sulfate, and neomycin (triple antibiotic)

Polymyxin B Sulfate

Polymyxin B sulfate is effective against several Gram-negative bacteria but not against Gram-positive bacteria or fungi. Fewer resistant organisms develop with polymyxin B sulfate than with neomycin. It is presumed to accomplish its antibacterial action by altering the permeability of the bacterial cell wall. Toxicity rarely occurs with topical therapy. Concentrations of 5,000 units per gram and 10,000 units per gram are available in nonprescription combination preparations. Applications are usually made one to three times a day. Because Gram-negative organisms may secondarily invade a Gram-positive infection, polymyxin B sulfate serves to minimize growth of these organisms.

Tetracyclines

Tetracycline, chlortetracycline, and oxytetracycline are broad-spectrum antibiotics. They are presumed to exert their bacteriostatic effects by binding to the 30S ribosomal subunit and thus inhibiting bacterial protein synthesis. Three-percent ointments of tetracycline and chlortetracycline are available as nonprescription agents; toxicity is rare when they are applied topically. Long-term use may lead to overgrowth of nonsusceptible bacteria or fungi. Oxytetracycline is included by the Food and Drug Administration (FDA) in its final monograph for nonprescription use only in combination with polymyxin B sulfate. These products are usually applied one to three times a day. Because tetracycline products oxidize in the presence of light on human skin, they may turn the skin a reversible yellow-brown color that is not cosmetically pleasing to most patients. They may also trigger hypersensitivity reactions in allergic patients, some of whom may have severe reactions even if exposure is by topical application only.

Antiseptic Products

Antiseptic products, which are subject to FDA's ongoing review of nonprescription topical antimicrobial drug products, encompass three groups of products that may contain the same active ingredients but are labeled and marketed for different intended uses. These products include health care

TABLE 1 Summary of FDA's proposed classification of first-aid antiseptic active ingredients

Category I[a]	Category II[b]	Category III[c]
Single ingredients	**Single ingredients**	**Single ingredients**
Alcohol (48–95%)	Ammoniated mercury	Benzyl alcohol
Benzalkonium chloride (0.1–0.13%)	Cloflucarban	Calomel (mercurous chloride)
Benzethonium chloride (0.1–0.2%)	Fluorosalan	Chlorobutanol
Hexylresorcinol (0.1%)	Mercuric chloride (mercury chloride)	Chloroxylenol
Hydrogen peroxide topical solution (USP)	Mercuric oxide, yellow	Merbromin
Iodine tincture (USP)	Mercuric salicylate	Mercufenol chloride (orthohydroxyphenylmercuric chloride, orthochloromercuriphenol)
Iodine topical solution (USP)	Mercuric sulfide, red	Phenylmercuric nitrate
Isopropyl alcohol (50–91.3%)	Mercury	Secondary amyltricresols
Methylbenzethonium chloride (0.13–0.5%)	Mercury oleate	Triclocarban
Phenol (0.5–1.5%)	Mercury sulfide	Triclosan
	Nitromersol	
Combinations	Parachloromercuriphenol	**Combinations and/or complexes**
Eucalyptol (0.091%), menthol (0.042%), methyl salicylate (0.055%), and thymol (0.063%) in alcohol (26.9%)	Thimerosal	Iodine complex (ammonium ether sulfate and polyoxyethylene sorbitan monolaurate)
	Tribromsalan	Iodine complex (phosphate ester of alkylaryloxy polyoxyethylene glycol)
Complexes	Vitromersol	
Camphorated metacresol (3–10.8% camphor and 1–3.6% metacresol) in a ratio of 3:1	Zyloxin	Mercufenol chloride and secondary amyltricresols
	Combinations and/or complexes	
Camphorated phenol (10.8% camphor and 4.7% phenol) in a light mineral oil (USP) vehicle	None	Nonylphenoxypoly (ethyleneoxy) ethanoliodine
		Poloxamer–iodine complex
Povidone–iodine complex (5–10%)		Triple dye
		Undecoylium chloride iodine complex

[a]Ingredients generally recognized as safe and effective for over-the-counter first-aid use within the established concentration(s).
[b]Ingredients not generally recognized as safe for over-the-counter first-aid use.
[c]Ingredients for which the available data are insufficient to make a final determination for over-the-counter first-aid use.

antiseptics for consumer and professional use and first-aid antiseptics discussed below.

First-Aid Antiseptics.

In 1991, FDA issued a proposed rule for first-aid antiseptic drug products. Table 1 summarizes FDA's proposed classification of first-aid antiseptic ingredients.[19]

Ethanol Ethanol has good bactericidal activity in a 20–70% concentration. It acts relatively quickly but has little residual effect. In concentrations above 80%, however, its bactericidal effect is low. It rapidly denatures cellular protein of microorganisms, lowers the surface tension of bacteria to assist in their removal, and has a solvent effect on sebum. It is not an effective antiviral agent, nor does it kill spores. It is not a desirable wound antiseptic because it irritates already damaged tissue. The coagulum formed may, in fact, protect the bacteria.

Ethanol usually contains denaturants. Exposure to high concentrations will dehydrate the stratum corneum. Excessive systemic ingestion usually produces alcoholic intoxication and severe gastrointestinal distress. The gastrointestinal symptoms will be exacerbated if denatured alcohol is ingested.

Isopropyl Alcohol Isopropyl alcohol has somewhat stronger bactericidal activity and lower surface tension than ethanol. It is generally used for its cleansing and antiseptic effects on the skin. It can be used undiluted or as a 70% aqueous solution. Denaturants are not added because isopropyl alcohol itself is not potable. Isopropyl alcohol has a greater potential for drying the skin (astringent action) because its lipid solvent effects are stronger than those of ethanol.

Iodine Solutions of elemental iodine or those that release iodine from chemical complexes are used as presurgical skin antiseptics and as wound antiseptics. Their antimicrobial effect is attributed to their ability to oxidize microbial protoplasm. Strong iodine solution (Lugol's) must not be used as an antiseptic. An iodine solution (USP) of 2% iodine and 2.5% sodium iodide is used as an antiseptic for superficial wounds. An iodine tincture (USP) of 2% iodine, 2.5% sodium iodide, and about 50% alcohol is less preferable than the aqueous solution because it is irritating to the tissue.

In general, bandaging should be discouraged after iodine application to avoid tissue irritation. Iodine solutions stain skin, may be irritating to tissue, and may cause allergic sensitization in some people. These agents may also be absorbed through the skin in amounts sufficient to inhibit thyroid activity if used chronically. Therefore, prolonged use should be monitored carefully.

Iodophors Iodophors are organic complexes of iodine. Two of these complexes are povidone–iodine (Betadine®) and poloxamer iodine. Free iodine, released slowly from the iodophor complex, is responsible for the antiseptic effects of these agents. The percentage of active ingredient varies according to the product type, from 0.5 to 1% in ointments to 0.75% in shampoos and antiseptics. Iodophors are less irritating, less staining, and less sensitizing than iodine solutions. They may inhibit thyroid activity after percutaneous absorption, but such occurrences are rare with limited use.

Chlorhexidine Gluconate Chlorhexidine gluconate is a biguanide and resembles quaternary ammonium salts.[20] It is effective against both Gram-positive and Gram-negative bacteria and some fungi. It exhibits residual adherence to skin surfaces.

Some surfactants and serum proteins can reduce the antiseptic potential of chlorhexidine gluconate; it exhibits low potential for sensitization and irritation.[20] A prominent warning against use in the ear appears on the labels of nonprescription products containing this compound.

Mercurial Compounds Several mercurial compounds have antiseptic properties. In general, however, they are considered poor antiseptics for skin wounds because serum and tissue proteins reduce their antimicrobial potency. If these compounds are used extensively on areas of abraded skin, mercury may be absorbed in significant amounts and systemic poisoning may result. The use of mercurial compounds for extensive abrasions should be discouraged.

Inorganic salts of mercury are tissue irritants. This toxic property is reduced when mercury is incorporated into an organic compound. Some investigators believe that the alcoholic component of mercurial tinctures has a greater antimicrobial effect than the mercurial component.[21]

Merbromin Merbromin is less effective as a skin antiseptic than most other organic mercurials. However, it is used in some cases as a preoperative germicide (2%, aqueous). Serous fluids reduce its antimicrobial potency.

Nitromersol Nitromersol is a more effective antiseptic than soluble inorganic compounds of mercury, but it is less effective than ethanol or isopropyl alcohol. It is not a serious tissue irritant and it is available as a tincture in a dilution of 1:200.

Thimerosal Thimerosal has antibacterial and antifungal properties, but it is less effective than ethanol or isopropyl alcohol. It is found in several types of topical products, including aqueous solutions, tinctures, ointments, creams, and aerosols. Systemic toxicity occurs less frequently with thimerosal than with other mercurials because the mercury in thimerosal is tightly bound to the organic configuration. However, allergic contact dermatitis is a relatively high risk with thimerosal. Thimerosal is a common preservative in ophthalmic products and injectable products, including some vaccines. Patients with a history of allergic contact dermatitis to mercurials should avoid products containing thimerosal. The usual concentration is 0.1%.

Hydrogen Peroxide Hydrogen peroxide (topical solution, USP) is the most widely used first-aid antiseptic. It is an antimicrobial oxidizing agent; sodium and zinc peroxides are also used. Enzymatic release of oxygen from hydrogen peroxide occurs when it comes into contact with blood and tissue fluids. Mechanical release (fizzing) of the oxygen has a cleansing effect on a wound, but organic matter reduces its effectiveness. The duration of action is only as long as the period of active oxygen release. Using hydrogen peroxide on intact skin is of minimal value, because the release of nascent oxygen is too slow.

Hydrogen peroxide should be used where released gas can escape; therefore, it should not be used in abscesses, nor should bandages be applied before the compound dries.

Phenolic Compounds In very dilute solutions, phenol is an antiseptic and disinfectant. It has local anesthetic activity and is claimed to be an antipruritic in concentrations of 1:100 to 1:200 (e.g., phenolated calamine lotion). In aqueous solutions of more than 1%, it is a primary irritant and should not be used on the skin except as a keratolytic or peeling agent.

Oleaginous Phenolic Solutions Oily solutions of phenol and camphor are often used as nonprescription antiseptics in the treatment of minor cuts, insect bites, athlete's foot, fever blisters, and cold sores. Such products contain relatively high concentrations of phenol (4%) and must be used with caution. If oleaginous phenolic solutions are applied to moist areas, partitioning of the phenol out of the vehicle into water results in caustic concentrations of phenol on the skin. To avoid such damaging effects, these products should be applied only to dry skin.

Triclosan Triclosan is used as a deodorant in soap bars at concentrations up to 0.5%,[21] although the usual concentration is 0.3%.[22] It has been placed by the FDA in Category III for use as a first-aid antiseptic.[19] The FDA has proposed that it may be effective and has placed it in Category III for use as a handwash, patient preoperative skin preparation, and surgical hand scrub

Hexylresorcinol Hexylresorcinol (0.1%) is more effective than phenol as an antibacterial agent and is less toxic. It has been used in mouthwashes. The FDA has judged it safe and effective (Category I) as a first-aid antiseptic.[23] Even though it is used in low concentrations, it may be irritating.

Parachlorometaxylenol Parachlorometaxylenol is another name for chloroxylenol.

Quaternary Ammonium Compounds Quaternary ammonium compounds are cationic surfactants that have antimicrobial effects on Gram-positive and Gram-negative bacteria, but not on spores. Gram-negative bacteria are more resistant than Gram-positive ones; thus, they need a longer period of exposure. Quaternary ammonium compounds are sometimes included in topical anti-infective products. In addition to their antiseptic properties, these agents are used for their cleansing properties. Quaternary ammonium compounds emulsify sebum and have a detergent effect that assists in removing dirt, bacteria, and desquamated epithelial cells. Their antimicrobial activity consists of disrupting cell membranes and denaturing the lipoproteins of microbes. The "quats" can be inactivated by various anionic adjuvant ingredients (e.g., soaps and viscosity-building agents).

The FDA's proposed monograph for first-aid antiseptics includes benzalkonium chloride, benzethonium chloride, and methylbenzethonium chloride.[19] These compounds are formulated as creams, dusting powders, and aqueous or alcoholic solutions. Concentrates are available for dilution to proper concentration for topical use.

If used undiluted, these concentrates may cause serious skin irritation. Quaternary compounds are irritating to the eyes, so caution must be used when applying them to skin near the eyes. For use on broken or diseased skin, concentrations of 1:5,000 to 1:20,000 may be used. For use on intact skin and minor abrasions, a concentration of 1:750 is recommended.

Treatment of Fungal Skin Infections

Agents used for cutaneous fungal infections are found in ointments, creams, powders, and aerosols. Clioquinol (3%), clotrimazole (1%), haloprogin (1%), miconazole nitrate (2%), clotrimazole (1%), povidone–iodine (10%), tolnaftate (1%), and various undecylenates (10–25%) are considered safe and effective by the FDA.[24] The FDA has issued a proposed notice of rulemaking, effective February 26, 1993, that has determined that certain topical antifungals should not be generally recognized as safe and effective for nonprescription use (Table 2).[25]

Creams or solutions are the most efficient and effective antifungal dosage forms for delivery of the active agent into the epidermis. Sprays and powders are less effective because they are often not rubbed into the skin. They are probably more useful as adjuncts to a cream or solution dosage form or as prophylactic agents in preventing new or recurrent infections.

When a cream or solution is used to treat an active fungal infection, it is important that the patient understand that the product needs to be massaged into the entire area. For example, in treating tinea pedis, the patient must apply the product between all toes, to the skin around

TABLE 2 Nonprescription topical antifungal ingredients

Topical nonprescription antifungal drug products generally recognized as safe and effective

Clioquinol	Povidone–iodine
Clotrimazole	Tolnaftate
Haloprogin	Undecylenates
Miconazole nitrate	

Topical nonprescription antifungal drug products not generally recognized as safe and effective[a]

Alcloxa	Phenol
Alum, potassium	Phenolate sodium
Aluminum sulfate	Phenyl salicylate
Amyltricresols, secondary	Propionic acid
Basic fuchsin	Propylparaben
Benzethonium chloride	Resorcinol
Benzoic acid	Salicylic acid
Benzoxiquine	Sodium borate
Boric acid	Sodium caprylate
Camphor	Sodium propionate
Candicidin	Sulfur
Chlorothymol	Tannic acid
Coal tar	Thymol
Dichlorophen	Tolindate
Menthol	Triacetin
Methylparaben	Zinc caprylate
Oxyquinoline	Zinc propionate
Oxyquinoline sulfate	

[a]Effective February 26, 1993.

every toenail, and to the entire sole of the foot. Because the infection almost always includes both feet, the patient should treat both feet with identical thoroughness, even if erythema and scaling are predominant on one foot.

In a final rule published December 18, 1992, the FDA established "that any over-the-counter (OTC) topical antifungal drug product for use in the treatment and/or prevention of diaper rash is not generally recognized as safe and effective and is misbranded." (See *Federal Register* 1992; 57: 60429–31). This final rule becomes effective June 18, 1993.

Chloroxylenol

In 0.5–3.75% concentrations, chloroxylenol (parachlorometaxylenol) is classified as safe for use for up to 13 weeks for the treatment of athlete's foot, jock itch, or ringworm. However, additional safety data (for long-term, repeated use) and clinical efficacy data are needed before the FDA can place chloroxylenol in Category I.[24]

Undecylenic Acid

Undecylenic acid has the greatest antifungal activity of the fatty acids. It is a fungistatic agent, requiring prolonged exposure at relatively high concentrations to be effective.

It is used as a zinc, calcium, or copper salt in ointment, cream, powder, and aerosol forms (2–5% acid, 20% salt) for an additive antifungal effect.

Haloprogin

Haloprogin products include haloprogin 1% cream and solution. Haloprogin is an effective alternative for the treatment of athlete's foot, jock itch, and ringworm. The compound has significant antibacterial activity against several species of *Trichophyton* as well as *Streptococcus*, *Staphylococcus*, and *Candida*.[26]

Haloprogin has been shown to be superior to placebo[27] and equal in effectiveness to tolnaftate.[27,28] One investigator found higher cure rates and fewer relapses with haloprogin than with tolnaftate when laboratory criteria were used (potassium hydroxide slide preparations and cultures), although clinical cure rates were equal.[29] Side effects of the topically applied drug are relatively rare and minor. They include burning, itching, and scaling of the skin. Should these side effects occur, use of the preparation should be discontinued.

Miconazole and Clotrimazole

Miconazole nitrate and clotrimazole are imidazole-structured topical antifungals originally approved for prescription use but now reclassified as nonprescription agents. They are active against fungi and some Gram-positive bacteria but not against Gram-negative bacteria.[30] Their broad spectrum includes common dermatophytes, the organism causing tinea versicolor, and *Candida albicans*.

Treatment with miconazole and clotrimazole results in a low rate of recurrent infection when therapy is continued for 2 weeks or more, depending on the clinical disorder.[31,32] However, the onset of recurrence may simply be delayed in several cases. Allergic contact sensitization is rare and other side effects are usually self-limiting on discontinuation of the preparation.

Selenium Sulfide

Selenium sulfide is usually effective in the treatment of tinea versicolor. It is a potential irritant, and contact with the eyes and sensitive skin areas should be avoided. Although selenium sulfide is not absorbed in significant amounts when applied to the skin, it is hazardous if swallowed, producing central nervous system effects and respiratory and vasomotor depression. Areas affected by tinea versicolor should be lathered with the agent for 5 minutes only and washed off thoroughly. This treatment should be repeated daily for 2 weeks or until a response is noted, then tapered to twice weekly and then once weekly according to response. Patients with recurrent tinea versicolor may use the product on a weekly basis indefinitely.

Tolnaftate

Tolnaftate is a topical antifungal agent that is effective against most superficial dermatophytes but ineffective in the treatment of tinea versicolor and *Candida albicans*. Complete clearing of cutaneous lesions may take more than a month of therapy. The mechanism of action appears to be inhibition of squalene epoxidation.[33] Topically, applied tolnaftate has a low incidence of toxicity; however, if local irritation occurs, treatment should be discontinued. (See Chapter 37, "Foot Care Products.")

Clioquinol

Clioquinol, formerly called iodochlorhydroxyquin, has both antifungal and antibacterial properties. Its antibacterial properties have been used to treat infectious dermal conditions such as pyoderma, folliculitis, and impetigo; its antifungal properties have been used to treat mucocutaneous mycotic conditions such as athlete's foot, jock itch, ringworm (tinea), and moniliasis.[34] Clioquinol is an irritant and allergen and may cause transient stinging or pruritus as well as allergic contact dermatitis. If these effects persist, discontinuation of the product is recommended. Several prescription dosage forms (lotion, cream, and ointment) contain both clioquinol and hydrocortisone. The FDA requires the special warning statements "Do not use on children under 2 years of age" and "Do not use for diaper rash."[24]

Treatment of Viral Skin Infections

There are currently no nonprescription products specifically used as antiviral agents for cutaneous viral infections. Most of the products used are antiseptic products used to relieve symptoms and prevent secondary bacterial infection.

Topical antibacterial and antifungal products are used both to treat and to help prevent infection. Topical antiseptic drug products are used to help prevent cutaneous infections.

Vaginal Infections

Vaginal discharge is a common complaint and a frequent reason for women to seek medical care. It has been estimated that more than 25% of women's visits to sexually transmitted disease clinics are due to infectious vaginitis or vulvovaginitis.[35] In addition, approximately 10% of office visits to primary care physicians are due to vaginal symptoms.[36] Infectious vaginitis is characterized by inflammation of the vagina, with vulvar involvement in some cases. Most episodes of infectious vaginitis are attributed to bacterial infection, trichomoniasis, or candidiasis. In 40–50% of cases, bacterial vaginosis (the commonly accepted term for noninflammatory vaginal infections) is the most common etiology, whereas candidiasis is responsible for approximately 20–30% of all episodes.[37,38] In view of the large number of women seeking diagnosis and treatment for vaginal infections and the recent FDA approval of nonprescription antifungal compounds for vaginal use, it is imperative that the pharmacist understand current therapeutic strategies for the treatment of infectious vaginitis.

The Normal Vagina

Some vaginal discharges are a normal physiologic response to vaginal irritants such as feminine hygiene deodorant products, vaginal douches and other cleansing products, contraceptive products and devices, or tampons. In addition, it is normal to observe an increase in mucus production during ovulation, sexual excitement, or emotional flares. Such physiologic discharges are referred to as leukorrhea. These normal vaginal discharges are odorless and clear or white; they consist of endocervical mucus, endogenous vaginal flora, and epithelial cells.[38,39]

The mature vagina is colonized by a variety of organisms, including certain species of *Lactobacillus*, *Streptococcus*, *Staphylococcus*, and *Gardnerella vaginalis*. Other organisms, including *Candida albicans* and anaerobic bacteria, may also be isolated in the absence of active infection. Various factors determine the number and type of endogenous organisms. These factors include vaginal pH, glycogen concentration, and glucose content. The normal vagina has an acidic pH (usually between 3.8 and 4.2). This relatively acid environment is maintained by lactic acid production from bacteria and vaginal epithelial cells that use glycogen and glucose as substrates. Growth of *Lactobacillus* species aids both in maintaining a low pH and in preventing overgrowth by potential vaginal pathogens. Pregnant women have a higher vaginal pH and may therefore be more prone to candidal infection. Vaginal pH also increases during menstruation, and this increase may predispose menstruating women to cyclic fungal vaginal infections. Estrogens are thought to maintain the glycogen content and thickness of vaginal epithelial cells and hence to ensure the integrity of the protective lining of the vaginal tract.[37,39]

In summary, normal vaginal physiologic mechanisms maintain an environment that discourages the overgrowth of pathogenic organisms. When this environment is altered, the potential for infection is increased.

Causes of Vaginal Infections

The three major types of infectious vaginitis are bacterial vaginosis (bacterial infection without inflammation), trichomoniasis, and candidiasis. Historically, bacterial vaginosis has been referred to as "nonspecific vaginitis." The organisms responsible for this infection are not well defined but probably include *Gardnerella vaginalis* and other anaerobic bacteria. Trichomoniasis is caused by *Trichomonas vaginalis* and is thought to be sexually transmitted. Eighty percent of all cases of candidal vaginitis are associated with *Candida albicans*; the remainder are caused by *Candida* (*Torulopsis*) *glabrata* and other *Candida* species.[38,40–42]

Candidiasis is also referred to as a "yeast infection" or moniliasis. The physician uses clinical presentation, physical examination, and specific diagnostic methods to distinguish among the three major causes of vaginal infection.

Signs and Symptoms

Vaginitis can be characterized by the following general symptoms:

- Vaginal and vulvar pruritus;
- An increase in vaginal discharge, together with a change in color and consistency;
- Malodorous discharge;
- Dysuria (pain on urination);
- Dyspareunia (pain during sexual intercourse).

Not all patients will have all of these symptoms. The symptoms reported may help to identify the most likely etiologic agent. Patients with bacterial vaginosis generally complain of a moderate to profuse thin vaginal discharge that is malodorous (fishy smelling) and clear, white, or gray. Trichomoniasis is associated with a profuse purulent discharge that appears yellow-green or brown. This discharge may have an unpleasant odor and a thin and frothy consistency. Vaginal candidiasis produces intense vaginal and vulvar itching. The discharge associated with candidal infections is typically white or whitish-gray and without any noticeable odor. Because of its thick consistency, it is often referred to as "curdlike" or "cottage cheese-like." Patients with candidal infections may also complain of dysuria, dyspareunia, or both.[38,39]

Diagnosis

Physical examination by a physician is an important component in defining the cause of vaginitis. A medical exam with a speculum is typically required to determine the source of the discharge, to examine the vaginal mucosa, and to obtain a specimen for microscopic evaluation. Patients with bacterial vaginosis show no signs of vaginal inflammation. Conversely, trichomoniasis and candidal vaginitis induce erythema and inflammation of the vaginal mucosa. Vulvar involvement is conspicuous with candidal vaginitis, and clumped, adherent plaques can be seen on the vaginal wall.[38,39]

Specific characteristics of the vaginal discharge are important in diagnosis. The discharge in bacterial vaginosis uniformly coats the vaginal walls and a microscopic examination will reveal clue cells (vaginal epithelial cells that are abnormal in appearance owing to the attachment of microorganisms to the cell surface). A Gram's stain of the discharge in bacterial vaginosis may reveal an absence of normal vaginal flora. In addition, the pH of this discharge is usually ≥ 4.5. If a sample of the discharge is mixed with 10% potassium hydroxide, it emits a fishy odor. Trichomonal discharge is characterized by the presence of motile trichomonads and polymorphonuclear leukocytes in a fresh sample of the discharge mixed with normal saline (a so-called wet-mount). Approximately 80% of symptomatic patients can be diagnosed using this wet-mount technique. If tested, the pH of vaginal secretions from women with trichomonal infection is usually ≥ 5.0. As previously mentioned, candidal infection produces a typical cottage cheese-like discharge, and a mixture of vaginal secretions with 10% potassium hydroxide often reveals fungal elements or pseudohyphae under microscopic examination. The pH of vaginal secretions from women with vaginal candidiasis is usually < 4.5, and the discharge emits no odor when mixed with 10% potassium hydroxide.[38,39,41]

Trichomoniasis and Bacterial Vaginosis

The treatment of trichomoniasis and bacterial vaginosis usually requires prescription medications. Currently, the standard therapy for trichomoniasis is oral metronidazole (Prostat® [Ortho]; Flagyl® [Searle]). For optimal efficacy, sexual partners must be treated concurrently. Metronidazole should be avoided during the first trimester of pregnancy, and its use in the second or third trimester is controversial. Patients treated with metronidazole should be instructed to avoid alcohol because of the "disulfiram-like" reaction noted when the two are taken together.

Metronidazole 0.75% vaginal gel (Metrogel-Vaginal®) and clindamycin 2% vaginal cream (Cleocin®) have recently been approved for treatment of bacterial vaginosis. Sultrin® Triple Sulfa Cream is another product previously approved for the treatment of bacterial vaginosis (nonspecific vaginitis). Alternatively, ampicillin, amoxicillin, and ampicillin/clavulanic acid have been used to treat bacterial vaginosis and clotrimazole vaginal tablets have been used for treatment of trichomoniasis, but unfortunately, these therapies for bacterial vaginosis and trichomoniasis are less successful.[37–39,41]

Candidiasis

Predisposing Factors

Candida albicans can be cultured from vaginal secretions in up to 50% of asymptomatic women.[40,42] Certain predisposing factors have been associated with the development of candidal vulvovaginitis, among them the taking of certain medications, the presence of certain underlying diseases, and pregnancy. The medications most often associated with an increased risk of candidal infection include corticosteroids, broad-spectrum systemic antibiotics, cytotoxic or immunosuppressant drugs, and oral contraceptives.

Virtually any antibacterial agent has the potential for promoting fungal overgrowth. Those most frequently implicated are the tetracyclines, ampicillin, and the cephalosporins. Systemic antibiotic therapy of long duration may alter the body's natural flora and result in increased candidal colonization and growth. Corticosteroids and immunosuppressant drugs alter the patient's immune status and thereby predispose the patient to infection. The association of increased candidal vaginitis with oral contraceptive use is controversial. Although older contraceptives with greater estrogen activity have been shown to increase candidal colonization, more recent studies involving low-estrogen agents have not supported this observation.[38–40,42]

Increased candidal colonization has been noted in patients with diabetes mellitus, and this increased colonization may increase the risk of symptomatic infection in this population. Candidiasis is also seen with increased frequency in immunocompromised patients with impaired cellular immunity, especially organ transplant patients and those with acquired immunodeficiency syndrome (AIDS).[42]

The higher incidence of candidiasis in pregnant women is well documented. It has been proposed that the increased vaginal glycogen content in pregnant women results in an increase in candidal growth. In addition, some researchers have demonstrated an increase in the adherence of *Candida* organisms to the vaginal epithelium during pregnancy.[42]

Other factors that may increase the risk of vaginal candidiasis include excessive douching, tight-fitting clothing, and "nonbreathing" nylon undergarments.[42]

Recurrent Vaginal Fungal Infections

Recurrent vaginal candidiasis (the occurrence of at least four episodes within 12 months) affects a large number of women. It is estimated that 45% of patients have more than one candidal infection after the first. Physicians may attempt to determine the cause of recurrences but such efforts are often unsuccessful. Although the predisposing factors discussed earlier may be present, most women with recurrent candidiasis exhibit no particular risk characteristics. Resistant subpopulations of fungal organisms may result in treatment failure. It has also been theorized that women who experience recurrent vaginal candidiasis may have an intestinal reservoir of *Candida* that leads to chronic reinfection from fecal–vaginal cross-contamination. This hypothesis is controversial. Sexual transmission may also promote recurrent infections, although this explanation appears to be unlikely, inasmuch as treatment of sexual partners has little effect on the incidence of recurrence.[40]

What should be done for patients with recurrent infections? Simple measures such as avoiding nylon underwear and tight-fitting clothing should be suggested. Patients taking oral contraceptives might consider an alternative method of birth control. Recurrent infections may need to be treated with longer courses of therapy. In addition, some practitioners advocate the prophylactic administration of antifungal agents, for example, topical antifungal agents or oral ketoconazole administered during menstrual cycles. Other practitioners have proposed concomitant antifungal therapy during courses of broad-spectrum antibiotic treatment. Further studies are needed to document the efficacy of these prophylactic regimens.[38,39,43]

Treatment

Topical intravaginal products are the currently recommended therapies for vulvovaginal candidiasis. Before the discovery of imidazole compounds, nystatin was the treatment of choice. Nystatin (available by prescription only) is a polyene antifungal available in cream and tablet form for topical use. Nystatin damages the cytoplasmic membrane of fungi and is effective in approximately 80% of all cases of vaginal candidiasis.[37]

There are currently four topical imidazole derivatives available in the United States for treating candidal vaginitis: miconazole, clotrimazole, butoconazole, and tioconazole. Terconazole (a recently approved antifungal) is often grouped with the imidazoles but is more appropriately classified as a triazole. These products are available as vaginal creams, suppositories, and tablets. Studies have shown the imidazoles to be effective and without major toxicities; effectiveness rates are approximately 90%.[37–39] Clinical studies have demonstrated that terconazole possesses comparable efficacy in the treatment of candidal vaginitis.[44,45] At this time both miconazole and clotrimazole are available as nonprescription intravaginal medications.

Other topical agents that have been used to treat candidiasis include povidone–iodine, 1% gentian violet, boric acid powder and capsules, and *Lactobacillus* preparations. A number of nonprescription preparations offer symptomatic

TABLE 3 Product information and dosage guidelines for vaginal antifungals

Generic name	Brand name	Dosage form and strength	Dosing regimen	Status
Clotrimazole	Gyne-Lotrimin; Mycelex-7	100-mg vaginal tablet	Insert 1 vaginal tablet at bedtime for 7 days	OTC
Clotrimazole	Gyne-Lotrimin; Mycelex-7	1% vaginal cream	Insert 1 applicatorful (≈ 5 g) at bedtime for 7 days	OTC
Miconazole	Monistat 7	100-mg vaginal suppository	Insert 1 vaginal suppository at bedtime for 7 days	OTC
Miconazole	Monistat 7	2% vaginal cream	Insert 1 applicatorful (≈ 5 g) at bedtime for 7 days	OTC
Clotrimazole	Mycelex-G	100-mg vaginal tablet	Insert 1 vaginal tablet at bedtime for 7 days or 2 tablets at bedtime for 3 days in nonpregnant women only	Rx
		500-mg vaginal tablet	Insert 1 vaginal tablet at bedtime (one dose)	Rx
Clotrimazole	Mycelex-G	1% vaginal cream	Insert 1 applicatorful (≈ 5 g) for 7 to 14 days	Rx
Miconazole	Monistat 3	200-mg vaginal suppository	Insert 1 vaginal suppository at bedtime for 3 days	Rx
Butoconazole	Femstat	2% vaginal cream	If nonpregnant, insert 1 applicatorful (≈ 5 g) at bedtime for 3 days. This therapy may be extended to 6 days if necessary. If pregnant, use during 2nd or 3rd trimester only and insert 1 applicatorful (≈ 5 g) at bedtime for 6 days	Rx
Terconazole	Terazol 3	80-mg vaginal suppository	Insert 1 vaginal suppository at bedtime for 3 days	Rx
Terconazole	Terazol 7	0.4% vaginal cream	Insert 1 applicatorful (≈ 5 g) at bedtime for 7 days	Rx
Tioconazole	Vagistat	6.5% vaginal ointment	Insert 1 applicatorful (≈ 4.6 g) at bedtime for 1 time only	Rx
Nystatin	Generic; Nilstat; Mycostatin	100,000-unit vaginal tablet	Insert 1 vaginal tablet at bedtime for 14 days	Rx

Adapted with permission from *Facts and Comparisons Drug Newsletter* 1992 June; 11: 41–44.

relief, including Vagisil® and Vaginex®. Use of these agents has decreased owing to the obvious advantages of the imidazole derivatives; these advantages include superior efficacy and improved patient compliance associated with ease of use, less frequent local reactions, and shorter treatment durations. Home remedies such as vaginal douches of yogurt or vinegar have also been used to treat vaginal candidiasis, although they are generally not effective.[37,46]

Although the FDA has not yet reviewed antimicrobial drug products for the treatment of candidal infections, it has reviewed several ingredients for the relief of minor irritation. The panel recommended the following ingredients as safe and effective: calcium and sodium propionate (20% gel), potassium sorbate (20% gel), and povidone–iodine (10–12% diluted to 0.30% solution for douche). Combination drug products (e.g., benzocaine plus resorcinol) have not been demonstrated to be effective.[47]

Pharmacology of Vaginal Antifungals The major antifungal effect of the imidazole and triazole compounds is accomplished by altering the membrane permeability of the fungi. These agents inhibit cytochrome P-450 enzymes in the fungal cell membrane, thereby decreasing synthesis of the essential fungal sterol ergosterol. The reduced membrane ergosterol content is accompanied by a corresponding increase in lanosterol-like methylated sterols. These lanosterol-like sterols cause structural and functional damage to fungal membranes, resulting in loss of normal membrane function.[46,48]

The topical intravaginal agents are not appreciably absorbed. One pharmacokinetic study with vaginal application of clotrimazole found that between 3% and 10% of a dose was systemically absorbed. This study also revealed that fungicidal clotrimazole concentrations were detectable in the vaginal fluid for up to 3 days after a single 500-mg intravaginal dose.[49] A study of intravaginally administered radiolabeled miconazole demonstrated that approximately 1% of the dose was excreted in the urine and found that the radioactivity of whole blood was too low for measurement.[50]

Side Effects of Vaginal Antifungals Toxicity from topical therapy is minimal. Topical imidazoles and triazoles have been associated with vulvovaginal burning, itching, and irritation; abdominal cramps; and (rarely) allergic reactions. Adverse effects form systemic antifungal therapy may, however, be more significant. The most common side effects of oral ketoconazole (available by prescription only) are nausea and vomiting. Hepatotoxicity has also been reported, and liver enzymes should be monitored in patients receiving chronic ketoconazole therapy. Fluconazole is also associated with nausea and vomiting. Other adverse effects reported include headache, skin rash, diarrhea, and abdominal pain.[51]

Specific Treatment Regimens for Vaginal Candidiasis The success rates of the topical imidazoles and triazoles in the treatment of candidal vaginitis are similar. Different treatment durations have been studied. Initially, 14-day antifungal treatment regimens were used, and this duration is still recommended for nystatin therapy. Recommended durations of treatment for other therapies include 7 days (6 days for prescription-only butoconazole), 3 days, and a single-dose regimen (approved only for the 500-mg clotrimazole vaginal tablet or tioconazole vaginal ointment). Some of the prescription-only 3-day and single-dose regimens demonstrate equivalent efficacy. However, these regimens have not been extensively studied in pregnant women or complicated hosts and thus should not be routinely used in these patient

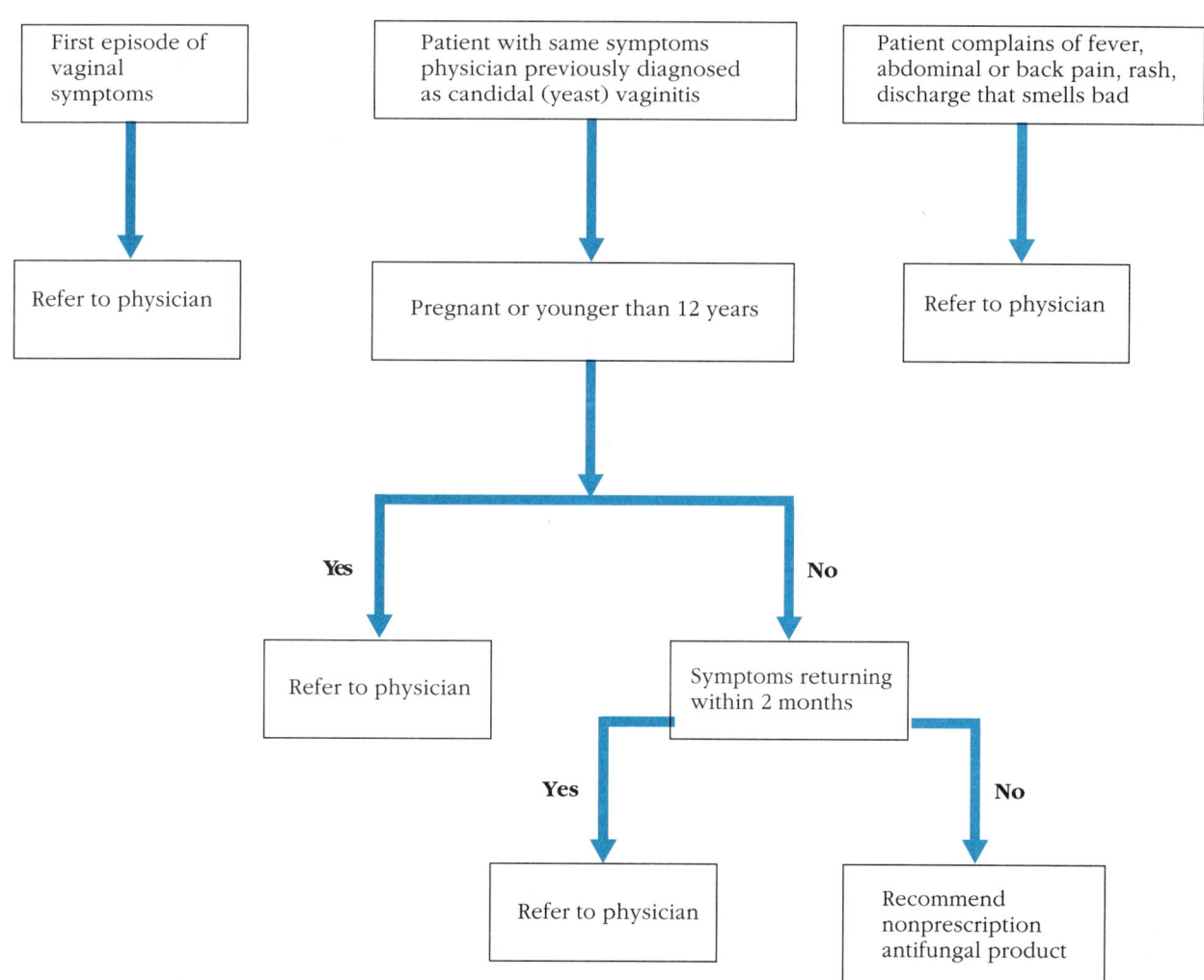

FIGURE 3 Algorithm for managing patient with symptoms of a vaginal infection.

populations. Currently, only the 7-day regimens are available without a prescription. A summary of recommended prescription and nonprescription regimens is presented in Table 3.

Systemic prescription therapy with ketoconazole or fluconazole for vaginal candidiasis has been investigated. Studies of 200-mg doses of ketoconazole taken one or two times daily for 3–6 days and single doses of 150-mg fluconazole have demonstrated efficacy comparable to that of topical therapy. Fluconazole can be given as a single oral dose because of its long elimination half-life. Oral therapy may increase compliance because of the relative ease of administration. However, neither ketoconazole nor fluconazole appears to be more effective than the topical imidazoles (i.e., clotrimazole, miconazole, butoconazole, and tioconazole), and they possess a greater potential to induce systemic toxicity. Further studies will be required to define the precise role of systemic therapy in the treatment of vaginal candidiasis.[52–54]

As discussed previously, pregnant women have both an increased risk of candidal vaginitis and a decreased response to therapy. Most short-course (1-day or 3-day) treatment has not yet been shown to be as efficacious in pregnant women as in nonpregnant women; therefore, the duration of therapy during pregnancy should be at least 7 days. Limited safety data are available on the use of these products during the first trimester, and risk versus benefit must be weighed.[37,46]

Patient Information Who should receive a nonprescription antifungal vaginal product? The patient should be certain that she has a vaginal fungal infection because she experienced the same symptoms at an earlier time and received a diagnosis of candidal vaginitis from her physician. If the patient has fever (above 100°F [38°C] orally), pain in the lower abdomen, back, or shoulder, or a vaginal discharge that smells bad, she should be referred to her physician immediately. These signs and symptoms may be indicative of a systemic and more severe infection. Women whose vaginal symptoms return within 2 months should also be referred to a physician. Pregnant women should never take nonprescription antifungal products without consulting their physicians. The vaginal antifungals should not be used for girls under 12 years of age unless directed by a physician.

The pharmacist should try to determine whether the patient has any of the underlying risk factors that predispose a woman to vaginal candidiasis. By obtaining a complete medication history, the pharmacist will be able to determine whether the patient is receiving any medication that may increase her risk of developing candidiasis (e.g., broad-spectrum antibiotics, corticosteroids, and cytotoxic or immunosuppressant agents). A medication history may also alert the pharmacist to specific disease states associated with an increased risk of candidiasis, such as diabetes mellitus, cancer, or AIDS.

Each patient should also be questioned about the possibility of pregnancy. The incidence of candidal vaginitis is almost twice as high in pregnant women as in nonpregnant women. Symptomatic pregnant women should be referred to a physician before beginning any treatment for vaginal candidiasis.

The selection of antifungal treatment should be based on efficacy, safety, patient acceptance, and cost of therapy. If specific products have been shown to be equally effective, the choice of a vaginal suppository, tablet, or cream should be discussed with the patient.

Directions for proper use should be discussed with the patient. This is best accomplished in a private counseling area. Appropriate directions for proper use are listed in Table 4. The pharmacist should also inform the patient of potential local reactions, including temporary burning, itching, and irritation. The patients must be instructed to

---

TABLE 4 Directions for vaginal antifungal products

1. It is advisable to start the treatment at night before going to bed. A supine position will reduce leakage of the product from the vagina.
2. Wash the entire vaginal area with mild soap and water and dry completely before applying the product.
3. To open the tube, unscrew the cap; place the cap upside down on the end of the tube. Push down firmly until the seal is broken. (For vaginal tablets/suppositories, remove the protective wrapper.)
4. Attach the applicator to the tube by turning the applicator clockwise. (For vaginal tablets/suppositories, place the product into the end of the applicator barrel.)
5. Squeeze the tube from the bottom to force the cream into the applicator. Do this until the inside piece of the applicator is pushed out as far as possible and the applicator is completely filled with cream. Remove the applicator from the tube.
6. While standing with your feet slightly apart and your knees bent or lying on your back with your knees bent, gently insert the applicator into the vagina as far as it will go comfortably. Push the inside piece of the applicator in and place the cream as far back in the vagina as possible. (For vaginal tablets/suppositories, insert the applicator into the vagina and press plunger until it stops to deposit the product.) Remove the applicator from the vagina. You may want to wear a sanitary napkin or pad during the time you are using the vaginal product, because some leakage will likely occur. Do not use a tampon to prevent leakage.
7. After use, recap the tube (if using cream) and clean the applicator. The applicator can be cleaned by pulling the two pieces apart and washing them with soap and warm water.
8. Continue using the product according to product instructions.
9. Complete the full course of therapy and use on consecutive days, even during menstrual flow.
10. Avoid sexual contact during treatment or suggest that your partner use protection to decrease the risk of infection.
11. If no improvement is noted after 3 days, if a worsening of symptoms is noted after 3 days, or if symptoms are still present after you have completed the course of therapy, contact your physician.

stop using the antifungal product and call her physician if she develops abdominal cramping, headache, urticaria, hives, or skin rash.

Nonprescription antifungals should not be used by pregnant women or women with a history of sensitivity to any of the product ingredients without consultation with a physician. The pharmacist must advise a patient with any of the following symptoms to seek medical advice: fever, abdominal or back pain, or foul-smelling discharge. A patient should also be referred to a physician if there has been no improvement after 3 days of therapy, if symptoms are incompletely resolved after the 7-day course, or if symptoms recur within 2 months of stopping therapy.

In October 1992 the FDA approved new statements in the labeling for currently marketed nonprescription vaginal candidiasis treatments (i.e., miconazole and clotrimazole), effective in 1993. The revised "warnings" section now includes the following statements:

> If you may have been exposed to the human immunodeficiency virus and are now having recurrent vaginal yeast infections, especially infections that don't clear up easily with proper treatment, see your doctor promptly to determine the cause of your symptoms and to receive proper treatment.

> If your symptoms return within two months, or if you have infections that do not clear up easily with proper treatment, consult your doctor. You could be pregnant or there could be a serious underlying medical cause for your infections, including diabetes or a damaged immune system (including damage from infections by HIV, the virus that causes AIDS).

Nonprescription topical imidazole therapy requires that the pharmacist counsel the patient on the proper selection and use of these products (drugs and dosage forms). The pharmacist must also be able to identify symptomatic patients who should be referred to a physician. An algorithm for an appropriate approach to the patient with vaginitis is listed in Figure 3. With advice and consultation from the pharmacist, many patients with uncomplicated infectious vaginitis can be safely and appropriately managed.

References

1. Bruinsma W. *The Guide to Drug Eruptions*. Oosthuizen, The Netherlands: 1990: The File of Medicines. 32–35, 62–98.
2. Odland GF. Structure of the skin in physiology. In: Goldsmith, LA, ed. *Physiology, Biochemistry, and Molecular Biology of the Skin*. New York: Oxford University Press; 1991: 3–62.
3. Jellinek JS. *Formulation and Function of Cosmetics*. 2nd ed. New York: John Wiley; 1970: 4–14.
4. Guy RH, Hadgraft J. In: Bronaugh RL, Maibach HI, eds. *Percutaneous Absorption*. 2nd ed. New York: Marcel Dekker; 1989: 13–26.
5. Roth RR, James WD. *J Am Acad Dermatol* 1989 20: 367–390.
6. Cascella PJ, Powers JE. *US Pharm* 1988 13 (12): 26.
7. Hojyo-Tomoka MT et al. *Arch Dermatol* 1973 107: 723.
8. Montes LF, Wilborn WH. *Br J Dermatol* 1969 81; 23.
9. Leyden JJ. In: Soter NA, Baden HP, eds. *Pathophysiology of Dermatologic Diseases*. 2nd ed. New York: McGraw-Hill; 1991: 427–440.
10. Maibach HI, Aly R. In: Moschella SL, Hurley HJ, eds. *Dermatology*. 3rd ed. Philadelphia: W. B. Saunders; 1992: 710–50.
11. Hay RJ, Roberts SOB, MacKenzie DWR. In: Campion RH, Burton JL, Ebling FJG, eds. *Textbook of Dermatology*. 5th ed. Oxford, England: Blackwell Scientific Publications; 1992: 1127–1216.
12. Goslen JB, Kobayashi GS. In: Fitzpatrick TB et al., eds. *Dermatology in General Medicine*. 3rd ed. New York: McGraw-Hill; 1987: 2193–2248.
13. Stone MS, Lynch PJ. In: Sams WM Jr, Lynch PJ, eds. *Principles and Practice of Dermatology*. New York: Churchill Livingstone; 1990: 119–27.
14. Elliott GW, Sams WM Jr. In: Sams WM Jr, Lynch PJ, eds. *Principles and Practice of Dermatology*. New York: Churchill Livingstone; 1990: 99–112.
15. Dillon HC. *Int J Dermatol* 1980 19: 443.
16. *Federal Register* 1990 55: 9721–22.
17. *Federal Register* 1987 52: 47312–24.
18. Sande MA, Mandell GL. In: Gilman AG et al., eds. *The Pharmacological Basis of Therapeutics*. 8th ed. New York: Pergamon Press; 1990: 1112.
19. *Federal Register* 1991 56: 33644.
20. Ward DR. Personal communication. FDA's Summary for Basis of Approval, NDA 17–768 (Hibiclens); laboratory data developed as part of NDA requirements. Stuart Pharmaceuticals; Wilmington, Del.
21. *Drug Evaluations Annual 1992*. Chicago: American Medical Association; 1992: 1515.
22. Spainhour S. Personal communication. CIBA-Geigy Corporation; Greensboro, NC; 1989.
23. *Federal Register* 1978 43: 1210–49.
24. *Federal Register* 1989 54: 51136.
25. *Federal Register* 1992 57: 38568.
26. Seki S et al. "Antimicrobial Agents Chemotherapy." 1963: 569.
27. Hermann HW. *Arch Dermatol* 1972 106: 839.
28. Katz R, Cahn B. *Arch Dermatol* 1972 106: 837.
29. Carter VH. *Curr Ther Res* 1972 14: 307.
30. Hildrick-Smith G. *Adv Biol Skin* 1972 12: 303.
31. Mandy SJ, Garrott TC. *JAMA* 1974 230: 72.
32. Fulton JE Jr. *Arch Dermatol* 1975 111: 596.
33. Barrett-Bee KJ et al. *J Med Vet Mycol* 1986 24: 5–160.
34. Harvey SC. In: Gennaro AR, ed. *Remington's Pharmaceutical Sciences*. 18th ed. Easton, Pa: Mack Publishing; 1990: 1236.
35. Centers for Disease Control. Nonreported sexually transmitted diseases. *MMWR* 1979 28: 61–63.
36. Paavonen J, Stamm WE. Lower genital tract infections in women. *Infect Dis Clin North Am* 1987 1: 179–98.
37. Rein MF. Vulvovaginitis and cervicitis. In: Mandell GL, Douglas RG, Bennett JE, eds. *Principles and Practice of Infectious Diseases*. New York: Churchill Livingstone; 1990: 953–65.
38. Eschenbach DA. Vaginal infection. *Clin Obstet Gynecol* 1983 26: 186–202.
39. McCue JD. Evaluation and management of vaginitis: an update for primary care practitioners. *Arch Intern Med* 1989 149: 565–68.
40. Sobel JD. Epidemiology and pathogenesis of recurrent vulvovaginal candidiasis. *Am J Obstet Gynecol* 1985 2: 924–35.
41. Holmes KK, Handsfield HH. Sexually transmitted diseases. In: Wilson JD, Braunwald E, Isselbacher KJ, et al., eds. *Harrison's Principles of Internal Medicine*. New York: McGraw-Hill; 1991: 524–33.
42. Sobel JD. Pathogenesis and epidemiology of vulvovaginal candidiasis. *Ann N Y Acad Sci* 1988 544: 547–57.
43. Sobel JD. Management of recurrent vulvovaginal candidiasis with intermittent ketoconazole prophylaxis. *Obstet Gynecol* 1985 65: 435–40.
44. Thomason JL. Clinical evaluation of terconazole: United States

experience. *J Reprod Med* 1989 34 (suppl): 597–601.
45. Kjaeldgaard A. Comparison of terconazole and clotrimazole vaginal tablets in the treatment of vulvovaginal candidosis. *Pharmatherapeutica* 1986 4: 525–31.
46. Koerign PL, Santiago TM. Drugs for treatment of vulvovaginal candidiasis: comparative efficacy of agents and regimens. *DICP Ann Pharmacother* 1990 24: 1078–83.
47. *Federal Register* 1983 48: 47694–47729.
48. Cauwenbergh G, Bossche HV. Terconazole pharmacology of a new antimycotic agent. *J Reprod Med* 1989 34(suppl): 588–92.
49. Ritter W, Patzschke K, Krause U, Stettendorf S. Pharmacokinetic fundamentals of vaginal treatment with clotrimazole. *Chemotherapy* 1982 28 (suppl 1): 37–42.
50. Abrams LS, Weintraub HS. Disposition of radioactivity following intravaginal administration of ^{3}H-miconazole nitrate. *Am J Obstet Gynecol* 1983 147: 970–71.
51. Antifungals. In: Mcevoy GK, Litvak K, Welsh OH, et al., eds. *AHFS Drug Information 92*. Bethesda, Md: American Society of Hospital Pharmacists; 1992: 2094–2122.
52. Bingham JS. Single blind comparison of ketoconazole 200mg oral tablets and clotrimazole 100mg vaginal tablets and 1% cream in treating acute vaginal candidosis. *Br J Venereal Dis* 1984 60: 175–77.
53. Puolakka J, Tuimala R. A comparison between oral ketoconazole and topical miconazole in the treatment of vaginal candidiasis. *Acta Obstet Gynecol Scand* 1983 62: 575–77.
54. Herzog RE, Ansmann EB. Treatment of vaginal candidosis with fluconazole. *Mycoses* 1989 32: 204–8.

CHAPTER 29

Acne Products

Joye Ann Billow

Questions to ask in patient assessment and counseling

- How old are you?
- How long have you had acne?
- Is the acne a problem on areas other than your face (e.g., neck, shoulders, chest, or back)?
- Have you consulted a physician about your acne? If so, what treatment was suggested? Are you currently following it?
- Are you currently using any medications, either prescription or nonprescription? If so, what are they?
- Have you already tried acne treatments? If so, which ones? How did you use them? How effective were they?
- Do you prefer one type of acne treatment product (e.g., lotion, cream, gel, or soap) over another?
- What type of cosmetics, including makeup, after-shave lotions, or hair preparations, do you use? Do they seem to aggravate the acne?
- How often do you wash your face? What type of soap do you use?
- How often do you shampoo your hair? What type of shampoo do you use?
- Do you notice a seasonal change in the number or severity of acne lesions?
- Are you routinely exposed to environmental conditions such as heat or humidity or cooking oils in the air?

Acne vulgaris is the most common adolescent skin disorder, and it is often linked to the onset of puberty. Involving the oil glands and hair follicles of the skin, primarily on the face and trunk, the disease is characterized by whiteheads, blackheads, acne pimples, and acne blemishes (Table 1).[1] If untreated, the cysts appearing in the more severe cases of acne may lead to pitting, which in turn may cause both physical and psychologic scars.

The incidence of acne is nearly universal; approximately 85% of people between the ages of 12 and 25 will develop it to some degree.[2] Although it may occur earlier, recognizable acne will typically develop in males aged 16–18 and in females aged 15–17 years old. Acne may occur in females as young as 10 years of age, or it may not occur until the 20s. It may also occur in prepubertal children and in older persons, and it may be exacerbated by cosmetics (acne cosmetica) at any age.[3]

Although acne is not a physical threat, it may have a significant negative psychosocial impact on an adolescent during a time when physiologic changes necessitate emotional and social adjustments. Adolescence is also a period when self-image and peer acceptance become of paramount importance. It is estimated that more than 60% of U.S. teenagers use nonprescription products to treat acne and that more than 65% of reported sales of acne remedies occur in pharmacies.[4] Thus, the pharmacist can be instrumental in assisting teenagers to make informed choices about a treatment that may greatly affect their cosmetic and psychosocial well-being. This contact also represents a tremendous opportunity for pharmacists to introduce a new group of consumers to the value of patient counseling.

Etiology and Pathophysiology of Acne

Acne vulgaris has its origin in the pilosebaceous units in the dermis (Figure 1A). These units, consisting of a hair follicle and the associated sebaceous glands, are connected to the skin surface by a duct (the infundibulum) through which the hair shaft passes. The sebaceous glands produce sebum, a mixture of fats and waxes. The sebum passes to the skin surface through the infundibulum, and then spreads over the skin to retard water loss and maintain hydration of the skin and hair. Because the sebaceous glands are more common on the face, back, and chest, acne tends to occur most often in these areas. (See Chapter 28, "Topical Anti-Infective Products.")

At puberty, the production of androgenic hormones increases in both sexes. The increase of circulating testosterone is taken up, in part, by the sebaceous glands and converted to dihydrotestosterone, which is considered to be the tissue androgen responsible for acne. The sebaceous glands, under the influence of increased androgen levels, increase in size and activity, producing larger amounts of sebum. At the same time, keratinization of the follicular walls increases and causes mechanical blockage of sebum flow, resulting in the dilation of the follicle and the entrapment of sebum and cellular debris. This results in a microcomedo, the initial pathologic lesion of acne (Figure 1B).

Although androgens are the major stimulus to sebaceous gland development and sebum secretion, patients with acne do not necessarily have abnormal androgen levels. It is theorized that acne-prone patients have

TABLE 1 Definition and classification of selected acne terms

Term	Definition	Comment
Whitehead	A condition of the skin that occurs in acne, characterized by a small, firm, whitish, closed elevation of the skin	Also known as a closed comedo; is a noninflammatory lesion
Blackhead	A condition of the skin that occurs in acne, characterized by a black coloration at the skin surface	Also known as an open comedo; is a noninflammatory lesion
Acne pimple	A small, prominent, inflamed elevation of the skin resulting from acne	May occur as a papule or pustule; is an inflammatory lesion; may progress to a nodulocystic lesion

increased end-organ sensitivity to normal levels of androgens, facilitating the hypertrophic changes.[5]

The epithelial tissue, an extension of the surface epidermis, forms the lining of the infundibulum and becomes thinner as it extends into the deeper portions of the duct. Normally, the epithelial tissue continually sheds cells, which are carried to the skin surface by the flow of sebum. However, in acne, the shed epithelial cells are more distinct and durable, and they stick together to form a coherent horny layer that blocks the follicular channel.[6] This impaction may plug and distend the follicle to form a microcomedo.

As more cells and sebum are added, the microcomedo enlarges and becomes visible; it is called a closed comedo (whitehead) because its contents do not reach the surface of the skin (Figure 1C). Two processes may then follow, one leading to noninflammatory acne and the other leading to inflammatory acne. Most individuals experience a combination of the two types.

If the plug enlarges and protrudes from the orifice of the follicular canal, it is called an open comedo (blackhead) because its contents open to the surface (Figure 1D). The tip of the plug of the open comedone may darken because of melanin (not dirt or oxidized fat) produced by the epithelial cells lining the infundibulum. Open comedones may be carefully expressed with a clean comedo extractor. To prevent infection, care should be taken to avoid using dirty extractors or squeezing with dirty fingers. Acne characterized by the presence of closed or open comedones is called noninflammatory acne. (See color plates, photograph 17.)

Inflammatory acne is characterized by inflammation around the comedo, which may rupture to form a papule (Figure 1E). Papules are inflammatory lesions appearing as raised, reddened areas on the skin. These lesions may enlarge to form pustules, which also appear as raised, reddened areas but are filled with pus (Figure 1F). The pustules can rupture spontaneously. More extensive penetration into surrounding and underlying tissue produces nodulocystic lesions.

Inflammatory acne typically begins with closed comedones. As the microcomedo develops, it distends the follicle so that the cellular lining of the walls is spread and thinned. Primary inflammation of the follicle wall may develop with the disruption of the epithelial lining and lymphocyte infiltration into and around the follicular wall.[7] If the follicle wall ruptures spontaneously or is ruptured by picking or squeezing, and if the contents are discharged into the surrounding tissue, a more severe inflammatory reaction results. The epithelial cells, sebum, and any microorganisms present represent foreign substances capable of eliciting an inflammatory reaction. The results may be abscesses, which, in the process of healing, may cause scars or pits.

Theories explaining the development of inflammatory acne suggest that the initial inflammation of the follicle wall results from the presence of free fatty acids derived from the sebum.[7] In the presence of bacterial lipolytic enzymes in the sebaceous glands, triglycerides in the sebum are split, releasing the free fatty acids.

The main microorganisms found in the sebaceous duct are an anaerobic rod, *Propionibacterium acnes* (*Corynebacterium acnes*), and one or two species of *Staphylococcus*, which are among the predominant flora normally inhabiting the skin. These microorganisms are not considered to be pathogens, and they die rapidly if the follicle wall is ruptured and they are released into the surrounding tissues. *P. acnes* is generally regarded as the primary source of the lipolytic enzymes responsible for free fatty acid formation in the sebum. The effectiveness of oral antibiotics (e.g., tetracycline or doxycycline) and topical antibiotics (e.g., tetracycline, erythromycin, or clindamycin) in treating inflammatory acne is possibly due to their ability to suppress the normal bacterial population of the sebaceous duct, thus reducing free fatty acid formation and concentration.[8]

The hair in the follicle may play a significant role in comedo development. If the hair shaft is thin and small, it may become entrapped in the plug. The heavier hair of the scalp and beard typically push the developing plug to the surface, thus preventing comedo formation. In adults, acne may disappear spontaneously for reasons that are not readily apparent.

Picking or squeezing inflamed follicles or attempting to express closed comedones may rupture the follicle walls and thus produce inflammatory lesions. The pustules or

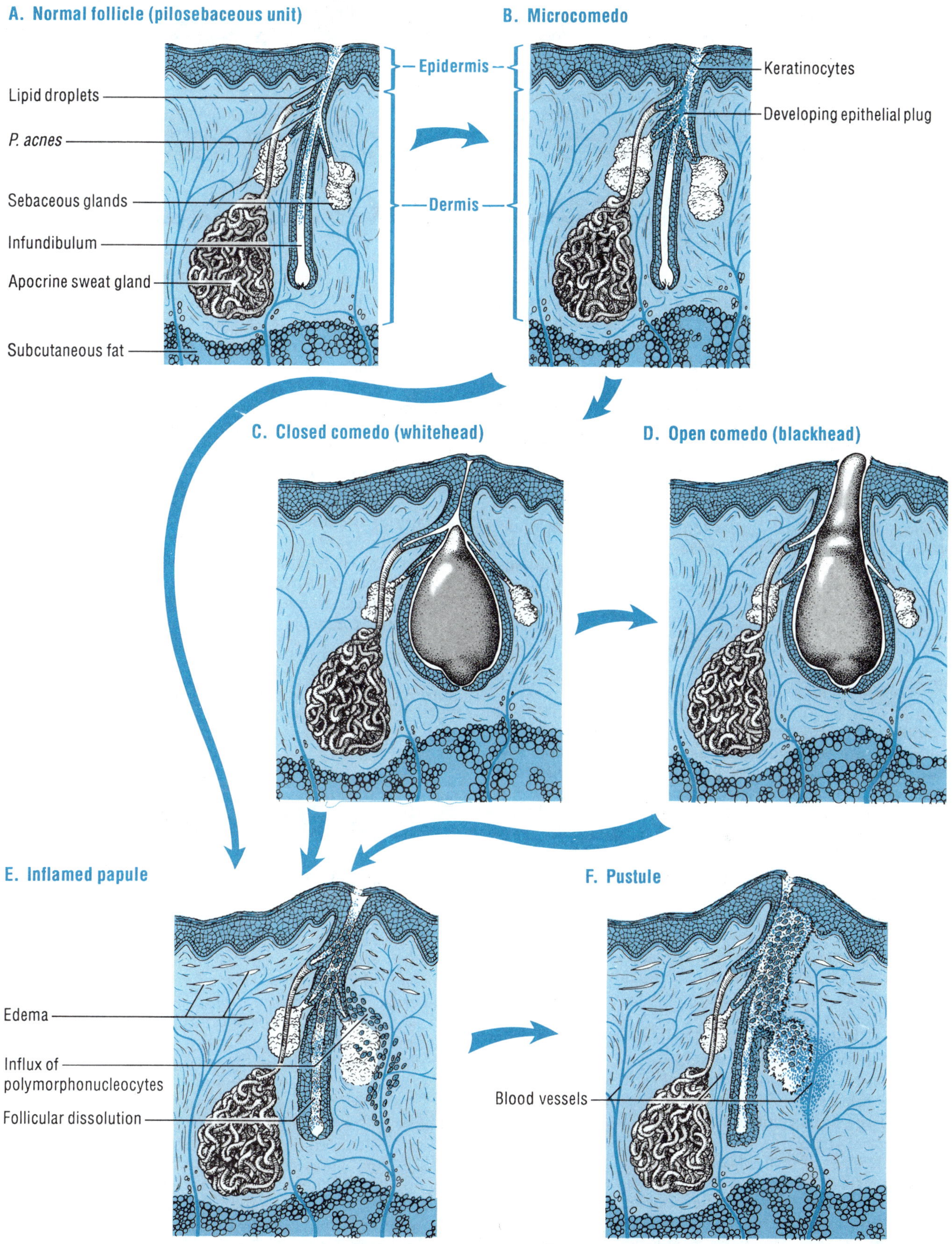

A. Normal follicle (pilosebaceous unit)

- Lipid droplets
- *P. acnes*
- Sebaceous glands
- Infundibulum
- Apocrine sweat gland
- Subcutaneous fat
- Epidermis
- Dermis

B. Microcomedo

- Keratinocytes
- Developing epithelial plug

C. Closed comedo (whitehead)

D. Open comedo (blackhead)

E. Inflamed papule

- Edema
- Influx of polymorphonucleocytes
- Follicular dissolution

F. Pustule

- Blood vessels

FIGURE 1 Pathogenesis of acne. Adapted with permission from Fulton JE, Bradley S. *Cutis* 1976; 17: 560.

cysts of inflammatory acne are much more likely to cause permanent scarring than those of noninflammatory acne. (See color plates, photograph 18.) Thus, inflammatory acne should be treated by a physician. Treatment typically requires both nonprescription and prescription medication. Prescription drugs such as tretinoin and isotretinoin, as well as the possible excision and drainage of inflammatory lesions, may be required.

Rosacea ("adult acne," acne rosacea) is a generalized disorder of the blood vessels. It can be differentiated from acne vulgaris in various ways. Onset is not typically linked to endocrine changes associated with surges in androgen levels, which occur from adolescence to the early to mid-20s. The condition may occur in early adulthood or at any time later. Symptoms may be progressive and may consist of sensitivity to touch, reddening of the face, enlarged blood vessels, and formation of solid red papules or pustules. Factors that may aggravate symptoms include alcohol ingestion, overexposure to sunlight, spicy foods, smoking, hot drinks, temperature extremes, friction, irritating cosmetics, and systemic steroid use. Symptoms tend to diminish and flare in a somewhat cyclic pattern. Lesions tend to be localized to the central portion of the face (e.g., center of forehead, nose, and chin). Comedones are not typically present.

There is no cure for rosacea. Medical referral is required, and treatment is directed toward relieving symptoms. If untreated, the symptoms may progressively worsen. Oral antibiotics (e.g., tetracycline), topical metronidazole (0.75%), or isotretinoin may be required to treat the lesions.[9]

Classification

Various systems have been used to classify the severity of acne vulgaris although none is universally accepted. In the Pillsbury grading scale, Roman numerals from I to IV indicate the level of severity. Grade I, the mildest form of acne, consists of primarily comedones with a small number of inflamed pustules and is often localized on one portion of the face. Grade II acne is confined mainly to the face but displays a marked increase in the number of inflammatory lesions. In grade III acne, the lesions can be found on the upper torso (e.g., chest, upper back, and shoulders) as well as one the face; papules and pustules predominate and some scar formation is likely. Grade IV acne is the most severe and is often called cystic acne, nodulocystic acne, or acne conglobata. Moderate to severe scarring is likely.[10,11]

One problem with the Pillsbury classification system is that the number of acne lesions is not considered. This may result in a person with several pustules being classified as having a more severe case of acne than the person with a large number of comedones and only a few or no pustules.

The issue of acne classification was addressed by a Consensus Conference on Acne Classification convened by the American Academy of Dermatology in 1990. The consensus panel concluded that a strictly quantitative classification of acne cannot be established and that "acne grading can best be accomplished by the use of a pattern–diagnosis system, which would include a global (total) evaluation of lesions as well as their complications such as drainage, hemorrhage, and pain."[12] The division of acne into inflammatory and noninflammatory types has not been changed. However, the opinion is that noninflammatory acne, presenting as comedones only, can rarely be classified as severe, even if the comedones are present in large numbers.

Inflammatory acne is defined as the presence of one or more of the following lesions: papules, pustules, and nodules or cysts. The parameters for defining the lesions are as follows:

- Papules are inflammatory lesions smaller than 5 mm in diameter.
- Pustules are similar in size to papules but have a visible central core of purulent material.
- Nodules are inflammatory lesions with a diameter of 5 mm or greater.[12]

The consensus panel's proposed classification of severity grades for inflammatory acne, based on a lesion count approximation, is presented in Table 2. A designation of "very severe" is recognized for the most destructive forms of acne, such as cystic acne.

TABLE 2 Severity grading of inflammatory acne lesions

Severity	Papules/Pustules	Nodules
Mild	Few to several	None
Moderate	Several to many	Few to several
Severe	Numerous and/or extensive	Many

Predisposing Factors

Many women with acne experience a premenstrual flare-up of symptoms. Hormonal changes associated with ovulation and pregnancy are also related to flare-ups. Oral contraceptives containing androgenic progestins have been implicated in the production of acne, as have certain menopausal hormone replacements. It is also possible that severe or prolonged stress or other emotional extremes may exacerbate the condition.

Hydration decreases the size of the pilosebaceous duct orifice, which explains why acne is exacerbated in conditions of high humidity or in situations that induce frequent and prolonged sweating.

Local irritation or friction may increase the incidence of acne symptoms. Rough or occlusive clothing, headgear straps, athletic equipment, and other friction-producing devices can aggravate acne (acne mechanica). Even resting the chin or cheek on the hand often or for long periods creates localized conditions conducive to lesion formation in acne-prone individuals.[6]

Acne cosmetica is a low-grade, mild form of acne on the face, cheek, and chin. The lesions of acne cosmetica typically are closed, noninflammatory comedones and cannot easily be distinguished from similar lesions of acne vulgaris. This form of acne is more common in women than in men because women are more likely to use cosmetics. Some products may contain oils that are comedogenic (e.g., lanolin, mineral oil, or cocoa butter). Oil-based cosmetics may be occlusive and plug the follicles, thus exacerbating or even initiating acne.

Pomade acne, most often seen in African-Americans and manifested by comedones along the hairline on the forehead and temples, is reported to be caused directly by the long-term use of hair dressings that contain occlusive petrolatum or liquid petrolatum.

Drug-induced acne is not a true acne. Drugs can exacerbate preexisting acne vulgaris. Corticosteroids, both systemic and topical, may also induce hypertrophic changes by sensitizing the follicle and producing "steroid acne." Other systemic drugs known to precipitate acne eruptions include androgens, oral contraceptives containing norgestrel or norethindrone, iodides, bromides, ethionamide, azothioprine, dantrolene, haloperidol, halothane, isoniazid, lithium, phenytoin, thyroid preparations, and trimethadione.[2,13]

Occupational exposure to certain industrial chemicals such as coal tar and petroleum derivatives may cause acne. The term "McDonald's" or "french fryers" acne refers to acne initiated or exacerbated by vaporized oils present as air contaminants.[14]

There is little evidence to support a direct relationship between diet and acne. Several studies have demonstrated that chocolate does not affect acne even though some clinicians and patients remain unconvinced. Other clinicians think that dietary restrictions are unwarranted because no convincing evidence has been presented to implicate nuts, fats, colas, or carbohydrates. However, an indirect relationship has been proposed between acne and a diet that is high in fat and refined carbohydrates and low in fiber, suggesting that dietary habits may be a risk factor in acne as well as in more serious illnesses.[15] The practical approach is for people to avoid any particular food that seems to exacerbate their acne.

As with many other medical conditions, heredity may predispose a person to the development of acne. Not unexpectedly, the chances are higher that offspring will develop acne if both parents suffered from acne, than if only one parent had it.[16]

Goals of Treatment

Acne is rarely cured, but its symptoms can be controlled to varying degrees. In most cases, available therapeutic regimens and patient compliance will reduce symptoms and minimize permanent scarring. Because acne persists for long periods, often from adolescence to the early 20s or beyond, treatment must be long-term and consistent.

Goals

The objectives of acne treatment should include the following:
- Ensuring patient compliance;
- Relieving physical and social discomfort;
- Removing excess sebum from the skin with proper cleansing;
- Preventing closure of the pilosebaceous orifice;
- Using irritants to unblock ducts;
- Reducing lipase activity;
- Minimizing conditions conducive to the development of acne, such as the presence of physical irritants and the use of oil-based cleansers and cosmetics;
- Educating the individual in the proper use of and need for patience with both the nondrug and drug portions of the treatment regimen.

Self-Treatment Versus Physician Referral

Self-treatment should be limited to patients who experience noninflammatory acne of mild to moderate severity that is limited to observed whiteheads and blackheads. Self-treatment is most appropriate if lesions are not extensive (fewer than 10 on one side of the face). Self-treatment should include attention to exacerbating factors such as cosmetic use, humidity, and overexposure to irritating chemicals. Self-treatment is most effective in patients who are mature enough to understand that acne treatment will be long-term and that acne symptoms can be controlled to varying degrees but cannot be cured.

Depending upon the answers provided in response to the patient assessment and counseling questions that introduce this chapter, the pharmacist may find the following pointers useful when advising the patient about self-treatment.

- If acne lesions are present where clothes, headbands, helmets, or other devices cause friction, preventing friction-induced irritation should be discussed with the patient. Irritation may also occur as a result of routinely resting the face on the hand; this habit should be avoided or minimized if it is problematic.
- If oil-based cosmetic products are used, water-based products should be considered. If the hair is oily, frequent shampooing with a water-based shampoo is encouraged.
- If face washing is frequent or if a drying soap is used, gentle washing two to three times daily with a mild facial soap is generally recommended.
- If exposure to environmental factors (e.g., dirt, dust, oil, or chemical irritants) seems to exacerbate the acne, the patient should be counseled on how to minimize or avoid these exposures.
- Regardless of the degree of acne severity, the patient should be advised against squeezing, pinching, or picking at acne lesions, especially inflammatory ones. Such behavior aggravates the condition and may result in scarring.

There are numerous situations in which self-treatment is inadequate and physician referral is required. For example, inflammatory acne consisting of observed papules, pustules, nodules, and cysts that are extensive (more than 10 lesions on one side of the face) should be referred to a physician, preferably a dermatologist. If the acne is thought to be associated with the use of a drug with comedogenic (e.g., androgenic) activity, a physician should be contacted. If acne lesions persist beyond the mid-20s or develop in the mid-20s or later, the symptoms may signal rosacea rather than acne vulgaris. These conditions need to be medically differentiated because the approach for treating rosacea, though similar to that for treating acne vulgaris in some ways, also has unique elements.

Suppressing or altering hormonal activity, correcting disfiguring effects, and using prescription drugs to treat acne must be directed by a physician.

Nondrug Approaches

The starting point in treating acne is proper skin hygiene. The preferred method of removing excess sebum from the skin is a conscientious program of daily washing. The purpose of washing is to produce a mild drying of the skin and, perhaps, mild erythema. The affected areas should be thoroughly but gently washed at least twice daily with warm water, medicated or unmedicated soap, and a soft washcloth; they should then be patted dry. More frequent washing is appropriate if the skin is oily. Washing should not be excessively vigorous because it may worsen the condition and cause acne mechanica. Washing should cause barely noticeable peeling that can loosen comedones. If it produces a feeling of tautness in the skin, the intensity and frequency of washings should be reduced and switching to a less drying soap should be considered.

Ordinary facial soaps that do not contain moisturizing oils are usually satisfactory. Soaps containing antibacterial agents have been suggested for controlling acne, but no conclusive evidence of their clinical value has been presented. Although salicylic acid, sulfur, and sulfur in combination with resorcinol or resorcinol monoacetate are safe and effective for self-treating acne, their benefit as ingredients in soaps is questionable because little, if any, residue is left on the skin after thorough washing.[17]

Soap substitutes containing surfactants (ionic or nonionic) have been suggested for acne because they are less drying to the skin. However, because a mild degree of drying is desirable, an ordinary facial soap should be tried first. Some cleansing preparations contain pumice, polyethylene, or aluminum oxide particles to add abrasive action. For example, there are polyester cleansing sponges that assist in removing the outer layer of dead skin cells by gentle abrasion. Used gently, these abrasive agents may be helpful in treating noninflammatory acne. Abrasives should be avoided in inflammatory acne, however, because of increased irritation. If it is inconvenient to wash during the day, a cleansing pad that contains alcohol, acetone, and a surfactant may be used.

Because acne treatment begins with removing excess sebum from the skin, topically applied products such as cosmetics and hair dressings should be water-based rather than oil-based. Hair should be shampooed often because acne is usually accompanied by an oily scalp.

Topical Nonprescription Products

The Category I (generally recognized as safe and effective by the Food and Drug Administration [FDA]) active topical antiacne ingredients include 0.5–2% salicylic acid, 3–8% sulfur, and a combination of 3–8% sulfur with either 2% resorcinol or 3% resorcinol monoacetate.[1] Benzoyl peroxide, although proposed and initially classified as a Category I ingredient, was temporarily reclassified to Category III (more data needed) because of concern over its tumorigenic potential. Safety studies are ongoing to determine whether benzoyl peroxide enhances the ability of ultraviolet (UV) radiation to produce skin cancer. In the meantime, the product remains on the market as an effective product.

Salicylic Acid

Salicylic acid is a mild comedolytic agent that is available in various nonprescription acne products in concentrations of 0.5–2%. Pharmacologically, it acts as a surface keratolytic.[2] The keratolytic effect and possible enhanced absorption of other agents provide the rationale for the topical use of salicylic acid; however, its safety is questionable when used over large areas for prolonged periods of time.[17]

The use of salicylic acid in cleansing preparations is considered adjunctive acne treatment in reducing comedonal lesions and in improving the overall condition.[18]

Sulfur

Sulfur has met the criteria of the FDA Advisory Review Panel for Over-the-Counter Topical Acne Products although the claim for antibacterial effects was disallowed.[1] Alternate forms of sulfur, such as sodium thiosulfate, zinc sulfate, and zinc sulfide, are not recognized in the monograph as safe and effective.

Sulfur, in a precipitated or colloidal form, is included in acne products as a keratolytic in concentrations of 3–10%.

Sulfur is generally accepted as being an effective agent for promoting the resolution of existing comedones, but on continued use it may have a comedogenic effect.

Sulfur-containing products are applied in a thin film to the affected area once or twice daily. They have a noticeable color and odor, characteristics that must be considered when their selection and use are being recommended. Compliance may be enhanced by recommending fleshtone products or suggesting usage after school and at bedtime.

Resorcinol and Resorcinol Monoacetate

Although resorcinol and resorcinol monoacetate are not regarded as efficacious as single agents in the treatment of acne, they have been offered in concentrations of 1 to 2%. There is some question as to whether percutaneous resorcinol absorption may precipitate systemic toxicity when these agents are applied to extensive areas of the body. The FDA advisory review panel concluded that, when used alone, the lower concentrations of these agents are safe but not effective in the topical treatment of acne. Therefore, the FDA placed such products in Category II (not generally recognized as safe and effective, or unacceptable indications).[11]

Sulfur Combined with Resorcinol and Resorcinol Monoacetate

The FDA includes the combination of 3–8% sulfur with either 2% resorcinol or 3% resorcinol monoacetate in the Category I list of active ingredients for nonprescription acne products.[1] The precise mechanism by which this combination helps to resolve acne lesions has not been determined. The agents function primarily as keratolytics fostering cell turnover and desquamation.

The sulfur–resorcinol products have the characteristic color and odor noted for the sulfur-only products. Additionally, resorcinol may produce a dark brown scale on some darker skinned individuals, who should be forewarned and reassured that the reaction is reversible when the medication is discontinued.

Benzoyl Peroxide

Having determined that additional studies are needed to address concerns about benzoyl peroxide's possible tumor-initiating and promotion potential, the FDA has delayed final action on benzoyl peroxide pending such further study.[1,19,20] Part of the reason for this uncertainty is attributed to reports that benzoyl peroxide is a tumor promoter and progressor, but is neither an initiator nor a complete carcinogen.[21,22] Thus, the FDA is unable to state that this ingredient is unsafe for use while studies are being conducted and analyzed. The FDA acknowledges that this research, as well as a final determination on benzoyl peroxide's safety, may take several years.[23] In the meantime, benzoyl peroxide has been placed in Category III because insufficient data are currently available to classify it as safe as well as effective.

Benzoyl peroxide, one of the most effective and widely used topical nonprescription medications available for treating acne, may act in several ways. It causes irritation and desquamation, which prevents closure of the pilosebaceous orifice. The irritant effect causes an increased turnover rate of the epithelial cells lining the follicular duct, which increases sloughing and promotes resolution of the comedones. The oxidizing potential may contribute to bacteriostatic and bactericidal activity, suppressing the local population of *P. acnes* and reducing the formation of irritating free fatty acids. It also exhibits irritant, drying, and sensitizing effects and may bleach hair and fabrics.

Benzoyl peroxide is available in concentrations of 2.5%, 5%, and 10% as lotions, gels, creams, cleansers, masks, and soaps. Clinical response to all concentrations is similar in terms of reducing the number of inflammatory lesions. However, the different formulations are not equivalent. The drying effect of the alcohol gel base enhances its effectiveness; therefore, it is superior to a lotion of the same concentration. Some products, mainly the gels, are available by prescription only. Although the washes and cleansers containing benzoyl peroxide are widely used as acne treatment adjuncts, they have been found to have little or no comedolytic effect.[18]

Instructions for the proper use of topical nonprescription benzoyl peroxide include the following:

- The affected area should be gently cleansed with a nonmedicated soap and patted dry, and a small quantity of the preparation should be smoothed over the area once or twice daily.
- Because some individuals are sensitive to benzoyl peroxide, the initial applications may be limited to one or two small areas at the 2.5% or 5% concentration to determine whether discomfort will occur.
- The initial application should be left on the skin for only 15 minutes and washed off. The time benzoyl peroxide is left on the skin should then be increased in 15-minute increments as tolerance allows. Once it is tolerated for 2 hours, it can be left on the skin overnight. The once-a-day application may be all that is needed. A morning dose may be applied if tolerated.
- Fair-skinned individuals should initiate therapy with the 5% strength and apply it only once daily during the first few weeks of therapy.
- Benzoyl peroxide should be used with great care near the eyes, mouth, lips, and nose because it is highly irritating.
- The drug should not be used concurrently with other topical products unless instructed by a physician.
- The drug should be used externally only.
- Excessive dryness, marked peeling, some skin sloughing, erythema, or edema suggests that lower concentrations should be used for shorter periods of time. Cool compresses may relieve the discomfort of inflamed skin.
- Use of the drug may bleach hair and clothing.
- Use of the drug may cause transient stinging and burning, but this is not generally a cause for alarm unless it persists or becomes worse.
- If excessive stinging and burning occur after application, the preparation should be removed with soap and water and not reapplied until the next day.
- Other sources of irritation, such as sunlamps and excessive exposure to the sun, should be avoided.
- The full therapeutic effect may not be experienced for 4–6 weeks, so users should be encouraged to be patient and compliant.

Other Combination Products

Assorted nonprescription combinations of benzoyl peroxide, sulfur, salicylic acid, and resorcinol have been used to treat acne. The efficacy of these combination products over the single-ingredient products has not been clearly demonstrated. However, these combination products, as well as an extensive list of other acne product ingredients, may soon be of only historical interest if the FDA does not recognize them as safe and effective for acne self-therapy.

Topical Prescription Products

Tretinoin

Tretinoin (all-*trans*retinoic acid) is a topical medication proven effective in treating acne. It is available, in order of increasing irritation, as a cream (0.025%, 0.05%, 0.1%), a gel (0.01%, 0.025%), and a liquid (0.05%). Tretinoin (Retin-A®) acts to normalize the follicular epithelium, promote drainage of comedones, and inhibit formation of new comedones. It is more irritating than benzoyl peroxide, particularly in the early stages of treatment.[2] Tretinoin should be reserved for use in moderate to severe acne after treatment with milder agents has failed. It may be used alone to treat comedonal acne; as an adjunct in the treatment of inflammatory papulopustular acne; or as an adjunct in treating acne secondary to steroid use, ionizing radiation, tars, and chlorinated hydrocarbons.

Individuals using tretinoin for the first time should be cautioned that the skin will become red and peel, usually within a week of initiating therapy. This condition will last approximately 3 or 4 weeks. Severe irritation may require alternate day therapy instead of the recommended daily use. The acne can be expected to become exacerbated during the initial 4–6 weeks of therapy, and patients should be reassured that this is normal and temporary. Eight to 12 weeks of treatment is generally required before the effectiveness of therapy can be fully assessed. Because tretinoin can increase susceptibility to sunburn, prolonged exposure to the sun should be avoided and an effective sunscreen should be used. (See Chapter 34, "Sunscreen and Suntan Products.")

Antibiotics

Topical antibiotics are useful in controlling the symptoms of acne although they are generally considered to be less effective than benzoyl peroxide.[2] They act by decreasing the follicular population of *P. acnes*, which reduces the production of comedogenic, inflammatory free fatty acids from the sebum. The fat soluble formulations of clindamycin, erythromycin, and tetracycline are able to diffuse through the fatty contents of the sebaceous follicle to reach *P. acnes* in the lower segments of the follicle. The products are formulated as either dilute solutions in organic solvents or as creams.

Systemic Prescription Products

Isotretinoin

Isotretinoin (13-*cis*retinoic acid) is an oral medication that is effective in treating severe nodulocystic acne that is resistant to all other forms of therapy. The precise mechanism of action has not been elucidated. Effects observed include inhibition of sebum production and follicular keratinization with a consequent reduction in the concentration of *P. acnes* on the skin surface. The condition may worsen temporarily when therapy is initiated, but resolution occurs with continued therapy. The severity of the disease should determine the dosage. Because severe, recalcitrant cystic acne is likely to flare up after treatment, higher doses are indicated for patients with this type of acne. Prolonged remission may persist following the course of therapy.[24]

Adverse reactions, which reportedly occur in more than 90% of patients treated, include severe mucocutaneous, musculoskeletal, and teratogenic effects. Many patients experience inflammation and dryness of the eyes, which may decrease their tolerance to contact lenses. Some patients should be advised not to wear contact lenses during treatment.

Because isotretinoin appears to share many of the toxicities observed with other retinoids, the patient should be advised not to take vitamin A or vitamin supplements containing vitamin A without consulting the prescriber.[25]

A significant portion of the patient population likely to use isotretinoin consists of women of reproductive age. Retrospective studies clearly show a link between use of isotretinoin in pregnancy and a high risk of either spontaneous abortion or severe congenital malformations.[26] Recognizing the hazards, the manufacturer introduced the Pregnancy Prevention Program for Women on Accutane®, which includes patient education brochures and a consent form for the prescribing physician. The pharmacist who dispenses isotretinoin should make every effort to ensure that female patients understand the dangers of becoming pregnant both while taking the drug and for several months after treatment ceases.

A thorough presentation of the side effect profile and guidelines for the proper use of isotretinoin is beyond the scope of this chapter. However, the reader is strongly encouraged to be fully aware of the risks, as well as the benefits, of isotretinoin therapy, for they are profound.

Anti-Infectives

Oral doxycycline, erythromycin, minocycline, tetracycline, and trimethoprim–sulfamethoxazole are effective in treating inflammatory acne. These drugs probably suppress the growth of normal cutaneous flora (*P. acnes*), which decreases formation of free fatty acids and consequently decreases inflammation.

Oral antibiotics are usually started at the full dose (e.g., 1 g of tetracycline per day in four equally divided doses) and then decreased to a maintenance dose after maximal improvement has occurred. Most of the adverse effects are limited in duration and are easily treated. Gastrointestinal upset is the most common side effect. Tetracycline is the drug of choice because it is effective and inexpensive, and it exhibits few side effects. Compliance may be a problem with tetracycline, however, because it should be taken between meals to maximize absorption. Minocycline has the disadvantage of causing occasional ototoxicity and rare pigmentary changes in the skin, as well as of being more expensive. Trimethoprim–sulfamethoxazole is the most likely to produce allergic reactions.

Once clearing is achieved with oral antibiotic therapy, maintenance therapy with topical agents may suffice.

Estrogen

Very severe or otherwise unresponsive cases of acne in young women may be treated with estrogen therapy. The effectiveness of estrogen therapy varies significantly from patient to patient and may be due to suppression of androgen production or competition with androgenic receptors in the sebaceous cells. The most commonly used estrogen products were the high-estrogen oral contraceptives, which are no longer available. There is currently no evidence that low-dose oral contraceptives offer a significant therapeutic advantage in managing acne in women.[27]

Investigational Therapies

The combination of oral ibuprofen and tetracycline for the treatment of acne vulgaris is under investigation.[28] Ketoconazole, an antifungal agent that inhibits testosterone synthesis, is being investigated as a treatment for acne in women.[3] Spironolactone is also used as an antiandrogen in some cases of female hyperandrogenism.[2] Applied topically, the alpha hydroxy acids (e.g., "fruit acids" such as lactic, malic, and glycolic acid) smooth the skin by facilitating the loosening and shedding of stratum corneum cells and may be useful in the removal of comedones.[29] The success of isotretinoin has led to the synthesis of isotretinoin derivatives in an attempt to retain the beneficial effects of the drug while reducing or eliminating the serious adverse effects.[3]

Other Treatments

Although sunlight and artificial UV radiation were once thought to be beneficial in acne treatment by virtue of their drying and peeling effect, they are largely ineffective and are not currently recommended. Sunlight can, in fact, aggravate acne. Additionally, excessive exposure to UV radiation hastens skin aging and wrinkling and contributes to an increased risk of skin cancer.

Both topical and systemic steroids have been used in acne treatment.[2] Systemic prednisone therapy is effective but rarely used because of the risks involved in long-term steroid therapy. Topical corticosteroid application has been found to be ineffective. Direct injections of corticosteroids may be used judiciously to reduce large inflammatory lesions.[2] Inflamed cysts may also be treated by cryotherapy using liquid nitrogen.[30]

Some patients whose acne has caused severe scarring and pitting may seek cosmetic repair. The initial approach in the past has been dermabrasion. Intralesional injection of bovine-derived collagen has been used with moderate success in selected cases.[30] Silicone implants have also been used with some degree of effectiveness.[3]

Formulation Considerations

The formulation that carries topical acne medication to the skin can influence the drug's effectiveness. Therefore, particular attention should be paid to this aspect of product selection when advising a patient.

Suspensions, lotions, creams, and gels are the vehicles generally used for antiacne preparations. Lotions and creams should have a low fat content so that they do not counteract drying and peeling. Nonfatty gels dry slowly if formulated in a completely aqueous base. Ethyl or isopropyl alcohol added to liquid preparations and gels hastens their drying to a film. The astringent (drying) effect of the volatile solvents may enhance the effectiveness of the various preparations, but it may be unacceptable to the patient.

Thickening agents in preparations should not dry to a sticky film. The solids in most preparations leave a film that is not noticeably visible and does not need coloring to blend in with the skin. However, some products are intended to hide blemishes by depositing an opaque film of insoluble masking agents such as zinc oxide on the skin. These products are tinted to improve their cosmetic effect; however, they rarely produce a satisfactory color match.

A general guideline might be to recommend cream formulations for individuals with fair complexions and gels for those with dark complexions.

Counseling Guidelines

Various therapeutic approaches may be used to treat acne. Familiarity with these approaches will help in advising individuals.

The questions at the beginning of this chapter provide an overview of baseline information to aid the pharmacist in advising and counseling an acne patient. Before counseling the patient on treatment, the pharmacist should try to determine whether the patient is suffering from acne vulgaris or another dermatological condition. The pharmacist should then decide whether the condition merits self-treatment or warrants physician referral.

Before recommending self-treatment, the pharmacist should evaluate the patient's attitude toward treatment and willingness to comply with a skin care program that involves a continued daily regimen of washing affected areas and applying or ingesting medication. The pharmacist should clearly explain the basis for the recommendation. Comedonal and mild papular acne can usually be successfully self-treated, whereas moderately severe papular acne and pustular and cystic acne require the attention of a physician.

Once the decision has been made as to which approach to recommend, the pharmacist should explain the treatment program and acne process, and correct any misconceptions the patient might have. The patient should be advised about scalp and hair care; the use of cosmetics; and, above all, the need for long-term, conscientious care. (See the appendix at the end of the chapter for sources of patient brochures on skin care, acne vulgaris, and acne rosacea.) The patient should also be advised of the following points when appropriate:

- Diet is important in maintaining health, but many of the myths about diet and acne are unfounded.
- Stressful situations may play a role in acne flare-ups but do not cause acne.
- Sexual activity plays no role in the occurrence or worsening of acne.

Because acne cannot be cured but only controlled, reassurance and emotional support is often necessary to reduce patient concern.

Summary

Acne vulgaris occurs almost universally in young adults from their early teens to their mid-20s, and it occasionally appears in prepubertal and older people. Generally, acne cannot be cured; however, it may be controlled enough to improve cosmetic appearance and prevent the development of severe acne with its resultant scarring. With empathy and reassurance, acne patients may understand that the condition will not exist forever but that care must be given to the affected areas for a long time for improvement to occur.

References

1. *Federal Register* 1991 Aug 16; 56 (9): 41018–20.
2. Leyden JJ, Shalita AR. Rational therapy for acne vulgaris: an update on topical treatment. *J Am Acad Dermatol* 1986 Oct; 15 (4 pt 2): 907–15.
3. Bennett RW, Popovich NG. Treatment of acne vulgaris. *US Pharm* 1989 Jan; 14: 40–51.
4. Gossel TA. OTC anti-acne medications. *US Pharm* 1990 Oct; 15: 24–34.
5. Arndt KA, ed. *Manual of Dermatologic Therapeutics with Essentials of Diagnosis.* 2nd ed. Boston: Little, Brown and Co; 1978: 3–15.
6. Kligman AM. An overview of acne. *J Invest Dermatol* 1974; 62: 268–87.

7. Frienkel RK. Pathogenesis of acne vulgaris. *N Engl J Med* 1969 May 22; 280: 1161–2.
8. Frienkel RK, Strauss JS, Yip SY, et al. Effect of tetracycline on the composition of sebum in acne vulgaris. *N Engl J Med* 1965 Oct 14; 273: 850–4.
9. Patient counseling. Facial skin problems may be rosacea. *Am Pharm* 1992 Jan; NS32 (1): 9–10.
10. Pillsbury DM. *A Manual of Dermatology*. Philadelphia: W. B. Saunders Co; 1971: 173–174.
11. *Federal Register* 1982 Mar 23; 47 (56): 12430–77.
12. Pochi PE, Shalita AR, Strauss JS, et al. Report of the consensus conference on acne classification. *J Am Acad Dermatol* 1991 Mar; 24 (3): 495–500.
13. Pochi PE. The pathogenesis and treatment of acne. *Annu Rev Med* 1990, 41: 187–98.
14. Popovich NG. Acne: control is a slow process. *US Pharm* (skin care supplement) 1991 Jun; 16: 20–7.
15. Rosenberg EW, Kirk BS. Acne diet reconsidered. *Arch Dermatol* 1981 Apr; 117: 193–5.
16. Pochi PE. Treatment of teenage acne. *Drug Therapy* 1991 Jan; 21: 56–62.
17. *Federal Register* 1985 Jan 15; 50 (10): 2172–82.
18. Shalita AR. Comparison of a salicylic acid cleanser and a benzoyl peroxide wash in the treatment of acne vulgaris. *Clin Ther* 1989; 11 (2): 264–7.
19. Slaga TJ, Klein-Szanko AJP, Triplett LL, et al. Skin tumor-promoting activity of benzoyl peroxide, a widely used free radical-generating compound. *Science* 1981; 213: 1023–5.
20. Kurokawa Y, Takamura N, Matsushima Y, et al. Studies on the promoting and complete carcinogenic activities of some oxidizing chemicals in skin carcinogenesis. *Can Let* 1984; 24: 299–304.
21. Schweizer J, Loehrke H, Edler L, et al. Benzoyl peroxide promotes the formation of melanotic tumors in the skin of 7,12-dimethyl benz[a]antracene-initiated syrian golden hamsters. *Carcinogenesis* 1987; 8 (3): 479–82.
22. Swauger JE, Dolan PM, Zweier JL, et al. Role of the benzoyloxyl radical in DNA damage mediated by benzoyl peroxide. *Chem Res Toxicol* 1991 Mar–Apr; 4 (2): 223–8.
23. *Federal Register* 1991 Aug 7; 56 (152): 37622–35.
24. Shalita AR. *Treatment Challenges in Acne Therapy*. Paper presented at Atlanta: 49th Annual Meeting of the American Academy of Dermatology; December 1990.
25. *USP DI—Drug Information for the Health Care Professional*, Vol IB. 12th ed. Rockville, Md: United States Pharmacopeial Convention, Inc; 1992: 1666–1669.
26. Pochi PE. Isotretinoin for acne: the experience broadens. *N Engl J Med* 1985 Oct 17; 313 (16): 1013–4.
27. Pochi PE. *Treatment Challenges in Acne Therapy*. Paper presented at Atlanta: 49th Annual Meeting of the American Academy of Dermatology; December 1990.
28. Wong RC, Kang S, Heezen JL, et al. Oral ibuprofen and tetracycline for the treatment of acne vulgaris. *J Am Acad Dermatol* 1984; 11: 1076.
29. Van Scott EJ. Reversing the signs of the times. *Wellcome Trends Dermatol* 1987 Nov; 2–3.
30. Popovich NG. Current acne therapy. *Pharm Int* 1986 Mar; 7: 68–71.

Appendix: Acne Information Sources

- National Rosacea Society
  18-3 East Dundee Road, Suite 206
  Barrington, IL 60010
  Patient brochures on acne rosacea.

- Dermatological Division
  Ortho Pharmaceutical Corporation
  U.S. Route 2
  Raritan, NJ 08869
  Patient brochures on tretinoin therapy.

- Roche Laboratories
  340 Kingsland Street
  Nutley, NJ 07110
  Patient brochures on isotretinoin therapy.

- The Skin Ecology Council
  P.O. Box 5096
  New York, NY 10185
  Patient brochures on skin care.

- The Upjohn Company
  Adult Acne
  P.O. Box 307
  Coventry, CT 06238
  Patient brochures on acne rosacea.

- The Upjohn Company
  7000 Portage Road
  Kalamazoo, MI 49001
  Patient brochures on acne vulgaris.

- Westwood Pharmaceuticals Inc.
  100 Forest Avenue
  Buffalo, NY 14213
  Patient brochures on acne vulgaris.

CHAPTER 30

Dermatologic Products

Joye Ann Billow

> **Questions to ask in patient assessment and counseling**
>
> ■ *How long have you had this skin problem? Has it changed since you have had it? Does it seem to come and go?*
> ■ *What areas are involved? What does the skin look like (for those areas covered by clothing)?*
> ■ *How does the skin feel (itchy, painful)? Is it dry or wet?*
> ■ *Do you scratch your skin? How often? When?*
> ■ *Do others in your family have a similar skin condition? Do allergies, asthma, or hay fever run in your family?*
> ■ *Do you notice a seasonal change in the skin problem?*
> ■ *Is there anything such as work activities; household cleaning; changing soaps, deodorants, or shampoos; or wearing jewelry that seems to make the skin condition worse?*
> ■ *Have you consulted a physician about your skin problem? If so, what treatment was suggested? Are you currently following the treatment?*
> ■ *Are you currently using any prescription or nonprescription medications? If so, what are they?*
> ■ *Have you already tried some skin care products? If so, which ones? How effective were they?*
> ■ *Do you prefer one type of product—lotion, cream, gel, etc.—over another?*
> ■ *How old are you or how old is the patient (if a child)?*

The skin is the body's largest organ. Although it is exposed to a wide variety of chemical and environmental insults, it demonstrates remarkable resiliency and recuperative ability. Nevertheless, skin problems are common, with an estimated 1 in 20 people suffering from a chronic skin disorder and millions of others encountering acute or seasonal problems. The pharmacist is often the first health care professional the patient consults concerning conditions such as dermatitis, dry skin, dandruff, seborrheic dermatitis (seborrhea), and psoriasis. Therefore, in addition to the underlying pathology, the pharmacist must consider the cosmetic, psychologic, and work- or recreation-related aspects of the dermal affliction before referring the patient to a physician or recommending the use of an appropriate nonprescription product. Moreover, because the person suffering from a symptomatic skin disorder will rarely consider it minor, this area of patient counseling offers the pharmacist a major opportunity to provide critical information to the patient.

Physiology of the Skin

Normal skin has a variety of functions, the most important being to serve as a protective barrier between the body and the environment. It is also important in controlling fluid and electrolyte balance, in regulating heat, and in mediating sensation.

The skin is composed of three basic layers: epidermis, dermis, and subcutaneous fat or hypodermis. The epidermis is the outer portion of the skin. It consists of several types of cells and has no blood supply. The deepest, or basal, layer of the epidermis consists of cells that divide and move upward. These cells produce keratin, which is an insoluble protein. As the cells move upward, the keratin becomes granular and the cells lose water and their nuclei, and finally die. The dead cells eventually reach the outermost layer, called the stratum corneum, where they are normally shed as invisible scales. Because the keratinized or "horny" layer of the stratum corneum is constantly being shed and regenerated, the epidermis is maintained at a uniform thickness. The complete cycle, from basal cell formation to shedding, is 28–45 days.

The dermis lies between the epidermis and the layer of subcutaneous fat. About 40 times thicker than the epidermis, the dermis supports the epidermis physically and contains blood vessels, nerves, and elastic and connective tissue. Its main constituent, other than water, is the fibrous protein collagen. Because this layer of skin contains nerve fibers, it is responsible for cutaneous sensations. The sensation of itching arises in the upper portion; that of stinging, in the middle portion; and that of pain, in the portion closest to the layer of subcutaneous fat.

The layer of subcutaneous fat is responsible for the pliability of the skin. It also provides insulation, serves as a nutritional reserve, and cushions against minor trauma.

The stratum corneum is the primary barrier to insults from the environment. The lipid components of the cells of the stratum corneum may store fat-soluble materials rather than allow them to pass into the systemic circulation. Keratin can absorb many times its weight in water, and so it retains water to maintain the flexibility and

---

This chapter is based in part on the chapter with a similar title that appeared in the 9th edition but was written by Joseph R. Robinson.

TABLE 1 Selected dermatologic terms useful in the assessment of skin lesions

Term	Type of lesion[a]	Definition
Crust (scab)	Secondary	Dried exudate containing proteinaceous and cellular debris from erosion or ulceration of primary lesions
Erythema	Primary	Reddened skin
Fissure	Secondary	A split in the epidermis extending into the dermis
Lichenification	Secondary	Thickening and hardening of the skin into an irregular plaque due to excessive rubbing or scratching
Macule	Primary	Flat, nonpalpable, discolored lesion less than 1 cm in diameter. Lesions larger than 1 cm are termed *patches*
Necrosis	Secondary	Dead cells or groups of cells caused by severe trauma or an infectious process
Papule	Primary	A solid, circumscribed, elevated lesion less than 1 cm in diameter
Plaque	Primary	A palpable, papular, relatively flat lesion more than 1 cm in diameter
Pustule	Primary	A circumscribed, elevated lesion less than 1 cm in diameter containing pus. A larger lesion is termed an *abscess* or *furuncle*
Scale	Secondary	Accumulation of loose, desquamated, hyperkeratitic epidermal cells
Ulcer	Secondary	An erosion of the epidermis exposing the dermis. Deep ulcers may result in destruction of the dermis
Vesicle	Primary	A sharply circumscribed, elevated lesion containing fluid. Diameter of a vesicle may be up to 1 cm. A fluid-filled cavity of diameter greater than 1 cm is termed a *blister* or *bulla*

[a]Primary lesions are changes in the skin as a result of the undisturbed disease process. Secondary lesions are the result of external influences on the primary lesion. Primary and secondary lesion frequently co-exist.
Adapted from Cahn RL, Longe RL. *The Skin: Assessment.* Palo Alto, Calif: Syntex Laboratories; 1986: 4–5.

integrity of the skin. The intracellular spaces of the stratum corneum contain a complex mixture of hygroscopic substances (free amino acids, pyrrolidine carboxylic acid, urea, uric acid, ammonia, creatinine, sodium, calcium, potassium, magnesium, phosphate, chloride, lactate, citrate, formate, sugars, organic acids, and peptides) called the natural moisturizing factor, which holds water and allows absorption of water-soluble drugs.

The flexibility of the stratum corneum depends on its water content, which is normally between 10 and 20% by weight. A variety of factors, including humidity, temperature, surfactants, and physical and chemical trauma, influence the water content of the stratum corneum.[1] When the water content drops below 10%, chapping occurs and the stratum corneum becomes brittle and cracks easily. This allows irritants and bacteria to penetrate and leads to inflammation and even infection.

Dermatitis and Dry Skin

Dermatitis is a nonspecific term that describes a number of dermatologic conditions that are inflammatory and generally characterized by erythema. Dermatitis may be either acute or chronic. The terms *eczema* and *dermatitis* are often used interchangeably to describe a group of inflammatory skin disorders of unknown etiology. When the cause of a particular skin condition is elucidated, the disease is given a specific name. Known causes of dermatitis include allergens, irritants, and infections. However, there are several distinct forms of dermatitis for which the causes are still unknown.

Initially, the signs and symptoms are very similar for all forms of dermatitis. These signs may include pruritus (itching), erythema (redness), and edema (swelling). Edema may be accompanied by fluid-filled vesicles, which often break and cause weeping or oozing from the skin. Evaporation of water from the exudate results in crusting and scaling. Over time, the weeping may diminish, giving way to a dry, scaly condition; at no time does the epidermal tissue appear normal. The lesions may be patchy in distribution. In the acute stages, there is a uniform pattern of papular vesicles on an erythematous base[2] (Table 1).

If the dermatitis becomes chronic, weeping may subside, the skin may become dry, and fissures may appear. If the itching results in excessive scratching, the epidermis may thicken owing to a process called lichenification. Infections may occur as sequelae to pruritus-induced scratching. Either hyperpigmentation or hypopigmentation may occur.[1]

The most common forms of dermatitis include atopic dermatitis, contact dermatitis (irritant or allergic), hand dermatitis ("dishpan hands"), and dry skin. Table 2 lists the primary characteristics of these conditions.

Specific Conditions

Atopic Dermatitis

The primary symptom of atopic dermatitis is intense itching that is often intermittent, leading to vigorous itch-scratch cycles. The areas affected are commonly the face and the skin folds on the inside of the knees and elbows. The skin is inflamed with vesicles that may weep and produce scales. Atopic dermatitis occurs primarily in children and young adults, and is the most common dermatologic problem seen in children. It is often accompanied by other skin conditions such as dry skin, contact dermatitis, and hand dermatitis.

Atopic dermatitis is not contagious but is genetically predetermined. If one parent has the condition, the child has greater than a one-in-four chance of developing it also. If both parents have atopic dermatitis, the child has greater than a 50% chance of developing it. Although the etiology of the condition is unknown, the patients and their families often have associated asthma, hay fever, or chronic allergic rhinitis. Because skin sensitivity to a wide range of agents is common, skin tests are not reliable diagnostic aids. Also, normal prevention and treatment of allergy, such as avoiding contact with allergens and administering antihistamines, seldom bring relief to the patient with this disease.

Although atopic dermatitis often develops in infancy, it is rarely present at birth. If it does develop early, it occurs in the first year of life in approximately 80% of the cases—often beginning at 2 to 3 months of age—with another 10% of cases developing before age 5. It initially appears as redness and chapping of the infant's cheeks and may not resolve for several years. Remission usually occurs between the second and fourth year with recurrences often diminishing in intensity or even disappearing as the child approaches adulthood.[1]

TABLE 2 Characteristics of selected forms of dermatitis and dry skin

Condition	Symptoms	Location	Signs
Atopic dermatitis	Itching, scratching	2 mo: chest, face	Red, raised vesicles; dry skin; oozing
		2 yr: scalp, neck, and extremities	Less acute lesions; edema; erythema
		2–4 yr: neck, wrist, elbow, knee	Dry, thickened plaques; hyperpigmentation
		12–20 yr: flexors, hands	
Contact dermatitis (irritant and allergic)	Acute: itching Chronic: stiffness, dry	Irritant: contact areas Allergic: exposed contact areas (transferable by touch)	Irritant (mild, acute): red, oozing blisters Irritant (mild, chronic): dry, thick, fissured skin Irritant (severe): blisters, ulcers Allergic: unusual pattern of lesions; sharp margins with angles and straight lines
Hand dermatitis	Itching, dry	Sides of fingers; occasionally palms	Red, dry, chapped, fissured skin
Dry skin (chapped)	Often none; moderate to severe itching	Lower legs, backs of hands, forearms; occasionally entire body	Dry, fine scale; patches, diffuse or round; if severe, fissures

Adapted from Ricciatti–Sibbald DJ. In: Clark C, ed. *Self-Medication: A Reference for Health Professionals*. 4th ed. Ottawa: Canadian Pharmaceutical Association; 1992: 65.

Because atopic dermatitis is primarily a disease of the young, the age of the patient is important in assessment. By taking a medical history, the pharmacist may determine whether the patient has a history of atopic disorders. Inquiries should be made regarding the onset and duration of the eruption. If the child is under 1 month of age, the disease may be seborrheic dermatitis, a condition that may be present from birth. If the disease presents in a child over 5 years of age, other conditions, including the possibility of contact dermatitis, should be considered. Finally, the location and distribution of the lesions should be taken into account. Atopic dermatitis does not usually involve the groin or the scalp, and the lesions are typically symmetric in distribution. The classic case of childhood atopic dermatitis involves the cheeks and extensor surfaces of the forearms and legs. (See color plates, photographs 19A, B, and C.)

Various factors may exacerbate atopic dermatitis including irritants, allergens, extremes of temperature and humidity, dry skin, and emotional stress. Advice to the patient should be directed toward identifying these factors so they may be avoided.

Irritants, if sufficiently strong, may cause burning, itching, or redness on the skin. Patients with atopic dermatitis are hypersensitive to low concentrations of irritants that would not generally cause a reaction on normal skin. Identified irritants include solvents, industrial chemicals, some fragrances, soaps containing a fragrance or other irritant, fumes, tobacco smoke, paints, bleach, wool, nylon, acidic foods, astringents, and various alcohol-containing skin products.[3]

Allergens may aggravate atopic dermatitis in a small number of patients who have had prior exposure. The allergens usually involved are plant or animal proteins from food, pollens, or pets. However, the role of food allergies in exacerbating atopic dermatitis is controversial. It is claimed that up to 20% of children with the disease are affected by allergic reactions to foods through either ingestion or skin contact during food preparation.[3] Although specific hypersensitivities to high-acid foods, milk products, and eggs have been identified, the dietary management needed to achieve strict avoidance poses tremendous compliance problems. The studies using dietary restriction showed a significant improvement in the condition initially, with decreasing long-term benefit. In none of the cases did the condition completely resolve. When the compliance problems are combined with the possibility of malnutrition in children on allergen-elimination diets, it is probably best to reserve that approach for those patients who have severe symptoms and are unresponsive to other treatments.[1,4]

Patients with atopic dermatitis are often intolerant to sudden changes and extremes of temperature and humidity. High humidity may result in increased perspiration, which may aggravate the condition. The low humidity often found in heated buildings during the winter dries the skin and increases the itching. Use of humidifiers may be of some help, especially if accompanied by lower thermostat settings.

Secondary or associated infections are common, are often difficult to prevent, and can make the condition worse. Patients should be counseled to seek medical attention promptly when signs of infection are noted. These signs include increased redness, pustules, fever blisters, and cold sores.[3]

If the atopic dermatitis is not extreme and the patient is not a child under 2 years of age, initial treatment may be attempted with nonprescription measures. There is a general proscription against topical products for children under 2 years of age except on the advice and supervision of a physician. Part of the rationale is that very young children have a higher body surface area–to–weight ratio than older individuals and are therefore at increased risk for systemic toxicity from topically applied drugs. This reason is accentuated by the fact that infants under 6 months of age have underdeveloped hepatic enzyme systems for metabolizing many absorbed drugs.

Because the stratum corneum in patients with atopic dermatitis contains less moisture than normal skin, frequent bathing with soap and water may increase the dryness of the skin and aggravate the dermatitis. Therefore, the first step is to decrease the frequency of bathing, preferably to once a week, substituting sponge baths for full-body bathing on most days. Because of the drying effect of most soaps, a mild soap (e.g., Neutrogena®) or a soapless cleanser (e.g., Cetaphil®) should be recommended.

Treatment of acute or wet dermatitis is directed toward drying the lesions. Wet compresses using an astringent such as Burow's solution should be applied for 20 minutes, four to six times daily. Bathing with warm water containing colloidal oatmeal may aid the drying. Hydrocortisone in an oil-in-water base may be used. If the condition does not resolve or if it involves a large area of the body, a physician should be consulted. The next treatment step is usually a more potent topical steroid.[1]

Treatment of chronic or dry dermatitis focuses on measures to maintain hydration of the skin. Colloidal oatmeal may be used for bathing, or a water-miscible bath oil may be added to the water near the end of the bath. The skin should be patted dry because rubbing can increase irritation. An emollient should be applied while the skin is still damp. Ointments with a petrolatum or water-in-oil base maintain hydration best. However, patients usually do not like the greasy, staining characteristics of these products. Oil-in-water preparations find greater acceptance, but they must be applied more often, and care must be taken to avoid products with potentially irritating ingredients such as lanolin. The next step is to use topical hydrocortisone, preferably in an ointment base. If the condition persists, medical help should be sought because further treatment may involve more potent steroids.[4]

Simply telling a child not to scratch an itch is generally not effective. Therefore, some adjunctive measures may be tried to minimize scratching and the damage that it produces. The patient's fingernails should be cut as short as possible and kept clean. Scratching may increase at night when there are minimal distractions, and it may even become automatic while the patient is sleeping; therefore, wearing cotton gloves or socks on the hands at night helps lessen the resultant mechanical damage. For some patients, the itching may disrupt sleep. Antihistamines are of little value in decreasing the itching, but those with a significant sedative effect (e.g., diphenhydramine) may be used to promote sleep. The major limitation with antihistamine use is the undesired drowsiness or residual sedation or "hangover" effect that may be experienced the following morning.[4]

Contact Dermatitis

Contact dermatitis refers to a rash that results from a chemical or allergen touching susceptible skin. It is one of the most common ailments pharmacists see. It may be further separated into irritant and allergic contact dermatitis. Although the cause of each type is different, the signs, symptoms, and treatment are essentially the same. As with other forms of dermatitis, itching is the primary symptom. The acute phase is often red, vesicular, and oozing. The chronic phase is likely to be dry, thickened, and fissured. The degree of inflammation is used to assess severity. Lesions are often asymmetric in distribution and reflect where contact with the insulting substance occurred.

Although many cases of contact dermatitis involve exposed skin such as the hands and face, the lesions may appear practically any place on the body. An accurate assessment is made on the basis of the character, configuration, and location of the rash and itching. Seborrhea also must be considered in cases of genitoanal or eyelid involvement.

Asking questions about the patient's environment (e.g., home, work, recreation, medication use, and clothes) may allow a possible irritant or allergen to be identified. Patch testing by a physician is also useful in diagnosing allergic reactions. It is important to identify the offending substance because its removal will result in improvement of the condition. Unfortunately, the cause may be elusive. For example, chemicals such as a host of airborne pollutants may function as sensitizers.

Accurate diagnosis also may be difficult if the contact dermatitis is superimposed over another dermatologic condition. Moreover, once the skin reacts to one substance, it may be more vulnerable to other substances, making diagnosis and treatment more complicated. Allergic or irritant dermatitis may be a secondary eruption caused by an agent used in therapy, complicating one of the other forms of dermatitis. For example, a minor topical infection may produce a rash and itching and be treated with a topical antibiotic product containing neomycin, which in turn causes further irritation and inflammation. The infection itself may heal, but the contact dermatitis produced by the neomycin may worsen. Not recognizing that the initial condition has resolved, the patient may continue to use the offending neomycin-containing product, thus setting up a vicious cycle that produces increased inflammation and itching.[2,5]

Irritant contact dermatitis is a nonimmunologic irritation. Inflammation may be produced by exposure to many substances if concentration and duration of contact are sufficient. Irritants account for 70–80% of all cases of contact dermatitis. A primary or strong irritant, such as a strong acid or alkali, generally elicits a response on first exposure; the injury it causes to the skin may not be limited to erythema and may result in ulceration and tissue necrosis. Mild or secondary irritants such as soaps, cosmetics, topical medications, and detergents generally require repeated or extended contact to cause an inflammatory response. Concomitant topical administration of more than one substance may also induce skin irritation. A secondary irritant that is not irritating to the skin when applied alone may cause irritation in combination with an agent that promotes absorption, such as a surfactant or keratolytic. Damaged skin also encourages skin irritation.[2,6]

Factors influencing skin irritation include the chemical itself, the climate, and biologic variation in the host. The degree of skin irritation from an applied substance is a function of the test material's intrinsic irritation potential, concentration, and ability to remain bound to the skin, as well as of the texture of the exposed skin. The irritant properties of topical drugs such as camphor, coal tar, menthol, and resorcinol are well known, but classification of these agents as primary or secondary irritants is largely a function of their concentration. Very high camphor concentrations are needed to produce the same degree of irritation as that achieved with relatively low coal tar concentrations. Agents such as hexachlorophene, which are bound to the epidermal layer, may cause irritation with repeated application. Some substances used to treat certain skin conditions such as psoriasis may be irritating to the affected and unaffected skin.

Environmental conditions play a role in skin texture and its resistance to irritant substances. High humidity allows greater skin hydration and thus faster penetration. Occlusion also keeps the skin hydrated.[2]

Allergic contact dermatitis is immunologically mediated and represents a delayed hypersensitivity reaction to contact allergens. It involves penetration of a chemical called a haptene into the skin, where it becomes attached to protein carriers on specific cells in the epidermis. An initial sensitizing exposure is necessary for the reaction to occur. On subsequent contact with the allergen, exposed areas will typically become dry and mildly inflamed and will look chapped. This reaction usually appears within 12–48 hours after subsequent exposure. Susceptibility to allergic contact dermatitis may last a lifetime.[6]

The most common contact allergens come from the *Rhus* genus of plants (e.g., poison ivy, oak, and sumac). The offending agent is urushiol, which is found in the leaves, stems, and roots of the plants. It is estimated that 70% of those exposed to urushiol will be sensitized to it. In addition, particles in smoke and indirect contact from pets may cause dermatitis in very sensitive persons.[1,6] (See Chapter 35, "Poison Ivy and Poison Oak Products.")

A number of metals (e.g., cobalt, chromium, and nickel) may cause allergic contact dermatitis. This sensitivity is important to keep in mind because nickel, often with cobalt as a contaminant, is widely used in costume jewelry, watches, and blue jean studs. Chromium is present in cement and may pose an occupational hazard to construction workers and masons.[6] Rubber has often been implicated as an allergenic substance; however, it is not the rubber or latex itself that causes the reaction, but rather the chemical accelerators and antioxidants used in processing the rubber.

To those patients who have experienced topical allergic reactions to cosmetics (particularly those containing lanolin or parabens), fragrances, hair care products, nail polish, hair dyes, deodorants, and soaps, a wide range of hypoallergenic cosmetics and soapless cleansers may be recommended. Many topical skin preparations used for medicinal effect may also be a source of allergens, including some used for itching and skin rashes. (See color plates, photograph 20.) Local anesthetics containing esters such as benzocaine, which is commonly used topically for pruritis, local pain, and sunburn, can sensitize individuals. Benzocaine can also react with related chemicals such as hair dyes and para-aminobenzoic acid–containing sunscreens. Products containing pramoxine may be recommended for patients sensitive to benzocaine.

Topical antihistamines such as diphenhydramine may also cause sensitization. Sensitization does not occur from oral use; however, once a patient has become sensitized, oral administration may produce dermatitis.[7]

Other agents that may act as sensitizers include iodine-containing products, sulfonamides, mercury-containing antiseptics, and ethylenediamine. Antibiotics that are used topically, such as neomycin, may also function as allergens. (See Chapter 28, "Topical Anti-Infective Products.") Health care workers may also be sensitized by glutaraldehyde, which is used in the sterilization process of some medical instruments.

In contact dermatitis, the patient may be sensitive to a wide variety of chemical agents. The duration of therapy is relatively short because the condition improves upon withdrawal of the allergen or irritant. Therefore, before recommending any product for the treatment of contact dermatitis, the pharmacist should encourage the patient to try to identify the offending substance(s). Prevention of further exposure is the best approach to effective therapy.

The choice of treatment of contact dermatitis depends on the severity of the condition. Mild to moderate dermatitis allows treatment with nonprescription agents. A person with a severe reaction or involvement of large areas of the body should be referred to a physician. In all cases, the involved area should be washed thoroughly to remove traces of the offending agent.

If the area is oozing, astringent compresses of Burow's solution applied for 20 minutes, four to six times daily, may be recommended to aid in drying. Application of calamine lotion between compress applications and use of colloidal oatmeal baths may help relieve the itching. Topical hydrocortisone to reduce inflammation and itching may be added to the regimen. If the condition does not resolve in a short time or if it worsens, a physician should be consulted.[1,5]

Hand Dermatitis

Hand dermatitis is not truly a specific disease but is rather the simplest and most localized form of contact dermatitis. It often occurs in individuals whose occupation requires frequent hand washing or contact with moisture and mild irritants (e.g., hairdressers, bartenders, food handlers, and medical personnel). It is marked by erythema, dryness, chapping, and, in severe cases, oozing vesicles that form crusts and pruritus of the dorsa of the hands. In severe, untreated cases, fissures may allow infection that can proceed to tissue necrosis.[1,6]

Hand dermatitis often begins under a ring that traps a residue of irritant. It may then spread to the adjacent fingers, the palm, and the other hand. Because the dermatitis is often related to occupational exposure to irritants, it may be chronic and recurrent.

Acute hand dermatitis (i.e., red, oozing, and edematous) and subacute hand dermatitis (i.e., red and scaling but no weeping) are usually treated in the same manner. Wet dressings may be applied, followed by a hydrocortisone cream or lotion.

Treatment of chronic hand dermatitis (i.e., dry, scaling, and fissured) initially focuses on maintaining skin hydration by applying emollients often, especially after immersion in water. A water-in-oil hand lotion or cream may be tried first, progressing to a hydrocortisone-containing preparation, if necessary. Because skin deterioration leading to infection can occur in all types of hand dermatitis, medical attention should be sought if the condition does not resolve within 1 to 2 weeks.[1]

A number of adjunctive measures, such as wearing vinyl (not rubber) gloves while doing "wet work," can be recommended in the management of hand dermatitis. Patients should be reminded, however, that wearing a glove with a hole in it will trap irritants next to the skin and is worse than wearing no glove at all. Thin cotton liners worn under vinyl gloves may prevent irritation from the vinyl and absorb perspiration. When washing the hands, the patient should use lukewarm water and a minimal amount of soap. The patient should also avoid hand creams and lotions that contain lanolin, parabens, or fragrances. After the acute condition subsides, a nonmedicated moisturizer or hydrocortisone ointment should continue to be applied at least four times a day until the skin condition has healed or resolved completely.

Dry Skin

Almost everyone has experienced dry or chapped skin. In some people, it is a seasonal occurrence; in others, the condition is chronic. Although dry skin is not life-threatening, it is annoying and uncomfortable because of the attendant pruritus and, in some cases, pain and inflammation. In addition, dry skin is more prone to bacterial invasion than is normal skin.

Dry skin (xerosis) is characterized by one or more of the following symptoms: roughness, scaling, loss of flexibility, fissures, inflammation, and pruritus. The condition tends to appear most often on the lower legs, the back of the hands, and the forearms. Dry skin is especially prevalent during the winter months and is often referred to as "winter itch." It may occur secondary to prolonged detergent use, malnutrition, or physical damage to the stratum corneum. It may also signal a systemic disorder such as hypothyroidism or dehydration.

It is a common misconception that dry skin is caused by a lack of natural skin oils; on the contrary, dry skin is caused by a lack of water in the stratum corneum. The pathophysiology of dry skin, therefore, can be described by examining the factors involved in skin hydration. Frequent bathing and the excessive use of soap will increase the dryness of the skin. Soap will remove the skin's natural oils, and the length of contact with the water is usually insufficient to hydrate the skin. Low relative humidity allows the outer skin layer to lose moisture, become less flexible, and crack when flexed, thus leading to an increased rate of moisture loss. High wind velocity also causes skin moisture loss. Physical damage to the stratum corneum dramatically increases the transepidermal water loss; however, within 1 or 2 days, a temporary parakeratotic barrier consisting of incompletely keratinized, nucleated cells provides approximately 50% of normal function. Total function is usually restored in 2 to 3 weeks. Also, keratin cross-linking induced by long-term overexposure to ultraviolet (UV) radiation causes skin to harden.[2]

Elderly people represent a subgroup within the general population in whom dry skin occurs with an increased incidence. With advancing age, the epidermal layer changes because of abnormal maturation or adhesion of the keratinocytes, which results in a superficial, irregular layer of corneocytes. This may be described as a thinning of the entire epidermis, which produces a roughened skin surface. The skin's hygroscopic substances also decrease in quantity with advancing age. Hormonal changes that accompany aging result in lowered sebum output and therefore lowered skin lubrication.[8]

Two dermatologic conditions difficult to differentiate from simple dry skin are asteatotic eczema and ichthyosis vulgaris. Asteatotic eczema is characterized by dry and fissured skin, inflammation, and pruritus. Sebaceous secretions are scanty or absent. It is more common during dry winter weather and in elderly individuals as an extension of the dry skin condition.

Ichthyosis vulgaris affects 0.3–1.0% of the population. It is a genetic disorder (autosomal dominant) that should be suspected when a patient complains of a familial tendency to excessive dryness and chapping. Patients may also have an associated history of atopic disease. Symptoms include dryness and roughness of the skin, accompanied by small, fine, white scales. The condition tends to appear on the extensor aspects of the arms and legs. Dryness of the cheeks, heels, and palms may also be noted. In severe forms of the disease, a classic fish scale appearance of the stratum corneum is noted. Extreme cases may be seen, even today, in large traveling side shows of fairs or circuses where individuals are billed as "alligator," "porcupine," or "lizard" people.[2,9]

Ichthyosis vulgaris may be placed at the most extreme end on a continuum of dermatitis conditions, with common dry skin at the least severe end. It should be noted that ichthyosis vulgaris and related ichthyoses do not respond to steroid therapy although the use of topical steroids may relieve the pruritus.[9]

The key to treating all degrees of dry skin is maintaining skin hydration. The first step is to decrease the frequency of full-body bathing, substituting sponge baths or quick showers with warm rather than hot water. The use of bath products to enhance skin hydration follows a progression of colloidal oatmeal, oilated oatmeal, or bath oil added near the end of the bath. Emollients should be applied while the skin is damp and should be reapplied frequently. The more severe cases of dry skin may require a urea or lactic acid–containing product to enhance hydration. Topical hydrocortisone may be applied on a short-term basis to reduce inflammation and itching. If resolution does not occur within 1 or 2 weeks, a physician should be consulted. Adjunctive measures are similar to those recommended for other forms of dermatitis that involve dry skin.[1]

Pharmacologic Agents

Nonprescription products for dermatitis and dry skin include bath products, emollients, hydrating agents, astringents, antipruritics, protectants, keratin-softening agents, and hydrocortisone. Keratolytics are usually avoided in dermatitis unless extensive lichenification has occurred; these agents and those that reduce the mitotic activity of the epidermis, such as tars and anthralin, should be used cautiously, if at all, because of their irritant properties.

Bath Products

Bath Oils Bath oils generally consist of a mineral or vegetable oil plus a surfactant. Mineral oil products are adsorbed better than vegetable oil products. Adsorption onto and absorption into the skin increase as temperature and oil concentration increase. Bath oils, which are applied at a relatively high temperature, are minimally effective in improving a dry skin condition because they are greatly diluted in water. The major effect is caused by the slip or lubricity they impart to the skin, which may be more important to the patient than the occlusive properties. This effect may be maximized by adding the oil near the end of the bath and patting the skin dry rather than rubbing it. When applied as wet compresses, however, bath oils (1 tsp in one-quarter cup of warm water) are effective in treating dry skin and allow a decrease in the frequency of full-body bathing.[1,10]

Bath oils make the tub and floor slippery, creating a safety hazard, especially for elderly patients. They also make cleansing the skin with soaps more difficult. There is no clear superiority of one type of bath oil product over another; however, scented products should be avoided if allergy to the product is suspected.

Oatmeal Products Colloidal oatmeal bath products contain starch, protein, and a small amount of oil. They are less effective than bath oils; however, oilated oatmeal products combine the effect of oatmeal and a bath oil. Colloidal oatmeal is claimed to be soothing and antipruritic, and it does have a lubricating effect.

Cleansers Bath soaps generally contain salts of long-chain fatty acids (commonly oleic, palmitic, or stearic acid), and alkali metals (e.g., sodium and potassium). Combined with water, they act as surfactants and will remove many substances from the skin, including the lipids that normally keep the skin soft and pliable. Some authorities recommend special soaps containing extra oils to minimize the drying effect of washing; however, these soaps lather and clean poorly. Cold cream has been added to some soaps for the same effect only with better lathering characteristics. Although its utility is controversial, Dove® has been cited as an excellent soap to recommend for patients with dry skin.[1,8]

Glycerin soaps have a higher oil content than standard toilet soaps because of the addition of castor oil. They also are transparent and more water soluble. They are closer to a neutral pH and therefore are regarded as less drying than soaps, which are alkaline. Although there is little objective proof of their superiority, the glycerin soaps are advertised for and well accepted by people with skin problems.

Soapless cleansers such as Cetaphil® may be recommended if soap should be avoided. These products consist primarily of surfactants and may contain an oil. They foam on application, and on removal they leave a thin layer of lipid material on the skin, which aids in retaining water in the stratum corneum.

Emollients/Moisturizers

Emollients, also called occlusive agents or moisturizers, are used to prevent or relieve the signs and symptoms of dry skin. They act primarily by leaving an oily film on the skin surface that promotes water retention because the moisture in the skin cannot readily pass through the occlusive barrier. These agents are often used in combination with a humectant (hydrating agent) in dry skin formulations. The most commonly used occlusives include petrolatum, lanolin, mineral oil, and silicones such as dimethicone.

Some researchers believe that preventing normal transepidermal water loss is not enough to maintain normal hydration. Therefore, the patient may be advised to hydrate the skin by soaking the affected area in water for 5–10 minutes, patting it dry, and applying the occlusive agent while the skin is still damp. In this way, more moisture will be trapped in the skin.

Cosmetically, emollients make the skin feel soft and smooth by helping to reestablish the integrity of the stratum corneum. The lipid materials make the scales on the skin translucent and flatten them against the underlying skin. This eliminates the air between the scales and the skin surface, which is responsible for the dry, flaky appearance.[11]

Frequency of application depends on the severity of the dry skin condition as well as on the hydration efficiency of the occlusive agent. In the case of dry hands, the patient may need to apply the occlusive agent after each hand washing and at numerous other times during the day. Care must be exercised to avoid excessive hydration or maceration. In addition, although most commercial formulations generally are bland, contact with the eye or with broken or abraded skin should be avoided because formulation ingredients may cause irritation. This is especially true with emulsion systems because the surfactants in these systems may denature protein.

Petrolatum seems to be the most effective occlusive agent and has been given Category I status by the Food and Drug Administration (FDA) as a skin protectant. Mineral oil is not as effective a barrier, and silicones are even less effective than mineral oil. Unfortunately, petrolatum is not well accepted by patients because of its greasiness and staining properties. Moreover, petrolatum should not be applied over puncture wounds, infections, or lacerations because its high occlusive ability may lead to maceration and further inflammation. Application to intertriginous areas, mucous membranes, and acne-prone areas should also be avoided. The same precautions should be taken with dimethicone.

Lanolin, a natural product derived from sheep wool, is found in many nonprescription moisturizing products. Some patients develop an allergic reaction to this substance, presumably because of its wool wax fraction. Patients with a previous history of allergic reactions to topical medications have a greater risk of developing an allergic reaction to lanolin and should generally avoid lanolin-containing products.

Emollient products are available in a wide variety of formulations. The ointments containing petrolatum are very greasy and generally lack consumer appeal because of the texture, difficulty of spreading and removing, and staining properties. The emollient ointments are inappropriate for an oozing dermatitis. The lotions and creams are either water-in-oil or oil-in-water emulsions. The higher the lipid content, the greater the occlusive effect. In most cases, the less effective but more aesthetic oil-in-water emulsions are preferred. These agents help alleviate the pruritus associated with dry skin by virtue of their cooling effect as the water evaporates from the skin surface. Moreover, there is enough oil in most oil-in-water emulsions to form a continuous occlusive film on the skin surface.[1,11]

Attempts have been made to formulate products that serve as sebum replacements. Although their efficacy has not been proven, these products are available as cosmetics. Because sebum and skin surface lipids contain a relatively high concentration of fatty acid glycerides, vegetable and animal oils such as avocado, cucumber, mink, peanut, safflower, sesame, turtle, and shark liver are included in dry skin products, presumably because of their unsaturated fatty acid content. However, although use of these oils contributes to skin flexibility and lubricity, their occlusive effect is less than that of petrolatum.

The prevention and care of dry skin may become a major focus for the pharmacist as the population continues to age. Facial moisturizer purchases have already surpassed sales of hand and body lotions. This is attributed to the baby boomers' increasing interest in facial skin care as they age. There is also an increasing awareness by those caring for elderly people that prophylactic dry skin care can reduce the risks, misery, and expense of treating preventable dermatologic conditions.[11,12]

Humectants

Humectants or hydrating agents are hygroscopic materials that may be added to an emollient base. Their function is to draw water into the stratum corneum to hydrate the skin. The water may come from the dermis or from the atmosphere although high relative humidity (80% or greater) is necessary for the latter to occur. Humectants are distinct from emollients, which serve to retain water already present. Commonly used hydrating agents are glycerin, propylene glycol, and phospholipids.

Because of glycerin's hygroscopic properties, high concentrations of it may actually increase the water loss by drawing water from the skin rather than from the atmosphere. However, at concentrations of 50% or less, humectants such as glycerin and rose water help decrease water loss by keeping the water in close contact with the skin and accelerating moisture diffusion from the dermal tissue to the epidermal surface. In addition, glycerin provides lubrication to the skin surface.

Propylene glycol is a viscous, colorless, odorless solvent with hygroscopic properties. It is less viscous than glycerin and is included in many skin care formulations for its humectant action. However, it can cause skin irritation.

Phospholipid products contain lecithin, which is a water-binding compound normally present in the skin. Each phospholipid molecule can complex with up to 15 molecules of water. Hydrolysis yields fatty acids, which help retain the water.

Keratin-Softening Agents

Chemically altering the keratin layer softens the skin and cosmetically improves the skin's appearance. This treatment approach does not need the substantial addition of water, but all the attendant dry skin symptoms may not be alleviated unless water is added to the keratin layer. Agents used as keratin softeners in nonprescription dry skin products are urea, lactic acid, and allantoin.

Urea Urea (carbamide) in concentrations of 10–30% is mildly keratolytic and increases water uptake in the stratum corneum, giving it a high water-binding capacity. Urea has a direct effect on stratum corneum elasticity because of its ability to bind to skin protein. It accelerates fibrin digestion at about 15% and is proteolytic at 40%. It is considered safe and has been recommended for use on crusted necrotic tissue. Concentrations of 10% have been used on simple dry skin; 20–30% formulations have been used for treating difficult dry skin conditions. Urea-containing creams are claimed to produce good hydration and help remove scales and crusts. They are also less greasy than some occlusive preparations. In some instances, however, urea preparations cause stinging and burning and may be irritating to sensitive patients.

Alpha-Hydroxy Acids Lactic acid is an alpha-hydroxy acid that has been useful in concentrations of 2–5% for treating dry skin conditions. Lactic acid increases the hydration of human skin and may act as a modulator of epidermal keratinization rather than as a keratolytic agent. Lactic acid may be added to urea preparations for both its stabilizing and its hydrating effects.

Other alpha-hydroxy acids, found in many fruits, are under investigation for a number of common skin conditions such as dry skin, acne, and fine age wrinkles. These acids include malic acid (apples), citric acid (oranges and lemons), glycolic and gluconic acid (sugar cane), and tartaric acid (grapes).[13]

Allantoin Allantoin and allantoin complexes are claimed to soften keratin by disrupting its structure. Allantoin is a product of purine metabolism and is considered to be a relatively safe compound. However, it is less effective than urea. The FDA has recommended that allantoin be considered safe and effective as a skin protectant for adults, children, and infants when applied in concentrations of 0.5–2.0%.[2]

Astringents

Astringents are substances that retard the oozing, discharge, or bleeding of dermatitis when applied to the unhealthy skin or mucous membranes. They work by coagulating protein. When applied as a wet dressing or compress, they cool and dry the skin through evaporation. They cause vasoconstriction and reduce blood flow in inflammation. They also cleanse the skin of exudates, crust, and debris. Because they generally have a low cell penetrability, their activity is limited to the cell surface and interstitial spaces. The protein precipitate that forms may serve as a protective coat, allowing new tissues to grow underneath.[2]

The FDA has identified two astringent solutions as being safe and effective. These are aluminum acetate (Burow's solution) and witch hazel (*Hamamelis* water). Numerous other ingredients, including alum and zinc oxide, have been promoted as astringents. However, data demonstrating their safety and effectiveness for use as astringents are lacking.[14]

Aluminum acetate solution (USP) contains approximately 5% aluminum acetate. The solution must be diluted 1:10 to 1:40 with water before use. It is commercially available as tablets and powders.

Witch hazel is no longer listed in the official compendia, but it has been used for centuries as an astringent solution. A natural product prepared from the twigs of *Hamamelis virginiana*, it contains tannins, trace amounts of volatile oils (which give it a characteristically pleasant odor), and 14 to 15% alcohol, all of which contribute to its astringent activity. The product may be applied as often as necessary in the treatment of minor skin irritations.

The patient may soak the affected area in the astringent solution two to four times daily for 15–30 minutes, or may loosely apply a compress of washcloths or small towels soaked in the solution and then wrung gently so they are wet but not dripping. The dressings should be rewetted and reapplied every few minutes for 20–30 minutes, four to six times daily. Isotonic saline solution, tap water, or diluted white vinegar (one-quarter cup per pint of water) may also be used in this fashion.[1,2]

Antipruritics

The itching associated with dermatitis may be mediated through several different mechanisms, which may explain how three major classes of pharmacologic agents—local anesthetics, antihistamines, and steroids—are useful as antipruritics. Cooling the area through application of a soothing, bland lotion may also reduce the extent of the pruritus, but this action is only transitory in its effect.

The itching sensation is mediated by the same nerve fibers that carry pain impulses. Local anesthetics block conduction along axonal membranes, thereby relieving itching as well as pain. Agents such as benzocaine (5–20%) may be applied to the affected area three or four times daily. Local anesthetics may cause systemic side effects and should not be used in large quantities or over long periods of time, particularly if the skin is raw or blistered. Nonprescription topical anesthetics that appear to be safe and effective are dyclonine and benzocaine; however, they may have a sensitizing effect in a small number of persons.

Itching may be mediated by various endogenous substances, including histamine. Topical antihistamines such as diphenhydramine, tripelennamine, and pyrilamine are effective in alleviating this symptom. Their activity stems from an ability to compete with histamine at H_1-receptor sites and to exert a topical anesthetic effect. Local anesthesia may be the more important mechanism of action because the cause of itching in many conditions (e.g., atopic dermatitis) has not been established and may not be related to histamine release at all. Antihistamines are considered safe and effective for use as nonprescription external analgesics. However, because of their significant sensitizing potential, the FDA does not recommend topical use of these agents for more than 7 consecutive days except under the advice and supervision of a physician.[6,15]

Oral antihistamines have been used to treat the itching of dermatologic disorders with variable results. Some researchers claim that the antipruritic effect is a result of the sedative side effect. Others claim the efficacy is owing to antihistaminic activity, although with a delay in onset of several days. If histamine is involved, it has already reached and stimulated the receptor sites to produce itching, and a finite time is required for the antihistamine to displace it. In either case, central nervous system depression may be a problem, as may the anticholinergic side effects in patients with conditions such as prostatic hypertrophy or glaucoma.[5,6]

Protectants

Skin protectants are substances that protect injured or exposed skin surfaces from harmful or annoying stimuli. Zinc oxide (1–25%) is one of the most widely used and clinically accepted skin protectants, and it is claimed to be mildly astringent and antiseptic as well. It may be applied as a paste (Lassar's), ointment, or lotion (calamine). Other protectants in general use include aluminum hydroxide and bismuth subnitrate. Patients should be cautioned that covering the lesions or applying a product with an occlusive barrier may increase the degree of tissue maceration and prevent heat loss, resulting in discomfort. Any powder-based aqueous product that dries weeping through water adsorption or astringency should be used with caution. These agents have a tendency to crust, and removing the crusts may cause bleeding and infections.[2,6]

Topical Hydrocortisone

Hydrocortisone is the only steroid anti-inflammatory agent available without a prescription for the topical treatment of dermatitis. It relieves the redness, heat, pain, swelling, and itch associated with various inflammatory dermatologic conditions. In addition, its immunosuppressive activity may account for some of its efficacy in any dermatitis involving a cell-mediated immune reaction. The official indications for its use include temporary relief of itching associated with minor skin irritations, inflammation, and rashes caused by dermatitis, seborrheic dermatitis, insect bites, poison ivy, poison oak, poison sumac, soaps, detergents, cosmetics, and jewelry.

There is a dose–response relationship seen in the use of topical hydrocortisone. The efficacy of preparations of less than 0.5% concentration has not been established. Concentrations of 0.5–1% are regarded as appropriate for the treatment of localized dermatitis. Hydrocortisone should be applied sparingly three or four times a day. If the emollient effect of the steroid vehicle is desired or if the agent is likely to be washed off, such as in hand dermatitis, more frequent applications may be necessary. An ointment formulation is best for chronic dry forms of dermatitis. Application to the scalp may be made once a day because the drug usually is not rubbed off.[1,2,6]

Before recommending a hydrocortisone-containing product, the pharmacist should be certain that the area of application is not infected. Signs of bacterial infection include redness, heat, pus, and crusting. Fungal infections may be marked by erythema and scaling; vaginal infections may be accompanied by a discharge. Topical hydrocortisone may mask the symptoms of these dermatologic infections while the infection progresses in severity.

Topical hydrocortisone generally will not produce systemic complications because absorption is minimal. Approximately 1% of a hydrocortisone solution applied to normal skin on the forearm is absorbed systemically. Absorption increases in the presence of skin inflammation or with the use of occlusive dressings. Certain local adverse effects such as skin atrophy may arise with prolonged use because of the antimitotic/antisynthetic effect of hydrocortisone on cells. In practice, however, clinically detectable atrophy rarely occurs with hydrocortisone in the concentrations available without a prescription. This problem may occur more often with the newer, fluorinated products available by prescription only. Because response to topical steroids decreases with continued use, intermittent courses of therapy are advised.[1]

When hydrocortisone was initially switched from prescription to nonprescription status in 1980, the concentrations available were 0.25 and 0.5%. In August 1991, the FDA approved the nonprescription marketing of hydrocortisone in strengths up to 1%.[16]

Product Selection Guidelines

When deciding on which product to recommend for the control of dermatitis or dry skin, the pharmacist must evaluate both the active ingredients and the vehicle. Primary active ingredients contained in nonprescription skin products are water and oil. However, a wide variety of secondary ingredients are added to enhance product elegance and stability, and many of them have the potential for producing contact dermatitis through either an irritant or sensitizing effect. These agents may include:

- *Emulsifiers*: cholesterol, magnesium aluminum silicate, polyoxyethylene lauryl ether (Brij®), polyoxyethylene monostearate (Myrj®), polyoxyethylene sorbitan monolaurate (Tween®), propylene glycol monostearate, sodium borate plus fatty acid, sodium lauryl sulfate, sorbitan monopalmitate (Span®), or triethanolamine plus fatty acid;
- *Emulsion stabilizers (thickening agents)*: carbomer, cetyl alcohol, glyceryl monostearate, methylcellulose, spermaceti or stearyl alcohol;
- *Preservatives*: cresol or the parabens.

The type of vehicle (e.g., ointment, cream, lotion, gel, solution, or aerosol) may have a significant effect on dermatitis. The following guidelines may be used to choose an appropriate vehicle:

- "If it's wet, dry it." If a drying effect is desired, solutions and gels should be recommended. It must be noted, however, that components of these systems may quickly diffuse into the underlying tissue and possibly cause irritation.
- If slight lubrication is needed, creams and lotions are preferred.
- "If it's dry, wet it." If the lesion is very dry and fissured, ointments are the vehicle of choice. However, they should be avoided in intertriginous areas because of

TABLE 3 Amount of topical medication needed for three times daily application for 1 week.

Part of the body	Cream/ointment (g)	Lotion/solution/gel (mL)
Face	5–10	100–120
Both hands	25–50	200–240
Scalp	50–100	200–240
Both arms or both legs	100–200	240–360
Trunk	200	360–480
Groin and genitalia	15–25	120–180

Adapted from Bingham EA. Topical dermatologic therapy. In: Rook A, Parish LC, Beare JM, eds. *Practical Management of the Dermatologic Patient.* Philadelphia: J. B. Lippincott; 1986: 227–8.

TABLE 4 Distinguishing features of dandruff, seborrhea, and psoriasis

	Dandruff	Seborrhea	Psoriasis
Location	Scalp	Adults and children: head and trunk Children only: back, intertriginous areas	Scalp, elbows, knees, trunk, and lower extremities
Exacerbating factors	Generally a stable condition, exacerbated by inadequate washing, dry climate	Exacerbated by many external factors, notably stress and low relative humidity	Exacerbated by mechanical irritation, stress, climate, drugs, infection, endocrine factors
Appearance	Thin, white, or grayish flakes; even distribution on scalp	Patchy lesions with margins; mild inflammation; oily, yellowish scales	Usually symmetrical, red, patchy plaques with sharp border; silvery-white scale; small bleeding points when removed. Difficult to distinguish from seborrhea in early stages or in intertriginous zones
Inflammation	Absent	Present	Present
Epidermal hyperplasia	Absent	Present	Present
Epidermal kinetics	Turnover rate is two times faster than normal	Turnover rate is about five to six times faster than normal	Turnover rate is about five to six times faster than normal
Percentage of incompletely keratinized cells	Rarely exceeds 5% of total corneocyte count	Commonly makes up 15–25% of corneocyte count	Commonly makes up 40–60% of corneocyte count

Information extracted from:
Wright DE. In: Clark C, ed. *Self-Medication: A Reference for Health Professionals*. 3rd ed. Ottawa: Canadian Pharmaceutical Association; 1988: 87.
McGinley KJ et al. *J Invest Dermatol* 1969; 53: 107.
Kligman AM et al. *J Soc Cosmet Chem* 1974; 25: 73.

their maceration potential. Also, in an acute process, ointments may cause further irritation because of their occlusive effect.
- Aerosols, gels, or lotions may be recommended when the dermatitis affects a hair-covered area of the body.

A large number of cosmetic dry skin formulations are commercially available. These may contain natural oils, vitamins, or a variety of fragrances that have a psychologic appeal. However, the fragrances and dyes found in many of these formulations may be irritating or allergenic to sensitive dry skin and should be avoided.

Efficacy of any skin care product may need to be sacrificed or compromised somewhat to achieve patient acceptance. The most efficacious product that the patient will accept should be recommended.

Topical nonprescription products come in various package sizes and strengths. Table 3 lists the amount of drug needed to cover a given area of the body three times daily over a 1-week period. By being aware of such details, the pharmacist can serve the patient economically as well as therapeutically.

Dandruff, Seborrheic Dermatitis, and Psoriasis

Dandruff, seborrheic dermatitis (seborrhea), and psoriasis are described as chronic, scaly dermatoses. They may be placed on a spectrum ranging from dandruff, a minor problem that is primarily cosmetic, to psoriasis, a clinical condition that can have significant physical, psychologic, and economic consequences. (See Table 4 for the distinguishing features of these three dermatoses.) Nonprescription products are appropriate for all degrees of dandruff. Many cases of seborrheic dermatitis will respond to the same nonprescription drug regimen used to treat dandruff. Mild, chronic cases of psoriasis that do not involve inflammation may be responsive to nonprescription treatment. However, most cases of psoriasis require the attention of a physician.[17]

Specific Conditions

Dandruff

Dandruff is a chronic, noninflammatory scalp condition that results in excessive scaling of scalp tissue. It occurs in approximately 20% of the population. Severity declines in the summer and is not aggravated by emotional states. Authorities disagree over whether inadequate shampooing exacerbates dandruff; however, there is agreement that frequent washing is important in managing the condition.[17,18]

Dandruff is not a disease; rather, it is a physiologic event and condition much like the growth of hair and nails, except that the end product is visible on the scalp and has a substantial cosmetic and social stigma associated with its presence. The process correlates with the proliferative lifetime activity of the epidermis. Dandruff generally appears at puberty (when many skin activities are altered), reaches a peak in early adulthood, levels off in middle age, and declines in advancing years (occurring only rarely after age 75).

Dandruff is characterized by accelerated epidermal cell turnover, an irregular keratin breakup pattern, and the shedding of cells in large flakes. It is normal for epidermal cells on the scalp to continually slough off just as they do on other parts of the body. However, the epidermal cell turnover rate in normal individuals is greater on the scalp than on other parts of the body. In dandruff patients, the epidermal cell turnover rate is about twice that in individuals without the condition.[2]

Dandruff is diffuse rather than patchy, it is not inflammatory, and pruritus is common. Flaking, the only visible manifestation of dandruff, is the result of an increased rate of horny substance production on the scalp and the sloughing of large scales. Dandruff flakes often appear around a hair shaft because of the epithelial growth at the base of the hair. This phenomenon does not occur on the normal scalp because the horny substance breaks up in a much more uniform fashion. The horny layer of the scalp normally consists of 25–35 fully keratinized, closely coherent cells per square millimeter arranged in an orderly fashion. However, in dandruff, the intact horny layer has fewer than 10 normal cells per square millimeter, and nonkeratinized cells are common. With dandruff, crevices occur deep in the stratum corneum, resulting in cracking, which generates large flakes. If the large clumps or flakes can be broken down to smaller units, the dandruff becomes less visible.

As the rate of keratin cell turnover increases, so too does the number of incompletely keratinized cells. This situation is characterized by the retention of nuclei in keratin layer cells. The number of these cells assists in distinguishing dandruff from psoriasis or seborrhea; there are more cells in psoriasis and seborrhea than in dandruff. Incompletely keratinized cells in dandruff appear in clusters, possibly as a result of tiny inflammatory foci that are incited when capillaries discharge a load of inflammatory cells into the epidermis, causing accelerated epidermal growth in a small area. These microfoci are found in all scalps but are increased proportionately in dandruff.[2]

The specific cause of the accelerated cell growth seen in dandruff is unknown. The debate over whether dandruff is a result of elevated microorganism levels—particularly of the yeast, *Pityrosporum ovale*—on the scalp continues. However, whether the yeast causes the dandruff or proliferates because the presence of dandruff provides a favorable environment for growth is immaterial.[18]

Dandruff is more of a cosmetic than a medical problem, and treatment is fairly straightforward. The patient needs to understand that there is no cure for dandruff but that the condition can be controlled. Total removal of hair eliminates dandruff, but this approach is rather drastic and generally unacceptable. Washing the hair and scalp frequently with a nonmedicated shampoo three times a week or even daily is often sufficient to control dandruff. If it is not, medicated nonprescription antidandruff products may be recommended. With the medicated shampoos, contact time improves effectiveness. The patient should be counseled to allow medicated shampoo to remain on the hair for approximately 5–10 minutes before rinsing. Thorough rinsing is important in the use of all shampoo products.

The first medicated shampoo to recommend is generally one containing a cytostatic agent, such as pyrithione zinc or selenium sulfide. These agents reduce the epidermal turnover rate. Next, a keratolytic shampoo containing salicylic acid or salicylic acid with sulfur may be used. Finally, a coal tar–containing shampoo may be tried; however, these products tend to stain light-colored hair and clothes and do not appeal to many patients. If the dandruff proves resistant to these agents, the patient should be referred to a physician for treatment with prescription agents.[17,19]

Seborrheic Dermatitis

Seborrheic dermatitis is a general term for a group of eruptions that occur predominantly in the areas of greatest sebaceous gland activity (e.g., the scalp, face, and trunk). This condition affects approximately 12 million Americans. Seborrhea occurs mostly in middle-aged and elderly persons, particularly men. It is often found in persons with parkinsonism, endocrine states associated with obesity, zinc deficiency, and human immunodeficiency virus infection. Quadriplegics and persons who have experienced a cerebrovascular accident (stroke) or a myocardial infarct (heart attack) also seem prone to seborrhea. Nonprescription therapy is effective in most cases. The pharmacist plays a key role in the management of seborrhea.[20]

Seborrhea is marked by accelerated epidermal proliferation and sebaceous gland activity. The distinctive characteristics of the disorder are its common occurrence in hairy areas (especially the scalp); the appearance of dull yellowish-red lesions, which are well demarcated; and the associated presence of oily-appearing, yellowish scales. Pruritus is common. The most common form, seborrhea capitis, is characterized by greasy scales on the scalp that often extend to the middle one-third of the face with subsequent eye involvement. (See color plates, photograph 21.) Lesions may also appear in the external auditory canal and around the ear. When seborrhea capitis occurs in newborns and infants during the first 12 weeks of life, it is referred to as cradle cap and is treated primarily by gentle but thorough washing. Pruritus does not appear to accompany cradle cap, and the condition often clears spontaneously by 8–12 months of age.[4,17,20]

The cause of seborrhea is unknown although predisposition appears to be a genetic trait. Emotional or physical stress serves as aggravating factors. Proposed etiologic factors have included vitamin B-complex deficiency, food allergies, autoimmunity, climate changes, and low relative humidity. The characteristic accelerated cell turnover and enhanced sebaceous gland activity give rise to the prominent scale displayed in the condition; however, there is no clear-cut quantitative relationship between the degree of sebaceous gland activity and susceptibility to seborrhea.

It is almost universally accepted that seborrhea is merely an extension of dandruff, and the controversy regarding the involvement of *P. ovale* extends to seborrhea. Some researchers, however, dispute the link with dandruff, offering evidence that seborrhea is a separate condition. Incompletely keratinized cells commonly make up 15–25% of the corneocyte count in seborrheic dermatitis but rarely exceed 5% in dandruff.[2,20]

The differential diagnosis of seborrheic dermatitis is not always simple. Other disorders that need to be considered include dandruff, psoriasis, atopic dermatitis, and fungal infections. Fortunately, misdiagnosis of seborrhea as dandruff is not of great consequence because both involve accelerated epidermal turnover with scaling as the principal manifestation; therefore, treatment is generally the same in both cases. However, some unique aspects of seborrhea capitis are worth noting. Dandruff is considered a relatively stable condition whereas seborrhea fluctuates in severity, often as a result of stress. Involvement of eyebrows and eyelashes with associated eyelid problems, such as blepharitis, is common in seborrhea but not in dandruff. And dandruff is a noninflammatory condition whereas seborrhea may be accompanied by erythema and sometimes by crusting.

The best distinguishing characteristic to differentiate seborrhea from psoriasis is the location of the lesions. Seborrhea commonly involves the face and generally is not found on the extremities whereas psoriasis is rarely found on the face but tends to appear on the elbows and knees. The scalp is generally involved in both conditions, and if this is the only site of involvement, differential diagnosis is difficult. The term *sebo-psoriasis* has been coined to describe this condition. However, the physical appearance of scales may help to differentiate the two disorders. Seborrhea is usually marked by greasy, thick, yellow scales whereas psoriatic scales are generally dry and silvery in appearance.

Atopic dermatitis, like psoriasis, can be distinguished from seborrhea on the basis of scale appearance and location of the lesions. Atopic dermatitis commonly occurs in the folds of the arms or knees. Itching from this disorder is generally more intense than it is from seborrhea. Moreover, patients presenting with atopic dermatitis often have a history of atopic disease such as asthma or hay fever. Thus, a medical history may help determine the probable etiology of the dermatologic condition.

Fungal infections may be mistaken for seborrhea. Proper diagnosis is important because seborrhea therapy using hydrocortisone may worsen fungal infections. If the lesion is located in the groin, tinea cruris (jock itch) must be considered, especially during warm weather. Scalp lesions must be evaluated for the possibility of tinea capitis (ringworm of the scalp).[2]

The treatment of seborrhea capitis is generally the same as that of dandruff, but with exceptions. Frequent cleansing with a nonmedicated shampoo should be tried first. If that is ineffective, seborrhea generally responds to shampoos containing pyrithione zinc, selenium sulfide, salicylic acid, or coal tar. The keratolytic combination of salicylic acid and sulfur is not recommended for seborrhea;[21] frequent use of selenium sulfide tends to make the scalp oily and may actually exacerbate the seborrheic condition.

A primary difference between the treatment of dandruff and seborrhea is the use of topical steroids in managing seborrhea. Hydrocortisone lotions for scalp dermatitis are available without a prescription. These products are not indicated for dandruff, but they may be used in the management of seborrhea.

The use of topical hydrocortisone in seborrhea capitis should be reserved for those cases that do not respond to therapy with shampoos. The patient should be instructed to apply the hydrocortisone product once a day until symptoms subside, and then intermittently to control acute exacerbations. The patient should also be instructed in the proper technique of applying hydrocortisone lotion to the scalp. The hair should be parted and the product applied directly to the scalp and massaged in thoroughly. This process should be repeated until the desired coverage of the affected area is achieved. The absorption of the medication into the scalp will be enhanced if the lotion is applied after shampooing; skin hydration will promote drug absorption.

Frequent and continued use of hydrocortisone in the treatment of seborrhea capitis is discouraged because topical steroids can produce a rebound dermatitis when therapy is discontinued. If the condition worsens or if symptoms persist for more than 7 days, a physician should be consulted. At this point, a more potent topical steroid may be indicated. The patient should be instructed to rely primarily on shampooing to control the condition and to use topical steroids only when necessary.[2]

If the seborrhea spreads to the ear canal, eyebrows, eyelashes, or eyelids, a physician should be consulted for appropriate therapy. Control of the scalp condition as well as use of prescription otic and ophthalmic agents may be warranted.

Nonprescription products used to treat seborrhea should not be used on children under 2 years of age, except under the advice and supervision of a physician.[22]

Psoriasis

Psoriasis is estimated to afflict 1–3% of the U.S. population. Lesions typically appear on small areas of the body for short periods of time. Remissions and exacerbations are unpredictable. Approximately 30% of persons with psoriasis find that the disease disappears spontaneously. However, chronic psoriasis may occur over extensive areas of the body and may cause enough psychologic distress to affect lifestyle and career choice adversely. In the form of psoriatic arthritis, it may even result in disability and deformity. Treatment of chronic, severe psoriasis can also produce a significant economic burden.[17,23]

Psoriasis is a papulosquamous skin disease marked by the presence of small elevations of the skin as well as scaling. Lesions are flat topped, pink or dull red in color, and covered with silvery scales. The edges of the lesions are sharply delineated, and individual diameters may vary from a few millimeters to 20 cm or more. When psoriatic scales are removed mechanically, small bleeding points appear (Auspitz sign). Psoriatic skin is more permeable to many substances than is normal skin; for example, it may lose water 8–10 times faster. In fact, when large areas of the body surface are involved, whole body skin water loss may be as much as 2 to 3 L per day in addition to normal perspiration loss. Evaporation of this volume of water requires more than 1,000 calories. For this reason, psoriatic patients may show increased metabolic rates at the expense of tissue catabolism, and muscle wasting may occur.[2]

Psoriatic lesions tend to appear on the scalp, elbows, knees, fingernails, and the genitoanal region. Lesions may develop in sites of vaccination or skin tests, scratch marks, or surgical incisions and have been reported to be produced by shock and noise. In fact, the response to skin trauma is so predictable that it can be used in diagnosis in up to 40% of persons afflicted. For example, when scaling is not evident, diagnosis is difficult. However, scales may be induced by light scratching. It has been shown that both the epidermis and dermis must be damaged before the reaction occurs, and the reaction generally occurs within 6–18 days following the injury.[2]

Many patients and clinicians do not mention pruritis as a symptom of psoriasis. However, several surveys indicate that itching is a significant manifestation of the disease in 30–70% of cases.[23]

Psoriasis assumes several different pathologic forms, the most common being psoriasis vulgaris. This is the chronic, plaque-type psoriasis of the general description. The plaques may be any size and may be quite extensive.[17]

Guttate psoriasis accounts for about 17% of psoriatic cases. It is characterized by many small, tear-shaped lesions distributed more or less evenly over the body. These lesions may later coalesce to form large characteristic plaques. (See color plates, photographs 22A, B, and C.) Psoriasis in children is usually of the guttate variety and may be precipitated by various systemic diseases such as streptococcal tonsillitis. Acute attacks of guttate psoriasis have also been noted to occur at puberty and following childbirth. When the psoriatic condition is initiated by a guttate attack, the disease carries a better prognosis than that of a slower and more diffuse onset.[2]

Another type of psoriasis is known as pustular psoriasis. It is marked by localized, sterile pustules on the palms and soles. In severe or generalized cases (von Zumbusch's type), the entire skin may be involved and the condition may become life-threatening.[23]

Flexural psoriasis involves the intertriginous folds. Often no other lesions are present, which makes it difficult to distinguish from seborrheic dermatitis. Because of moisture and friction associated with the affected areas, treatment is often difficult as well.[17]

Erythrodermic psoriasis is a severe complication that can be life-threatening. The entire skin surface can become red with little evidence of scales. Massive shunting of blood to the skin surface can cause heat and water loss extensive enough to cause cardiac failure.[17,23]

Psoriasis is basically a disease of the skin; mucous membranes are rarely involved. The only tissues besides skin known to be clinically involved are the synovium and nails. In many patients with coexisting joint disease and psoriasis, the arthritic component is not easily distinguishable from rheumatoid arthritis. Certain psoriatic patients, however, have a unique form of arthritis, psoriatic arthritis, which is recognized as a distinct clinical entity. Psoriatic arthritis is distinguished from rheumatoid arthritis in several respects. Its onset is often in the distal rather than the proximal joints of the fingers or toes, and this involvement is associated with psoriasis of the nails in 80% of persons affected. Nail involvement includes onycholysis (separation from the nail bed), pitting, and yellow discoloration. Differentiation from a fungal infection requires laboratory analysis. Unfortunately, there is no effective treatment for nail psoriasis. Psoriatic arthritis is often asymmetric in its joint involvement. Usually the rheumatoid factor is absent and prognosis is better than it is with rheumatoid arthritis. The psoriatic lesions are treated topically; the joint involvement is usually treated with nonsteroidal anti-inflammatory agents.[17,23]

The duration of psoriasis is variable. Lesions may last a lifetime or may disappear quickly. When they disappear, they may leave the skin either hypopigmented or hyperpigmented. The disease course is marked by spontaneous exacerbations and remissions, and it tends to be chronic and relapsing.

When one examines the natural history of psoriasis in patients, several points of interest emerge. For example, there seems to be an inherited predisposition to psoriasis, given that about 30% of psoriatic patients show an associated family history. Evidence supports an autosomal dominant mode of inheritance, and genetic markers as determined by the major histocompatibility locus antigen system have been identified. Persons with psoriasis also have a higher than usual incidence of occlusive vascular episodes, which seems to correlate with the extensiveness of the lesions. Environmental factors are not to be underestimated. Hot weather and sunlight have been noted to improve the condition; cold weather worsens it. However, sunlight worsens psoriatic conditions in a small number of patients. This photosensitive variant is more common with increasing age and in women. Many investigators agree that emotional stress also affects psoriasis adversely. Another factor involved in the pathogenesis of psoriasis is endocrine function; for example, psoriasis has been noted to improve or clear during pregnancy and reappear after parturition. It is well documented that antimalarial agents, beta blockers, and lithium can exacerbate or even precipitate psoriasis. Abrupt withdrawal of corticosteroids in psoriatic patients may precipitate the severe pustular form.[17,23] The bulk of information supports multiple factors in the genesis of psoriasis because both genetic and environmental components play a role in the disease.

No age group is exempt from psoriasis; incidence of initial onset peaks in the late 20s and then declines with advancing age. It is also distributed almost equally between men and women. Psoriasis is most prevalent in Caucasians; its incidence is lower in people living in countries close to the equator and in Japanese and Native Americans. Incidence in dark-skinned races is extremely low at 0.7%.[23]

The pathophysiology of the psoriatic lesion is very complex, involving not only the epidermis but also the dermis and the body's immune system. The major pathophysiologic events involved in the disease process are accelerated epidermal proliferation and metabolic activity, proliferation of capillaries in the dermal region, and invasion of the dermis and epidermis by inflammatory cells.

Accelerated epidermal proliferation is one hallmark of psoriasis, leading to excessive scaling of the skin. Normal epidermal turnover is 25–30 days; in psoriatic plaque it is 3 to 4 days. There are two schools of thought on this phenomenon. The first theory is that the accelerated epidermal proliferation is due to a shortening of cell division cycle time. Data have been collected showing that the germinative cell cycle of the psoriatic cell is 12 times faster than normal (37.5 versus 457 hours). These data, however, have been disputed. The second theory is that the germinative layer in human epidermis is composed of three distinct populations of epidermal cells. In normal skin, only one of these populations may be actively cycling, but in psoriasis all three epidermal cell populations may be involved in active proliferation.[2]

Accelerated epidermal proliferation is aided by the fact that psoriatic lesions demonstrate extensive infolding of the dermal–epidermal junction. The greatly expanded surface area that results and the presence of two or three basal cell layers lead to a greatly exaggerated mitotic growth and epidermal thickness. The keratin produced has many incompletely keratinized cells, and the granular layer is absent in severe cases.

When one considers the extent of epidermal proliferation in psoriasis, it logically follows that an expanded vascular system is needed to satisfy increasing metabolic requirements. In psoriasis, proliferation of capillaries in the dermal region occurs. The resultant capillary loops are arranged vertically at the center of the plaque and are responsible for the bleeding (Auspitz sign). It has been postulated that psoriatic plaque may generate an angiotactic substance responsible for this capillary proliferation, enabling the lesion to expand.[2]

The third major pathophysiologic event in psoriasis is invasion of the dermis and epidermis by inflammatory cells. Mononuclear cells and polymorphonuclear (PMN) leukocytes can be found in the dermis; PMN leukocytes also tend to infiltrate the epidermis. Extracts of psoriatic scale have been shown to contain factors that can induce directed migration (chemotaxis) of these inflammatory cells. Moreover, mononuclear cells and PMN leukocytes from psoriatic patients have been shown to exhibit enhanced responsiveness to chemoattractants. Lithium carbonate increases the total mass of circulating PMN leukocytes and is therefore associated with an induction or exacerbation of psoriatic symptoms. The presence of inflammatory cells in psoriatic skin may induce epidermal proliferation and has led to many theories about the possible role of the immune system in the pathogenesis of psoriasis.[2]

The mononuclear infiltrate found in psoriatic dermal tissue is largely composed of T lymphocytes and macrophages. The T lymphocytes are thought to be responsible for cell-mediated immunity and may also suppress or assist in the stimulation of antibody production. It has been postulated that there is a T-cell defect in psoriasis. More specifically, there may be a lack of suppression of the humoral immune system, leading to autoantibody production against skin antigens. Various data have been collected in support of an autoimmune theory of psoriasis.[2]

Although much research has been conducted on the causes of psoriasis, the specific biochemical event triggering psoriatic skin formation remains unknown. Prostaglandins and polyamines, as well as cyclic nucleotides, are being investigated as having a possible etiologic role. It is possible that cyclic adenosine 3', 5'-monophosphate (cAMP) mediates the regulation of epidermal proliferation and that there is a defect in the adenylcyclase–cAMP system in psoriatic skin. It originally was thought that cAMP levels were lowered in the psoriatic lesion and that this contributed to enhanced epidermal proliferation. Conflicting data, however, have been obtained, and the precise role of cAMP in the pathogenesis of psoriasis has yet to be clarified.[2]

Diagnosis usually is straightforward for simple psoriasis. Sites of involvement, the dry silvery appearance of the scale, and a small area of bleeding after scale removal are characteristic. Pruritus and joint involvement may also be present. Information regarding precipitating factors such as disease, pregnancy, a recent vaccination, emotional stress, or physical trauma is useful in a preliminary diagnosis.

It is important to differentiate psoriasis from other diseases that may have similar symptoms but call for different treatment. When the scalp or the flexural and intertriginous areas are involved, psoriasis must not be mistaken for a fungal infection or seborrhea. A fungal organism may be identified from lesion scrapings. Seborrhea and psoriasis of the scalp may be distinguished by the difference in scale appearance and color. Also, in psoriasis the plaque has a full, rich, red color with a depth of hue and opacity not normally seen in seborrhea or dermatitis. In dark-skinned races, this quality is lost. If lesions are present in the groin, axilla, and inframammary region, diagnosis based on visual inspection may be difficult, and a physician may need to conduct more elaborate histologic and pathologic diagnoses.

Other skin diseases whose symptoms resemble those of psoriasis are localized neurodermatitis, particularly in the genitoanal region, and fungal conditions with circular or annular lesions. When psoriasis alternates with or is complicated by other diseases such as seborrhea, diagnosis is more difficult.

Careful questioning of the patient and examination of the lesions, when feasible, are essential in determining whether the complaint is simple psoriasis and recommendation of a nonprescription product is appropriate. If a nonprescription product is used, the pharmacist should counsel the patient to consult a physician if the condition does not improve in 1 to 2 weeks or if it worsens. Also, if the pharmacist can help the patient to gain some understanding and acceptance of the condition, it may reduce the patient's emotional stress and therefore decrease psychogenic exacerbations.

There is no cure for psoriasis, only a reduction in its severity. The patient should be reassured that, in most cases, control is possible. Such reassurance tends to increase compliance with treatment regimens that may prove inconvenient and will usually be prolonged. Prophylaxis, achieved by avoiding identified precipitating factors such as skin irritation, emotional stress, and physical trauma, should be emphasized.

Because dry skin, often accompanied by pruritus, is very common in psoriasis, the starting point in treatment focuses on relieving those symptoms. Emollients, with or without hydrating agents, are appropriate for dry skin. Oatmeal baths may ease the pruritus. Gentle rubbing with a soft cloth following the bath will help remove the scales. Vigorous rubbing, which can aggravate the lesions, should be avoided. If this therapy is insufficient, self-treatment may

TABLE 5	Concentrations of approved nonprescription ingredients for products for the treatment of dandruff, seborrheic dermatitis, and psoriasis		
Ingredient	Dandruff[a]	Seborrheic dermatitis	Psoriasis
Coal tar	0.5–5%	0.5–5%	0.5–5%
Pyrithione zinc (brief exposure)	0.3–2%	0.95–2%	—
Pyrithione zinc (residual)	0.1–0.25%	0.1–0.25%	—
Salicylic acid	1.8–3%	1.8–3%	1.8–3%
Selenium sulfide	1%	1%	—
Sulfur	2–5%	—	—

[a]For control of dandruff, salicylic acid may be combined with sulfur, provided each ingredient is present within the approved concentrations.
Reprinted from *Federal Register* 1982; 47: 54646–84.

progress to the use of keratolytics, coal tar, and topical hydrocortisone.[17]

Different stages of the disease are treated differently. Acute psoriatic onset characterized by severely erythematous lesions calls for soothing local therapy with emollients. Tars, salicylic acid, and aggressive UV radiation therapy must be avoided at this stage because of the potential irritant effect. As the acute process subsides and the usual thick-scaled plaques appear, however, more potent therapy with agents such as keratolytics may be used. Many patients respond well to simple measures, but other patients are refractory to the most aggressive treatment.[2]

There is consensus that "guerrilla tactics are better than a frontal assault," with the more powerful agents held in reserve. In eruptive or unstable forms of the disease, even mild sunlight may provoke a Koebner-type exacerbation. The FDA recommends that only mild cases of psoriasis be self-treated. Individuals with severe cases involving large areas of the body should be under a physician's care.[2]

Nonprescription drugs may be an efficacious part of the physician's armamentarium; therefore, the pharmacist must be a knowledgeable consultant. In addition to nonprescription products, several prescription-only medications are available. The use of these medications sometimes necessitates day care or hospitalization of the patient.

The FDA final monograph on nonprescription dandruff, seborrheic dermatitis, and psoriasis products was published on December 4, 1991 and became effective on December 4, 1992.[21] Active ingredients cited as Category I (generally recognized as safe and effective) include the following:

- *Dandruff:* coal tar preparations, pyrithione zinc, salicylic acid, selenium sulfide, sulfur, and sulfur in combination with salicylic acid;
- *Seborrheic dermatitis:* coal tar preparations, pyrithione zinc, salicylic acid, and selenium sulfide;
- *Psoriasis:* coal tar preparations and salicylic acid (Table 5). Topical hydrocortisone is also found useful in the self-treatment of seborrhea and psoriasis.

Twenty eight additional nonprescription ingredients commonly found in dandruff, seborrhea, and psoriasis products were not found to be effective for these uses and were designated as nonmonograph (Table 6). These ingredients should soon be of historic interest only as products are reformulated. Emollients and humectants that may be useful have been described above.

High-potency topical steroids may be used to treat seborrhea and psoriasis under medical supervision. Prescription drug treatment for psoriasis also includes anthralin, antimetabolites (such as methotrexate), psoralens combined with long-wave UV phototherapy (PUVA), retinoids (such as etretinate), and systemic steroids.

Pharmacologic Agents

Cytostatic Agents

By increasing the time necessary for epidermal cell turnover, it is possible to bring about a dramatic decline in visible scales. Thus, cytostatic agents represent the most direct approach to controlling dandruff and seborrhea. However, cytostatic activity is not restricted to conditions in which the rate of epidermal turnover is great.

Pyrithione Zinc Pyrithione zinc's action is likely due to a nonspecific toxicity for epidermal cells. The pyrithione moiety is apparently the active part of the molecule. Product effectiveness is influenced by several factors. Pyrithione zinc is strongly bound to both hair and the external skin layers; the extent of binding correlates with clinical performance. The drug does not penetrate into the dermal region. Its absorption increases with contact time, temperature, concentration, and frequency of application. Some consider

TABLE 6	Nonmonograph ingredients commonly found in nonprescription dandruff, seborrhea, and psoriasis products[a]
Alkyl isoquinolinium bromide	Lauryl isoquinolinium bromide
Allantoin	Menthol
Benzalkonium chloride	Mercury oleate
Benzethonium chloride	Methylbenzethonium chloride
Benzocaine	Methyl salicylate
Boric acid	Phenol
Calcium undecylenate	Phenolate, sodium
Captan	Pine tar
Chloroxylenol	Povidone–iodine
Colloidal oatmeal	Resorcinol
Cresol, saponated	Sodium borate
Ethohexadiol	Sodium salicylate
Eucalyptol	Thymol
Juniper tar	Undecylenic acid

[a]These ingredients were classified as nonmonograph in FDA's final action on the categorization and uses of dandruff, seborrheic dermatitis, and psoriasis active ingredients for nonprescription products.

Reprinted from *Federal Register* 1982; 47: 54646–84.

pyrithione zinc to be slower acting than selenium sulfide.[2]

For pyrithione zinc products intended to be applied and washed off after a brief exposure, the FDA allows concentrations of 0.3–2% for treating dandruff and 0.95–2% for treating seborrhea. Concentrations for products to be applied and then left on the skin or scalp are 0.1–0.25% for both dandruff and seborrhea.[21] Shampoos and soaps are currently available in 1 and 2% concentrations. Lower concentration residual products are anticipated.[24]

Before using one of these products, the patient should be advised to shampoo with a nonmedicated product to remove scalp and hair dirt, oil, and scale. This may be followed by a pyrithione zinc shampoo worked into the scalp vigorously for at least 5 minutes, followed by thorough rinsing. This treatment should be repeated twice weekly for 2 weeks and then once weekly as needed.[17]

Long-term use of 1 to 2% pyrithione zinc products has not been associated with toxicity. This may be because zinc pyrithione is relatively insoluble in water and is not easily absorbed through the skin or mucous membranes. Nevertheless, patients should be cautioned against using this agent on broken or abraded skin. Rare cases of contact dermatitis have been reported.

Selenium Sulfide Selenium sulfide is thought to have a direct antimitotic effect on epidermal cells. Like zinc pyrithione, it is more effective with longer contact time and should be applied in a similar manner. The product must be rinsed from the hair thoroughly or discoloration may result, especially in blond, gray, or dyed hair. Frequent use of selenium sulfide tends to leave a residual odor and an oily scalp.

Selenium sulfide has been approved in a 1% concentration as an active ingredient in nonprescription products to treat dandruff and seborrhea.[21] A higher concentration is available by prescription for use in resistant cases.

Cytostatic toxicity is minimal. Selenium sulfide, however, can cause sensitization of scalp and adjacent skin areas and should be avoided if sensitization occurs. Contact with the eyes should be avoided because of the potential for irritation. If contact does occur, the patient should flush the eyes with copious amounts of water. Selenium sulfide is highly toxic if ingested. Because of the risk of systemic toxicity, it should never be applied to damaged skin.[25]

Keratolytic Agents

Keratolytic agents are used in dandruff and seborrhea products to loosen and lyse keratin aggregates, thereby facilitating their removal from the scalp in smaller particles. These agents act by dissolving the cement that holds epidermal cells together. The keratolytic concentrations in nonprescription scalp products are not sufficient to impair the normal skin barrier but do affect the abnormal, incompletely keratinized stratum corneum.

Keratolytic agents may produce several adverse effects, and the patient should be counseled accordingly. These agents have a primary, concentration-dependent irritant effect, particularly on mucous membranes and the conjunctiva of the eye. They also have the potential of acting on hair keratin as well as on skin keratin. Thus, hair appearance may suffer as a result of extended use. Vehicle composition, contact time, and concentration are important factors in the success of a keratolytic. The directions and precautions for the use of keratolytic shampoos are essentially the same as for shampoos containing cytostatic agents.

Salicylic Acid Salicylic acid lowers skin pH, causing increased hydration of keratin and thus facilitating its loosening and removal. Salicylic acid functions best as a keratolytic when used in an oil-in-water emulsion base. Contact time is minimal in a shampoo. Therefore, significant absorption/adsorption of the agent by the skin should not occur. Ointments applied a few times per day and left on are much more effective. Because ointments and pastes are difficult to use on the hairy scalp, aqueous and alcoholic preparations are preferred for those locations.

Salicylic acid in cream or ointment form is useful in psoriasis when very thick scales are present. The patient should soak the psoriatic area in warm water for 10–20 minutes before application. The preparation should be applied several times a day and may be covered by an occlusive dressing. However, application over extensive areas should be avoided because of the potential for systemic toxicity. Initially, low concentrations should be used because it is always possible that the irritant effect may worsen the condition.[2]

Salicylic acid has been approved in concentrations of 1.8–3% for the self-treatment of dandruff, seborrhea, and psoriasis.[21] At these concentrations, the keratolytic effect typically takes 7–10 days. In higher concentrations for other uses, the keratolytic effect may be evident in 2–3 days. This difference in time may be important information for the patient who may have used keratolytics for other purposes, such as callus removal.

Sulfur Sulfur is believed to function by an inflammatory process, causing increased sloughing of cells and reduced corneocyte counts.[26] Sulfur shows its best activity in a nonemulsion base.

Sulfur has been approved in concentrations of 2–5% for the self-treatment of dandruff only. Although it is approved as a single-entity active ingredient, sulfur is usually combined with salicylic acid. For the control of dandruff, the sulfur–salicylic acid combination is useful if both ingredients are present within the approved concentrations.[21] While not an official indication, many authorities recommend this combination for the self-treatment of seborrhea.[20]

Coal Tar

Coal tar products have long been popular for the treatment of dandruff, seborrhea, and psoriasis. Many nonprescription products are available. Crude coal tar, which consists of a heterogeneous mixture of more than 10,000 different compounds, is produced by the destructive distillation of bituminous coal. Its composition varies depending on the source of the coal and the process used. Crude coal tar is the most active; the refined tars, less so; and liquor carbonis detergens, the least active.[17]

Its mechanism of action is not known, but coal tar has been attributed with being antiseptic, antipruritic, keratoplastic, antiparasitic, antifungal, antibacterial, vasoconstrictive, and photosensitizing. The beneficial activity in the conditions under consideration seems to depend on dispersion of scales and an ability to reduce the number and size of epidermal cells produced.

Crude coal tar (1–5%) and UV radiation therapy have been used in the treatment of psoriasis since 1925 in a method known as the Goeckerman regimen. A therapeutic benefit of both the tar alone and the irradiation alone has been demonstrated, but the combination is more effective than either agent by itself. Remissions lasting up to 12 months have been reported after 2–4 weeks of therapy. The coal tar is removed from the skin before irradiation takes place. Otherwise, the UV radiation will not reach the skin. For many years, the therapeutic response to this form of therapy was believed to be caused by phototoxicity, but this theory has been challenged. Now it is thought that the beneficial effect of coal tar may lie in its ability to cross-link with deoxyribonucleic acid (DNA). Coal tar in combination with UV radiation may also increase prostaglandin synthesis in the skin, which may be related to its beneficial effect. Combinations of 1% crude coal tar with long-wave UV (UV-B) radiation and of 6% crude coal tar with UV-B radiation have been shown to be equally effective. Hence, only modest levels of coal tar are needed.[2]

Coal tar is available in creams, ointments, pastes, lotions, bath oils, shampoos, soaps, and gels. This wide variety of products has partly resulted from an attempt to develop a cosmetically acceptable product, one that masks the unpleasant odor, color, and staining properties of crude coal tar that most patients find aesthetically unappealing. Liquor carbonis detergens is a 20% tincture of coal tar that has been useful in the development of acceptable tar products. It is used in concentrations of 3–15%.

Tar gels represent a unique dosage form that appears to deliver the beneficial elements of crude coal tar in a form both convenient to apply and cosmetically acceptable. These gels are nongreasy, nonstaining, and nearly colorless. The pharmacist should caution the patient, however, that these gels may have a drying effect on the skin, necessitating the use of an emollient.

Certain side effects are associated with the use of coal tar. These include folliculitis, particularly of the axilla and groin; staining of the skin and hair, particularly blond, gray, and dyed hair; photosensitization; and dermatitis due to irritation.[27] Certain patients may even show a worsening of the condition being treated when they are exposed to coal tar products. This is particularly of concern in the acute phase of psoriasis, when topical steroids are recommended to reduce inflammation prior to the use of coal tar preparations.[17]

The active photosensitizers of coal tar include acridine, anthracene, and pyridine. If the patient is currently using other photosensitizing drugs such as tetracyclines, phenothiazines, thiazides, or sulfonamides, the pharmacist should give appropriate warnings. Moreover, the patient should not use extensive exposure to sunlight or sunlamps to simulate the Goeckerman regimen. This procedure requires careful monitoring of UV radiation exposure by a physician. Generally, patients should be cautioned that the use of coal tar may increase their tendency to sunburn for up to 24 hours after application. However, before advising the patient to avoid sun exposure, the pharmacist should ask what directions were given by the physician because patients are commonly told to apply the coal tar in the evening and then spend time in the sunlight on the following day.

Crude coal tar and UV radiation are both thought to have carcinogenic potential, particularly in the anogenital area. However, there have been no reports of an increased frequency of skin cancer in psoriatic patients treated for many years with coal tar and UV radiation. The FDA considers the benefits to outweigh the risks for use in shampoo formulations for dandruff and seborrhea because of the short contact time.

The FDA approves coal tar in concentrations of 0.5–5% for the self-treatment of dandruff, seborrhea, and psoriasis.[21] In the past, coal tar has been combined with various other agents such as menthol, salicylic acid, allantoin, benzocaine, and hydrocortisone. These products cannot now be marketed unless the manufacturer proves the efficacy and safety of the additional agents for the claimed use.[23]

Topical Corticosteroids

Topical hydrocortisone (0.25–1%) is available without a prescription and has been promoted for the temporary relief of itching due to body and scalp dermatoses. Hydrocortisone is generally efficacious as an antipruritic agent when used in concentrations of 1% or more. However, it is not indicated, nor is there evidence that it is effective, in the treatment of dandruff. It may be useful for seborrhea accompanied by inflammation and should be reserved for scalp seborrhea unresponsive to medicated shampoos.[20]

Nonprescription hydrocortisone products play an important role in the management of psoriasis. A major problem with hydrocortisone and all topical steroids is that there is usually a prompt rebound when topical steroid therapy is discontinued and the psoriasis may reappear as the more severe pustular form. Relapse occurs more quickly after use of topical corticosteroids than after tar or anthralin therapy. Nevertheless, these agents are more appealing to the patient on cosmetic grounds, which are a consideration in long-term therapy.[23]

Topical corticosteroids have several effects (e.g., antiinflammatory, antimitotic/antisynthetic, antipruritic, vasoconstrictor, and immunosuppressive) on cellular activity. Efficacy may be enhanced by an occlusive dressing. However, continued use of topical steroids beyond 2 or 3 weeks may render the drug less effective. If the patient does not respond adequately to hydrocortisone, physician referral is appropriate because the use of more potent steroids may be in order. Selection of the proper prescription steroid may be complex owing to the common assumption that potency and adverse effects are linked directly to halogenation.[28,29]

Adverse effects associated with the use of topical steroids include local atrophy of the skin after prolonged use and the aggravation of certain cutaneous infections. The possibility of systemic sequelae exists and is enhanced by the use of the more potent compounds, occlusive dressings, or application to large areas of the body. Because children have a greater surface area–to–body mass ratio, they are at greater risk of developing systemic complications. In general, however, the concentrations of hydrocortisone available in nonprescription preparations are unlikely to cause systemic sequelae.[28,29]

Pharmacists may play a vital role in patient care by prudently advising patients about the safe and appropriate use of nonprescription topical hydrocortisone preparations. This role has become especially important since the FDA has allowed marketing of the 1% concentration, which is deemed effective in treating seborrheic dermatitis and some forms of psoriasis.[16] The patient may be instructed to apply the hydrocortisone as a thin film two to four times a day at the onset of therapy and intermittently thereafter to control exacerbations. The medication should be massaged into the skin thoroughly. Continued and frequent use of hydrocortisone is to be discouraged because topical steroids may become less effective with prolonged use, may promote local rebound, may cause adverse local effects, and, most importantly, may not induce remissions of psoriasis. The patient should be instructed to rely primarily on other treatments and to use topical hydrocortisone only when necessary.

Anthralin

Anthralin (dithranol) is a synthetic anthroquinone that is available for the treatment of psoriasis by prescription only. It is an effective topical agent that may cause a more rapid resolution of psoriatic plaques than crude coal tar, with few patients failing to respond. Anthralin is structurally related to acridine, a component of crude coal tar, and is thought to act by hydrolyzing to biologically active free radicals.[17] It is irritating to the skin and should not be applied to normal skin, the face, genitalia, or areas of acute eruption. It also has a propensity to stain clothing and skin. Anthralin (0.2–0.8%) is used in combination with a daily coal tar bath and UV radiation exposure in a procedure known as the Ingram technique. It is most effective when incorporated into a stiff paste allowing prolonged (24-hour) adherence to the affected skin and minimizing contact with normal skin.[17] These pastes, however, can be difficult to apply, and because they are not water soluble, their removal from the skin is difficult. Skin irritation and a burning sensation are common, so a short-contact regimen (20–30 minutes) has been developed as an alternative to the 24-hour Ingram method.[23]

Methotrexate

Because a characteristic of psoriasis is accelerated epidermal proliferation, methotrexate has been used in the therapy of psoriasis because it serves as an antimitotic agent. Specifically, it is thought to inhibit DNA synthesis by blocking dihydrofolate reductase. The serious potential side effects and toxicity of systemic methotrexate are well known. Because of its potential toxicity, methotrexate is used primarily as an antineoplastic agent. Its use in psoriasis is generally reserved for psoriatic arthritis or for severe cases of psoriasis vulgaris and pustular psoriasis that are not responsive to more conventional therapy. Strict supervision of patients receiving methotrexate, including frequent blood analysis and regular liver function tests, is essential.

PUVA therapy

PUVA therapy, a photochemotherapeutic process, stands for psoralen (P) and long-wave UV radiation (UV-A). The most common psoralen used in this process is methoxsalen (8-methoxypsoralen, 8-MOP), administered in oral doses of 0.65 mg/kg, followed 2 hours later by carefully monitored exposure to long-wave UV radiation. Treatments are repeated two or three times weekly for a mean of 10–20 treatments. Patients then receive weekly or biweekly maintenance therapy.[17]

PUVA therapy has demonstrated its efficacy in the treatment of psoriasis. However, the safety of the procedure must also be considered. Immediate side effects that may occur include nausea, pruritus, erythema, and occasional blistering. Concomitant use of other dermal irritants may aggravate dermal toxicity, and special precautions have been called for in treating patients who are using other photoactive drugs such as sulfonamide-based diuretics. Long-range side effects that may occur include the development of cataracts or cutaneous carcinoma. Therefore, PUVA therapy should be restricted to patients with severe, recalcitrant, disabling psoriasis that is not adequately responsive to other forms of therapy.[31] Topical use of psoralens combined with phototherapy has largely been abandoned.

Retinoids

Etretinate, a synthetic vitamin-A analog, has been shown to be an effective oral antipsoriatic agent. Side effects associated with its use include alopecia on withdrawal of therapy; elevated serum transaminase levels; and dryness of the lips, mouth, and nose, which occurs in approximately 80% of those receiving the drug. Etretinate shares its teratogenic potential with other retinoids and so is contraindicated in women of childbearing age. Because the risks outweigh the benefits for mild psoriasis, etretinate should be reserved for severe, recalcitrant psoriasis vulgaris; erythrodermic psoriasis; and pustular psoriasis.

Systemic Steroids

The systemic use of corticosteroids is contraindicated in all but the most severe forms of psoriasis. This restriction is owing to the undesirable side effects that accompany systemic use of steroids as well as to the fact that, after therapy is stopped, the disease is almost certain to be worse than it was initially.[23] Intralesional injections of steroids have a limited use in treating isolated lesions and nail psoriasis.[17]

Miscellaneous

Many other ingredients have been included in nonprescription products for the treatment of dandruff, seborrhea, and psoriasis that were claimed to have antimicrobial or antipruritic effects (Table 6). Because of their ineffectiveness in controlling these conditions, as well as their potential for irritation and other adverse effects, these ingredients received nonmonograph status.[21]

Detergents are not generally considered to be active ingredients in nonprescription dandruff products. However, for mild forms of dandruff, frequent and vigorous washing with a nonmedicated shampoo may help control excess scaling. Massaging the scalp produces a dispersion of scales into smaller, less visible subunits. Detergents may contribute to this effect by virtue of their surfactant activity. Detergents found in shampoos include sodium lauryl sulfate, polyoxyethylene ethers, triethanolamine, and quaternary ammonium compounds such as benzalkonium chloride, benzethonium chloride, and isoquinolinium bromides.[2]

Vitamin D_3, both topical and oral, has been investigated in the treatment of psoriasis with inconclusive results. One major reason for pursuing the investigation of D_3 as a possible therapeutic agent is that no adverse effects were reported when it was administered by either route.[32,33] However, the use of vitamin D_3 in psoriasis is currently not included in the FDA-approved labeling.[34]

Other agents under investigation for the treatment of psoriasis include gamma interferon, neuropeptides, fish oil, hydroxyurea, acetazolamide, ranitidine, halobetasol propionate, clobetasol propionate, cyclosporine, and piritrexim. The use of ultrasound to produce localized heating (hyperthermia) has been applied in the treatment of isolated psoriatic lesions. An external osmotic pump has also been developed to deliver medication to the psoriatic lesions.[35–37]

Product Selection Guidelines

Dandruff and Seborrheic Dermatitis

When deciding on which product to recommend, the pharmacist may follow these simple guidelines:

- The patient first should increase the frequency of shampooing, using the usual product and rinsing the hair thoroughly after shampooing.
- If increased frequency of shampooing does not control the condition, a pyrithione zinc–containing product may be used. Selenium sulfide is a suitable alternative. Improvement may be noted within several weeks.
- Shampoos containing keratolytic agents and coal tar may also be tried.
- The patient should be reassured that dandruff is a normal physiologic event and cautioned that total control using therapeutic agents may not be possible. If the patient has tried one medicated product, the next one recommended should have a different mechanism of action.
- If the condition fails to respond to traditional cytostatic or keratolytic agents, a coal tar–containing shampoo may be used. Alternatively, a coal tar gel or a tar oil bath additive may be applied sparingly to the lesions 3–8 hours before shampooing.
- If the condition is still refractory, a hydrocortisone lotion or gel may be applied sparingly once a day and worked into the scalp thoroughly. Improvement should be seen within 7 days.
- Recalcitrant cases, cases involving large areas of the body, and cases in children under 2 years of age should be referred to a physician for evaluation.

Psoriasis

Psoriasis is not a trivial medical problem, and psoriatic patients should be under a physician's care. The pharmacist's role in the management of psoriasis is that of a knowledgeable consultant. When deciding which product to recommend for a psoriatic condition, the pharmacist must consider the area to which the agent is going to be applied. The response to topical medications shows striking regional variation.

Scalp Psoriasis Elaborate psoriasis shampoos are not necessary to control psoriasis of the scalp. Frequency of shampooing rather than the product itself is the key to effective therapy. The resultant removal of scales is the goal of therapy. The patient may be instructed to shampoo using any type of product. Tar oil bath additives or coal tar solutions may be painted sparingly on the lesions 3–12 hours before each shampoo. Tar gels also may be useful in this approach. Hydrocortisone has been claimed to have little impact on psoriasis of the scalp.

Psoriasis of the Body, Arms, and Legs Because dry skin often accompanies psoriasis, emollients may be the first course of therapy if the condition is mild. Emollients may also be a useful adjunct to more aggressive therapy.

Salicylic acid products may be tried before progressing to the coal tar products because they are more cosmetically acceptable to most patients and may encourage better compliance. Such products may be useful if thick scales are present. Salicyclic acid may be applied several times during the day. The patient may be instructed to soak the affected area in warm water for 10–20 minutes before applying the medication.

Coal tar products may be applied to the body, arms, and legs at bedtime. Because coal tar often stains clothing, the patient should be advised to use old sheets and bed clothing. This therapy may be followed by a bath in the morning to help remove the coal tar as well as the psoriatic scale.

Topical hydrocortisone may be applied sparingly to the lesions several times during the day and massaged into the skin thoroughly. Continued and frequent use of hydrocortisone should be discouraged.

Intertriginous Psoriasis Intertriginous areas such as the armpits and genitoanal region are sensitive to irritants such as coal tar and salicylic acid. Therefore, these agents should not be used to treat psoriasis in these areas. Rather, hydrocortisone cream may be applied sparingly two or three times a day and should be used less often as improvement occurs.

Summary

Many patients are afflicted with dermatitis, dry skin, dandruff, seborrhea, and psoriasis. It is important that these patients be assessed properly before self-treatment is recommended. Therapy effective in one disorder may exacerbate another. The pharmacist can perform a valuable service either by helping patients to determine the nature of their problem and choose the most effective therapy or by providing an appropriate referral.

References

1. Ricciatti–Sibbald DJ. Dermatitis. In: Clark C, ed. *Self-Medication: A Reference for Health Professionals*. 3rd ed. Ottawa: Canadian Pharmaceutical Association; 1988: 67–85.
2. Robinson JR. Dermatitis, dry skin, dandruff, seborrheic dermatitis, and psoriasis products. In: *Handbook of Nonprescription Drugs*. 9th ed. Washington, DC: American Pharmaceutical Association; 1990: 811–40.
3. Pearce M. Atopic dermatitis. *Pharm Times* 1990 May: 88–92.
4. David TJ, Devlin J, Ewing CI. Atopic and seborrheic dermatitis: practical management. *Pediatrician* 1991; 18: 211–7.
5. Gossel TA. Therapeutic relief of contact dermatitis. *US Pharm* 1990 May: 12–6.
6. Keefner KR, DeSimone EM. Contact dermatitis: skin reactions to irritants. *US Pharm* 1991 Jun; Skin Care Supplement: 36–9.
7. Fisher AA. Allergic contact dermatitis associated with OTC topical anesthetics and antihistamines. *Pharm Times* 1991 May: 65–8.
8. Fitzpatrick JE. Common inflammatory skin diseases of the elderly. *Geriatrics* 1989 Jul; 44 (7): 40–6.
9. Shwayder T, Ott F. All about ichthyosis. *Pediatr Clin North Am* 1991 Aug; 38 (4): 835–57.
10. Gossel TA. Dry skin. *US Pharm* 1990 Jan: 20–4.
11. Lazar AP, Lazar P. Dry skin, water, and lubrication. *Dermat Clin* 1991 Jan; 9 (1): 45–51.
12. DP Hamacher. Facial moisturizers. *NARD* 1991 Aug: 63.
13. Van Scott EJ. Reversing the signs of the times. *Wellcome Trends in Dermatology* 1987 Nov: 2–3.
14. *Federal Register* 1982; 47: 39444–8.
15. *Federal Register* 1979; 44: 69768–866.
16. *Federal Register* 1991; 56: 43025–6.
17. Wright DE. Psoriasis, seborrheic dermatitis and dandruff. In: Clark C, ed. *Self-Medication: A Reference for Health Professionals*. 3rd ed. Ottawa: Canadian Pharmaceutical Association; 1988: 87–98.
18. Dolnick E. A flaky concern. *Hippocrates* 1989 Jan–Feb; 3 (1): 28–30.
19. Cauwenbergh G, De Doncker P, Schrooten P, et al. Treatment of dandruff with a 2% ketoconazole scalp gel: a double-blind placebo-controlled study. *Int J Dermatol* 1986 Oct; 25 (8): 541.
20. Gossel TA, Slattery CD. Self-treatment of seborrhea. *US Pharm* 1991 Mar: 24–34.
21. *Federal Register* 1991; 56: 63554–69.
22. *Federal Register* 1982; 47: 54646–84.
23. Pray WS. Psoriasis: it can be dangerous. *US Pharm* 1991 Jun; Skin Care Supplement: 28–34.
24. *Drug Facts and Comparisons*. St. Louis: J. B. Lippincott; 1992 Oct: 567a.
25. *AHFS Drug Information 92*. Bethesda, Md: American Society of Hospital Pharmacy; 1992: 2136–7.
26. *AHFS Drug Information 92*. Bethesda, Md: American Society of Hospital Pharmacy; 1992: 2165–6.
27. *AHFS Drug Information 92*. Bethesda, Md: American Society of Hospital Pharmacy; 1992: 2168–70.
28. Vonderweidt J. Sorting out topical corticosteroids. *US Pharm* 1988 Jul: 54–65.
29. Trozak DJ. Topical corticosteroid therapy in psoriasis vulgaris. *Cutis* 1990 Oct; 46: 341–50.
30. *AHFS Drug Information 92*. Bethesda, Md: American Society of Hospital Pharmacy; 1992: 577–83.
31. *AHFS Drug Information 92*. Bethesda, Md: American Society of Hospital Pharmacy; 1992: 2189–93.
32. Araujo OE, Flowers FP, Brown K. Vitamin D therapy in psoriasis. *DICP, the Annals of Pharmacotherapy* 1991 Jul–Aug; 25: 835–9.
33. McQueen KD. Is vitamin D effective in treating psoriasis? *DICP, the Annals of Pharmacotherapy* 1991 Jul–Aug; 25: 753–4.
34. *AHFS Drug Information 92*. Bethesda, Md: American Society of Hospital Pharmacy; 1992: 2231–3.
35. McCarthy G. Fish oil and psoriasis. *Lancet* 1991 Sep 28; 338 (8770): 824.
36. Gawkrodger DJ. Acetazolamide for psoriasis. *Lancet* 1991 Mar 2; 337 (8740): 558–9.
37. Farber EM. 10 years of progress: 1980–1990. *Psoriasis newsletter* 1990; 10 (2): 1–2.

CHAPTER 31

Diaper Rash and Prickly Heat Products

Gary H. Smith

> **Questions to ask in patient assessment and parental counseling**
>
> **Diaper Rash**
>
> - *Do you use disposable diapers or a diaper service?*
> - *Do you use cloth diapers? How do you launder them?*
> - *Do you use double diapers or plastic pants?*
> - *How often do you change the baby's diapers?*
> - *How do you clean the baby's skin during a diaper change?*
> - *What products have you tried for the rash?*
> - *Does the baby have a fever?*
> - *Has the baby had diarrhea recently?*
> - *Has the baby ever had a yeast infection in the diaper area?*
> - *Is there a family history of allergic disorders?*
> - *Has any new type of food recently been added to the baby's diet?*
> - *Is the baby being given any medication? If so, what and by what route?*
>
> **Prickly Heat**
>
> - *Where is the rash located and what does it look like?*
> - *How long has the rash been present?*
> - *Does the patient sleep in a warm and humid room?*
> - *How much clothing does the patient wear during the day and night?*
> - *What products have you already tried for the rash?*

Diaper rash and prickly heat (miliaria rubra) are acute, transient, inflammatory skin conditions that occur in many infants and young children. Both conditions cause burning and itching that can result in restlessness, irritability, and sleep interruptions. Prevention is the best treatment.

The skin of most adults is about 2 mm thick, but infants' skin is only about 1 mm thick and therefore is more delicate and susceptible to injury. The epidermis (the outermost skin layer) represents about 5% of the total skin thickness; therefore, the external barrier that protects the infant from the environment is very thin and vulnerable.[1] For skin to function efficiently, it should remain dry, smooth, and slightly acidic.

Diaper Rash

Diaper rash, or diaper dermatitis, is one of the most common dermatitides in infants. A survey of 1,089 infants 1–20 months of age showed a frequency of diaper rash approaching 65%; the majority of cases were mild or of minor severity. Only about 5% of the infants had severe dermatitis; the remainder of the cases were classified as moderate. The incidence of diaper rash peaked between 9 and 12 months of age.[2]

In 1982, the Food and Drug Administration (FDA) reopened four administrative records (antimicrobial, external analgesic, skin protectant, and antifungal) for drug product ingredients used in the treatment of diaper rash or prickly heat. In 1990, the FDA modified the definition of diaper rash and issued four notices of proposed rulemakings.[3–7] The FDA defined diaper rash or diaper dermatitis as:

> An inflammatory skin condition in the diaper area (perineum, buttocks, lower abdomen, and inner thighs) caused by one or more of the following factors: moisture, occlusion, chafing, continued contact with urine or feces or both, or mechanical or chemical irritation. Mild conditions appear as simple erythema. More severe conditions include papules, vesicles, oozing, and ulceration.

Etiology

Urine and feces have long been implicated as contributors to the development of diaper rash. Normal newborns begin urinating within 24 hours after birth. Urination occurs up to 20 times daily until approximately 2 months of age and as often as eight times daily from 2 months to 8 years of age. Defecation also occurs several times daily in infants. Breast-fed infants tend to urinate less frequently and have a lower incidence of diaper-area dermatitis than bottle-fed infants. Furthermore, urine and feces of nursing infants tend to be less alkaline and therefore less irritating than those of bottle-fed infants.[2,8]

The distribution of diaper rash may be positional. If the baby lies on the stomach, the rash may be ventral; if the baby lies on the back, the rash may be dorsally located. It may spread to the entire diaper area, depending on the promptness of therapy and the cause of the rash. The diaper area is vulnerable to inflammation because the skin is thin, warm, and moist and is exposed to irritants and bacteria. Ammonia probably plays a role in irritating a preexisting inflammatory condition. Certain foods in the baby's diet may also be contributing factors. High-protein foods may make the urine and stools more acidic and produce an "acid scald."[9] Complications may occur, including secondary infections caused by various microorganisms.

The pathologic changes vary with the causative factors and the severity of the dermatitis. Diaper rash may range from mild erythema with or without maceration and chafing to vesicles, pustules, or bullae. Deeper nodular and infiltrated lesions may develop, depending on the primary cause of the dermatitis. Seborrhea, psoriasis, and atopic dermatitis may predispose to irritation and infection.

Ammonia

Until recently, it was widely accepted that diaper rash was caused by the presence of ammonia and other irritating end products of the enzymatic breakdown of urine. More recent studies have not confirmed this relationship. The FDA believes that the ammonia theory of diaper rash, although perhaps not yet totally disproven, has been discredited by recent studies. None of the data submitted to the FDA are sufficiently compelling to allow claims that are based on the activity of antimicrobials against specific urea-splitting bacteria. Any claims concerning the ammonia theory need to be justified by clinical studies on infants that include bacteriological studies to correlate a reduction in ammonia-producing bacteria with a clinical improvement in diaper rash.

It has been confirmed that infant urine does not cause significant skin irritation for up to 48 hours, but that skin damage can occur after 10 days of continuous exposure. Although specific irritants have not been identified, the ammonia found in the diaper area may promote irritation by increasing the pH of the area, which in turn may increase the activity of fecal proteases and lipases, which may damage skin. Feces in the absence of urine or ammonia have been shown to cause skin irritation. The presence of feces in the diaper area is substantially more likely to promote diaper rash than is the presence of urine. This explains the increased occurrence of diaper rash in infants with diarrhea or frequent stools.[2,10–12] The role of urine in the genesis of diaper rash may simply be a function of overhydration of the skin in the diaper area. Wet skin is more permeable than dry skin to low-molecular-weight compounds and therefore is more susceptible to irritation.[13]

Retention of Moisture

If a soiled diaper is not changed promptly, the stratum corneum in the diaper area becomes waterlogged. This saturation causes keratotic plugging of the sweat glands, which results in sweat retention and may produce vesicles and irritation.

Mechanical and Chemical Irritants

Tightly fitting diapers covered with plastic pants increase moisture and temperature in the diaper area and prevent air from circulating around the skin. This environment is conducive to irritation and secondary infection. Irritation results from the diaper's constant rubbing against the skin. Eroded skin is more susceptible to infection. Frequent changing of diapers may prevent or minimize irritation.

Chemical irritants from various sources may precipitate a rash in the diaper area. Feces remaining in contact with the skin cause irritation, especially if the infant's diet promotes the elimination of irritating substances and unabsorbed foodstuffs or causes diarrhea. (See color plates, photograph 23.) Preparations applied to the diaper area, such as proprietary antiseptic agents and harsh soaps containing phenol, tars, salicylic acid, or sulfur, also may cause diaper rash. Diapers rinsed inadequately after washing may retain residues from detergents or bleach that can irritate the diaper area or cause allergic reactions. Precautions should be taken to avoid exposing the sensitive skin of infants and young children to these irritating substances.

Complications

Fungal and bacterial infections are the most common complications of diaper rash. These cutaneous infections are often secondary to untreated or improperly treated diaper dermatitis. The moist, warm, alkaline environment created by unchanged diapers is conducive to the development and multiplication of pathogenic bacteria and fungi.[10] If the skin is eroded or macerated or if the normal balance of the skin's bacterial flora is disturbed, these organisms may become pathogenic and cause infection in the diaper area.[8]

Fungal infections are caused most commonly by *Candida albicans*, an organism that may be part of the normal colonic flora. Infections caused by *C. albicans* are the most frequent cause of diaper rash complications. *C. albicans* has been cultured from the feces of up to 20% of normal infants;[8,14,15] a strong correlation exists between the presence of *C. albicans* in the stool and the severity of the diaper dermatitis.[8] Fungal infections of the diaper area have been believed to be a secondary complication of diaper dermatitis, but recent evidence suggests that they may be a primary cause. Therefore, fungal infections should be considered in all cases of severe diaper dermatitis.[2,14] The only precise method of diagnosis is culturing from scrapings or swabs of the skin lesions. A potassium hydroxide prep from skin scrapings may be highly suggestive of *C. albicans* infection.[12]

In newborns younger than 2 weeks, candidal diaper dermatitis is usually accompanied by oral thrush. Both conditions probably result from a maternal candidal vaginal infection before and during delivery. The lesions are usually erythematous and are surrounded by characteristic satellite pustules. They may become eroded and begin weeping. A physician should be consulted for appropriate treatment of this condition.

The relatively long-term systemic use of some broad-spectrum antibiotics may predispose the infant to diaper candidiases caused by overgrowth of *C. albicans* in the stool. Infants with severe diaper dermatitis who are concurrently receiving a broad-spectrum antibiotic should be evaluated for candidiasis by a physician.[16] Infectious complications of diaper rash caused by other dermatophytes have also been reported, including *Epidermophyton floccosum*[17–19] and *Trichophyton rubrum*.[20]

Bacterial infection of the diaper area is caused most commonly by *Staphylococcus aureus* and is often seen as a form of folliculitis. Classic lesions are follicular micropustules that coalesce with adjacent lesions to form lakes or pustules. Occasionally, bullous or encrusted impetigo, characterized by large blister-like lesions or honeycomb crusting, may occur. In some cases, group A *Streptococcus pyogenes* may be the pathogen. An infant with a suspected bacterial infection in the diaper area should be referred to a physician for appropriate diagnosis and treatment.[3]

Herpetiform diaper dermatitis has recently been reported and should be considered when a parent of an infant has an active herpes simplex infection.[21] Cytomegalovirus diaper rash has now been reported in infants born with congenital human immunodeficiency virus disease and therefore should be considered in such patients.[22] Other rare complications include granuloma gluteale infantum[23] and Kawasaki syndrome.[24] Kawasaki syndrome should be suspected if an erythematous, desquamating perineal rash appears in diapered infants or young children who also have symptoms such as fever, lymphadenopathy, or a rash elsewhere, especially on the ears and fingertips.

Ulceration of the penile meatus may be a painful complication of diaper rash in babies who are circumcised. The pain associated with this condition may lead to reflex inhibition of micturition and secondary distention of the bladder.

The FDA's review of products used to treat diaper rash includes the following statements regarding diaper rash and its complications. The skin under the diaper is macerated by prolonged wetness. Disposable diapers with a plastic backing, or plastic pants used over regular diapers, hold in heat and moisture, causing miliaria (prickly heat) and more maceration than occurs with the use of cloth diapers alone. Bacteria may proliferate in this warm, moist environment, thrive on nutrients in feces, and metabolize urine by-products to produce ammonia, an irritant. *C. albicans*, often present in feces, also proliferates to produce a characteristic, bright red, sharply marginated rash with satellite pustules and erosions. Other exacerbating factors are mechanical irritation (chafing), which is caused by rough cloth or tight or stiff plastic diapers, and chemical irritation, which is caused by detergent or bleach in diapers, by soap used to cleanse the baby, and by diarrhea.

Prickly Heat (Miliaria)

The lesions associated with prickly heat (miliaria) result from obstruction of the sweat gland pores. Retained sweat causes the dilation and rupture of the epidermal sweat pores, producing swelling and inflammation. (See color plates, photograph 24.) The term "prickly heat" was coined because the lesions usually produce itching and stinging. Prickly heat occurs primarily during hot, humid weather or during a febrile illness with profuse sweating. It may also occur as a result of excessive clothing, polyester clothing, and overcovering, especially at night in warm, humid rooms. Prickly heat may occur during infancy, childhood, or adulthood.

In infants, the lesions most often appear in intertriginous areas and under plastic pants, diapers, and adhesive tape. In children and adults, the dermatitis is seen on areas of skin that have been heavily occluded with clothing. The lesions, which are erythematous papules, may become pustular and are usually localized to the sites of occlusion.

Patient Assessment

In general, if diaper dermatitis is confined to the diaper area and does not present symptoms of fungal or bacterial infection, the pharmacist may recommend a nonprescription protectant product. If the infant has had diaper rash for only a few days, treatment by the parent may be recommended. The pharmacist should determine whether nondisposable cloth diapers are used and whether diapers are laundered with detergents containing irritants. If diaper rash persists 1 week or more after the infant has been treated with protectants and diapers have been changed frequently, or if the rash recurs frequently, the rash may be caused by a problem other than the diaper and a physician should be consulted. If the infant has had persistent diarrhea, appears irritable, or has a fever, or if the rash is resistant to nonprescription treatment, a physician should be consulted because the problem may be more serious than simple diaper rash.

If the rash occurs on areas outside the diaper area (groin, intergluteal fold, and lower abdomen), a condition such as atopic dermatitis, psoriasis, seborrheic dermatitis, allergic contact dermatitis, or scabies may be present; infants with such a rash should be diagnosed and treated by a physician. If the lesions are follicular micropustules or bullous or if they look like impetigo, a bacterial infection may be the cause.

The pharmacist may be able to determine the cause of many conditions by questioning the parents. In addition to explaining the steps that must be taken to prevent diaper rash and prickly heat, the pharmacist may recommend several nonprescription products suited to the child's condition. If the pharmacist ascertains that the rash has persisted and appears to be complicated by infection or another process, it should be suggested that the child be taken to a physician.

Treatment

Primary Treatment

The treatments for diaper rash and prickly heat may be considered together, but modifications and additional measures may be required for each condition. The active treatment of diaper rash involves (1) removing the source of irritation, (2) reducing the immediate skin reaction, (3) relieving discomfort, and (4) preventing secondary infection and other complications. The treatment plan should be individualized for both diaper rash and prickly heat. The area should be kept as dry and clean as possible. The diaper should be loose and well ventilated and should be changed as quickly as possible after becoming soiled. Plastic pants should be avoided. Products helpful in treatment include skin protectant products. The FDA has stated[4-7] that ordinary mild diaper rash, characterized by erythema of the buttocks, perineum, and lower abdomen, responds to very frequent diaper changes, cleansing with water, and removal of plastic occlusion. Most protectant treatments, such as talc and zinc oxide ointment and paste, help by protecting the skin, acting as a physical barrier to irritants, and absorbing moisture. The pharmacist should be able to advise parents about which products should be used for a particular kind of dermatitis and the specific care required. As with most forms of therapy, the simplest regimen is the one most likely to be followed consistently. A baby's skin is sensitive, and many babies may be irritated by or allergic to some available products.

The best treatment for mild forms of diaper rash is to change diapers as soon as they are soiled and to dry the diaper area completely before a new diaper is used. Plain water should be used to cleanse the diaper area to avoid sensitizing chemicals in soaps and commercial wipes. Cornstarch is a safe and effective dusting powder; it does not promote the growth of bacteria or fungi, as was once thought.[25] Careful use of a hair blow-dryer on a low setting to dry the area is effective and safer than a heat lamp. The use of a good protective agent, such as zinc oxide paste (Lassar's paste), Desitin®, or white petrolatum, provides a barrier to protect the skin from moisture.

In the treatment of prickly heat, the primary goal is to reduce sweating. Clothing should be made of light material and should not cause any rubbing of the skin. Light clothing and coverings are recommended to allow air to reach the skin. Air-conditioning the environment helps to lower humidity and temperature. Maceration and irritants may be reduced by frequent baths or sponge baths at least two times a day and the use of a bland talc dusting powder. Frequent diaper changes and the elimination of excessive soap or chemical irritants help to reduce discomfort associated with prickly heat.

Because occlusive dressings facilitate the absorption of topically applied steroids, they should not be used in the diaper area. When steroids are applied topically to inflamed or abraded skin, systemic levels may be higher than when they are applied to normal skin because of increased absorption. Also, chronic use of steroids (e.g., 0.1% triamcinolone cream) can cause thinning of the skin, with resultant striae and easy bruising.[4-7]

The medical community's recognition of the value of topical hydrocortisone for diaper dermatitis does not warrant its use for infants on a nonprescription basis. Because 0.25%, 0.5%, and 1.0% hydrocortisone ointments and creams are available for nonprescription use, pharmacists should caution parents concerning the use of this product for diaper rash. Hydrocortisone is not recommended for use on children under 2 years of age except under the advice and supervision of a physician. Furthermore, it has been suggested that hydrocortisone should be reserved for cases in which zinc oxide ointment or similar products and standard preventive measures have not been sufficient. The topical use of hydrocortisone for the infant patient without a physician's intervention does not appear to be warranted.

Pharmacological Agents

As stated earlier in this chapter, in 1990 the FDA issued notices of proposed rulemakings for the four types of product ingredients used in the treatment of diaper rash and prickly heat. These products included antimicrobials, external analgesics, skin protectants, and antifungals.[4-7] Guidelines for study protocols to demonstrate safety and efficacy in clinical trials were provided by the FDA.

In a December 18, 1992, final rule, the FDA declared that diaper rash claims should be removed from all nonprescription antifungals and external analgesics because of lack of adequate evidence of safety and efficacy. After June 18, 1993, any claim that such products are safe or efficacious in treating or preventing diaper rash will be considered misbranding. The FDA has encouraged the voluntary removal of such products from the market as soon as possible.

External Analgesics Regarding external analgesics, the FDA considered clinical data deficient in demonstrating that nonprescription external analgesics are safe and effective in treating or preventing diaper rash. The FDA further noted that the target population for these drugs (0–24-month-old infants and young children) could not adequately communicate symptoms to a parent or caregiver, so objective assessment of need could not be appropriately determined.

Antifungals Regarding antifungals, safety and efficacy data were considered deficient. Further, the FDA determined that antifungal active ingredients should not be included in nonprescription diaper rash products because fungal infections associated with diaper rash are not suitable for diagnosis and treatment by parents or caregivers and should be diagnosed and treated by a physician. Diagnosis and treatment of an infectious process associated with diaper rash is challenging even for the physician at times.

Antimicrobials The FDA currently classifies no nonprescription antimicrobial ingredients in diaper rash products as Category I (safe and effective). The FDA has further stated that manufacturers are encouraged to remove all ingredients in diaper rash products that are not classified as Category I. Category II products include boric acid, hexachlorophene, p-chloromercuriphenol, phenol, and resorcinol. One or more Category III products may eventually receive Category I classification, but this remains to be determined. Category III products include benzalkonium chloride, benzethonium chloride, calcium undecylenate, chloroxylenol, methylbenzethonium chloride, oxyquinoline sodium propionate, and triclosan.

Protectants Protectants help prevent or treat diaper rash by protecting from or sealing out moisture. Several protectants are classified as Category I. These include allantoin, calamine, and cod liver oil (in combination); dimethicone, kaolin, and lanolin (in combination); mineral oil; petrolatum; talc; topical cornstarch; white petrolatum; and zinc oxide. Category II products include bismuth subnitrate, boric acid, sulfur, and tannic acid. Category III products include aldioxa, aluminum acetate, aluminum hydroxide, microporous cellulose, cholecalciferol, cocoa butter, colloidal oatmeal, cysteine hydrochloride, dexpanthenol, glycerin, live yeast cell derivative, peruvian balsam oil, protein hydrolysate, racemethionine, shark liver oil, sodium bicarbonate, vitamin A, zinc acetate, and zinc bicarbonate.

Zinc oxide, an excellent protectant found in many products used to treat diaper rash, is a mild astringent with weak antiseptic properties. Many preparations contain various concentrations of zinc oxide and petrolatum. Zinc oxide paste (USP), the simplest of these formulations, contains 25% zinc oxide, 25% cornstarch, and 50% white petrolatum. Parents should be informed that this paste is most easily removed with mineral oil. This combination serves as a highly protective and water-absorptive base. Many preparations contain zinc oxide in a higher concentration than that contained in Lassar's paste (Desitin® contains 40% zinc oxide). Most of the preparations also contain one or more of various other protectant medications, such as cod liver oil, vitamins A and D, lanolin, peruvian balsam, and silicone.

In general, these products are popular and are promoted primarily for the treatment of diaper rash. Only recently have there been controlled studies with these products.[26] Reports from Leeming/Pacquin[26] showed Desitin® Ointment to be superior to bland soap and unmedicated talcum powder in the treatment of diaper rash. Only two reports have compared one diaper rash product with another: Lantiseptic Ointment® (Corona) (*p*-chloromercuriphenol [1:1,500] in a lanolin and petrolatum base) was shown in a controlled study to be equal or superior to vitamin A and D ointment in the treatment of diaper rash.[27,28] Although several anecdotal reports indicate that vitamin A and D ointment or ointments containing cod liver oil may be beneficial in preventing and treating diaper rash, no evidence exists that any of these products is superior to zinc oxide paste or white petrolatum. Zinc oxide paste or white petrolatum can be used alone as a protectant and as initial treatment for diaper rash. Use of these products avoids subjecting the infant to compounds that may cause skin sensitization, such as peruvian balsam. Zinc oxide paste is absorptive because of the powders in its base and is thus able to take up moisture, keeping the skin dry, whereas white petrolatum is oleaginous and hydrophobic and cannot absorb any moisture. Therefore, petrolatum may trap moisture beneath it and keep the diaper area hydrated, a condition that is not desirable in cases of prickly heat. White petrolatum is also more irritating to the skin than zinc oxide paste. Of the two products, the one that will keep the diaper area driest and cause the least irritation is zinc oxide paste.

The powdered protectant agents that have been used most often in treating diaper rash and prickly heat are talc, cornstarch, calcium carbonate, kaolin, zinc stearate, microporous cellulose, and magnesium stearate. Talc is a natural hydrous magnesium silicate that allays irritation, prevents chafing, and absorbs sweat. Talc is similar to ointments and creams in that it adheres well to the skin. It is a finely milled powder that will not cake in the folds and cause maceration by friction. Magnesium stearate has been included in some dusting powders promoted for use in infants because of its ability to adhere to the skin and to serve as a mechanical barrier to irritants. Calcium carbonate, cornstarch, kaolin, zinc stearate, and microporous cellulose are also included in diaper rash products for their moisture-absorbing properties. When applied after each diaper change, these products serve primarily to keep the diaper area dry. However, they should be used cautiously because inhalation of the dust by the infant may be harmful and could lead to chemical pneumonia. A recent report substantiates the potential hazards of powders.[29] They should be applied with a cotton fluff to spread evenly. Powders should never be applied to an acute oozing dermatitis because they may promote secondary crusting and infection.

Although it recognized that powdered dosage forms had been extensively used for many years, the FDA proposed an additional warning for diaper rash products in a powdered dosage form because of the numerous reported incidents of accidental inhalation of baby powders that had appeared in the literature.[6] Powders should be used cautiously and parents should be instructed to apply these products carefully. The FDA has proposed the following warnings for products containing talc: "Do not use on broken skin." "Keep powder away from child's face to avoid inhalation, which can cause breathing problems." In addition, the FDA has proposed directions for applying powder products: "Apply powder close to the body away from child's face. Carefully shake the powder into the diaper or into the hand and apply to diaper area."

Treatment of Secondary Complications

Various topical antiseptic agents have been used to treat staphylococcal and streptococcal infections. The FDA believes that antimicrobial (antiseptic) drug products have significant limitations in treating the secondary infections that may accompany irritation caused by diaper rash.[4] A rash in the diaper area that does not clear up in a reasonable amount of time may indicate the presence of a secondary bacterial or fungal skin infection. These conditions should not be treated with nonprescription drugs. The infant with a suspected bacterial or fungal infection in the diaper area or with diaper rash that has persisted for a week or more should be taken to a physician for appropriate diagnosis and treatment. Some physicians will recommend treating bacterial or fungal infections in the diaper area with systemic antibiotics or topical antifungals.

Nonprescription topical antibiotics have an adjunctive role, at best, in the treatment of these bacterial infections. Systemic antibiotics are the treatment of choice for impetigo. Quaternary ammonium compounds, such as benzalkonium chloride, are included as antibacterial agents in commercial products; however, their effectiveness has been questioned because these cationic surfactants are inactivated by organic matter included in urine and feces. In addition, these antibacterial compounds may act as irritants in some cases, exacerbating the inflammation and causing discomfort when applied.[11] Antibiotic ointments should be used only when clearly indicated because they may cause hypersensitivity reactions and foster the evolution of resistant organisms. Because of the high incidence of adverse reactions to neomycin, which is a dermal sensitizer; the increased probability of absorption through inflamed and occluded skin; and the availability of more appropriate topical antibiotics, use of topical neomycin for diaper rash should be avoided. Secondary infections that may be caused by bacteria or species of *Candida* or other fungi should be diagnosed and treated by a physician.

Topical 2% miconazole cream and 1% haloprogin cream have been shown to be effective in treating candidal diaper rash.[30,31] Hydroxyquinoline can be applied topically for its antibacterial and antifungal activity. A combination of nystatin (100,000 units per gram), chlorhexidine (1%), and hydrocortisone (1%) has been favorably evaluated for both fungal and bacterial infections.[32] Calcium undecylenate is used for its antifungal activity. Nystatin, amphotericin B, haloprogin cream, and hydroxyquinoline are prescription-only products; aluminum acetate solution, miconazole, clotrimazole, chlorhexidine, and calcium undecylenate are available without prescription. The FDA, however, has not yet approved any of these nonprescription antifungals for the treatment or prevention of diaper rash. Tioconazole cream 1% has been shown to compare favorably with topical miconazole or econazole for the treatment of candidal diaper rash.

Prevention

Good prophylactic practices depend on parental cooperation and responsibility. A diaper should be changed as soon as it is soiled; leaving a wet diaper on for several hours increases the chances of diaper rash. The apparently unsoiled part of the diaper should never be used to wipe the baby. This practice spreads microorganisms over the skin that may proliferate when the child next urinates or defecates. If frequent changes are impossible, the infant should be kept belly down to reduce the tendency for feces and urine to become compressed under the gluteal area. Nondisposable cloth diapers should be made of soft material and should be fastened loosely to prevent rubbing. Plastic pants should be used as seldom as possible because they are occlusive and impede air flow through the diaper. The use of plastic pants at night and for extended periods should be discouraged, and daily baths should be encouraged.

Infants often urinate soon after they are put to bed for the night. Parents can reduce the time a child is exposed to a wet diaper and the amount of urine accumulated at night by changing the diaper within several hours after putting the child to bed.

The diaper area should be cleaned at each diaper change. Mild soap should be used for cleaning the diaper area and for bathing. It is important that skin folds that entrap perspiration and feces be cleaned thoroughly and rinsed well with clean water. The various diaper wipe products now available may contain antiseptics, soap, and lanolin that may contribute to the rash. Convenience may dictate their use, but caution should be exercised because of the possible presence of irritants and because a hypersensitivity reaction may occur. Therefore, if the use of such products is necessary, unscented, hypoallergenic wipes should be used. The diaper area should be completely dry before a clean diaper is put on. Exposing the diaper area to warm, dry air for a few minutes between changes helps to keep the skin dry. A bland ointment or dusting powder (such as zinc oxide ointment, cornstarch, or talcum powder) may be recommended after washing.

Diapers should be washed with mild soap. The use of harsh detergents and water softeners should be avoided. After they are washed, the diapers should be rinsed thoroughly. Air drying diapers in the sun helps kill bacteria. Ironing dry, washed diapers will reduce any surviving bacteria or fungi.

The addition of a disinfectant during the washing process is an effective means of reducing the bacterial count. Adding ordinary laundry bleach to the wash may reduce the number of organisms substantially. The use of clorophene (o-benzyl-p-chlorophenol) in the first rinse water in a concentration of 1 part clorophene to 2,500 parts water also is effective in treating and preventing diaper dermatitis. Acidification of diapers may also be helpful. Acidification can be accomplished by a final rinsing of the diapers in a solution made by adding one cup of vinegar to a half-filled washing machine tub. The diapers are then added and soaked for 30 minutes.

Over the past 10–15 years, there has been a trend away from the use of cloth diapers. Market research and surveys of parents have shown that 53–71% use only disposable diapers, 22–42.7% use both, and less than 7% use cloth diapers exclusively.[2,33,34] About 16 billion disposable diapers are bought each year in the United States. The majority of these are Pampers® or Luvs® from Procter & Gamble or Huggies® from Kimberly-Clark.[34]

Several studies have been conducted to compare the incidence of diaper rash in infants diapered with cloth and those diapered with the different types of disposable diapers.[2,35–42] Cloth diapers cleaned by a diaper service were associated with the lowest incidence of diaper rash, disposable diapers showed a similar low incidence, and home-laundered diapers were associated with the highest incidence. The home-laundered diapers were not rinsed with a bacteriostatic agent. These reports show the necessity of using a bacteriostatic agent either in the rinse water or in the diaper pail. Diapers containing fecal material should be rinsed well in the toilet before being placed in the diaper pail. Commercial diaper services provide essentially sterile diapers.

Over the last 10 years there has been considerable effort on the part of disposable diaper manufacturers to improve their products. Since it has been shown that major causes of diaper rash are skin wetness, skin damage from fecal protease and lipase enzymes, and pH increase from ammonia production when urine and feces are together in the same area, the focus has been on the development of diapers that control skin wetness and pH.[10,12]

The disposable diaper Ultra Pampers® contains absorbent gelling material (AGM) consisting of cross-linked sodium polyacrylate. Diapers containing AGM are designed to absorb moisture and bind it tightly to a gel matrix, to provide a buffering system with the AGM's partially neutralized carboxylic acid structure, and to reduce the potential for urine and feces to mix, thereby providing better pH control. Infants who wear the AGM diapers have been found to be substantially drier and to have significantly less diaper rash and less severe diaper rash than do infants wearing either conventional disposable or home-laundered diapers. Cloth diapers do not appear to be superior to the improved disposable diapers.[33,36,37–41]

In a study in day-care centers, 180 children wearing conventional disposable or AGM disposable diapers were evaluated for frequency of diarrhea, antibiotic use, and diaper dermatitis. The children with diarrhea and diapered with AGM diapers had a statistically significantly lower grade of diaper rash than infants diapered with conventional diapers. Diaper dermatitis in children taking antibiotics and in children with diarrhea and taking antibiotics was less with the AGM diapers than the conventional diapers, but in neither case was the difference statistically significant.[38]

Atopic dermatitis occurs in about 10% of children as an inherited skin disease. The erythematous and pruritic nature of the skin in children with atopic dermatitis makes the skin very sensitive to substances that irritate or dry it.

Infants with atopic dermatitis need to maintain epidermal hydration to prevent the skin from becoming brittle and more sensitive to toxins and infections. A randomized study of 1,800 infants was conducted to evaluate the effects on infants with atopic dermatitis of the AGM diapers in comparison with conventional cellulose disposable diapers and cloth diapers. There were no differences between AGM diapers and conventional cellulose disposable diapers. Infants in the cloth-diaper group had consistently worse diaper rash than did the other two groups. Diaper rash in the control group (infants without atopic dermatitis) did not differ with the type of diaper. However, a comparison of all infants in the atopic dermatitis group with all infants in the control group showed that the control group had less rash at all times during the 30 weeks of the study, indicating that any type of diaper increases the risk of rash or makes it more severe in infants with atopic dermatitis.[42]

Overall, studies appear to favor AGM diapers but fail to reveal any statistical difference between conventional disposable diapers and home-laundered cloth diapers. No comparison was made with commercial diaper services, nor were mothers of the infants in the cloth-diaper groups given any specific washing instructions. The cost of the more expensive AGM diapers must be weighed against the slightly increased benefit in the prevention of diaper dermatitis. Over a 2-year period the cost for home-laundered cloth diapers is approximately $526; the cost for a diaper service, $1,268; and the cost for disposable diapers, $1,352.[34]

In 1991 the Consumers Union evaluated the various disposable and cloth diapers. Ratings were consistently higher for disposable diapers than for cloth diapers in the areas of leakage, dryness, and fastening quality. However, it was noted that all disposables were subject to padding shifts (i.e., the padding sags or clumps when it is wet and leaves some area of the diaper without padding), which was not the case with the cloth diapers. Improved design and placement of elastic barriers make disposable diapers more resistant to leakage. Absorbent gel in the padding improves the diaper's ability to keep the infant dry.[34]

An additional concern is that disposable diapers, for the most part, are not biodegradable and may present an ecological hazard. Even those that are promoted as biodegradable (e.g., green label Nappies® and Tender Care®) are really not, because they depend on air, water, and sunlight to degrade. Most landfills would not provide these ingredients. Composting may be an alternative method for disposal of these diapers, but further research is needed.[34]

Prophylaxis with powders and ointments is not necessary for all babies. Just because an infant wears diapers does not mean that powders and ointments should be applied. If a problem occurs, it should be treated. If it recurs, prophylaxis is warranted. In clinical practice, a significant number of infants with a history of diaper rash will fall into this category. This is especially true in those cases induced by antibiotics or specific food groups. However, most babies who develop diaper rash will respond to treatment and will not need prophylaxis. Babies who require continued prophylaxis should have it stopped periodically to determine whether it is still necessary.[6]

The prompt changing of soiled or wet diapers is still the best method of preventing diaper rash, irrespective of the type of diaper used.

Product Selection Guidelines

Pharmacists should advise parents about the correct use of any product they recommend. Some general precautions should be mentioned, such as use of products prior to their expiration dates (when dated) and precautions to observe in applying topical preparations that might sting already irritated skin. If powders are recommended, parents should be instructed to apply them carefully to prevent the infant from inhaling the powder, which could lead to chemical pneumonia. When soaks and solutions (such as aluminum acetate solution) are used, the unused portion should be discarded after each use; that is, only a fresh preparation should be used each time.

Above all, pharmacists should caution parents about the general use of any medication for a baby's skin. The best therapy for diaper dermatitis is to keep the skin clean and dry.

Few infants escape diaper rash. The pharmacist may help by teaching parents the proper procedures for preventing diaper rash and prickly heat. Parents should understand that using medications indiscriminately is not the proper way to treat either condition and is ill-advised. Drugs alone cannot stop or prevent diaper rash or prickly heat. Many newborns, infants, and young children may be hypersensitive to various medications, and more harm than good can result from their use.

Summary

Pharmacists should be prepared to offer sound advice on a good prophylactic program and to recommend therapy for uncomplicated, uninfected cases of diaper rash and prickly heat. They should also be prepared to assess the severity of the rash and be able to recommend appropriate action, whether referral to a physician or a treatment plan.

Diaper dermatitis and prickly heat are the two most common dermal afflictions of newborns, infants, and young children, but their incidence and severity may be reduced by following proper procedures. If the dermatitis does not respond within 1 week to frequent diaper changes, frequent exposure to air, and application of a protectant, such as zinc oxide paste, a physician should be consulted.

References

1. Weston WL. *Practical Pediatric Dermatology*. Boston, Mass: Little, Brown and Company; 1979: 1–2.
2. Jordan WE et al. Diaper dermatitis: frequency and severity among a general infant population. *Pediatr Dermatol* 1986 Jun; 3: 198–207.
3. Leyden JJ, Kligman AM. The role of microorganisms in diaper dermatitis. *Arch Dermatol* 1978 Jan; 114: 56–9.
4. *Federal Register* 1990; 55: 25246.
5. *Federal Register* 1990; 55: 25234.
6. *Federal Register* 1990; 55: 25204.
7. *Federal Register* 1990; 55: 25240.
8. Berg RW. Etiologic factors in diaper dermatitis: a model for development of improved diapers. *Pediatrics* 1987; 14 (suppl 1): 27.

9. Brown CP et al. Diaper region irritations. *Clin Pediatr* 1964 Jul; 3 (7): 409–13.
10. Berg RW. Etiologic factors in diaper dermatitis: the role of urine. *Pediatr Dermatol* 1986 Feb; 3 (2): 102–6.
11. Buckingham KW, Berg RW. Etiologic factors in diaper dermatitis: the role of feces. *Pediatr Dermatol* 1986 Feb; 3 (2): 107–12.
12. Benjamin L. Clinical correlates with diaper dermatitis. *Pediatrician* 1987; 14 (suppl 1): 21–6.
13. Zimmerer RE et al. The effects of wearing diapers on skin. *Pediatr Dermatol* 1986 Jan; 3: 95–101.
14. Rebora A, Leyden JJ. Napkin (diaper) dermatitis and gastrointestinal carriage of *Candida albicans*. *Br J Dermatol* 1981 Mar; 105: 551–5.
15. Sevim A et al. Relation between the intestinal flora and diaper dermatitis in infancy. *Trop Geogr Med* 1990 Jun 27; 42: 238–40.
16. Honig PJ et al. Amoxicillin and diaper dermatitis. *J Am Acad Dermatol* 1988 Aug; 19 (2): 275–9.
17. Hayden GF. Dermatophyte infection in the diaper area: report of two cases. *Pediatr Infect Dis J* 1985 May; 4 (3): 289–91.
18. Congly H. Infection of the diaper area caused by *Epidermophyton floccosum*. *Can Med Assoc J* 1983 Sep 1; 129: 410–1.
19. Kahana M et al. Dermatophytosis of the diaper area. *Clin Pediatr* 1987 Mar; 26 (3): 149–51.
20. Cavanaugh RM, Greeson JD. Infection of the diaper area. *Arch Dermatol* 1982 Jun; 118: 446.
21. Jenson HB, Shapiro ED. Primary herpes simplex virus infection of a diaper rash. *Pediatr Infect Dis J* 1987 Dec; 6 (12): 1136–8.
22. Thiboutot DM et al. Cytomegalovirus diaper dermatitis. *Arch Dermatol* 1991 Mar; 127: 396–8.
23. Bluestein J et al. Granuloma guteale infantum: case report and review of the literature. *Pediatr Dermatol* 1990 Sep; 7 (3): 196–8.
24. Friter BS, Lucky AW. The perineal eruption of Kawasaki syndrome. *Arch Dermatol* 1988 Dec; 124: 1805–10.
25. Leyden JJ. Corn starch, candida albicans, and diaper rash. *Pediatr Dermatol* 1984 Apr; 1 (4): 322–5.
26. Research report. New York, NY: Leeming/Pacquin Pharmaceutical Co; 1974.
27. James WS. A new use for an old ointment: Lantiseptic ointment as a treatment for diaper dermatitis. *J Med Assoc Ga* 1975 May; 64: 133–4.
28. Bosch-Banyeras JM et al. Diaper dermatitis: value of vitamin A topically applied. *Clin Pediatr* 1988 Sep; 27 (9): 448–50.
29. Mofenson HC et al. Baby powder—a hazard! *Pediatrics* 1981 Aug; 68 (2): 265–6.
30. Mackie RM, Scott E. Topical miconazole cream in infantile napkin dermatitis. *Practitioner* 1979 Jan; 222: 124–6.
31. Montes LF, Hermann HW. Clinical and antimicrobial effects of haloprogin cream in diaper dermatitis. *Cutis* 1978 Mar; 21: 410–2.
32. Grimshaw JJ, Rivlin RS. An evaluation of nystaform-hc cream in napkin dermatitis. *Br J Clin Pract* 1982 Mar; 36: 363–6.
33. Lane AT et al. Evaluations of diapers containing absorbent gelling material with conventional disposable diapers in newborn infants. *Am J Dis Child* 1990 Mar; 144: 315–8.
34. Diaper Decisons: which are best for the baby? *Consumer Reports* 1991 Aug; 551–6.
35. Stein H. Incidence of diaper rash when using cloth and disposable diapers. *J Pediatr* 1982 Nov; 101 (5): 721–3.
36. Seymour JL et al. Clinical effects of diaper types on the skin of normal infants and infants with atopic dermatitis. *J Am Acad Dermatol* 1987 May 14; 17 (6): 988–97.
37. Campbell RL et al. Clinical studies with disposable diapers containing absorbent gelling materials: evaluation of effects on infant skin condition. *J Am Acad Dermatol* 1987 Dec; 17 (6): 978–87.
38. Campbell RL et al. Effects of diaper types on diaper dermatitis associated with diarrhea and antibiotic use in children in daycare centers. *Pediatr Dermatol* 1988; 5 (2): 83–7.
39. Austin AP et al. A survey of factors associated with diaper dermatitis in thirty-six pediatric practices. *J Pediatr Health Care* 1988 Nov–Dec; 2 (6): 295–9.
40. Campbell RL. Clinical tests with improved disposable diapers. *Pediatrician* 1987; 14 (suppl 1): 34–8.
41. Davis JA et al. Comparison of disposable diapers with fluff absorbent and fluff plus absorbent polymers: effects on skin hydration, skin pH, and diaper dermatitis. *Pediatr Dermatol* 1989 Jun; 6 (2): 102–8.
42. Seymour JL. Clinical and microbial effects of cloth, cellulose core, and cellulose core/absorbent gel diapers in atopic dermatitis. *Pediatrician* 1987; 14 (suppl 1): 39–43.

CHAPTER 32

External Analgesic Products

Arthur I. Jacknowitz

Questions to ask in patient assessment and counseling

- How long has the pain been present? How did it first appear? How often does it occur?
- Can you relate the pain to any specific event, such as overwork, an accident, or a sports-related activity?
- Is the pain in a joint or in the muscle? If in a joint, is the joint red, swollen, or warm to the touch?
- Is the pain worse when you get up in the morning? Does it tend to subside as the day goes on?
- Does the pain move to other areas of the body?
- Do you have a fever or any flulike symptoms?

Painful injuries as a result of our active lifestyles and the prevalence of arthritis have led to increased use of external analgesics. In fact, 40% of adults over the age of 50 are regular users of external pain relievers, and arthritis patients account for more than 75% of total usage. In 1990, external analgesics were the undisputed nonprescription drug growth leader, with sales increasing by more than 25% over the previous year. No other category came close.[1]

External analgesics are topically applied substances that may have either local analgesic, local anesthetic, local antipruritic, or counterirritant effects. It is important to differentiate these four groups. The topical analgesic, anesthetic, and antipruritic agents depress cutaneous sensory receptors for pain, burning, and itching, and act directly on the skin to diminish or obliterate these symptoms caused by burns, cuts, abrasions, insect bites, and other cutaneous lesions. (See Chapters 36, "Insect Sting and Bite Products," and 33, "Burn and Sunburn Products.") Topical counterirritants are included among the external analgesics because they are applied to the intact skin to relieve pain. They differ from the other three types of agents, however, in that the pain relief they produce results from stimulation of cutaneous receptors to induce sensations such as cold, warmth, and sometimes itching.[2] These induced sensations distract from the deep-seated pain in muscles, joints, and tendons, which are distant from the skin surface where the ingredient is applied. In this manner, deep-seated pain is indirectly relieved. Some counterirritant agents, when present in low concentrations, actually depress cutaneous receptors in a manner similar to local anesthetics, analgesics, and antipruritics. For example, menthol in concentrations below 1.0% depresses cutaneous receptors and stimulates them in concentrations above 1.25%. Counterirritants are a distinct class of external analgesic products because percutaneous absorption of active ingredients is not desired with them.

Etiology of Muscular Pain

Pain is one of the most common ailments for which people seek advice and help from health care providers. Although everyone is familiar with the sensation of pain, the International Association for the Study of Pain developed a definition of it a little more than a decade ago that is accepted by pain clinicians and researchers: an "unpleasant sensory and emotional experience associated with actual or potential tissue damage or described in terms of such damage."[3] Pain is a multidimensional experience that involves both a discriminative capacity and an interpretation of a stimulus in terms of present and past encounters.

More than a quarter century ago, the gate-control theory of pain integrated physiologic components of pain.[4] It postulated that a neural mechanism in the spinal cord acts like a gate that can control the transmission of pain impulses to the brain. According to this theory, pain signals are carried from specialized pain receptors to the spinal cord via two types of nerve fibers: small nonmyelinated fibers (type C fibers) and large myelin-containing nerve cells (type A delta fibers). The small fibers conduct impulses slowly and are associated with dull, aching, and lingering pain. The large fibers are linked with immediate pain, characterized as sharp and precise with a pricking sensation.

Small and large nerve fiber impulses can oppose each other. In fact, mild stimulation of large fibers can attenuate pain felt from activation of small fibers, a finding that helps to explain the efficacy of topical counterirritants. An example is the effect of applying an external analgesic (stimulating large fibers) to diminish the pain caused by a sports-related knee injury (activating small fibers).

Pain receptors are present in most areas of the body, including skeletal muscles. Stimuli activating these receptors cause sensory impulses to be transmitted via the nerve fibers to the brain, which may integrate and evaluate the signals as a perception of pain.[5]

Skeletal muscle pain is quite common, especially among persons who are not accustomed to strenuous exercise. Motivated by a heightened awareness of the beneficial effects of exercise, more Americans than ever are exercising regularly. With this increased participation, exercise-induced injuries have become more common. Such injuries are caused by equal and opposite reactions, which result either in macrotrauma or microtrauma.[6] Macrotrauma, a sudden catastrophic injury, occurs when an equal and opposite force exceeds the inherent tensile strength of a body structure such as a bone, ligament, muscle, or tendon, causing the structure to collapse. In contrast, microtrauma is a microscopic subclinical injury that results from repeated activity that, over a period of time, overwhelms the tissue's ability to repair itself. By definition, this pain and dysfunction is described as "overuse syndrome" and is most often encountered in the form of tendinitis.[7] In addition, bursae, cartilage, bone, and nerve can break down because of repetitive microtrauma from exercise-related activities.

Another overuse injury described as the new industrial epidemic,[8] involves occupational repetition strain injuries. These muscle and tendon injuries of the upper limbs, shoulder girdles, and neck are caused by an overload on particular muscles due to awkward working postures or repeated use; the overload on these muscles causes pain, fatigue, and a decline in work performance. Assembly line workers and typists are likely candidates for this type of strain injury, which has become a major cause of disability in industry and has had considerable social and economic consequences.[9]

Sprain, bruise, and *strain* are terms used to characterize injury to soft tissue. Specifically, a sprain is defined as a partial or complete rupture of a ligament; a bruise, a rupture of tissue resulting in a hematoma; and a strain, a partial tear of muscles.[10] Sprains occur as a result of a joint being forced beyond its normal range of motion (e.g., a hyperextended knee) or forced in a plane through which little or no motion actually existed (e.g., a lateral ankle sprain). The abnormal forces producing the sprain can be rapid, as exemplified by a clipping injury in football, or slow, as observed with a slow, twisting fall in skiing. Although ligaments behave differently, depending on how quickly or slowly they are stretched, either mechanism can induce injury. Most strains, on the other hand, occur during forceful muscle action. The injury might occur soon after an activity has begun, such as coming out of the blocks when a race has just started, or with an interruption of some motion, such as momentarily losing one's footing on a slippery surface.[11] When these injuries occur, the muscles become sore and painful, and movement becomes difficult.

Acute, temporary stiffness and muscle pain can also result from cold, dampness, rapid temperature changes, and air currents. In some cases, visceral stimuli resulting from cardiovascular disease (such as angina pectoris) or gastrointestinal complaints (such as disorders of the gallbladder and esophagus) are felt as referred pain in the skeletal muscles of the shoulder. These episodes tend to be sudden in onset but are self-limiting (i.e., the condition will resolve with or without treatment in a short time). Elimination of the cause or symptomatic treatment generally provides relief.[5]

Because of its pendulous structure, the shoulder area is subject to continuous gravitational pull and therefore endures more stress and strain than any other articulation of the body. Thus, the prehensile grasp, which raised humans above their ancestors, has resulted in the development of a shoulder girdle that sacrifices stability for mobility and is a major cause of muscular pain.[12] Although painful conditions affecting the shoulder are more prevalent in elderly persons, they often occur in athletes[13] and in those engaged in certain occupations in which the arms are used vigorously and repetitively.[14]

Tendinitis, resulting from a strain or injury of tendons, is often seen at times of maximum physical effort, such as during an athletic competition. There are three distinct pathologic phases.[15] The first phase includes the development of the acute inflammatory response. As inflammation continues and remains untreated, excessive proliferation of connective tissue occurs. Microscopically, the tissue changes in this second phase are characterized by the development of young, vascular elements with fibroblastic growth. In the third phase, persistent and chronic inflammation results in further overgrowth of connective tissue plus tendon degeneration, which may lead to rupture. The pathologic changes occurring in each of the three phases appear to be related primarily to repetitive intrinsic tension overload in the muscle–tendon unit.

Although tendinitis in the shoulder area is a major cause of pain, athletes often suffer injury of tendons in other areas of the body. In fact, it has been said that Achilles tendinitis is the most common injury in sports.[7] (See Chapter 37, "Foot Care Products.") Other examples of this common injury include biceps tendinitis, which occurs in the throwing athlete, such as a football quarterback or baseball pitcher; patellar tendinitis, which occurs in the volleyball and basketball player; and iliotibial-band tendinitis, which occurs in the runner. In a recent prospective study of sports injuries in elderly athletes (those over 60 years of age),[16] the investigators found that shoulder as well as Achilles tendon and calf complaints were significantly more common in elderly athletes than in younger ones. Although for both groups the knee joint was the area most often affected, young athletes suffered this injury more often than elderly persons. Most of the injuries in the elderly (70%) were overuse injuries, but these accounted for less than half of the injuries (41%) in the young.[16]

Many factors contribute to producing an overuse injury such as tendinitis. In industry, these factors include poorly designed equipment, awkward working positions, lack of job variation, long work hours, inadequate rest breaks, and bonuses for high work rates and overtime.[17] In athletics, contributing factors can include the athlete's age, poor technique, exercise of prolonged intensity or duration, improper conditioning, and poorly designed equipment for specific activities (such as poor cushioning of athletic shoes).[6]

Bursae are sacs formed by two layers of synovial tissue that are located at sites of friction between tendon and bone or skin and bone. The bursae enable the tendons and muscles to move over bony prominences. With overuse, repetitive trauma from either friction of the overlying tendon or external pressure may cause the bursa to become inflamed, with resultant fluid buildup in the bursal wall. This condition, termed *bursitis*, is a common cause of localized pain, tenderness, and swelling, which is worsened by any movement of the structure adjacent to the bursa. It may be an acute pain due to either macro- or microtrauma, or it may be chronic pain, in which case an infectious cause should be suspected. Infection or trauma can be documented by appropriate studies of aspirated fluid. Most cases of bursitis are due to overuse. This is particularly true in sports that involve repetitive overhead throwing motions, such as baseball, swimming, gymnastics, skiing, and weight lifting. Runners commonly are afflicted

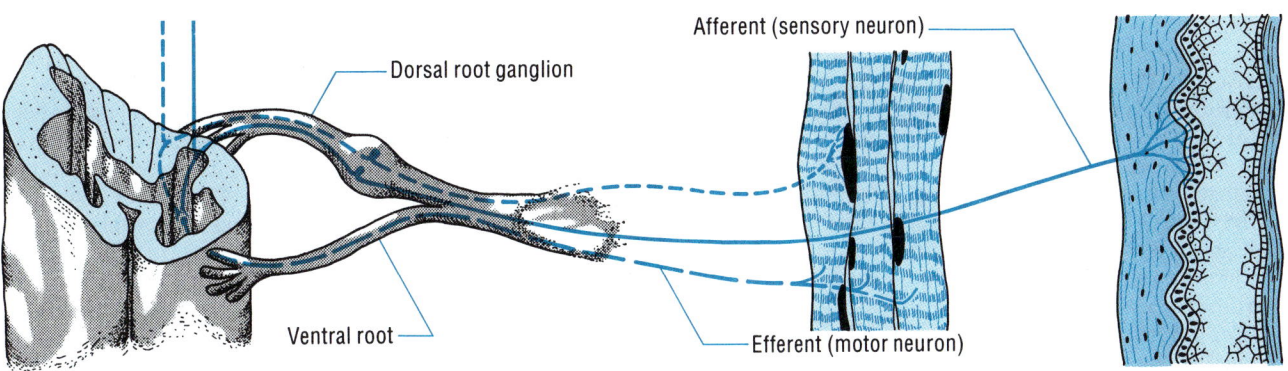

FIGURE 1 Reflex pathways showing the afferent (sensory) fibers, efferent (vasometer) fibers, and their synapse in the spinal cord. Adapted from Netter FH. *The Ciba Collection of Medical Illustrations.* New York: Ciba Pharmaceutical Company; 1962: 65.

with bursitis of the knees, hips, ankles, and feet.[18]

Bursitis is a common cause of joint pain and often results in limited motion of adjacent joints, especially when the inflamed bursa is superficial and obvious redness and swelling are present. Symptoms of bursitis that mimic those of arthritic pain can be distinguished by a physical examination. For instance, direct pressure over the joint capsule of the shoulder does not cause pain in bursitis although it does in arthritis. (See Chapter 5, "Internal Analgesic Products.")

Arthritic pain may be caused by rheumatoid arthritis, which may involve almost all peripheral joints, tendons, bursae, and the cervical spine; or by osteoarthritis, which involves degeneration of cartilage with secondary changes in joints. Although both types of rheumatic disorders are chronic systemic diseases, local treatment of painful joints coupled with rest may give temporary symptomatic relief.

Just as the prehensile grasp has imposed a stress upon the shoulder girdle of humans, so has erect posture predisposed their lower spine to the painful twinge of an aching back. At least 70% of the population experiences lower back pain at some time in their lives. Lower back pain rivals the common cold as the leading cause of absenteeism from work.[19] However, this regional musculoskeletal disorder, unlike the overuse injuries described previously, is due primarily to a sedentary lifestyle (particularly one disrupted by bursts of activity), as well as to poor posture, improper shoes, excess body weight, poor mattresses and sleeping posture, and improper technique in lifting heavy objects. Thus, back pain is primarily a disease of living. Although most victims recover within a few days to a few weeks with conservative treatment, lower back pain is significantly likely to recur if the initial episode of pain is severe; advancing age also increases the risk of recurrence.

In addition to injuries, the causes of backache include congenital anomalies, osteoarthritis, spinal tuberculosis, and referred pain from diseased kidneys, pancreas, liver, or prostate. Emotional factors, including tension, anxiety, repressed anger, and other manifestations of "psychosocial prestress," have been postulated to correlate with the occurrence of lower back pain, but a comprehensive review of the literature could not confirm a relationship between lower back pain and temperament.[20]

Mechanism of Counterirritant Action

Counterirritation, the paradoxical pain-relieving effect achieved by producing less severe pain to counter a more intense one, has been known for centuries. The Greeks and probably the Egyptians knew about these effects and referred to them in numerous manuscripts.[21] Today, to counter pain of pathologic origin, pain sufferers produce bearable pain by biting their lips, clenching their fists, digging their nails into the palms of their hands,[22] or using counterirritant preparations.

Pharmacologic Methods of Counterirritation

Counterirritants are medications applied to the skin at pain sites to produce a mild local inflammatory reaction. The objective is to provide relief at another site usually adjacent to, or underlying, the skin surface being treated. The intensity of response depends on the irritant used, its concentration, the solvent in which it is dissolved, and the duration of its contact with the skin.[22]

Pain is only as intense as it is perceived to be, and the perception of other sensations caused by the counterirritant or its application, such as massage, warmth, or redness, causes the sufferer to disregard the sensation of pain. Several theories have been proposed to explain the action of irritant drugs:

- Stimulation of sensory nerve endings in the skin causes reflexive stimulation of vasomotor fibers to the viscera. These reflexes are mediated through the cerebrospinal axis and dilate the visceral vasculature.[23]
- Stimulation of sensory nerve endings in the skin causes axon reflexes, resulting in stimulation of the nerves enervating branches of arterioles to produce vasodilation in the muscles. This action produces an increase in the blood flow to the muscles.[24]
- Summation of pain stimuli produces intense stimulation of the areas of pain interpretation in the brain, partly abating visceral pain stimuli.

According to this last theory, stimuli originating in the viscera or muscles are transmitted, along with sensations from the skin, over fibers in a common pathway and are referred to the same area of the spinal cord as the stimuli from the skin (Figure 1). If the intensity of the stimulation from the skin is increased by a drug's irritant action, the character of the visceral or muscle pain is modified. With intense skin stimulation, the referred pain stimuli may be partly or completely obliterated insofar as the sensorium is concerned. The patient's attention is diverted from the muscular or visceral structure by the application of the counterirritant drug.[25]

An additional effect of some products is to produce vasodilatation of cutaneous vasculature. These drugs, known as rubefacients, produce reactive hyperemia; it is hypothesized that this increase in blood pooling and/or flow is accompanied by an increase in localized skin temperature, which then may act by the counterirritant effect. This positive thermal response for some agents has been documented by thermography.[26] Although not considered a rubefacient, a topical analgesic containing menthol and methyl salicylate has reportedly produced a three- to fourfold increase in blood flow to the skin in five subjects.[27] Unpublished data from the same study reported subsequently indicated that the warming effect may go deeper than the skin.[28] Indeed, a temperature-sensitive needle inserted into the lateral thigh muscle of three of the subjects recorded a 38.5°F (3.6°C) rise in temperature after the counterirritant was applied. However, the author cautioned that the massage alone may have caused the muscle temperature to rise. The degree of irritation must be controlled, however, because strong irritation may cause erythema and blistering. There is no evidence that the risk of adverse reactions to counterirritants increases when the application site is lightly bandaged. However, there is an increased risk of irritation, redness, or blistering with tight bandaging or occlusive dressing.[29]

Undoubtedly, the action of counterirritants in relieving pain has a strong psychologic component; indeed, these agents may exert a placebo effect through pleasant aromatic odors or the sensation of warmth or coolness they produce on the skin.

Some topical analgesics act by overcoming the stimulus that causes the pain. To do this, they must first be percutaneously absorbed. The effects following this absorption are then systemic in nature, resulting in the relief of any deep-seated pain provided that the interstitial fluid drug concentration obtained is sufficiently high.[30] The action is the same as that produced by an internal analgesic. (See Chapter 5, "Internal Analgesic Products.")

Current clinical investigations are ongoing with topical nonsteroidal anti-inflammatory agents which have been marketed for a number of years in Europe.[31] These preparations presumably act locally in a manner analogous to their systemic mechanism of action. In a recent communication, the FDA Arthritis Advisory Committee discussed problems associated with the evaluation of these products and offered recommendations to enhance the ability to discriminate between the topical nonsteroidal anti-inflammatory and the comparison topical placebo.[32]

Physical Methods of Counterirritation

Although the nonprescription preparations described in this chapter have their own merit as therapeutic agents, there are simple physical methods of inducing counterirritation. Perhaps the most often used method is heat applied with a heat lamp, hot-water bottle, heating pad, or moist steam pack. Under normal conditions, collagen recoils like a spring once the load is released. After a stretching injury, the collagen tissue does not return to its resting length. Heat helps to restore the elastic property of collagen by increasing the viscous flow. Heat also acts selectively on free nerve endings in the tissue and on peripheral nerve fibers to increase the pain threshold; this results in an analgesic effect.[33] However, the application of heat should be used with extreme caution, if at all, in conjunction with a counterirritant preparation. Severe burning or blistering of skin; muscle and skin necrosis; and interstitial nephritis have resulted from the simultaneous use of a counterirritant preparation and heat.[34]

Massaging the painful area is another method of producing counterirritation. The therapeutic benefits of massage have been known for centuries. It is possible that the beneficial effects of some counterirritants used in treating musculoskeletal disorders may be owing largely to the rubbing and massage involved in applying the medication. Massage increases the flow of blood and lymph in the skin and underlying structures.

Studies comparing massage with other modalities are nonexistent because it is difficult to prepare protocols for conducting controlled objective clinical studies documenting the therapeutic effectiveness of massage techniques. Many clinicians have found that massage is therapeutically beneficial in select situations and use it extensively.

Patient Assessment and Treatment

To assess the patient's condition accurately before recommending a nonprescription counterirritant preparation, the pharmacist should ask the patient the following questions:

TABLE 1 Relative potencies of counterirritants

Group	Characteristics	Ingredients
A	Cause redness, irritation; are relatively more potent than other counterirritants	Allyl isothiocyanate, stronger ammonia water, methyl salicylate, turpentine oil
B	Produce cooling sensation; have organoleptic properties	Menthol, camphor
C	Vasoactive substances; vasodilator	Histamine dihydrochloride, methyl nicotinate
D	Produce irritation without rubefaction, although approximately equal in potency to Group A	Capsaicin, capsicum, capsicum oleoresin

Reprinted from the *Federal Register* 1979; 44: 69784.

- How long has the pain been apparent? What kind of pain is it? Is it debilitating? Conditions amenable to nonprescription treatment are self-limiting. Pain that has been apparent for longer than 7 days may indicate a more serious underlying condition. These patients should be evaluated by a physician. Furthermore, prolonged use of external analgesics can increase the sensitivity to and decrease the effectiveness of these products.[35]
- Is there any apparent cause of the pain? Often, muscular or joint pain can be brought on by simple overexertion, such as unaccustomed exercise or other physical activity; such pain is a valid indication for these agents.
- Can the patient specifically locate and describe the pain? If so, and if the pain is of mild intensity, it may be appropriate to recommend a nonprescription product. However, if the patient has difficulty locating the origin of the pain, it may be referred pain. For example, pain in the lumbar area may be referred from pelvic viscera and may be an early manifestation of disease in these organs. If the pain is of severe intensity, nonprescription treatment should not be recommended.
- If the pain is in a joint, is the joint red, swollen, and tender to the touch? If so, there may be a fracture or rupture of ligaments or tendons, or there may be arthritic involvement. Nonprescription products used in this condition would delay an accurate diagnosis.
- Has the patient been diagnosed by a physician as having any type of arthritic condition? If so, and if the patient is under medical supervision for any type of arthritic condition, it may be appropriate to recommend only a counterirritant preparation as adjunctive treatment. The rationale for this therapy is that the topical analgesic helps the patient over intermittent painful episodes, thus reducing the patient's intake of oral medications, which may pose a greater risk of adverse reactions.

Topical analgesics are very inexpensive when compared with many oral anti-arthritic agents. Therefore, a positive economic factor may also exist. Arthritic conditions should not be self-diagnosed or self-treated. (See Chapter 5, "Internal Analgesic Products.")

If the pharmacist determines that the condition is minor and that there are no serious underlying conditions, it may be appropriate to recommend a nonprescription preparation. The pharmacist should advise the patient that if the symptoms persist or are not relieved by the preparation within 7 days, or if the symptoms clear up and occur again within a few days,[35] the medication should be discontinued and a physician should be consulted.

The pharmacist should arrange a follow-up consultation to review the patient's condition. This may prevent prolonged ineffective self-treatment that allows a more serious underlying disease to progress.

Pharmacologic Agents

The following ingredients have been recognized as safe and effective counterirritants by the Food and Drug Administration (FDA) Advisory Review Panel on Over-the-Counter Topical Analgesic Products. Table 1 classifies these agents by their relative potencies.

Allyl Isothiocyanate

Allyl isothiocyanate, also known as volatile oil of mustard and essence of mustard, is derived from powdered seeds of the black mustard plant and other species of mustard. It can also be prepared synthetically or by distillation after expression of the fixed oil.

In high concentrations, allyl isothiocyanate is absorbed rapidly from intact skin as well as from all mucous membranes. Because penetration into the skin is rapid, ulceration may occur if the agent is not removed soon after application. A poultice, erroneously termed a *mustard plaster*, has often been used as a home remedy. It is prepared by mixing equal parts of powdered mustard and flour and moistening with water to form a paste. The paste is then spread on a towel or piece of material and placed on the affected area. The person who is preparing a mustard plaster should take care to avoid inhaling this powerful irritant. The continuous release of allyl isothiocyanate by the presence of water and body heat may cause the inflammatory action to go beyond redness to blistering; therefore, the poultice should not remain on the skin for more than a few minutes.

Allyl isothiocyanate is considered to be safe and effective for nonprescription use in concentrations of 0.5–5.0% applied to the affected areas no more than three or four times a day. This dosage is for adults and children over 2 years of age. There is no recommended dosage for children under 2 years of age except under the advice and supervision of a physician.[29] In February 1983, the FDA issued a proposed ruling on external analgesic products, indicating that, although it is true that by 6 months of age a child's skin is similar to an adult's with regard to any absorption, there are enough other differences between adults and children under 2 years of age to require different standards of practice in the use of drugs.[29]

Stronger Ammonia Water

Stronger ammonia water is also known as strong ammonia solution. Because it is caustic and the vapors are irritating, this product should be handled with care and the vapors should not be inhaled. Inhalation of ammonia vapor causes sneezing and coughing and, in high concentrations, can cause pulmonary edema. Asphyxia has been reported following edema or spasm of the glottis. In addition, ammonia vapor is an eye irritant and can cause weeping, conjunctival swelling, and temporary blindness.[36] Stronger ammonia water is an aqueous solution of ammonia containing 27–30% by weight of ammonia (NH_3). It must be diluted before use as a topical agent because of its caustic nature. To be safe and effective for topical use by adults and children over 2 years of age, the concentration used is a 1.0–2.5% solution of available ammonia, which should be applied to the affected area no more than three or four times a day.[37]

Methyl Salicylate

Methyl salicylate occurs naturally as wintergreen oil or sweet birch oil, gaultheria oil and teaberry oil are other names for the natural compound. Synthetic methyl salicylate is prepared by the esterification of salicylic acid with methyl alcohol. In either form, methyl salicylate is the most widely used counterirritant and has been categorized as safe and effective for use as a nonprescription analgesic when applied in the appropriate dosage.[38] At very low concentrations (0.04%), methyl salicylate is used in oral preparations for its pleasant flavor and aroma. Indeed, it has been used as a flavoring agent in candies, cough drops, lozenges, chewing gum, toothpastes, and mouthwashes. However, ingestion of more than small amounts of the substance is hazardous because of its high salicylate content. Although the average lethal dose of methyl salicylate is estimated to be 10 mL for children and 30 mL for adults,[39] as little as 4 mL has caused death in infants and 5 mL has caused death in children.[40]

A survey by the FDA advisory review panel considering methyl salicylate found that oral ingestion of this ingredient from products formulated as ointments caused no deaths and that few cases manifested severe symptoms.[41] Nevertheless, regulations require the use of child-resistant containers for liquid preparations containing more than 5% methyl salicylate.[42] Even though the agent possesses a high degree of safety for topical use and has had a long marketing history, a single case report[34] emphasizes the importance of avoiding the use of a heating pad in conjunction with counterirritants containing methyl salicylate. The heating pad produced the elevated temperature, vasodilation, and occlusion necessary to greatly enhance percutaneous absorption of menthol and methyl salicylate, which causes full-thickness skin and muscle necrosis as well as persistent interstitial nephritis.

In addition, a clinical study was undertaken to determine the effects of exercise and heat exposure on the percutaneous absorption of methyl salicylate in six healthy volunteers.[43] The results indicated that a threefold increase in systemic availability of salicylate occurred under heat exposure and exercise as judged by plasma and urine data. The authors cautioned that if individuals were subjected to extreme heat or strenuous physical activity, the resultant increase in the absorption of topically applied preparations could lead to adverse systemic reactions. Therefore, patients should be told not to use heating pads in conjunction with topically applied external analgesics and not to apply these products after strenuous exercise, especially during hot and humid weather. Rather, these products should be applied after the body has cooled down.

The rate and extent of percutaneous absorption of various commercially available methyl salicylate preparations were studied after the agents were left in place for 10 hours under occlusive dressing.[44] It was found that only about 12–20% of the amount of salicylate applied to the skin was absorbed into the systemic circulation during this period. Furthermore, both the skin permeability coefficient for methyl salicylate and the percentage of salicylate absorbed decreased when the agents were applied to different areas of the body in this order: abdomen > forearm > instep > heel > plantar. The slower absorption from the foot regions was primarily attributed to fewer hair follicles and a thicker stratum corneum. The authors concluded that topical application of products containing methyl salicylate results in low plasma salicylate concentrations and that the usefulness of these preparations is limited to their local effects.

The recommended topical dosage of methyl salicylate for adults and children over 2 years of age is a 10–60% concentration applied to the affected area no more than three or four times a day.[45] Because of its etiologic role in Reye's syndrome, methyl salicylate should not be used on infants, children, or adolescents during or following a flulike illness. Also, because percutaneous absorption can occur, this product should be used with caution in individuals who are sensitive to aspirin or who suffer from severe asthma or nasal polyps. In an isolated case report, a patient sensitive to aspirin experienced allergic symptoms when exposed to various products containing methyl salicylate, including candy, toothpaste, and liniment.[46] The patient reacted to all products, experiencing throat discomfort and soreness with the oral products, and marked swelling and itching with the topical preparation. However, because the patient did not previously report allergic reactions when methyl salicylate and aspirin were used together, the author concluded that the case was a coincidence rather than the result of cross-reactivity. Nevertheless, patients who report an allergy to aspirin should be cautioned to avoid products containing methyl salicylate.

Turpentine Oil

Turpentine oil is commonly misnamed "turpentine." Turpentine oil for medicinal use must be of higher quality than commercial turpentine oil. Medicinal turpentine oil, known as spirits of turpentine or rectified turpentine oil, is prepared by steam distillation of turpentine oleoresin collected from various species of pine trees.

Turpentine oil is both a primary irritant and a sensitizer. As an irritant, it usually acts by defatting the skin, causing dryness and fissuring. It is often used as a cleanser for removing paints and waxes and can cause hand eczema by irritating sensitive skin.

Turpentine oil has been used as an ingredient in counterirritant preparations with a long history of safety and efficacy. The recommended dosage for adults and children over 2 years of age is a 6–50% concentration applied to the affected area no more than three or four times a day.[47] Application of turpentine liniments to the skin in greater amounts may cause vesicular eruption, urticaria, and vomiting in susceptible individuals.[48] Several human fatalities from the ingestion of turpentine oil have been reported. An oral dose of 140 mL in adults (15 mL in children) may be fatal. A case report has been reviewed of a man known to be sensitive to turpentine who applied a liniment containing turpentine oil to a bruised neck and trunk and who subsequently developed erythema multiforme.[49] The authors of the original report concluded that immune complexes were formed with the antigen, resulting in a severe contact dermatitis.

Menthol

Menthol is extracted from peppermint oil or prepared synthetically. The fatal dose of menthol in humans is approximately 2 g.[50] However, it may be used safely in small quantities as a flavoring agent and has found wide acceptance in candy, chewing gum, cigarettes, cough drops, toothpaste, nasal sprays, and liqueurs. Additionally, menthol has had extensive use in inhalant preparations for the relief of nasal congestion.

Menthol causes sensitization in certain individuals although the sensitization index is low.[51] Signs and symptoms include urticaria, erythema, and other cutaneous lesions such as contact dermatitis.[52]

When menthol is used in topical preparations in concentrations of 0.1–1.0%, it depresses sensory cutaneous receptors and acts as an antipruritic. When used in higher concentrations of 1.25–16%, it acts as a counterirritant. When applied to the skin, menthol stimulates the nerves for the perception of cold while depressing those nerves that perceive pain. Topical application of counterirritant concentrations of menthol initially produces a feeling of coolness that is soon followed by a sensation of warmth. An experimental study demonstrated that exposure to 2.0% menthol solution caused the threshold for warmth to rise significantly whereas the threshold for heat pain remained unchanged.[53] Although menthol-induced sensations of cold masking sensations of warmth may explain the results, the author considered a direct effect of the menthol molecule on warmth receptors (i.e., inhibition or desensitization) to be a more likely explanation.

Menthol is usually combined with other ingredients with antipruritic or analgesic properties, such as camphor.[54]

The recommended dosage for menthol when used as a counterirritant for adults and children over 2 years of age is 1.25–16% applied to the affected area no more than three or four times a day.[55]

Camphor

Although camphor is naturally occurring and is obtained from the camphor tree, approximately three-fourths of the camphor used is prepared synthetically. The natural product is dextrorotatory; the synthetic product is optically active. In concentrations exceeding 3% and particularly when combined with other counterirritant ingredients, camphor stimulates the nerve endings in the skin and induces relief of pain and discomfort by masking moderate to severe deeper visceral pain with a milder pain arising from the skin at the same level of innervation.[56] When applied vigorously, it produces a rubefacient reaction.

The recommended concentration for external use as a counterirritant for adults and children over 2 years of age is 3–11%. Higher concentrations are not more effective as counterirritants and can cause more serious adverse reactions if accidentally ingested.[57] In concentrations of 0.1–3.0%, camphor depresses cutaneous receptors and is used as a topical analgesic, anesthetic, and antipruritic. The FDA Review Panel on External Analgesic Drug Products has recommended that camphor products for external use be limited to 2.5% concentrations due to camphor toxicity concerns and the agent's low benefit-to-risk ratio.[58] However, FDA has yet to take final action on this panel recommendation.

Application of topical camphor products should be made no more than three or four times a day. In children under 2 years of age, there is no recommended dosage except under the advice and supervision of a physician.

Because of its systemic toxicity in high concentrations when taken internally, preparations with camphor concentrations exceeding 11%, such as camphorated oil (camphor liniment), which is a solution of 20% camphor in cottonseed oil, are not considered safe for nonprescription use and have been removed from the market.[59]

Histamine Dihydrochloride

As a Category I external analgesic agent, histamine dihydrochloride in a 0.025–0.10% concentration is considered to be a safe and effective counterirritant when applied no more than three or four times a day. Application of products containing histamine dihydrochloride results in vasodilatation and causes percutaneous absorption of histamine from an ointment vehicle containing other medicinal agents. Aqueous vehicles seem to be superior to ointments for percutaneous absorption.[60]

Methyl Nicotinate

Methyl nicotinate, when used in a 0.25–1.0% concentration, is a safe and effective counterirritant when applied no more than three or four times a day. As noted with other counterirritants, methyl nicotinate is not indicated in children under the age of 2 years. Although nicotinic acid is inactive topically, this ester possesses a marked power of diffusion and readily penetrates the cutaneous barrier. Vasodilation and elevation of skin temperature result from very low concentrations. It has been shown that indomethacin, ibuprofen, and aspirin significantly depress the skin's vascular response to methyl nicotinate. Because these three drugs suppress prostaglandin biosynthesis, it was concluded that the vasodilator response to methyl nicotinate is mediated at least in part by prostaglandin biosynthesis.[61] Susceptible persons who apply methyl nicotinate over large areas may experience a drop in blood pressure and pulse rate and syncope due to generalized vascular dilatation.[45] In this regard, a study was undertaken to explore the possibility of age and racial differences in methyl nicotinate–induced vasodilation of human skin.[62] The results indicated an equivalent response among young Caucasian and African-American subjects (26–30 years of age) and elderly Caucasian subjects (63–80 years of age) when calculating time-to-peak response, the area under the time–response curve, and the time for the response to decline to 75% of its maximum value. These results were unexpected because differences in percutaneous absorption between black and white human skin have been described in several studies.[63]

Capsicum Preparations

Capsicum preparations (capsaicin, capsicum, and capsicum oleoresin) are derived from the fruit of various species of plants of the nightshade family. Capsicum contains about 1.5% of an irritating oleoresin, the major component of which is capsaicin (0.02%). Capsaicin is the major pungent ingredient of hot pepper. It has been noted that the more tropical the climate, the more pungent the fruit.[64] Sweet peppers contain the same compounds as the pungent peppers but with little or no pungent properties. When applied to normal skin, capsaicin elicits a transient feeling of warmth. More concentrated solutions produce a sensation of burning pain. However, as a result of tachyphylaxis, this local effect diminishes with repeated applications. Capsicum preparations do not cause blistering or reddening of the skin, even when applied in high concentrations, because they do not act on capillaries or other blood vessels.

To determine the reason for this feeling of warmth, investigators applied a solution of capsaicin to the skin, followed by an intradermal injection of histamine to test for chemical responsiveness.[65] Although the capsaicin-treated sites responded by developing a wheal and itch, the flare response did not occur. This latter response, also known as axon reflex vasodilation, is postulated to be under the control of substance P, a neurotransmitter that is thought to function in the passage of painful stimuli from the periphery to the spinal cord and higher structures.[66] High concentrations of substance P are also present in sensory nerves supplying sites of chronic inflammation.[67]

Capsaicin appears primarily to affect substance P by depleting it from sensory neurons that have been implicated in mediating cutaneous pain. Local application of capsaicin to the peripheral axon results in depletion of substance P, both peripherally and centrally—presumably, the result of impulse initiation. When substance P is released, the initial burning pain and redness occurs, but this phenomenon abates with repeated applications. The net effect may be analogous to cutting a nerve or ligating it, which also depletes the substance P content of the neuron.[68]

Substance P is one of the many neuropeptides that have been isolated from peripheral nerve cells; its depletion by capsaicin has assumed an increasing role in the treatment of certain cutaneous disorders, including postherpetic neuralgia,[69,70] psoriasis,[71] postmastectomy pain,[72] reflex sympathetic dystrophy, and diabetic neuropathy.[66,73] It has also been used to relieve posttraumatic amputation stump pain[74,75] as well as to alleviate intractable itching associated with hemodialysis.[76]

Capsaicin in concentrations of 0.025% and 0.075% is indicated both for relief of pain of rheumatoid arthritis and osteoarthritis and for relief of postherpetic neuralgia or painful diabetic neuropathy. Although both concentrations share the same indications, the more concentrated formula has been recently studied in diabetic neuropathy[77-80] and has also been reported in a single case study to alleviate the constant aching and burning foot pain that accompanies Guillain–Barré syndrome;[81] studies using the 0.025% concentration have primarily focused on the arthritis pain[82,83] and postherpetic neuralgia indications.[69,70]

The recommended dosage for adults and children over 2 years of age is a concentration of capsicum preparation that yields 0.025–0.25% capsaicin, applied to the affected area no more than three or four times a day.[84] It appears that efficacy decreases and local discomfort increases when capsaicin is applied less often because the drug's duration of action is 4–6 hours. Interruption of the therapy results in reaccumulation of substance P. Pain relief is usually noted within 14 days after therapy is begun, but occasionally relief will be delayed by as much as 4–6 weeks. It should also be noted that, because of variations between lots of capsicum, the concentration range for this drug cannot be expressed as a percentage and must be calculated for each lot. Several recently published reviews have discussed the use of topical capsaicin in the treatment of cutaneous disorders.[85-87]

Ingredients of Unproven Effectiveness or Safety

Eucalyptus Oil

Eucalyptus oil is a naturally occurring volatile oil with a characteristic, aromatic, camphoraceous odor. One of the chief constituents of eucalyptus oil is eucalyptol. Both have been categorized as flavors and have mild irritant and rubefacient actions causing a sensation of warmth. Marketing experience of a topical analgesic product containing small amounts of eucalyptus oil revealed no evidence of toxicity. Nevertheless, a case report emphasized the profound central nervous system depression experienced after accidental ingestion.[88] In a recent status report of certain Category II and III active ingredients in external analgesic products, the FDA advised that eucalyptus oil "had not been shown to be generally recognized as safe and effective" for its intended use and that it should be eliminated from nonprescription counterirritant products.[89] However, a product has been recently introduced containing natural eucalyptus oil as an "inactive" ingredient. The recommended topical dosage for adults and children over 2 years of age is a 0.5–3.0% concentration applied to the affected area not more than three or four times a day.

Trolamine Salicylate

Trolamine salicylate, formerly known as triethanolamine salicylate, although a salicylate salt, is not a counterirritant analgesic. The exact mechanism by which salicylates produce their analgesic effect is not known, but it is generally conceded that they act in part centrally and in part peripherally as anti-inflammatory agents that inhibit prostaglandins with subsequent relief of pain. Data exist to show that trolamine salicylate is absorbed from the skin;[90] 10g of a 10% cream, applied topically, may result in a concentration of salicylate in synovial fluid of approximately 60% of that obtained from a 500-mg oral dose of aspirin. However, the FDA concluded after a comprehensive review of submitted documents that the data were still insufficient to support a general recognition of the effectiveness of trolamine salicylate as a nonprescription external analgesic.[91]

Although the FDA's review of the data in 1983 indicated that then-current trolamine salicylate studies did not show any significant differences between active drug and placebo, several reports published after the review suggest that trolamine may be effective in alleviating neuralgia caused by unaccustomed strenuous exercise[92] and muscle soreness induced by a reproducible program of weight training.[93] A study documenting a unique use of trolamine was designed to evaluate the degree of pain relief and the increase in playing time among musicians with moderate or severe localized pain in the arms, wrists, hands, and fingers. After 750 mg of trolamine given over a 6-hour period was compared with placebo in a double-blind crossover trial, the investigators concluded that topical use of trolamine was associated with a diminution of pain and an increase in playing time.[94] Additional studies should help clarify the use of this agent as an external analgesic.

Rationale for Combining Ingredients

Two or more safe and effective active ingredients may be combined when each active ingredient contributes to the claimed effect and when the combination does not decrease the safety or effectiveness of any of the individual active ingredients. There are four separate chemical and/or pharmacologic groups of counterirritants that provide four qualitatively different types of irritation. Many marketed preparations use at least two such effects when greater potency is desired. Table 1 lists the individual ingredients and classifies them according to their relative potency. Many products will combine active ingredients from one group of counterirritants with one, two, or three other active ingredients, provided that each active ingredient is from a different group. General guidelines for nonprescription drug combination products state that Category I active ingredients from the same therapeutic category should not ordinarily be combined unless there is some benefit over the single ingredient in terms of enhancing effectiveness, safety, patient acceptance, or quality of formulation.[95] In this case, combination products containing only camphor and menthol as the active ingredients have been identified.[54]

It is irrational to combine counterirritants with local anesthetics, topical antipruritics, or topical analgesics. These latter agents depress sensory cutaneous receptors, and their effects would be opposed by the counterirritants, which stimulate cutaneous sensory receptors. It is also irrational to combine counterirritants with skin protectants because the protectants act in opposition to the counterirritants and may nullify their effects.[96]

Dosage Forms

The vehicles used to formulate the finished product containing counterirritants are important because percutaneous absorption of counterirritant drugs is generally undesirable. The finished product should consist of ingredients and vehicles that keep skin penetration at or near zero. The ideal topical drug vehicle should be:[97]

- Easy to apply;
- Easy to remove;
- Nontoxic;
- Nonirritating;
- Nonallergenic;
- Chemically stable;
- Homogenous;
- Bacteriostatic;
- Cosmetically acceptable;
- Nondehydrating;
- Nongreasy;
- Pharmacologically inert.

The FDA urged manufacturers to list all inactive ingredients voluntarily,[98] and this listing has been for the most part implemented. The nonprescription counterirritant preparations are usually available as liniments, gels, lotions, and ointments. (See also Chapter 28, "Topical Anti-Infective Products.")

Liniments
Solutions or mixtures of various substances in oil, alcoholic solutions of soap, or emulsions are called liniments. They are intended for external application and should be so labeled. They are applied to the affected area with friction and rubbing of the skin, the oil or soap base providing ease of application and massage. Liniments with an alcoholic or hydroalcoholic vehicle are useful when rubefacient or counterirritant action is desired; oleaginous liniments are used primarily when massage is desired. By their nature, oleaginous liniments are less irritating to the skin than alcoholic liniments.[99]

Liniments should not be applied to skin that is broken or bruised. The vehicle for a liniment is selected on the basis of the kind of action of the desired components.[99]

Gels
Gels used for the delivery of counterirritants are more appropriately classified as jellies because they are generally clear, composed of water-soluble ingredients, and of a more uniform and semisolid consistency. A greater sensation of warmth is experienced with a gel than with equal quantities of the same product in a dosage form such as lotion or ointment. Products formulated as gels promote a more rapid and extensive penetration of the medication into the skin and hair follicles. Patients should be advised against using excessive amounts of gels or vigorously rubbing them into the skin because increased penetration may cause an unpleasant burning sensation.[99]

Lotions
Lotions, liquid suspensions, or dispersions are applied to the skin, usually without friction, for the protective or therapeutic value of the constituents. Depending on the ingredients, they may be alcoholic or aqueous and are often emulsions. Their fluidity allows rapid and uniform application over a wide surface area and makes them especially suited for application to hairy body areas. Lotions are intended to dry on the skin soon after application, leaving a thin layer of their active ingredients on the skin's surface. Because lotions tend to separate while standing, the label should include the instruction to shake the product before each use.

Ointments

Ointments are semisolid preparations intended for external application to the skin or mucous membranes. Ointments are applied to the skin to elicit one of these general effects: a surface activity, an effect within the stratum corneum, or a more deep-seated activity requiring penetration into the epidermis and dermis. These semisolid dosage forms are particularly desirable for counterirritation because these agents are applied with massage.[100]

Clinical Considerations

The dosage forms referred to as "greaseless" are oil-in-water formulations, are therefore "water washable," and are usually preferred for daytime use. In the past, many formulations contained lanolin or anhydrous lanolin as a vehicle. However, because both of these vehicles are obtained from wool fat (to which many people are allergic), these animal waxes are no longer used in contemporary formulations.

The longer any dosage form remains in contact with the skin, the longer its duration of action. There seems to be little agreement on how long the preparations should be left in contact with the skin for optimal results; however, a practical guideline is that preparations should be used no more than three or four times a day. Although it is desirable to protect clothing from stains by covering the application site, the covering should not be tightly applied. Tight bandages increase the risks of irritation, redness, and blistering.

Labeling of Counterirritant Preparations

Labeling approved by the FDA panel on topical analgesics identifies the product as an "external analgesic," "topical analgesic," or "pain relieving" cream, lotion, or ointment and may not necessarily be similar to advertising claims.[101] By evaluating product information, the pharmacist can provide patients with accurate and unbiased information about specific products.

Labeling of preparations must list the active ingredients, including their concentrations, and identify them by their officially recognized "established" names. Recently, manufacturers have voluntarily listed inactive ingredients on the label. The manner of usage and the frequency of applications should also be indicated.[101]

The labeling for indications states that these preparations should be used "for the temporary relief of minor aches and pains of muscles and joints." In addition, the labeling recommended by most of the panel includes claims for "simple backache, strains, bruises, and sprains."[102] These terms were selected because they would be readily and easily understood by the general population.

It is acceptable to use terms describing certain physical or chemical qualities of the counterirritant preparations as long as these terms do not imply that any therapeutic effects occur. Terms such as *nongreasy, soothing, cooling action, penetrating relief, warming relief,* and *cool comforting relief* are considered acceptable in labeling.

As with all nonprescription drug products, external analgesics are intended to achieve a beneficial effect within a reasonable period of time. However, claims related to product performance are unacceptable unless they can be substantiated by scientific data. Claims such as "fast," "quick," "prompt," "swift," "immediate," and "remarkable" are misleading and would not signal any property that is important to the safe and effective use of these products.[103]

Label warnings on counterirritant preparations are as follows:[104]

- This product is for external use only. Do not use it near the eyes or apply it to mucous membranes. If some of the liquid is accidentally swallowed, contact a regional poison control center or physician immediately.
- Discontinue use of this product if your condition worsens or if there is only a transient improvement. If symptoms persist for more than 7 days or if the pain is constant and felt in any position, consult a physician.
- Do not apply this product to open wounds or to broken or damaged or sunburned skin.
- Do not apply this product more often than three or four times a day, except under the advice and supervision of a physician.
- Avoid excessive exposure to sunlight or sunlamps after using this product. Do not use a hot-water bottle or electric heating pad at the same time as this product.
- If you apply a covering over this product, do not bandage it tightly.
- Do not apply this product on children under 2 years of age, except under the advice and supervision of a physician.
- Keep this and all other medications out of the reach of children.

Safety of Counterirritants

The oral toxicity of the counterirritant preparations is variable; some agents such as capsicum preparations have a low oral toxicity whereas other agents such as methyl salicylate and camphor are highly toxic when ingested orally. Although some percutaneous absorption occurs when counterirritants are applied topically, the amounts absorbed are insignificant if the ingredients do not exceed the maximum recommended effective concentrations and the environmental conditions are normal (i.e., the counterirritant is not applied after strenuous exercise in high outdoor heat).

Self-treatment with nonprescription counterirritant preparations may result in harm if directions are not followed exactly. Some individuals overreact to the irritant properties of counterirritants and develop rashes and blisters. In addition to irritation, counterirritants also may produce sensitization, in which case immune complexes are involved. It may be difficult to distinguish between direct topical irritation and topical sensitization. Therefore, the labeling of preparations must indicate prompt discontinuation if excessive skin irritation develops. Skin in sensitive areas (e.g., behind the knees) may be particularly susceptible to irritation.

A letter to the editor in a recent issue of *JAMA* described two patients who were receiving maintenance warfarin therapy and who experienced marked prolongation of the prothrombin time due to concomitant use of salicylate-containing external analgesics (both methyl salicylate and trolamine salicylate were implicated).[105]

Summary

Counterirritant external analgesic agents provide a method of decreasing the pain and discomfort associated with many minor aches and pains of muscles and joints. However, they must be used correctly to be safe and effective.

Pharmacists can play an important role in patient education by instructing patients on the proper use of these agents. Because external analgesic drug products temporarily relieve only minor pain, patients should understand the degree of relief that can reasonably be expected and the amount of time that it takes for relief to occur. Patients should also be advised when self-treatment is not indicated and a physician should be consulted.

References

1. Hammacher DP and Associates. *NARD* 1991; 133 (12): 47–8.
2. *Federal Register* 1983; 48: 5867.
3. Merskey H. *Pain* 1979; 6: 249–52.
4. Melzack R, Wall PD. *Science* 1965; 150: 971–9.
5. Lipman AG. In: Herfindal ET et al., eds. *Clinical Pharmacy and Therapeutics*. 4th ed. Baltimore, Md: Williams and Wilkins; 1988: 945–9.
6. Puffer JC, Zachazewski MS. *Am Fam Physician* 1988; 38: 225–32.
7. Herring SA, Nilson KC. *Clin Sports Med* 1987; 6: 225–39.
8. Ferguson D. *Med J Aust* 1984; 140: 318–9.
9. Brown CD et al. *Med J Aust* 1984; 140: 329–32.
10. Anon. *Drug Ther Bull* 1976; 14: 66–7.
11. Garrick JG, Webb DR. *Sports Injuries—Diagnosis and Management*. Philadelphia: W. B. Saunders Co; 1990: 14–22.
12. Booth RE Jr, Marvel JP Jr. *Orthop Clin North Am* 1975: 353–79.
13. Jobe FW, and Jobe CM. *Clin Orthop* 1983; 173: 117–24.
14. Hadler NM. *Arthritis Rheum* 1977; 20: 1019–25.
15. Nirschl RP. In: *Symposium on Upper Extremity Injuries in Athletes*. Petron FA, ed. St. Louis: C. V. Mosby; 1986: 322–36.
16. Kannus P et al. *Age Ageing* 1989; 18: 263–70.
17. Evans G. *Br Med J* 1987; 294: 1569–70.
18. McCarthy P. *Physician Sports Med* 1989; 17 (11): 115–25.
19. Quinet RJ, Hadler NM. *Semin Arthritis Rheum* 1979; 8: 261–87.
20. Crown S. *Rheumatol Rehabil* 1978; 17: 114–24.
21. Kane K, Taub A. *Pain* 1975; 1: 125–38.
22. Gossel TA. *US Pharm* 1987; 12 (8): 26.
23. Swinyard EA, Pathak MA. In: Goodman AG et al., eds. *The Pharmacological Basis of Therapeutics*. 7th ed. New York: Macmillan; 1985: 950.
24. Post BS. *Arch Phys Med Rehabil* 1961; 42: 791–8.
25. Aviado DM. *Krantz and Carr's Pharmacological Principles of Medical Practice*. 8th ed. Baltimore, Md: Williams and Wilkins; 1972: 891–3.
26. Lewis DW, Verhonick PJ. *Appl Radiol* 1977; 6: 114.
27. Shellock FG. *Med Sci Sports Exerc* 1987; 19: S49.
28. Barone J. *Physician Sports Med* 1989; 17 (2): 162–8.
29. *Federal Register* 1983; 48: 5864.
30. *Federal Register* 1979; 44: 69784.
31. Anon. *Lancet* 1989; 2: 779–80.
32. Weisman MH et al. *Arthritis Rheum* 1991; 34: 931.
33. Sherman M. *Am Pharm* 1980; NS20: 470–3.
34. Heng MCY. *Cutis* 1987; 39: 442–4.
35. *Federal Register* 1983; 48: 5865.
36. Reynolds JEF, ed. *Martindale: The Extra Pharmacopoeia*. 29th ed. London: Pharmaceutical Press: 1989: 1542.
37. *Federal Register* 1979; 44: 69792–3.
38. *Federal Register* 1979; 44: 68930.
39. Budauari S, ed. *The Merck Index*. 11th ed. Rahway, NJ: Merck and Co; 1989: 6038.
40. Reynolds, JEF, ed. *Martindale: The Extra Pharmacopoeia*. 29th ed. London: Pharmaceutical Press; 1989: 27.
41. *Federal Register* 1979; 44: 68831.
42. Trapnell K. *J Am Pharm Assoc* 1976; NS16: 147.
43. Danon A et al. *Eur J Clin Pharmacol* 1986; 31: 49–52.
44. Roberts MS et al. *Aust N Z J Med* 1982; 12: 303–5.
45. *Federal Register* 1979; 44: 69830.
46. Speer F. *Ann Allergy* 1979; 43: 36–7.
47. *Federal Register* 1979; 44: 69840–1.
48. Reynolds JEF, ed. *Martindale: The Extra Pharmacopoeia*. 29th ed. London: Pharmaceutical Press; 1989: 1067.
49. Fisher AA. *Cutis* 1986; 37: 101–2, 104.
50. Reynolds JEF, ed. *Martindale: The Extra Pharmacopoeia*. 29th ed. London: Pharmaceutical Press; 1989: 1586.
51. Blondeel A et al. *Contact Dermatitis* 1978; 4: 270–6.
52. Fisher AA. *Cutis* 1986; 38: 17–8.
53. Green BG. *Physiol Behav* 1986; 38: 833–8.
54. *Federal Register* 1983; 48: 5857.
55. *Federal Register* 1979; 44: 69828.
56. Phelam WJ III. *Pediatrics* 1976; 57: 428–31.
57. *Federal Register* 1983; 48: 5854.
58. *Federal Register* 1980; 45: 63878.
59. Gossel TA. *US Pharm* 1983; 8 (4): 12, 14, 16.
60. *Federal Register* 1979; 44: 69812–3.
61. Wilkin JK et al. *Clin Pharmacol Ther* 1985: 38: 273–7.
62. Guy RH et al. *J Am Acad Dermatol* 1985; 12: 1001–6.
63. Andersen KE, Maibach HI. *J Am Acad Dermatol* 1979; 1: 276–82.
64. Tyler VE. *Pharmacognosy*. 3rd ed. Philadelphia: Lea and Febiger; 1981: 155–6.
65. Bernstein JE et al. *J Invest Dermatol* 1981; 76: 394–5.
66. Bernstein JE. *Semin Dermatol* 1988; 7: 304–9.
67. Lembeck F et al. *Neuropeptides* 1981; 1: 175–80.
68. Fitzgerald M. *Pain* 1983; 15: 109–30.
69. Bernstein JE et al. *J Am Acad Dermatol* 1987; 17: 93–6.
70. Watson CPN et al. *Pain* 1988; 33: 333–40.
71. Bernstein JE et al. *J Am Acad Dermatol* 1986; 15: 504–7.
72. Watson CPN et al. *Pain* 1989; 38: 177–86.
73. Todd FT, Varipapa RJ. *N Engl J Med* 1989; 321: 474–5.
74. Weintraub M et al. *Lancet* 1990 Oct 20; 336: 1003–4.
75. Rayner HC et al. *Lancet* 1990 Nov 25; 336: 1276–7.
76. Breneman DL et al. *J Am Acad Dermatol* 1992; 26: 91–4.
77. Donofrio PD et al. *Arch Intern Med* 1991;151: 2225–9.
78. Dailey GE et al. *Diabetes Care* 1992; 15: 159–65.
79. Tandan R et al. *Diabetes Care* 1992; 15: 15–8.
80. Tandan R et al. *Diabetes Care* 1992; 15: 8–14.
81. Morgenlander JC et al. *Ann Neurol* 1990; 28: 199.
82. Deal CL et al. *Clin Ther* 1991; 13: 383–95.
83. McCarthy GM, McCarthy DJ. *J Rheumatol* 1992; 19: 604–7.
84. *Federal Register* 1979; 44: 69804–5.
85. Rumsfield JR, West DP. *DICP: Ann Pharmacother* 1991; 25: 381–7.
86. Carter RB, *Drug Devel Res* 1991; 22: 109–23.
87. Gossell TA. *US Pharm* 1990; 15 (12): 27, 28, 30, 32.
88. Patel S, Wiggins J. *Arch Dis Child* 1980; 55: 405–6.
89. *Federal Register* 1990; 55: 46918.
90. Rabinowitz JI et al. *J Clin Pharmacol* 1982; 22: 42–8.
91. *Federal Register* 1983; 48: 5855.
92. Politino V et al. *Curr Ther Res* 1985; 38: 321–7.
93. Hill DW, Richardson JD. *J Orthop Sports Phys Training* 1989; 11: 19–23.

94. Hochberg FH et al. In: *Medical Problems of Performing Artists.* Philadelphia: Hanley and Belfus; 1988: 9–14.
95. *Federal Register* 1983; 48: 5856.
96. *Federal Register* 1979; 44: 69786–7.
97. Carr DS, Bennett TA. *Pharm Times* 1991; 57 (3): 112–9.
98. *Federal Register* 1983; 48: 5859.
99. Nairn JG. In: *Remington's Pharmaceutical Sciences.* 18th ed. Easton, Pa: Mack; 1990: 1519–44.
100. Block LH. In: *Remington's Pharmaceutical Sciences.* 18th ed. Easton, Pa: Mack; 1990: 1602–9.
101. *Federal Register* 1979; 44: 69784.
102. *Federal Register* 1979; 44: 69841.
103. *Federal Register* 1983; 48: 5861.
104. Gossell TA. *US Pharm* 1992; 17 (9): 22–4, 26.
105. Littleton F Jr. *JAMA* 1990 Jun 6; 263: 2888.

CHAPTER 33

Burn and Sunburn Products

Robert H. Moore III

Questions to ask in patient assessment and counseling

- *What caused the burn—chemicals, sun exposure, electricity, or heat?*
- *How severe is the burn? Is the skin broken and/or blistered?*
- *When did the burn occur?*
- *Where is the burn? Does it affect the eyes, genitalia, face, hands, or feet?*
- *Is the burn oozing?*
- *Is the burn painful?*
- *How large is the burned area?*
- *Do you have any other injuries?*
- *What treatments have you used on the burn?*
- *How long have you been using this treatment?*
- *What effect has this treatment had?*
- *Do you have any other medical problems?*
- *Are you currently taking any oral prescription or nonprescription medication?*
- *Are you currently or have you recently been using any topical medication for a condition other than the burn?*

Burns of all types and degrees of severity account for approximately 2.3% of all injuries in the United States each year, affecting about 1.75 million people. However, because of the effectiveness of fire control measures, flame-retardant clothing, and improved safety standards for housing, this number is decreasing each year. Additionally, improved therapy, better understanding of burn pathophysiology, and the availability of burn centers have reduced morbidity and mortality associated with severe burns. More than 92% of the people with burn injuries receive medical attention. Of these, 22.8% have injuries that confine the patients to bed and 46.2% have injuries that restrict their activity. Burn injuries occur much more often in persons under 17 years of age, persons with low income, and persons with less than 12 years of formal education.[1]

The pharmacist will encounter a large number of patients with minor burns and sunburns amenable to outpatient treatment and should have the knowledge and skills necessary to advise those patients about treatment. The pharmacist should also know, however, when the severity of the injury requires referral to a physician.

Etiology

More than 80% of minor burns occur in the home. Sixty-three percent of household burns are on the hands and arm, and 34% are on the face and legs. Most of these minor burns do not require medical intervention, and symptoms may be managed by the patient with appropriate care and nonprescription products. Of the minor burns that occur outside the home, sunburn is the most common. The importance of sunburn has been underrated, and the injury goes unreported in most burn surveys because the public often does not consider sunburn in the same context as thermal, electrical, and chemical burns.

Anatomy and Physiology of the Skin

The skin is the largest organ of the human body, accounting for approximately 17% of the body weight of an average person. Physiologically, the skin performs a number of vital functions. It protects the body from injury, serving as a barrier against many foreign bodies, including microorganisms. By synthesizing melanin, the skin protects the underlying tissues from certain forms of irradiation. The skin is also a sense organ, receiving sensory input from the proximal environment, especially regarding touch and temperature. Oil, which lubricates and prevents excessive drying of the skin, is produced in the sebaceous glands. Fat deposits in the subcutaneous tissue play a role in lipid biotransformation. Cholecalciferol (vitamin D_3), which is involved in calcium regulation, is produced in the skin through exposure to ultraviolet (UV) radiation. The skin plays a major role in thermoregulation because cutaneous blood flow and perspiration are important in maintaining the core temperature of the body at a normal level. These two factors are also involved with maintaining water balance in the body.

A cross section of the anatomy of the skin is depicted in Figure 1. Also illustrated are the depths of injury caused by thermal burn damage.

Editor's Note: This chapter is based in part on the chapter with the same title that appeared in the 9th edition but was written by Chester A. Bond.

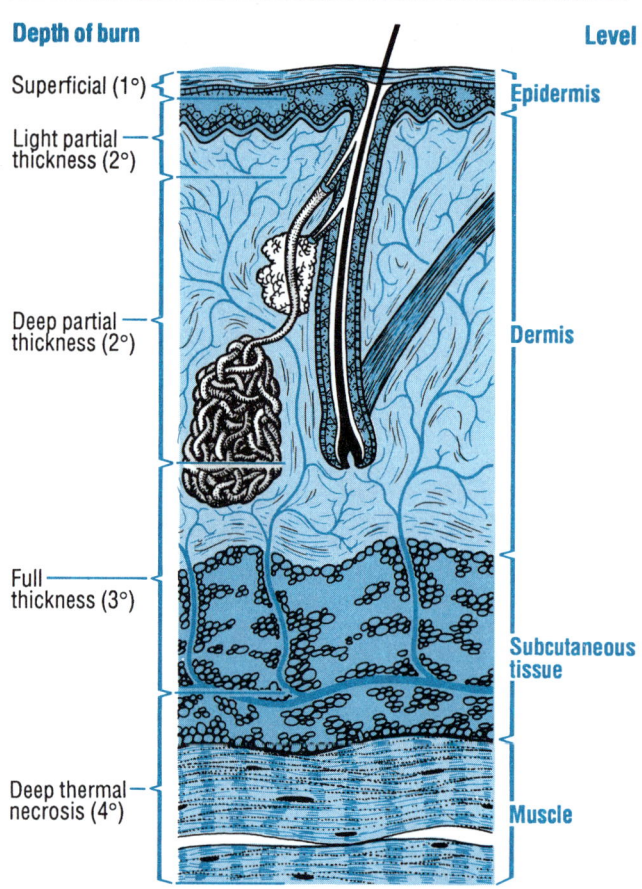

FIGURE 1 Cross section of skin showing depth of burns.

Categorization of Burns

Burns are tissue injuries caused by thermal (flame and scalding), electrical (flash and contact), chemical, and irradiation contacts. Injury to the skin results in denaturation of proteins, localized edema, and a loss of fluid (both intravascular and extravascular).

Determining the area and degree of a burn is not simple, even for burn specialists. The American Burn Association currently identifies three major categories of burn injuries:

- *Major* burn injuries are second-degree burns over a body surface area (BSA) greater than 25% in adults or 20% in children; all third-degree burns over a BSA of 10% or greater; all burns involving hands, face, eyes, ears, feet, and perineum; all inhalation injuries; electrical burns; complicated burn injuries involving fractures or other major trauma; and burns on all high-risk patients (i.e., those who are elderly or who have debilitating diseases).
- *Moderate*, uncomplicated burn injuries are second-degree burns over a BSA of 15–25% in adults or 10–20% in children; third-degree burns over a BSA of 2–10%; and burns not involving eyes, ears, face, hands, feet, or perineum.
- *Minor* burn injuries are second-degree burns over a BSA of 15% or less in adults or 10% or less in children; third-degree burns over a BSA of less than 2%; and burns not involving eyes, ears, face, hands, feet, or perineum. Minor burns exclude electrical injuries, inhalation injuries, and burns on all high-risk patients.

The severity of a burn is determined quantitatively by the percentage of BSA affected and by the depth of the burn (Figure 1).

The percentage of the adult body that has been burned can be estimated by the rule of nines (Figure 2). The total BSA is divided into 11 areas, each accounting for 9% or a multiple of 9. The head accounts for 9% of the BSA (the front and the back of the head are each considered 4.5%); the arms are 9% each; the legs are 18% each; and the trunk is 36% (18% front, 18% back). The perineum is considered 1%. The rule of nines is reliable for adults but is inaccurate for children and persons with small body surfaces. Table 1 illustrates how the distribution of BSA changes with age. This table allows for the quick estimation of the BSA of a burn on a child. If the burn is second degree or greater and covers more than 1% of the BSA, a physician should be consulted.

The depth of a burn has traditionally been described as first, second, or thrird degree (Table 2). A classification of fourth degree is currently being used to describe burns affecting all layers of the skin as well as underlying muscle. The terms *superficial, partial thickness,* and *full thickness* are being used with greater frequency. Further differentiation of burn severity is in evolution (e.g., superficial–partial thickness and partial thickness–full thickness).

First-degree burns are superficial, involving only the epidermis (partial thickness). In most circumstances, there is no blistering. Redness, warmth, and slight edema are present. The burn may be painful because the sensory nerve endings are intact. First-degree burns tend to heal spontaneously within 3–10 days with no scarring. Symptomatic relief of pain and fever and avoidance of additional injury are usually the only treatment required. Sunburn is classified most often in this category.

Second-degree burns involve the entire depth of the epidermis and may extend into the dermis (deep partial

TABLE 1	Changes in body surface area with age (%)					
			Age			
Surface	Birth	1 yr	5 yr	10 yr	15 yr	Adult
Head	19	17	13	11	9	7
Neck	2	2	2	2	2	2
Trunk (anterior)	13	13	13	13	13	13
Trunk (posterior)	13	13	13	13	13	13
Buttocks	5	5	5	5	5	5
Perineum	1	1	1	1	1	1
Arms	8	8	8	8	8	8
Forearms	6	6	6	6	6	6
Hands	5	5	5	5	5	5
Thighs	11	13	16	17	18	19
Legs	10	10	11	12	13	14
Feet	7	7	7	7	7	7

thickness). Second-degree burns are characterized by erythema, blistering, and oozing. Pain is usually more intense than in first-degree burns because of the irritation to the nerve endings. With superficial second-degree burns, healing is generally spontaneous, occurring within about 3 weeks, and there is minimal or no scarring. Deep second-degree (partial-thickness) burns involve more of the dermis. These burns take longer to heal (up to 6 weeks) and may cause thick scar formation.

Third-degree (full-thickness) burns destroy both the dermis and epidermis and may extend into underlying tissues. Usually the burn is not edematous because the vascular supply to the area has been destroyed. The affected area will have a leathery, white, or charred appearance. Because nerve terminals are destroyed, pain will be absent or diminished in comparison with the other degrees of burns. Healing occurs slowly over months, and grafting may be required to achieve wound closure. Scarring usually results.

The term *fourth-degree burn* is used to describe burn wounds that are full skin thickness with damage to underlying tissue, including muscle. The damaged tissue is dry and charred, and there is a high risk of infection. Healing takes months and usually requires skin grafting. Scarring is prominent.

Flame burns are usually partial-thickness or full-thickness burns, or a mixture of the two. Scald burns are usually partial-thickness burns but can be full-thickness burns, especially in children. Superheated steam can cause full-thickness burns, and chemical injury should be considered. Many steam cleaners contain chemicals that can produce a chemical injury as well. Thermal damage to the respira-

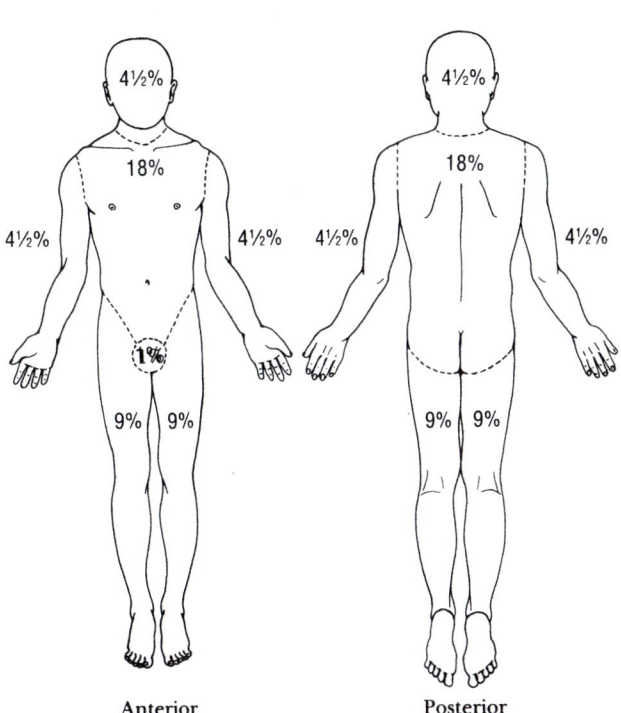

FIGURE 2 Rule-of-nine method for quickly establishing the percentage of adult body surface burned. Adapted with permission from *The Guide to Fluid Therapy.* Deerfield, Ill: Baxter Laboratories; 1969: 111.

TABLE 2 Classification of burn by depth

Type	Tissue affected	Characteristics
First degree	Epidermis	Superficial, erythematous, local pain, no blistering, no scarring, little epidermal alteration. Heals within 3–10 days
Second degree	Epidermis and the most superficial portion of dermis	Erythematous, local pain, elevated vesicle (blister) formation, little or no irreversible damage to dermis, depigmentation in some cases. Usually heals fully in 3 to 4 weeks with no scarring. Considered a partial-thickness burn.
Third degree	Entire depth of dermis and epidermis; may penetrate into subcutaneous tissue	Extensive and partially irreversible damage to entire depth of dermis and epidermis (and possibly subcutaneous tissue), too severe to blister, leathery/white mottled appearance. Less painful than some first- or second-degree burns because of destruction of nerve endings. Infection a significant risk. Heals over several months. Scarring probable, skin grafting may be necessary to minimize scarring. Considered a full-thickness burn.
Fourth degree	All layers of skin (full thickness) and underlying tissue, including muscle	Charred, dry. Great risk of severe Gram-positive or Gram-negative infection. Takes months to heal. Skin grafting necessary.

TABLE 3 Selected groups of medications associated with photosensitivity reactions

Antidepressants
Amitriptyline
Amoxapine
Desipramine
Doxepin
Imipramine
Isocarboxazid
Maprotiline
Nortriptyline
Protriptyline
Trimipramine

Antihistamines
Astemizole
Azatadine
Brompheniramine
Buclizine
Carbinoxamine
Chlorpheniramine
Clemastine
Cyclizine
Cyproheptadine
Dexchlorpheniramine
Dimenhydrinate
Diphenhydramine
Doxylamine
Hydroxyzine
Meclinzine
Methapyrilene
Methdilazine
Pheniramine
Promethazine
Pyrilamine
Terfenadine
Trimeprazine
Tripelennamine
Triprolidine

Antipsychotics
Acetophenazine
Chlorpromazine
Fluphenazine
Haloperidol
Mesoridazine
Methdilazine
Perphenazine
Prochlorperazine
Promazine
Thioridazine
Thiothixene
Trifluoperazine
Triflupromazine
Trimeprazine

Coal tar and derivatives (selected brand name products)
Alphosyl®
Aquatar®
Denorex Medicated Shampoo®
DHS Tar Gel Shampoo®
DOAK Shampoo®
Estar®
Ionil T Plus®
LAVATAR®
Medotar®
T/Derm Tar Emollient®
Tegrin Shampoo®
T/Gel Therapeutic Shampoo®
Zetar Shampoo®

Diuretics (thiazides)
Bendroflumethiazide
Benzthiazide
Chlorothiazide
Chlorthalidone
Cyclothiazide
Hydrochlorothiazide
Hydroflumethiazide
Methyclothiazide
Polythiazide
Trichlomethiazide

Estrogens/progestins (includes ingredients in oral contraceptives)

Estrogens
Chlorotrianisene
Diethylstilbestrol
Estradiol
Estrogens, conjugated
Estrogens, esterified
Estropipate
Ethinyl estradiol
Megestrol

Progestins
Norethindrone
Norgestrel
Medroxyprogesterone

Nonsteroidal anti-inflammatory drugs
Dioclofenac
Diflunisal
Fenoprofen
Flurbiprofen
Ibuprofen
Indomethacin
Ketoprofen
Meclofenamate
Naproxen
Phenylbutazone
Piroxicam
Sulindac
Tolmetin

Psoralens
Methoxsalen
Trioxsalen

Sulfonamides
Sulfadiazine
Sulfamethizole
Sulfamethoxazole
Sulfapyridine
Sulfasalazine
Sulfinpyrazone
Sulfisoxazole

Sulfonylureas (oral)
Acetohexamide
Chlorpropamide
Glipizide
Glyburide
Tolazamide
Tolbutamide

continued

tory tract can also result from exposure to steam. Inhalation of hot gases can lead to immediate upper airway obstruction as well as to obstruction due to slowly developing edema. Small airway alveolar capillary injury can cause progressive respiratory failure. Flash burns are most often partial-thickness injuries to exposed areas. Chemical burns can be partial or full thickness. If not properly treated, chemical burns will occasionally extend slowly for several hours after exposure; thus, all efforts should be made to remove the chemical to prevent further injury. Electrical burns result from exposure to heat of up to 9,000°F (5,000°C). Most of the resistance to an electrical burn is at the skin. However, electrical burns can cause extensive damage to underlying tissues and may be of any size and depth. Progressive necrosis and sloughing are usually greater than the initial lesion indicates.

The pharmacist should feel confident in recommending treatment for minor first-degree burns that do not cover an extensive area and do not involve the eyes, ears, face, feet, or perineum, and for minor second-degree burns that cover less than 1% of the BSA. All burns greater than first degree should generally be evaluated by a physician to prevent complications, particularly infections. Any second-degree burn covering a more extensive area should always be referred to a physician. Extreme care should be taken when the burn is electrical or occurs by inhalation or in a high-risk patient. If the degree or severity of the burn is difficult to determine, the patient should be referred to a physician immediately.

Infection as a Complication of a Burn

Infection secondary to burns is dangerous and difficult to treat because the burned dead skin may serve as a growth medium for certain bacteria. The avascular burned tissue hinders effective delivery of systemic or topical

TABLE 3 continued

Tetracyclines
Chlortetracycline
Demeclocycline
Doxycycline
Methacycline
Minocycline
Oxytetracycline
Tetracycline

Other agents

Anticancer drugs
Dacarbazine
Fluorouracil
Flutamide
Methotrexate
Procarbazine
Vinblastine

Anti-infectives (other)
Ciprofloxicin
Ethionamide
Flucytosine
Gentamicin
Griseofulvin
Nalidixic acid
Norfloxacin
Other fluoro-quinolones
Pyrazinamide
Trimethoprim

Antiparasitic drugs
Bithionol
Quinine

Diuretics (other)
Acetazolamide
Amiloride
Furosemide
Metolazone
Triamterene

Sunscreens
Benzophenones
Cinnamates
Oxybenzone
PABA esters
Para-aminobenzoic acid

Miscellaneous
Amiodarone (antiarrhythmic)
Benzocaine (local anesthetic)
Carbamazepine (anticonvulsant)
Disopyramide (antiarrhythmic)
Enalapril (antihypertensive)
Etretinate (antipsoriatic)

Gold salts (antiarthritic)
Isotretinoin (antiacne)
Labetalol (antihypertensive)
Lisinopril (antihypertensive)
Lovastatin (antihyperlipidemic)
Nabilone (antiemetic)
Nifedipine (antihypertensive, antianginal, calcium channel blocker)
Phenytoin (anticonvulsant)
Quinidine sulfate (antiarrhythmic)
Selegiline (antiparkinsonism)
Tretinoin (antiacne)

Sources: *Med Lett* 1986; 18: 713.
Medications That Increase Sensitivity to Light: A 1990 Listing. FDA Pub. No. 91–8280. Washington, DC: U.S. Department of Health and Human Services, Public Health Service.
Drug Facts and Comparisons. St. Louis, Mo: J.B. Lippincott Co., 1992.

---

antimicrobials. The following sequence of events can lead to clinically significant infections in burn injuries. For a very brief period immediately after a severe burn, the wound surface is sterile. Shortly thereafter, colonization occurs by mixed flora, in which Gram-positive organisms (e.g., *Staphylococcus* and *Streptococcus*) predominate. By the third postburn day, this bacterial population becomes dominated by Gram-negative organisms (e.g., *Pseudomonas aeruginosa*, *Klebsiella*, *Enterobacter*, and *Proteus*) and the fungi, *Candida*.[2] By the fifth postburn day, invasion of tissue well beneath the burn surface may occur. These organisms can then proliferate and eventually invade adjacent unburned tissue, causing burn-wound sepsis.

Sunburn

Excessive exposure to sunlight (especially those rays between 290 and 320 nm) can lead to an acute dermatologic reaction known as sunburn.[3] (See Chapter 34, "Sunscreen and Suntan Products.") Several endogenous vasoactive agents have been suggested as mediators of the erythema seen in sunburn, but none has been definitively shown to cause the reaction. However, there is evidence that the prostaglandins and leukocytes are involved.[3–5]

Sunburn-producing UV radiation is filtered out somewhat by window glass, smoke, and smog but readily passes through light clouds, fog, and clear water. Exposure to UV rays may be enhanced by reflection off snow and sand.

As a normal protective response, the epidermis thickens and melanin production increases when the skin is exposed to sunlight. People vary tremendously in their individual responses to such exposure. For example, many fair-haired individuals will freckle because of uneven melanin deposition. Blonds and redheads are particularly susceptible to sunburn because of a low population of melanocytes. Blacks and other darker-skinned persons can also burn with prolonged exposure to the sun.

Signs and symptoms of sunburn are seen in 1–24 hours following excessive exposure (see color plates, photograph 25). With mild exposure, erythema with subsequent scaling and exfoliation of the skin occurs. Pain and low-grade fever may accompany the erythema. More prolonged exposure causes pain, edema, skin tenderness, and possibly blistering. Systemic symptoms similar to those of thermal burn, such as fever, chills, weakness, and shock, may be seen in persons in whom a large portion of the BSA has been affected.

TABLE 4	Nonprescription oral analgesics for minor burn pain (adult)	
Drug	**Dose (mg)**	**Frequency of administration**
Aspirin (e.g., Bayer®)	325–650	Every 3 to 4 hr, as needed
Acetaminophen[a] (e.g., Tylenol®)	325–650 1,000	Every 4–6 hr, as needed Three to four times a day, as needed
Ibuprofen[b] (e.g., Advil®, Motrin IB®, Nuprin®)	200–400	Every 4–6 hr, as needed

[a]Daily dosage should not exceed 4 g. The recommended dose should not be exceeded. Consult physician if use extends beyond 10 consecutive days for adults or beyond 3 days in the presence of fever.

[b]Daily dose of ibuprofen should not exceed 1,200 mg. Should not be taken for pain that persists beyond 10 days or for fever that persists beyond 3 days unless directed by a physician.

Following exfoliation and for several weeks thereafter, the skin will often be more susceptible than normal to burning.

Photosensitization

Some drugs can produce photosensitivity reactions. The drugs alone pose no hazard, but when the patient comes into contact with UV radiation, photosensitivity reactions may occur (see color plates, photographs 26 and 27). These can be manifested as photoallergy or phototoxicity.

Photoallergic reactions, which are immunologic, are most commonly caused by exposure to UV radiation in the UV-A range (320–400 nm).[6] (Chapter 34, "Sunscreen and Suntan Products," provides detailed information on the various bands of UV radiation associated with sunburn and photosensitivity.) With photoallergy, a drug or other chemical absorbs UV radiation. This combination is then acted upon by the immune system as an antigen, eliciting antibody formation. With future use of the drug and exposure to UV radiation, a hypersensitive immunologic response can occur. Usual reactions include erythema, edema, and warmth. Eczema may occur. Topical preparations cause more photoallergic responses than do systemic agents. Table 3 lists 12 groups of medication including selected, specific drugs that are positively associated with photosensitivity reactions. It is important to remember, however, that not every individual taking these medications will experience an adverse reaction to UV light, and that those who do will not exhibit the same degree of symptomatic response.

Phototoxicity is more common than photoallergy. Phototoxicity does not produce an immune response, so it may occur the first time an offending or precipitating drug is used. Such a reaction occurs rapidly (within minutes to hours) following exposure to UV radiation, especially UV-A radiation. An exaggerated erythema, relative to the time of exposure, is seen. The effects are maximal within a few hours to a few days. Areas exposed to UV radiation are the only areas of involvement.[6]

Patient Assessment

The pharmacist must accurately assess the status of the patient before intervening with therapy. Of utmost importance is determining whether the burn is amenable to self-medication or calls for referral to a physician. The cause, depth, and location of the burn; the surface area involved; and when the burn occurred should all be taken into consideration.

Age should also be taken into account. Newborns, young children, and elderly people do not tolerate the effects of burns as well as young adults. Individuals with chronic illnesses (diabetes, cardiovascular disease, or renal disease) also exhibit a poorer tolerance to the trauma and complication of burns than do normal healthy adults.

Patients who have received burns to the genitalia, the perineum, and the eye are prone to more serious symptoms and complications. These patients should be routinely referred to a physician. Facial burns may be

TABLE 5	Topical protectant agents used in the treatment of minor burns
Ingredient	**Approved concentrations (%)**
Allantoin	0.5–2
Cocoa butter	50–100
Petrolatum	30–100
Shark liver oil	3
White petrolatum	30–100

Adapted from *Federal Register* 1983; 48: 6832.

associated with respiratory injuries due to inhalation, and those that are greater than first degree may also result in permanent scarring. Burns of the hands and feet also deserve special attention, not only because they are often quite painful but also because healing may be delayed in these areas, particularly in patients with a circulatory disorder. In all these cases, patients should be referred to a physician.

Outpatient Treatment of Minor Burns

Thermal Burns

The initial treatment of minor thermal burns is to cool the affected area in cool tap water for 10–30 minutes. This phase of treatment does not apply when the depth and extent of the burn is serious because such action would delay emergency treatment. However, immersion has been shown to decrease the area of redness associated with the burn, perhaps owing to decreased vasodilation, and thus edema, in the surrounding tissue. This treatment may help to prevent blister formation. If blisters form, medical referral should be made. Aspirin, ibuprofen, or acetaminophen can be given to reduce pain (Table 4).

Electrical Burns

The only visible signs of electrical burns may be the points of entrance and exit. The superficial extent of these points may mask extensive underlying tissue damage. Only when an electrical burn is very minor should self-medication be attempted. Otherwise, electrical burns should be routinely referred to a physician.

Chemical Burns

In the case of a chemical burn, any clothing on or near the affected area should be immediately removed. The affected area should then be washed with tap water for anywhere from 15 minutes to 2 hours until the offending agent has been removed. If the eye is involved, the eye, with the eyelid pulled back, should be irrigated with tap water for at least 15–30 minutes. The irrigation fluid should flow from the nasal side of the eye to the outside corner to prevent washing the contaminant into the other eye. In most cases of chemical contact with the eye, further medical attention is encouraged and should be sought as soon as possible. (See Chapter 20, "Ophthalmic Products.")

No attempt should be made to antagonize or neutralize a chemical burn chemically. Such an action can produce an exothermic chemical reaction, which can damage the eye more than the original offending agent. An example of an inappropriate approach would be to treat a burn caused by an acid by applying a base, such as sodium bicarbonate.

Sunburn

Initial treatment for minor sunburn is to get out of the sunlight and avoid further exposure. Minor sunburn can be relieved to some extent with cool compresses or a cool bath. Administration of nonprescription analgesics (e.g., aspirin, ibuprofen, or acetaminophen) for treatment of pain is recommended (Table 4).

Heat stroke may occur with excessive exposure to sunlight in a hot and/or humid environment. Because of the complications of heat stroke, patients exhibiting hyperpyrexia, confusion, weakness, or convulsions should be referred to their physician or to an appropriate medical facility immediately.

Cleansing of Burns

The goals in treating first- and second-degree burns are to (1) relieve pain associated with the burn, (2) protect the area from air, (3) prevent dryness, and (4) provide a favorable environment for healing that minimizes the chances of infection. After cool moisture is applied to the burned area to help stop the progression of the burn injury, reduce local edema, and relieve pain, the area should be gently cleansed with water and a bland soap. After the burn is cleansed, a nonadherent, hypoallergenic burn dressing may be applied if the area is small. A skin protectant/lubricant may be applied if the burn is extensive or in an area that cannot be dressed easily (Table 5). If the burn is weeping, soaking it in warm tap water three to six times a day for 15–30 minutes will provide a soothing effect and diminish the weeping. Minor burns usually heal without additional treatment.

Dressings for Burns

Sterile, nonadherent gauze dressings are the most convenient way to cover a small burn on an area of the body that is easily bandaged, such as the arm or leg. The following is the recommended sequence for dressing a small burn (normally necessary only with second-degree burns):[7]

- First, a nonadherent primary layer of sterile, fine-mesh gauze lightly impregnated with sterile petrolatum should be applied over the burn. Petrolatum gauze does not stick to the wound and allows burn exudate to flow freely through the dressing, thus avoiding tissue maceration. Commercially prepared nonadhering petrolatum dressings (e.g., Xeroflow® or Adaptic®) incorporate hydrophilic petrolatum into the gauze to aid permeability.
- Second, an absorbent intermediate layer of piled-up gauze should be applied over the petrolatum gauze. This layer draws and stores exudate away from the wound, protecting the wound against maceration. Cotton or other nonlubricated products should not be applied directly to the burn because they often stick to the burn and are painful and difficult to remove. This layer should be applied loosely to accommodate edema, should it occur.

- Finally, a supportive layer of rolled gauze bandage should be applied over the primary and intermediate gauze layers to hold these layers in place and mildly restrict movement. Elastic or other expandable bandages that tighten after being applied should not be used because they could restrict circulation if edema develops.

The dressing should be changed every 24–48 hours. If the dressing sticks to the wound, soaking in warm water will loosen the gauze from the burn with minimal pain and trauma. Also, removing the sticking gauze slowly will protect the regenerating epithelium and minimize pain. The wound should be examined for signs of infection at each dressing change. The earliest signs of infection may be inflamed wound edges, new blistering, or intensified pain. If the affected skin begins to become macerated (i.e., if it feels or looks wet, wrinkled, or fissured), dressing the wound should be temporarily discontinued, and the wound should be exposed to air. Once the pain subsides and healing begins (usually in 4–10 days), wound dressings may be discontinued.

Soaks

The inflammation from first- and minor second-degree burns may be reduced by having the patient soak the affected area in water, normal saline, or Burow's solution (diluted 1:20–1:40) for 15–30 minutes three to six times a day. Soaking is particularly applicable with weeping lesions because it provides a cooling, soothing treatment that promotes drying and prevents crusting. All soaking solutions should be freshly prepared. If allowed to sit open, soaking solutions become concentrated and can cause irritation; they may also serve as a growth medium for bacteria and could promote the development of infections. Once weeping subsides, a skin protectant may be applied to the skin.

Depending on burn size and location, the patient may immerse the affected areas directly in the soak, apply a towel or cloth soaked in the solution (lightly wrung), or draw a bath and soak in it for the prescribed time. The temperature of the soak should be cool to warm (not cold or hot), depending on the patient's preference. If maceration occurs, soaks should be discontinued. To dry the affected area after the soak, care must be taken not to irritate the burn by rubbing with a towel. The proper technique for drying a burned area (or other irritated areas of the skin) is patting gently with a dry, clean towel.

Pharmacologic Agents

As previously mentioned, most first- and minor second-degree burns heal readily by themselves without complications. The purpose of pharmacotherapy in managing minor burns is to make the patient more comfortable and symptom free, and to allow the skin to heal normally. Pharmacists should generally limit their treatment recommendations to patients with such burns (those affecting <1% of the BSA). The pharmacist should not recommend a product for extensive or deep second-, third-, or fourth-degree burns because this may cause the patient to delay appropriate medical evaluation and treatment. Additionally, inappropriate applications of topical preparations to severe burns must be removed (usually with considerable discomfort) when the patient seeks medical treatment. The pharmacist should also be aware that damaged skin secondary to burns loses some of its barrier function, thus enhancing percutaneous absorption of drugs and other chemicals. This factor increases the possibility of systemic, drug-induced adverse effects.

Protectants

Based on recommendations of its advisory review panel on over-the-counter (OTC) skin-protectant drug products, the Food and Drug Administration (FDA) has recognized the agents in Table 5 as safe and effective

TABLE 6 Topical ingredients approved by the FDA in the treatment of minor burns

Types	Approved concentrations (%)
Amine and "caine"-type local anesthetics	
Benzocaine	5–20
Butamben picrate	1
Dibucaine	0.25–1
Dibucaine hydrochloride	0.25–1
Dimethisoquin hydrochloride	0.3–0.5
Dyclonine hydrochloride	0.5–1
Lidocaine	0.5–4
Lidocaine hydrochloride	0.5–4
Pramoxine hydrochloride	0.5–1
Tetracaine	1–2
Tetracaine hydrochloride	1–2
Alcohol and ketone counterirritants	
Benzyl alcohol	10–33
Camphor	0.1–3
Camphor	3–10.8[a]
Camphorated metacresol	
Camphor	3–10.8
Metacresol	1–5
Juniper tar	1–5
Menthol	0.1–1
Phenol	4.7[a]
Phenolate sodium	0.5–1.5
Resorcinol	0.5–3
Antihistamines	
Diphenhydramine hydrochloride	1–2
Tripelennamine hydrochloride	0.5–2

[a] When combined in a light mineral oil, USP vehicle.
Adapted from *Federal Register* 1983; 48: 5867–8.

(Category I) for the temporary protection of minor burns and sunburn. Skin protectants benefit patients with minor burns by making the wound area less painful. They provide their therapeutic effects by protecting the burn from mechanical irritation caused by friction and rubbing and by preventing drying of the stratum corneum. Rehydrating the stratum corneum assists in relieving the symptoms of irritation and permits normal healing to continue. Skin protectants provide only symptomatic relief. The FDA has revised labeling for the indications of skin protectants as follows: "For the temporary protection of minor cuts, scrapes, burns, and sunburn."[8]

In selecting a skin protectant for burns, the pharmacist should choose products that prevent dryness and provide lubrication. The FDA has proposed that bismuth subnitrate, boric acid, sulfur, and tannic acid not be generally recognized as safe and effective when used as skin protectants.

Based on advisory panel recommendations, the FDA has also proposed that products with labeling claims of "cures any irritation" or "prevents formation of blisters" not be generally recognized as safe and effective (Category II). The FDA has not recognized claims that certain substances (e.g., allantoin, live yeast cell derivatives, or zinc acetate) contained in many skin protectants are effective in accelerating wound healing. There are no controlled studies that conclusively demonstrate that minor wounds treated with any nonprescription treatment can be healed faster with these products.

The provisional FDA-approved skin protectants (Table 5) are considered safe. The FDA recommended that the restriction preventing their use on children under 2 years of age be waived for most such products except those containing live yeast cell derivatives, shark liver oil, and zinc acetate, for which the age limit applies. Generally, the patient with minor burns may apply a skin protectant as often as needed; if the burn has not improved in 7 days or if it worsens during or after treatment, the patient should consult a physician immediately.

Analgesics

Aspirin and ibuprofen may be used to help alleviate the pain associated with minor burns. As prostaglandin inhibitors and anti-inflammatory agents, these drugs may decrease the erythema and edema in the burned area. For patients who cannot tolerate aspirin or ibuprofen, acetaminophen can provide pain relief. The dose of acetaminophen should not exceed 4 grams per day (Table 4). Acetaminophen is a weak prostaglandin inhibitor and is not an anti-inflammatory agent, but it may still produce beneficial analgesia. Further guidelines for the proper use of internal analgesic agents are included in Chapter 5.

The use of various systemic nonsteroidal anti-inflammatory drugs has been shown to decrease inflammation caused by exposure to UV radiation. However, this effect has been found to last only about 24 hours.[9] This may be because the initial inflammation of sunburn is mediated by prostaglandins, whereas the later, ensuing inflammation is primarily associated with leukocytes. The combined use of a topical corticosteroid and topical ibuprofen has been found to produce more effective sunburn relief than either agent used alone.[10] The ibuprofen may decrease the early inflammation by inhibiting prostaglandin formation, and later relief is produced by the corticosteroid decreasing leukocyte infiltration into the area. The use of oral aspirin combined with a topical hydrocortisone-containing preparation may also produce an anti-inflammatory as well as an analgesic effect.

Local Anesthetics

The pain of minor burns and sunburn can be attenuated by the judicious use of local anesthetics. The agents that have been approved as safe and effective in providing temporary relief of pain associated with minor burns are found in Table 6.

Benzocaine (5–20%) and lidocaine (0.5–4%) are the two amine local anesthetics that are most often used in nonprescription drug preparations. Dibucaine (0.25–1%), tetracaine (1–2%), butamben (1%), and pramoxine (0.5–1%) are also found in topical anesthetic preparations. The higher concentrations of the local anesthetics are appropriate for burns in which the skin is intact; the lower concentrations are better for skin that has been broken.

Benzocaine produces a hypersensitivity reaction in about 1% of the patients on whom it is used. This is a higher incidence than that seen with lidocaine. In contrast, benzocaine is essentially devoid of systemic toxicity, whereas systemic absorption of lidocaine can lead to a number of side effects if serum concentrations are high enough. Systemic toxicities due to lidocaine are rare, however, if it is used on intact skin, on localized areas, and for short periods.

The local anesthetics should be applied no more than three or four times daily. Their duration of action is short, ranging from about 15 to 45 minutes. Continuous pain relief cannot be obtained with these agents, however; increasing the number of applications increases the risk of a hypersensitivity reaction or, more important, the chance for systemic toxicity. Local anesthetics should not be used to treat serious burns because their use may delay the seeking of appropriate medical treatment.

Topical Hydrocortisone

Although not approved for use in treating minor burns, 1% topical hydrocortisone is often used in first-aid treatment of minor burns covering a small area. Hydrocortisone is an anti-inflammatory agent. It should be used with caution if the skin is broken because its use may allow infections to develop.

Antimicrobials

Antimicrobial therapy is crucial in major burns; however, nonprescription first-aid antiseptic drugs are of extremely limited value, especially on burns in which the skin is intact. For minor burns in which the skin has been broken, these drugs have some limited value. Based on data and information submitted to the rule-making panel for OTC topical antimicrobial drug products, the FDA issued an amended proposed rule for first-aid antiseptics. Those preparations that may be used to help prevent infection in minor burns or sunburn are presented in Chapter 28, "Topical Anti-Infective Products."[11]

Moderate to severe burn wounds are particularly susceptible to infection. Because the effects of infection can be serious and devastating, any patient in whom infection is evident or whose burn is so severe that the risk of a bacterial infection is likely should be referred to a physician immediately. Prophylactic application of a triple antibiotic ointment to minor burns is not a routine component of treatment.

Counterirritants

Although counterirritants, such as camphor, menthol, and ichthammol, are currently approved for use in minor burn treatment, the FDA is still evaluating these agents and they should not generally be used for such purposes. They do reduce pain by stimulating sensory nerve fibers. However, they increase blood flow to the area, which will cause further development of edema in the area. They also further irritate the already sensitized and damaged skin.

The ability of agents such as aloe vera, vitamin E, and shark liver oil to aid in the healing of minor burns and sunburns has not been substantiated. These agents are not approved as healing aids.

Product Formulation

Rarely will a product that is intended to treat minor burns contain only one ingredient. The FDA Advisory Review Panel on Over-the-Counter Skin-Protectant Drug Products concluded that two or more skin-protectant ingredients may be combined, provided that:

- Each is present in sufficient quantity to act additively or synergistically to produce the claimed therapeutic effect when the ingredients are within the effective concentration range specified for each in the monograph;
- The ingredients do not interact with or reduce the effectiveness of each other by precipitation, change in acidity or alkalinity, or some other manner that hinders the claimed therapeutic effect;
- The partition of the active ingredients between the skin and the vehicle in which they are incorporated is not impeded, and the therapeutic effectiveness of each ingredient remains as claimed or is not decreased.[11]

Additionally, this panel recognized that skin protectants are suitable vehicles for delivering active ingredients classified in other categories, such as external analgesics (Chapter 32) and sunscreens (Chapter 34). Under these circumstances, the skin protectant may serve a different purpose and is expected to meet the criteria established for this other purpose (analgesic or sunscreen).

Product Selection Guidelines

An initial step in treating the patient with a minor burn is to recommend the administration of an oral analgesic, preferably one with anti-inflammatory activity, such as aspirin or ibuprofen. If the patient cannot tolerate these agents, acetaminophen would be an alternative. Aspirin or ibuprofen may be especially beneficial in the patient with mild sunburn, especially in the first 24 hours after overexposure to UV radiation.

If a local anesthetic or topical hydrocortisone is appropriate therapy, the pharmacist should determine the type of preparation to suggest. Such products are available as ointments, creams, solutions (lotions), and sprays (aerosols).

Ointments are oleaginous-based preparations that provide a protective film that impairs the passage of water from the wound area. This helps keep the skin from drying. However, if the skin is broken, an ointment may not be so appropriate because its impermeability and the presence of moisture may promote bacterial growth. Thus, ointments would be more appropriate for minor burns, in which the skin is intact. Creams are emulsions that allow some fluid to pass through the film, so they provide less of a medium for bacterial growth and are best applied to broken skin. Generally, creams are also a little less messy and less difficult to apply than ointments. To prevent contamination of the preparation, ointments and creams should not be applied directly onto the burns from the container.

Emulsion lotions are easily spreadable and may be more easily applied when the area of the burn is large. Lotions that produce a powdery cover should not be used on a burn. These tend to dry the area, are difficult (and possibly painful) to remove, and provide a medium for bacterial growth under the caked particles.

Generally, sprays are more costly than the other topical preparations. But sprays offer the advantage of precluding the need to touch the injured area physically, so there is less pain associated with applying the medication. Application requires holding the container approximately 6 inches from the burn and spraying for 1–3 seconds. This method decreases the chances of chilling the area. However, sprays are not usually protective in that the aerosol is water or alcohol based and will evaporate. Sprays usually do not contain oleaginous substances.

Summary

To be able to assess the burn patient accurately and recommend appropriate treatment, the pharmacist should be able to:

- Understand the etiology and pathophysiology of burns and sunburns;
- Recognize the complications associated with burns and sunburns;
- Deliver initial care to the patient with a minor burn;
- Recommend appropriate nondrug therapy for the burn patient;
- Recommend appropriate pharmacotherapy for the burn patient;
- Recommend referral to a physician, if necessary.

In addition to providing accurate information and product recommendations, the pharmacist should be able to instruct the burn patient on how to care for the burn to optimize healing, manage symptoms, and minimize complications.

References

1. Types of injuries by selected characteristics: United States 1985–97. *Vital and Health Statistics.* Pub. No. 10–175 NCHS. Washington, DC: U.S. Department of Health and Human Services; Dec 1990: 9–35.
2. Macmillan BC. Ecology of bacteria colonizing the burned patient given topical and systemic gentamicin therapy: a five-year study. *J Infect Dis* 1971 Dec; 124 (suppl): 278–83.
3. Fitzpatrick TB, Freedberg IM. *Dermatology in General Medicine.* 3rd ed. New York: McGraw-Hill; 1987: 1425.
4. Greaves MW, Sondergaard J. Pharmacologic agents released in ultraviolet inflammation studied by continuous skin perfusion. *J Invest Dermatol* 1970 May; 54 (5): 365–7.
5. Mathur GP, Gandhi VM. Prostaglandins in human and albino rat skin. *J Invest Dermatol* 1972 May; 58 (5): 291–5.
6. Pathak MA, Fitzpatrick TB, Parrish JA. Photosensitivity and other reactions to light. In: Braunwald E et al., eds. *Principles of Internal Medicine.* 11th ed. New York: McGraw-Hill; 1987: 254–62.
7. Epstein MF, Crawford JD. Cooling in the emergency treatment of burns. *Pediatrics* 1973 Sep; 52 (3): 430–2.
8. Skin protectant drug products for over-the-counter human use: tentative final monograph. *Federal Register* 1983 Feb; 48: 6820–33.
9. Greenberg RA, Eaglestein WH, Turnier H, et al. Orally given indomethacin and blood flow responses to UVL. *Arch Dermatol* 1975 Mar; 111 (3): 328–30.
10. Eaglestein WH, Ginsberg LD, Mertz PM. Ultraviolet irradiation-induced inflammation: effects of steroids and nonsteroidal anti-inflammatory agents. *Arch Dermatol* 1979 Dec; 115 (12): 1421–3.
11. Topical antimicrobial drug products for over-the-counter human use: tentative final monograph for First Aid Antiseptic Drug Products. *Federal Register* 1991 July; 56 (140): 33644–80.

CHAPTER 34

Sunscreen and Suntan Products

Edward M. DeSimone II

> **Questions to ask in patient assessment and counseling**
>
> - *Do you sunburn easily?*
> - *How long can you stay in full sun without your skin turning red?*
> - *Is it difficult for you to tan?*
> - *Do you normally spend much time in the sun because of your job, sports, or other activities?*
> - *Are you currently using a sun protection product?*
> - *What products have you used in the past?*
> - *Have you ever had a growth on your skin or lip caused by sun exposure?*
> - *Have you ever had a reaction to a prescription or nonprescription drug?*
> - *Have you ever had a reaction to any sunscreen products?*
> - *Are you taking any medications such as a tetracycline, diuretic, or sulfa drug?*
> - *Will you be using the product while swimming, skiing, participating in strenuous activities, or working?*

For most Americans, sunbathing is a popular recreational activity. In addition, many Americans are exposed to the sun for extended periods as a normal part of their occupations. Most people erroneously associate tanned skin with good health, and many use a variety of methods to obtain a bronze or tanned complexion. These methods include the application of pigmenting agents or sun-attracting oils to the skin or the use of tanning booths or beds. Whether sun exposure is recreational or occupational, sunburn often occurs, with its pain, swelling, and tenderness. The severity of a sunburn depends on an individual's natural skin type as well as on the measures used to protect the skin, such as wearing protective clothing (e.g., hats) and applying sunscreens properly.

Most people consider sunburn a minor, albeit painful, inconvenience. However, repeated exposure to ultraviolet (UV) radiation is cumulative and can produce serious, long-term problems such as premature aging of the skin. In addition, cumulative exposure from childhood to adulthood, even without a serious sunburn ever developing, may cause both precancerous and cancerous skin conditions. The mortality rate from certain types of skin cancer (e.g., malignant melanoma) is high. An apt warning is "fry now, pay later."

A large variety of sunscreen and suntan products are available to help darken as well as protect the skin from the harmful effects of exposure to the sun. Applied properly, these products physically or chemically block some or most of the sun's harmful UV rays. Unfortunately, the average consumer shows a considerable lack of understanding of both the process of tanning and the necessity of using sunscreens properly. Thus, pharmacists need to educate the public on the safe and effective use of sunscreen and suntan products. To perform this function, they must be aware of many important factors.

Ultraviolet Radiation

UV radiation is commonly referred to as UV light. However, *light* technically refers to only the visible spectrum; thus, the correct terminology in this context is *radiation*.[1] The UV spectrum is divided into three major bands: UVC, UVB, and UVA.

UVC Band

The wavelength of UVC, also known as germicidal radiation, is within the 200- to 290-nm band. Little UVC radiation from the sun reaches the surface of the earth because it is screened out by the ozone layer of the upper atmosphere. However, UVC is emitted by some artificial sources of UV radiation, and most of the UVC that strikes the skin is absorbed by the dead cell layer of the stratum corneum.[2] Although UVC does not stimulate tanning, it can cause some erythema (redness) of the skin.[2]

UVB Band

The wavelength of the UVB band is between 290 and 320 nm. This is the most active UV radiation wavelength for producing erythema, which is why it is called sunburn radiation. Cutaneous UVB exposure is responsible for vitamin D_3 synthesis in the skin. Current consensus suggests that this is the only true therapeutic effect of UVB.[3] For infants in the United States who receive vitamin D–fortified milk, vitamin D deficiency does not seem to be a problem. However, it may be a problem for chronic shut-ins or for elderly individuals who spend little time outdoors if they do not receive adequate vitamin D in their diet or as a vitamin supplement. UVB is considered to be primarily responsible for inducing skin cancer. The carcinogenic effects of UVB are believed to be augmented by UVA.[4]

UVA Band

The wavelength of UVA radiation ranges from 320 to 400 nm. Although most of the concerns regarding the hazards of sun exposure to date have focused specifically on UVB, a slowly developing concern about the adverse effects of UVA has emerged since the early 1980s.[5] It is now known that UVA radiation penetrates deeper into the skin than UVB, thereby having a greater effect on the dermis than on the epidermis. This deeper penetration can cause vascular damage.[6,7] Evidence suggests that subsequent UVA exposure may cause further and more serious damage to the underlying tissue.

Based on current research into the effects of UVA on the skin, researchers have proposed dividing the UVA band into two subsets: UVA II (320–340 nm) and UVA I (340–400 nm).[8] It has been suggested that, after UVB, UVA II is the most damaging to the skin.[9] This has significant implications for sunscreen products and the type of protection they offer.

Erythemogenic activity is relatively weak in the UVA band, requiring from 800 to 1,000 times more UVA energy than UVB energy. The irradiance (intensity of the radiation reaching the surface) of UVB is more intense from late morning to early afternoon. However, the irradiance of UVA is relatively constant throughout the day, and at least 10 times more UVA reaches the earth's surface than UVB.[10] UVA represents the range in which most photosensitizing chemicals such as 8-methoxypsoralen (8-MOP) are active. This is true throughout the UVA range but especially above 360 nm.

The Process of Burning and Tanning

The degree to which an individual will develop a sunburn or a tan depends on a number of factors, including (1) the type and amount of radiation received, (2) the thickness of the epidermis and stratum corneum, (3) the pigmentation of the skin, (4) the hydration of the skin, and (5) the distribution and concentration of peripheral blood vessels.[11] Most UV radiation that strikes the skin is absorbed by the epidermis.

A tan is produced when UV radiation stimulates the melanocytes in the germinating skin layer to generate more melanin and oxidizes the melanin already in the epidermis. Both processes serve as protective mechanisms by diffusing and absorbing additional UV radiation. Both UVB and UVA contribute to the tanning process. UVA radiation also produces an immediate pigment darkening (IPD) reaction followed by delayed tanning or melanogenesis.[10] This contributes to the development of a slow natural tan.

Although the exact mechanism is not fully understood, it is believed that UVB radiation produces erythema by first causing damage to cellular deoxyribonucleic acid, or DNA.

A sunburn is the result of an inflammatory reaction involving a number of mediators, including histamine, lysosomal enzymes, kinins, and at least one prostaglandin. These mediators produce peripheral vasodilatation as the UV radiation penetrates the epidermis; an inflammatory reaction involving a lymphocytic infiltrate develops. Swelling of the endothelium and leakage of red blood cells from capillaries also occur. The intensity of the UVB-induced erythema peaks at 12–24 hours after exposure.[11]

Sunburn is, in fact, a burn. It is most often seen as a first-degree (superficial) burn with a reaction ranging from mild erythema to tenderness, pain, and edema. Severe reactions to excessive UV exposure can sometimes produce a second-degree (partial thickness) burn with the development of vesicles (blisters) or bullae (many large blisters), as well as the constitutional symptoms of fever, chills, weakness, and shock. Shock caused by heat prostration or hyperpyrexia can lead to death. (See Chapter 33, "Burn and Sunburn Products.")

Sunscreen Products
Indications

Sunscreens are used primarily to prevent sunburn and to aid in the development of a tan. They are also used to protect exposed areas of the body from the long term hazards of skin cancer and premature photoaging. Sunscreens are also effective in protecting against drug-related UV-induced photosensitivity and other types of photodermatoses.

Photosensitivity

Photosensitivity encompasses two types of conditions: photoallergy and phototoxicity. Drug photoallergy, a relatively uncommon immunologic response, involves an increased, chemically induced reactivity of the skin to UV radiation and/or visible light. UV radiation (typically UVA) triggers an antigenic reaction in the skin, which is characterized by urticaria, bullae, and/or sunburn. This reaction, which is not dose related, is usually seen after at least one prior exposure to the involved chemical agent or drug.

Phototoxicity is also an increased, chemically induced reactivity of the skin to UV radiation and/or visible light. However, this reaction is not immunologic in nature. It is often seen upon first exposure to a chemical agent (drug); it is dose related; and it usually exhibits no drug cross-sensitivity. It is most likely to appear as an exaggerated sunburn.[12] Some of the drugs associated with phototoxicity are tetracyclines (especially demeclocycline), sulfonamides, antineoplastics (e.g., 5-fluorouracil), hypoglycemics, thiazides, phenothiazines (especially chlorpromazine), and the psoralens. This type of reaction is not limited to drugs but is also associated with plants, cosmetics, and soaps. (For an additional reference to photosensitivity, see Chapter 33, "Burn and Sunburn Products.")

The efficacy of sunscreen agents in preventing photosensitization has been questioned by some investigators and is apparently under discussion between manufacturers and the Food and Drug Administration (FDA). Although the issue has yet to be resolved, it seems reasonable to assume that,

TABLE 1 Skin types and recommended sunscreen products[a]

Skin type	Sunburn and tanning history	Recommended sun protection factor (SPF)	Recommended product category designation
I	Always burns easily; never tans (sensitive)	8 or more	Maximal, ultra
II	Always burns easily; tans minimally (sensitive)	6–7	Extra
III	Burns moderately; tans gradually (light brown–normal)	4–5	Moderate
IV	Burns minimally; always tans well (moderate brown–normal)	2–3	Minimal
V	Rarely burns; tans profusely (dark brown–insensitive)	2	Minimal
VI	Never burns; deeply pigmented (insensitive)	—	—

[a]This table is based on the most recent recommendations of the FDA advisory panel, published in 1978. Additional data regarding the danger of overexposure to ultraviolet radiation suggest the need for a higher SPF.
Adapted from the *Federal Register* 1978; 43: 38213.

because UVA radiation is primarily responsible for triggering a photosensitivity reaction, a sunscreen effective throughout the entire UVA range, especially above 360 nm, would be effective in preventing photosensitivity.

Photodermatoses
Photodermatoses are idiopathic skin eruptions that are initiated or exacerbated by radiation of varying wavelengths, including UVA and some visible light. UVB, however, is most often responsible for the reaction. The most common of the photodermatoses is polymorphic light eruption. This condition usually manifests itself in a single morphologic form that includes erythema, vesicles, or plaques on skin exposed to sunlight. It appears to affect approximately 10% of the population, with a first occurrence usually before the age of 30.[12] It affects women more often than men and is most often seen in persons of skin types I–IV, as shown in Table 1.[13]

In addition to the various photodermatoses, sunlight can precipitate or exacerbate more than 20 other dermatologic conditions, including psoriasis, herpes simplex labialis (cold sores), rosacea, lupus erythematosus (and skin lesions of systemic lupus erythematosus), erythema multiforme, chloasma (which may affect pregnant women and women taking oral contraceptives), atopic and contact dermatitis, and a variety of solar lesions.

Avoidance of sunlight is the best way to prevent the occurrence or exacerbation of photodermatoses. It is generally believed that sunscreens with a wide range of UV absorbance may afford some protection.

Premature Aging
One of the long-term hazards of radiation is premature photoaging of the skin. This type of aging is genetically determined; Caucasians are more susceptible than African-Americans. The condition, which is most easily characterized by wrinkling and yellowing of the skin, is called premature photoaging because the obvious physical findings are similar to those seen in natural aging. However, histologic and biochemical differences distinguish these degenerative changes from those associated with normal aging. Conclusive evidence reveals that prolonged exposure to UV radiation in susceptible individuals results in elastosis (degeneration of the skin due to breakdown of the skin's elastic fibers). Pronounced drying, thinning, and wrinkling of the skin may also result. Other physical changes include cracking, telangiectasia (spider vessels), solar keratoses (growths), and ecchymoses (subcutaneous hemorrhagic lesions).[14]

As with normal aging of the skin, solar damage has been generally believed to be irreversible. However, there is some evidence that, in certain cases, sun protection allows for true repair of existing damage.[15] In addition, one of the most promising areas in the treatment of photoaged skin is the use of topical retinoids, especially tretinoin (Retin-A®). Investigators have reported significant reversal of minor photodamage to the skin with the use of tretinoin.[16] Additional studies are being conducted to measure the long-term effects of such treatment.

Skin Cancer

Numerous epidemiologic studies have been conducted since the 1950s that demonstrate a strong relationship between chronic, excessive, and unprotected sun exposure and human skin cancer. Skin cancer is the most common type of cancer by far, accounting for approximately 33% of all malignancies. Chronic, unprotected sun exposure accounts for up to 90% of skin cancer. The two most common types of skin cancer are basal cell epithelioma and squamous cell carcinoma. About 80% of both cancers occur on the most exposed areas of the body. Other UV-induced disorders include premalignant actinic keratosis (which usually develops into squamous cell carcinoma if left untreated), keratoacanthoma, and malignant melanoma. It is estimated that approximately 400,000 individuals developed basal cell and squamous cell carcinomas in the United States in 1988.[17] The rate at which these carcinomas grow and invade tissue is relatively low, and 95% are curable with early detection and treatment. By contrast, it is estimated that there were 32,000 cases of malignant melanoma in 1991, representing 5% of all skin cancers. The mortality rate from malignant melanoma is estimated to be as high as 20–25% of all those who develop the condition.[18]

Although the evidence linking sun exposure to malignant skin changes is strong, there are several other contributory factors, including age, sex, occupation, and skin pigmentation. In a frequently cited study, the incidence of skin cancer among Caucasian adults in a rural Tennessee county was found to be a function of both age and sex. The rate ranged from 0.7/100 for males under 44 years of age to 13.6/100 for males between the ages of 65 and 74; for females, the incidence was 0.4/100 and 6.8/100, respectively.[19] The exposed areas of the body (the hands, arms, head, and neck) are most prone to the development of skin cancer. This finding is supported by the relationship between occupation and skin cancer. Some of the more susceptible occupational groups have been identified as farmers, sailors, and construction workers. The three factors of age, sex, and occupation appear to be interrelated. The findings related to age suggest a cumulative effect from UV radiation; those concerning sex and occupation seem to be exposure related because, traditionally, fewer women have worked in these at-risk occupations.

The fourth contributory factor is skin pigmentation. Studies have shown conclusively that skin cancer occurs more often in Caucasians than in other ethnic groups.[2] This is believed to be because individuals with darker pigmentation have more melanin in the skin; melanin functions to absorb UV radiation, thereby preventing the radiation from penetrating into the tissue.

Another factor is the relationship between skin cancer and latitude. It has been shown that the incidence of skin cancer increases steadily in populations closer to the equator. The quantity of harmful UV radiation that reaches the earth's surface increases as the angle of the sun to a reference point on earth approaches 90° and the distance of the sun to the earth decreases.[20] In the United States as elsewhere, a constant rate of increase in the incidence of skin cancer is found as one approaches the equator from north to south; the incidence approximately doubles for every 3°48' reduction in latitude.[21]

Sunscreen Efficacy

Minimal Erythemal Dose

It is difficult to ascertain the efficacy of sunscreens on humans because individual responsiveness to UV radiation varies greatly. One standardized measure that is used is the minimal erythemal dose (MED), defined as the "minimum UV radiation dose that produces clearly marginated erythema in the irradiated site, given as a single exposure."[11] It is a dose of radiation and not a grade of erythema. The MED is indicative not only of the amount of energy reaching the skin but also of the responsiveness of the skin to the radiation. For instance, 2 MEDs will produce a bright erythema, 4 MEDs will produce a painful sunburn, and 8 MEDs will produce a blistering burn. There may also be different MEDs on different parts of the body because of variations in the thickness of the stratum corneum. In addition, the MED for African-Americans with heavy pigmentation has been estimated to be up to 33 times higher than that for Caucasians with light pigmentation.

Sun Protection Factor

Another important measure is the sun protection factor (SPF), derived by dividing the MED of protected skin by the MED of unprotected skin. For example, if an individual requires 25 mJ/cm^2 of UVB radiation to experience 1 MED on unprotected skin but requires 250 units of radiation to produce 1 MED after applying a given sunscreen, the product would be given an SPF rating of 10. The higher the SPF, the more effective the agent in preventing sunburn. If it normally takes 60 minutes for someone to experience 2 MEDs (a bright erythematous sunburn), a sunscreen with an SPF of 6 will allow that individual to stay in the sun six times longer (or 6 hours) before receiving this same sunburn (assuming the sunscreen is reapplied at the recommended intervals).

Table 1 illustrates the proposed classification and relationship of skin types to SPF and product category designations. Since the SPF recommendations in this table were published, a consensus has developed for the use of higher SPF products.

Measures of UVA Protection

With concern about the long-term adverse effects of UVA growing, the utility of the SPF value has been questioned. The SPF provides a measure of the relative amount of UVB striking the skin (i.e., the erythemogenic response). However, UVA is 1,000 times less likely than UVB to produce erythema, and its effect is different from that produced by UVB.[22] Recent investigations have shown that sunscreens with similar SPFs show significant differences in their abilities to protect against UV-induced immunologic injury to the skin.[23] Current data suggest that high SPF products block significant amounts of UVA. However, among products of equal SPF, UVA blockade varies considerably. At present, SPF is not considered to be a reliable measure of UVA protection.

Phototoxic Protection Factor Studies have been conducted using topical or systemically administered photosensitizers such as 8-MOP or anthracene to elicit erythema with small UVA exposures.[24] Photosensitizing chemicals have been used because UVA is extremely weak in its ability to produce erythema. Determining the minimal dose of UVA that causes erythema in sensitized individuals allows for the minimal phototoxic dose to be calculated. Comparing the minimal phototoxic dose of sunscreen-protected skin with that of unprotected skin enables the phototoxic protection factor (PPF) of a sunscreen to be determined.

UVA Protection Factor UVA protection in sensitized skin (PPF) creates an artificial state of photosensitivity to certain regions of the UV spectrum and may not provide an accurate index of protection for normal skin in outdoor conditions. A method that measures the UVA protection factor (APF) in unsensitized skin has been described.[25] This measure of UVA protection, which is defined as the sunscreen-protected threshold dose for each UVA effect divided by the unprotected threshold dose and is analogous to SPF, is determined on the basis of three separate measures: IPD, delayed melanogenesis, and delayed erythema. It is currently recommended that an APF range of 3–6 provides protection similar to that provided by a product of SPF-15 for UVB.[26] Other investigators have suggested that the measurement of IPD protection is the best measure of UVA sunscreen efficacy.[27] APF and IPD need further definition before they can be used generally.

Other Measures of UVA Protection A number of researchers and manufacturers are currently involved in a significant debate about the best approach to measuring UVA protection accurately. They are collaborating with the FDA to develop an informative, accurate, and useful UVA protection indicator. Some researchers have proposed the use of a UVA-protection percent (APP).[28] The APP is intended to represent the fraction of UVA in the 320- to 400-nm range that is blocked by a sunscreen product. A product could conceivably then have an SPF value and an APP on the same package label. It is also possible that an APP could be determined for each product specifically for UVA II and/or UVA I. Other UVA protection factors have also been proposed. Currently, the FDA allows only claims for SPF to be used for commercial sunscreen products.

Substantivity

The efficacy of a sunscreen is related to its substantivity—that is, its ability to remain effective during prolonged exercise, sweating, and swimming. This property appears to be a function of both the active sunscreen and the vehicle. Generally speaking, products with cream-based (water in oil) vehicles appear more resistant to removal than those with alcohol bases and will reduce desquamation of the skin. It should be remembered, however, that part of a sunscreen's effectiveness may relate to the ability of the active agent to bind with constituents of the skin. This binding characteristic may be independent of the vehicle. Oil-based products have traditionally been the most popular and are the easiest to apply. However, they tend to have lower SPF values.

Proposed guidelines for sunscreen product substantivity are:[13]

- *Sweat resistant*: protects for up to 30 minutes of continuous heavy perspiration;
- *Water resistant*: protects for up to 40 minutes of continuous water exposure;
- *Waterproof*: protects for up to 80 minutes of continuous water exposure.

Formulation Factors

Although a pharmacist cannot control the formulation of the various commercially available sunscreen products, a knowledge of the specific active and inactive ingredients and their concentrations may help differentiate a good product from a mediocre one. Several factors affecting the efficacy of nonprescription sunscreen products are related to the vehicle/solvent system. For example:

- The partition coefficient relative to the skin should favor passage of the sunscreen to the skin.
- The pH of the solvent can vary the fraction of ionized and nonionized sunscreen agent, thereby rendering it less effective or even ineffective.
- The solvent system should provide a high degree of substantivity.
- The sunscreen must remain stable for the desired period of protection.

According to the FDA's Advisory Review Panel on Over-the-Counter (OTC) Topical Analgesic, Antirheumatic, Otic, Burn, and Sunburn Prevention and Treatment Products:

> An ideal sunscreen vehicle would be stable, neutral, nongreasy, nondegreasing, nonirritating, nondehydrating, nondrying, odorless, and efficient on all types of human skin. It should also hold at least 50% water, be easily compounded of known chemicals, and have infinite stability during storage.[13]

The panel stated that an ideal vehicle does not exist and recommended that all inactive ingredients be included on product labels. This labeling would allow evaluation by the consumer, pharmacist, and physician for several factors, including sensitivity to any product ingredients.

Sunscreen Agents

The advisory review panel issued its proposed monograph concerning sunscreen products in 1978.[13] The FDA has yet to issue a tentative final monograph in response. In the absence of such a response, the panel's recommendations continue to serve as the primary guidelines for nonprescription sunscreen products.

Three definitions for therapeutic sunscreen types have been proposed:

- *Sunscreen–suntanning agent*: an active ingredient that absorbs at least 85% of the radiation in the UVB

range at wavelengths from 290 to 320 nm but that transmits UVA wavelengths longer than 320 nm (thereby permitting tanning in the average individual and also some erythema without pain).
- *Sunscreen–sunburn preventive agent:* an active ingredient that absorbs 95% or more of the radiation in the UVB range at wavelengths from 290 to 320 nm and thereby removes the primary sunburning rays.
- *Sunscreen–opaque sunblock agent:* an opaque agent that reflects or scatters all radiation in the UV and visible range from 290 to 760 nm and thereby prevents or minimizes suntan and sunburn.

Most products on the market contain a combination of the first two types of agents. The primary differences between the suntanning agent and the preventive agent may involve distinct sunscreen agents with different UV absorbances or may be as simple as the same agent with a different concentration or in a different formulation.

The advisory review panel has recommended that 21 distinct chemical agents be classified as safe and efficacious for nonprescription use as topical sunscreens. These tentative recommendations are included in Table 2. Those sunscreen agents that have not been judged to be both safe and efficacious are listed in Table 3. Prior to the OTC review, sunscreens were considered to be cosmetics. However, the FDA now considers them to be drugs with specific therapeutic indications.

Sunscreens may be generally classified as either oral or topical. The FDA panel recommendations deal strictly with topical sunscreen agents and do not address the issue of oral tanning agents. Topical sunscreens can be divided into two major subgroups: chemical and physical. Chemical sunscreens work by absorbing and thus blocking the transmission of UV radiation to the epidermis. Physical sunscreens are generally opaque and act by reflecting and scattering UV radiation rather than by absorbing it.

Chemical Sunscreens

Aminobenzoic Acid and Derivatives

For many years, aminobenzoic acid (ABA; formerly known as para-aminobenzoic acid, or PABA) has been used in many sunscreen products. ABA is an effective UVB sunscreen, especially when formulated in a hydroalcoholic base (maximum of 50–60% alcohol). The SPF of such formulations increases proportionally as the concentration of ABA increases from 2 to 5%. There is evidence that some UVA is also blocked at the 5% or higher level.[29]

One advantage of ABA is its ability to penetrate into the horny layer of the skin and provide lasting protection. It has significant substantivity on skin that is sweating although not so much on skin that is immersed in water. The primary advantage of ABA derivatives is that they do not stain clothing.

The disadvantages of alcoholic solutions of ABA include (1) contact dermatitis, (2) photosensitivity, (3) stinging and drying of the skin, and (4) yellow staining of clothes upon exposure to the sun.[30] It is perhaps ironic that certain sunscreen agents such as ABA, which are intended to prevent photosensitivity reactions, can themselves induce photosensitivity and contact dermatitis. Some of the drugs that may induce cross-sensitivity to ABA and its derivatives include thiazide diuretics, sulfonamides, and "caine" anesthetics such as lidocaine and benzocaine. Patients who have experienced a photosensitivity reaction to any of these drugs should not use a sunscreen containing ABA or any of its derivatives.

Two of the ABA derivatives listed in Table 2 have received official nonproprietary names from the United States Adopted Names (USAN) Council. Lisadimate is the name for glyceryl para-aminobenzoate and roxadimate is the name for ethyl 4-[bis(hydroxypropyl)]aminobenzoate. Of all the available sunscreens, lisadimate is associated with the highest risk of inducing allergic contact dermatitis. Because of this risk and because it is a very irritating substance, lisadimate is not currently found in any commercially available nonprescription sunscreen product.

There have been recent reports of significant phototoxic reactions to padimate A. Based on these reports, the Office of OTC Drug Evaluation has announced its intention to recommend that the FDA place padimate A in Category III at concentrations of less than 5% and in Category II at concentrations of 5% or more.[31] As a result, no commercially available sunscreen products currently contain padimate A.

Anthranilates

The anthranilates are ortho-ABA derivatives. Menthyl anthranilate, the menthyl ester of anthranilic acid, is a weak UV sunscreen with maximal absorbance in the UVA range. It is usually found in combination with other sunscreen agents to provide broader UV coverage.

Benzophenones

There are three agents in the benzophenone group: dioxybenzone, oxybenzone (benzophenone-3), and sulisobenzone (benzophenone-4). As a group, these agents are primarily UVB absorbers with maximum absorbance between 282 and 290 nm. However, their absorbance extends well into the UVA range, with oxybenzone up to 350 nm and dioxybenzone up to 380 nm. Because of their extended spectrum of action, benzophenones are often found in combination with other sunscreens to provide a very broad spectrum of coverage.

Cinnamates

There are four sunscreens in this group. Three of the four agents have virtually identical absorbance ranges as well as maximum absorbances; the exception is octocrylene, which is the new official nonproprietary (USAN) name given to 2-ethylhexyl 2-cyano-3, 3-diphenylacrylate. Octocrylene has an absorbance range of 250–360 nm, which is well into the UVA range. Octocrylene is currently found in many more commercial sunscreen preparations than it was in the past, possibly reflecting its broader spectrum of absorbance. Unfortunately, cinnamates do not adhere well to the skin and must rely on the vehicle in a given formulation for their substantivity.

Salicylates

Salicylic acid derivatives are weak sunscreens and must be used in high concentrations. They do not adhere well to the skin and are easily removed by perspiration or swimming.[32]

Physical Sunscreens

Physical sunscreens scatter rather than absorb UV and visible radiation (290–760 nm). They are most often used on small and prominently exposed areas by people who cannot limit or control their exposure to the sun (e.g., lifeguards). The nose and tops of the ears are often coated

TABLE 2 Sunscreens considered to be safe and effective by the FDA advisory review panel

Sunscreen	Absorbance range (nm)	Maximum range (nm)	Approved concentration (%)
Anthranilates			
Menthyl anthranilate	260–380[a]	340[a]	3.5–5
Benzophenones			
Dioxybenzone	260–380[b]	282[c]	3
Oxybenzone	270–350	290[d]	2–6
Sulisobenzone	260–375	285[e]	5–10
Cinnamates			
Cinoxate	270–328	310	1–3
Diethanolamine *p*-methoxy-cinnamate	280–310	290	8–10
Ethylhexyl *p*-methoxy-cinnamate	290–320	308–310	2–7.5
Octocrylene	250–360	303	7–10
Dibenzoylmethane derivatives			
Avobenzone[f,g]	320–400	360	3
ABA and Derivatives			
Aminobenzoic acid	260–313	288.5	5–15
Lisadimate	264–315	295	2–3
Padimate A	290–315	310	1–5
Padimate O	290–315	310	1.4–8
Roxadimate	280–330	308–311	1–5
Salicylates			
2-Ethylhexyl salicylate	280–320	305	3–5
Homosalate	295–315	306	4–15
Triethanolamine salicylate	260–320	298	5–12
Miscellaneous			
Digalloyl trioleate	270–320	300	2–5
Lawsone with dihydroxyacetone (DHA)	290–400	—	0.25 lawsone; 3 DHA
2-Phenylbenzimidazole-5-sulfonic acid	290–320	302	1–4
Red petrolatum[h]	290–365	—	30–100
Titanium dioxide[i]	290–700	—	2–25
Zinc oxide	290–700	—	—

[a]Values are for concentrations higher than normally found in nonprescription drugs.
[b]Values available when used in combination with other screens.
[c]Second peak at 327 nm.
[d]Second peak at 329 nm.
[e]Second peak at 324 nm.
[f]Currently marketed through a new drug application.
[g]Commercially available as 3% in combination with 7% padimate O.
[h]A 0.03-mm film absorbs UV radiation below 320 nm. At 334 nm, 16% of radiation is transmitted; at 365 nm, 58% is transmitted.
[i]Scatters radiation from 290 to 700 nm rather than absorbs it.
Adapted from the *Federal Register* 1978; 43: 38223 and from Shaath NA. Encyclopedia of UV absorbers for sunscreen products. *Cosmet Toiletries* 1987 Mar; 102: 21–36.

TABLE 3 Agents cited to lack safety and/or efficacy data by the FDA advisory review panel

Agent	Safe	Effective
Category II		
2-Ethylhexyl 4-phenylbenzophenone-2′-carboxylic acid	Insufficient data	Insufficient data
3-(4-methylbenzylidene) camphor	Insufficient data	No data
Sodium 3,4-dimethyl-phenylglyoxylate	Insufficient data	No data
Category III		
Allantoin with aminobenzoic acid (AL-PABA)	Safe	Insufficient data
5-(3,3-Dimethyl-2-norboryliden)-3-penten-2-one	Safe	Insufficient data
Dipropylene glycol salicylate	Insufficient data	Insufficient data

Adapted from the *Federal Register* 1978; 43: 38219–53.

---

with a white or colored substance containing zinc oxide or titanium dioxide. Manufacturers have not yet developed a way to make physical sunscreens transparent while maintaining similar efficacy. The effectiveness of physical sunscreens is related to the thickness with which they are applied. Their disadvantages are that they can discolor clothing and may occlude the skin to produce miliaria (prickly heat) and folliculitis.

Zinc oxide was inadvertently skipped when the review panel initially evaluated the various sunscreen agents, and it will be most likely recommended for inclusion in Category III in the tentative final monograph.[33] Meanwhile, because titanium dioxide increases the effective SPF of a product and extends the spectrum of protection well into the UVA range, the number of commercial products containing this agent has increased.

UVA Sunscreens

Dibenzoylmethane derivatives are the first of a new class of full-spectrum sunscreen agents effective throughout the UVA range. The first of these new agents is avobenzone (butyl methoxydibenzoylmethane), which has maximum absorbance at approximately 360 nm.[25] Although avobenzone absorbs UV radiation through all the UVA spectrum, its absorbance falls off sharply at 370 nm. There is still the possibility of a photosensitivity reaction from those chemicals that are reactive in the 370–400 nm range. Clinical trials have demonstrated that optimal sunscreen protection can be obtained by using a combination of 3% avobenzone and 7% padimate O. This combination produced the highest PPF when compared in two studies with avobenzone alone, padimate A alone, and a combination of padimate O, oxybenzone, and octyl salicylate.[24,34] The mean PPF for the combination in each study was 4.5 and 4.8 using artificial light indoors.

Combination Products

The FDA has not recommended any limits on the number of sunscreen agents that may be used together in a nonprescription product. The advisory review panel made only the following two major recommendations in this area:

- Any additional sunscreen agents must contribute to the efficacy of the product and not be included merely for marketing promotion purposes.
- Any combination of sunscreens with active nonsunscreen agents must meet the requirements for safety and efficacy.

Suntan Products

Two types of products fall under the general heading of suntan products: those that contain a sunscreen and those that do not. Products without a sunscreen are easily identified by the absence of an SPF value on the label. These products are considered cosmetics and are used for coloring the skin rather than for any therapeutic indications. Thus, they are formulated with oily vehicles that tend to concentrate UV radiation onto the skin. Although they are also formulated with emollients, this type of suntan product provides no protection whatsoever against all the short- and long-term hazards of overexposure to UV radiation.

The second type of suntan product is actually a low SPF sunscreen product. It can differ from high SPF products in one of two ways. First, the formulation may consist of a sunscreen agent in an oily vehicle, which concentrates UV radiation, rather than in a lotion-type of vehicle, which aids in the penetration of sunscreens into the skin. Second, a simple reduction in the concentration of certain sunscreen agents may lower the product's effective SPF without changing any other aspects of the product's formulation.

Although suntan products without a sunscreen can make various claims of tanning, sunscreen products cannot. The advisory review panel has stated that "claims such as promoting tanning for sunlight protective agents are unsubstantiated," and the FDA does not allow them.

Pigmenting Agents

Oral Agents

During the past several years, a number of products have claimed to be effective oral tanning compounds. Their active ingredients are the dyes canthaxanthin and beta carotene, which are chemically similar to one another. Beta carotene and canthaxanthin are approved by the FDA as color additives in foods and drugs, and beta carotene is also approved for use in cosmetics. Canthaxanthin is a synthetic dye that is similar to those dyes found naturally in fruits, vegetables, and flowers. Both agents are used to enhance the appearance of foods such as pizza, barbecue and spaghetti sauces, soups, salad dressings, fruit drinks, baked goods, pudding, cheese, ketchup, and margarine. However, they are used in food in lower concentrations than those found in oral products that claim to produce tanning. For example, the daily dietary intakes of beta carotene and canthaxanthin as food colorants are about 0.3 mg and 5.6 mg, respectively;[35] in one brand of tanning tablet, however, the daily intakes are 12 mg and 100 mg, respectively.

The dyes alter skin tone by coloring the fat cells under the epidermal layer. Because of variations in fat cells and epidermal thickness, the extent of the tan varies from person to person. Canthaxanthin is dosed by body weight, with a 20-day schedule necessary to achieve a significant change in skin tone. This process is followed by doses of 1 to 2 capsules per day to maintain the color. The promotional literature cautions the user that if the palms turn orange, too much of the product is being consumed.

According to the 1960 Color Additive Amendment, any new use of a color additive must be submitted to the FDA for approval.[36] The FDA has not yet approved either compound for artificial tanning. One major concern is the discoloration of the feces to brick red, which could mask gastrointestinal bleeding. A second concern is the long-term adverse effects that may be associated with the large doses recommended. Although beta carotene is used on a prescription basis to help prevent photosensitivity in patients with erythropoietic protoporphyria, there is no evidence documenting the safety of canthaxanthin at the high doses found in oral tanning products. In fact, a recent case has been reported of fatal aplastic anemia associated with canthaxanthin ingestion from an oral tanning product. Reported cases of retinopathy, hepatitis, and urticaria associated with the use of oral tanning agents has prompted the FDA to issue further warnings on such products.[37] In addition, Canada, which previously allowed the nonprescription sale of canthaxanthin for tanning purposes, has decided that there is insufficient evidence of safety, and no longer allows such sales.

Topical Dyes

Another type of available pigmenting agent is dihydroxyacetone (DHA). For years, DHA has been the major ingredient in products that claim to tan without sun. DHA produces a reddish-brown color by binding with specific amino acids in the stratum corneum. The intensity of the tan is related to the thickness of the skin. If the product is not washed off the hands immediately after application, however, the palms may also develop this tan. In addition, dry areas such as elbows and kneecaps will absorb the DHA more readily, resulting in uneven coloration. The color fades after 5–7 days with desquamation of the stratum corneum.

The advisory review panel has determined that DHA alone is ineffective as a sunscreen and that it should be classified as a cosmetic. However, in combination with lawsone, a major dye component of henna, the product is classified as a weak sunscreen as well as a cosmetic. This combination will not directly affect melanin production, and in one study, the SPF of such products was calculated to be less than 2.[30] Several sunless tanning products combine DHA with various sunscreen agents, which at least helps prevent photodamage for those persons who intend to spend some time in the sun.

Tan Accelerators

Tan accelerators are cosmetic products that claim to stimulate a faster and deeper tan. There are a number of these products currently on the market. The major ingredient in these products is tyrosine, an amino acid necessary for the production of melanin. Product literature recommends application of these products once daily for at least 3 days before sun exposure. However, one study that tested two commercial products using indoor UV radiation found no evidence of benefit.[38] Although the FDA advisory review panel did not evaluate tan accelerators, the tentative final monograph is expected to address these types of products as drugs rather than as cosmetics.

Melanotropins

A hormone known as alpha-melanotropin or alpha-melanocyte–stimulating hormone (ALPHA-MSH) has been located within the human central nervous system. The role of ALPHA-MSH in humans, if any, has not yet been identified. However, this hormone is produced by the pituitary gland of numerous vertebrates and has been shown to affect skin color through its action on melanocytes. Alpha-melanotropin is currently under investigation to determine whether it can affect skin tanning.[39]

Tanning Booths and Beds

The availability of tanning booths and beds may prompt questions from patients concerning their safety. The newer types of tanning devices use UV light sources composed of more than 96% UVA and less than 4% UVB, a considerably different mix of UV radiation than that obtained from natural sunlight.[8]

It would appear that UVA, if used properly, could generate a tan without producing an erythematous sunburn. However, there is a concern about UVB contamination of UVA lamps. It is believed that even 1% UVB emission can cause a significant increase in the incidence of skin cancer. In addition, some UVA lamps produce more than five times as much UVA per unit of time than does sunlight.[9]

UVA also presents other hazards, such as deeper tissue penetration than UVB, as described earlier. UVA radiation may trigger the eruption of cold sores. In addition, it can produce a photosensitivity reaction in patients who have ingested or applied photosensitizing agents. Moreover, because UVA is less likely to produce the overt burning (erythema) of UVB, patients may become complacent and forgo the use of eye goggles; this practice will produce eye burns and may increase the risk of subsequently developing cataracts.

The FDA sets standards for UVA and UVB emissions and specific wave lengths. For example, tanning booth timers cannot be set to exceed 4 MEDS for type II skin. In addition, FDA regulations include the use of goggles with specified transmittance limits. Despite all these precautions and warnings, however, patients should be advised that the possibility of long-term hazards related to UVA has not yet been fully assessed.

Sunglasses

Concern has been expressed regarding the relationship between UV radiation and eye damage such as cataracts or long-term retinal damage.[40] UV radiation may also cause temporary injuries such as photokeratitis (a painful type of snow blindness associated with highly reflective surfaces). This concern is all the more serious because of the erroneous belief that all sunglasses screen out UV radiation. In response, the FDA has developed a voluntary labeling program with manufacturers of sunglasses. Abbreviated information concerning the UV radiation screening properties is directly attached to each pair of sunglasses. In addition, brochures describing the appropriate use of each type of lens are available at outlets selling sunglasses.[41] Based on its UV radiation filtration properties, each pair of sunglasses is placed in one of three categories:

- *Cosmetic* sunglasses block at least 70% of UVB, 20% of UVA, and less than 60% of visible light. They are recommended for activities in nonharsh sunlight, such as shopping.
- *General purpose* sunglasses block at least 95% of UVB, at least 60% of UVA, and 60–92% of visible light. With shades that range from medium to dark, they are recommended for most activities in sunny environments, such as boating, driving, flying, or hiking.
- *Special purpose* sunglasses block at least 99% of UVB, 60% of UVA, and at least 97% of visible light. They are recommended for activities in very bright environments such as ski slopes and tropical beaches.

Product Selection Guidelines

Questions To Ask

The most important thing a pharmacist needs to know before recommending a sunscreen product is the patient's natural skin type (Table 1) and tanning history. Other important information includes both the active and inactive ingredients in the various products (Table 2) as well as the products' SPF. The pharmacist should find out from the patient how much time is normally spent out of doors in occupational and recreational pursuits. Other questions the pharmacist might ask are presented at the beginning of this chapter. Using this information, the pharmacist can feel comfortable in recommending a sunscreen product.

SPF

Patients with less natural skin protection should use products with higher SPFs. A product with an SPF of 15 or greater will prevent sunburn while also allowing for a gradually developing tan. This type of product should be recommended for patients who burn easily, cannot tan, or cannot afford any degree of sunburn or overexposure to UV radiation of any type. Patients who have a personal or family history of certain dermatologic problems, such as atopic dermatitis or sunburn with short exposure, or who have any type of skin cancer or precancerous dermatologic lesion should use a total blocking agent or a sunscreen with an SPF of 15 or higher when prolonged exposure to sunlight is expected. Studies have shown that even low protective sunscreens (SPF-2) can reduce the incidence of nonmelanoma skin cancers from 36 to 54% if properly used beginning in childhood.[42] However, some investigators and clinicians have suggested that products with an SPF of less than 6 not be recommended routinely to patients;[30] because of the hazards associated with UV radiation, they recommend instead the selection of a product with an SPF of 15 or higher.

Although products beyond an SPF of 15 do not appear to have a markedly superior advantage over SPF-15 products, this recommendation may be moderated on the basis of the patient's natural skin color. Patients with type I and type II skin, as well as those with a history of skin disease or malignancies and those taking photosensitizing drugs, should use a sunscreen with an SPF of at least 30. There are even commercial products currently available with SPFs up to 50. However, any product in the 15–50 SPF range will significantly reduce the total amount of UV radiation received, virtually blocking out all UVB and a significant amount of UVA radiation.

Substantivity

A very important factor in product selection is the product's substantivity. Given three products of equal SPF, but varying substantivity, the best and most cost-effective selection is the product that is most substantive. A waterproof product needs to be reapplied only after 80 minutes of swimming or continuous water exposure, whereas a sweat-resistant product requires reapplication after every 30 minutes of perspiration and a water-resistant product must be reapplied after 40 minutes of swimming or continuous water exposure.

Damage to Clothing, Vinyl, and Fiberglass

There has been some concern about sunscreen products staining clothing or the vinyl and fiberglass found in boats. This is no longer a major concern because staining is primarily associated with ABA, which currently exists in only a few commercial products and whose esters (e.g., padimate O) do not cause staining. However, to be used safely, sunscreen products containing ABA should be allowed to dry before the skin comes into contact with clothing, vinyl, or fiberglass. This is probably a good rule to follow regardless of the sunscreen used. The only other sunscreen that has potential for staining is DHA, which is found in some tanning products. Again, product labels warn that, to prevent staining, the skin should be allowed to dry thoroughly before coming into contact with clothing.

Broad-Spectrum Sunscreens

The question of what constitutes a broad-spectrum sunscreen remains. A number of commercial products claim to be broad spectrum; the FDA allows such claims as long as the ingredients in the sunscreen absorb in both the UVA and UVB ranges. It appears that products with equal SPFs may still differ significantly in total UV protection, depending on the absorbances of the various sunscreens they contain. Most currently available broad-spectrum products have a minimum of two sunscreen ingredients while many others incorporate three or even four sunscreens.

Although UVA II is more damaging to the skin than UVA I, the lack of a standardized UVA protection factor does not allow such considerations to be taken into account in product selection. Thus, there is no one generally accepted measure to evaluate the actual efficacy of a product that claims to provide UVA protection. The best recommendation would be to select a product that contains a combination of sunscreen agents that protect across the widest possible UVB and UVA ranges. There are several explanations for this recommendation. First, although most photosensitizing chemicals are active in the UVA range from 320 to 400 nm, UVB can also trigger such a reaction. Second, the UVB sunscreen can be effective in preventing sunburn and can help to reduce the long-term hazards of skin cancer and premature aging of the skin. A very broad spectrum of coverage can be obtained by using an ABA derivative combined with one of the benzophenones. There are a number of such combinations on the market. A commercial product that contains avobenzone, a true UVA sunscreen, in combination with an ABA derivative (e.g., padimate O) would be a reasonable recommendation for maximal protection.

Contact Dermatitis and Other Skin Considerations

Photosensitivity and contact dermatitis are more likely to occur with ABA and its esters. Other sunscreens have also been reported to produce both conditions, although to a lesser degree. These sunscreens include the benzophenones, the cinnamates, homosalate, avobenzone, and menthyl anthranilate. In addition, patients who are allergy prone and have allergies to various drugs, such as benzocaine, thiazides, or sulfonamides, may also develop an allergic reaction to either ABA or its esters.

Other general cosmetic considerations also need to be taken into account because anything that will motivate an individual to use a sunscreen is a welcome consideration. For example, at least one-third of the commercial products currently available are labeled noncomedogenic, fragrance-free, and hypoallergenic. Products that are noncomedogenic are those that do not plug the pores and therefore do not exacerbate acne. This is especially important for teenagers, who generally spend more time out of doors than other age groups and would generally prefer to not use comedogenic sunscreens. Regarding fragrance-free and hypoallergenic properties, many individuals are sensitive to various ingredients, including fragrances, emulsifiers, and preservatives. It is very possible that some cases of contact dermatitis that were attributed to a sunscreen may actually have been due to excipients in the formulation. Thus, patients who have a history of sensitivity to these types of ingredients would do well to use a fragrance-free, hypoallergenic product.

Many commercial formulas contain glyceryl monostearate, carbowaxes, fragrances, and other potentially sensitizing ingredients to increase the cosmetic appeal and acceptability. These ingredients may, in fact, enhance product appeal and increase its use. However, ethyl and isopropyl alcohols, which are included in a number of commercial sunscreen products, can dry the skin.

A product that promises sunless tanning and has an SPF rating contains DHA with a sunscreen, whereas a product that promises sunless tanning and has no SPF most likely contains DHA alone. Such products may create a false sense of security. The individual might look tan, but these products provide no sunscreen protection, and overexposure to UV radiation may thus result in a serious burn.

Lip Protection

Several products are on the market in stick or lipstick form. These products prevent burning of the lips (or nose). Although they differ in ingredients and UVA and UVB spectrum, these products carry the same labeling, including the SPF, as do the sunscreen lotions. The SPF of these products is usually at least 15. Studies have shown that lip protection not only helps prevent drying and burning of the lips but also helps prevent the development of cold sores (fever blisters) triggered by the herpes simplex virus in patients who are susceptible to recurrent cold sores. This type of product is convenient to carry and use, and it can be reapplied as often as necessary. Lipsticks are perhaps the most often neglected sunscreen product.

Sunscreens and Children

Special consideration is needed when recommending a sunscreen for young children. The consensus is that the absorptive characteristics of human skin in children under 6 months of age are different from those of adult skin. Related to this is the belief that the metabolic and excretory systems of children under 6 months of age are not fully developed to handle any drug absorbed through the skin. Therefore, the advisory review panel has recommended that only persons over 6 months of age be considered to have adult human skin. The panel has made two specific, age-related recommendations regarding the labeling of nonprescription sunscreens:[13]

- Sunscreen products should not be used on children under 6 months of age.
- Products with an SPF as low as 2 or 3 are not to be used on children under 2 years of age.

This second recommendation was made because this SPF range does not supply adequate protection.

Caregivers should be extremely careful regarding sun exposure in children, especially those under 6 months old. Regular use of an SPF-15 product starting after 6 months of age and continuing through 18 years can reduce the incidence of skin cancer over a lifetime by as much as 78%.[42] Such usage would also result in a reduction in sunburn and a reduced risk of premature skin aging and other skin problems.

Patient Education and Counseling

Pharmacists can provide a great service by counseling consumers about the suntanning process and the proper selection and use of sunscreens. In one study involving almost 500 persons, a considerable amount of misinformation was found to exist concerning sunscreen use. For example, 51% of those surveyed did not know the definition of SPF or its significance, 26% were not even aware of the existence of sunscreens before the study, and of the 41% who used sunscreens, one-third thought those products would promote tanning.[43]

The rays of the sun are the most direct and damaging between 10 AM and 2 PM. It is best to avoid sunning during this period, especially at the beginning of the season before any protective tan has developed. Closely related to this is the misconception that one cannot burn on an overcast or cloudy day. Although varying amounts of visible sunlight may not pass through cloud cover and the clouds tend to filter out the infrared radiation that contributes to the sensation of heat, this reduction in heat sensation provides a false sense of security against a burn.[44] In fact, very little UV radiation is filtered and most (60–80%) will penetrate clouds. In addition, the intensity of exposure increases as one moves closer to the equator. People in the southern part of the United States are at greater risk from the harmful effects of UV radiation than those in northern areas. Also, the irradiance of UVB increases by 4% for every 1,000 feet of altitude. This may be of particular concern to skiers and individuals living and working in higher elevations.

Another potential problem is that UV radiation reflects off surfaces. Fresh snow will reflect 85–100% of the light and radiation that strikes it, creating the need for sunglasses when one is skiing on a sunny day. This reflected radiation is also why a skier can receive a significant sunburn, even on a cloudy day, and thus should use a sunscreen. Similarly, sand and white-painted surfaces, while not as reflective as snow, nevertheless reflect a significant amount of the radiation striking them. Therefore, a person sitting in the shade of a beach umbrella may still be bombarded by UV radiation reflecting off the sand. This contributes to the overall radiation received, and a severe sunburn may result. Water reflects no more than 5% of UV radiation and allows the remaining 95% to penetrate and burn the swimmer. Therefore, time in the water, even if the swimmer is completely submerged, should be considered as part of the total time spent in the sun. In addition, although dry clothes reflect almost all UV radiation, wet clothes allow transmission of approximately 50% of UV radiation. However, if light passes through dry clothing when held up to the light, UV radiation will also penetrate that clothing. Tightly woven material offers the greatest protection.

If properly applied, products with an SPF of 8–15 allow an individual to stay out in the sun for long periods and slowly develop a tan over several days. It is important to remember, however, that as an individual tans, a natural protection against burning also develops. Therefore, an individual who begins the summer using a product with an SPF of 15 may want to switch to a product with a lower SPF (e.g., 12, then 10, then 8, etc.) as the natural tan progresses. This change will allow a more rapid deepening of the tan. The person can, however, continue to use the product with the SPF of 15; it will simply take longer to achieve the desired tan.

Patients should be advised that, although tanning and thickening of the skin serve as protective mechanisms against future injury, peeling of the skin removes part of this protection. The amount of exposure to the sun as well as the SPF of the product being used must be reevaluated as tanning and peeling occur.

Other specific information relating to the safe and effective use of sunscreen agents has been reviewed by the advisory review panel. The panel concluded that two major causes of poor sun protection with sunscreen use are application of inadequate amounts and infrequent reapplication. Sunscreens must be liberally applied to all exposed areas of the body and reapplied as often as the label recommends for maximum effectiveness. Although these two factors drive up the cost of sunscreen use, the long-term benefits of proper sunscreen use far outweigh the costs. The panel recommended that the directions for use state: "Apply liberally before sun exposure and reapply after swimming or after excessive sweating." The panel also recommended that labeling of all sunscreens contain the following warnings:

- For external use only, not to be swallowed.
- Avoid contact with eyes.
- Discontinue use if signs of irritation or rash appear.

The FDA standard for application of sunscreens is 2 mcL/cm² of body surface area. This means that, for sufficient protection, the average adult in a bathing suit should apply nine portions of sunscreen of approximately one-half teaspoon each, or approximately four and one-half teaspoons in total. The sunscreen should be distributed as follows:[45]

- Face and neck: one-half teaspoon;
- Arms and shoulders: one-half teaspoon to each side;

- Torso: one-half teaspoon each to front and back;
- Legs and top of feet: one teaspoon to each side.

Because of the cost of sunscreen products and the need to apply it often and in sufficient amounts, people may use far less sunscreen than necessary to provide adequate protection. One study demonstrated, however, that the effective SPF of commercial products was only 50% of the labeled value when subjects were allowed to apply sunscreen according to their own assessment of need.[46] One simple way to find out if patients are using sunscreen properly is to ask how long the current bottle they are using has lasted. When applied properly, according to the above-suggested dosing guidelines and in accordance with the appropriate substantivity of the product, a sunbather could easily use about 1 oz every 80–90 minutes. This would amount to several ounces a day and several bottles per week. Incredibly, many frequent sunbathers use only one bottle in an entire season. This demonstrates the importance of individuals receiving adequate counseling from pharmacists to get the protection they desire.

Reapplying a sunscreen does not extend the amount of time a person can spend in the sun. Outdoor exposure to UV radiation should be within the limits of the SPF value of the sunscreen. Moreover, although some sunscreen products now have an SPF of 50, the use of an SPF over 15 offers little advantage to the average person.[47] The best all-purpose, general recommendation for providing optimal protection from immediate as well as long-term injury from sun exposure is to recommend a product with an SPF of at least 15. This will allow the development of a slow tan with safety. Children should use SPF-15 sunscreens daily whenever they play outdoors, not just when swimming. Pharmacists should emphasize these recommendations during consultation.

Recently, questions have arisen as to whether the substantivity of a sunscreen may affect the temperature-regulating ability of the body. One study reported that exercising in hot weather after applying a sunscreen product may increase the risk of overheating.[48] Under hot, humid conditions, there is increased sweating but poor evaporation. When the humidity is low, overheating during exercise may still occur, possibly because the oily vehicle of the sunscreen may block the pores. Therefore, sunbathers should be cautious when exercising in hot weather after applying a sunscreen product.

There has been one report of individuals ingesting ABA orally in doses of up to 1 g daily to prevent phototoxic reactions.[49] However, there is no evidence demonstrating the safety or efficacy of ABA when so used. Moreover, oral ingestion of ABA has been associated with a lowered white blood cell count, drug fever, and organ damage, and thus should be vigorously discouraged.

Consumers should be advised that if itching, redness, or a rash develops while using a particular product, they should discontinue using the product and contact a pharmacist.

Summary

Tanning or burning of the skin can result from recreational sunbathing or outdoor activities such as yard work or sports; it can also be an occupational hazard. Whatever the circumstances, the hazards of long-term exposure to UV radiation are well documented, and sustained efforts to educate the public are needed to minimize these hazards.

The key to proper protection is the identification of skin type and tolerability to UV exposure. With this information, an individual can select a product with the appropriate SPF. Because products with the same SPF provide equivalent efficacy against sunburn, other factors that may help determine product selection may then be taken into account. These factors are skin sensitivity, product substantivity, ability of product to damage fabrics, price, and the intended use of the product.

Current evidence strongly suggests that a broad-spectrum product is best for most people. This is especially true for patients taking photosensitizing drugs and those at risk for developing skin cancer. Many authorities recommend products containing ABA or its esters in combination with a benzophenone. A better option may be a product containing avobenzone. However, avoidance of unnecessary exposure to UV radiation is the primary preventive measure.

Once a product is selected, it should be applied at least 30 minutes before exposure to the sun (up to 2 hours before with ABA and its esters) to allow binding to the skin. The product should be applied often, especially after heavy sweating and swimming.

If the individual's ultimate goal is to develop a deep tan, the best approach is slow and cautious. Increasing exposure to the sun gradually while avoiding peak sun times provides natural protection to the skin through melanin formation and thus allows for gradual tanning with minimal burning. With proper use of sunscreen products and judicious tanning, both the short- and long-term hazards of exposure to the sun can be minimized.

Editor's Note: As this edition of the *Handbook* went to press, the FDA published a tentative final monograph on suntan and sunscreen products dated May 12, 1993.

References

1. Kochevar IE, Pathak MA, Parrish JA. In: Fitzpatrick TB, Eisen AZ, Wolff K, et al., eds. *Dermatology in General Medicine*. 3rd ed. New York: McGraw-Hill; 1987: 1441–51.
2. Patnak MA, Fitzpatrick TB, Parrish JA. In: Fitzpatrick TB, Eisen AZ, Wolff K, et al., eds. *Dermatology in General Medicine*. 3rd ed. New York: McGraw-Hill; 1987: 254–62.
3. Forbes PD, Davies RE, Urbach F, et al. In: Jackson EM, ed. *Photobiology of the Skin and Eye*. New York: Marcel Dekker; 1986: 67–84.
4. Willis I, Menter JM, Whyte HJ. The rapid induction of cancer in the hairless mouse utilizing the principle of photoaugmentation. *J Invest Dermatol* 1981 May; 76 (5): 404–8.
5. Kligman LH. In: Urbach F, Gange RW, eds. *The Biological Effects of UV-A Radiation*. New York: Praeger; 1986: 98–110.
6. Gilchrest BA, Soter NA, Hawk JLM, et al. Histologic changes associated with ultraviolet A–induced erythema in normal human skin. *J Am Acad Dermatol* 1983 Aug; 9: 213–9.
7. Staberg B, Worm AM, Brodthagen H, et al. Direct and indirect effects of UVA on skin vessel leakiness. *J Invest Dermatol* 1982 Dec; 79 (6): 358–60.
8. Mutzhas MF, Cesarini JP. In: Passchier WF, Bosnjakovic BFM, eds. *Human Exposure to Ultraviolet Radiation: Risk and Regulations*. Amsterdam: Elsevier Science Publishers; 1987: 345–52.

9. *Consensus Development Conference Statement on Sunlight, Ultraviolet Radiation, and the Skin.* Bethesda, Md: National Institutes of Health; 1989 May 8–10.
10. Pathak MA. In: Urbach F, Gange RW, eds. *The Biological Effects of UV-A Radiation.* New York: Praeger; 1986: 156–67.
11. Gange RW. In: Fitzpatrick TB, Eisen AZ, Wolff K, et al., eds. *Dermatology in General Medicine.* 3rd ed. New York: McGraw-Hill; 1987: 1451–7.
12. Bernhard JD, Pathak MA, Kochevar IE, et al. In: Fitzpatrick TB, Eisen AZ, Wolff K, et al., eds. *Dermatology in General Medicine.* 3rd ed. New York: McGraw-Hill; 1987: 1480–507.
13. *Federal Register* 1978 Aug 25: 38206–69.
14. Kligman LH, Kligman AM. In: Fitzpatrick TB, Eisen AZ, Wolff K, et al., eds. *Dermatology in General Medicine.* 3rd ed. New York: McGraw-Hill; 1987: 1470–5.
15. *Consensus Conference Statement on Photoaging/Photodamage.* St. Louis: American Academy of Dermatology; 1988 Mar 3–4: 10.
16. Kligman AM. The treatment of photoaged human skin by topical tretinoin. *Drugs* 1989 Jul; 38 (1): 1–8.
17. Lindley CM, Cronquist SE. Skin cancers: detection, prevention and therapeutics. *Am Pharm* 1988 Apr; NS28 (4): 244–53.
18. Rigel DS. Malignant melanoma in the 1990s. *Pharm Times* 1991 May; 57 (5): 33–9.
19. Zagula-Mally ZW, Rosenberg EW, Kashgarian M. *Cancer* 1974 Aug; 34: 345–9.
20. Urbach F, et al. *Tenth International Cancer Congress* (Abstracts). Philadelphia: Lippincott; 1970: 109–10.
21. Averbach H. Geographic variation in incidence of skin cancer in the United States. *Public Health Rep* 1961 Apr; 76 (4): 345–8.
22. Breit R, Endres L. In: Urbach, F, Gange RW, et al., eds. *The Biological Effects of UV-A Radiation.* New York: Praeger; 1986: 68–78.
23. Mommaas AM, van Praag MCG, Bavinck JNB, et al. Analysis of the protective effect of topical sunscreens on the UVB-radiation-induced suppression of the mixed-lymphocyte reaction. *J Invest Dermatol* 1990 Sep; 95: 313–6.
24. Lowe NJ, Dromgoole SH, Sefton J, et al. Indoor and outdoor efficacy testing of a broad-spectrum sunscreen against ultraviolet A radiation in psoralen-sensitized subjects. *J Am Acad Dermatol* 1987 Aug; 17 (2): 224–30.
25. Kaidbey K, Gange RW. Comparison of methods for assessing photoprotection against ultraviolet A in vivo. *J Am Acad Dermatol* 1987 Feb; 16 (2): 346–53.
26. Stanfield JW, Feldt PA, Csortan ES, et al. Ultraviolet A sunscreen evaluations in normal subjects. *J Am Acad Dermatol* 1989 May; 20 (5): 744–8.
27. Kaidbey KH, Barnes A. Determination of UVA protection factors by means of immediate pigment darkening in normal skin. *J Am Acad Dermatol* 1991 Aug; 25 (2): 262–6.
28. Sayre RM, Agin PP. A method for the determination of UVA protection for normal skin. *J Am Acad Dermatol* 1990 Sep; 23 (3): 429–40.
29. Roelandts R, Vanhee J, Bonamie A, et al. A survey of ultraviolet absorbers in commercially available sun products. *Int J Dermatol* 1983 May; 22: 247–55.
30. Pathak MA. Sunscreens: topical and systemic approaches for protection of human skin against harmful effects of solar radiation. *J Am Acad Dermatol* 1982 Sep; 7 (3): 285–312.
31. Gilbertson, WE. Letter to Howard Iserman, June 6, 1989, Freedom of Information, Comment No. C00058, Docket No. 78N–0038.
32. Gossel TA. Use of sunscreens to prevent sun-damaged skin. *U.S. Pharm* 1989 May; 14 (5): 67–88.
33. Ripere J. Personal communication of status of zinc oxide. Bethesda, Md: FDA, Office of OTC Drug Evaluation; April 1, 1992.
34. Gange RW, Soparkar A, Matzinger E, et al. Efficacy of a sunscreen containing butyl methoxydibenzoylmethane against ultraviolet A radiation in photosensitized subjects. *J Am Acad Dermatol* 1986 Sep; 15 (3): 494–9.
35. Fenner L. The tanning pill, a questionable dye job. *FDA Consumer* 1982 Feb; 23–4.
36. Tanning pills. Talk paper. Rockville, Md: U.S. Department of Health and Human Services, FDA; 1981 Jul 6.
37. Bluhm R, Branch R, Johnston P, et al. Aplastic anemia associated with canthaxanthin ingested for "tanning" purposes. *JAMA* 1990 Sep 5; 264 (9): 1141–2.
38. Jaworsky C, Ratz JL, Dijkstra JWE. Efficacy of tan accelerators. *J Am Acad Dermatol* 1987 Apr; 16 (4): 769–71.
39. Levine N, Sheftel SN, Eytan T, et al. Induction of skin tanning by subcutaneous administration of a potent synthetic melanotropin. *JAMA* 1991 Nov 20; 266 (19): 2730–6.
40. Taylor HR, West SK, Rosenthal FS, et al. Effect of ultraviolet radiation on cataract formation. *N Engl J Med* 1988 Dec 1; 319 (22): 1429–33.
41. New labeling for sunglasses. *HHS News.* Rockville, Md: U.S. Department of Health and Human Services; 1989 May 15.
42. Stern RS, Weinstein MC, Baker SG. Risk reduction for nonmelanoma skin cancer with childhood sunscreen use. *Arch Dermatol* 1986 May; 122: 537–45.
43. Johnson EY, Lookingbill DP. Sunscreen use and sun exposure: trends in a White population. *Arch Dermatol* 1984 Jun; 120: 727–31.
44. Pathak MA, Fitzpatrick TB, Greiter F, et al. In: Fitzpatrick TB, Eisen AZ, Wolff K, et al., eds. *Dermatology in General Medicine.* 3rd ed. New York: McGraw-Hill; 1987: 1507–77.
45. Sunscreens. *Consumer Rep* 1980 Jun; 45: 353–6.
46. Stenberg C, Larko O. Sunscreen application and its importance for the sun protection factor. *Arch Dermatol* 1985 Nov; 121: 1400–2.
47. Sunscreens. *Med Lett* 1988 Jun 17; 30 (768): 61–3.
48. Wells TD, Jessup GT, Langlotz KS. Effects of sunscreen use during exercise in the heat. *Physician Sportsmed* 1984 Jun; 12 (6): 132–42.
49. Letter to the editor. *JAMA* 1984 May 11; 251 (18): 2348.

CHAPTER 35

Poison Ivy and Poison Oak Products

Henry Wormser

> **Questions to ask in patient assessment and counseling**
>
> - *How long have you had the rash?*
> - *Have you recently been exposed to any poisonous plants or to pets, sports equipment, or other items that may have been in contact with a poisonous plant?*
> - *Have you recently been walking in the woods, camping, or working in the garden?*
> - *Have you ever had a rash from poison ivy, poison oak, or poison sumac?*
> - *When did you notice the rash?*
> - *Where is the rash located? How extensive is it?*
> - *Would you describe the rash or affected skin?*
> - *Do the skin lesions contain fluid? Are the skin lesions oozing?*
> - *What treatments have you tried? Were they effective?*
> - *Are you allergic to any medication or product ingredient?*

Poison ivy, poison oak, or poison sumac dermatitis is a seasonal, allergic contact dermatitis that is often assessed by pharmacists and treated with nonprescription drugs. It may be acute or chronic, depending on the extent of the patient's exposure and the degree of the patient's sensitivity to the allergens.

Etiology

Causative Plants

There are more than 60 plants and parts of plants that may cause allergic reactions in hypersensitive individuals.[1]

The Anacardiaceae family of trees and shrubs, which contains both noxious and useful plants, grows in many parts of the world. It includes the Japanese lacquer tree (*Rhus verniciflua*), which grows in Japan, China, and Indochina and from which a rich furniture lacquer is obtained; the cashew nut tree (*Anacardium occidentale*), which grows in India, Pakistan, the East Indies, Africa, and Central and South America; and the mango tree (*Mangifera indica*), which grows in tropical areas. Cross-sensitivity may occur on skin contact with parts of or products from these plants, such as cashew nut shells or oil, mango rinds, and furniture painted with natural lacquer.

Four species of the Anacardiaceae family are most commonly encountered in the United States and cause the more severe cases of allergic contact dermatitis: poison ivy (*Toxicodendron radicans*), western poison oak (*Toxicodendron diversilobum*), eastern poison oak (*Toxicodendron quercifolium*), and poison sumac (*Toxicodendron vernix*).[2] Poison ivy, which grows as either a shrub or a trailing vine, is identified by its characteristic clusters of three lobe-shaped leaflets arranged on stalks; its white, ball-shaped berries that appear in the fall; and its usual climbing nature and hair roots when it appears as a vine (Figure 1). Abundant in North America, the plant grows everywhere in the United States except at altitudes above 4,000 feet and in Alaska, Hawaii, and desert areas of California and Nevada.

Poison oak has blunt-tipped leaflets, hairy on both sides, that cluster in threes. It commonly appears as either an unsupported, erect bush or a vine, and the center leaf of the cluster resembles an oak leaf. Western poison oak grows along the Pacific Coast from New Mexico to Canada. Eastern poison oak ranges from New Jersey to Florida and from central Texas to Kansas, growing in sandy soil (Figure 2).

Poison sumac, also known as poison dogwood or poison elder, has pointed, pale green leaves in 7- to 13-leaf clusters arranged on each side of a red-ribbed leaf stalk[3] (Figure 3). A coarse, woody shrub or small tree, it is commonly found in swamps and along ponds and streams of the southern and eastern United States.[4,5]

Formerly the species were assigned to the genus *Rhus*; hence, the term *rhus dermatitis* is used to describe the topical reactions caused by exposure to these plants. In the United States, poison ivy and poison oak are the main causes of rhus dermatitis. In England and western Europe, primrose dermatitis is more common than poison ivy dermatitis.[6]

Irrespective of the etiology (i.e., poison ivy, poison oak, or poison sumac), the dermatitides and treatments discussed in this chapter generally pertain to reactions to all three plants. Accordingly, unless otherwise noted, the following discussions of poison ivy also pertain to poison oak and poison sumac.

Allergenic Constituents

Toxicodendrol, a phenolic oily resin, is present in all the poisonous species and contains a complex active principle, urushiol. Urushiol is distributed widely in the roots, stems, leaves, and fruit of the plant, but not in the flowers, pollen, or epidermis.[7] Contact with the intact epidermis of

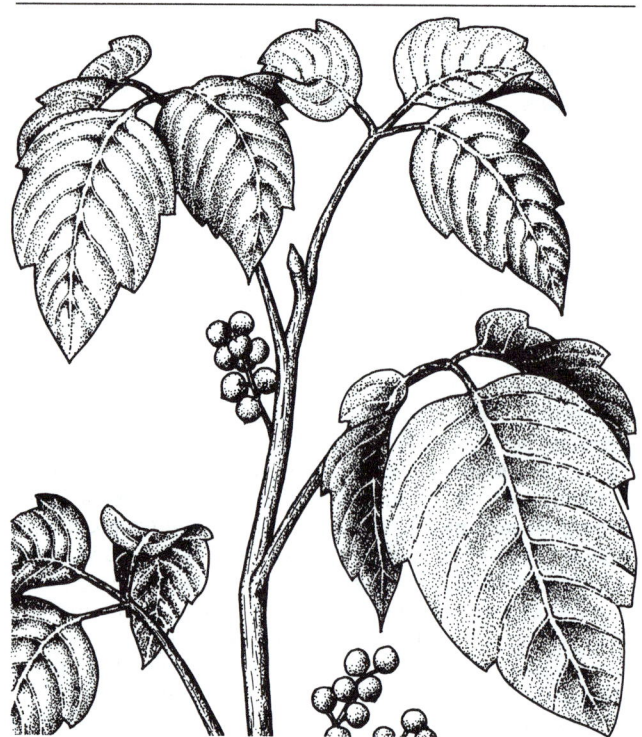

FIGURE 1 Poison ivy.

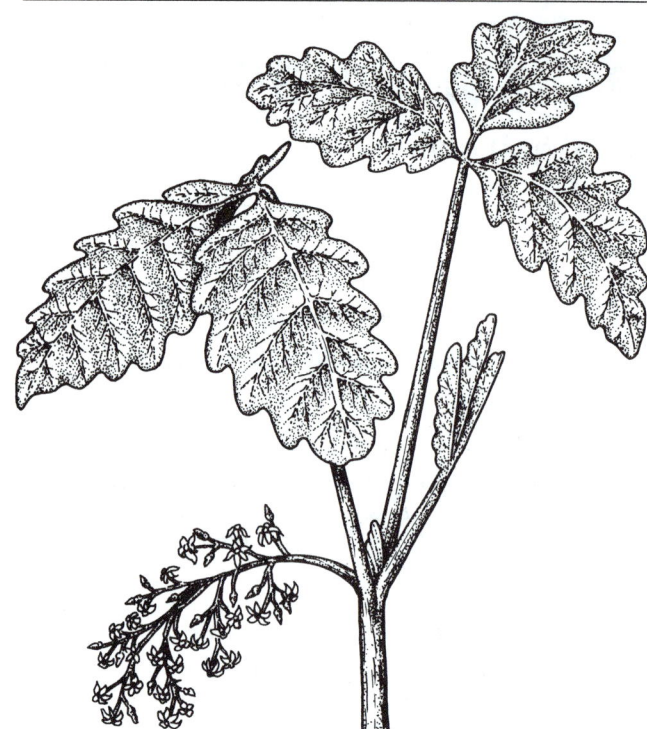

FIGURE 2 Poison oak.

the plant is harmless; dermatitis occurs only after contact with an injured plant or its sap. However, the epidermis of these plants is very fragile, and relatively minor friction or force will injure the plant. Dead and dried plants may be dangerous as well because their leaves and vines are also easily damaged.

Because neither toxicodendrol nor urushiol is volatile, the dermatitis cannot be contracted through the air unless the plants are burned. Smoke from burning plants carries a substantial amount of the irritating oleoresin and may cause serious external and systemic reactions in susceptible individuals. Inhalation may produce severe trauma to the oral and nasal mucosa and lung tissue.

Researchers have identified four allergens in poison ivy, the chemical structures of which have been identified and elucidated.[8–10] Although all four allergens possess a 1,2-dihydroxybenzene or pyrocatechol nucleus with either a 15- or a 17-carbon atom side chain at position 3, their chemical structures differ primarily by the degree of unsaturation of the alkyl side chains. The allergens include a saturated component (3-pentadecylcatechol, or 3-PDC); a mono-olefin; a diolefin; a triolefin; and a tetraolefin. The concentrations and ratios of these compounds vary considerably among species of toxicodendrol-containing plants and within different growing environments. The most reactive compounds are those containing one or more double bonds.[11] Certain individuals who are hypersensitive to 3-PDC show cross-reactivity with other compounds such as resorcinol, hexylresorcinol, and the hydroquinones, but not with phenol itself.[12]

As little as 1 mcg of crude urushiol may cause dermatitis in hypersensitive individuals.[13] Direct contact with the plant is not necessary; contact may be made with the allergens via an article that injured the plant or soot particles that contain allergenic material from the plant. The urushiol may be active for months on tools, sports equipment, shoes, and clothing, especially in a dry atmosphere. Stroking a pet whose fur is contaminated is also a common cause of allergic reaction.

Although the highest incidence of rhus dermatitis occurs in spring and summer, when the plant leaves are young, soft, and more easily injured, the dermatitis also occurs in autumn and winter.[3] In autumn, yellow leaves on the plant still have allergenic properties. Once they wither and fall, the leaves are much less allergenic. Winter episodes of the dermatitis often occur around Christmas in tree nursery employees and in people who cut their own trees; such episodes are caused by contact with the roots or vines of toxicodendron plants growing on the trees.

Mechanism of Contact Dermatitis

Development of a plant contact dermatitis requires that an individual be sensitized to the toxic agent by a previous exposure; therefore, an allergic reaction does not occur on first contact with the plant. Accordingly, contact dermatitis has two phases: a *sensitization* phase, during which a specific hypersensitivity to the allergen is acquired, and an *elicitation* phase, during which subsequent contact with the allergen elicits a visible dermatologic response.[14]

In the sensitization phase, components of the allergen urushiol are presumably oxidized to the o-quinone derivatives, which react readily with human epidermal proteins by nucleophilic addition to form complete antigens. More

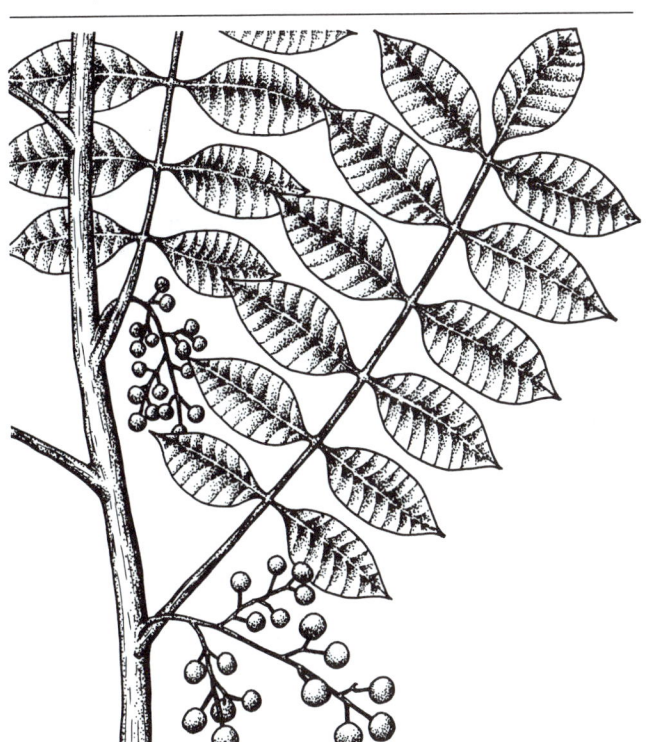

FIGURE 3 Poison sumac.

recent research suggests that the urushiol components go through a process of redox cycling and depletion of reducing equivalents to form reactive radical species, which serve as the ultimate haptenes.[15] Each allergen then leaves the skin through the lymphatic system and is carried to the reticuloendothelial system. There, in response to the antigenic stimulus, special globulins and antibodies are synthesized and T-lymphocytes are sensitized.

In the elicitation phase, repeated contact with the allergen again produces the antigenic conjugate, this time causing a noticeable reaction with the activated T-lymphocytes. The reaction appears to be triggered by the association of specific immunologic elements (effector cells and lymphokines) carried by the blood to the skin.

The degree of hypersensitivity to the toxic agent varies. Dark-skinned people seem less susceptible to the dermatitis. Young people are more susceptible than the elderly, and newborns are readily sensitized if they come in contact with sap from the plants.[1] The interval between contact with the allergen and the appearance of the rash and associated symptoms varies with the individual's degree of sensitivity, as well as with the amount of allergen contacted and the thickness of the skin at the site of contact. Reaction time—the time between contact with the allergen and the first sign of reaction—is usually 2 to 3 days but not less than 12 hours. This interval is characteristic of delayed hypersensitivity reactions involving cell-mediated immunity.

Dermatologic lesions vary from simple maculae to vesicles and bullae. Contrary to popular belief, fluid in the vesicles and bullae is not antigenic. Thus, patch tests with the fluid give negative results. Histologically, nonspecific inflammatory changes occur in the dermis; and edema, followed by intraepidermal vesicles, develops in the epidermis in the acute stage of the disease. Premature bursting of the vesicles may lead to secondary bacterial infection.

Symptoms and Assessment

Although the limbs, face, and neck are common sites of the dermatitis, all skin areas that come in contact with the allergen may be affected. Distribution of lesions may be bizarre, especially if the allergen is in the clothes or is transferred to various parts of the body by the fingers. The dermatitis may appear early in one area of the body and later in another. Often, parts of the body that are in contact with a heavy concentration of the antigen show more severe reactions and remain hypersensitive for several years. Similarly, areas where the skin is thicker (e.g., the palms of the hands or the soles of the feet) may take longer to erupt.

Poison ivy produces an allergic eczematous contact dermatitis. The initial reaction after exposure to the antigen is erythema or rash. The development of raised lesions (erythematous maculae and papules) follows, and finally, fluid accumulates in the raised lesions of the epidermis, forming vesicles and bullae. (See color plates, photographs 28A and B.) The lesions are more severe than those of dermatitides caused by other plants. The initial lesions are usually marked by mild to intensive itching and burning because of the fine nerve endings in the epidermis. The affected area, often hot and swollen, oozes and eventually dries and crusts.[16] Secondary bacterial infections may occur.

Most cases of the dermatitis are self-limiting and disappear in 14–20 days. Again, the duration of the dermatitis depends on the degree of sensitization and on the frequency and degree of reexposure to the allergen.

Chewing poison ivy leaves may result in edematous swelling and pain of the tongue, cheeks, palate, and pharynx. If the leaves are then swallowed, swelling and pain may occur in the anal region.[17] Very rare complications include eosinophilia, kidney damage, toxic shock syndrome, urticaria, erythema multiforme, dyshidrosis, marked pigmentation, and leukoderma (loss of melanin pigmentation occurring in patches).

Rhus dermatitis may be assessed not only from the morphologic appearance of its lesions but also from their distribution. Linear streaking is common and occurs naturally as the skin brushes against the poisonous plant. Because toxicodendron plants are not photosensitizers, the dermatitis can occur on covered and uncovered parts of the body.

Diagnostic patch testing is a valuable tool in investigating allergic contact dermatitis;[18-20] however, substances used in patch testing may sensitize the patient during testing. The currently accepted device for patch testing is a small aluminum disk, 8 mm in diameter, known as the Finn chamber. The Finn chamber is charged with a small ribbon of a petrolatum-based allergen or, if the allergen is a liquid, a small disk of filter paper containing one to several drops of the test allergen. (In the case of rhus oleoresin, a 1:50 solution in absolute alcohol is used.) The Finn chamber is then applied to the patient's back for 2 days with an adhesive, nonallergenic tape.[21] Patch testing should be performed only by allergists or other individuals thoroughly familiar with accepted techniques. It should never be done during the acute phase of any dermatitis. Furthermore, because approximately 75% of the U.S. population has been sensitized to urushiol, patch testing should not be a routine procedure. Also, patch testing results alone are not diagnostic. To interpret test results properly, practitioners must also consider the patient's history of exposure to the causative plants and any physical findings, as well as their own clinical experience.

Treatment

Prophylaxis

The best way to prevent any allergic contact dermatitis is to avoid the allergen completely. People should learn to recognize and avoid poison ivy and related plants. They should observe and search surrounding terrain carefully when hiking and before choosing a picnic area or campsite. Susceptible individuals should wear protective clothing (e.g., long sleeves, long pants, socks, and shoes) when exposure to the offending agents is probable. After an outing, they should carefully launder their clothing with a detergent and hot water. They should also wash with alcohol or another suitable organic solvent any object that may have come in contact with the plants to remove the oleoresin. As previously noted, any unremoved oleoresin will remain potent on the object's surface for a considerable time.

When a poisonous plant is in a garden or yard, it should be destroyed chemically or removed physically. Herbicide sprays may be used any time poison ivy is in full leaf, but June and July are the preferred months. Ordinarily, spraying should begin no later than mid-August because poison ivy begins to go dormant then and the herbicides are ineffective. At least three to four sprayings at intervals of 2–8 weeks are necessary to kill all the plants.[22] The herbicides most effective against poison ivy include amitrole (aminotriazole); ammonium sulfamate; (2,4-dichlorophenoxy) acetic acid (2,4-D); (2,4,5-trichlorophenoxy) acetic acid (2,4,5-T); ammonium thiocyanate; borax; carbon disulfide; coal tar; creosote oils; fuel oil and similar petroleum distillates (e.g., kerosene and diesel fuel); sodium chlorate; and sodium arsenite.

Applying herbicides is the easier and less dangerous method, but there are areas where they cannot be used (e.g., around some grasses, hedges, and shrubbery). In such situations, digging and pulling up the plants by the roots is the only satisfactory method of removal. Whichever method is chosen, individuals should always wear appropriate protective gear.

Should contact with poison ivy be made, however, its antigen enters the skin very rapidly. Thus, thorough washing with an alkaline soap or an organic solvent such as alcohol within 5–10 minutes of exposure is necessary to prevent absorption of the antigen. Another topical prophylactic measure includes the application of barrier creams prior to contact.[12] However, many investigators and clinicians question the effectiveness of barrier creams.[23–25]

Thirty-four barrier preparations were tested over a 2-year period on a group of people highly susceptible to rhus dermatitis.[12] The preparations contained substances such as potassium permanganate, hydrogen peroxide, sodium perborate, iodine, and iron and silver salts. The investigator concluded that none of the preparations could prevent the dermatitis. This suggests that the antigen reacts rapidly and quite selectively with the skin and that the antigen–antibody reaction occurs and progresses before effective preventive action can be taken. Although enthusiastic anecdotal claims have been made for zirconium oxide, an agent found in some nonprescription products, tests found it to be completely ineffective.[12] In addition, several researchers found that extensive, sarcoid-like granulomas of glabrous skin developed because of allergic hypersensitivity to insoluble zirconium oxide.[26–28] More recently, some success has been obtained with some formulations of organoclay (a quaternary ammonium salt of bentonite),[29] polyamine salts of linoleic acid dimer[30] (Stokoguard®), and a product marketed under the name Ivy Shield®.[31]

Hyposensitization Therapy

Specific hyposensitization may be tried by administering repeated doses of toxicodendron antigens. Various forms of these antigens, administered either by mouth or by intramuscular injection, have been used in hyposensitization therapy. For equivalent effects, however, larger amounts of the antigen are required orally than parenterally. Moreover, when taken orally, the antigen may undergo partial inactivation and imperfect absorption. Sustained release is probably the major factor in the superior efficacy of intramuscular antigen injection. Nevertheless, such prophylaxis is neither complete nor permanent, nor is it approved by the Food and Drug Administration (FDA). The original sensitivity returns approximately 6 months after the therapy ends.[32,33]

Hyposensitizing by administering crude extracts or oleoresins from the plants has also been generally ineffective. This is because potency of the extracts varies, and recommended dosages of the antigens are usually far below those required. Three or four injections cannot provide the clinical protection needed for moderately or extremely hypersensitive persons.

Because hyposensitization is temporary, maintenance doses of the antigen should be administered at predetermined intervals. Hyposensitization, if successful, results in milder and shorter reactions that are less likely to spread to other parts of the body. In fact, the only objective proof of successful hyposensitization is a negative or weak positive reaction to the antigens at a site that previously gave a strong positive reaction.

Administering an antigenic substance to hypersensitive individuals involves great risk. The exact course of treatment must be individualized to the person's sensitivity level and capacity to tolerate the antigen without serious allergic reactions. Further, the dermatitis must be diagnosed by a dermatologist before hyposensitization can begin. Prophylactic administration of toxicodendrol antigens has no effect on contact dermatitis caused by other substances. Finally, if the dermatitis appears during prophylactic treatment, the treatment should be stopped for the duration of the eruption.

Topical Treatment

The initial symptoms of the dermatologic reaction may be discomforting and alarming, and the temptation to treat them is strong. However, simplicity and safety are key elements of treatment. Many claims for products used for self-medication take credit for the body's own natural reparative and homeostatic processes; in most cases, the contact dermatitis is self-resolving. Thus, the major treatment objectives of therapy are to:

- Provide protection to the damaged tissue until the acute reaction has subsided;
- Prevent both excessive accumulation of debris and complications resulting from oozing, scaling, and crusting, without disturbing normal tissue;
- Relieve itching and thus prevent scratching, excoriation, and secondary bacterial infection.

Mild Dermatitis

Linear streaks of papules and vesicles often characterize mild poison ivy dermatitis. These lesions and their accompanying pain and itching can be treated by an antipruritic lotion such as calamine or zinc oxide. A combination of 1% menthol and equal parts of calamine, zinc oxide, and rubbing alcohol can be soothing.[34]

Soaks, baths, or wet dressings can also be effective in soothing pain and itching. A diluted (1:40) aluminum acetate solution (Burow's solution), a saline solution, or a sodium bicarbonate solution can be used in this manner for 30 minutes, three or four times a day. Burow's solution for topical use (USP) is usually a 1:10 or 1:40 dilution of aluminum acetate solution in water.[35] In addition, the application of either warm or very cold water may provide relief.

Topical preparations containing local anesthetics or antihistamines are available; however, their routine use is somewhat controversial because of their sensitizing capabilities. Nonprescription topical steroids, such as hydrocortisone 0.5–1%, are also available and have proven safe and effective for use in mild dermatitis.[36] Greasy ointments should not be used when vesicles are present and oozing.

Moderately Severe Dermatitis

Moderately severe poison ivy dermatitis is characterized by the presence of bullae and edematous swelling of affected body parts, in addition to the papules and vesicles present in milder cases. To reduce discomfort, large bullae may be drained by puncturing their edges with a sterilized needle; this should preferably be done by a trained medical professional. The tops of the lesions should be kept intact because they protect the underlying, denuded epidermis of the lesions as they dry. The patient should be reassured that fluid from the lesions will *not* spread the dermatitis and that the dermatitis is *not* contagious. Application of cool compresses of Burow's solution (1:10) to edematous areas may be helpful.

Lesions on the face can be treated by applying wet dressings. If the eyelids are affected, cold compresses of a dilute boric acid solution can be used.[1] Lotions should be avoided because they tend to cake, causing discomfort. Men may find that shaving, although uncomfortable, is more comfortable and aesthetic than accumulation of crust and debris in the beard.

During the healing phase, application of a soothing cream (e.g., Allercreme® or Aveeno Moisturizing Cream®) helps prevent crusting, scaling, and thickening of the lesions. It is important, however, that any such cream be neutral. Following exposure to a plant sensitizer, some patients may have a heightened sensitivity to various ingredients (e.g., dye, perfume, or preservatives) of a certain formulation; this may be particularly true of emulsions. In such cases, the patient reacts to the medication but may assume it is the poison ivy that is responsible. The response is to apply still more medication, which perpetuates the cycle.

Tepid tub baths using potassium permanganate, oatmeal, or a commercially available colloidal preparation (e.g., Aveeno®) may be soothing. After vesicles or bullae are opened, potassium permanganate is effective in drying the lesions and preventing secondary bacterial infection. However, the tendency of potassium permanganate solution to stain the skin purple has prevented its widespread use. The patient who does use it should be instructed to sit for 15–20 minutes in a tub full of lukewarm water to which 1 tsp of potassium permanganate crystals has been added.[1] To avoid skin burns, the crystals should be completely dissolved before the patient gets into the tub.

Colloidal oatmeal baths, two to six times daily, may be very soothing. However, because these preparations make the bathtub very slick, patients who use them should be warned to place a nonskid mat in the tub.

Severe Dermatitis

When the reaction is widespread over the body or is associated with major swelling or other reactions on or around the eyes, systemic treatment is recommended and the patient should be referred to a physician.

Topical treatment of severe poison ivy dermatitis is basically similar to that recommended for moderately severe dermatitis.[1] Physicians will often prescribe topical corticosteroids such as 0.1% betamethasone valerate (Valisone®), 0.05% betamethasone dipropionate (Diprosone®), 0.01% fluocinolone acetonide (Synalar®), or 0.1 or 0.5% triamcinolone acetonide (Aristocort® or Kenalog®). For facial lesions, however, a less potent drug such as 0.5–1.0% hydrocortisone is preferred because it is less likely to cause steroid-induced acne or atrophic changes in the skin with short-term use.

Systemic treatment usually involves prescription drugs such as anti-inflammatory steroids. Corticosteroids such as prednisone and methylprednisolone are commonly administered orally over 7 days to 3 weeks in a gradually descending dosage schedule. The starting dose should be based on the patient's age and ideal body weight. The tapering regimen is relatively safe because it is short term and does not lead to significant hypothalamic-pituitary-adrenal suppression.

Oral antihistamines such as diphenhydramine, chlorpheniramine, or tripelennamine may be useful for their systemic antipruritic effects.[1,37] However, the anticholinergic side effects of antihistamines could exacerbate preexisting conditions of patients who have prostatic hypertrophy, narrow-angle glaucoma, stenosing peptic ulcer, bladder neck obstruction, and a tendency toward constipation.

Respiratory emergencies resulting from inhalation of dust or smoke from burning plants are extremely rare except among forest firefighters, but such occurrences require immediate attention. Patients may experience shortness of breath, dyspnea, or stridor as a result of pharyngeal or laryngeal edema. Treatment should be directed toward maintaining a patent airway and administering intravenous corticosteroids.

Pharmacologic Agents

Four major types of pharmacologic agents—local anesthetics, antipruritics, antiseptics, and astringents—are used in topical nonprescription products for poison ivy dermatitis.

Local Anesthetics

Local anesthetics affect sensation by interfering with the transmission of impulses along sensory nerve fibers. Many nerve fibers, specialized endings (receptors), and free nerve endings are present in the epidermis. The topically applied anesthetics act only at the application site.

Benzocaine, diperodon hydrochloride, pramoxine hydrochloride, dibucaine, and tetracaine hydrochloride are the most common local anesthetics found in nonprescription products for poison ivy and poison oak. Poorly soluble local anesthetics (e.g., benzocaine) are less likely to be absorbed and to produce systemic toxicity than are more soluble local anesthetics (e.g., tetracaine hydrochloride). The high serum concentrations necessary to produce systemic toxicity are difficult to achieve with nonprescription topical anesthetics. If a contact dermatitis worsens after the topical application of a local anesthetic, the affected area should be washed thoroughly with mild soap and water, and use of the anesthetic should be discontinued. Side effects of topically applied local anesthetics can include dermatitis (characterized by cutaneous lesions), urticaria and edema, and anaphylactic reactions. (See Chapter 33, "Burn and Sunburn Products.")

Antipruritics

Topically applied antipruritics, including antihistamines, counterirritants, and hydrocortisone, are agents that help to alleviate itching.

Antihistamines
Antihistamines such as diphenhydramine (Benadryl®), pyrilamine, and tripelennamine (PBZ®) relieve the discomfort of itching by competing with histamine at the H_1 receptor (one of two broad classes of histamine receptors). They also produce a mild local anesthetic effect if applied topically. For instance, application of a 1 to 2% concentration of topical diphenhydramine to the affected area three times a day should relieve itching to a significant extent. The topical use of antihistamines does not produce anticholinergic adverse effects or systemic toxicity. However, like the "caine" anesthetics, antihistamines may, on rare occasions, act as sensitizers and aggravate a contact dermatitis.

Antihistamines are more effective as antipruritics when taken orally, particularly when itching is generalized. However, an individual who is sensitized to a topical agent should not take it orally.

Counterirritants
Counterirritants, which contain products such as menthol, phenol, and camphor, produce a sensation of coolness and reduce irritation. The sensation is difficult to explain because these chemicals produce local hyperemia and, when applied to severely damaged skin, may actually cause irritation. However, low concentrations of these drugs, particularly menthol, relieve irritation by the depression of cutaneous receptors. (See Chapter 32, "External Analgesic Products.")

Hydrocortisone
Hydrocortisone is a naturally occurring glucocorticoid manufactured endogenously in the adrenal cortex. Although topical corticosteroids are useful for a variety of dermatitides, their effectiveness on poison ivy dermatitis is equivocal. Steroids applied topically were previously implicated in the exacerbation of bacterial infections. However, the FDA's Advisory Review Panel on Over-the-Counter External Analgesic Drug Products reported that short-term topical use of 0.5–1% hydrocortisone is unlikely to exacerbate cutaneous bacterial, fungal, or viral infections. The panel also reported that allergic reactions to hydrocortisone at these concentrations are rare. Additionally, the panel found evidence that prolonged administration of 0.5–1% hydrocortisone did not appear to cause toxic effects by systemic absorption, even when applied to large areas of damaged or abraded skin.[38]

Nonprescription hydrocortisone products approved by the FDA for use on rashes and minor skin irritations carry the following label: "For the temporary relief of minor skin irritations, itching, and rashes due to eczema, dermatitis, insect bites, poison ivy, poison oak, poison sumac, soaps, detergents, cosmetics, and jewelry and for itchy genital and anal areas but not for ophthalmic use." The dosage for adults and children 2 years of age and above is 0.5–1% hydrocortisone applied to the affected area three or four times a day. Children under 2 years of age should be treated only under the advice and supervision of a physician.

Antiseptics

Antiseptics contained in poison ivy and poison oak products are intended for prophylaxis against secondary bacterial infections, but their effectiveness is questionable. Of the available antiseptics (e.g., phenols, alcohols, and oxidizing agents) and quaternary ammonium compounds (e.g., benzalkonium chloride), the latter seem to be more effective. Unfortunately, their activity is decreased by anionic compounds such as soaps.[39]

Astringents

Astringents, which include witch hazel, aluminum acetate, tannic acid, zinc and iron oxides, and potassium permanganate, are mild protein precipitants that are used to stop oozing, reduce inflammation, and promote healing of the dermatitis. They accomplish this either by forming a thick coagulum on the surface of lesions or by coagulating and removing overlying debris. The astringent action may be accompanied by contraction, wrinkling, and blanching of tissue. The cement substance of the capillary endothelium is hardened so that pathologic transcapillary movement of plasma proteins is inhibited, thus reducing local edema, inflammation, and exudation.

As noted previously, Burow's solution is generally diluted with water to produce a 1:10 or 1:40 solution and used as a wet dressing three or four times a day. Therapy may be continued for approximately 5–7 days. However, continuous or prolonged use for extended periods may be inflammatory. Because application of the concentrate can cause skin damage and pain, the pharmacist should make sure that the patient understands how to dilute Burow's solution.

Zinc oxide lotion (15–25%) has mild astringent, protective, and antiseptic actions. Calamine plus zinc oxide is often preferred over zinc oxide alone.

Potassium permanganate is most effective when applied as a dilute solution (1:10,000) on opened vesicles or bullae; however, it leaves an objectionable purple stain and may be very irritating if highly concentrated.[34]

Product Selection Guidelines

Selection of products depends on the severity of the dermatitis. Patients with severe cases of poison ivy dermatitis should consult a physician. However, mild to moderately severe cases can usually be treated with one or more topical products. Systemic use of antihistamines may be combined with application of topical agents to relieve itching. Preparations that contain benzocaine or other local anesthetics should be used with caution. Products that contain zirconium oxide should be avoided.

Lotions, which may contain phenol or menthol, provide prompt relief from itching. However, the pharmacist should caution against their frequent or excessive use. Lotions pile masses of plaster-like material on the skin, which may produce discomfort and can be difficult and painful to remove.

Finally, the pharmacist should inform individuals who are sensitive to toxicodendron plants that certain cosmetics, hair dyes, bleaches, and other commercial products contain compounds related to 3-PDC and could cause cross-sensitivity.

Summary

Every year poison ivy, poison oak, and poison sumac produce contact dermatitides in thousands of people. The best approach to treatment is prevention—avoiding contact with the offending plant. Once the dermatitis develops, symptomatic relief is the only therapy. A better understanding of the mechanism of the allergic reaction, cross-sensitivity, and hyposensitization will help in formulating products that are more effective in treating and in possibly eradicating this annoying and often serious disorder.

References

1. Fisher AA, Adams RM. *Contact Dermatitis*. 3rd ed. Philadelphia: Lea and Febiger; 1986: 405–17.
2. Lesser MA. Poison ivy. *Drug Cosmet Ind* 1952 May; 70: 610–1.
3. Dawson CR. The chemistry of poison ivy. *Trans NY Acad Sci* 1956; 18: 427–43.
4. Marderosian AHD. Poison ivy and related dermatitis. *Drug Ther* 1977 Aug; 112: 57–74.
5. Vietmeyer N. Science has got its hands on poison ivy, oak and sumac. *Smithsonian* 1985; 16: 89–95.
6. Rook A, Wilson HTH. Primula dermatitis. *Brit Med J* 1965 Jan 23; 5429: 220–2.
7. Doyle JH. Poison ivy dermatitis. *Pediatr Clin N Amer* 1961; 8: 259–63.
8. Sunthankar SV, Dawson CR. The structural identification of the olefinic components of Japanese lac urushiol. *J Am Chem Soc* 1954; 76: 5070–4.
9. Symes WF, Dawson CR. Poison ivy "urushiol." *J Am Chem Soc* 1954; 76: 2959–63.
10. Loev B, Dawson CR. The geometrical configuration of the olefinic components of poison ivy urushiol. The synthesis of a model compound. *J Am Chem Soc* 1956; 78: 1180–3.
11. Gross M et al. Urushiols of poisonous Anacardiaceae. *Phytochemistry* 1975; 4: 2263.
12. Kligman AM. Poison ivy (rhus) dermatitis. *Arch Dermatol* 1958; 77: 149–80.
13. Stevens FA. Status of poison ivy extracts. *JAMA* 1945 Apr 7; 127: 912–21.
14. Epstein, WL. In: Fitzpatrick TB et al., eds. *Dermatology in General Medicine*. New York: McGraw-Hill; 1979: 1373–83.
15. Schmidt RJ, Khan L, Chung LY. Are free radicals and not quinones the haptenic species derived from urushiols and the other contact allergenic mono- and dihydric alkylbenzenes? The significance of NADH, glutathione, and redox cycling in the skin. *Arch Dermatol Res* 1990; 282 (1): 56–64.
16. Selfon PM. The treatment of acute poison ivy dermatitis among our military field personnel. *Milit Med* 1963 Sep; 128: 895–900.
17. Silvers SH. Stomatitis venenata and dermatitis of anal orifice from chewing poison ivy leaves (Rhus toxicodendron). *JAMA* 1941 May 17; 116: 2257.
18. Kligman AM. The identification of contact allergens by human assay: I. A critique of standard methods. *J Invest Dermatol* 1966 Nov; 47: 369–74.
19. Kligman AM. The identification of contact allergens by human assay. II. Factors influencing the induction and measurement of allergic contact dermatitis. *J Invest Dermatol* 1966 Nov; 47: 375–92.
20. Kligman AM. The identification of contact allergens by human assay: III. The maximization test: a procedure for screening and rating contact sensitizers. *J Invest Dermatol* 1966 Nov; 47: 393–409.
21. Rietschel RL. Contact dermatitis and diagnostic techniques. *Allergy Proc* 1989 Nov–Dec; 10 (6): 403–11.
22. Crooks DM, Kephart LW. *Farmers' Bulletin*. Pub. No. 1972. Washington DC: U.S. Department of Agriculture; 1951: 30.
23. Shelmire B. Contact dermatitis from weeds; patch testing with

their oleoresins. *JAMA* 1939 Sep 16; 113: 1085–90.
24. Gisvold O. Effect of some absorbents, precipitants and oxidants upon resin of Rhus toxicodendron. *J Am Pharm Assoc, Scientific Edition* 1941 Jan; 30: 17–8.
25. Howell JB. Evaluation of measures for prevention of ivy dermatitis. *Arch Dermatol & Syph* 1943 Oct; 48: 373–8.
26. LoPresti PJ, Hambrick GW Jr. Zirconium granuloma following treatment of rhus dermatitis. *Arch Dermatol* (Chicago) 1965 Aug; 92: 188–91.
27. Epstein WL, Allen JR. Granulomatous hypersensitivity after use of zirconium-containing poison oak lotion. *JAMA* 1964 Dec 7; 190 (10): 940–2.
28. Hall NA. O-T-C products for rhus dermatitis—zirconium-containing topical application. *J Am Pharm Assoc* 1972 Nov; 12: 576–7.
29. Epstein WL. Topical prevention of poison ivy/oak dermatitis. *Arch Dermatol* 1989 Apr; 125 (4): 499–501.
30. Orchard SM, Fellman JH, Storrs FJ. Poison ivy/oak dermatitis: Use of polyamine salts of a linoleic acid dimer for topical prophylaxis. *Arch Dermatol* 1986; 122: 783–9.
31. Basiliere D. Personal communication of unpublished research on Ivy Shield. Haverhill, Mass: Interpro, Inc; 1989.
32. Kligman AM. Hyposensitization against rhus dermatitis. *Arch Dermatol* 1958; 78: 47–72.
33. Kligman AM. Cashew nut shell oil for hyposensitization against rhus dermatitis. *Arch Dermatol* 1958; 78: 359–63.
34. Fowler JF. In: Rakel RE, ed. *Conn's Current Therapy*. Philadelphia: W. B. Saunders Co; 1992: 786–7.
35. Skin protectant drug products for over-the-counter human use; astringent drug products. *Federal Register* 1989 Apr 3; 54: 13480–99.
36. du Vivier AWP. Over-the-counter hydrocortisone. *Practitioner* 1986; 230: 897–900.
37. Bond CA. In: Young LY, Koda-Kimble MA, eds. *Applied Therapeutics: The Clinical Use of Drugs*. 4th ed. Vancouver, Wash: Applied Therapeutics Inc; 1988: 1413–4.
38. Hydrocortisone: Marketing status as external analgesic drug product for over-the-counter human use; notice of enforcement policy. *Federal Register* 1991 Aug 30; 156: 43025.
39. Apted JH. Poison ivy dermatitis in Victoria [letter]. *Australas J Dermatol* 1978 Apr; 19 (1): 35–6.

CHAPTER 36

Insect Sting and Bite Products

Farid Sadik

> **Questions to ask in patient assessment and counseling**
>
> ■ *How extensive are the bites or stings on your body?*
> ■ *Have you developed hives, excessive swelling, dizziness, vomiting, or difficulty in breathing since being bitten or stung?*
> ■ *Have you previously had severe reactions to insect bites or stings?*
> ■ *What have you tried so far, if anything, to treat the reaction?*
> ■ *Have you ever had adverse reactions to topically applied products?*
> ■ *Do you have a personal or family history of allergic reactions such as hay fever?*
> ■ *If a child, what is the patient's age and approximate weight?*

Summertime outdoor activists such as gardeners, beach goers, hunters, fishermen, and hikers, as well as individuals whose occupation requires them to remain outdoors and even those who spend time in their back yard are at risk of insect bites and stings. An insect bite or sting is an injury to the skin caused by penetration of the biting or stinging organ of an insect. The reactions are produced mainly by substances contained in the saliva of biting insects or in the venom of stinging insects. Although the pain associated with the skin penetration is brief, the aftereffects vary according to the degree of exposure and hypersensitivity. For the vast majority of Americans, the reactions to these injuries are mild and local in nature, and may compel those who have been injured to seek their pharmacist's advice in selecting a nonprescription product that provides symptomatic relief from the resultant local reactions. However, for more than 2 million persons who are allergic to the insect venom, the reaction can be severe and possibly life-threatening.

Types of Injuries

Biting Insects/Arachnids

Insects such as mosquitoes, fleas, bedbugs, arachnids such as ticks and chiggers ("red bugs"), and lice bite their prey. They insert their biting organs into the skin to feed by sucking blood from their hosts (see color plates, photograph 29).

Mosquitoes

Mosquitoes usually attack exposed parts of the body (face, neck, forearms, and legs). They can, however, bite through thin clothing. When a mosquito alights on the skin, it cuts through the skin with its mandibles and maxillae. A fine, hollow, needle-like, flexible structure (proboscis) is introduced into the cut and probes the tissue for a blood vessel. Blood is sucked directly from a capillary lumen or from previously lacerated capillaries with extravasated blood. During feeding, the mosquito injects into the wound a salivary secretion containing an anticoagulant and antigenic components, which cause the itching.

Fleas

Fleas are tiny (1.5–4 mm long), bloodsucking, wingless, laterally compressed parasites with strongly developed posterior legs used for leaping. Fleas parasitize various avian and mammalian hosts. Most people are bitten about the legs and ankles. Bites usually are multiple and grouped and cause intense itching. Each lesion is characterized by an erythematous region around the puncture. Fleas not only are annoying but are responsible for transmitting diseases such as bubonic plague and endemic typhus. Fleas are found throughout the world (including arctic regions) but breed best in warm areas with relatively high humidity. They may survive and multiply without food for several weeks. Places that have been vacant for weeks may be heavily infested, partly because of the hatching of eggs, which are usually deposited in floor crevices or on rugs, particularly those on which pets have been sleeping.

Bedbugs

Bedbugs have a short head and a broad, flat body (4 to 5 mm long and 3 mm wide). Their mouth parts consist of two pairs of stylets used to pierce the skin. The outer part has barbs that saw the skin, and the inner part is used to suck blood and to allow salivary secretions to flow into the wound. Depending on the severity of the reaction and subsequent bullous papules, itching on an occasional small dermal hemorrhage is present at the puncture site. Bedbugs usually hide and deposit their eggs in crevices of walls, floors, picture frames, bedding, and other furniture. They normally hide during the day, become active at night, and bite their sleeping victims. Persons may also be bitten in subdued light by day while sitting in theaters or other public places. A bedbug can engorge itself with blood within 3–5 minutes, and then typically seeks its hiding place.

This chapter is based in part on the chapter with the same title that appeared in the 9th edition but was written by Farid Sadik and Jeffrey C. Delafuente.

Chiggers

Chiggers are very annoying pests. Only the chigger larvae, which are nearly microscopic, attack the host by attaching to the skin and sucking blood. Once in contact with the skin, the larvae insert their mouth parts into the skin and secrete a digestive fluid that causes cellular disintegration of the affected area and intense itching. Chiggers do not burrow in the skin; however, as a result of the injected fluid, the skin hardens and a tube is formed. The chigger lies in this tube and continues to feed until engorged, after which it drops off and changes into an adult. Chiggers are prevalent in southern parts of the United States mainly during summer and fall. They usually live in wooded areas, grass, and brush.

Lice

Lice are wingless parasites with well-developed legs. They do not jump like fleas and do not fly. Each leg has a claw that helps the louse cling firmly to hair or clothing fibers while sucking blood. An adult louse inserts its mouth in the skin and injects anticoagulant saliva to allow the flow of blood into the mouth. It feeds for 30–45 minutes every 3 to 4 hours. Thus, depending on the extent of the infestation, the host may receive hundreds of bites each day.

Lice infestations (pediculosis) in the United States are common.[1] Three types of lice infest humans: head lice (*Pediculus humanus capitis*), body lice (*Pediculus humanus corporis*) and pubic lice (*Phthirus pubis*).

Head Lice

Head lice is the most common lice infestation,[2] affecting more than 10 million Americans annually. The vast majority of cases involve children 1–12 years of age, and the outbreaks usually occur between the months of August and November.[3] Outbreaks of lice infestations are common in crowded places such as schools, day care centers, and nursing homes, particularly if hygienic conditions are poor.

Head lice usually infest the head and live on the scalp (see color plates, photographs 30A and B).[4] The female deposits 10–150 eggs (nits), which become glued to the hair and hatch in 5–10 days. The nit is about 5 mm in diameter and has yellowish or grayish-white color. Once hatched, the louse must begin the feeding process within 24 hours or it dies. The nymph (newly hatched immature louse) resembles an adult and matures within 8 to 9 days. The lifespan of an adult is about 1 month. The nymph is active and tends to move about the head, whereas the adults are less active.

Transmission of head lice occurs directly through physical contact with an infested individual or indirectly through the sharing of articles such as combs, brushes, towels, caps, and hats.[5] Awareness and action by health officials, school authorities, and parents is essential in stopping the spread of lice. Pharmacists can be effective in this regard and can obtain information on safe treatments and preventive measures for head lice from the National Pediculosis Association, P.O. Box 149, Newton, MA 02161, (617-449-NITS).

Head lice may be diagnosed by examining the hair for nits, nymphs, or crawling adults. Examination is best done under strong light,[6] and a magnifying glass may be used. Parting the hair with a comb or with fingers protected by gloves may help reveal the nits that are found attached to the hair and will not brush or comb off with a regular comb. The nits are laid on the hair shaft close to the scalp. Because hair grows at a relatively constant rate of approximately one-half inch per month, the duration of infestation may be estimated by measuring the distance of the nit from the scalp surface.

Head lice infestation often causes itching, a reaction to the bites or fecal deposits of the lice. Scratching the irritation may result in excoriation of the scalp tissue and, possibly, a secondary bacterial or fungal infection. In some instances, pyoderma results, characterized by erythema, crusting, and oozing on the scalp and hair margins. In severe cases, the patient may suffer from swollen glands and mild fever. Prolonged and frequent exposure to bites may lead to immunity, and the infected person may experience little or no reaction to bites.

Treatment is initiated following diagnosis. Currently, there are pediculicides that are available in both prescription and nonprescription products.

In 1986 the Food and Drug Administration (FDA) approved 1% permethrin cream rinse as a prescription drug[7] and has recently approved it as a nonprescription drug. The 1% permethrin cream rinse is the drug of choice for treating head lice in adults and in children 2 years of age and older, and it may be used in treating pubic lice.[8,9] A study has shown that the cure rate following its application is higher than that following application of 1% gamma benzene hexachloride (lindane). Permethrin is a synthetic pyrethroid that acts on the nerve cell membrane of the lice, causing delayed repolarization and paralysis.[10] Its pediculicidal and ovicidal activities as well as its residual persistence on the hair result in eradicating the head lice and preventing reinfestation. There is a cure rate of up to 99% in patients with head lice following a single application. Some patients may require a second application 7 days after the initial treatment.

Before permethrin cream rinse is applied, the hair should be shampooed with regular shampoo, rinsed, and dried. Enough of the undiluted liquid (25–30 mL) is then applied to saturate the hair and scalp and allowed to remain there for 10 minutes. Next, the medication is rinsed out with water, and the hair is towel dried. A specially designed comb, which is included in the package, may be used to remove the nits and nits' shells. The main adverse reaction to permethrin is transient pruritus, burning, stinging, and irritation to the scalp. Permethrin should not be used on infants under 2 years of age or on individuals who are sensitive to pyrethroid, pyrethrin, or chrysanthemums.

Gamma benzene hexachloride possesses pediculicidal and ovicidal activities and is available as a 1% shampoo for treating head and pubic lice. However, extreme caution should be exercised in its use because accidental oral ingestion or overdosing may cause central nervous system stimulation and seizures. The shampoo should not be applied to the face, eyelashes, or eyebrows. Because of its neurotoxicity, the shampoo should not be used on a daily basis. When used according to directions, a single shampooing poses no health hazard because the level of gamma benzene hexachloride in the blood is very low.

The proper use of the shampoo requires that any oil-based hair dressing be removed before applying the shampoo because oil may enhance absorption of the drug. Enough shampoo (30–60 mL) is applied to the hair along with enough water to form good lather. The lather is allowed to remain for 4 minutes, after which the hair is rinsed thoroughly and towel dried. When the shampoo is used to treat pubic lice, simultaneous treatment of sexual contacts is recommended.

The pyrethrins are insecticides extracted from *Chrysanthemum cinerariafolium*, and they exert their paralyzing effect by disrupting the nervous transmission in the insect. Pyrethrins are effective in concentrations ranging from 0.17%–0.33%, but they lose their potency within 12–24 hours owing to their instability in light. Pyrethrins are usually combined with 2–4% piperonyl butoxide, a chemical that has no insecticidal activity but potentiates the lethal action of the pyrethrins by blocking detoxification of the drug by the insect. These pediculicides are available in gel, liquid, and shampoo formulations. The medication is applied to the infested area and allowed to remain in place for no less than 10 minutes; it is then thoroughly washed out with warm water. Pyrethrins rarely produce any adverse reactions. However, contact with eyes and mucous membranes should be avoided.

Malathion is an organophosphorous compound that acts as a cholinesterase inhibitor. In addition to being an effective pediculicide and ovicide, it slowly bonds to the hair to provide enough residual effect to prevent reinfestation. It is available in 0.5% lotion containing 78% isopropyl alcohol. Consequently, caution must be exercised not to apply the medication near open flames or hair dryers. Malathion is recommended for adults and children 2 years of age and older. However, pregnant women and nursing mothers should avoid using the medication. The lotion is applied to the hair until the hair is moistened, and it is allowed to remain in place for 8–12 hours, after which the hair is shampooed, rinsed, and towel dried. A fine-toothed comb may be used to remove dead lice and nits. The main disadvantage of malathion is its unpleasant odor and the long contact time required with the scalp to exert its activity.

Body Lice Body lice live, hide, and lay their eggs in clothing, particularly in seams and folds of underclothing. These insects are larger than head lice and twice as long. Consequently, more eggs (300) are laid by the female body louse. Diagnosis of body lice can be made by identifying the adult lice and nits in the seams of clothing. Intense body itching and the scratching it triggers should also provide a clue for the presence of the infestation. Treatment of body lice is similar to that of head lice. However, body lice may be eradicated by measures other than medications. Washing clothing with hot water (125°F [52°C]) or disinfecting them with dry cleaning is effective. Changing clothing and underclothing daily as well as bathing daily should then rid the body of these lice. To relieve itching, an antipruritic lotion may be applied.

Pubic Lice Pubic lice, commonly called crab lice because of their crablike appearance, may be encountered in all persons, even those with high standards of hygiene. An infestation of pubic lice is identified by the presence of the parasite and its nits. The lice are usually found in the pubic area but may infest armpits and occasionally eyelashes, mustaches, beards, and eyebrows. They may be transmitted through sexual contact, toilet seats, or shared undergarments and sheets. A female adult pubic louse deposits 50 eggs during her lifetime. Treatment of pubic lice is similar to that of head lice.

Sarcoptes scabiei

Scabies, commonly called "the itch," is a contagious parasitic skin infestation caused by the arachnid mite *Sarcoptes scabiei*, which burrows beneath the stratum corneum but neither bites nor stings. Characterized by secondary inflammation and intense itching, this infestation is often associated with poor hygiene, crowded conditions, and venereal disease. Scabies is transmitted through bodily contact with an infested host, clothing, or bed linen. An infected person may easily spread the disease to other family members. It is also possible to acquire scabies from a toilet seat. The female mite, which is responsible for causing scabies, is transmitted readily by close personal contact with an infected person. Once on the skin, the impregnated female burrows into the stratum corneum with her jaws and the first two pairs of legs, forming tunnels in which she lays eggs and excretes fecal matter. In a few days, the hatched larvae form their own burrows and develop into adults. The adult mites copulate, and the impregnated females burrow into the stratum corneum to start a new life cycle. The most common infestation sites are the interdigital spaces of the fingers, the flexor surface of the wrists, the external male genitalia, the buttocks, and the anterior axillary folds (see color plates, photograph 31). The head and neck are not affected, except in infants. Intense itching caused by scabies, especially at night, occurs at the infestation site. Unrestrained scratching may cause secondary bacterial infections, such as excoriation and impetigo, furuncles, or cellulitis. Scabies diagnosis may be made by identifying the mite under a microscope and the burrow in the skin. The burrow (<1 cm long) is visible to the naked eye and appears as a narrow, slightly raised dark line.

Scabies may be controlled by using any of the following treatments: 25% benzyl benzoate lotion, 1% gamma benzene hexachloride cream or lotion, 5% permethrin cream, or 10% crotamiton lotion or cream. Before applying the medication, the patient should bathe, vigorously scrubbing the infested area. The preparation should then be applied to the entire body except the face and should remain in place for a specified period of time, after which the patient should bathe again. A second application is usually unnecessary but may sometimes be required.

Ticks and Lyme Disease

Ticks are arachnid parasites that feed on the blood of humans and of both wild and domesticated animals. During feeding, the tick's mouth parts are introduced into the skin, enabling it to hold firmly. If the tick is removed, the mouth parts are torn from the tick and remain embedded, causing intense itching and nodules (see color plates, photograph 32). If the tick is left attached to the skin, it becomes fully engorged with blood and remains for as long as 10 days before it drops off.

Certain species of ticks can transmit systemic disease such as Lyme disease. This disease was first recognized in 1975 when a number of juvenile rheumatoid arthritis cases occurred in Lyme, Connecticut; it was described and named by Dr. Allen Steere in 1977.[11] Five years later, Dr. Willy Burgdorf recognized that Lyme disease is a systemic infection caused by a spirochete found in *Ixodes dammini* (deer ticks) and is transmitted into the victim following tick bites. The spirochetes, which were named *Borrelia burgdorferi*, appear as irregular coils that range from 10–30 microns in length and 0.18–0.25 microns in diameter.

TABLE 1	Properties of Hymenoptera venom components					
	Histamine	**Melitin**	**Apamin**	**MCD-peptide**	**Hyaluronidase**	**Phospholipase A**
Pain production	+	+	?	?	0	?
Increased capillary permeability	+	+	+	+	I	+
Smooth muscle contraction	+	+	0	0	0	+
Histamine release	0	+	0	+	0	+
Cellular damage	0	+	?	+	0	+
Antigenic	0	+	?	?	+	+

Key:
+ means indicated reaction occurs.
0 means indicated reaction does not occur.
? means indicated reaction is not demonstrated.
I means indicated reaction occurs indirectly.

The deer tick lives in wooded areas and parasitizes white-tailed deer (the primary carrier), mice, dogs, squirrels, and other mammals including humans. *I. dammini* is very small compared with dog ticks; it is about one-eighth of an inch in diameter and thus is difficult to find when it parasitizes animals. (See Figure 1 for the life cycle of the deer tick.) The tick inserts its mouth piece into its prey to suck blood. During the feeding process, *B. burgdorferi* are released at the bite site and spread throughout the body hematogenously to initiate the infection.[12]

Most of the acute stages of the infection are heralded by a skin rash known as erythema migrans and by flu-like symptoms. The rash appears first as a papule at the bite site and gradually spreads to various parts of the body. The lesions are usually urticarial in nature and tender. They disappear spontaneously within 3 to 4 weeks, but when they are treated with antibiotics, remission occurs within several days. The flulike symptoms include fever, muscle and joint pain, and, in severe cases, conjunctivitis. If left untreated, neurologic (aseptic meningitis, headache, stiff neck, paresis, paresthesias), cardiac (tachycardia), and musculoskeletal symptoms may develop and may last up to several months. The last symptoms and the most durable ones are arthritis and the appearance of red discoloration of the skin of the hands, wrists, feet, or ankles.

Lyme disease can be diagnosed by studying the medical history of the patient and conducting laboratory examinations such as enzyme-linked immunosorbent assays, immunoblotting technique, and indirect fluorescent antibody. Early diagnosis and prompt treatment of Lyme disease can prevent the development of neurologic, cardiac, and rheumatologic manifestations. The disease is treated with antibiotics such as tetracycline, doxycycline, amoxicillin, and cephalosporins. Lyme disease can be prevented by (1) avoiding areas that may be infested with deer ticks, especially during the spring and summer months; (2) applying insect repellent containing *N,N*-diethyl-*m*-toluamide (DEET) on the skin as well as on shoe tops and socks; (3) applying the pesticide permethrin only on clothes; and (4) treating pets regularly with insecticides.

Stinging Insects/Hymenoptera

Stinging insects belonging to the order Hymenoptera (membranous wings) are most often responsible for insect sting hypersensitivity. Among the three families commonly involved are the Apidae, including honeybees (genus *Apis*); the Vespidae, including paper wasps (genus *Polistes*), yellow jackets, and hornets (genus *Vespa*); and the Formicidae, including imported fire ants (genus *Solenopsis*) and harvester ants (genus *Pogonomyrmes*). Although they are small, these insects have a venom as potent as that of snakes. However, death from an insect sting is the result of an anaphylactic reaction and usually occurs within 5–30 minutes, whereas death from a snakebite usually is not associated with hypersensitivity and occurs within 3 hours to several days. In the United States more people die from insect stings than from bites of other poisonous animals combined.

The stinging insects are nonparasitic and attack only to defend themselves or to kill other insects. They inject the venom into their victims through a piercing organ (stinger), a modified ovipositor delicately attached to the rear of the female's abdomen. (Males do not have an ovipositor and consequently are stingless.) The stinger consists of two lancets made of highly chitinous material and separated by the poison canal. The venom flows through the canal from the venom sac attached to the stinger's dorsal section. The tip of the stinger, which is directed posteriorly, has sharp barbs, and the base enlarges into a bulblike structure. Most species of bees and wasps have two types of venom glands under the last abdominal segment. The larger gland secretes an acidic toxin directly into the venom sac; the smaller one, at the base of the sac, secretes a less potent alkaline toxin. The injected venom is usually a mixture of the two toxins.

When the honeybee stings, it attaches firmly to the skin with tiny, sharp claws at the tip of each foot, arches its abdomen, and immediately jabs the barbed stinger into the skin. The barbs firmly embed the stinger, and when the honeybee pulls away or is brushed off, the entire stinging apparatus (stinger, appendages, venom sac, and glands) is detached from the bee's abdomen. The disemboweled bee later dies. The abandoned stinger, driven deeper into the skin by rhythmic contractions of the venom sac's smooth muscle wall, continues to inject venom. Honeybees are most commonly found in the western and midwestern United States. Wild honeybees usually nest in hollow tree trunks.

The stinging mechanism of wasps, hornets, and yellow jackets resembles that of the honeybee except that the stingers are not barbed. The stingers can be withdrawn easily after the venom is injected, enabling these insects to survive and sting repeatedly. Paper wasps, hornets, and yellow jackets are more commonly found in the southcentral and southwestern United States. Paper wasps tend to nest in high places, under eaves of houses, or on branches of high trees, whereas hornets prefer to nest in hollow spaces, especially hollow trees. Yellow jackets, considered the most common stinging culprits, usually nest in low places such as burrows in the ground, cracks in walls, or small shrubs.

Some ants only bite; others bite and sting simultaneously. Stinging ants (fire ants) use their mandibles to cling to the skin of their prey; then they bend their abdomen, sting the flesh, and empty the contents of their poison vesicle into the wound. Because they use their mandibles, it is often believed that the bite causes the reaction. Fire ants, commonly found in the southern and western United States, live in underground colonies.

Types of Reactions

Reactions to Biting Insects

Reactions to biting insects are usually local although the pathogenesis of these reactions has not been well characterized. Some species of mosquitoes have agglutinin and anticoagulant agents in their salivary secretions; others have neither.

Many attempts have been made to identify the antigenic factors in mosquito bites by studying whole mosquito extracts. Extracts from *Aedes aegypti* were shown by paper chromatography to contain at least four fractions that can produce skin reactions. Eluates of each constituent caused positive reactions in sensitized individuals. Eighteen amino acids have been identified in the extracts of all species of mosquitoes.

Reactions to mosquito bites vary in intensity. Wheal formation, erythema, papular reaction, and itching are characteristic. Hypersensitivity to mosquito bites aggravated by scratching causes papule and nodule formations that may persist and lead to secondary infections such as impetigo, furunculosis, or infectious eczematoid dermatitis. The bite site may influence reaction intensity; bites on the ankles and legs are more severe than bites elsewhere on the body because of the relative circulatory stasis in the legs. Consequently, the tendency toward vesiculation, hemorrhage, eczematization, and ulceration is greater in these areas. Systemic reactions such as fever and malaise also are common.

Allergic Reactions to Stinging Insects

In the past decade, significant progress has been made in understanding the pathogenesis of allergic reactions to the Hymenoptera order of insects. Venoms from these insects have been purified and analyzed. Their mechanisms for causing severe reactions have been investigated, and they are now being used to diagnose and treat allergic reactions to insect stings.

Hymenoptera venom contains a number of allergenic proteins as well as several pharmacologically active molecules. The contents of venoms vary among different families within the Hymenoptera order. Therefore, venoms are discussed here in general terms.

The major antigenic proteins are the enzymes hyaluronidase and phospholipase A. Hyaluronidase breaks down hyaluronic acid, which is the binding agent in connective tissue. By altering tissue structure, hyaluronidase acts as a spreading factor, allowing for enhanced penetration of venom substances. Phospholipase A attacks phospholipids in cell membranes. It also contracts smooth muscle, causes hypotension, increases vascular permeability, and destroys mast cells.

Studies have shown that 50–100% of individuals with a history of local or systemic reactions to insect stings will have demonstrable immunoglobulin E (IgE) antibody to venom constituents. The variability among studies in detecting IgE may be due to differences in laboratory techniques and the lack of positive identification of the insect eliciting the reaction. Studies further show that the presence of venom-specific IgE in the sera of patients who have local reactions correlates with the duration of the reaction.

Other venom components include histamine, melitin, apamin, and mast cell degranulating peptide. Of these, only melitin is antigenic, and not all individuals make antibodies against it. Although these mediators do not directly contribute to insect sting anaphylaxis, they do affect the rate at which venom antigens become available to the systemic circulation following a sting. These molecules have direct and indirect effects on mast cell mediator release, vascular permeability, and smooth muscle contractions. Table 1 summarizes the pharmacologic actions of the venom constituents.

Reactions to insect stings range from small local reactions limited to the sting site to systemic reactions leading to death. Several theoretical factors may explain why a local reaction occurs in one instance and a systemic reaction occurs in another. The dose of venom injected at each sting may vary, thereby varying the amount of antigen entering the body. The location of the sting may also influence the type of reaction. Head and neck stings may cause more laryngeal edema, whereas stings on extremities may produce only local reactions. A sting that limits the venom to the intradermal space may present as a local reaction; a sting on a capillary or venule would allow for

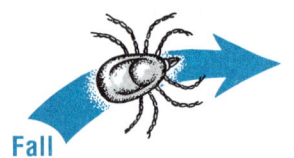
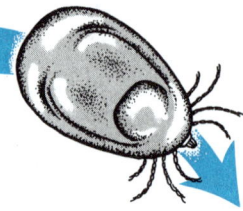

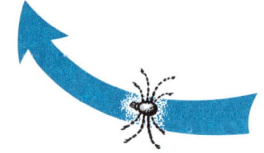
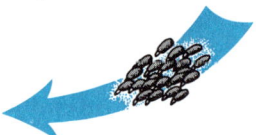

Fall/Winter/Spring
Adult ticks feed on deer and other large mammals.

Fall
Nymphs molt and become adult ticks. Adults may feed on dogs, people, and other mammals such as deer.

Early Spring
Female ticks drop off large mammals and lay eggs.

Spring/Summer
Nymphs emerge and feed on small mammals. While taking a blood meal, the tick may inject the Lyme disease bacteria into the small mammal. Later in the spring, newly hatched larvae will feed on these animals and become infected with the Lyme disease bacteria. Nymphs are likely to attach to people from May through July, making this the period in which most people acquire infections.

Late Spring/Summer
Larvae hatch from eggs and attach to mice and other small mammals and birds. Larvae may ingest Lyme disease bacteria as they feed. Before larvae find their first host, they are unlikely to carry Lyme disease bacteria.

Late Summer/Fall/Winter
Larvae molt and become nymphs. Nymphs overwinter without feeding.

FIGURE 1 Life cycle of the deer tick (*Ixodes dammini*). Reprinted from *Lyme Disease in Wisconsin: An Update*. Madison, Wisc: Wisconsin Department of Natural Resources and Department of Health and Social Services; 1989.

systemic injection of the venom and may present as a systemic reaction. Reactions may be divided into three categories: local, unusual, and anaphylactic.

Local Reactions

These reactions occur at the sting site. The manifestations are erythema and varying amounts of pain with symptoms lasting from several hours to several days. Swelling may extend from the sting site and cover an extensive area. Immune mechanisms have been implicated as the cause of the reaction in some patients. However, not all patients studied have shown evidence of immunologically mediated reactions.[13]

Unusual Reactions

Occasionally, unusual reactions follow insect stings. Neurologic reactions, renal involvement, serum sickness reactions, encephalopathy, and delayed hypersensitivity skin reactions have been reported. The mechanisms for these reactions have not been clearly elucidated, but immunologic causes have been implicated in some cases.

Anaphylactic Reactions

These reactions are immunologically mediated, usually occurring within 15 minutes after the sting. Most allergic reactions from insect stings are cutaneous. Symptoms include erythema, pruritus, urticaria (hives), or angioedema. The most serious sequelae from stings are systemic anaphylactic reactions. In severe reactions, hypotension, laryngeal edema, bronchospasm, and respiratory distress may occur, leading to a shocklike state. If not treated promptly, death may ensue. Less common anaphylactic reactions may produce nausea, vomiting, or diarrhea.

Anaphylactic reactions are mediated by IgE antibodies that bind to the specific antigens (allergens) causing the reaction. The insect sting antigens are proteins and glycoproteins contained in insect venom. After an initial exposure to certain antigens, the body responds by making IgE antibodies against the antigens. These IgE antibodies bind to tissue mast cells and blood basophils. Mast cells are primarily located in lung tissue, bronchial smooth muscle, and vascular endothelium. Once these IgE antibodies are bound to the cells, the person is considered sensitized.

When sensitized persons are exposed to antigens to which they are sensitive, under the appropriate circumstances, IgE on mast cells or basophils will bind the antigens. When this occurs, IgE receptors on the cells are bridged together and the cells release active substances from their granules.[14] Active substances released or immediately generated by degranulation include histamine, serotonin, eosinophil chemotactic factor of anaphylaxis (ECF-A), leukotrienes, and bradykinin.

Histamine is a bioactive amine that increases capillary permeability, contracts bronchial and vascular smooth muscle, and increases nasal and bronchial mucous gland secretion. Serotonin increases vascular permeability in mice, but its role in human anaphylaxis is unknown. Leukotrienes contract smooth muscle. Unlike histamine, which is preformed in the cell granules, leukotrienes are formed after the IgE–antigen interaction occurs and are then released. Antihistamines are ineffective at reversing the effects of leukotrienes, but epinephrine will terminate muscle contractions induced by them. ECF-A is also released by mast cells and causes eosinophils to accumulate in the area of the allergic reaction. Eosinophils can release an enzyme, arylsulfatase B, which inactivates leukotrienes. Bradykinin contracts vascular and bronchial smooth muscle, increases vascular permeability, increases mucus secretion, and stimulates pain fibers.

The severity and type of anaphylactic reaction depends on the location and number of cells degranulating their mediators. Degranulation in specific target organs produces local anaphylaxis. If the reaction is limited to the gastrointestinal tract, diarrhea may occur; if mast cell mediators are released in the nasal mucosa, rhinorrhea may occur; if the mediators are limited to the skin, hives may be the only prominent sign.

Systemic degranulation of mast cells and basophils leads to severe systemic symptoms and is responsible for shock and death occurring after an insect sting. Release of large amounts of mediators can cause a marked increase in capillary permeability, leading to leakage of intravascular fluids and hypotension. This shocklike state can be further compounded by mediator-induced laryngeal edema and bronchoconstriction, resulting in respiratory distress or failure.

may be severe, the sooner medical attention is given, the better the chances for recovery.

Systemic reactions caused by insect stings and bites are considered emergencies for which aqueous epinephrine (1:1,000; 0.3–0.5 mL) should be injected immediately, either subcutaneously or intramuscularly; it may also be injected directly into the sting site to delay absorption of the venom. Sublingual isoproterenol should not be administered simultaneously because it may induce serious arrhythmia. Parenteral antihistamines may be used for persistent urticaria, angioedema, or laryngeal edema in patients who do not respond to epinephrine. Pressor agents may be used if shock persists. Parenteral corticosteroids administered through the systemic route may be used for patients with protracted anaphylaxis and delayed reactions. Respiratory support should be available if needed; in severe cases, a tracheotomy may be necessary.

The pharmacist should advise hypersensitive individuals of the following:

- If symptomatic, the victim must seek medical attention immediately after an insect sting or bite.
- Basic first aid, such as applying ice to the sting and removing the stinger, is generally helpful.
- Emergency kits for insect stings are available by prescription. Kits containing epinephrine are preferable to those containing antihistamines for treating allergic reactions to stings.
- Receiving injections of venom extract for protection against systemic reactions (desensitization) is useful.
- Insect repellents are not effective against stinging insects.

Preventive Measures

Individuals who are hypersensitive to insect stings should take precautions to avoid exposure to these insects. Foods and odors tend to attract insects; therefore, outdoor activities such as picnicking should be engaged in cautiously. Keeping garbage contained and food covered will help keep insects away. Shoes should always be worn in grass and fields. In addition, perfumes and brightly colored clothes attract stinging insects and should not be worn outdoors. A common sense approach will lower the risk of stings and subsequent adverse reactions.

Active Treatment

Because of the wide range of reactions to insect stings and bites, treatment usually depends on the symptoms. For local reactions, a nonprescription product that minimizes scratching by relieving discomfort, itching, and pain may be recommended. Prophylactic products, such as insect repellents, also are available. However, nonprescription drugs are of no value in systemic reactions; such cases need prompt medical attention.

Physician-directed medical treatment (acute or prophylactic) is important in many cases. Because hypersensitive reactions to insect stings and bites occur rapidly and

First Aid

Basic first aid is helpful until medical help is available. Prompt application of ice packs to the sting site helps to slow absorption and reduce itching, swelling, and pain. Removal of the honeybee's stinger and venom sac, which usually are left in the skin, is another measure that should be explained, particularly to allergic individuals. The stinger should be removed before all venom is injected; it takes approximately 2 to 3 minutes to empty all the contents from the honeybee's venom sac. The sac should not be squeezed; rubbing, scratching, or grasping it releases more venom. Scraping the stinger with tweezers or a fingernail minimizes the venom flow. After the stinger is removed, an antiseptic should be applied.

Emergency Kits (Prescription Only)

Emergency kits for individuals hypersensitive to insect stings are available by prescription. In addition to tweezers for removing the honeybee stinger, the typical kit includes epinephrine hydrochloride and antihistamines. Also, kits containing autoinjectable epinephrine syringes are now available.

Emergency kits for insect stings no longer require refrigeration but must be stored in the dark at room temperature. A kit should not be left in the glove compartment of a car. The pharmacist should carefully explain the directions for and the benefits of using an emergency kit for insect stings, emphasizing that epinephrine is the drug of choice for anaphylactic reactions.

Epinephrine Hydrochloride

Because of its potent and rapid action, epinephrine hydrochloride (1:1,000) injection is preferred to counteract the bronchoconstriction associated with anaphylaxis. It should be administered subcutaneously immediately after stinging. Some insect sting emergency kits have a preloaded (0.3 mL) sterile syringe. Generally, a 0.25-mL dose is injected subcutaneously and, after 15 minutes, another dose is injected if necessary. For individuals with cardiovascular disease, diabetes, hypertension, or hyperthyroidism, the injection should be administered with caution.

The FDA encourages physicians to prescribe kits containing epinephrine injections for patients who are allergic to insect stings and for individuals responsible for those who may be exposed to insect stings, such as scout leaders, camp counselors, and paramedical personnel. These individuals should be trained to administer epinephrine injections. In some states, specially trained nonphysicians may legally administer epinephrine to individuals suspected of having an anaphylactic reaction to insect stings (localized or generalized urticaria, difficult breathing, wheezing, abdominal pain, weakness, confusion, lowered blood pressure, cyanosis, collapse, and unconsciousness). The FDA opposes the nonprescription sale of epinephrine kits because of possible misuse or deliberate abuse of the material in the kit.[15]

Antihistamines

Although they are slow in onset of action and may be ineffective in severe reactions, antihistamines often are used in conjunction with epinephrine hydrochloride. They are administered orally or parenterally.

Venom Immunotherapy

Hymenoptera venom is used prophylactically to treat patients who have had reactions to stings. Venom immunotherapy, also known as desensitization, is done by subcutaneous injection of small amounts of venom at regularly scheduled intervals. The dose of the venom is gradually increased over many weeks until a predetermined maintenance dose is reached. The optimal doses, frequency of injections, and duration of maintenance therapy are still being investigated.

Immunotherapy causes a decrease in venom-specific serum IgE levels, with a rise in venom-specific serum IgG (blocking antibodies) levels. It is believed that production of blocking antibodies offers protection against anaphylactic reactions although unequivocal proof is lacking. Blocking antibodies compete with IgE antibodies for binding of venom antigens, preventing the antigens from reacting with mast cell–bound IgE. Other factors may also be responsible for successful immunotherapy.

Lyophilized venom extracts are now available for diagnosis and treatment of hypersensitivity to insect stings. More than 95% of patients treated with these venoms in recommended doses and regimens are protected against serious reactions when stung again. The remaining 5% are partially protected. Before the use of venom extracts, whole-body extracts of insects were used for immunotherapy, but these have been shown to be no better than placebo treatment and should not be used.

A kit of individual venoms of stinging insects is available to diagnose hypersensitivity by skin testing. The same individual venoms or fixed venoms from yellow jackets and white-faced hornets are used for immunotherapy. Mixed venoms are used because some individuals develop cross-sensitivity among vespids. These injections can be dangerous if improperly administered. Thus, the following warning is stated in the package insert.[16]

> **WARNING** Hymenoptera venom preparations should be used only by physicians experienced in administering allergens to the maximum tolerated dose and/or after allergy consultation.

Because severe systemic reactions are possible, the patients should be fully informed by the physician of the risks involved and should be under constant supervision. The venom preparations should be used only in settings where emergency resuscitative equipment and trained personnel are immediately available to treat such reactions. Treatment with Hymenoptera venom preparations should be restricted to patients who have previously experienced a potentially life-threatening systemic reaction following the sting of the honeybee, yellow jacket, hornet, or wasp, and should be given only after venom hypersensitivity has been confirmed by venom skin testing. All patients receiving venom immunotherapy should have instruction on emergency self-injection of subcutaneous epinephrine and should be advised to carry an emergency epinephrine kit during the Hymenoptera season, even while receiving immunotherapy. Before administering these venom preparations, physicians should be thoroughly familiar with the information concerning adverse reactions, treatment of overdosage, and precautions for use during pregnancy. After stopping venom immunotherapy, patients may again be at high risk for anaphylaxis following a sting.

Nonprescription Pharmacologic Treatment

Most nonprescription products used for symptomatic relief of insect stings and bites contain one or more pharmacologic agents, which fall into one of three main categories: external analgesics/antipruritics, skin protectants, and antibacterials.

External Analgesics/Antipruritics

This category is subdivided further into three groups: agents with analgesic activity derived from (1) the stimulation of cutaneous sensory receptors (counterirritants), (2) the depression of cutaneous sensory receptors (anesthetics and antihistamines), and (3) the reduction of inflammation (hydrocortisone). These agents are considered safe and effective when used as recommended for adults and children over 2 years of age. They are not recommended for children under 2 years of age except under the advice or supervision of a physician.

Insect Bite Neutralizers

Ammonium Hydroxide and Trimethanolamine

Ammonium hydroxide and trimethanolamine have been claimed to have a neutralizing effect on insect bites and stings. The FDA now regards ammonium hydroxide as Category I. Although there has not yet been a public announcement of this classification, manufacturers have been informed.

Counterirritants

Counterirritants reduce pain and itching by stimulating cutaneous sensory receptors to provide a feeling of warmth, coolness, or milder pain, which obscures the more severe pain of the injury. The activity of these agents depends on the concentration. In low concentrations, they may depress the cutaneous receptors and result in an anesthetic effect.

Camphor At concentrations of 0.1–3%, camphor depresses cutaneous receptors, thereby relieving itching and irritation. At higher concentrations of 3–11%, camphor stimulates cutaneous receptors and therefore acts as a counterirritant. Camphor is safe and effective for use as an external analgesic at these concentrations when applied to the affected area no more than three or four times a day. However, camphor-containing products can be very dangerous if ingested. Patients should be warned to keep these (and all drugs) out of the reach of children and to contact a physician or poison control center immediately if ingestion is suspected.

Cresol Camphor complex (camphorated metacresol) is used to reduce pain. Although the drug is not classified by the FDA as effective in treating insect bites and stings, it is classified as Category I for use as an external analgesic in treating poison ivy.

Ichthammol Ichthammol has bacteriostatic and irritant properties. However, its effectiveness for insect stings is difficult to assess in concentrations used in nonprescription products.

Menthol In concentrations of more than 1.25%, menthol acts as a counterirritant and excites cutaneous sensory receptors. However, in concentrations of less than 1%, it depresses cutaneous receptors and exerts an analgesic effect. Menthol is considered a safe and effective antipruritic when applied to the affected area in concentrations of 0.1–1%.

Methyl Salicylate Methyl salicylate stimulates cutaneous receptors when used in concentrations of 10–60%.

Peppermint and Clove Oils When applied externally, peppermint and clove oils act as mild counterirritants, causing a sensation of warmth.

Local Anesthetics

The FDA Advisory Review Panel on Over-the-Counter External Analgesic Drug Products concluded that benzocaine and dibucaine, the local anesthetics used in insect sting and bite products, are safe and effective when used according to label directions. Dermatitis has reportedly resulted from topically applied local anesthetics, including benzocaine. Any dermatitis that may occur is caused by frequent contact, and patients should be warned against continued applications for prolonged periods. Although adverse reactions from topical applications are often blamed on allergy to local anesthetics, allergy is an infrequent cause of reaction.

Benzocaine Benzocaine was found to be safe and effective for use by adults and children over 2 years of age when applied to the affected area no more than three or four times a day. The concentrations of benzocaine available in nonprescription products range from 5–20%.

Cyclomethycaine Sulfate The FDA panel on external analgesic products concluded that cyclomethycaine sulfate is safe and effective but that available data are insufficient to permit final classification of its effectiveness for use as a nonprescription external analgesic.

Dibucaine Dibucaine is another local anesthetic found in insect sting and bite products. Although in the same class as benzocaine, dibucaine products carry specific additional labeling:

> **WARNING** Do not use in large quantities, particularly over raw surfaces or blistered areas.

This is because of the danger of systemic toxicity. Convulsions, myocardial depression, and death have been reported from systemic absorption. The recommended dosage for adults and children over 2 years of age is a 0.25–1% solution applied to the affected area no more than three or four times a day.

Phenol Phenol exerts topical anesthetic action by depressing cutaneous sensory receptors. It is caustic when applied in undiluted form to the skin. Phenol aqueous solutions of greater than 2% are irritating and may cause sloughing and necrosis. Phenol is considered safe and effective as a nonprescription external analgesic when applied to the affected area no more than three or four times a day in concentrations of 0.5–1.5% for adults and children 2 years of age and older. Nonprescription products that contain phenol should include the following specific warning:

> Do not apply this product to extensive areas of the body or under compresses or bandages.

Antihistamines

Topical antihistamines are considered to be safe and effective external analgesics. These ingredients relieve pain and itching by depressing cutaneous sensory receptors. Although some absorption occurs through the skin, these ingredients are not absorbed in sufficient quantities to cause systemic side effects even when applied to damaged skin. However, antihistamines are capable of acting as haptenes, producing hypersensitivity reactions.

Continued use of these agents over 3 to 4 weeks increases the possibility of allergic contact dermatitis. In addition, their continued antipruritic action over a period of time is questionable. With this in mind, the FDA panel on external analgesic products recommended that these agents be used for no longer than 7 days except under the advice of a physician. These agents are not recommended for children under 2 years of age.

Both local anesthetics and antihistamines carry the following labeling as recommended by the FDA panel:

> For temporary relief of pain and itching due to minor burns, sunburn, minor cuts, abrasions, insect bites, and minor skin irritations.

Diphenhydramine Products containing diphenhydramine in concentrations of 1 to 2% may be applied three or four times a day.

Tripelennamine Tripelennamine in concentrations of 0.5–2% may be applied three or four times a day.

Hydrocortisone

Hydrocortisone is an anti-inflammatory agent that is capable of preventing or suppressing the development of edema, capillary dilation, swelling, and tenderness accompanying inflammation. It relieves pain and itching by reducing inflammation. Preparations containing hydrocortisone in concentrations of up to 1% have been approved by the FDA and are considered relatively safe and effective for use as nonprescription products. These preparations should be applied three or four times a day for adults and children 2 years of age and older. Patients should be warned against using topically applied hydrocortisone in the presence of scabies, tinea, bacterial infections, and moniliasis. Not only may the underlying condition be worsened, but hydrocortisone may also mask these disorders, making accurate diagnosis difficult. Products containing hydrocortisone or its acetate salts carry specific labeling as follows:

> For the temporary relief of minor skin irritations, itching, and rashes due to eczema, dermatitis, insect bites, poison ivy, poison oak, poison sumac, soaps, detergent, cosmetics, and jewelry, and for itchy genital and anal areas.

Aspirin

The topical use of aspirin for insect stings has been reported to be effective in reducing the wheal reaction and its subsequent itching and irritation. The FDA panel on external analgesic products concluded that aspirin is safe, but available data are insufficient to permit final classification of its effectiveness for use as a nonprescription external analgesic. Aspirin possesses no direct topical anesthetic activity; therefore, it exerts no anesthetic, analgesic, or antipruritic effect on the skin.

Skin Protectants

Aluminum Acetate

Aluminum acetate solutions in concentrations of 2.5–5% are used as an external astringent.

Glycerin

The FDA Advisory Review Panel on Over-the-Counter Skin Protectant Drug Products concluded that glycerin is safe and effective for nonprescription use as a skin protectant because of its absorbent, demulcent, and emollient properties. In addition, glycerin is widely used for its solvent properties.

Hamamelis Water

Hamamelis water (witch hazel) possesses astringent properties and may act as a hemostatic for small superficial wounds.

Titanium Dioxide

Titanium dioxide has an action similar to that of zinc oxide (see the following section). The FDA has classified titanium dioxide as Category I for use as a skin protectant in sunscreen agents. However, the agency has not addressed the safety and effectiveness of this ingredient in insect bite and sting products.

Zinc Oxide and Calamine

Zinc oxide and calamine are used in lotions, ointments, creams, and sprays for their cooling, slightly astringent, antiseptic, antibacterial, and protective actions. Calamine is a mixture of zinc and ferrous oxide. The ferrous oxide acts only as a coloring agent and is not an active ingredient. Zinc oxide and calamine tend to absorb fluids from weeping rashes. The FDA panel on skin protectant products concluded that zinc oxide and calamine are safe and effective in the nonprescription concentration range of 1–25% and for use as a nonprescription skin protectant. Topical dosage for adults, children, and infants is application of the preparation to the affected areas as needed.

Antibacterials

The most commonly used antibacterial agents in nonprescription products for insect stings and bites are benzalkonium chloride, benzethonium chloride, and methylbenzethonium chloride. These medications are included to prevent and treat secondary infection that may result from scratching. These quaternary ammonium compounds are classified as safe and effective for first-aid use.

Chlorothymol

Chlorothymol acts as an antibacterial and antifungal agent. However, it is irritating to mucous membranes.

Chloroxylenol

Chloroxylenol is a bacteriostatic agent that primarily acts against Gram-positive bacteria. The FDA Advisory Review Panel on Over-the-Counter Antimicrobial Drug Products could not evaluate the safety and effectiveness of chloroxylenol in topical preparations because of insufficient data.

Cresol

Cresol has a similar action to phenol. It is often used as a preservative.

8-Hydroxyquinoline Sulfate

The 8-hydroxyquinoline sulfate chemical is included in topical preparations for its antibacterial effect.

Salicylic Acid

At concentrations ranging from 2–20%, salicylic acid acts as a keratolytic. In addition, it exerts a slight antiseptic action.

Insect Repellents

Insect repellents do not kill insects. Most repellents are volatile, however, and when they are applied to skin or clothing, their vapor tends to discourage the approach of insects and prevent them from alighting. Thus, repellents protect the skin against insect bites.

Oils of citronella, turpentine, pennyroyal, cedarwood, eucalyptus, and wintergreen were previously used in insect repellent formulations. However, after World War II, investigations showed that these agents were relatively ineffective. Although more than 15,000 compounds have been tested, only a few have been found to be effective and safe enough to use on the skin. An insect repellent should have an inoffensive odor, protect for several hours, be effective against as wide a variety of insects as possible, be relatively safe, withstand all weather conditions, and have an aesthetic feel and appearance.

The best all-purpose repellent is *N,N*-diethyl-*m*-toluamide, commonly called DEET. Use of products containing DEET is discouraged in children under 2 years of age because of possible toxicity to the central nervous system. Ethohexadiol dimethyl phthalate, dimethyl ethyl hexanediol carbate, and butopyronoxyl are effective repellents, but they are not as effective against as many kinds of insects as DEET. However, a mixture of two or more of these repellents is more effective against a greater variety of insects than a single repellent.

Repellents may be toxic if taken internally. People who are sensitive to these chemicals may develop skin reactions such as itching, burning, and swelling. Repellents cause smarting when they are applied to broken skin or mucous membranes. They should be applied carefully around the eyes because they may cause a burning sensation. Even though permethrin is a pesticide, it may be used as a clothing spray for protection against mosquitoes and ticks.[17]

The FDA's final rule on insect repellents for nonprescription oral use in humans indicates that these products are not generally recognized as safe and effective and are misbranded.[18] Thiamine hydrochloride (vitamin B_1) has been marketed as an ingredient in nonprescription drug products for oral use as an insect repellent. Oral sulfur tablets have also been suggested. However, there are no data to establish the effectiveness of these or any other ingredients for nonprescription oral use as a systemic insect repellent. Labeling claims for such products—for example, "oral mosquito repellent," "mosquitoes avoid you," "bugs stay away," "keep mosquitoes away for 12–24 hours," and "the newest way to fight mosquitoes"—are either false, misleading, or unsupported by scientific data.

Product Selection Guidelines

Medication is often requested after symptoms appear; thus, it is important to determine what symptoms appeared following the sting or bite, how soon the symptoms appeared, how severe the symptoms are, and what other drugs are being used concurrently.

Nonprescription products are of minimal value to hypersensitive individuals. The pharmacist should record all information on hypersensitive individuals and should recommend that the person wear a tag or carry a card showing the nature of the allergy. If the symptoms, such as localized irritation, itching, or swelling, are minor, an appropriate nonprescription product may be recommended. Topical lotions, creams, ointments, and sprays are the main nonprescription products used for symptomatic relief of local reactions to insect stings and bites. The main considerations in product selection are reducing the possibility of additional stings or bites, providing proper protection to the affected skin, preventing secondary infection in the affected area, and relieving itching and irritation. The pharmacist may also suggest several measures to relieve itching and irritation:

- Avoiding rough and irritating clothing, especially wool, over the affected area;
- Avoiding strong soaps, highly perfumed soaps, or harsh detergents;
- Applying an occlusive skin protectant to the affected area after bathing;
- Bathing in cool (never warm) water for 10–20 minutes;
- Avoiding scratching the affected area; also, keeping fingernails trimmed short and filed smooth to minimize possible skin damage of the affected area if scratching occurs.

Although they are capable of producing topical or systemic adverse reactions, external analgesics and antipruritics are considered to be relatively safe and effective. These nonprescription products are for adults and children 2 years of age and older and should be applied no more than three or four times a day. For children under 2 years of age, there is no recommended dosage except under the advice and supervision of a physician.

The labels on external analgesic nonprescription products should indicate the ingredients and their concentrations, the manner of usage and frequency of applications, and the indications for use. The FDA panel on external analgesic products recommended that the labels should also include the following warnings:

- For external use only.
- Avoid contact with eyes.
- If condition worsens or if symptoms persist for more than 7 days, discontinue use of this product and consult a physician.
- Do not use for children under 2 years of age except under the advice and supervision of a physician.

Summary

Stings of honeybees, bumblebees, yellow jackets, hornets, wasps, and ants cause pain, discomfort, illness, and severe local and systemic reactions. In normal individuals, insect stings and bites cause local irritation, inflammation, swelling, and itching that provoke rubbing and scratching. In hypersensitive individuals, anaphylactic reactions may pose serious emergency problems.

People sensitized to insect venom may react violently when stung. They need immediate, active treatment such as the administration of epinephrine hydrochloride. Partial desensitization may be accomplished by insect venom immunotherapy. The pharmacist can play a significant role by advising hypersensitive individuals on emergency procedures for insect stings. The pharmacist should also advise and educate patients in the treatment and prevention of lice infestation, tick-induced diseases, and other insect bites.

A wide variety of nonprescription products are available to treat stings and bites. These include external analgesics and antipruritics (e.g., antihistamines, local anesthetics, counterirritants, hydrocortisone, and aspirin), skin protectants, and antibacterials.

References

1. Fusia AF, Marek WJ, Puerini A. et al. *Curr Ther Res* 1987; 41: 881.
2. Sause RB Galizia VJ. *Pharm Times* 1989 Sep; 132.
3. Robinson DH, Shephard DA. *Curr Ther Res* 1980; 27: 1.
4. Zack R. *RN* 1987 Sep; 30.
5. Rasmussen J. *NARD J* 1987 Sep; 32.
6. Covington TR. *Facts and Comparisons Drug Newsletter* 1990; 9: 65.
7. Hussar DA. *Am Pharm* 1987; 27: 26.
8. Abramowicz M., ed. *Med Lett Drugs Ther* 1990; 32: 23.
9. Abramowicz M., ed. *Med Lett Drugs Ther* 1990; 32:21.
10. Phipps MV. *Am Pharm* 1991; 31: 53.
11. Steere AC. *N Engl J Med* 1989; 321: 9, 586.
12. Carlstedt BC, Johnson RC, Kreter B. *US Pharm* 1990 Apr; 33.
13. Green AW, et al. *J Allergy Clin Immunol* 1980; 66: 186.
14. Ishizaka T. *J Allergy Clin Immunol* 1981; 67: 90.
15. *FDA Drug Bull* 1980; 10: 2, 12.
16. *FDA Drug Bull* 1979; 9: 3, 15.
17. Abramowicz M., ed. *Med Lett Drug Ther* 1989; 31: 45.
18. *Federal Register* 1985; 50: 25170.

Chapter 37

Foot Care Products

Nicholas G. Popovich

Questions to ask in patient assessment and counseling

General Foot Conditions

- Where is the lesion located (on or between the toes or on the sole of the foot)? Is the toenail involved?
- Is there any redness, itching, blistering, oozing, scaling, or bleeding from the lesion?
- Is the condition painful? Is it too uncomfortable to walk? Do your feet hurt or ache at the end of the day?
- During which activities is the pain noticed?
- How long have you had the problem?
- Did the problem begin with the use of new shoes (sandals or enclosed shoes, jogging or tennis shoes, flat or high heels), socks, or soaps? Do your new shoes seem tighter than they have been in the past or tight at the end of the day?
- Do your feet sweat excessively? Do you notice a foot odor when you take off your shoes? Do your feet sweat more when you wear nylons or synthetic hosiery?
- Do you have allergies, asthma, or skin problems?
- What is your occupation?
- Do you participate in a daily or regular exercise program such as jogging or aerobics?
- Is there any history of injury to the foot?
- How often and in what manner do you trim your toenails?
- Have you tried to treat this problem yourself? If so, how?
- Did you see your physician about this problem? If so, what did he or she tell you to do? What have you done? Did it help?
- Is a physician treating you for any other medical condition, such as diabetes, heart trouble, or circulatory problems?
- Do you take insulin? What other prescription or nonprescription medications do you take on a routine basis?
- Have you ever had vascular surgery or been treated for circulatory problems?

Foot Conditions Related to Running/Jogging

- Is the discomfort getting progressively worse?
- Has the discomfort plateaued at a level that continues to affect your performance?
- Is the discomfort more frequent and severe while running? Is it present while not running?
- Is the discomfort causing you to compensate and develop additional injuries?
- Have attempts at self-treatment (e.g., new shoes, a change of running surface, or change in training intensity) failed to relieve the symptoms?

Orthotic Devices

- Is there a symptom that requires treatment?
- Did the symptom occur gradually?
- Do you have a history of a fracture, dislocation, or surgery in the legs or feet?
- Did you wear corrective shoes or braces on the legs or feet as a child?
- Have you significantly increased repetitive weight-bearing activity? Do you plan to continue this activity?
- Have attempts at self-treatment with nonprescription inserts failed?

A 1988 Gallup survey of family/general practitioners, dermatologists, and podiatrists identified the foot problems most often encountered and how patients deal with them.[1] The five most common foot complaints were sore, aching feet; ingrown toenails; corns and calluses; and plantar warts. The survey identified harmful foot practices, such as scraping or cutting corns and calluses, improperly trimming toenails, opening blisters or removing the skin cover, and inappropriately using hot water. The survey also identified potentially harmful home remedies for foot problems, including the application of caulk plaster, WD 40® lubricant, Crisco® or butter, Clorox® or other bleach products, and gasoline or kerosene. Obviously, there is a significant need to educate patients about proper foot care, including self-treatment measures; the pharmacist can serve as a valuable resource in this regard.

Instruction in proper foot care should begin at an early age when good health habits can be nurtured. At

TABLE 1   Mycotic infection

Type	Site(s) of invasion	Example
Superficial	Outermost layer of skin and appendages	Tinea versicolor (caused by *Malassezia furfur*)
Cutaneous	Skin lesion and/or nail	Tinea pedis (caused by *Trichophyton rubrum*)
Subcutaneous	Cutaneous and subcutaneous tissue	Sporotrichosis (caused by *Sporotrichum schenckii*)
Intermediate	Skin, mucous membranes, internal viscera	Vaginal candidiasis (caused by *Candida albicans*)
Deep systemic	Viscera, bone, nerve, skin	Blastomycosis (caused by *Blastomyces dermatitidis*)

Reprinted with permission from Raskin J. In: Conn HF, ed. *Current Therapy*. Philadelphia: W. B. Saunders; 1976; 611–4.

birth, an infant's foot has 35 joints, 19 muscles, more than 100 ligaments, and cartilage that will develop into 26 bones. These small components continue to develop and mature until the age of 14–16 for females and 15–21 for males. Women will generally begin to notice changes in their feet in their 30s; men will begin to notice changes in their 40s. The feet tend to broaden and flatten after years of bearing the body's weight, thus stretching ligaments and causing bones to shift positions. These changes subject the feet to stress, which is compounded by prolonged standing: an estimated 40% of the U.S. population spend about 75% of their workday on their feet. Such stresses increase the potential for painful foot conditions. Thus, the simplest rule of foot care is routine daily inspection of the feet to note any overt signs of early problems.

There are three distinct groups of patients who often encounter foot problems. The first is the pediatric patient whose difficulty is a congenital malformation or deformity or a specific disease that affects the foot (e.g., juvenile arthritis). These patients need special shoes and foot care provided with the oversight of an orthopedic surgeon. The second group are adolescents who experience rapid growth. Growth plates in their feet may become stressed and irritated. Athletic activity at this age can also contribute to problems, especially if there are associated injuries to the feet that are not properly treated. Osteoarthritis, for example, can occur secondary to a foot injury. Third, geriatric patients encounter foot problems due to aging (as the foot assumes its final shape) and disease. In particular, diabetes mellitus and arthritis can cause secondary foot problems.

Prevention of foot problems begins with the purchase of comfortable, well-fitted shoes of proper width and length (i.e., the toes should not bump into the front of the shoe or be cramped in the toe box). The heel support in the shoe should fit snugly and help hold the foot straight. Depending on the activity level of the person, the midsole should provide adequate cushioning and support. Because shoes are mass produced, a person should try both shoes on at the time of purchase, preferably wearing a pair of socks or stockings of the type that will be worn normally with the new pair of shoes. If people are prone to edema, shoe selection should occur at the end of the day.

Geriatric persons should be advised to wear shoes that are comfortable and provide support, even around the home. A real danger for such patients around the home occurs with slippers. Although slippers are comfortable and easy to get on and off, they tend to get caught on carpeting, throw rugs, or stairs. Consequently, the elderly person may slip or fall, risking serious injury (e.g., broken hip or bone fracture).

In the past two decades, society's attitude toward physical fitness and body awareness has changed dramatically. Millions of people exercise every day; jogging, running, and aerobic exercising are methods used most often to remain or get "in shape." Unfortunately, however, if people do not take adequate precautions, problems can arise, particularly involving the feet. Appropriate footwear is one of several factors that should be addressed by joggers and runners to prevent foot problems.

Although foot conditions are generally not life-threatening, except perhaps to persons with diabetes (PWDs), severely arthritic patients, and those with impaired circulation, such problems may cause a substantial measure of discomfort and impaired mobility and may even indicate a serious disease condition. Corns, calluses, and ingrown toenails are common and may contribute to impairment. Hardening of the skin may signal a biomechanical problem and cause abnormal weight distribution in a particular area of the foot. In this case, a podiatric examination is warranted to determine whether an imbalance is present. Human mycotic (fungal) infections may be subdivided into five categories based on the site of invasion (Table 1).[2] The superficial and cutaneous types, such as athlete's foot, usually warrant the pharmacist's advice. (See Chapter 28, "Topical Anti-Infective Products.")

Common Foot Problems

Corns and Calluses

Corns and calluses are similar in one respect: each produces a marked hyperkeratosis of the stratum corneum. Besides this feature, however, there are marked differences.

A corn (clavus) is a small, sharply demarcated, hyperkeratotic lesion having a central core (Figure 1). It is raised, has a yellowish-gray color, and ranges from a few millimeters to 1 cm or more in diameter. The base of the corn is on the skin surface; the apex of the corn points inward and presses on the nerve endings in the dermis, causing pain.

Corns may be either hard or soft. Hard corns occur on the surface of the toes and appear shiny and polished. Soft corns are whitish thickenings of the skin, usually found on the webs between the fourth and fifth toes. Accumulated perspiration macerates the epidermis and gives the corn a soft appearance; soft corns are often mistaken for fungal infections. This situation occurs because the fifth metatarsal is much shorter than the fourth, and the web between these toes is deeper and extends more proximally than the webs between the other toes.

Hard corns (usually) and soft corns (less frequently) are caused by underlying bony prominences. A bony spur, or exostosis (a bony tumor in the form of an ossified muscular attachment to the bone surface), nearly always exists between long-lasting hard and soft corns. A lesion located over non–weight-bearing bony prominences or joints—such as metatarsal heads, the bulb of the great toe, the dorsum of the fifth toe, or the tips of the middle toes—is usually a corn.[3]

A callus may be broad based or have a central core with sharply circumscribed margins and diffuse thickening of the skin. It has indefinite borders and ranges from a few millimeters to several centimeters in diameter. It is usually raised and yellow, and it has a normal pattern of skin ridges on its surface. Calluses form on joints and weight-bearing areas, such as the palms of the hands and the sides and soles of the feet. (See color plates, photograph 33.)

Pathophysiology

During corn or callus development, the cells in the basal cell layer undergo accelerated mitotic division, leading to the migration of maturing cells through the prickle cell (stratum spinosum) and the granular (stratum granulosum) skin layer. The mitotic rate is normally equal to that of the continual surface cellular desquamation. Normal mitotic activity and subsequent desquamation lead to the complete replacement of the epidermis in about 1 month. In the case of a callus, friction and pressure increase mitotic activity of the basal cell layer,[4] producing a thicker stratum corneum as more cells reach the outer skin surface. When the friction or pressure is relieved, mitotic activity returns to normal, causing remission and disappearance of the callus.

Symptoms

Pressure from tight-fitting shoes is the most frequent cause of pain from corns. As narrow-toed or high-heeled shoes crowd toes into the narrow toe box, the most lateral toe,

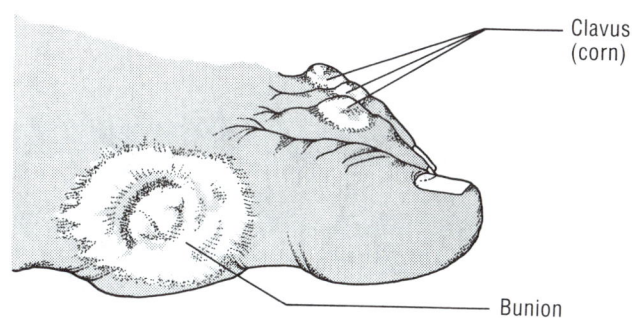

FIGURE 1 Conditions affecting the top of the foot.

the fifth, experiences the most pressure and friction and is the usual site of a corn. The resultant pain may be severe and sharp (when downward pressure is applied) or dull and discomforting.

Friction (caused by loose-fitting shoes or tight-fitting hosiery), walking barefoot, and structural biomechanical problems contribute to the development of calluses. Structural problems include improper weight distribution, pressure, and the development of bunions with age. Calluses are usually asymptomatic, causing pain only when pressure is applied. Individuals who suffer from calluses on the sole of the foot often liken their discomfort to that of walking with a pebble in the shoe.

Treatment

Successful treatment of corns and calluses with nonprescription products depends on eliminating the causes: pressure and friction. This process entails using well-fitting, nonbinding footwear that evenly distributes body weight. For anatomical foot deformities, orthopedic corrections must be made. These measures relieve pressure and friction to allow normal mitosis of the basal cell layer to resume, the stratum corneum to normalize after total desquamation of the hyperkeratotic tissue, and topical products to take effect. Before instituting a self-treatment program, however, a patient should secure a medical opinion; this should definitely be done if circulatory problems are present or if the patient has diabetes.

In the final monograph for drug products that remove corns and calluses, the Food and Drug Administration (FDA) adopted the advisory review panel's recommendations that only salicylic acid be categorized as safe and effective for this purpose.[5] The final monograph dictates that products containing salicylic acid in a plaster, pad, disk, or collodion vehicle must be classified as Category I.[5] The FDA recognized that use of the term *plaster* includes "disk" and "pad" because these dosage forms are similar in nature. It also indicated that these products were to be advertised to consumers "for the removal of corns and calluses."

In some experiments, corns have been treated with a subdermal injection of fluid silicone.[6] The injected silicone, at times, seems to augment digital and plantar

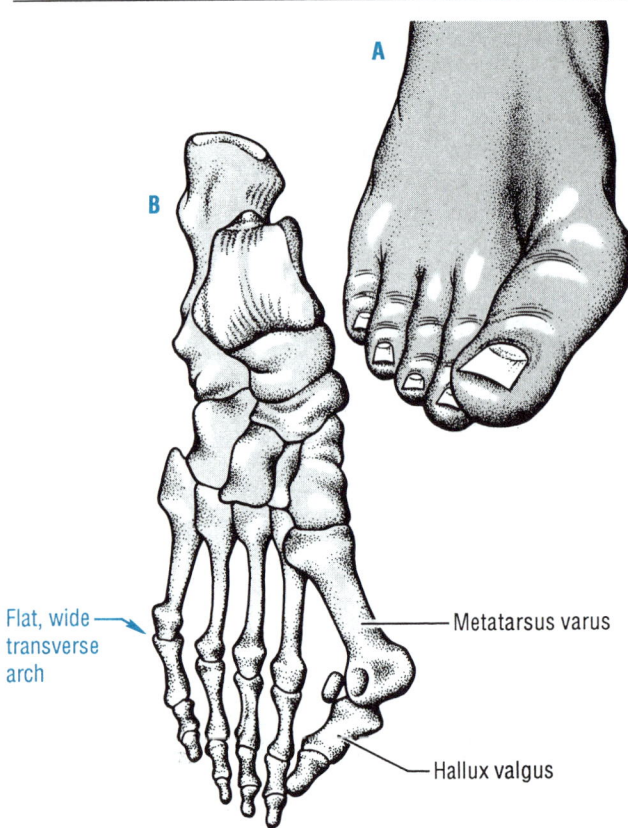

FIGURE 2A and B Two views of hallux valgus. A, gross representation of hallux valgus. B, bone structure of hallux valgus.

tissues using a cushioning effect, reducing pain, and decreasing the need for regular palliative treatment.

There are no clinical studies to indicate whether prescription products are superior to nonprescription products for the removal of corns and calluses. Conclusions are based only on subjective physician evaluation reports. Again, salicylic acid in a plaster or collodion-like dosage form appears to be most effective for self-treatment of corns and calluses.

Bunions

The hallux, or great toe, along with the inner side of the foot, provides the elasticity and mobility needed to walk or run. Thus, the hallux is a dynamic body part. However, this mobility causes several anatomical disorders associated with the foot, such as hallux valgus, which is the deviation of the great toe toward the lateral (outer) side of the foot. Prolonged pressure caused by hallux valgus may result in pressure over the angulation of the metatarsophalangeal joint of the big toe, causing inflammatory swelling of the bursa over that joint (Figure 2). This may result in bunion formation (Figure 1).

Bunions, which are swellings of the bursae and/or exostoses, can be caused by various conditions. Pressure may result from the manner in which a person sits, walks, or stands, but pressure from a tight-fitting shoe over a period of time generally aggravates the condition. Friction on the toes from bone malformations (wide heads or lateral bending) is also a major factor in bunion production. Some individuals have a hereditary predisposition to the development of bunions.

Corrective steps to alleviate bunions often depend on the degree of discomfort. Bunions are usually asymptomatic but may become quite painful, swollen, and tender. The bunion itself usually is covered by an extensive keratinous overgrowth.

Bunions are not amenable to topical drug therapy. Nor is the routine, chronic use of oral nonprescription analgesics, particularly ibuprofen, suggested. The patient should correct the etiologic condition by wearing properly fitting shoes or seek the advice of a podiatrist or orthopedist.

Topical nonprescription padding (e.g., moleskin) can be helpful and may be all that is necessary to decrease the irritation of footwear. Eventually, padding can help decrease inflammation around the bunion area.

If the pharmacist recommends the use of topical adhesive cushioning to alleviate the pressure on a bunion, instructions should be given on proper use. Before the protective pad is applied, the foot should be bathed and thoroughly dried. The pad should then be cut into a shape that conforms to the bunion. If the intent is to relieve the pressure from the center of the bunion area, the pad should be cut to surround the bunion. Precut pads are available for immediate patient use. Constant skin contact with adhesive-backed pads should generally be avoided, however, unless under the recommendation of a podiatrist or physician.

Larger footwear may be necessary to compensate for the space taken up by the pad; not increasing shoe size appropriately may cause pressure in other areas. Also, protective pads should not be used on bunions when the skin is broken or blistered. Abraded skin should receive palliative treatment before pads are applied. If conditions persist, particularly in diabetic patients, the pharmacist should recommend that these patients consult a podiatrist or orthopedist. Ultimately, surgical treatment may be necessary.

Warts (Verrucae)

Warts, or verrucae, are common viral inflections of the skin and mucous membranes. Approximately 9 million U.S. citizens contract them each year. They are caused by human papillomaviruses (HPVs), which contain deoxyribonucleic acid (DNA).[7]

Papillomavirus particles assemble in the nuclei of upper-layer keratinocytes and are subsequently released into the milieu within the stratum corneum. It has been demonstrated that HPVs do not bud from the cell membrane and thus lack a thermosensitive lipid envelope like that found in the herpes viruses and the human retroviruses. It is thought that the presence of this stable protein coat allows the HPV to remain infectious outside the host cells for substantial periods of time.

Types

Because warts were induced when extracts from common warts and anogenital warts were injected into different sites, it was hypothesized that all warts were caused by a single agent. In the past decade, however, immunologic techniques in conjunction with DNA purification and restrictive endonuclease digestion have identified at least 50 HPV types,[8] each with its own characteristic histopathology and cytopathology.

Past studies showed that HPV-6 and HPV-11 were responsible for anogenital warts, and that these strains were different from other HPVs in serologic molecular hybridization.[7,9] This prompted the belief that HPV type dictated the kind of wart and that these viruses were confined to specific body locations. Evidence now suggests that HPV types are not restricted to a specific site, but that, for unknown reasons (perhaps epithelial cell receptor specificity), viral particles function in keratinocytes only in specific locations and will induce warts only in these locations.

Common virogenic warts are defined according to their location. Common warts (verruca vulgaris) are usually located on the hands and fingers but may also occur on the face. They are recognized by their rough, cauliflower-like appearance. These warts are slightly scaly, rough papules or nodules; they appear alone or grouped; and they can be found on any skin surface although they most often appear on the hands. (See color plates, photograph 34.) Periungual and subungual warts occur around and underneath the nail beds, especially in nail biters and cuticle pickers.[7] Juvenile, or flat, warts (verruca plana) are small (usually 2–4 mm in diameter), slightly elevated, flat-topped papules that usually occur in groups on the face, neck, and dorsa of the hands, wrists, and knees of children. Venereal warts (condyloma lata and condyloma acuminata) occur near the genitalia and anus. Condyloma acuminatum present as flesh to gray-colored hyperkeratotic, exophytic papules; they either have a broad base of attachment or are attached by a short, broad stem (or stalk). They range in size from less than a millimeter in diameter to several square centimeters when they merge into plaques. The penile shaft is the most common site of lesions in men. Plantar warts (verruca plantaris) are common on the soles of the feet.[7] (See color plates, photograph 35.)

Plantar warts, hyperkeratotic lesions generally associated with pressure, are more common in older children and adolescents but also occur in adults. They may be confined to the weight-bearing areas of the foot (the sole of the heel, the great toe, the areas below the heads of the metatarsal bones, and the ball), or they may occur in non–weight-bearing areas of the sole of the foot (Figure 3). Calluses are also commonly found on weight-bearing areas of the foot, and because of their smooth keratotic surfaces, they resemble isolated plantar warts. Therefore, the distinction between a wart and a callus or corn is sometimes unclear. However, unlike a callus, a plantar wart is tender with pressure and interrupts the footprint pattern. Optimally, a podiatrist or dermatologist will have the opportunity to assess the condition and make a differential diagnosis. To do this, the physician may shave away the outer keratinous surface to expose thrombosed capillaries in the papilloma, which appear as black dots or seeds.

Plantar warts, if located on weight-bearing portions of the foot, are under constant pressure and are usually not raised above the skin surface. The wart itself is in the center of the lesion and is roughly circular with a diameter of 0.5–3.0 cm. The surface is grayish and friable, and the surrounding skin is thick and heaped. Several warts may coalesce and fuse, giving the appearance of one large wart (mosaic wart).

Susceptibility

Three criteria must be met for an individual to develop a wart:

- The papillomavirus must be present.
- There must be an open avenue such as an abrasion through which the virus can enter the skin.
- The individual's immune system must be susceptible to the virus (probably the key reason that certain individuals develop warts and others do not).

Indeed, immunodeficient patients (e.g., those maintained on systemic or topical glucocorticoids), once infected, develop widespread and highly resistant warts.[10]

Warts are most common in children and young adults and usually appear on exposed areas of the fingers, hands, face, and soles of the feet. The peak incidence of warts occurs between 12 and 16 years of age; as many as 10% of schoolchildren under age 16 have one or more warts.[11]

Warts may spread by direct person-to-person contact, by autoinoculation to another body area, or indirectly through public shower floors or swimming pools. It is thought that swimming, especially in warm water with a pH greater than 5, swells and softens the horny skin layer cells on the sole of the foot. The abrasive surface of the pool and diving board contributes to tissue debridement, and inoculation in the area of heavy foot traffic around the pool is likely, especially when running and springing contribute to stress on the soles of the feet. Scrapings of the horny layer of plantar warts contain virus particles; therefore, it is conceivable that a heavy traffic area of a pool can be easily contaminated by one person with a plantar wart. The incubation period after inoculation is 1–20 months, with an average of 3 to 4 months.

Mechanism

Warts begin as minute, smooth-surfaced, skin-colored lesions that enlarge over time. Repeated irritation causes the wart to continue enlarging. Plantar warts are usually asymptomatic when small and may not be noticed. However, if they are large or occur on the heel or ball of the foot, there may be discomfort and limitation of function.

Warts are not usually permanent; approximately 30% clear spontaneously in 6 months, 65% clear in 2 years, and most warts clear in 5 years.[12] The mechanism of spontaneous resolution is not fully understood.

Treatment

Many practitioners believe that early and vigorous treatment of warts is best. Prolonged treatment with nonprescription products may increase the chance of autoinoculation. The urgency for treatment is based on such considerations as the cosmetic effect (facial warts), the number of warts present in an area, the site of the wart (weight-bearing area of the foot), and the age of the patient.

No specific effective medication for treating warts is available although topical agents and procedures can sometimes help in their removal and relieve the pain. But topical therapy might not always be indicated. The FDA Advisory Review Panel on Over-the-Counter Miscellaneous

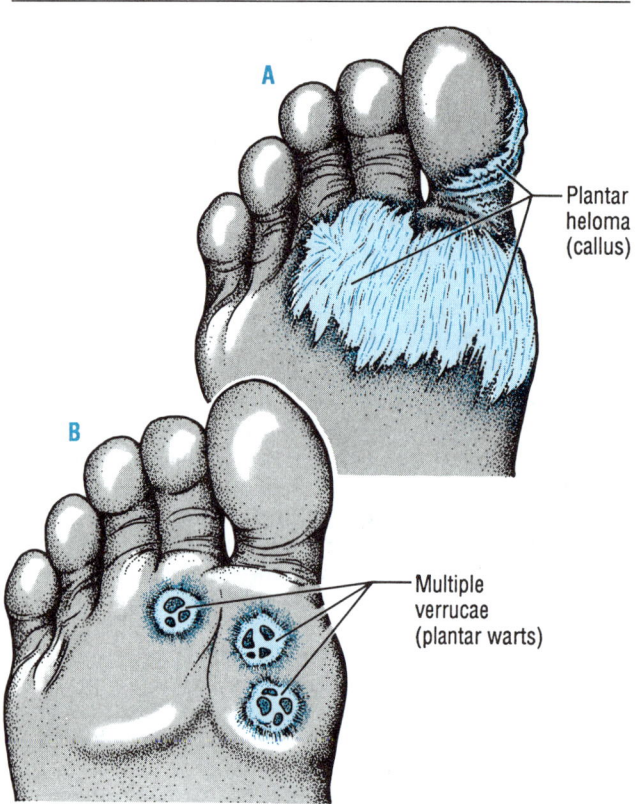

FIGURE 3A and B Conditions affecting the sole of the foot. A, plantar heloma (callus). B, multiple verrucae (plantar warts).

External Drug Products recommended that these products be labeled for treating only common and plantar warts.[13] This panel excluded the other wart types from self-therapy because of the difficulty in recognizing and treating them without the supervision of a physician.[13] Indeed, painful plantar warts, multiple flat warts, facial warts, periungual warts, and venereal warts should all be treated by a physician. Because of the latency factor, warts may reappear several months after they have been "cured."

Choice of treatment type depends on the location, size, and type of wart, and on the extent and number of lesions present. It should also take into account the patient's age, immunologic status, and expected compliance with treatment. The pain, inconvenience, risk of scarring, and experience of the physician or dermatologist are important considerations prior to initiation of treatment. Topical salicylic acid in three different vehicles has been recognized as the only drug safe and effective for self-treatment of common or plantar warts.[13] As mentioned earlier, all wart types other than plantar and common warts, including those that may occur on the face or eyelids or along nail beds, should be diagnosed and treated by a physician.[12]

Evaluation of Corns, Calluses, and Warts

Many foot conditions require a physician's attention, especially those accompanying chronic, debilitating diseases such as diabetes mellitus or arteriosclerosis. Without proper supervision, nonprescription products may induce more inflammation, ulceration, or possibly gangrene, particularly in cases of vascular insufficiency in the foot. In addition, simple lesions may mask more serious abscesses or ulcerations. If exostoses associated with corns are not excised by a physician, the corns will persist. Sites with many corns, many calluses, or lesions that ooze purulent material (a sign of a secondary bacterial infection) should also be examined by a physician.

Most patients with rheumatoid arthritis eventually have foot involvement; painful metatarsal heads, hallux valgus, and clawfoot are the major forefoot deformities in these patients. Corrective surgical procedures are often indicated to reduce pain and improve function and mobility. There is little evidence supporting the effectiveness of conventional nonsurgical therapy (e.g., orthopedic shoes, metatarsal inserts, conventional arch supports, and metatarsal bars) in these cases.

The patient's medical history and medication profile are extremely valuable, particularly in cases in which self-medication has been tried. Again, warts, calluses, and corns can mask more serious abscesses and ulcerations; if left medically unattended, they may lead to such conditions as osteomyelitis, which may require hospitalization and aggressive parenteral antibiotic therapy. Because circulation is impaired in chronic, debilitating diseases, treatment with nonprescription products may easily cause inadvertent injury. Such injury may heal slowly. PWDs and patients not properly screened for ischemic changes are susceptible to gangrene. (See Chapter 16, "Diabetes Care Products and Monitoring Devices.")

The pharmacist must be aware that warts may occasionally be confused with more serious conditions, such as squamous cell carcinoma and deep fungal infections. A squamous cell carcinoma may develop rapidly, attaining a diameter of 1 cm within 2 weeks. The lesion generally appears as a small, red, conical, hard nodule that quickly ulcerates. Subungual verrucae, which occur under the nail plate, may exist in conjunction with periungual verrucae. A long-standing subungual verruca may be difficult to differentiate from a squamous cell carcinoma, especially in elderly patients. Condyloma acuminata, which are moist and often cauliflower-like in appearance, must be differentiated from condyloma lata (secondary syphilis), which have a smooth, whitish surface. Because of the possible link between this wart type and the development of cervical cancer, the female patient must be advised to consult a physician.

In addition to responses to some of the questions suggested in the patient assessment and counseling section at the beginning of this chapter, the patient's medical history and medication profile should include the following information:

- Characteristics (particularly oozing and bleeding of warts) and duration of the condition;
- Similar problems that may have occurred in other family members;
- Any medical treatment being given for the problem or for other conditions (e.g., immunosuppressive therapy, diabetes mellitus, or rheumatoid arthritis);
- Any drug allergies.

Medical referral is indicated if:

- A peripheral circulatory disease, diabetes mellitus, or a medical condition already under a physician's care exists;
- Hemorrhaging or oozing of purulent material occurs;
- Corns and calluses indicate an anatomical defect or fault in body weight distribution;
- Corns and calluses on the foot are extensive or are painful and debilitating;
- Facial warts, plantar warts on weight-bearing areas, periungual warts, perianal or venereal warts, or extensive warts at one site exist;
- Proper self-medication for warts has been tried for an adequate period without success;
- Patient has a history of rheumatoid arthritis and complains of painful metatarsal heads or deviation of the great toe.

Self-treatment is appropriate if:

- Chronic, debilitating diseases do not contraindicate the use of foot care products;
- The patient is not diabetic;
- The directions for use of the products can be followed with no difficulty;
- No concurrent medication (e.g., immunosuppressives) is being taken that contraindicates the use of these products;
- Corns and calluses are minor;
- Predisposing factors (e.g., ill-fitting footwear and hosiery) of corns and calluses are removed;
- Neither an anatomical defect nor faulty weight distribution is indicated by corns or calluses;
- Plantar warts have not spread extensively over the sole of the foot.

Treatment of Corns, Calluses, and Warts

As previously stated, salicylic acid is the only nonprescription drug found by the FDA to be both safe and effective as a keratolytic agent for the treatment of corns, calluses, and plantar warts.[5] Although several prescription products (e.g., cantharidin, podophyllum, and podofilox) and/or cryotherapy may also be used to treat warts, discussion of these treatments is outside the scope of this chapter.

Pharmacologic Agents

Salicylic Acid Salicylic acid is the oldest of the keratolytic agents and is formulated in many strengths (0.5–40%), depending on its intended use. For the self-treatment of corns, calluses, and warts, its approved concentration ranges in the various topical dosage forms are listed in Table 2.

Salicylic acid is thought to act on hyperplastic keratin in two ways: it decreases keratinocyte adhesion, and it increases water binding, which leads to a hydration of keratin. Because of the latter effect, the presence of moisture had been thought to be an important component of salicylic acid's therapeutic efficacy, and soaking the area in a warm water bath for 5 minutes before applying salicylic acid was recommended. However, evidence submitted to the FDA indicated that presoaking produced no significant positive effects for any efficacy parameter assessed.[13] In its final rule, the FDA proposed to allow the manufacturers of these products to state as an optional direction to the consumer: "May soak corn/callus (or wart) in warm water for 5 minutes to assist in removal."

Significant percutaneous absorption may occur when salicylic acid is applied over large body areas—for example, during therapy for extensive psoriasis on the face, trunk, or extremities. Absorbed salicylic acid is largely metabolized in the liver and excreted in the urine; patients with impaired liver or kidney function are therefore predisposed to accumulation and salicylate toxicity. However, although occlusive vehicles can enhance the percutaneous absorption of salicylic acid, it is highly unlikely that salicylism will result during corn, callus, or wart therapy. Further, it is not necessary to encircle surrounding healthy skins with a film of white petrolatum to protect it from inadvertent salicylic acid application during treatment. Thus, the FDA has deleted the necessity of this instruction on salicylic acid product packaging.

In years past, packaging and labeling for corn, callus, or wart removal products warned patients with diabetes or peripheral vascular disease not to use the products except under direct physician supervision. This was because any acute inflammation or ulcer formation caused by the topical salicylic acid could be dangerous. In its final monograph, the FDA determined that the warning should be stronger and should caution against using the product under certain conditions rather than including an "except under" condition for use. Consequently, the revised warning is as follows:

> **WARNING** Do not use this product on irritated skin, on any area that is infected or reddened, if you are diabetic, or if you have poor blood circulation.[13]

Salicylic acid is usually applied to a corn, callus, or common wart in a collodion or collodion-like vehicle. The patient should thoroughly wash and dry the affected area before applying the product. For corns and calluses, the solution is applied once or twice daily as needed for up to 14 days, or until the corn or callus is removed. For warts, the salicylic acid–containing product is applied once or twice daily as needed for up to 12 weeks, or until the wart is removed. For all three conditions, the

---

TABLE 2   **FDA final monographs on foot care products for corns, calluses, and warts**

Corn and callus remover drug products[a]

Salicylic acid, 12–40% in a plaster vehicle
Salicylic acid, 12–17.6% in a collodion-like vehicle

Wart remover drug products[b]

Salicylic acid, 12–40% in a plaster vehicle
Salicylic acid, 5–17% in a collodion-like vehicle
Salicylic acid, 15% in a karaya gum, glycol plaster vehicle

[a] *Federal Register* 1990 Aug 14; 55 (157): 33258–62.
[b] *Federal Register* 1990 Aug 14; 55 (157): 33246–56.

product is applied one drop at a time until the affected area is well covered. The patient should be advised not to overuse the product.

The liquid dosage form is often the easiest for the patient to apply. However, this treatment mode requires patience and persistence because of the length of time it requires to resolve the problem. It is suggested that the patient keep the adjacent healthy skin dry and clean and that the collodion film be peeled away every 2 or 3 days to remove keratotic debris.[11]

Salicylic acid may also be delivered to the skin through the use of a plaster disk or pad. This delivery system provides direct and prolonged contact of the drug with the affected area. Salicylic acid plaster is a uniform solid or semisolid adhesive mixture of salicylic acid in a suitable base, spread on appropriate backing material (e.g., felt, moleskin, cotton, or plastic), which may be applied directly to the affected area. The usual concentration of salicylic acid in the base is 40%. A small piece of the 40% plaster may be cut to the size of the wart and held in place by waterproof tape. More convenient, however, are corn or callus pads that have small salicylic acid disks for direct application to the skin. The patient selects the appropriately sized disk, places it directly on the affected area, and then covers it with the pad.

For corns and calluses, salicylic acid plasters or disks are generally applied and removed within 48 hours, with a maximum of five treatments over a 2-week period. For warts, salicylic acid plasters or disks are applied and removed every 48 hours, with a maximum treatment period not to exceed 12 weeks. The karaya-gum, glycol plaster with 15% salicylic acid for wart removal is specifically designed to be applied at bedtime and left on for at least 8 hours; in the morning, it is removed and discarded. This procedure is repeated every 24 hours as needed for up to 12 weeks. If the wart remains, a physician should be consulted.

Collodion Vehicles Topical keratolytics used in treating corns, calluses, and warts generally are formulated in flexible collodion-like delivery systems containing pyroxylin; various combinations of volatile solvents such as ether, acetone, or alcohol; and a plasticizer, usually castor oil. Pyroxylin is a nitrocellulose derivative that, after evaporation of the volatile solvents, remains on the skin as a water-repellent film. The advantages of collodions are that they form an adherent flexible or rigid film and they prevent moisture evaporation; these qualities aid penetration of the active ingredient into the affected tissue and result in sustained local action of the drug. The systems are water insoluble, as are most of their active ingredients such as salicylic acid. They are less apt to run than are aqueous solutions.

The disadvantages of collodions are that they are extremely flammable and volatile and that, by occluding normal water transport through the skin, they may be mechanically irritating. Also, the collodion's occlusive nature allows systemic absorption of some drugs. Some patients may abuse these vehicles by sniffing their volatile aromatic solvents.

Historically Used Unapproved Agents In its final monograph, the FDA classified drugs used historically for corn, callus, or wart removal as nonmonograph ingredients.[5,13] These drugs include acetic acid, glacial acetic acid, allantoin, ascorbic acid, belladonna extract, benzocaine, calcium pantothenate, camphor, castor oil, chlorobutanol, diperodon hydrochloride, ichthammol, iodine, lactic acid, menthol, methylbenzethonium chloride, methyl salicylate, panthenol, phenoxyacetic acid, phenyl salicylate, vitamin A, and zinc chloride. These ineffective drugs are no longer approved for self-treatment of corns, calluses, or warts and cannot be marketed for either use unless they are the subject of a specifically approved application.

Folk Remedies

Some folk remedies are occasionally recommended for wart treatment with beneficial effects claimed.[14] There is a long list of such remedies, but a few are worth sharing:

- Rub a dusty, dry toad on warts, and they will disappear.
- Rub the gizzard of a chicken on warts during the decrease of the moon; bury the gizzard in the center of a dirt road.
- Cut a potato and rub it on the warts; then throw the potato over the fence.
- Steal a used washcloth, rub it over the warts, bury it, and the warts disappear as the cloth rots.
- Rub the wart with castor oil every day.

The perceived beneficial effects of these remedies is most likely due to the coincidental and spontaneous resolution of the wart in response to natural immune functions. Nonetheless, the pharmacist may be asked about their usefulness.

Adjunctive Therapy

In addition to nonprescription drugs, self-therapy measures include daily soaking of the affected area throughout treatment for at least 5 minutes in warm (not hot) water to remove dead tissue. Dead tissue should be removed gently rather than forcibly after normal washing because further damage could result. A rough towel, callus file, or pumice stone effectively accomplishes this purpose. Sharp knives or razor blades that have not been properly sterilized should not be used because they may cause bacterial contamination and infection. Petroleum jelly need not be applied to healthy skin surrounding the affected area before corrosive products are applied. However, this precaution should be suggested to persons with poor eyesight or other conditions that increase the likelihood of misapplication or accidental spillage.

To relieve painful pressure emanating from inflamed underlying tissue and irritated or hypertrophied bones directly underneath a corn or callus, patients may use a pad such as a Dr. Scholl's® with an aperture for the corn or callus. If the skin can tolerate the pads, they may be used for up to 1 week or longer. To prevent the pads from adhering to hosiery, patients may wax them with paraffin or a candle and then powder them daily with a hygienic foot powder or cover them with an adhesive bandage. If, despite these measures, friction causes the pads to peel up at the edge and stick to hosiery, the pharmacist may recommend that patients cover their toes with the forefoot of an old stocking or pantyhose before putting on hosiery.

Pharmacists should advise patients that if at any time the pad begins to cause itching, burning, or pain, it should be removed and a physician or podiatrist be consulted. Pharmacists should also advise patients that these pads will provide only temporary relief and will rarely cure a corn or callus.

To avoid the spread of warts, which is contagious, patients should wash their hands before and after treating or touching wart tissue. A specific towel should be used only for drying the affected area after cleaning. Patients should not probe or poke the wart tissue. If warts are present on the sole of the foot, patients should not walk in bare feet unless the wart is securely covered.

Patient Education and Consultation: Corns, Calluses, and Warts

Remission of corns, calluses, and warts does not happen quickly; it can take several days to several months. Thus, adherence to the dosage regimen and selection of a convenient time to apply the product are important. Topical products should be applied no more than twice daily; the most convenient times are generally in the morning and evening. If the wart remains after a full course of treatment, a physician should be consulted.

The pharmacist should counsel the patient on how to use the medication. Because many products contain corrosive materials, they must be applied only to the corn, callus, or wart. If a plaster or pad is used, the pharmacist should first explain how to trim the pad to follow the contours of the corn or callus. The pharmacist should then instruct the patient how to apply the plaster to the skin and cover it with adhesive occlusive tape; how to remove the dressing the next day and soak the foot in warm water; how to remove the macerated, soft white skin of the corn or callus by scrubbing gently with a rough towel, pumice stone, or callus file; and how to reapply the plaster. Patients must be careful not to debride healthy skin when using a pumice stone or callus file.

If a solution is used, the pharmacist should instruct the patient to apply one drop at a time directly to the corn, callus, or wart; to allow the drops to dry and harden so the solution does not run; and to continue the procedure until the entire affected area is covered. Adjacent areas of normal healthy skin should not come in contact with the drug. If they do, the solution should be washed off immediately with soap and water. If the solution is being used on a soft corn between the toes, the toes should be held apart until the solution has dried. The solution should solidify before a dressing is applied. This treatment is to be followed for 3–6 days.

Pharmacists should remind patients that these products are keratolytic and cause skin tissue to slough off, leaving an unsightly pinkish tinge to the skin; nevertheless, they should continue to be used. These products should be discontinued only when a severe inflammatory response (swelling or reddening) or irritation occurs, or when pain occurs immediately upon application.

Because liquid nonprescription preparations contain volatile and irritating ingredients, the patient should be cautious in using them. After use, the container should be tightly capped to prevent evaporation and to prevent the active ingredients from assuming a greater concentration. The volatile delivery systems are quite flammable, and the product should be stored in amber or light-resistant containers away from direct sunlight or heat.

Pharmacists should alert patients that the products that contain collodions are poisonous when taken orally and that these products, as well as all other corn, callus, and wart removal products, should be stored out of children's reach. Collodion-containing products are volatile, have an odor similar to that of airplane glue, and may be subject to abuse by inhalation.

Nonprescription corn, callus, and wart removal products are not generally recommended for patients with diabetes or circulatory problems. Pharmacists should reinforce contraindications, warnings, and precautions with all patients to avoid the inadvertent use of these products by other family members who have such conditions.

Athlete's Foot

The most prevalent cutaneous fungal infection in humans is athlete's foot (dermatophytosis of the foot, or tinea pedis). Athlete's foot afflicts approximately 26.5 million people in the United States every year, and of every 10 sufferers, 7 are male. It is estimated that 70% of the population will be afflicted with athlete's foot in their lifetime and that approximately 45% will suffer with it episodically for more than 10 years. When exposure to infectious environments is equal, the incidence of tinea infections in women approaches that of men.

The clinical spectrum of athlete's foot ranges from mild itching and scaling to a severe, exudative inflammatory process characterized by fissuring and denudation. The prevalent type of athlete's foot, midway between these two extremes, is characterized by maceration, hyperkeratosis, pruritus, malodor, itching, and a stinging sensation of the feet (see color plates, photograph 36).

Etiology

Tinea pedis is an infection type of relatively recent onset. It was not common until humans began wearing occlusive footwear, and it was not reported in the medical literature until 1888. Because ringworm fungi (dermatophytes) are generally the causative or initiating organisms, athlete's foot is often synonymous with a ringworm infection.[15] Tinea pedis is most commonly caused by *Trichophyton rubrum*, *Trichophyton mentagrophytes*, or *Epidermophyton floccosum*. *T. rubrum* often causes a dry, hyperkeratotic, involvement of the feet; *T. mentagrophytes* often produces a blister-like or vesicular pattern; and *E. floccosum* is capable of producing both of these patterns.

In addition to specific microorganisms, other environmental factors contribute to the disease's development. Footwear is a key variable, as illustrated by the incidence of the disease in any population that wears occlusive footwear with little ventilation. Occlusion with a nonporous material increases temperature and hydration of the skin and interferes with the barrier function of the stratum corneum. The climatic conditions of the area and the customs of the resident population also play roles in the dermatophytosis infection. The infection is common in the summer or in tropical or semitropical climates among individuals who customarily wear occlusive footwear that promotes overhydration of the skin.

The type of dermatophytosis present varies with geographic location.[16] In Vietnam, U.S. soldiers often acquired a disabling, inflammatory *T. mentagrophytes* infection, although South Vietnamese soldiers did not. In a resident population, dermatophytosis infection is often observed as chronic and noninflammatory whereas the same infection in virgin hosts is markedly inflammatory and self-limited.[16]

Species of dermatophytes that infect humans (e.g., *T. rubrum* and *T. mentagrophytes*) are transmitted either directly by human contact or indirectly by exposure to inanimate objects. It is thought that this infection is acquired most often by walking barefoot on infected floors (e.g., hotel bathrooms, swimming pools, or locker rooms) and may be spread within families by exposure to bathroom floors, mats, or rugs. Therefore, tinea pedis is considered to be an exogenously transmitted infection in which cross-infection among susceptible individuals readily occurs.[16]

Pathophysiology

After being inoculated into the skin under suitable conditions, the infection progresses through several stages. These stages include periods of incubation and then enlargement, followed by a refractory period and a stage of involution.

During the incubation period, the dermatophyte grows in the stratum corneum, sometimes with minimal signs of infection. After the incubation period and once the infection is established, two factors appear to play a role in determining the size and duration of the lesions. These factors are the growth rate of the organism and the epidermal turnover rate.[16] The fungal growth rate must equal or exceed the epidermal turnover rate, or the organism will quickly shed.

Dermatophytic infestations remain within the stratum corneum. This resistance to the spread of infection seems to involve both immunologic and nonimmunologic mechanisms. For example, the substance serum inhibitory factor (SIF) appears to limit the growth of dermatophytes beyond the stratum corneum. SIF is not an antibody but a dialyzable, heat-labile component of fresh sera. It appears that SIF binds to the iron that dermatophytes need for continued growth.[16]

Once into the stratum corneum, dermatophytes produce keratinases and other proteolytic enzymes. U.S. combat personnel in Vietnam demonstrated a particularly inflammatory type of *T. mentagrophytes* infection associated with elastase production. This indicated that enzymes or toxins produced by these microorganisms account for some of the severe clinical reactions.

Types

Clinically, there are four accepted variants of tinea pedis; two or more of these types may overlap. The most common is the chronic, intertriginous type,[16] characterized by fissuring, scaling, or maceration in the interdigital spaces. Typically, the infection involves the lateral toe webs, usually between the fourth and fifth or third and fourth toes. From these sites, the infection spreads to the sole or instep of the foot but rarely to the dorsum. Warmth and humidity aggravate this condition. Consequently, hyperhidrosis (excessive sweating) becomes an underlying problem and must be treated along with the dermatophyte infestation.

It is also known that normal resident aerobic diphtheroids may become involved in the athlete's foot process. After initial invasion of the stratum corneum by dermatophytes, enough moisture may accumulate to trigger a bacterial overgrowth. Increased moisture and temperature then lead to bacterial proliferation and the release of metabolic products, which diffuse easily through the underlying horny layer already damaged by fungal invasion. In the more severe cases, Gram-negative organisms intrude and may exacerbate the condition, causing skin maceration, white hyperkeratosis, or erosions with increased patient symptomatology.

The second variant of athlete's foot is known as the chronic, papulosquamous pattern.[16] It is usually found on both feet and is characterized by a mild inflammation and a diffuse scaling on the soles of the feet. Tinea unguium (i.e., ringworm of the nails, or onychomycosis) of one or more toenails may also be present. Toenail involvement may continue to fuel the infection. The toenails must first be cured with oral drug therapy, such as griseofulvin or ketoconazole, or removed surgically to rid the area of the offending fungus. Surgery is preferred because oral antifungal therapy is not always effective.

The third variant of tinea pedis is the vesicular type, usually caused by *T. mentagrophytes* var. *interdigitale*.[16] Small vesicles or vesicopustules are observed near the instep and on the midanterior plantar surface. Skin scaling is seen on these areas as well as on the toe webs. This variant is symptomatic in the summer and clinically quiescent during the cooler months.

The acute ulcerative type is the fourth variant of tinea pedis. It is often associated with macerated, denuded, weeping ulcerations of the sole of the foot. Typically, white hyperkeratosis and a pungent odor are present. This type of infection, which is complicated by the presence of an overgrowth of opportunistic, Gram-negative bacteria such as *Proteus* and *Pseudomonas*, has been called dermatophytosis complex or Gram-negative athlete's foot, and it may produce an extremely painful, erosive, purulent interspace that can be disabling.

Susceptibility

Although there are many pathogenic fungi in the environment, the overall incidence of actual superficial fungal infections is remarkably low. Many degrees of susceptibility produce a clinical infection—from instantaneous "takes" by a single spore to severe trauma with massive exposure. It appears, however, that trauma to the skin, especially that which produces blisters (from wearing ill-fitting footwear), may be significantly more important to the occurrence of human fungal infections than is simple exposure to the offending pathogens.

Although tinea pedis may occur at all ages, it is more common in adults, presumably because of their increased opportunities for exposure to pathogens. However, tinea pedis should not be ignored as a possibility in children. Individual susceptibility is also affected by other disease processes the patient may have. For example, dermatophytosis infections may be more severe and difficult to ameliorate in patients with diabetes mellitus, lymphoid malignancies, immunologic compromise, and Cushing's syndrome.[16]

Evaluation

The most common complaint of patients suffering from tinea pedis is pruritus. However, if fissures are present, particularly between the toes, painful burning and stinging may also occur. If the foot area is abraded, denuded, or inflamed, there may be weeping or oozing in addition to pain. Some patients may merely remark on the bothersome scaling of dry skin, particularly if it has progressed to the sole of the feet. Small vesicular lesions may combine to form a larger bullous eruption marked by pain and irritation. The only symptoms may be brittleness and discoloration of a hypertrophied toenail.

The only true determinant of a fungal foot infection is clinical laboratory evaluation of tissue scrapings from the foot. This process involves a potassium hydroxide mount preparation of the scrapings and cuttings on a special growth medium to show the actual presence and specific identity of fungi. The procedure can be ordered and performed only at the direction of a physician, and microscopic confirmation probably will be possible only in the dry, scaly type of tinea pedis. The recovery of fungi for diagnosis decreases as athlete's foot becomes progressively more severe. In typical cases of dermatophytosis complex, fungus recovery rates are only about 25–50%.

The pharmacist should question the patient thoroughly as to the condition and its characteristics to determine symptoms, the extent of disease, previous patient compliance with medications, and any mitigating circumstances, such as diabetes or obesity, that might render the patient susceptible. PWDs, for example, may present with a mixed dermatophytic and monilial infection.

The pharmacist should seek to distinguish tinea pedis from diseases with similar symptoms such as dermatitis, allergic contact dermatitis, and atopic dermatitis. In children, peridigital dermatitis or atopic dermatitis is more common than tinea pedis. Shoe dermatitis is perhaps the most common form of allergic contact dermatitis from clothing. Since 1950, the increased use of rubber and adhesives in footwear has paralleled the increase in reports of shoe dermatitis in the dermatologic and podiatric literature. Contact allergy to accelerators—the chemical compounds used to speed up the processing of rubber used in sponge-rubber insoles for tennis shoes—has also been reported.[17] In addition to accelerators, antioxidants have been implicated as major chemical allergens, and various phenolic resins used in adhesives are also troublesome. The patient is usually unaware that the footwear may be causing the problem.

Hyperhidrosis of interdigital spaces and the sole of the foot is common, as is infection of toe webs by Gram-negative bacteria. In hyperhidrosis, tender vesicles cover the sole of the foot and toes and may be quite painful. The skin generally turns white, erodes, and becomes macerated. This condition is accompanied by a foul foot odor. Infection by Gram-negative bacteria is characterized by a soggy wetness of the toe webs and immediately adjacent skin. The affected tissue is damp, softened, and soggy.

The last toe web (adjacent to the little toe) is the most common area of primary or initial involvement because it is deeper and extends more proximally than the web between the other toes. Furthermore, abundant exocrine sweat glands, a semiocclusive anatomical setting, and the added occlusion provided by footwear enhance development of the disease at this site. The pharmacist must be careful not to confuse this condition with soft corns, which also appear between the fourth and fifth toes.

Severe forms of tinea pedis may progress to disintegration and denudation of the affected skin and to profuse, serous, purulent discharge. Denudation may involve all the toe webs, the dorsal and plantar surfaces of the toes, and an area about 1 cm wide beyond the base of the toes on the plantar surface of the foot. When the disease is out of control, its progression is observed on the dorsum of the foot and the calf in the form of tiny red follicular crusts. Paradoxically, this condition may be caused by the use of reputed germicidal soaps such as pHisoHex®, Dial®, and Safeguard®. It was hypothesized that these soaps reduce the presence of harmless saprophytes and thus promote overgrowth of resistant pathogens (e.g., *Pseudomonas aeruginosa* and *Proteus mirabilis*) by removing their competitors.

If the patient has used a nonprescription antifungal product appropriately for several weeks without relief, a disease other than tinea pedis may be involved. Therapeutic failure may be due to Gram-negative athlete's foot, which no nonprescription antifungal product will ameliorate. Persons suffering from hyperhidrosis, allergic contact dermatitis, atopic dermatitis, or a possible Gram-negative infection of the toe should see a podiatrist or physician for treatment.

The pharmacist should be aware of the implications of the following conditions and be able to recommend to the patient the appropriate course of action:

- If the toenail is involved, topical treatment is ineffective and will not allay the condition until the disease's primary focus is treated with oral griseofulvin or ketoconazole or until other preventive measures are instituted (e.g., surgical avulsion of the nail).
- If vesicular eruptions are oozing purulent material that could indicate a secondary bacterial infection, topical astringent therapy and/or antibiotic therapy may be appropriate.
- If the interspace between the toes is foul smelling; whitish; painful; soggy; or characterized by erosions, oozing, or serious inflammation, and especially if the condition is disabling, the patient should be referred to a physician.
- If the foot is seriously inflamed or swollen and a major portion of the foot is involved, supportive therapy must be instituted before an antifungal agent may be applied.
- If the patient is a child who presents with an eczematous eruption of the feet, including that complicated by blisters and/or pyoderma, self-treatment should not be recommended.
- If the patient is under a physician's supervision for a disease such as diabetes or asthma, in which normal host-defense mechanisms may be deficient, nonprescription products should not be recommended before medical consultation.

Pharmacologic Treatment

Before self-medication can be effective, the correct type of tinea pedis and the correct treatment must be determined. Self-treatment of an acute, superficial tinea foot infection may be effective if certain conditions are met. In acute, inflammatory tinea pedis, characterized by reddened, oozing, and vesicular eruptions, the inflammation must be counteracted before antifungal therapy can be instituted. This step is especially important if the eruptions are caused by a secondary bacterial infection.

Hydrocortisone, in conjunction with clioquinol (formerly iodochlorhydroxyquin), has demonstrated favorable results toward resolving uncomplicated cutaneous fungal infections (tinea cruris, tinea pedis, and moniliasis). Erythema and itching were relieved more with the combination of these two drugs than with either drug alone or the placebo cream. However, with the availability of nonprescription topical hydrocortisone products, it is conceivable that their indiscriminate use to relieve the itching and redness of athlete's foot could complicate and delay appropriate medical care. Topical hydrocortisone by itself is contraindicated in the presence of fungal infections.

Self-treatment is effective only if the patient understands the importance of compliance with all facets of the treatment plan. Specific antifungal products must be used appropriately in conjunction with other treatment measures, including general hygienic measures and local drying. Local hygienic measures should not be minimized as a useful adjunct to specific antifungal therapy.

The pharmacologic agents used to treat athlete's foot have been evaluated for safety and efficacy by the FDA Advisory Review Panel on Over-the-Counter Antimicrobial Drug Products.[18] Table 3 lists these agents according to their assigned category. The panel concluded that, to best serve all consumers, a nonprescription product must provide more than temporary symptomatic relief of athlete's foot, jock itch, and ringworm. Such products must contain a Category I antifungal ingredient capable of killing the fungus. The panel required each antifungal ingredient to have at least one well-designed clinical trial demonstrating its effectiveness in the treatment of athlete's foot to be classified as Category I.

Carbol–Fuchsin Solution

Basic fuchsin (NF XIII) dye is a mixture of rosaniline and pararosaniline hydrochloride. It is used only in superficial fungal foot infections in the form of carbol–fuchsin solution (NF XIII) or Castellani's paint. The solution is dark purple but appears red when painted onto the affected area in a fine film. It has local anesthetic, drying, and antimicrobial properties.

The use of carbol–fuchsin solution in tinea pedis is indicated in the subacute or chronic stages of infection when there is little or no inflammation. Before the solution is applied, the affected area should be cleaned thoroughly with soap and water and dried. The solution is then applied to the area with an applicator and reapplied once or twice daily for 1 week. If the condition has not improved after this time, the choice of medication as well as the assessment of the actual condition should be reevaluated.

Because the preparation contains several volatile components, the bottle cap should be securely tightened to avoid evaporation. Otherwise, volatile ingredients will escape, causing other nonvolatile components (e.g., resorcinol) to become more concentrated, and irritation may result with subsequent applications.

Carbol–fuchsin solution should not be applied to an area greater than 10% of the foot or to a severely inflamed or denuded foot because systemic toxicity can result if the solution is percutaneously absorbed. This limitation, the medication's staining properties, its poisonous nature, and possible patient sensitivity to its ingredients limit the appeal and usefulness of carbol–fuchsin solution for tinea pedis. This is unfortunate because carbol–fuchsin solution suppresses fungi and bacteria and simultaneously produces a local drying or astringent effect; these properties are necessary for effective therapy of uncomplicated athlete's foot. Carbol–fuchsin solution has demonstrated efficacy equivalent to that of 30% aluminum chloride solution for interdigital dermatophytosis. Anecdotal reports suggest, however, that the extemporaneous preparation and use of the paint without the fuchsin dye may be just as effective and more aesthetically acceptable. The FDA Advisory Review Panel on Over-the-Counter Antimicrobial Drug Products placed basic fuchsin into Category III.[18]

Clioquinol

Clioquinol has demonstrated efficacy in treating athlete's foot and jock itch. The FDA classified it as Category I—safe and effective for topical nonprescription use in the treatment of both conditions. Evaluations of clioquinol used alone and in combination with hydrocortisone indicate the following effectiveness: clioquinol–hydrocortisone combination > clioquinol alone > hydrocortisone alone > placebo.

Clioquinol has a low incidence of side effects; however, it may cause itching, redness, and irritation. Even though the possibility of its percutaneous absorption is low, clioquinol may interfere with thyroid function tests. Thus, patients undergoing these tests must be questioned carefully to assess their prior use of iodine-containing clioquinol.

Clioquinol is also used to treat diaper rash; however, concerns for its safety in this regard have been raised. Those who use topical clioquinol should be monitored for any signs or symptoms of neurologic toxicity, abdominal pain, weakness or paralysis of the legs, or muscle twitching.

Clotrimazole and Miconazole Nitrate

Clotrimazole and miconazole nitrate are imidazole derivatives that demonstrate fungistatic/fungicidal activity (depending upon concentration) against *T. mentagrophytes, T. rubrum, E. floccosum,* and *Candida albicans*. These agents act by inhibiting the biosynthesis of ergosterol and other steroids, and by damaging the fungal cell wall membrane and altering its permeability. As a result, essential intracellular elements may be lost. These drugs have also been shown to inhibit oxidative and peroxidative enzyme activity, which results in intracellular buildup of toxic concentrations of hydrogen peroxide; this may then contribute to degradation of subcellular organelles and cellular necrosis. In *C. albicans*, these drugs have been shown to inhibit the transformation of blastospores into invasive mycelial form.

Both of these prescription drugs have been reclassified as nonprescription. Both are suggested for application

TABLE 3 FDA classification of topical antifungals and ingrown toenail relief products

FDA OTC panel	Category assignment		
	Category I	Category II	Category III
Topical antifungal drug products; establishment of a monograph[b]	Haloprogin Clioquinol Miconazole nitrate Nystatin Tolnaftate Undecylenic acid and its salts	Camphor Candicidin Coal tar Menthol Phenolates Resorcinol Tannic acid Thymol Tolindate	Aluminum salts[a] Basic fuchsin Benzethonium chloride Benzoic acid Borates Caprylates Chlorothymol Chloroxylenol Oxyquinolines Povidone–iodine Salicylic acid Triacetin
Ingrown toenail relief drug products; tentative final monograph[c]	None	Chloroxylenol Urea	Sodium sulfide Tannic acid

[a] Partial listing only.
[b] *Federal Register* 1982 Mar 23; 47.
[c] *Federal Register* 1982 Sep 3; 47.

twice daily, once in the morning and once in the evening. Controlled studies have demonstrated their efficacy for jock itch and athlete's foot; they have also been approved for self-treatment of previously diagnosed vaginal yeast (i.e., candidal) infections. (See Chapter 28, "Topical Anti-Infective Products.") Both would be expected to demonstrate efficacy comparable to that of tolnaftate (see next section) for tinea pedis, and in the event of treatment failure in which patient factors (e.g., noncompliance or improper foot hygiene) have been ruled out as a cause, both can be suggested as alternative treatment modalities. Rare cases of mild skin irritation, burning, and stinging have occurred with use of these agents.

Tolnaftate

Tolnaftate acts on typical fungi responsible for tinea pedis, including *T. mentagrophytes* and *T. rubrum*. It is also effective against *E. floccosum* and species of *Microsporum*. Although its exact mechanism of action has not been reported, it is believed that tolnaftate distorts the hyphae and stunts the mycelial growth of the fungi species. Tolnaftate is more effective in tinea pedis than it is in onychomycosis or tinea capitis; for those conditions, concomitant administration of oral griseofulvin or ketoconazole is necessary unless the condition is superficial.

Tolnaftate is well tolerated when applied to intact or broken skin in either exposed or intertriginous areas, although it usually stings slightly when applied. Delayed hypersensitivity reactions to tolnaftate are extremely unlikely. As with all topical medications, discontinuation is warranted if irritation, sensitization, or worsening of the skin condition occurs.

Tolnaftate (1% solution, cream, gel, powder, spray powder, or spray liquid) is applied sparingly twice daily after the affected area is cleaned thoroughly. Effective therapy usually takes 2–4 weeks although some individuals (patients with lesions between the toes or on pressure areas of the foot) may require treatment lasting 4–6 weeks. When medication is applied to pressure areas of the foot, where the horny skin layer is thicker than normal, concomitant use of a keratolytic agent may be advisable. Neither keratolytic agents nor wet compresses, such as aluminum acetate solution (Burow's solution), which promote the healing of oozing lesions, interfere with the efficacy of tolnaftate. If weeping lesions are present, the inflammation should be treated before tolnaftate is applied.

As a cream, tolnaftate is formulated in a polyethylene glycol 400–propylene glycol vehicle. The 1% solution is formulated in polyethylene glycol 400 and may be more effective than the cream. The solution solidifies when exposed to cold, but if allowed to warm, it will liquefy with no loss in potency. These vehicles are particularly advantageous in superficial antifungal therapy because they are nonocclusive, nontoxic, nonsensitizing, water miscible, anhydrous, easy to apply, and efficient in delivering the drug to the affected area.

The topical powder formulation of tolnaftate uses cornstarch–talc as the vehicle. This vehicle not only is an effective drug delivery system but also offers a therapeutic advantage because the two agents retain water. The topical aerosol formulation of tolnaftate includes talc and the propellant vehicle.

Tolnaftate has demonstrated clinical efficacy since its commercial introduction into the United States in 1965, and it has become the standard topical antifungal medication. In addition, irritation and hypersensitivity to tolnaftate has been consistently absent in its cream, solution, or powder form, thus enabling it to be approved for nonprescription use.

Tolnaftate is valuable primarily in the dry, scaly type of athlete's foot. Superficial fungal infection relapse has occurred after tolnaftate therapy was discontinued. Relapse may be caused by inadequate treatment time, patient noncompliance with the medication, or use of tolnaftate when oral griseofulvin or ketoconazole should have been employed. Because tolnaftate does not possess antibacterial properties, its value must be viewed with skepticism for use in the soggy, macerated type of athlete's foot in which bacteria are involved.

Organic Fatty Acids

The antifungal effect of various fatty acids and their salts on dermatophytes have produced encouraging clinical results. The sodium salt of caprylic acid (an eight-carbon fatty acid) was more effective than sodium undecylenate in treating dermatophytosis of the foot. However, both propionic and undecylenic acids are weakly fungistatic.

Whether organic fatty acids are more effective than sulfur or iodine preparations in treating superficial fungal infections is questionable. Organic acid preparations should be used, if at all, only for very mild or chronic forms of tinea pedis. The FDA advisory panel placed these agents into Category III.[18]

These organic fatty acids and their salts are available in various dosage forms. The cream or ointment form is usually used at bedtime; the powder is usually sprinkled into the socks and shoes in the morning. Solutions should be used for their soothing effects after a foot bath.

The concentration of organic fatty acids or their salt forms is usually too low to irritate the skin. Treatment should be discontinued if irritation or sensitivity develops with their use.

Acetic Acid

Acetic acid is delivered to the infected area as triacetin. The fungistatic activity of triacetin is based on the fact that, at the neutral or alkaline pH of infected skin, fungal esterase enzymes divide triacetin into acetic acid and glycerin. The acetic acid then affects antifungal activity by lowering the pH at the infection site. As the pH increases after the initial release of acetic acid, more acetic acid is generated by the enzymes, and the process is repeated.

The efficacy of products containing triacetin has not been proven in controlled clinical trials.[18] Because the ultimate efficacy of triacetin depends on the presence of moisture for conversion to acetic acid, the FDA Advisory Review Panel on Over-the-Counter Antimicrobial Drug Products placed this drug in Category III with the proviso that it be recommended and used only for the soggy, wet form of athlete's foot.[18]

Triacetin is relatively colorless and odorless. The small amount of acetic acid liberated is nonirritating to the skin in most cases. The incidence of sensitization is also low. The acetic acid formed may damage rayon fabrics, so the treated areas should be covered with a clean bandage if the medication is applied to an area exposed to fabric. Triacetin must not come into contract with the eyes.

Triacetin, which is available in a number of topical dosage forms, should be applied every morning and evening after the affected area is thoroughly cleaned. The product should be used until the infection has cleared entirely, and then once a week as a preventive measure.

Undecylenic Acid–Zinc Undecylenate

This combination is widely used and may be effective for various mild superficial fungal infections, excluding those involving nails or hairy parts of the body. It is fungistatic and effective in mild chronic cases of tinea pedis. Compound undecylenic acid ointment (USP XXI) contains 5% undecylenic acid and 20% zinc undecylenate in an ointment base. It is believed that zinc undecylenate liberates undecylenic acid (the active antifungal entity) on contact with moisture (perspiration). In addition, zinc undecylenate has astringent properties because of the presence of the zinc ion; this astringent activity decreases the irritation and inflammation of the infection.

Applied to the skin as an ointment, diluted solution, or dusting powder, the combination of undecylenic acid–zinc undecylenate is relatively nonirritating, and hypersensitivity reactions are rare. The undiluted solution, however, may cause transient stinging when applied to broken skin because of its alcohol content. Caution must be exercised to ensure that these ingredients do not come into contact with the eye or that the powder is not inhaled.

The vehicle in compound undecylenic acid ointment has a water-miscible base, making it nonocclusive, removable with water, and easy to apply. The powder uses talc as its vehicle and absorbent. The aerosol contains menthol, which serves as a counterirritant and antipruritic. The solution contains 10% undecylenic acid in an isopropyl alcohol vehicle with either an applicator or a spray pump container. The product is applied twice daily after the affected area is cleansed. The usual period required for therapeutic results depends on the severity of the infection. However, if improvement does not occur in 2–4 weeks, the condition should be reevaluated and an alternative medication used.

When the solution is sprayed or applied to the affected area, the area should be allowed to air dry; otherwise, water may accumulate and further macerate the tissue. The relatively high alcohol concentration in these solutions could cause some burning, and the strong odor of undecylenic acid may be objectionable to some patients, possibly promoting patient noncompliance.

The FDA Advisory Review Panel on Over-the-Counter Antimicrobial Drug Products classified undecylenic acid and its derivatives (10–25% total undecylenate content) as Category I for the treatment of athlete's foot.[18]

Phenolic Compounds and Derivatives

Phenol and resorcinol have been included in many topical antifungal products for their keratolytic or fungicidal effects. The fungicidal potency of resorcinol is about one-third that of phenol. Phenol is reported to be more effective in aqueous solutions than in glycerin or fats; it is relatively ineffective, however, when incorporated into soaps.

Applied to unabraded skin in low concentrations, phenol causes warmth and a tingling sensation. Its irritant qualities usually restrict its effectiveness in athlete's foot remedies; for phenol to be fungicidal in these preparations, concentrations irritating to human skin generally must be used.

Resorcinol in concentrations usually applied topically (<10%) is nonirritating; higher concentrations, however, may be irritating. Resorcinol rarely produces allergic reactions.

Phenol and resorcinol resemble each other with regard to systematic action, particularly on the central nervous system. Thus, preparations containing either agent should never be applied to large areas or to irritated or denuded skin because of possible absorption and systemic toxicity. Nonprescription phenol-containing products are limited to concentrations of not more than 1.5%. Local and systemic toxicity may occur following the use of such products covered with bandages or occlusive dressings; therefore, these products should be used with caution for athlete's foot because occlusive footwear could enhance its absorption. Percutaneous absorption would seem more probable from the top of the foot rather than the bottom of the foot, where the thick outer layer of skin would seem to inhibit penetration. With inherent safety problems and insufficient data regarding phenol's efficacy for treating athlete's foot in concentrations of not more than 1.5%, the FDA Advisory Review Panel on Over-the-Counter Antimicrobial Drug Products classified phenol as Category II.[18]

Chloroxylenol, a substituted phenol, is an antiseptic agent. Chloroxylenol (0.5% solution) has been reported to be effective in treating and preventing athlete's foot. It is included in some topical liquid, cream, and powder dosage forms. However, its limited water solubility makes its efficacy in powder delivery systems questionable. If the inert agents of the vehicle are effective in adsorbing moisture, the effect of the chloroxylenol may be diminished. Chloroxylenol causes no cutaneous irritation in concentrations of up to 5%. It is less toxic than phenol, but eczematous reactions have followed its use. Because efficacy data are lacking, the FDA placed chloroxylenol in Category III.[18]

Salicylic Acid

The basic criterion for evaluating the efficacy of salicylic acid products as keratolytic agents is the concentration of salicylic acid. In high concentrations, salicylic acid is a keratolytic agent, causing the keratin layer of the skin to shed and thereby facilitating penetration of other drugs. Lower concentrations (<2%) are keratoplastic; they aid normal keratinization. Salicylic acid (5–10%) softens the stratum corneum by increasing the endogenous hydration of this layer. This effect probably results from a lowering of the pH, which causes the cornified epithelium to swell, soften, macerate, and then desquamate.[16] If no moisture is present, the cornified epithelium is not softened significantly by tolerable amounts of salicylic acid. Because salicylic acid accelerates exfoliation of the infected keratin tissue, its use in conjunction with topical antifungals may be very beneficial in appropriate conditions.

Salicylic acid alone has little or no antifungal activity. It is usually applied to the skin as a combination of 3% salicylic acid and 6% benzoic acid in a polyethylene glycol base (Whitfield's ointment). Benzoic acid alone is alleged to have some fungistatic activity, but this claim is debatable. This ointment is available in double strength and half strength. The half-strength formula (1.5% salicylic acid) does not have the keratolytic properties of the regular or double strength and should never be used when keratolytic activity is necessary. Thus, on the basis of current literature, to be keratolytic agents, these products should contain concentrations of more than 2% salicylic acid. Because of insufficient evidence to support either salicylic or benzoic acid in the treatment of athlete's foot, the FDA classified these agents as Category III.[18]

The pharmacist must recognize the irritant properties of topically applied salicylic acid. Many skin irritations have been reported following its unsupervised use.

Quaternary Ammonium Compounds

Quaternary ammonium compounds (benzethonium chloride and methylbenzethonium chloride) are contained in several antifungal products for their antiseptic and detergent properties. Solutions of these agents have emulsifying properties that favor wetting and penetrating the surfaces to which they are applied. The fungicidal activity of quaternary ammonium compounds is generally less than their bactericidal activity. (See Chapter 28, "Topical Anti-Infective Products.")

The disinfectant action of these compounds in concentrations used may not be as great as expected. Gram-positive microorganisms are generally more susceptible to them than are Gram-negative pathogens. A concern with quaternary ammonium compounds is that their misuse or overuse could lead to overgrowth of *Pseudomonas* sp. or of other poorly susceptible Gram-negative pathogens.

These agents are cationic and are incompatible with anionic compounds such as soaps. Thus, any residual soap or soap film on the skin may inactivate them. Patients who are told to clean their feet thoroughly every day must also be instructed to rinse the affected area completely before drying it. Otherwise, if the nonprescription product contains a quaternary ammonium compound, any beneficial effects may be negated. This precaution should also be considered for any formulations of products that contain anionic compounds (zinc undecylenate or sodium propionate) to prevent the germicide from being rendered ineffective.

A tincture delivery system of these cationic compounds is more effective as a skin disinfectant and is less affected by soap than is an aqueous solution. Accordingly, tincture forms of these agents are used in more dilute concentrations than aqueous solutions. In a liquid form, especially a tincture, quaternary compounds should be effective if appropriate concentrations are used. However, when applied topically in powder form with adsorbent agents included in the formulation, their efficacy is doubtful. If all moisture is removed effectively by the adsorbing material, the quaternary compound may be unable to exert germicidal activity.

Quaternary ammonium compounds are generally safe when applied topically. However, their assignment to Category III indicates a need for substantive additional data relevant to efficacy.[18]

Quinoline Derivatives

Of 24 quinoline derivatives investigated in vitro, only the benzoxiquine (8-hydroxyquinoline benzoate) salt was active in fungistatic and fungicidal testing. It has been postulated that the activity of 8-hydroxyquinoline is caused by the chelation of trace metals essential to the growth of fungi. A 3% benzoxiquine preparation in a vanishing cream base is fungicidal in vitro. An antifungal preparation containing 2.5% benzoxiquine has been used successfully to treat dermatophytosis.

Several proprietary powder antifungals use fungicidal 8-hydroxyquinoline sulfate in their formations. Because the sulfate is water soluble and forms an acidic solution in the presence of moisture, it may enhance the antifungal effect of 8-hydroxyquinoline. However, because there is no objective clinical evidence to support this hypothesis, these agents were classified as Category III.[18]

The quinoline antibiotics bear no chemical or pharmacologic similarity to the antifungal quinolines, and the two chemical classes should not be confused with one another.

Salts of Aluminum

Historically, the foremost astringent used for both the acute, inflammatory state and the wet, soggy type of tinea pedis has been aluminum acetate. Evidence also supports the use of aluminum chloride in treating the wet, soggy type of infection. The action and efficacy of the aluminum salts appear to be two-pronged. First, these compounds act as astringents. Their drying ability probably involves the complexing of the astringent agent with proteins, thereby altering the proteins' ability to swell and hold water. Astringents decrease edema, exudation, and inflammation by reducing cell membrane permeability and hardening the cement substance of the capillary epithelium. Second, aluminum salts in concentrations greater than 20% possess antibacterial activity. Aluminum chloride (20%) may exhibit that activity in two ways: by directly killing bacteria and by drying the interspaces. Solutions of 20% aluminum acetate and 20% aluminum chloride demonstrate equal in-vitro antibacterial efficacy.

Aluminum acetate solution for use in tinea pedis generally is diluted with about 10–40 parts of water. Depending on the situation, the patient may immerse the whole foot in the solution for 20 minutes up to three times a day (every 6–8 hours) or may apply the solution to the affected area in the form of a wet dressing.

For patient convenience, aluminum acetate solution (Burow's solution) or modified Burow's solution is available for immediate use (in solution) or for preparation with water (powder packets, powder, and effervescent tablets). These products are intended for external use only, are not to be ingested, and should be kept away from contact with the eyes. Prolonged or continuous use of aluminum acetate solution may produce necrosis. In the acute inflammatory state of tinea pedis, this solution should be used for less than 1 week. The pharmacist should instruct the patient to discontinue its use if inflammatory lesions appear or worsen.

Concentrations of 20–30% aluminum chloride have been the most beneficial for the wet, soggy type of athlete's foot.[6] Twice-daily applications are generally used until the signs and symptoms (odor, wetness, and whiteness) abate; after that, once-daily applications control the symptoms. In hot, humid weather, the original condition may return within 7–10 days after the application is stopped.

Aluminum salts do not entirely cure athlete's foot but are useful when combined with other topical antifungal drugs. Application of the aluminum salt merely shifts the disease process back to the simple dry type of athlete's foot, which then can be controlled with other agents such as tolnaftate. Safety and efficacy data were submitted to the FDA for only two aluminum compounds, alcloxa (aluminum chlorhydroxyallantoinate) and aluminum sulfate. Owing to a lack of sufficient efficacy data, both were classified as Category III.[18]

Because aluminum salts penetrate skin poorly, their toxicity, like that of aluminum chloride, is low. However, a few cases of irritation have been reported in patients where deep fissures were present. Thus, the use of concentrated aluminum salt solutions is contraindicated on severely eroded or deeply fissured skin. In such a case, the salts must be diluted to a lower concentration (10% aluminum chloride) for initial treatment.

Used appropriately, aluminum acetate solution or aluminum chloride solution is valuable in the wet, soggy, macerated form and the acute, inflammatory states of athlete's foot. However, each solution has potential for misuse (accidental childhood poisoning by ingesting the solutions or the solid tablets), and precautions must be taken to prevent this occurrence.

Other Ingredients and Dosage Forms

The primary drug delivery systems used in treating tinea pedis are creams, solutions, and powders. Powders, including those in aerosol dosage forms, generally are indicated for adjunctive use with solutions and creams. In very mild conditions, powders may suffice as the only therapy.

Solution and cream forms should be formulated in a vehicle that is:

- Nonocclusive (i.e., it should not retain moisture or sweat, which exacerbates the condition);
- Water miscible or water washable (i.e., removable with minimal cleansing efforts) because hard scrubbing of the affected area further abrades the skin;
- Anhydrous, because including water in the formulation introduces a variable that is one of the primary causes of the condition;
- Spreadable with minimal effort and without water;
- Capable of efficient drug delivery (i.e., it must not interact with the active ingredient but allow it to penetrate to the seat of the fungal infection);
- Nonsensitizing and nontoxic when applied to intact or denuded skin, especially if it is absorbed into the systemic circulation.

Most vehicles used to deliver topical solutions and creams are polyethylene glycol and alcohols, which meet these criteria. Polyethylene glycol bases deliver water-insoluble drugs topically and do it more efficiently than water-soluble agents. This feature is an added advantage because most topical antifungal drugs (e.g., tolnaftate) are largely water insoluble.

Criteria for the powder dosage form (shaker or aerosol) are basically the same as those for creams or solutions. Certain agents in power forms are therapeutic and also serve as vehicles (talc and cornstarch). Powders inhibit the propagation of fungi by adsorbing moisture and preventing skin maceration; thus, they actually alter the ecologic conditions of the fungi. The adsorbing material within the powder, rather than the intended active ingredient, may be responsible for much of the disease remission.

Many authorities consider cornstarch superior to talc for these formulations. This is because cornstarch is virtually free of chemical contamination and does not tend to produce granulomatous reactions in wounds as readily as talc. Moreover, cornstarch adsorbs 25 times more moisture from moisture-saturated air than talc.

Product Selection Guidelines

Patient compliance is influenced by product selection. Therefore, the pharmacist should recommend an appropriate drug and dosage form designed to cause the least interference with daily habits and activities without sacrificing efficacy. Product selection should be geared to the individual patient. For example, elderly patients may require a preparation that is easy to use; obese patients, in whom excessive sweating may contribute to the disease, should use topical talcum powders as adjunctive therapy.

Before recommending a nonprescription product, the pharmacist should review the patient's medical history. For example, PWDs should have their blood glucose levels moderately controlled because increased glucose in perspiration may promote fungal growth. Patients with allergic dermatitides are extremely sensitive to most oral and topical agents; such patients usually have a history of asthma, hay fever, or atopic dermatitis. By acquiring a good history, the pharmacist may be able to distinguish a tinea infection from atopic dermatitis and avoid recommending a product that may cause skin irritation.

The pharmacist should bear in mind that in some cases prescription drugs may be more beneficial than nonprescription products. In the soggy, macerated athlete's foot complicated by bacterial infection, the broad-spectrum antifungal agents (e.g., econazole nitrate) are preferable to both tolnaftate and the prescription drug haloprogin.

Patient Education and Consultation

Pharmacists should advise patients not to expect dramatic remission of the condition. The onset of symptomatic relief may take several days. Patients should be advised that, depending on certain factors (e.g., the extent of the affected area and variable patient response to medication), medication should be used for a minimum of 2–4 weeks. The FDA advisory panel recommended that products used for athlete's foot effect improvement within 4 weeks.[18] If there is no improvement within these time frames, the patient should consult a physician. Patients should also be told of the necessity to adhere strictly to the physician-prescribed dosage regimen or to the directions for use on the product label. Patient noncompliance contributes significantly to the failure of topical products in treating tinea pedis. Pharmacists may advise patients to continue the medication for a few days beyond the recommended time to decrease risk of relapse.

All topical antifungal products may induce various hypersensitivity reactions. Although the incidence of hypersensitivity is small, patients should be advised to discontinue the product if itching, swelling, or exacerbation of the disease occurs. In addition, patients should avoid contact of the product with the eyes. After applying the product, patients should thoroughly wash their hands with soap and water.

Pharmacists should emphasize the need for proper hygiene before effective drug therapy for athlete's foot can begin. The feet should be cleaned and thoroughly dried each day and kept as dry as possible during the day. Patients should have their own washcloths and towels. After bathing, the feet should be dried last so the towel does not spread the infection to other sites. The affected area should be thoroughly patted dry.

General measures should be taken to eliminate the predisposing factors of heat and perspiration. Shoes and light cotton socks that allow ventilation should be worn. Wool and some synthetic fabrics interfere with foot moisture dissipation. Occlusive footwear, including canvas rubber-soled athletic shoes, should not be worn for prolonged periods. Shoes should be alternated as often as possible so that the inside can adequately dry, and they should be dusted with medicated or unmedicated foot powders. Socks should be changed daily and washed thoroughly after use.

Contaminated clothing and towels should be laundered well in hot water. The feet, particularly the area between the toes, should be dusted with a medicated or unmedicated drying powder at every change of socks. Whenever possible, the feet should be aired to prevent moisture buildup. Cotton balls or Dr. Scholl's Smooth Touch Pedi-spreads® may be placed between the tips of the toes to keep the web spaces open and less moist. Pencil erasers have sometimes been recommended for this purpose, but they may contain sensitizing accelerators or antioxidants. Nonocclusive protective footwear (e.g., rubber or wooden sandals) may be worn in areas of family or public use, such as home bathrooms or community showers.

Individuals whose feet perspire excessively may find odor-controlling insoles (e.g., Odor Attackers® and Sneaker Snuffers®) useful for casual dress or sports activities. These insoles absorb moisture and prevent the growth of odor-causing bacteria. They also provide some support and cushioning for the feet. Patients must be advised, however, to change insoles routinely (e.g., every 3 to 4 months).

Pharmacists should inform patients of the need for adjunctive protective measures that assist the topical antifungal product in eradicating the fungal infection. However, patients should be cautioned against overzealous cleansing with soap and water and vigorous drying between the toes; this practice may further irritate the area.

Other Potentially Serious Conditions

It is important for the pharmacist to realize that selected chronic diseases predispose certain patients to foot problems. Most noteworthy is the diabetic patient in whom poor circulation and diminished limb sensitivity exist. These factors make the PWD especially vulnerable to infectious foot problems. Other vulnerable patients include those with peripheral circulatory disease or arthritis. The pharmacist can identify these patients by asking appropriate questions about daily medication use or reviewing the patient's drug profile. Typical drug use patterns for high-risk patients include insulin, oral sulfonylureas, drugs for circulation (e.g., cyclandelate, isoxsuprine, nylidrin, papaverine, and pentoxifylline), and drugs for arthritic conditions (e.g., aspirin and nonsteroidal anti-inflammatory drugs).

Pharmacists are also in a position to advise patients with or without chronic conditions on self-treatment and prevention of ingrown toenails—a common foot problem. Frostbite—a less frequent but nonetheless potentially serious condition that often involves the feet—is another area in which pharmacists can educate patients and consumers about preventive measures.

Diabetes Mellitus

In terms of direct medical care and lost productivity, the annual health care costs associated with diabetes were an estimated $24 billion in 1989. Trend analysis demonstrates that, as the population and proportion of elderly persons grow, the number of persons exhibiting diabetes mellitus and the costs associated with its treatment can be expected to increase. During the decade of the nineties, it is anticipated that the incidence of diabetes will increase by 31% in people between the ages of 45 and 64, and that 85% of all newly diagnosed PWDs will be over 45 years of age.

Approximately 25% of PWDs will develop severe foot or leg problems within their lifetime. It is also estimated that these patients are 17 times more likely than people without this disease to develop gangrene of the extremities. About two-thirds of all nontraumatic amputations per year occur in PWDs. Data suggest that more than 50% of foot amputations could have been prevented through appropriate diabetes control and education. Effective patient education about appropriate foot care is the key, and when it is coupled with advances in microvascular surgical techniques, a decrease in the incidence of amputations in this population group in future years seems likely.

An estimated 20% of all hospitalizations for diabetes are due to unresolved foot infections, which account for more in-hospital days than any other complication of the disease. Angiopathies develop in these patients with time, and the likelihood of occurrence increases when blood glucose is poorly controlled. Microangiopathies occur in the small-caliber blood vessels of the feet; macroangiopathies occur in the larger blood vessels of the foot and leg. These angiopathies contribute to compromised circulation to the foot. Neuropathies may cause sensory deficits and diminished pain perception and, when combined with decreased blood flow to the foot, can contribute to the development of foot ulcers. Foot ulcers must be promptly and vigorously treated because they are easily infected, may lead to gangrene, may affect the loss of a limb, and could jeopardize the life of the patient. In the PWD who has a foot infection, the risk of limb loss remains substantial for up to 6 months after the infection.

One in two PWDs of greater than 10 years duration will exhibit peripheral neuropathy. The resultant decreased sensitivity of the feet makes it almost impossible for the patient to be aware of minor trauma without visual observation. In fact, some patients may concede that they walk on what feels like "peg legs" because they have diminished feeling below the knees. Thus, because any constant irritation of the foot in the PWD can cause an ulceration within 24 hours if measures are not taken to remove the irritation, even a small pebble in the shoe for a brief time can have devastating consequences. In addition, callus formation may occur from ill-fitting shoes. Ultimately, repeated and unrelieved pressure on the callus site can encourage ischemia and ulceration of the underlying tissue. This situation may go unnoticed until bleeding becomes significant or an odor is noticed from the wound.

Another mitigating factor in the development of diabetic foot ulcerations is peripheral vascular disease. This disease develops at an earlier age and is 20 times more prevalent in the diabetic population than in the general population. Arterial insufficiency, which is often in evidence below the knee, results in ischemia.

When diabetes is not well controlled, there may be an increase in low-density lipoprotein cholesterol and a decrease in high-density lipoprotein cholesterol. This nurtures arterial plaque development and further compromises circulation.

Diabetic foot ulceration may also occur if the patient becomes immunocompromised. Such an outcome may result from decreased ability to mobilize leukocytes, decreased phagocytic ability, and decreased oxygen-radical production. Collectively, these factors interfere with the patient's ability to localize and stave off infection. Decompensated peripheral circulation results in reduced clearance of metabolic waste, decreased pH, and greater susceptibility to anaerobic infection. Fungal and bacterial infections are distinct possibilities within the skin and nails of the diabetic foot.

Unfortunately, many PWDs simply do not view their condition as a disease as much as a nuisance. Consequently, they may minimize the potential consequences of a foot ulcer. If PWDs do not inspect their feet daily, they might not even know an ulcer exists until it is advanced. Further, because their touch sensation might be so minimal, these patients might not be aware that foreign objects are present within the ulcer(s). Tacks and pins are examples of foreign objects podiatrists have removed from these ulcers. PWDs should wear soft, well-fitting leather shoes that are comfortable, and they should never walk barefoot outside the house.

When counseling a PWD about a possible foot ulcer, the pharmacist should err on the side of safety and suggest that the patient consult a physician or podiatrist. Depending on the severity of the foot infection, the patient may be treated on an outpatient or an inpatient basis. On an outpatient basis, superficial foot ulcers are treated with topical antibiotic creams or ointments with a simple dressing. If the ulcer shows signs of a local infection, erythema, and swelling, appropriate oral anti-infective therapy may be prescribed. Such therapy should consist of at least 10 days of treatment and is subject to change when culture and microorganism susceptibility results become available.

Besides medication, an important nondrug measure is to have the patient keep his or her weight off the foot, especially if the foot is swollen or shows signs of a deep infection. As long as the patient keeps walking on it, even for as little as 10 minutes a day, an infected lesion simply may not heal. A wheelchair, cane, or crutches may be used when ambulatory activity is necessary. Pharmacists are strongly encouraged to reinforce these points.

Hospitalization may be required when the lesion shows signs of a deep infection, gas is present in the lesion, gangrenous patches are observed, or there are signs of systemic infection. About 70% of foot infections are polymicrobial and may involve between three and five organisms, with *Staphylococcus aureus, Staphylococcus epidermidis,* and *Streptococcus* sp. being the most common among those cultured from the lesion. Anaerobes (e.g., *Bacteroides* sp., *Peptococcus* sp., and *Clostridium perfringens*), Gram-negative aerobes (e.g., *Escherichia coli, Proteus* sp., and *Klebsiella* sp.), and Gram-negative bacilli can also be cultured. Limb-threatening infections dictate aggressive combination parenteral antibiotic therapy; total bed rest; and incision, drainage, and debridement of the foot ulcer.

Diabetic Patient Education: Foot Care
PWDs should understand the need to visually inspect their feet daily. One physician suggests to his patients, "If you look at your feet every day, they will stay attached to your ankles." This is scary to hear, but it gets the patient's immediate attention. Foot hygiene and proper foot care can never be overemphasized. Feet must be washed every day with mild soap and lukewarm water. After cleansing, they should be thoroughly dried, especially between the toes. The patient should not rub too vigorously because this may irritate and break the skin.

After drying the feet, the patient may apply a vegetable oil or moisturizing cream to the skin to keep it soft, to prevent excessive friction, to remove scales of dead skin, and to prevent dryness. Such products should not be applied between the toes, however, because they may promote the development of a bacterial or fungal infection.

Care should be taken to avoid dry and brittle toenails. To soften toenails, patients can soak their feet for one-half hour each night in lukewarm water containing 1 tbsp/qt of powdered borax (i.e., sodium borate). This can be followed by rubbing vegetable oil or a moisturizing cream around the nails. When the nails become too long, it is advisable to use an emery board to file them. The nails should be filed straight across, and patients should take care not to file them shorter than the underlying soft tissue of the toe. Care must also be taken to not cut the corners of the nails; otherwise, an ingrown toenail could develop.

PWDs should massage their feet every day. When doing so, they should rub their feet upward toward the tips of their toes. If patients have varicose veins, the feet should be massaged gently but the legs should not.

Diabetic patients should observe usual foot care measures when traveling. It is wise to take off the shoes for a time during prolonged travel. Frostbite is a distinct possibility if travel involves prolonged exposure to the cold.

In the case of poor circulation, or cold feet, diabetic patients should keep their feet warm by wearing warm hosiery. Cold air causes the blood vessels to constrict, thus reducing blood flow to the feet. Constricting clothing (e.g., elastic hosiery with a tight top band) will decrease blood flow to the feet and should be avoided by PWDs and others with poor circulation. When sitting down, PWDs should not cross their legs because they may compress leg arteries and impair or close off the blood supply to the legs.

If the weight of the bedclothes is uncomfortable for a patient, it helps to place a pillow under the covers at the foot of the bed. The patient should not apply heat in any form (e.g., hot water bottles or heating blankets and pads) without a physician's consent. Because of a sensory deficit, even moderate heat can injure the skin if the circulation is poor.

Footwear
PWDs who experience neuropathy should be instructed not to walk barefoot, even in the home. The need for properly fitted footwear cannot be overemphasized. Ill-fitting footwear can very easily cause friction and blister formation, particularly in these individuals because of their sensory deficit. As a preventive measure, after taking off their shoes, these patients should shake them out to remove any foreign objects, and they should also run their hand inside the shoes before putting them on again to ensure that no foreign object is present.

Fashion-conscious women with diabetes pose special problems related to footwear because a comfortable pair of shoes is often not stylish. In any case, it is suggested that the female PWD wear low-heeled shoes of soft leather that correctly fit the shape of the foot. The shoe should have adequate room in the toe box so there is minimal pressure between the toes; it should fit close in the arch and snugly grip the heel. It is important to find a salesperson who is conscientious and knowledgeable and a shoe store that provides good service. If lower extremity edema is a complicating condition, the PWD should purchase shoes at the end of the day. Shoes should then be "broken in"; that is, new shoes should be worn no longer than a half hour the first day, and that time should be increased by 1 hour each subsequent day.

Shoes and socks should be changed every day, and depending on the patient's tendency to retain moisture on the feet and in the shoes, changes may be required more than once a day. If foot moisture is present, the patient could develop athlete's foot. To prevent this, a prophylactic foot powder can be used on the feet and in the shoes daily. However, PWDs usually have dry skin.

Treatment for Corns and Calluses in the Diabetic Foot
Corns and calluses occur as a result of friction, usually from improperly fitting footwear. Prevention is the key, so a PWD should wear shoes that fit properly.

To help remove a bothersome callus or corn, the patient should soak the foot with mild soap in lukewarm water for about 15 minutes. The excess tissue can then be gently rubbed off with a towel, a file, or medium sandpaper. The excess skin should not be torn off, and under no circumstances should it be allowed to become irritated. Corns and calluses should *not* be trimmed with razor blades or paring knives. This may predispose the patient to an infection, which could have serious and even life-threatening consequences. If the corn or callus is particularly discomforting, a podiatrist should be consulted. The patient should not use one of the available nonprescription topical corn or callus removers, whose primary active ingredient is salicylic acid. These can irritate and injure the skin and predispose the patient to harm.

A common problem for some PWDs is the development of a callus under the ball of the foot. This can be avoided by wearing shoes that are not too short or that do not have high heels. Curling and stretching the toes several times during the day also helps to prevent this problem, as does finishing each step on the toes rather than on the ball of the foot.

Skin Disorders

Even with seemingly trivial injuries, proper first-aid treatment is a necessity. Any development of redness, blistering, pain, or swelling should be brought to the attention of the physician. Even the slightest break in the skin could become infected, ulcerated, or gangrenous unless properly treated. Patients should follow self-treatment measures suggested by their physician.

Athlete's foot in the PWD, which generally begins with peeling and itching around and between the toes, should be immediately treated by a physician or podiatrist. So, too, should tinea unguium, a fungal infection of the toenail that is characterized by a brittle and discolored nail bed.

The PWDs should avoid using strong antiseptics (e.g., tincture of iodine) to treat infection because these products can irritate and dry the skin. A mild disinfectant might be preferable to use. If it is necessary to cover the wound with a gauze bandage, only fine paper tape or cellulose tape (Scotch Tape®) should be used to secure the bandage to the skin. Ordinary adhesive tape can make the skin soggy, encourage the growth of microorganisms, and irritate the skin when removed.

Poor Circulation

Patients with poor circulation of the feet and legs may complain of persistent and unusual feelings of cold, numbness, tingling, burning, or fatigue. Other symptoms may include discolored skin, dry skin, absence of hair on the feet or legs, or a cramping or tightness in the leg muscles. The most discriminating questions a pharmacist can ask this type of patient are (1) Do you experience aching in your calves when you walk? and (2) Do you have to hang your feet over the edge of the bed during sleep to relieve the soreness in your calves? A yes response to either question warrants referring the patient to a physician.

If a patient complains of coldness in only one foot, the patient should be referred to a physician because of a possible blockage (clot) of circulation to the foot. Sometimes the involved foot or lower leg will appear physically larger than the other, be red or waxy in appearance, have no hair growth on the toes, and exhibit thickened nails. If a review of the patient's medication history does not indicate use of medications intended to relieve these symptoms, the patient with suspected circulatory problems should be advised to consult a physician or podiatrist for evaluation.

A daily foot bath is a simple measure that will assist these patients. After the foot is patted dry, an emollient foot cream can be applied to aid in retaining moisture and pliability. The foot bath also will soften brittle toenails for clipping and filing. The feet should be kept warm and moderately exercised every day.

Arthritis

Arthritic patients, particularly those with osteoarthritis or rheumatoid arthritis, are also vulnerable to foot problems. Osteoarthritis is a noninflammatory, degenerative joint disease that occurs primarily in older people. Degeneration of the articular cartilage and changes in the bone result in a loss of resilience and a decrease in the skeleton's shock absorption capability. This condition, however, is also experienced by individuals in their late teens and early twenties as a secondary complication of an old athletic injury (e.g., from basketball, football, or cheerleading). This might be evidenced by the development of hallux limitus or rigidus of the big toe (i.e., a stiff toe or painful flexion of the big toe due to stiffness and spur formation in the metatarsophalangeal joint). Subsequently, these patients have a lot of difficulty with their shoes not fitting properly. They may also develop an osteoarthritic condition in the ankle joint. Referral to an orthopedic physician or podiatrist is appropriate.

Proper foot care is especially important for arthritic patients and should include properly padding the shoes with insoles to protect the feet from the shock of hard surfaces. These patients should wear properly fitted shoes and undergo regular podiatric or medical examinations.

Ingrown Toenails

An ingrown toenail occurs when a section of nail presses into the soft tissue of the nail groove. The nail curves into the flesh of the toe corners and becomes embedded in the surrounding soft tissue of the toe, causing pain. Swelling, inflammation, and ulceration are secondary complications that can arise from this condition.

The frequent cause of ingrown toenails is incorrect trimming of the nails. The correct method is to cut the nail straight across without tapering the corners in any way. Nails that are left sharp or jagged-edged grow outward and eventually become embedded in the soft lip tissue of the nail bed. This process then results in microtears of the skin which, coupled with invasion by opportunistic resident foot bacteria, can cause a superficial infection. Wearing pointed-toe or tight shoes, as well as hosiery that is too tight, has also been implicated. In these instances, direct pressure can force the lateral edge of the nail into the soft tissue. The embedded nail may then continue to grow into the soft tissue. Bedridden patients may develop ingrown toenails because tight bed covers press the soft skin tissue against the nails. Nail curling, which can be hereditary or secondary to either incorrect nail trimming or a systemic, metabolic disease, can also result in ingrown toenails. Psoriatic arthritis is such a disease whose presence may be demonstrated in the nail.

Education is probably the best way to prevent the development of ingrown toenails. In the early stages of development, therapy is directed at providing adequate room for the nail to resume its normal position adjacent to soft tissue. This is accomplished by relieving the external source of pressure and applying medications that will harden the nail groove or help shrink the soft tissue. The patient should be referred to a podiatrist or physician if the condition is recurrent or gives rise to an oozing discharge, pain, or severe inflammation. Sometimes surgery is warranted, and even with subsequent systemic antibiotic therapy, the toe may take up to 3 to 4 weeks to heal.

The FDA, in a tentative final monograph, has classified two active ingredients in ingrown toenail products—sodium sulfide and tannic acid—as Category III (Table 2).[19] At present, data are insufficient to determine the effectiveness of these ingredients for this condition. In theory, sodium sulfide is intended to soften the keratin in the nail and the calloused skin surrounding the nail, thereby relieving the pressure and pain caused by the embedded nail. The claimed effect of tannic acid is that it hardens the skin surrounding the embedded nail and shrinks the soft tissue adjacent to it, providing enough room for the nail to resume its normal position adjacent to soft tissue.

Ingrown toenail products with these active ingredients should not be used for more than 7 days. If there is no improvement within this time, a podiatrist or physician should be consulted. These products should not be applied to open sores, and if swelling and redness increase or if there is a discharge around the nail, their use should be stopped and a physician consulted. Patients with diabetes mellitus and circulatory disease should not use these products without consulting their physician.

To enhance the effectiveness of these products, the FDA panel recommended that the directions for use include the statement, "Cleanse affected toes thoroughly. Place a small piece of cotton in the nail groove (the side of the nail where the pain is) and wet cotton thoroughly with the solution. Repeat several times daily until nail discomfort is relieved, but do not use more than 7 days." Daily foot soaks in warm water sometimes help to reduce inflammation and facilitate drainage.

To protect the toe temporarily while the ingrown nail is being treated, a patient may use a soft foam toe cap. However, continual use of a toe cap without removing the source of the problem merely delays inevitable corrective treatment. Infected ingrown toenails need prompt and appropriate attention.

Patients with ingrown toenails often fail to realize that they may be helped by oral medication intended to allay pain and inflammation. The pharmacist may recommend aspirin or ibuprofen, two proven analgesics with anti-inflammatory activity, provided there are no contraindications to their use for a particular patient. (See Chapter 5, "Internal Analgesic Products.")

Frostbite

Frostbite is defined as the actual freezing of tissues by excessive exposure to low temperatures. To maintain normal core temperature in cold weather, the body reflexly reduces the flow of blood to the skin surface and the extremities. Therefore, frostbite usually involves areas of the body that are the farthest from deep organs or large muscles (e.g., feet, hands, earlobes, nose, and cheeks). Minor frostbite may cause only blanching of the skin; severe frostbite may result in the loss of fingers and toes.

Predisposing factors to the development of frostbite include:

- Low temperatures (especially with high winds);
- Long periods of exposure to cold;
- Lack of proper clothing;
- Wet clothing;
- Poor nutrition, exhaustion, or dehydration;
- Circulatory disease;
- Immobility;
- Direct contact with metal or petroleum products at low temperatures;
- Individual susceptibility to cold.

Frostbite is not amenable to therapy with nonprescription drug products. The frostbitten part should be promptly and thoroughly rewarmed in water heated to 104–108°F (45.6–47.8°C). The water should *not* be hot to a normal hand at room temperature and should *not* be tested with the frozen part. The container of water should be large enough for the frozen part to move freely without bumping against the sides. Rewarming should be continued until a flush returns to the most distal tip of the thawed part. This usually takes about 20–30 minutes. Dry heat (e.g., a heating pad) should be avoided because it is difficult to control the temperature and rewarm the frozen part evenly; overapplication of heat could actually burn the skin without the patient being aware. Once the injured part has been properly warmed, it should be soaked for about 20 minutes in a whirlpool bath once or twice daily until the healing process is complete.

The best treatment for frostbite is prevention; pharmacists should be able to provide a few simple rules to follow:

- Dress to maintain body warmth, taking into account the face, neck, and head as well as the extremities.
- Avoid exposure to cold during times of sickness or exhaustion.
- Do not exceed the body's tolerance to cold exposure.
- Avoid tight-fitting garments; dress with layered clothing.
- Wear clothing that allows ventilation and prevents perspiration buildup (water enhances heat loss).
- Wear insulated boots or shoes and socks (preferably wool) that fit snugly but are not tight in spots.
- Wear mittens instead of gloves in severe cold; the thumb should be with the rest of the fingers and not by itself.
- Never touch objects (especially cold metal or petroleum products) that facilitate heat loss.

When given the opportunity, the pharmacist should seek to correct a few misconceptions. It is dangerous to rub the affected area with ice or snow even though it seems to provide warmth. This can result in prolonged contact with the cold, and the ice crystals may lacerate cells. In addition, persons should refrain from drinking alcohol for "antifreeze" purposes, at least until they are in a warm place. Alcohol can induce a loss of body heat even though it may give the person a feeling of warmth when ingested. Finally, frostbite victims should avoid smoking. Nicotine can induce peripheral vasoconstriction and further reduce the blood supply to the frostbitten extremity. Thus, it would also seem prudent to forewarn individuals who want to stop smoking and have been prescribed Nicorette® (i.e., nicotine polacrilex) or one of the topical transdermal nicotine patches (Habitrol®, Nicoderm®, Nicotrol®, or ProStep®) that they should avoid excessive exposure to the cold.

Exercise-Induced Foot Problems

The pharmacist should be aware of the problem of exercise-induced foot injuries, particularly those caused by running, jogging, or other high-impact physical activity (Figure 4). Often, individuals fail to take certain precautions in their rush to recapture physical fitness, and they dive headlong into a strenuous exercise program. Yet jogging, aerobics, and running are not without risk; one study documented that several exercise enthusiasts have died from heart attacks while jogging.[20] Some people, especially those over 35 years of age, should consult a physician before embarking on a fitness program. So, too, should patients with high blood pressure or a family history of heart disease or diabetes. Ultimately, a vigorous walking program may be a more prudent form of exercise for middle-aged, unconditioned individuals than jogging or running, and it may minimize potential orthopedic problems incurred from those more strenuous forms of exercise.

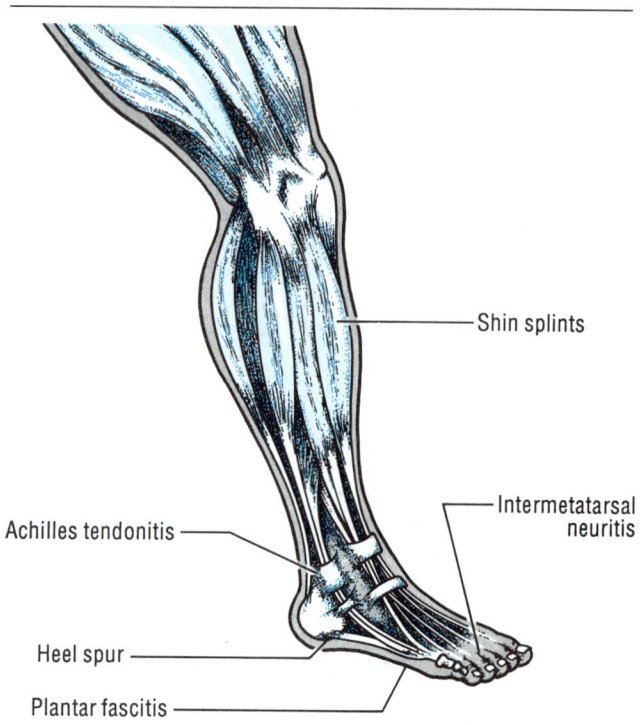

FIGURE 4 Selected foot and leg injuries associated with excessive impact shock.

Specific Injuries

Shin Splints

The term *shin splint* is used generically by some to describe all the pain emanating from below the knee and above the ankle. Shin splints are an overuse phenomenon that occurs in runners or walkers who use hard surfaces. This condition may also occur from running on a banked track or on the sloped shoulder of a road, wearing improper footwear, or overstriding.

The typical complaint of a runner with shin splints is pain in the medial lower third of the shin that seems to increase gradually with exercise. The patient may admit that soreness begins after running; with a continual running program, the pain will eventually occur during and after running. Complaints of pain when walking or climbing stairs may also indicate a serious case of shin splints. If the discomfort is located on the anterior lateral aspect of the skin; is described as a cramping, burning tightness; and occurs at the same distance or time during a run, the runner should be referred to a physician, podiatrist, or physical therapist.

Rest and application of ice (e.g., an ice bag or a cold compression wrap) to the painful area are good initial treatments. The cold anesthetizes the area and affects a decrease in pain. It is best to alternate compresses (10 minutes applied, 10 minutes off). To ensure greater contact with the injured part, the patient should be advised to use crushed or shaved ice. Aspirin or ibuprofen can also be used to relieve pain and reduce tissue inflammation. However, the use of analgesics to suppress pain or increase endurance during a workout is not recommended.

Stress Fracture

Stress fracture, also known as march, army, or fatigue fracture, may be encountered in runners, especially those who run repetitively on hard, inflexible surfaces. This injury usually involves the long bones of the foot or leg. It is not an overt break of the bone but rather an alteration in the architecture of the normal bone.

The onset of pain is associated with runners who drastically change aspects of their training routine (e.g., running surface, speed, or distance). Although the pain begins insidiously, the person suffering from a stress fracture will often complain of deep pain in the lower leg with an area of extreme tenderness. A misconception among runners is that they can "work out" the problem by continuing to jog. Individuals must be instructed that pain is the body's communication mechanism to indicate that enough is enough and that something is abnormal.

Treatment for stress fractures is complete rest from running, sometimes for 4–6 weeks, or longer if the tibia is involved.

Achilles Tendinitis

Running on hills or the beach, wearing improper footwear (e.g., running and jogging in shoes designed for racquet sports), and moving with excessive pronation (rolling in of the feet) are common causes of Achilles tendinitis. Yet it is not caused solely by running, and it may be an early sign of arthritis or rupture of a tendon; the exact cause of the problem is difficult to distinguish. Thus, Achilles tendinitis should be referred to a physician, podiatrist, or physical therapist.

By definition, Achilles tendinitis is a painful inflammation about the Achilles tendon. However, it may not show the classic signs of inflammation such as pain, erythema, increased skin temperature, or swelling. Typical symptoms are posterior heel pain, which is worse in the morning when getting out of bed, at the beginning of an exercise session, and when walking after prolonged sitting.

The best treatment is prevention with careful progression of training and replacement of worn footwear. Bony malalignments leading to excessive pronation should be accounted for with orthotic therapy. An orthotic device approximately positions the foot. The properties of shoe inserts vary (e.g., flexible or rigid); the choice of shoe insert should be based on specific treatment objectives. Shoe inserts can be custom-made or purchased off the shelf. Arch supports are intended to provide buttressing for the foot, and custom-made inserts are designed to account for specific bony malalignments.

Symptomatic self-treatment may consist of rest, new shoes, ice applications, appropriate nonsteroidal anti-inflammatory medication use, temporary heel lifts, and careful calf-stretching exercises.

Blisters

Ill-fitting footwear and inappropriate hosiery can often cause or contribute to the development of blisters. When shoes are worn while running, the shoe can place excessive pressure on a specific area on the skin between the stratum corneum and stratum lucidum. Fluid quickly accumulates at this site, often on the heel, the ball of the foot, and the ends or tops of the toes. Running barefoot can also cause blisters.

Again, prevention is the key to treating blisters. Cotton or woolen socks are preferred for running. The runner can wear two pairs of socks with ordinary talcum powder sprinkled between them. Some individuals with soft skin will continue to suffer from blisters until their skin toughens enough to withstand friction during running. Application of compound tincture of benzoin or of a flexible collodion product (e.g., New Skin®) will help toughen the skin.

Ankle Sprains

The typical mechanism of lateral ligament injury to the ankle is through rotation of the body over the fixed foot. This occurs most often in contact sports where the foot remains stationary while the body is unintentionally rotated. The incidence of ankle sprains during jogging and running is low because runners usually do not take sharp diagonal cuts.

The differential diagnosis of an ankle fracture from a sprained ankle is impossible without an X-ray. The immediate treatment of an ankle sprain involves applying a compressive bandage or wrap, elevating the ankle, and applying ice. If possible, the ankle should be bound with a wet elastic wrap while the cold is being applied. The wet wrap facilitates temperature transfer so that the ankle benefits most from the cold application. The recovery process can be made easier if the ankle is in a dorsiflexed position (foot toward the nose) when it is wrapped in the elastic bandage. Consistent with all sprains, including those of the neck and lower back, the use of alternating cold applications should continue for 24–72 hours, depending on injury severity.

Ice, compression, elevation (I.C.E.) therapy is well accepted as the most appropriate immediate treatment for an ankle sprain. It remains controversial whether cold application without elevation is helpful or harmful. Regardless, treatment for a sprained ankle should be initiated as soon as possible. Sometimes an ankle sprain is perceived as a minor problem, even by trained professionals; however, the severity of the ligament damage can vary widely, and an extensive ligament rupture that has been given insufficient treatment may result in a permanently unstable ankle.

Intermetatarsal Neuritis

Intermetatarsal neuritis is characterized by pain and numbness between the toes, most often within the third interspace. The cause is linked to the foot jamming forward into the shoe without enough space to accommodate the foot. Nerves become inflamed when compressed or caught in the area between the metatarsal heads and digital bases.

The solution is correct-fitting shoes with the addition of a metatarsal pad or orthotic. Lacing of the shoe can be modified by skipping the bottom two eyelets; this provides additional room for the ball of the foot.

Toenail Loss

Blisters under the toenail occur as a result of not keeping the toenails trimmed and of running in poorly fitted shoes. Long toenails catch on the sock or inside the shoe toe box, particularly when the individual is running downhill. This lifts the nail and separates it from the nail bed, and blood accumulates under the nail. This condition is very painful and can result in the temporary loss of the toenail.

Runner's Bunion

Bunion deformity and pain can increase in size. Management of the bunion should address the cause, such as tight-fitting shoes, high heel shoes, excessive pronation, or a previous injury. Thus, self-treatment includes properly fitted shoes, a wide toe box, avoidance of high heel shoes, and protective padding, as well as appropriate anti-inflammatory drug therapy. If shoe adjustments fail to alleviate pain, referral to a properly trained health care professional is indicated.

Heel Pain

Heel pain in runners is a common and insidious injury. The common diagnosis is plantar fascitis and/or heel spur. The cause is excessive running or rapid gain in body weight. Like Achilles tendinitis, heel pain can be an early sign of systemic arthritis. The pain is worse when getting out of bed in the morning or when standing up after sitting.

Self-treatment includes replacing worn shoes or heel pads, strapping or taping the arch, decreasing the amount of weight-bearing activity, and, if necessary, entering a weight reduction program. Anti-inflammatory treatment, including ice applications, is appropriate. When self-treatment fails, referral to an appropriate health care professional for evaluation of possible bony malalignments and possible orthotic therapy is indicated.

Treatment

The pharmacist may be called upon to play a triage role in treating an exercise-induced injury to the foot; that is, the pharmacist may have to decide whether the person should be referred to a physician or podiatrist, or whether a self-treatment program is advisable. When consulted by the patient for advice about foot injuries resulting from an exercise or jogging program, the pharmacist must ask appropriate questions. These questions are listed at the beginning of this chapter. Based on the individual's responses, the pharmacist can then refer the patient to a physician or recommend some form of nonprescription therapy.

Responses to questions may indicate that the person has had a number of continuous days of high-intensity workouts. It is essential that the body be allowed to recuperate after vigorous exercise; continual strenuous workouts cause accumulated fatigue and microtrauma. Some runners believe that the more mileage logged per week, the better their running ability; however, the incidence of acquired injuries among runners increases dramatically after 25–30 miles per week. An increased injury rate is also observed in runners who increase mileage too rapidly. A good training program entails "hard–easy" days, with extended mileage on 3 or 4 days per week and light, easy workouts on the remaining days.

If the runner or jogger has an injured leg or foot, that activity must occasionally be interrupted to allow the injured leg or foot to rest. Relative rest (i.e., avoiding activities that produce the symptoms) is often indicated, but some runners resist this suggestion. The pharmacist should encourage alternative exercise modes, such as swimming or bicycling (stationary or outdoor). This allows the serious runner to maintain aerobic conditioning despite missing regular exercise.

Prevention

Prevention is the best way to treat foot problems. This entails the use of proper footwear, running surface, and running posture. Most running injuries can be successfully treated with shoe modifications, in-shoe supports, correction for leg length discrepancies, modified training methods, ice applications, and stretching exercises.[21]

Proper Footwear

A number of manufacturers offer a variety of shoes for running. A good running shoe should provide the runner with cushioning, support, and stability. At the same time, it should maintain its flexibility, softness, and lightness. Running shoes usually have a waffle tread and a deep toe box. Basketball shoes, tennis shoes, and baseball shoes are not designed for running and should never be worn for this purpose. Unlike ice skates or ski boots, which have to be broken in, jogging and running shoes should fit immediately. The toes should have ample room, but there should be no slip in the heel. If the shoe is too loose, the foot tends to move forward when it strikes the running surface, contributing to callus formation on the plantar surface of the ball of the foot or to blood blisters under the toenail.

Pharmacists should advise patients to seek out sales personnel who have experience in the sport in which the patients are participating. Sales personnel with little or no experience or those who try to hurry through a sale should be avoided. The buyer should understand that service can be as important as the shoe.

The Running Surface

The convenience, safety, and preferences of the runner often dictate the running surface (e.g., concrete sidewalk, grassy surface, or dirt shoulder of roads). Because hard surfaces have no give and provide little shock-absorbing capacity, they cause intense shock to the legs, feet, and back; grassy surfaces, on the other hand, are often irregular, and the runner can easily incur a sprained ankle. Running on a sloping or banked surface may cause the foot to rotate excessively and may place additional stress on the tendons and ligaments of the leg and foot. Uphill running places a strain on the Achilles tendon and muscles of the lower back; downhill running places a lot of impact on the heel. The ideal running surface is relatively smooth, level, and resilient.

Patient Education and Consultation

A pharmacist can play an integral role in educating the exercise enthusiast, even if the pharmacist is not an enthusiast of the particular sport.

Hydration is crucial for joggers and runners, especially in the summer when perspiration can effect a loss of body water. The runner is advised to drink 6–8 oz of water before a workout. If participating in runs of 5 km or greater, the runner should drink 6–8 oz of water every 20 minutes or about every 2.5 miles of running. In the summer, joggers and runners should not overindulge in fluids but should at least attempt to keep the mouth moist. These athletes should avoid using salt (sodium chloride) tablets because they can induce an electrolyte imbalance by increasing potassium loss in perspiration.

When self-treatment is appropriate, the pharmacist can assist the patient in selecting nonprescription drugs (e.g., aspirin, ibuprofen, or topical antibiotic ointments) and can make recommendations for their administration. The pharmacist can also assist in selecting prescription accessories (e.g., a compression ice wrap, ice bags, Ace bandages®, arch supports, or heel cushions) that will alleviate injuries or problems.

Information and instructions about aspirin and ibuprofen use are found elsewhere in this book (see Chapter 5, "Internal Analgesic Products"), as is similar material about topical anti-infective ointments (see Chapter 28, "Topical Anti-Infective Products"). However, it is important to review some points about ice bags and cold wraps.

If an ice bag is used, the English type, which is identified by its commercial cloth material, is better because the patient does not have to wrap a towel around it to protect the skin. The ice should be broken into walnut-sized pieces with no jagged edges and should fill the bag to about one-half to two-thirds capacity. If the bag is overfilled, it will be difficult to apply because it will not rest on the contour of the body area. Once the bag has been filled, trapped air should be squeezed out, the outside dried, and the bag checked for leaks. The bag is then applied to the specific body area. Usually, the ice should be replaced every 2–4 hours, depending on patient preference. Alternate applications (30 minutes applied, 30 minutes off) up to three to four times per day are suggested to avoid tissue damage. Because maximal swelling from an ankle sprain occurs within 48 hours of the injury, patients should continue applying ice for 2 to 3 days. Unfortunately, many people do not continue ice application for this long because it is inconvenient to do so and the ankle starts to feel a little better. After the ice bag is used, the patient should be encouraged to drain it and allow it to air dry. If possible, the bag should be turned inside out for more efficient drying. After this, the cap should be placed on the bag and the whole accessory stored in a cool, dry place.

Cold wraps are also useful for cold application. These can be either one-use products (e.g., Faultless Instant Cold Pack®) or those intended for multiple use. The patient activates the one-use product by squeezing the middle of the pack to burst the bubble, which initiates an endothermic reaction of ammonium nitrate, water, and special additives. Reusable products consist of a cold pack or gel pack that is stored in the freezer and a cloth cover that is kept at room temperature. Once placed in the freezer, the cold pack will reach optimal temperature within 2 hours. The patient removes the cold pack from the freezer, inserts it in the cloth cover, and applies it to the specific body area. The patient should be instructed that the cold pack should not be uncomfortable. If it is, it should be removed for a minute or two and then reapplied. After use, the cold pack is stored in the freezer. Although some gel packs are nontoxic, all cold packs should be kept out of the reach of children.

Typically, an Ace bandage® is used for an ankle sprain or a knee sprain. However, the pharmacist must consider whether the patient will understand how to use the bandage in conjunction with an ice application so that additional damage is not incurred. If there is reason to believe the patient may cause further injury with a compression bandage through inappropriate use, the pharmacist should just recommend elevating the body part and applying an ice pack or, if warranted by the severity of the injury, consulting a physician.

If an Ace bandage® is to be used, the patient should be advised to unwind about 12–18 in. of bandage at a time and allow the bandage to relax. After the bandage is unwound, it can be soaked in water: when applied with ice, a wet elastic bandage facilitates the transfer of cold. The injured area should then be wrapped by overlapping the previous layer of bandage by about one-third to one-half its width. The point most distal from the ankle—that is, just above the toes—should be tightly wrapped, with decreasing tightness as the bandage is wrapped upward toward and past the ankle. The patient should assess the degree of discomfort after wrapping. If the bandage feels tight or uncomfortable, it should be removed and rewrapped. After use, the bandage should be washed—not scrubbed—in lukewarm, soapy water and thoroughly rinsed. It should be allowed to air dry on a flat surface and then rolled to prevent wrinkles. It should not be ironed.

The width of bandage needed depends on the injury site. For example, a foot or an ankle requires a 2.5- to 3-in. bandage. At the time of purchase, the pharmacist should review with the patient the correct procedure for wrapping, which is also described on the bandage package.

Summary

The nonprescription drug of choice in the treatment of corns, calluses, and warts is salicylic acid in a collodion-like vehicle or plaster dosage form, whichever is more convenient. Predisposing factors responsible for corns and calluses must be corrected. Plantar warts should be treated with a higher concentration of salicylic acid (20–40%); warts on thin epidermis require a lower concentration (10–20%). The effectiveness of salicylic acid in treating plantar warts is increased if the wart is pared to the point of near-bleeding or bleeding, or pain. This procedure should be performed only by a podiatrist or physician. Because warts are usually self-limiting, treatment should be conservative; vigorous therapy with salicylic acid may scar tissue.

Historically, the nonprescription drug of choice to treat the dry, scaly type of athlete's foot has been tolnaftate. Other agents such as clioquinol, clotrimazole, miconazole nitrate, and undecylenic acid and its derivatives are also efficacious for this purpose. Their effectiveness will be limited, however, unless the patient eliminates other predisposing factors to tinea pedis. These drugs are effective in all their delivery systems, but the powder form should be reserved only for extremely mild conditions or as adjunctive therapy. When recommended for suspected or actual dermatophytosis of the foot, these drugs should be used twice daily, morning and night. Because the vehicle forms of solution and cream are spreadable, they should be used sparingly. Treatment should be continued for 2–4 weeks, depending on the symptoms. After this time, the patient and pharmacist should evaluate the effectiveness of the drug.

The value of any topical nonprescription product for treating the soggy, macerated type of athlete's foot is dubious. The complex nature of the topical flora (resident aerobic diphtheroids) superimposed on the fungal infection dictates rigorous therapy with broader spectrum antifungals (e.g., ciclopirox olamine or econazole nitrate). In addition, oral therapy with either griseofulvin or ketoconazole may be indicated. Soaks and compresses of astringent agents (e.g., aluminum chloride) may be used as adjuvant therapy to dry the soggy, macerated tissue. Once this condition is converted to the dry form, appropriate use can be made of such agents as tolnaftate, clotrimazole, miconazole nitrate, and undecylenic acid derivatives.

To minimize noncompliance, patients should be advised that alleviation of the symptoms does not occur overnight. Patients should also be cautioned that frequent recurrence of any of these problems is an indication for consultation with a podiatrist or physician.

Patients with diabetes, circulatory problems, and/or arthritis pose special challenges to the pharmacist, who plays an important role in patient education. These patients should know not to self-medicate with any topical or oral nonprescription drug without first checking with their physician, podiatrist, or pharmacist. They should understand that there are certain ingredients in such products that may threaten the delicate balance that must be struck for their care. Misadventuring with nonprescription products could have devastating consequences and, at the least, may interfere with the attainment of intended patient outcomes.

Besides understanding concepts related to good foot care for patients with the above-mentioned chronic conditions, the pharmacist must be wary about drugs that can exacerbate these conditions or interact with other chronically used medications. Typically, PWDs, for example, have other therapy problems (e.g., hypertension, hyperlipidemia, or arthritis) and associated drug regimens. Thus, the pharmacist must monitor patient progress carefully and be attuned to patient comments that might indicate the occurrence of drug interactions.

In an era of physical fitness and health awareness, the pharmacist must be prepared to educate and assist patients who develop athletic injuries. With careful questioning, the pharmacist can help the patient determine whether the problem can be addressed through self-treatment or requires the assistance of a physician, podiatrist, or physical therapist. Most running injuries can be treated with shoe modifications, in-shoe supports, correction of leg length discrepancies, modified training methods, ice applications, and stretching exercises. It is important that the pharmacist be capable of providing informed recommendations to the sports enthusiast.

References

1. Brown JA, Scholl Inc. Personal communication. Memphis, Tenn; 1988.
2. Raskin J. Superficial fungal infections of the skin. Conn HF, ed. *Current Therapy 1976*. Philadelphia: W. B. Saunders; 1976: 611–4.
3. Gossel TA. The safe way to treat corns and calluses. *US Pharmacist* 1987 Mar; 12: 41–2, 47–53.
4. Stewart WD, Danto JL, Maddin S. Callus. In: *Dermatologic Diagnosis and Treatment of Cutaneous Disorders*. 4th ed. St. Louis, Mo: CV Mosby; 1978: 129.
5. *Federal Register* 1990 Aug 14; 55 (157): 33258–62.
6. Balkin SW. Treatment of corns by injectable silicone. *Arch Dermatol* 1975 Sep; 111: 1143–5.
7. Reichman RC, Bonnez W. Papillomaviruses. In: Mandell GL, Douglas RG Jr, Bennett JE, eds. *Principles and Practice of Infectious Diseases*. 3rd ed. New York: Churchill Livingstone; 1990: 1191–7.
8. Vance JC, Bart BJ, Hansen RC, et al. Intralesional recombinant alpha-2 Interferon for the treatment of patients with condyloma acuminatum or verruca plantaris. *Arch Dermatol* 1986 Mar; 122: 272–7.
9. Rock B, Shah KV, Farmer ER. A morphologic pathologic and virologic study of anogenital warts in men. *Arch Dermatol* 1992 Apr; 127: 495–500.
10. Melton JL, Rasmussen JE. Clinical manifestations of human papillomavirus infection in nongenital sites. *Dermatol Clin* 1991 Apr; 9: 219–33.
11. Jarratt M. Viral infections of the skin: herpes simplex, herpes zoster, warts, and molluscum contagiosum. *Pediatr Clin North Am* 1978 May; 25: 339–55.
12. Goldfarb MT, Gupta AK, Gupta MA, et al. Office therapy for human papillomavirus infection in nongenital sites. *Dermatol Clin* 1991 Apr; 9: 287–96.
13. *Federal Register* 1990 Aug 14; 55 (157): 33246–56.
14. Smith EL. The occult removal of warts: a continuing practice. *Int J Dermatol* 1979 Jan/Feb; 18: 89–91.
15. Hay RJ. Dermatophytosis and other special mycoses. In: Mandell GL, Douglas RG Jr, Bennett JE, eds. *Principles and Practice of Infectious Diseases*. 3rd ed. New York: Churchill Livingstone; 1990: 2017–28.
16. Goslen JB, Kobayashi GS. Dermatophytosis. In: Fitzpatrick TB, Eisen AZ, Wolff K, et al., eds. *Dermatology in General Practice*. 3rd ed. New York: McGraw-Hill; 1987: 2193–248.
17. Jung JH, McLaughlin JL, Stannard J, et al. Isolation, via activity-directed fractionation, of mercaptobenzothiazole and dibenzothiazyl disulfide as 2 allergens responsible for tennis shoe dermatitis. *Contact Dermatitis* 1988 Mar; 19: 254–9.
18. *Federal Register* 1982 Mar 23; 47 (56): 12480–566.
19. *Federal Register* 1982 Sep 3; 47 (172): 39120–5.
20. Thompson PD, Stern MP, Williams P, et al. Death during jogging or running. *JAMA* 1979 Sep 21; 242: 1265–7.
21. Pinshaw R, Atlas V, Noakes TD. The nature and response to therapy of 196 consecutive injuries seen at a runner's clinic. *South African Med J* 1984 Feb; 65: 291–8.

PRODUCT TABLES

About the Product Tables

For the first time in the history of the *Handbook of Nonprescription Drugs*, the product tables for the book have been produced from a computerized database. It is our hope and plan to revise and add to this database, thus continuing it as pharmacists' most current source of product information on nonprescription drugs.

How To Use the Ingredient and Formulation Flags

One significant new feature of the product tables are the codes, or "flags," that appear to the left of the product name. These flags represent the following designations:

AL = Alcohol Free	**LA** = Lactose Free
AF = Aspirin Free	**PR** = Preservative Free
CO = Cholesterol Free	**PU** = Purine Free
CA = Caffeine Free	**SO** = Dietetically Sodium Free
DY = Dye Free	**SL** = Sulfite Free
FL = Fluoride Free	**SU** = Dietetically Sugar Free
FR = Fragrance Free	**PE** = Pediatric Formulation
GL = Gluten Free	**GE** = Geriatric Formulation

Please note that these designations were provided by the manufacturers of the products and are not necessarily comprehensive. Because the flag information could not be independently verified, readers should use these flags only as guides to help them locate products that might meet special needs. Formulations change frequently, and pharmacists and patients should *always* carefully check the ingredients listed on packages.

Other Codes

In addition to the new flags, we use one other code and several editorial conventions in the tables.

- **NS = Not Specified.** This code is used in a number of places, especially when the column heading is an ingredient name and the manufacturer did not provide the quantity, strength, or concentration for that ingredient.
- **A blank column = No Information.** The manufacturer did not provide information for this column. Usually this means that the product has no ingredients that fit under that column head. However, especially in the "Other Ingredients" columns, the manufacturer may have chosen not to list those ingredients.
- ● = **Bullet.** This graphic symbol is used to divide the ingredients listed for each product.

Location and Order of the Tables

Responding to numerous requests from readers to make both the chapters and the product tables more accessible, we have created this special section for the product tables in the second half of the book. Each chapter's tables appear together, in the order of the chapters. Thumb tabs showing chapter titles and numbers help readers find information.

Scope of the Tables

Space limitations prevent us from making these tables comprehensive, although the database from which they are drawn is as complete as possible. Our goal in the *Handbook* is to present a broad scope of products in each category, including major and less-widely-known products. If a product line is large, our goal is to present a representative sampling of that line, including dosage forms, flavors, strengths, etc. Because of the size of some product lines, we cannot include every product submitted by every manufacturer.

Accuracy and Completeness of Entries

We have made every possible effort to ensure that the table entries are as accurate and complete as possible; however, the scope of the tables makes it impossible to verify all information independently. Some manufacturers listed all ingredients for their products; others concentrated on active or significant ingredients. We urge pharmacists and their patients to check package ingredient listings.

Special Thanks

APhA owes special thanks to the American Diabetes Association for help with the tables for Chapter 16, "Diabetes Care Products." We also thank pharmacist Joe Smith (APhA member and owner of The Medicine Shoppe Pharmacy, Falls Church, Virginia) for help with several product tables.

ELECTRONIC OSCILLOMETRIC BLOOD PRESSURE MONITOR PRODUCTS

Product & Manufacturer	Comments
Lumiscope Model 1081 Blood Pressure Monitor Lumiscope	extra large lcd display • oscillometric cuff design • fully automatic inflation and deflation • one button operation • error indicator • pre-set inflation pressure
Lumiscope Model 1083 Blood Pressure Monitor Lumiscope	takes readings from finger • adjusts for correct fit • record log
Lumiscope Model 1091 Blood Pressure Monitor with Printer Lumiscope	completely automatic • printout of systolic and diastolic measurements, time, and date • D-ring cuff • auto inflate and deflate • lcd panel • operates on two "AA" batteries (not included) • includes 2 rolls of printing tape
Lumiscope Model 1096 Blood Pressure Monitor with Printer Lumiscope	automatically inflates to pre-set level and cycles to deflation and measurement • jumbo digital display • prints date, time, blood pressure, and pulse • prints listing or bargraph of up to 7 memory entries • case
Marshall Model 91 Automatic Inflation B.P. Monitor Marshall	D-ring cuff automatically inflates and deflates • measures pulse and displays on lcd panel • error indicators signal incorrect testing procedures • automatic power-off • lightweight and portable • optional AC adapter • uses 4 "AA" batteries • battery life approx. 7 months when used once a day for two minutes • console weight approx. 14.5oz
Marshall Model 94 Pressure Valve Preset B.P. Monitor Marshall	pressure valve preset switch predetermines appropriate cuff inflation level • D-ring cuff • push-button inflate, and automatic deflate • automatic power-off • error indicators • carrying case • compatible with optional 85-LA cuff for arm circumference range 13" to 17" • optional AC adapter • uses 4 "AA" batteries, battery life approx. 200 times when used once a day for 2 minutes • console weight approx. 1lb
Marshall Model 97 Measurement Print-out B.P. Monitor Marshall	prints measurements, time and date • arm cuff inflates and deflates automatically • D-ring cuff • lcd panel • error indicators signal incorrect testing procedure • optional AC adapter • uses 4 "AA" batteries • battery life approx. 5 months when used for two minutes one time a day • console weight approx. 1lb, 1.6oz
Marshall Model F-89 Finger Blood Pressure Monitor Marshall	measures pulse in left index finger • adjustable finger cuff fits finger circumference range 2" to 3" • cuff inflates at the push of a button, automatically deflates • lcd panel • lightweight and portable
Omron Model HEM-601 Wrist Blood Pressure Monitor Omron	measures pulse • small, preformed wrist cuff • inflates automatically • pressure valve preset switch allows correct cuff inflation to be determined before measurement is taken • measurements alternately shown on an extra large lcd panel • error indicator • automatic power-off • built-in cuff storage • uses 4 "AA" batteries, battery life approx. 1 year when used once a day for two minutes • console weight approx. 1lb with batteries
Omron Model HEM-703CP Measurement Print-out B.P. Monitor Omron	prints measurements, time and date • arm cuff inflates and deflates automatically • D-ring cuff • lcd panel • error indicators signal incorrect testing procedure • optional AC adapter • uses 4 "AA" batteries • battery life approx. 5 months when used for two minutes one time a day • console weight approx. 1lb, 1.6oz
Omron Model HEM-704C Self-Storage Blood Pressure Monitor Omron	storage case holds monitor and cuff • D-ring cuff provides a uniform fit • automatic inflation/deflation • pressure valve preset switch allows the correct cuff inflation level to be determined before measurement is taken • large lcd panel • optional AC adapter • uses 4 "AA" batteries • battery life approx. 200 times when used once a day for 2 minutes • console weight approx. 2lbs
Omron Model HEM-705CP Memory/Printout/Graph B.P. Monitor Omron	retains up to 14 readings in memory • prints measurements in both digital and bar graph form • bar graph indicates blood pressure ranges: normal, borderline, hypertensive • large lcd panel • D-ring cuff • has printer storage case • optional AC adapter • uses 4 "C" batteries • battery life approximately 500 times when used for 2 minutes one time a day • console weight approx. 1lb, 2.3oz
Omron Model HEM-706 Fuzzy Logic Blood Pressure Monitor Omron	determines the ideal cuff inflation level according to the user's systolic blood pressure and arm size • D-ring cuff inflates and automatically deflates • large lcd panel • error indicators signal incorrect procedure testing • automatic power-off • built-in cuff storage • uses 4 "AA" batteries • battery life approx. 8 months when used once a day for two minutes • console weight approx. 1lb, 8oz
Omron Model HEM-713C Automatic Inflation B.P. Monitor Omron	D-ring cuff automatically inflates and deflates • measures pulse and displays on lcd panel • error indicators signal incorrect testing procedures • automatic power-off • lightweight and portable • optional AC adapter • uses 4 "AA" batteries • battery life approx. 7 months when used once a day for two minutes • console weight approx. 14.5oz

ELECTRONIC OSCILLOMETRIC BLOOD PRESSURE MONITOR PRODUCTS — continued

Product & Manufacturer	Comments
Omron Model HEM-815F Finger Blood Pressure Monitor Omron	measures pulse from left index finger • adjustable finger cuff fits finger 2" to 3" in circumference • inflates and deflates automatically • lcd panel • uses 2 "AA" batteries • battery life approx. 10 months when used once a day for two minutes • console weight approx. 8oz with batteries
Sunbeam Model 7650-10 Digital Blood Pressure Monitor Sunbeam	measures heart rate • auto inflate • over- or under-inflation indicator
Sunbeam Model 7655-10 Digital Finger B.P. Monitor Sunbeam	measures heart rate • adjustable finger cuff • over- or under-inflation indicator • auto inflate
Sunbeam Model 7656-10 Digital Finger B.P. Monitor Sunbeam	measures heart rate • adjustable finger cuff • auto inflate
Sunbeam Model 7657-10 Digital B.P. Monitor with Printer Sunbeam	measures heart rate • memory stores up to 7 blood pressure reading by date and time • prints current display information • history of measurements • graphic display of history • auto inflate

FECAL OCCULT BLOOD TEST KITS

Product & Manufacturer/Supplier	Sizes Available	Comments
ColoCARE Helena	3 tests per kit	use for three consecutive bowel movements • flush toilet twice before each bowel movement • pad is floated in toilet bowl with specimen • observe 30 seconds • pad check area on left will turn blue and/or green, the other will not • positive result is appearance of a blue cross on the test pad
EZ-Detect Biomerica	3 specimen pads	use for three consecutive bowel movements • flush toilet twice before each bowel movement • pad is floated in toilet bowl with specimen • observe for up to 2 minutes • positive result appears as a blue-green color on test pad • no diet restrictions (vitamin C and rare meat are okay) • avoid anti-inflammatory medications and those that cause internal bleeding
Hemoccult II SmithKline Diagnostic	3 slides per test	for in-home fecal collection • must be sent to lab or physician for results • patient kit includes flushable collection tissue, applicators, mailing pouch, and diet and test instructions • obtain 2 stool samples from 3 separate bowel movements • follow dietary restrictions for 48 hours prior to first specimen • avoid NSAIDS for 7 days prior to testing
Hemoccult Sensa SmithKline Diagnostic	3 slides per kit	for in-home fecal collection • must be sent to lab or physician for results • positive reaction a vivid blue • more sensitive than Hemoccult • patient kit includes flushable collection tissues, applicators, mailing pouch, and diet and test instructions • obtain 2 stool samples from 3 separate bowel movements • follow dietary restrictions for 48 hours prior to first specimen • avoid NSAIDS for 7 days prior to testing

OVULATION PREDICTION TEST KITS

Product & Manufacturer or Supplier	Sizes Available	Time for Procedure	Indication of Positive Result	Comments
Answer Ovulation Test Kit Carter-Wallace	5-day kit	3 minutes	when color in test well is similar or darker than example color	use first morning urine • do not shake stored sample • positive result indicates ovulation should occur within 12-24hrs
Clearplan Easy Whitehall	5-day kit	5 minutes	color of line in large window is similar or darker than line in small window	test any time during the day • positive result indicates ovulation should occur in next 24-36hrs • blue line in small window shows that the test is complete
Conceive Quidel	5-day kit	3 minutes	pink test line is darker than reference line	use first morning urine for best results (can use urine collected at any time) • collect urine at same time each day • positive result indicates ovulation should occur within 24-40hrs
First Response Ovulation Predictor Test Carter-Wallace	5-day kit	3 minutes	when color in test well is similar or darker than example color	use first morning urine • do not shake stored sample • positive result indicates ovulation should occur within 12-24hrs
Fortel Biomerica	9-day kit	30 minutes	color of liquid is significantly darker blue than the previous day	use first morning urine
OvuKIT Quidel	6-day & 9-day kits	1 hour	blue color on test stick is darker than the surge guide test	use urine collected between 10am and 8pm • do not use first morning urine • collect at the same time each day over the testing period • positive result indicates ovulation should occur within 24-40hrs
OvuQUICK Quidel	6-day & 9-day kits	4 minutes	color of test result area on test pad matches or is darker than the reference spot	use urine collected between 10am and 8pm • do not use first morning urine • collect at the same time each day over the testing period • positive result indicates ovulation should occur within 24-40hrs
Q-Test Quidel	5-day kit	35 minutes	markedly darker blue on test pad area as compared to previous day • error control pad should remain white or pale blue	collect urine at any time • positive result indicates ovulation should occur within 20-44hrs

PREGNANCY TEST KITS

Product & Manufacturer or Supplier	Sizes Available	Time for Procedure	Indication of Positive Result	Comments
Advance Ortho	1 test per kit	5 minutes	appearance of two bars "‖" on test stick is positive • negative result indicated by one bar "|" on test stick	can test on first day of missed period, any time of day • one step after collecting urine
Advance 2 Ortho	2 tests per kit	5 minutes	appearance of two bars "‖" on test stick is positive • negative result indicated by one bar "|" on test stick	can test on first day of missed period, any time of day • one step after collecting urine
Answer Plus Carter-Wallace	1 test per kit	1 minute	appearance of pink or purple color in test well	can be used as early as first day of missed period, at any time of day
Answer Plus 2 Carter-Wallace	2 tests per kit	1 minute	appearance of pink or purple color in test well	can be used as early as first day of missed period, at any time of day
Answer Quick & Simple 1-Step Pregnancy Test Carter-Wallace	1 & 2 tests per kit	as early as 3 minutes	appearance of a pink or purple line in result window	one-step test: hold test stick in urine stream • can be used as early as first day of missed period, at any time of day • product can be purchased as a single or a double test kit
Clearblue Easy Whitehall	1 & 2 tests per kit	3 minutes	blue line in large window	can test day period is due • one-step test • test stick is held in stream of first morning urine to wet tip • must hold stick upright during testing • blue line in small window indicates test is complete
Conceived Quidel	1 & 2 tests per kit	1 minute	pink test line appears	has blue control line • use first morning urine for best results (can use urine collected at any time) • can test first day after period has been missed
E.P.T. Stick Parke-Davis	1 & 2 tests per kit	4 minutes	color change from white to pink to light purple in window of stick	day 1 test: collect urine any time of day
Fact Plus Ortho	1 & 2 tests per kit	5-8 minutes	appearance of a "+" on plus cube is positive • negative result indicated by a dark "–" on plus cube	can test on first day of missed period • one step after collecting urine • instructions in English and Spanish
First Response 1-Step Pregnancy Test Carter-Wallace	1 & 2 tests per kit	as early as 3 minutes	appearance of a pink or purple line in result window	one-step test: hold test stick in urine stream • can be used as early as first day of missed period, at any time of day • product can be purchased as a single or a double test kit
First Response Pregnancy Test Carter-Wallace	1 & 2 tests per kit	1 minute	appearance of pink or purple color in test well	can be used as early as first day of missed period, at any time of day • product can be purchased as a single or a double test kit
Precise Becton Dickinson	1 test per kit	1 minute	blue checkmark appears • "error control" bar indicates test is correct	window turns pink when result is ready to read • test as early as first day of missed period • test any time of day or night
Q-Test Quidel	1 test per kit	9 minutes • results can be seen as early as 3 minutes	blue color change • error control feature	test any time of the day • add urine to a vial, add Q-Test strips for 5 minutes, rinse • negative results can be confirmed in 16 minutes and as early as 7 minutes

INTERNAL ANALGESIC PRODUCTS

	Product & Manufacturer	Dosage Form	Aspirin	Acetaminophen	Ibuprofen	Caffeine	Other Ingredients
	Acephen Suppositories G & W	suppository		120mg; 325mg; 650mg			hydrogenated vegetable oil • polysorbate 80
CA SO SL	Aceta Century	elixir		160mg/ 5ml			alcohol, 7%
	Aceta-Gesic Rugby	tablet		325mg			phenyltoloxamine dihy. citrate, 30mg • microcrystalline cellulose • powdered cellulose • starch • stearic acid • amorphous fumed silica • yellow #6 lake • orange oil
AF CA	Acetaminophen Various Manufacturers	suppository		120mg; 325mg; 650mg			
AF	Acetaminophen Various Manufacturers	tablet		325mg; 500mg; 650mg			
AL AF CA SU	Acetaminophen Oral Solution USP, cherry Roxane	solution		160mg/ 5ml			polyethylene glycol • propylene glycol • glycerin • sorbitol • methylparaben • propylparaben • FD&C red#40 • cherry flavoring • water
AF CA SU	Acetaminophen Oral Solution USP, lime Roxane	solution		160mg/ 5ml			polyethylene glycol • glycerin • sorbitol solution • methylparaben • propylparaben • D&C yellow#10 • FD&C blue#1 • FD&C yellow#6 • alcohol • lime flavoring • water
AF CA SO SU	Actamin Buffington	tablet		325mg		ns	
AF CA SO SU	Actamin Extra Buffington	tablet		500mg			
AF SO SU	Actamin Super Buffington	tablet		500mg		ns	
CA SO SU	Addaprin Dover	tablet			200mg		
AF CA GL PU SO	Advil Whitehall	caplet • tablet			200mg		
	Alka-Seltzer Extra Strength Miles Incorporated	effervescent tablet	500mg				sodium bicarbonate, 1985mg (sodium, 588mg) • citric acid, 1000mg
	Alka-Seltzer Flavored, lemon-lime Miles Incorporated	effervesent tablet	325mg				sodium bicarbonate, 1710mg (sodium, 506mg) • flavors • saccharin sodium
	Alka-Seltzer Original Miles Incorporated	effervescent tablet	325mg				sodium bicarbonate, 1916mg (sodium, 567mg) • citric acid, 1000mg
AF CA GL PR PU SO SU	Allerest Headache Strength CIBA Consumer	tablet		325mg			chlorpheniramine maleate, 2mg • pseudoephedrine hydrochloride, 30mg

Internal Analgesic Product Table

INTERNAL ANALGESIC PRODUCTS — continued

	Product & Manufacturer	Dosage Form	Aspirin	Acetaminophen	Ibuprofen	Caffeine	Other Ingredients
AF CA GL PR PU SO SU	Allerest, No Drowsiness CIBA Consumer	tablet		325mg			pseudoephedrine hydrochloride, 30mg
AF CA GL PR PU SO SU	Allerest, Sinus Pain Formula CIBA Consumer	tablet		500mg			chlorpheniramine maleate, 2mg • pseudoephedrine hydrochloride, 30mg
CA SO SU	Aminofen Dover	tablet		324mg			
AF CA SO SU	Aminofen Max Dover	tablet		500mg			
	Anacin A.H. Robins	tablet	400mg			32mg	
	Anacin Aspirin Free A.H. Robins	caplet • gelcap • tablet		500mg			
	Anacin Maximum Strength A.H. Robins	tablet	500mg			32mg	
	Anacin P.M. Aspirin Free A.H. Robins	caplet		500mg			diphenhydramine hydrochloride, 25mg
SO	Anodynos Buffington	tablet	ns			ns	salicylamide
SO SU	Arthriten Alva-Amco	tablet		250mg		32.5mg	magnesium salicylate, 250mg • magnesium carbonate • magnesium oxide • calcium carbonate
CA SO SU	Arthriten PM Alva-Amco	caplet		250mg			magnesium salicylate, 250mg • diphenhydramine hydrochloride, 25mg • magnesium carbonate • magnesium oxide • calcium carbonate
CA GL PR SO SU	Arthritis Pain Formula Whitehall	caplet	500mg				aluminum hydroxide, 27mg • magnesium hydroxide, 100mg
	Arthropan Liquid Purdue Frederick	liquid					choline salicylate, 174mg/ml (equivalent to 130mg of aspirin)
CA SO SU	Aspercin Otis Clapp	tablet	324mg				
CA SO SU	Aspercin Extra Otis Clapp	tablet	500mg				
	Aspergum, cherry and orange Schering-Plough	gum	227mg				flavor
CA SO SU	Aspermin Buffington	tablet	324mg				

INTERNAL ANALGESIC PRODUCTS — continued

	Product & Manufacturer	Dosage Form	Aspirin	Acetaminophen	Ibuprofen	Caffeine	Other Ingredients
CA SO SU	Aspermin Extra Buffington	tablet	500mg				
	Aspirin Various Manufacturers	suppository	125mg; 300mg; 600mg				
	Aspirin Paddock	tablet	325mg				
	Aspirin Enteric Coated Paddock	tablet	325mg; 650mg				
CA SO SU	Aspirtab Dover	tablet	324mg				
CA SO SU	Aspirtab Max Dover	tablet	500mg				
	Azo-Standard[a] PolyMedica	tablet					phenazopyridine hydrochloride, 95mg
CA SO SU	Back-Quell Otis Clapp	tablet	425mg				ephedrine sulfate • atropine sulfate
AF CA SO SU	Backaid PM Pills Alva-Amco	caplet		500mg			pamabrom, 25mg • pyrilamine maleate, 15mg
AF CA SO SU	Backaid Pills Alva-Amco	caplet		500mg			pamabrom, 25mg
	Banesin Forest	tablet		500mg			
CA GL PR PU SO SU	Bayer Aspirin, Genuine Sterling Health	caplet • tablet	325mg				
CA GL PR PU SO SU	Bayer Aspirin, Maximum Sterling Health	caplet • tablet	500mg				
CA GL PR PU SO SU PE	Bayer Children's Aspirin Sterling Health	tablet • chewable tablet	81mg				saccharin • flavor
	Bayer Delayed Release Enteric Aspirin Adult Low Strength Sterling Health	caplet	81mg				
	Bayer Delayed Release Enteric Aspirin Regular Strength Sterling Health	caplet	325mg				

INTERNAL ANALGESIC PRODUCTS — continued

	Product & Manufacturer	Dosage Form	Aspirin	Acetaminophen	Ibuprofen	Caffeine	Other Ingredients
CA GL PR PU SO SU	Bayer Extended Release 8-Hour Aspirin Sterling Health	timed-release tablet	650mg			ns	
	Bayer Plus Buffered Aspirin Sterling Health	tablet	325mg				calcium carbonate • magnesium carbonate • magnesium oxide
	Bayer Plus, Extra Strength Buffered Aspirin Sterling Health	caplet	500mg				calcium carbonate • magnesium carbonate • magnesium oxide
AF CA GL PR PU SO SU	Bayer Select Ibuprofen Pain Reliever/Fever Reducer Sterling Health	caplet			200mg		
AF GL PR PU SO SU	Bayer Select Maximum Strength Headache Sterling Health	caplet		500mg		65mg	
	Bayer Select Maximum Strength Menstrual Multi-Symptom Sterling Health	caplet		500mg			pamabrom, 25mg
	Bayer Select Maximum Strength Night Time Pain Relief Sterling Health	caplet		500mg			diphenhydramine hydrochloride, 25mg
	Bayer Select Maximum Strength Sinus Pain Relief Formula Sterling Health	caplet		500mg			pseudoephedrine hydrochloride, 30mg
AF CA GL PR PU	Bromo-Seltzer Warner-Lambert	granular effervescent		325mg/ capful			sodium bicarbonate, 2.78g/ capful • citric acid, 2.22g/ capful
CA SO SU	Buffaprin Buffington	tablet	325mg				magnesium oxide
CA SO SU	Buffaprin Extra Buffington	tablet	500mg				magnesium oxide
CA SO SU	Buffasal Dover	tablet	324mg				magnesium oxide
CA SO SU	Buffasal Max Dover	tablet	500mg				magnesium oxide
	Bufferin AF Nite Time Bristol-Myers	caplet		500mg			diphenhydramine citrate, 38mg
	Bufferin Arthritis Extra Strength, Tri-Buffered Bristol-Myers	caplet • tablet	500mg				calcium carbonate, 222.3mg • magnesium oxide, 88.9mg • magnesium carbonate, 55.6mg

INTERNAL ANALGESIC PRODUCTS — continued

	Product & Manufacturer	Dosage Form	Aspirin	Acetaminophen	Ibuprofen	Caffeine	Other Ingredients
	Bufferin, Tri-Buffered Bristol-Myers	caplet • tablet	325mg				calcium carbonate, 158mg • magnesium oxide, 63mg • magnesium carbonate, 39mg
CA SO SU	**Buffinol** Otis Clapp	tablet	325mg				magnesium oxide
CA SO SU	**Buffinol Extra** Otis Clapp	tablet	500mg				magnesium oxide
	Congespirin For Children Chewable Bristol-Myers	chewable tablet		81mg			phenylephrine hydrochloride, 1.25mg • fruit flavor • saccharin • sucrose
SU	**Cope** Mentholatum	tablet	421mg			32mg	magnesium hydroxide, 50mg • dried aluminum hydroxide gel, 25mg • corn starch • hydrogenated vegetable oil • microcrystalline cellulose • sodium lauryl sulfate • talc
AF CA GL PR PU SO SU	**Dapa** Ferndale	tablet		325mg			
AF CA GL PR PU SO SU	**Dapa Extra Strength Capsules** Ferndale	capsule		500mg			
AF CA GL PR PU SO SU	**Doan's Extra Strength** CIBA Consumer	tablet					magnesium salicylate, 500mg • magnesium stearate • microcrystalline cellulose • Opadry white • polyethylene glycol • stearic acid
AF CA GL PR PU SO SU	**Doan's Original** CIBA Consumer	tablet					magnesium salicylate, 325mg • magnesium stearate • microcrystalline cellulose • polyethylene glycol • stearic acid • Opadry light green
	Doan's P.M. Extra Strength CIBA Consumer	tablet					magnesium salicylate, 500mg • diphenhydramine hydrochloride, 25mg • carnauba wax • colloidal silicon dioxide • croscarmellose sodium • microcrystalline cellulose • magnesium stearate • Opadry blue • stearic acid • talc
	Duradyne Forest	tablet	230mg	180mg		15mg	
CA SO SU	**Dyspel** Dover	tablet		325mg			atropine sulfate, 0.06mg • ephedrine sulfate, 8mg
	Ecotrin Maximum Strength SmithKline Beecham	tablet	500mg				
	Ecotrin Regular Strength SmithKline Beecham	tablet	325mg				

INTERNAL ANALGESIC PRODUCTS — continued

	Product & Manufacturer	Dosage Form	Aspirin	Acetami-nophen	Ibuprofen	Caffeine	Other Ingredients
SO SU	Emagrin Otis Clapp	tablet	ns			ns	salicylamide
CA	Empirin Burroughs Wellcome	tablet	325mg				potato starch • microcrystalline cellulose
	Excedrin AF Dual Bristol-Myers	caplet		500mg			calcium carbonate, 111mg • magnesium carbonate, 64mg • magnesium oxide, 30mg
	Excedrin Caplets Aspirin Free Bristol-Myers	caplet		500mg		65mg	
	Excedrin Extra Strength Bristol-Myers	caplet • tablet	250mg	250mg		65mg	
	Excedrin IB Bristol-Myers	caplet • tablet			200mg		
	Excedrin P.M. Bristol-Myers	caplet • tablet		500mg			diphenhydramine citrate, 38mg
	Excedrin P.M. Bristol-Myers	liquid		1000mg/30ml			diphenhydramine hydrochloride, 50mg/30ml
	Excedrin Sinus Bristol-Myers	caplet • tablet		500mg			pseudoephedrine hydrochloride, 30mg
GL	Gemnisyn Schwarz Pharma	tablet	325mg	325mg			microcrystalline cellulose • starch • stearic acid
	Genapap Extra Strength Goldline	caplet • tablet		500mg			
	Genapap, Children's Chewable Goldline	chewable tablet		80mg			
	Genapap, Children's Elixir Goldline	elixir		32mg/ml			flavor
	Genapap, Infants' Drops Goldline	drops		100mg/ml			fruit flavor
	Genebs Goldline	tablet		325mg			
	Genebs Extra Strength Goldline	tablet		500mg			
	Genpril Goldline	tablet			200mg		
	Genprin Goldline	tablet	325mg				
	Gensan Goldline	tablet	400mg			32mg	
	Goody's Extra Strength Goody's	tablet	260mg	130mg		16.25mg	
	Goody's Headache Powder Goody's	powder	520mg	260mg		32.5mg	lactose • potassium chloride
AF CA PR PU SU	Ibufen-200 Ferndale	caplet			200mg		

INTERNAL ANALGESIC PRODUCTS — continued

Product & Manufacturer	Dosage Form	Aspirin	Acetaminophen	Ibuprofen	Caffeine	Other Ingredients
AF **Ibuprin Tablets** CA Thompson Medical GL PR SU	tablet			200mg		microcrystalline cellulose • sodium starch glycolate • sodium lauryl sulfate • hydroxypropyl cellulose • water • dicalcium phosphate • stearic acid • colloidal silicon dioxide • hydroxypropyl methylcellulose • titanium dioxide • polyethylene glycol • polysorbate 80 • magnesium stearate
Ibuprofen-200 Reese Chemical	tablet			200mg		
AF **Legatrin** CA Columbia	tablet					quinine sulfate, 162.5mg • calcium phosphate dibasic • cellulose • croscarmellose sodium • FD&C blue#2 aluminum lake • FD&C red#40 aluminum lake • gelatin • hydroxypropyl cellulose • hydroxypropyl methylcellulose • magnesium stearate • polyethylene glycol 400 • silica • starch • stearic acid • titanium dioxide
AL **Liquiprin Infants'** AF **Drops** CA Menley & James PE	drops		48mg/ml			dextrose • fructose • sucrose • fruit flavor • D&C red#33 • FD&C red#40 • propylparaben • methylparaben • glycerin
AF **Lurline PMS** CA **Tablets** GL Fielding PR PU SU	tablet		500mg			pyridoxine hydrochloride • pamabrom, 25mg
Magnaprin Rugby	tablet	325mg				magnesium hydroxide, 50mg • dried aluminum hydroxide gel, 50mg • calcium carbonate • corn starch • hydroxypropyl methylcellulose • magnesium stearate • microcrystalline cellulose • pregelatinized starch • stearic acid • triethyl citrate
Magnaprin Arthritis Strength Rugby	tablet	325mg				magnesium hydroxide, 75mg • dried aluminum hydroxide gel, 75mg • calcium carbonate • corn starch • hydroxypropyl methylcellulose • magnesium stearate • microcrystalline cellulose • pregelatinized starch • stearic acid • triethyl citrate
GL **McNess Pain** PR **Tablets** PU Furst-McNess SO SU GE	tablet	400mg			32mg	microcrystalline cellulose • starch
Menadol Ibuprofen, USP Rugby	caplet • tablet			200mg		
Midol IB, Cramp Relief Formula Caplets Sterling Health	caplet			200mg		

INTERNAL ANALGESIC PRODUCTS — continued

	Product & Manufacturer	Dosage Form	Aspirin	Acetaminophen	Ibuprofen	Caffeine	Other Ingredients
AF GL PR PU SO SU	**Midol Menstrual, Maximum Strength Multisymptom Formula** Sterling Health	caplet		500mg		60mg	pyrilamine maleate, 15mg
AF CA GL PR PU SO SU	**Midol Menstrual, Regular Strength Multisymptom Formula** Sterling Health	caplet		325mg			pyrilamine maleate, 12.5mg
AF CA GL PR PU SO SU	**Midol PM, Nighttime Pain Reliever/Sleep Aid Caplets** Sterling Health	caplet		500mg			diphenhydramine hydrochloride, 25mg
AF CA GL PR PU SO SU	**Midol PMS Capsules** Sterling Health	capsule		500mg			pamabrom, 25mg • pyrilamine maleate, 15mg
	Midol Teen, Multisymptom Formula Caplets Sterling Health	caplet		400mg			pamabrom, 25mg
AF SO SU	**Migranol** Otis Clapp	tablet		500mg		ns	phenylephrine hydrochloride
CA GL PR SO SU	**Momentum** Whitehall	caplet	500mg				phenyltolaxamine citrate, 15mg
AF CA GL PR PU SO SU	**Motrin IB** Upjohn	caplet • tablet			200mg		
	Neopap Suppositories PolyMedica	suppository		125mg			
CA	**Norwich Aspirin** Chattem Consumer	tablet	325mg				starch • hydroxypropyl methylcellulose • polyethylene glycol
CA	**Norwich Aspirin Caplets** Chattem Consumer	caplet	500mg				starch • hydroxypropyl methylcellulose • polyethylene glycol
CA SO	**Norwich Aspirin Enteric Coated** Chattem Consumer	tablet	325mg; 500mg				dioctyl sodium sulfonate • hydroxypropylcellulose • hydroxymethylcellulose • iron oxide • microcrystalline cellulose • pharmaceutical glaze • polyethylene glycol • polyvinyl acetate phthalate • pregelatinized starch • silicone dioxide • stearic acid • talc • titanium dioxide • triethyl citrate • yellow#6 • yellow#10

INTERNAL ANALGESIC PRODUCTS — continued

	Product & Manufacturer	Dosage Form	Aspirin	Acetaminophen	Ibuprofen	Caffeine	Other Ingredients
CA SO	Norwich Aspirin Enteric, Adult Low Strength Chattem Consumer	tablet	81mg				
	Nuprin Bristol-Myers	caplet • tablet			200mg		
AF	Ornex Menley & James	caplet		325mg			pseudoephedrine hydrochloride, 30mg • FD&C blue#1 • microcrystalline cellulose • povidone • starch
AF CA	Ornex Maximum Strength Menley & James	caplet		500mg			pseudoephedrine hydrochloride, 30mg • microcrystalline cellulose • povidone • starch
AF CA	Ornex Severe Cold Menley & James	caplet		500mg			pseudoephedrine hydrochloride, 30mg • dextromethorphan hydrobromide, 15mg • FD&C yellow#6 • D&C yellow#10 • microcrystalline cellulose • povidone • starch
	P-A-C Roberts Pharm.	tablet	400mg			anhydrous, 32mg	cellulose • corn starch • croscarmellose sodium • sucrose • FD&C blue #2 • FD&C yellow #5 (tartrazine)
	Pain Reliever Tablets Rugby	tablet	250mg	250mg		65mg	
	Pain-Eze + Reese Chemical	tablet		650mg			
AF CA GL PR PU SO SU	Panadol Caplets, Maximum Strength Sterling Health	caplet		500mg			
AF CA GL PR PU SO SU PE	Panadol Children's Chewable Tablets Sterling Health	chewable tablet		80mg			fruit flavor
AL AF CA PR SO SU SL PE	Panadol Children's Liquid Sterling Health	liquid		32mg/ml			saccharin • sorbitol • fruit flavor
AL AF CA PR PU SO SU SL PE	Panadol Children's and Infants' Drops Sterling Health	drops		80mg/0.8ml			fruit flavor • saccharin
PE	Panadol Junior Strength Sterling Health	caplet		160mg			

INTERNAL ANALGESIC PRODUCTS — continued

Product & Manufacturer	Dosage Form	Aspirin	Acetaminophen	Ibuprofen	Caffeine	Other Ingredients
AF CA GL PR PU SO SU **Panadol Maximum Strength** Sterling Health	tablet		500mg			
AF CA **Percogesic Coated Tablets** Procter & Gamble	tablet		325mg			phenyltoloxamine citrate, 30mg • cellulose • flavor • FD&C yellow #6 • hydroxypropyl methylcellulose • magnesium stearate • polyethylene glycol • povidone • silica gel • starch • stearic acid • sucrose
AF GL PU SO **Sinarest** CIBA Consumer	tablet		325mg; 500mg			chlorpheniramine maleate, 2mg • pseudoephedrine hydrochloride, 30mg
AF CA GL PR PU SO SU **Sinarest, No Drowsiness** CIBA Consumer	tablet		500mg			pseudoephedrine hydrochloride, 30mg
Sodium Salicylate Various Manufacturers	tablet					sodium salicylate, 325mg; 650mg
Sominex Pain Relief Formula SmithKline Beecham	tablet		500mg			diphenhydramine hydrochloride, 25mg
St. Joseph Aspirin-Free Tablets For Children Schering-Plough	tablet		80mg			flavor
St. Joseph Low Dose Adult Aspirin Schering-Plough	chewable tablet	81mg				
CA **Stanback AF Extra-Strength** Stanback	powder		1000mg			
Stanback Powder, Original Formula Stanback	powder	650mg			32mg	salicylamide • 200mg
AF CA GL PR PU SO SU **Synabrom** Ferndale	tablet		325mg			pamabrom, 25mg • cinnamedrine hydrochloride, 14.9mg
AL AF CA PR SU SL PE **Tempra 1 Drops** Mead Johnson Nutrit'l	drops		80mg/0.8ml			grape flavor
AL AF CA SU SL PE **Tempra 2 Syrup** Mead Johnson Nutrit'l	syrup		160mg/5ml			grape flavor

INTERNAL ANALGESIC PRODUCTS — continued

Product & Manufacturer	Dosage Form	Aspirin	Acetaminophen	Ibuprofen	Caffeine	Other Ingredients
AF CA GL PR SU PE **Tempra 3 Chewable Tablets** Mead Johnson Nutrit'l	chewable tablet		80mg			grape flavor • aspartame (3.3mg phenylalanine)
AF CA GL PR SU PE **Tempra 3 Chewable Tablets, Double Strength** Mead Johnson Nutrit'l	chewable tablet		160mg			grape flavor • aspartame (6.6mg phenylalanine)
AF CA SO SU **Tranquil Plus** Alva-Amco	caplet		250mg			diphenhydramine hydrochloride, 25mg • magnesium salicylate, 250mg • magnesium carbonate • magnesium oxide • calcium carbonate
PR SU **Tri-Pain Caplets** Ferndale	caplet	162mg	162mg		16.2mg	salicylamide, 162mg
AL AF CA SL PE **Tylenol Children's Elixir Cherry Flavor** McNeil	elixir		32mg/ml			sorbitol • sucrose • cherry flavor • benzoic acid • citric acid • glycerin • polyethylene glycol • propylene glycol • sodium benzoate • purified water • red #33 • red #40
AL AF CA SU SL PE **Tylenol Children's Suspension Liquid** McNeil	suspension		80mg/ 2.5ml			butylparaben • cellulose • citric acid • corn syrup • cherry flavors • glycerin • purified water • sodium benzoate • sorbitol • xanthan gum • FD&C red#40
AF CA SL **Tylenol Extra Strength Adult Liquid Pain Reliever** McNeil	liquid		500mg/ 15ml			alcohol, 7% • citric acid • flavors • glycerin • polyethylene glycol • purified water • sodium benzoate • sorbitol • sucrose • blue #1 • yellow #6 • yellow #10
AF CA GL PR PU SU **Tylenol Extra Strength Caplet** McNeil	caplet		500mg			cellulose • hydroxypropyl methylcellulose • magnesium stearate • polyethylene glycol • sodium starch glycolate • corn starch • red #40
CA GL PU SU **Tylenol Extra Strength Gelcap** McNeil	gelcap		500mg			benzyl alcohol • butylparaben • castor oil • cellulose • edetate calcium disodium • gelatin • hydroxypropyl methylcellulose • magnesium stearate • methylparaben • propylparaben • sodium lauryl sulfate • sodium propionate • sodium starch glycolate • corn starch • titanium dioxide • blue #1 • blue #2 • red #40 • yellow #10
GL **Tylenol Extra Strength Headache Plus** McNeil	caplet		500mg			calcium carbonate, 250mg • acacia • cellulose • cornstarch • croscarmellose sodium • hydroxypropyl methylcellulose • magnesium stearate • maltodextrin • propylene glycol • sodium starch glycolate • titanium dioxide • blue #1 • blue #2

Internal Analgesic Product Table

INTERNAL ANALGESIC PRODUCTS — continued

Product & Manufacturer	Dosage Form	Aspirin	Acetaminophen	Ibuprofen	Caffeine	Other Ingredients
AF GL PU **Tylenol Extra Strength PM** McNeil	gelcap		500mg			diphenhydramine hydrochloride, 25mg • benzyl alcohol • butylparaben • castor oil • cellulose • cornstarch • edetate calcium disodium • gelatin • hydroxypropyl methylcellulose • magnesium stearate • propylparaben • sodium lauryl sulfate • sodium citrate • sodium propionate • sodium starch glycolate • titanium dioxide • blue #1 • red #28
AF CA GL PR PU SU **Tylenol Extra Strength Tablet** McNeil	tablet		500mg			magnesium stearate • cellulose • sodium starch glycolate • cornstarch
AL AF CA SU SL PE **Tylenol Infants'** McNeil	drops		100mg/ml			saccharin • fruit flavor • butylparaben • citric acid • glycerin • polyethylene glycol • propylene glycol • sodium citrate • purified water • yellow #6
AL AF CA SU SL PE **Tylenol Infants' Suspension Drops** McNeil	drops		80mg/ 0.8ml			butylparaben • cellulose • citric acid • corn syrup • grape flavors • glycerin • propylene glycol • purified water • sodium benzoate • sorbitol • xanthan gum • D&C red#33 • FD&C blue#1
AF CA GL PR PU SO SU PE **Tylenol Junior Strength Grape Chewable Tablet** McNeil	chewable tablet		160mg			aspartame • cellulose • citric acid • cornstarch • ethylcellulose • grape flavors • magnesium stearate • mannitol • blue #1 • red #7
AF CA GL PR PU SU PE **Tylenol Junior Strength Swallowable** McNeil	caplet		160mg			cellulose • cornstarch • ethylcellulose • magnesium stearate • sodium lauryl sulfate • sodium starch glycolate
AF CA GL PR PU SU **Tylenol Regular Strength Caplet** McNeil	caplet		325mg			cellulose • hydroxypropyl methylcellulose • magnesium stearate • polyethylene glycol • sodium starch glycolate • corn starch • red #40
CA SO SU **Ultraprin** Otis Clapp	tablet			200mg		
AF GL PU SO **Unisom With Pain Relief** Pfizer	tablet		650mg			diphenhydramine, 50mg
AF CA SO SU **Valorin** Otis Clapp	tablet		325mg			
AF CA SO SU **Valorin Extra** Otis Clapp	tablet		500mg			

CHAPTER 5 — Internal Analgesics

INTERNAL ANALGESIC PRODUCTS — continued

Product & Manufacturer	Dosage Form	Aspirin	Acetami-nophen	Ibuprofen	Caffeine	Other Ingredients
AF **Valorin Super** SO Otis Clapp SU	tablet		500mg		ns	
CA **Valprin** SO Buffington SU	tablet			200mg		
GL **Vanquish Caplet** PR Sterling Health PU SO SU	caplet	227mg	194mg		33mg	magnesium hydroxide, 50mg • aluminum hydroxide gel, dried, 25mg

[a]Urinary tract analgesic.

ANTIPYRETIC PRODUCTS

Product & Manufacturer	Dosage Form	Aspirin	Acetaminophen	Ibuprofen	Caffeine	Other Ingredients
CA SO SL **Aceta** Century	elixir		160mg/5ml			alcohol, 7%
AF CA **Acetaminophen** Various Manufacturers	suppository		120mg; 325mg; 650mg			
AF **Acetaminophen** Various Manufacturers	tablet		325mg; 500mg; 650mg			
AL AF CA SU **Acetaminophen Oral Solution USP, cherry** Roxane	solution		160mg/5ml			polyethylene glycol • propylene glycol • glycerin • sorbitol • methylparaben • propylparaben • FD&C red #40 • cherry flavoring • water
AF CA SU **Acetaminophen Oral Solution USP, lime** Roxane	solution		160mg/5ml			polyethylene glycol • glycerin • sorbitol • methylparaben • propylparaben • D&C yellow #10 • FD&C blue #1 • FD&C yellow #6 • alcohol • flavoring • water
AF CA SO SU **Actamin** Buffington	tablet		325mg			
AF CA SO SU **Actamin Extra** Buffington	tablet		500mg			
AF SO SU **Actamin Super** Buffington	tablet		500mg		ns	
CA SO SU **Addaprin** Dover	tablet			200mg		
AF CA GL PU SO **Advil** Whitehall	caplet • tablet			200mg		
CA SO SU **Aminofen** Dover	tablet		324mg			
AF CA SO SU **Aminofen Max** Dover	tablet		500mg			
Anacin A.H. Robins	tablet	400mg			32mg	
Anacin Aspirin Free A.H. Robins	caplet • gelcap • tablet		500mg			
Anacin Maximum Strength A.H. Robins	tablet	500mg			32mg	
Anacin P.M. Aspirin Free A.H. Robins	caplet		500mg			diphenhydramine hydrochloride, 25mg
SO **Anodynos** Buffington	tablet	ns			ns	salicylamide

ANTIPYRETIC PRODUCTS — continued

	Product & Manufacturer	Dosage Form	Aspirin	Acetaminophen	Ibuprofen	Caffeine	Other Ingredients
CA GL PR SO SU	**Arthritis Pain Formula** Whitehall	caplet	500mg				aluminum hydroxide, 27mg • magnesium hydroxide, 100mg
	Arthropan Liquid Purdue Frederick	liquid					choline salicylate, 174mg/ml (equivalent to 130mg of aspirin)
	Ascriptin AD Rhone-Poulenc Rorer	caplet	325mg				magnesium hydroxide, 75mg • aluminum hydroxide, 75mg • calcium carbonate
	Ascriptin Extra Strength Rhone-Poulenc Rorer	caplet	500mg				magnesium hydroxide, 80mg • dried aluminum hydroxide gel, 80mg • calcium carbonate
	Ascriptin Regular Strength Rhone-Poulenc Rorer	tablet	325mg				magnesium hydroxide, 50mg • dried aluminum hydroxide gel, 50mg • calcium carbonate
CA SO SU	**Aspercin** Otis Clapp	tablet	324mg				
CA SO SU	**Aspercin Extra** Otis Clapp	tablet	500mg				
CA GL PU	**Aspergum** Schering-Plough	gum	228mg				cherry or orange flavor
CA SO SU	**Aspermin** Buffington	tablet	324mg				
CA SO SU	**Aspermin Extra** Buffington	tablet	500mg				
	Aspirin Various Manufacturers	tablet	325mg; 500mg; 650mg				
	Aspirin, Buffered Various Manufacturers	tablet	325mg				buffers
PE	**Aspirin, Children's** Various Manufacturers	chewable tablet	65mg; 75mg; 81mg				
CA SO SU	**Aspirtab** Dover	tablet	324mg				
CA SO SU	**Aspirtab Max** Dover	tablet	500mg				
	Banesin Forest	tablet		500mg			
CA GL PR PU SO SU	**Bayer Aspirin, Genuine** Sterling Health	caplet • tablet	325mg				

ANTIPYRETIC PRODUCTS — continued

Product & Manufacturer	Dosage Form	Aspirin	Acetaminophen	Ibuprofen	Caffeine	Other Ingredients
CA GL PR PU SO SU SL **Bayer Aspirin, Maximum** Sterling Health	caplet • tablet	500mg				
CA GL PR PU SU PE **Bayer Children's Chewable Aspirin** Sterling Health	chewable tablet	81mg				saccharin • orange flavor
CA GL PR PU SO SU **Bayer Extended Release 8-Hour Aspirin** Sterling Health	timed-release caplet • timed-release tablet	650mg				
Bayer Plus Buffered Aspirin Sterling Health	tablet	325mg				calcium carbonate • magnesium carbonate • magnesium oxide
Bayer Plus, Extra Strength Buffered Aspirin Sterling Health	caplet	500mg				calcium carbonate • magnesium carbonate • magnesium oxide
AF CA GL PR PU SO SU **Bayer Select Ibuprofen Pain Reliever/Fever Reducer** Sterling Health	caplet			200mg		
AF CA GL PR PU **Bromo-Seltzer** Warner-Lambert	granular effervescent		325mg/ capful			sodium bicarbonate, 3.78g/ capful • citric acid, 2.22g/ capful
CA SO SU **Buffaprin** Buffington	tablet	325mg				magnesium oxide
CA SO SU **Buffaprin Extra** Buffington	tablet	500mg				magnesium oxide
CA SO SU **Buffasal** Dover	tablet	325mg				magnesium oxide
CA SO SU **Buffasal Max** Dover	tablet	500mg				magnesium oxide
Bufferin AF Nite Time Bristol-Myers	caplet		500mg			diphenhydramine citrate, 38mg
Bufferin Arthritis Strength, Tri-Buffered Bristol-Myers	caplet	500mg				calcium carbonate, 222.3mg • magnesium oxide, 88.9mg • magnesium carbonate, 55.6mg
Bufferin Extra Strength, Tri-Buffered Bristol-Myers	tablet	500mg				calcium carbonate, 222.3mg • magnesium oxide, 88.9mg • magnesium carbonate, 55.6mg
Bufferin, Tri-Buffered Bristol-Myers	caplet • tablet	325mg				calcium carbonate, 158mg • magnesium oxide, 63mg • magnesium carbonate, 39mg

ANTIPYRETIC PRODUCTS — continued

	Product & Manufacturer	Dosage Form	Aspirin	Acetaminophen	Ibuprofen	Caffeine	Other Ingredients
CA SO SU	**Buffinol** Otis Clapp	tablet	325mg				magnesium oxide
CA SO SU	**Buffinol Extra** Otis Clapp	tablet	500mg				magnesium oxide
CA GL PU SU	**Cama Arthritis Pain Reliever & In-Lay tablets** Sandoz Pharm.	tablet	500mg				magnesium oxide, 150mg • aluminum hydroxide, 150mg • colloidal silicon dioxide • croscarmellose sodium • hydrogenated vegetable oil • methylcellulose • methylparaben • microcrystalline cellulose • polyethylene glycol • povidone • starch • yellow #6 • yellow #10
	Congespirin For Children, Aspirin Free Bristol-Myers	chewable tablet		81mg			phenylephrine hydrochloride, 1.25mg
AF CA GL PR PU SO SU	**Dapa** Ferndale	tablet		324mg			
AF CA GL PR PU SO SU	**Dapa, Extra Strength** Ferndale	capsule		500mg			
AF CA GL PR PU SO SU	**Dapa-500** Ferndale	caplet		500mg			
	Duradyne Forest	tablet	230mg	180mg		15mg	
	Ecotrin Maximum Strength SmithKline Beecham	caplet	500mg				
	Ecotrin Regular Strength SmithKline Beecham	caplet	325mg				
SO SU	**Emagrin** Otis Clapp	tablet	ns			ns	salicylamide
CA GL	**Empirin** Burroughs Wellcome	tablet	325mg				
	Excedrin AF Dual Bristol-Myers	caplet		500mg			calcium carbonate, 111mg • magnesium carbonate, 64mg • magnesium oxide, 30mg
	Excedrin Caplets Aspirin Free Bristol-Myers	tablet		500mg		65mg	
	Excedrin Extra Strength Bristol-Myers	caplet • tablet	250mg	250mg		65mg	

ANTIPYRETIC PRODUCTS — continued

	Product & Manufacturer	Dosage Form	Aspirin	Aceta-minophen	Ibuprofen	Caffeine	Other Ingredients
	Excedrin IB Bristol-Myers	caplet • tablet			200mg		
	Excedrin P.M. Bristol-Myers	caplet • tablet		500mg			diphenhydramine citrate, 38mg
	Excedrin P.M. Bristol-Myers	liquid		1000mg/30ml			diphenhydramine hydrochloride, 50mg/30ml
AF CA PE	**Feverall, Children's Suppositories** Upsher-Smith	suppository		120mg			
AF PE	**Feverall, Infant's Suppositories** Upsher-Smith	suppository		80mg			
	Feverall, Junior Strength Suppositories Upsher-Smith	suppository		325mg			
GL	**Gemnisyn** Schwarz Pharma	tablet	325mg	325mg			microcrystalline cellulose • starch • stearic acid
AF	**Genapap Extra Strength** Goldline	caplet • tablet		500mg			
	Genapap, Children's Chewable Goldline	chewable tablet		80mg			
	Genapap, Children's Elixir Goldline	elixir		160mg/5ml			cherry flavor
	Genapap, Infants' Drops Goldline	drops		100mg/ml			fruit flavor
	Genebs Goldline	tablet		325mg			
	Genebs Extra Strength Goldline	tablet		500mg			
	Genpril Goldline	tablet			200mg		
	Genprin Goldline	tablet	325mg				
	Gensan Goldline	tablet	400mg			32mg	
AL AF CA PE	**Liquiprin Infants' Drops** Menley & James	drops		48mg/ml			dextrose • fructose • sucrose • fruit flavor • D&C red #33 • FD&C red #40 • propylparaben • methylparaben • glycerin
	Mobigesic B.F. Ascher	tablet					phenyltoloxamine citrate, 30mg • magnesium salicylate, 325mg
AF CA GL PR PU SO SU	**Motrin IB** Upjohn	caplet • tablet			200mg		
CA	**Norwich Aspirin** Chattem Consumer	tablet	325mg				starch • hydroxypropyl methylcellulose • polyethylene glycol

ANTIPYRETIC PRODUCTS — continued

	Product & Manufacturer	Dosage Form	Aspirin	Acetaminophen	Ibuprofen	Caffeine	Other Ingredients
CA	Norwich Aspirin Caplets Chattem Consumer	caplet	500mg				starch • hydroxypropyl methylcellulose • polyethylene glycol
CA SO	Norwich Aspirin Enteric Coated Chattem Consumer	tablet	325mg; 500mg				dioctyl sodium succinate • hydroxypropylcellulose • hydroxymethylcellulose • iron oxide • microcrystalline cellulose • pharmaceutical glaze • polyethylene glycol • polyvinyl acetate phthalate • pregelatinized starch • silicone dioxide • stearic acid • talc • titanium dioxide • triethyl citrate • yellow #6 • yellow #10
CA SO	Norwich Aspirin Enteric, Adult Low Strength Chattem Consumer	tablet	81mg				
	Nuprin Bristol-Myers	caplet • tablet			200mg		
	P-A-C Roberts Pharm.	tablet	400mg			anhydrous, 32mg	cellulose • corn starch • croscarmellose sodium • FD&C #2 • FD&C yellow #5 (tartrazine)
	Pain-Eze + Reese Chemical	tablet		650mg			
CA	Pamprin Maximum Pain Relief Caplets Chattem Consumer	caplet		250mg			pamabrom, 25mg • magnesium salicylate, 250mg
AF CA	Pamprin Multi-Symptom Formula Chattem Consumer	caplet • tablet		500mg			pamabrom, 25mg • pyrilamine maleate, 15mg
AF CA GL PR PU SO SU	Panadol, Maximum Strength Sterling Health	caplet • tablet		500mg			
AF CA GL PR PU SO SU PE	Panadol Children's Chewable Tablets Sterling Health	chewable tablet		80mg			fruit flavor
AL AF CA PR SO SU SL PE	Panadol Children's Liquid Sterling Health	liquid		32mg/ml			saccharin • sorbitol • fruit flavor
AL AF CA PR PU SO SU SL PE	Panadol Children's and Infants' Drops Sterling Health	drops		80mg/ 0.8ml			fruit flavor • saccharin

ANTIPYRETIC PRODUCTS — continued

	Product & Manufacturer	Dosage Form	Aspirin	Aceta-minophen	Ibuprofen	Caffeine	Other Ingredients
PE	Panadol Junior Strength Sterling Health	caplet		160mg			
AF CA	Premsyn PMS Caplets Chattem Consumer	caplet		500mg			pamabrom, 25mg • pyrilamine maleate, 15mg
	Sodium Salicylate Various Manufacturers	tablet					sodium salicylate, 325mg; 650mg
AF CA PU SU	St. Joseph Aspirin-Free For Children And Infants Schering-Plough	chewable tablet		80mg			fruit flavor
	St. Joseph Low Dose Adult Aspirin Schering-Plough	chewable tablet	81mg				
AF CA PR SU SL PE	Tempra 1 Drops Mead Johnson Nutrit'l	drops		80mg/ 0.8ml			grape flavor
AL AF CA SU SL PE	Tempra 2 Syrup Mead Johnson Nutrit'l	syrup		160mg/ 5ml			grape flavor
AF CA GL PR SU PE	Tempra 3 Chewable Tablets Mead Johnson Nutrit'l	chewable tablet		80mg			aspartame (3.3mg phenylalanine) • grape flavor
AF CA GL PR SU PE	Tempra 3 Chewable Tablets, Double Strength Mead Johnson Nutrit'l	chewable tablet		160mg			grape flavor • aspartame (6.6mg phenylalanine)
GL PR PU SO SU	Tri-Pain Ferndale	caplet	162mg	162mg		16.2mg	salicylamide, 162mg
AL AF CA SL PE	Tylenol Children's Elixir Cherry Flavor McNeil	elixir		32mg/ml			sorbitol • sucrose • cherry flavor • benzoic acid • citric acid • glycerin • polyethylene glycol • propylene glycol • sodium benzoate • purified water • red #33 • red #40
AL AF CA SL PE	Tylenol Children's Elixir Grape Flavor McNeil	elixir		80mg/ 2.5ml			sorbitol • sucrose • grape flavors • benzoic acid • citric acid • glycerin • malic acid • polyethylene glycol • propylene glycol • sodium benzoate • purified water • blue #1 • red #40
AF CA GL PR PU SU PE	Tylenol Children's Fruit Flavor McNeil	chewable tablet		80mg			aspartame • cellulose • citric acid • ethylcellulose • fruit flavor • magnesium stearate • mannitol • cornstarch • red #7

ANTIPYRETIC PRODUCTS — continued

	Product & Manufacturer	Dosage Form	Aspirin	Aceta-minophen	Ibuprofen	Caffeine	Other Ingredients
AF CA GL PR PU SU PE	Tylenol Children's Grape Flavor McNeil	chewable tablet		80mg			aspartame • cellulose • citric acid • ethylcellulose • grape flavors • magnesium stearate • mannitol • starch • blue #1 • red #7
AL AF CA SU SL PE	Tylenol Children's Suspension Liquid McNeil	suspension		80mg/ 2.5ml			butylparaben • cellulose • citric acid • corn syrup • cherry flavors • glycerin • purified water • sodium benzoate • sorbitol • xanthan gum • FD&C red #40
AF CA SL	Tylenol Extra Strength Adult Liquid Pain Reliever McNeil	liquid		500mg/ 15ml			alcohol, 7% • citric acid • flavors • glycerin • polyethyleneglycol • purified water • sodium benzoate • sorbitol • sucrose • blue #1 • yellow #6 • yellow #10
AF CA GL PR PU SU	Tylenol Extra Strength Caplet McNeil	caplet		500mg			cellulose • hydroxypropyl methylcellulose • magnesium stearate • polyethylene glycol • sodium starch glycolate • corn starch • red#40
CA GL PU SU	Tylenol Extra Strength Gelcap McNeil	gelcap		500mg			benzyl alcohol • butylparaben • castor oil • cellulose • edetate calcium disodium • gelatin • hydroxypropyl methylcellulose • magnesium stearate • methylparaben • propylparaben • sodium lauryl sulfate • sodium propionate • sodium starch glycolate • corn starch • titanium dioxide • blue #1 • blue #2 • red #40 • yellow #10
AF CA GL PR PU SU	Tylenol Extra Strength Tablet McNeil	tablet		500mg			magnesium stearate • cellulose • sodium starch glycolate • cornstarch
AL AF CA SU SL PE	Tylenol Infants' McNeil	drops		100mg/ml			saccharin • fruit flavor • butylparaben • citric acid • glycerin • polyethylene glycol • propylene glycol • sodium citrate • purified water • yellow #6
AL AF CA SU SL PE	Tylenol Infants' Suspension Drops McNeil	drops		80mg/ 0.8ml			butylparaben • cellulose • citric acid • corn syrup • grape flavors • glycerin • propylene glycol • purified water • sodium benzoate • sorbitol • xanthan gum • D&C red#33 • FD&C blue#1

ANTIPYRETIC PRODUCTS — continued

	Product & Manufacturer	Dosage Form	Aspirin	Acetaminophen	Ibuprofen	Caffeine	Other Ingredients
AF CA GL PR PU SU PE	**Tylenol Junior Strength Fruit Chewable Tablet** McNeil	chewable tablet		160mg			aspartame • cellulose • citric acid • cornstarch • ethylcellulose • fruit flavors • magnesium stearate • mannitol • red#7
AF CA GL PR PU SO SU PE	**Tylenol Junior Strength Grape Chewable Tablet** McNeil	chewable tablet		160mg			aspartame • cellulose • citric acid • cornstarch • ethylcellulose • grape flavors • magnesium stearate • mannitol • blue#1 • red#7
AF CA GL PR PU SU PE	**Tylenol Junior Strength Swallowable** McNeil	caplet		160mg			cellulose • cornstarch • ethylcellulose • magnesium stearate • sodium lauryl sulfate • sodium starch glycolate
AF CA GL PR PU SU	**Tylenol Regular Strength Caplet** McNeil	caplet		325mg			cellulose • hydroxypropylmethylcellulose • magnesium stearate • polyethylene glycol • sodium starch glycolate • cornstarch • red #40
AF CA GL PR PU SU	**Tylenol Regular Strength Tablet** McNeil	tablet		325mg			magnesium stearate • cellulose • sodium starch glycolate • cornstarch
CA SO SU	**Ultraprin** Otis Clapp	tablet			200mg		
AF CA SO SU	**Valorin** Otis Clapp	tablet		325mg			
AF CA SO SU	**Valorin Extra** Otis Clapp	tablet		500mg			
AF SO SU	**Valorin Super** Otis Clapp	tablet		500mg		ns	
CA SO SU	**Valprin** Buffington	tablet			200mg		
GL PR PU SO SU	**Vanquish Caplet** Sterling Health	caplet	227mg			33mg	magnesium hydroxide, 50mg • aluminum hydroxide, 25mg

CHAPTER 6 Antipyretics

MENSTRUAL PRODUCTS

Product & Manufacturer	Analgesic	Diuretic	Antihistamine	Caffeine[a]	Other Ingredients
CA A-Nuric Alvin Last		buchu powdered extract, 65mg • couch grass powdered extract, 65mg • hydrangea powdered extract, 32.5mg • corn silk powdered extract, 32.5mg			
CA Addaprin SO Dover SU	ibuprofen, 200mg				
AF Advil Caplets CA & Tablets GL Whitehall PU SO	ibuprofen, 200mg				
AF Aqua-Ban GL Thompson PR Medical PU SU		ammonium chloride, 325mg		100mg	dibasic calcium phosphate • FD&C blue#1 aluminum lake • talc • titanium dioxide • ethylcellulose • zinc stearate • carnauba wax • cellulose acetate phthalate • diethyl phthalate • hydroxypropyl cellulose • microcrystalline cellulose • pharmaceutical glaze • propylene glycol • stearic acid • triacetin
AF Aqua-Ban GL Plus PR Thompson PU Medical SU		ammonium chloride, 650mg		200mg	iron, 6mg (as ferrous sulfate) • ethylcellulose • sodium starch glycolate • calcium phosphate dibasic • zinc stearate • cellulose acetate phthalate • diethyl phthalate • carnauba wax • FD&C blue#1 aluminum lake • calcium stearate • dibasic calcium phosphate • cellulose acetate phthalate • polyethylene glycol • triacetin • stearic acid
CA Arthritis GL Pain PR Formula SO Caplets SU Whitehall	aspirin, 500mg				aluminum hydroxide, 27mg • magnesium hydroxide, 100mg
Bayer Select Maximum Strength Menstrual Multi-Symptom Sterling Health	acetaminophen, 500mg	pamabrom, 25mg			
SO Diurex Long Acting Capsules Alva-Amco	potassium salicylate • acetaminophen			ns	

MENSTRUAL PRODUCTS — continued

Product & Manufacturer	Analgesic	Diuretic	Antihistamine	Caffeine[a]	Other Ingredients
AF CA SO SU **Diurex MPR Tablets** Alva-Amco	acetaminophen, 500mg	pamabrom, 25mg			
AF CA SO SU **Diurex PMS Tablets** Alva-Amco	acetaminophen, 500mg	pamabrom, 25mg	pyrilamine maleate, 15mg		
AF CA SO SU **Diurex Timed-Release Water Caplets** Alva-Amco	acetaminophen, 325mg	pamabrom, 50mg			
SO **Diurex Water Pills** Alva-Amco	potassium salicylate • salicylamide			ns	
AF CA SO SU **Diurex-2 Water Pills** Alva-Amco	acetaminophen, 162.5mg	pamabrom, 25mg			iron • calcium
CA SO SU **Dyspel** Dover	acetaminophen				ephedrine sulfate • atropine sulfate, 0.06mg
Excedrin IB Caplets & Tablets Bristol-Myers	ibuprofen, 200mg				
SO SU **Femcaps** Buffington	acetaminophen			32.5mg	ephedrine sulfate • atropine sulfate, 0.03mg
Haltran Tablets Roberts Pharm.	ibuprofen, 200mg				carnauba wax • cornstarch • hydroxypropyl methylcellulose • propylene glycol • silicon dioxide • pregelatinized starch • stearic acid • titanium dioxide
AF CA GL PR SO SU **Humphrey's No. 11** Humphrey's					cimicifuga, 3x • pulsatilla, 3x • sepia, 3x
AF CA GL PR PU SU **Lurline PMS Tablets** Fielding	acetaminophen, 500mg	pamabrom, 25mg			pyridoxine hydrochloride, 50mg
Menadol Ibuprofen Caplets & Tablets, USP Rugby	ibuprofen, 200mg				
AF CA GL PR SO SU **Midol 200** Sterling Health	ibuprofen, 200mg				

MENSTRUAL PRODUCTS — continued

Product & Manufacturer	Analgesic	Diuretic	Antihistamine	Caffeine[a]	Other Ingredients
AF GL PR SO SU **Midol For Cramps, Maximum Strength Caplets** Sterling Health	aspirin, 500mg			32.4mg	cinnamedrine hydrochloride, 14.9mg
Midol IB, Cramp Relief Formula Caplets Sterling Health	ibuprofen, 200mg				
AF GL PR PU SO SU **Midol Menstrual, Maximum Strength Multisymptom Formula** Sterling Health	acetaminophen, 500mg		pyrilamine maleate, 15mg	60mg	
AF CA GL PR PU SO SU **Midol Menstrual, Regular Strength & Multisymptom Caplets** Sterling Health	acetaminophen, 325mg		pyrilamine maleate, 12.5mg		
AF CA GL PR PU SO SU **Midol PM, Nighttime Pain Reliever/ Sleep Aid Caplets** Sterling Health	acetaminophen, 500mg		diphenhydramine hydrochloride, 25mg		
AF CA GL PR PU SO SU **Midol PMS Capsules** Sterling Health	acetaminophen, 500mg	pamabrom, 25mg	pyrilamine maleate, 15mg		
Midol Teen, Multisymptom Formula Caplets Sterling Health	acetaminophen, 400mg	pamabrom, 25mg			
Nuprin Caplets & Tablets Bristol-Myers	ibuprofen, 200mg				
AF CA **Odrinil** Fox		pamabrom, 25mg			
CA **Pamprin Maximum Pain Relief Caplets** Chattem Consumer	acetaminophen, 250mg • magnesium salicylate, 250mg	pamabrom, 25mg			
AF CA **Pamprin Multi-Symptom Formula Tablets** Chattem Consumer	acetaminophen, 500mg	pamabrom, 25mg	pyrilamine maleate, 15mg		

MENSTRUAL PRODUCTS — continued

	Product & Manufacturer	Analgesic	Diuretic	Antihistamine	Caffeine[a]	Other Ingredients
AF CA	**Premsyn PMS Caplets** Chattem Consumer	acetaminophen, 500mg	pamabrom, 25mg	pyrilamine maleate, 15mg		
CA SO SU	**Ultraprin** Otis Clapp	ibuprofen, 200mg				
CA SO SU	**Valprin** Buffington	ibuprofen, 200mg				

[a]Caffeine is also a diuretic.

COLD, COUGH, ALLERGY PRODUCTS

	Product & Manufacturer	Dosage Form	Decongestant	Antihistamine
AF	12-Hour Cold Tablets Goldline	tablet		dexbrompheniramine maleate, 6mg
	A.R.M. Menley & James	caplet	phenylpropanolamine hydrochloride, 25mg	chlorpheniramine maleate, 4mg
	Aceta-Gesic Rugby	tablet		phenyltoloxamine citrate, 30mg
	Actagen Goldline	syrup	pseudoephedrine hydrochloride, 30mg/5ml	triprolidine hydrochloride, 1.25mg/5ml
	Actagen Goldline	tablet	pseudoephedrine hydrochloride, 60mg	triprolidine hydrochloride, 2.5mg
AL LA SL	Actifed Burroughs Wellcome	syrup	pseudoephedrine hydrochloride, 30mg/5ml	triprolidine hydrochloride, 1.25mg/5ml
AF GL	Actifed Burroughs Wellcome	tablet	pseudoephedrine hydrochloride, 60mg	triprolidine hydrochloride, 2.5mg
AF GL	Actifed Plus Burroughs Wellcome	tablet	pseudoephedrine hydrochloride, 30mg	triprolidine hydrochloride, 1.25mg
AF GL GE	Actifed Sinus Daytime/ Nighttime Burroughs Wellcome	caplet • tablet	Daytime: pseudoephedrine hydrochloride, 30mg • Nighttime: pseudoephedrine hydrochloride, 30mg	Nighttime: diphenhydramine hydrochloride, 25mg
LA SU SL	Actifed With Codeine Burroughs Wellcome	syrup	pseudoephedrine hydrochloride, 30mg/5ml	triprolidine hydrochloride, 1.25mg/5ml
AF GL SO	Advil Cold and Sinus Whitehall	caplet	pseudoephedrine hydrochloride, 30mg	
	Afrin Tablets Schering-Plough	tablet	pseudoephedrine sulfate, 120mg	
	Alka-Seltzer Plus Cold Medicine Miles Incorporated	effervescent tablet	phenylpropanolamine bitartrate, 24.08mg	chlorpheniramine maleate, 2mg
	Alka-Seltzer Plus Cold and Cough Medicine Miles Incorporated	effervescent tablet	phenylpropanolamine bitartrate, 24.08mg	chlorpheniramine maleate, 2mg
	Alka-Seltzer Plus Maximum Strength Sinus Allergy Medicine Miles Incorporated	effervescent tablet	phenylpropanolamine bitartrate, 24.08mg	brompheniramine maleate, 2mg
	Alka-Seltzer Plus Night-Time Cold Medicine Miles Incorporated	effervescent tablet	phenylpropanolamine bitartrate, 20mg	brompheniramine maleate, 2mg
	Aller-Chlor Rugby	tablet		chlorpheniramine maleate, 4mg
	Allerchlor Rugby	syrup		chlorpheniramine maleate, 2mg/5ml
AF GL PU	Allerest CIBA Consumer	tablet	pseudoephedrine hydrochloride, 30mg	chlorpheniramine maleate, 2mg
AF GL PU PE	Allerest Children's CIBA Consumer	tablet	phenylpropanolamine hydrochloride, 9.4mg	chlorpheniramine maleate, 1mg

COLD, COUGH, ALLERGY PRODUCTS — continued

Analgesic	Expectorant	Cough Suppressant	Other Ingredients
pseudoephedrine sulfate, 120mg			
			D&C yellow#10 • FD&C yellow#6 • lactose • starch • magnesium stearate
acetaminophen, 325mg			
			sorbitol
			lactose • sucrose
acetaminophen, 500mg			
Daytime: acetaminophen, 325mg • Nighttime: acetaminophen, 500mg			
		codeine phosphate, 10mg/5ml[a]	alcohol, 4.3% • sorbitol
ibuprofen, 200mg			
aspirin, 325mg			citric acid • flavor • sodium bicarbonate (sodium, 506mg)
aspirin, 500mg		dextromethorphan hydrobromide, 10mg	aspartame • citric acid • flavor • sodium bicarbonate (sodium, 506mg)
aspirin, 500mg			aspartame • citric acid • flavors • sodium bicarbonate (sodium, 506mg)
aspirin, 500mg		dextromethorphan hydrobromide, 10mg	aspartame • citric acid • flavor • sodium bicarbonate (sodium, 506mg)
			alcohol, 7% • caramel coloring #100 • FD&C blue#1 • FD&C yellow#10 • flavors • glycerin • liquid sugar • menthol • methylparaben • propylene glycol • propylparaben • purified water • may also contain citric acid • sodium citrate
			blue #1 lake • dibasic calcium phosphate • magnesium stearate • microcrystalline cellulose • povidone • pregelatinized starch • sodium starch glycolate
			saccharin sodium • sorbitol • calcium stearate • citric acid • flavor • magnesium trisilicate

COLD, COUGH, ALLERGY PRODUCTS — continued

	Product & Manufacturer	Dosage Form	Decongestant	Antihistamine
AF GL PU SO	Allerest Headache Strength CIBA Consumer	tablet	pseudoephedrine hydrochloride, 30mg	chlorpheniramine maleate, 2mg
AF GL PU SO	Allerest No Drowsiness CIBA Consumer	tablet	pseudoephedrine hydrochloride, 30mg	
AF GL PU	Allerest Sinus Pain Formula CIBA Consumer	tablet	pseudoephedrine hydrochloride, 30mg	chlorpheniramine maleate, 2mg
	Allerfrim Rugby	syrup	pseudoephedrine hydrochloride, 30mg/5ml	triprolidine hydrochloride, 1.25mg/5ml
	Allerfrim Nasal Decongestant & Antihistamine Rugby	tablet	pseudoephedrine hydrochloride, 60mg	triprolidine hydrochloride, 2.5mg
	Allergy Cold Tablets Geneva	tablet	pseudoephedrine hydrochloride, 60mg	triprolidine hydrochloride, 2.5mg
	Allermed Maximum Strength Murdock	capsule	pseudoephedrine hydrochloride, 60mg	
	Ambenyl-D Decongestant Cough Formula Forest	liquid	pseudoephedrine hydrochloride, 30mg/5ml	
	Amonidrin Forest	tablet		
SO	Anodynos Forte Buffington	tablet	phenylephrine hydrochloride	chlorpheniramine maleate
LA SL	Anti-Tuss Century	syrup		
AF CA LA PU SL	Anti-Tuss DM Century	syrup		
	B.Q. Cold Bristol-Myers	tablet	phenylpropanolamine hydrochloride, 12.5mg	chlorpheniramine maleate, 2mg
LA SL	Benadryl Parke-Davis	elixir		diphenhydramine hydrochloride, 12.5mg/5ml
AF GL PU SO	Benadryl 25 Parke-Davis	capsule • tablet	diphenhydramine hydrochloride, 25mg	
LA SL	Benadryl Cold Nighttime Formula Parke-Davis	liquid	pseudoephedrine hydrochloride, 30mg/15ml	diphenhydramine hydrochloride, 25mg/15ml
AF GL PU	Benadryl Cold Tablet Parke-Davis	tablet	pseudoephedrine hydrochloride, 30mg	diphenhydramine hydrochloride, 12.5mg
LA PR SL	Benadryl Decongestant Parke-Davis	elixir	pseudoephedrine hydrochloride, 30mg/5ml	diphenhydramine hydrochloride, 12.5mg/5ml
LA PR SL	Benylin Parke-Davis	liquid		diphenhydramine hydrochloride, 12.5mg/5ml
LA PR SL	Benylin D Cough Syrup Parke-Davis	elixir	pseudoephedrine hydrochloride, 30mg/5ml	diphenhydramine hydrochloride, 12.5mg/5ml

COLD, COUGH, ALLERGY PRODUCTS — continued

Analgesic	Expectorant	Cough Suppressant	Other Ingredients
acetaminophen, 325mg			magnesium stearate • microcrystalline cellulose • povidone • pregelatinized starch
acetaminophen, 325mg			magnesium stearate • microcrystalline cellulose • povidone • pregelatinized starch
acetaminophen, 500mg			magnesium stearate • microcrystalline cellulose • povidone • pregelatinized starch • sodium starch glycolate
			povidone • microcrystalline cellulose • dibasic phosphate • stearic acid • magnesium stearate • colloidal silicon dioxide • starch
			golden seal root • eyebright herb • licorice root • cleavers herb • echinacea purpurea root • nettle herb • feverfew leaf • ma huang herb • dong quai root
	guaifenesin, 100mg/5ml	dextromethorphan hydrobromide, 15mg/5ml	alcohol, 9.5% • menthol • saccharin • sorbitol • sucrose
	guaifenesin, 200mg		
salicylamide • acetaminophen			caffeine
	guaifenesin, 100mg/5ml		alcohol, 3.5%
	guaifenesin, 100mg/5ml	dextromethorphan hydrobromide, 15mg/5ml	
acetaminophen, 325mg			sucrose
			alcohol, 5.6%
acetaminophen, 500mg/15ml			alcohol, 10% • saccharin • honey-lemon flavor
acetaminophen, 500mg			
			alcohol, 5%
	ammonium chloride, 112.5mg/5ml • sodium citrate, 50mg/5ml		alcohol, 5%
			alcohol, 5% • saccharin • sucrose • menthol

COLD, COUGH, ALLERGY PRODUCTS — continued

	Product & Manufacturer	Dosage Form	Decongestant	Antihistamine
AL LA SU SL PE	Benylin DM Pediatric Cough Syrup Parke-Davis	liquid		
LA SL	Benylin Expectorant Parke-Davis	liquid		
	Bromotap Goldline	elixir	phenylpropanolamine hydrochloride, 12.5mg/5ml	brompheniramine maleate, 2mg/5ml
LA SU SL	Bron Kote Parnell	solution		
AL LA SL PE	Cenafed Century	syrup	pseudoephedrine hydrochloride, 30mg/5ml	
AF GL PU	Cenafed Century	tablet	pseudoephedrine hydrochloride, 30mg or 60 mg	
AF GL PU	Cenafed Plus Century	tablet	pseudoephedrine hydrochloride, 60mg	triprolidine hydrochloride, 2.5mg
	Cheracol D Roberts Pharm.	liquid		
	Cheracol Plus Roberts Pharm.	liquid	phenylpropanolamine hydrochloride, 25mg	chlorpheniramine, 4mg
	Cheracol Sinus Roberts Pharm.	tablet	pseudoephedrine sulfate, 120mg	dexbrompheniramine maleate, 6mg
	Cheracol Sore Throat Spray Roberts Pharm.	spray		
	Chlor-Rest Rugby	tablet	phenylpropanolamine hydrochloride, 18.7mg	chlorpheniramine maleate, 2mg
	Chlor-Trimeton 12 hour Allergy Tablets Schering-Plough	tablet		chlorpheniramine maleate, 12mg
	Chlor-Trimeton 12 hour Allergy/Decongestant Tablets Schering-Plough	tablet	pseudoephedrine sulfate, 120mg	chlorpheniramine maleate, 8mg
AL	Chlor-Trimeton Allergy Syrup Schering-Plough	syrup		chlorpheniramine maleate, 2mg/5ml
AF	Chlor-Trimeton Allergy, Sinus, Headache Schering-Plough	caplet	phenylpropanolamine hydrochloride, 12.5mg	chlorpheniramine, 2mg
	Chlor-Trimeton Non-Drowsy 4 hour Tablets Schering-Plough	tablet	pseudoephedrine sulfate, 60mg	
AL	Chloraseptic Advanced Formula Sore Throat Gargle, cherry Procter & Gamble	liquid		

COLD, COUGH, ALLERGY PRODUCTS — continued

Analgesic	Expectorant	Cough Suppressant	Other Ingredients
	sodium citrate, 7.5mg/5ml	dextromethorphan hydrobromide, 7.5mg/5ml	glycerin • monoammonium glychrrhizinate • flavors
	guaifenesin, 100mg/5ml	dextromethorphan hydrobromide, 5mg/5ml	alcohol, 5%
			alcohol, 2.3% • saccharin • sorbitol • grape flavor
	guaifenesin, 100mg/5ml		xylitol • sorbitol • yerba santa • citric acid • ascorbic acid • sodium benzoate • sodium saccharin
	guaifenesin, 100mg	dextromethorphan hydrobromide, 10mg	alcohol, 4.75% • benzoic acid • fructose • glycerin • propylene glycol • sodium chloride • sucrose
		dextromethorphan hydrobromide, 20mg	alcohol, 8% • glycerin • methylparaben • propylene glycol • propylparaben • sodium chloride • sorbitol solution
			acacia • calcium carbonate • carnauba wax • gelatin • hydrogenated castor oil • magnesium stearate • methylparaben • povidone • propylparaben • sodium benzoate • titanium dioxide • shellac • confectioners sugar • D&C yellow#10 • FD&C blue#1 • FD&C yellow#6 • sucrose • talc
phenol, 1.4%			alcohol, 12.5% • glycerin • propylene glycol • sodium citrate • sodium saccharin • citric acid • sorbitol
acetaminophen, 500mg			
			phenol, 1.4% • FD&C red#40 • flavor • glycerin • purified water • saccharin sodium

COLD, COUGH, ALLERGY PRODUCTS — continued

	Product & Manufacturer	Dosage Form	Decongestant	Antihistamine
AL	Chloraseptic Advanced Formula Sore Throat Spray, mint Procter & Gamble	spray		
AL PE	Chloraseptic Sore Throat Spray Children's, grape Procter & Gamble	spray		
	Chlorpheniramine Maleate Geneva	tablet		chlorpheniramine maleate, 4mg
	Chlorpheniramine Maleate, Extended Release Geneva	timed-release capsule		chlorpheniramine maleate, 12mg/tablet
AF GL PU SO	Clemastine Fumarate Tablets, USP Lemmon	tablet		clemastine fumarate, 1.34mg
	Codimal Central	capsule	pseudoephedrine hydrochloride, 30mg	chlorpheniramine maleate, 2mg
AL	Codimal D.M. Central	syrup	phenylephrine hydrochloride, 5mg/5ml	pyrilamine maleate, 8.3mg/5ml
	Codimal P.H. Central	syrup	phenylephrine hydrochloride, 5mg/5ml	pyrilamine maleate, 8.3mg/5ml
SO	Coldonyl Dover	tablet	phenylephrine hydrochloride, 5mg	
	Comtrex Bristol-Myers	caplet • tablet	pseudoephedrine hydrochloride, 30mg	chlorpheniramine maleate, 2mg
	Comtrex Bristol-Myers	liqui-gel	phenylpropanolamine hydrochloride, 12.5mg	chlorpheniramine maleate, 2mg
	Comtrex Bristol-Myers	liquid	pseudoephedrine hydrochloride, 60mg/30ml	chlorpheniramine maleate, 4mg/30ml
	Comtrex Allergy-Sinus Bristol-Myers	caplet • tablet	pseudoephedrine hydrochloride, 30mg	chlorpheniramine maleate, 2mg
	Comtrex Day/Night Bristol-Myers	Day, caplet	pseudoephedrine hydrochloride, 30mg	
		Night, tablet	pseudoephedrine hydrochloride, 30mg	chlorpheniramine maleate, 2mg
	Comtrex Hot Flu Drink Bristol-Myers	individual packet	pseudoephedrine hydrochloride, 60mg	chlorpheniramine maleate, 4mg
	Comtrex Non-Drowsy Bristol-Myers	caplet	pseudoephedrine hydrochloride, 30mg	
	Comtrex Non-Drowsy Bristol-Myers	liqui-gel	phenylpropanolamine hydrochloride, 12.5mg	
	Conex Forest	liquid	phenylpropanolamine hydrochloride, 12.5mg/5ml	
	Conex D.A. Forest	tablet	phenylpropanolamine hydrochloride, 37.5mg	chlorpheniramine maleate, 4mg
	Conex Plus Forest	tablet	phenylpropanolamine hydrochloride, 25mg	chlorpheniramine maleate, 4mg
	Congespirin For Children, Aspirin Free Bristol-Myers	chewable tablet	phenylpropanolamine hydrochloride, 1.25mg/tablet	
AF	Congestac Menley & James	caplet	pseudoephedrine hydrochloride, 60mg	

COLD, COUGH, ALLERGY PRODUCTS — continued

Analgesic	Expectorant	Cough Suppressant	Other Ingredients
			phenol, 1.4% • FD&C blue#1 • flavor • glycerin • purified water • saccharin sodium
			phenol, 0.5% • FD&C blue#1 • FD&C red#40 • flavor • glycerin • purified water • saccharin sodium • sorbitol
			colloidal silicon dioxide • corn starch • lactose • povidone • pregelatinized starch • stearic acid
acetaminophen, 325mg			
		dextromethorphan hydrobromide, 10mg/5ml	
		codeine phosphate, 10mg/5ml[a]	
acetaminophen, 325mg			
acetaminophen, 325mg		dextromethorphan hydrobromide, 10mg	
acetaminophen, 325mg		dextromethorphan hydrobromide, 10mg	
acetaminophen, 650mg/30ml		dextromethorphan hydrobromide, 20mg/30ml	alcohol, 20% • sucrose
acetaminophen, 500mg			
acetaminophen, 325mg		dextromethorphan hydrobromide, 10mg	
acetaminophen, 325mg		dextromethorphan hydrobromide, 10mg	
acetaminophen, 500mg		dextromethorphan hydrobromide, 20mg	apple cinnamon or lemon flavor
acetaminophen, 325mg		dextromethorphan hydrobromide, 10mg	
acetaminophen, 325mg		dextromethorphan hydrobromide, 10mg	
	guaifenesin, 100mg/5ml		methylparaben, 0.13% • propylparaben, 0.03%
			sucrose, 20mg
acetaminophen, 325mg			
acetaminophen, 81mg/tablet			fruit flavor • saccharin • sucrose
	guaifenesin, 400mg		microcrystalline cellulose • croscarmellose sodium • starch • povidone

COLD, COUGH, ALLERGY PRODUCTS — continued

	Product & Manufacturer	Dosage Form	Decongestant	Antihistamine
	Contac 12 Hour SmithKline Beecham	timed-release capsule	phenylpropanolamine hydrochloride, 75mg	chlorpheniramine maleate, 8mg
	Contac Day & Night Allergy/Sinus SmithKline Beecham	caplet	pseudoephedrine hydrochloride, 60mg	diphenhydramine hydrochloride, 50mg
	Contac Day & Night Cold & Flu SmithKline Beecham	caplet	pseudoephedrine hydrochloride, 60mg	diphenhydramine hydrochloride, 50mg
	Contac JR SmithKline Beecham	liquid	pseudoephedrine hydrochloride, 15mg/5ml	
	Contac Maximum Strength 12 Hour SmithKline Beecham	caplet	phenylpropanolamine hydrochloride, 75mg	chlorpheniramine maleate, 12mg
	Contac Severe Cold & Flu SmithKline Beecham	caplet	phenylpropanolamine hydrochloride, 12.5mg	chlorpheniramine maleate, 2mg
	Contac Severe Cold & Flu Nighttime SmithKline Beecham	liquid	pseudoephedrine hydrochloride, 60mg	chlorpheniramine maleate, 4mg
AF	**Coricidin** Schering-Plough	tablet		chlorpheniramine maleate, 2mg
AF	**Coricidin D** Schering-Plough	tablet	phenylpropanolamine hydrochloride, 12.5mg	chlorpheniramine maleate, 2mg
AF	**Coricidin Demilets** Schering-Plough	chewable tablet	phenylpropanolamine hydrochloride, 6.25mg	chlorpheniramine maleate, 1mg
AF	**Coricidin Maximum Strength Sinus Headache** Schering-Plough	caplet	phenylpropanolamine hydrochloride, 12.5mg	chlorpheniramine maleate, 2mg
AL	**DM Syrup** Paddock	syrup		
AL AF GL PU	**Dallergy-D** Laser	capsule	pseudoephedrine hydrochloride, 120mg	chlorpheniramine maleate, 12mg
AL LA SL PE	**Dallergy-D** Laser	syrup	phenylephrine hydrochloride, 5mg/5ml	chlorpheniramine maleate, 2mg/5ml
AF	**DayQuil LiquiCaps** Procter & Gamble	capsule	pseudoephedrine hydrochloride, 30mg/capsule	
AL	**DayQuil Liquid Non-Drowsy Cold/Flu Medicine** Procter & Gamble	liquid	pseudoephedrine hydrochloride, 60mg/30ml	
	Dehist Forest	capsule	phenylpropanolamine hydrochloride, 75mg	chlorpheniramine maleate, 8mg

COLD, COUGH, ALLERGY PRODUCTS — continued

Analgesic	Expectorant	Cough Suppressant	Other Ingredients
			benzyl alcohol • butylparaben • carboxymethylcellulose sodium • colors • edetate calcium disodium • gelatin • methylparaben • pharmaceutical glaze • polysorbate 80 • propylparaben • sodium lauryl sulfate • sodium propionate • starch • sucrose
acetaminophen, 650mg			carnauba wax • colors • hydroxypropyl methylcellulose • magnesium stearate • microcrystalline cellulose • polyethylene glycol • polysorbate 80 • silicon dioxide • starch • stearic acid • titanium dioxide • white wax
acetaminophen, 650mg			carnauba wax • color • hydroxypropyl methylcellulose • polyethylene glycol • polysorbate 80 • silicon dioxide • starch • stearic acid • titanium dioxide • white wax
acetaminophen, 160mg/5ml		dextromethorphan hydrobromide, 5mg/5ml	saccharin • sorbitol • berry flavor
			acetylated monoglycerides • carnauba wax • colloidal silicon dioxide • ethylcellulose • hydroxypropyl methylcellulose • lactose • stearic acid • titanium dioxide
acetaminophen, 500mg		dextromethorphan hydrobromide, 15mg	
acetaminophen, 1000mg		dextromethorphan hydrobromide, 30mg	alcohol, 18.5% • colors • dibasic sodium phosphate • flavors • glycerin • hydrogenated glucose syrup • phosphoric acid • potassium sorbate • povidone • saccharin sodium • sorbitol • water
acetaminophen, 325mg			
acetaminophen, 325mg			
acetaminophen, 80mg			saccharin
acetaminophen, 500mg			
		dextromethorphan, 15mg/5ml	
			raspberry/vanilla flavor • sugar
acetaminophen, 250mg/capsule	guaifenesin, 100mg/capsule	dextromethorphan hydrobromide, 10mg/capsule	FD&C red#40 • FD&C yellow#6 • gelatin • glycerin • polyethylene glycol • povidone • propylene glycol • purified water • edible ink
acetaminophen, 650mg/30ml	guaifenesin, 200mg/30ml	dextromethorphan hydrobromide, 20mg/30ml	citric acid • FD&C yellow#6 • flavor • glycerin • polyethylene glycol • propylene glycol • purified water • saccharin sodium • sodium citrate • sucrose

COLD, COUGH, ALLERGY PRODUCTS — continued

Product & Manufacturer	Dosage Form	Decongestant	Antihistamine
AL **Delsym, Extended Release** Fisons	suspension		
AL **Demazin** Schering-Plough	syrup	phenylpropanolamine hydrochloride, 12.5mg/5ml	chlorpheniramine maleate, 2mg/5ml
Demazin Schering-Plough	timed-release tablet	phenylpropanolamine hydrochloride, 25mg	chlorpheniramine maleate, 4mg
Dimacol A.H. Robins	caplet	pseudoephedrine hydrochloride, 30mg	
Dimetane A.H. Robins	elixir		brompheniramine maleate, 2mg/5ml
Dimetane A.H. Robins	tablet		brompheniramine maleate, 4mg
Dimetane Decongestant A.H. Robins	caplet	phenylephrine hydrochloride, 10mg	brompheniramine maleate, 4mg
Dimetane Decongestant A.H. Robins	elixir	phenylephrine hydrochloride, 5mg/5ml	brompheniramine maleate, 2mg/5ml
Dimetapp A.H. Robins	elixir	phenylpropanolamine hydrochloride, 12.5mg/5ml	brompheniramine maleate, 2mg/5ml
Dimetapp A.H. Robins	tablet	phenylpropanolamine hydrochloride, 25mg	brompheniramine maleate, 4mg
Dimetapp 4-Hour Liqui-Gels A.H. Robins	liqui-gel	phenylpropanolamine hydrochloride, 25mg	brompheniramine maleate, 4mg
Dimetapp Cold & Allergy A.H. Robins	chewable tablet	phenylpropanolamine hydrochloride, 6.25mg	brompheniramine maleate 1mg
Dimetapp Cold & Flu A.H. Robins	caplet	phenylpropanolamine hydrochloride, 12.5mg	brompheniramine maleate, 2mg
Dimetapp DM A.H. Robins	elixir	phenylpropanolamine hydrochloride, 12.5mg/5ml	brompheniramine maleate, 2mg/5ml
Dimetapp Extentabs A.H. Robins	timed-release tablet	phenylpropanolamine hydrochloride, 75mg	brompheniramine maleate, 12mg
Dimetapp Sinus A.H. Robins	caplet	pseudoephedrine hydrochloride, 30mg	
Diphenhist Antihistamine Captabs Rugby	tablet		diphenhydramine hydrochloride, 25mg
Diphenhist Cough Syrup Rugby	syrup		diphenhydramine hydrochloride, 12.5mg/5ml
Disophrol Schering-Plough	tablet	pseudoephrine sulfate, 60mg	dexbrompheniramine maleate, 2mg
Disophrol Chronotabs, Sustained Action Schering-Plough	timed-release tablet	pseudoephedrine sulfate, 120mg	dexbrompheniramine maleate, 6mg

COLD, COUGH, ALLERGY PRODUCTS — continued

Analgesic	Expectorant	Cough Suppressant	Other Ingredients
		dextromethorphan polistirex (equivalent to 30mg/5ml dextromethorphan hydrobromide)	citric acid • ethylcellulose • FD&C yellow#6 • flavor • high fructose corn syrup • methylparaben • polyethylene glycol 3350 • polysorbate 80 • propylene glycol • propylparaben • purified water • sucrose • tragacanth • vegetable oil • xanthan gum
	guaifenesin, 100mg	dextromethorphan hydrobromide, 10mg	saccharin
			alcohol, 3% • saccharin
			alcohol, 2.3% • sorbitol • grape flavor
			alcohol, 2.3% • saccharin • sorbitol • grape flavor
			sorbitol
			aspartame • sorbitol
		dextromethorphan hydrobromide, 10mg/5ml	alcohol, 2.3% • sorbitol • saccharin
ibuprofen, 200mg			
			starch • microcrystalline cellulose • dibasic calcium phosphate • sodium starch glycolate • colloidal silicon dioxide • stearic acid • sodium lauryl sulfate • hydroxypropyl methylcellulose • titanium dioxide • FD&C red#3 aluminum lake • polyethylene glycol • polysorbate 80 • FD&C blue#2 aluminum lake
			alcohol, 5%/5ml • artificial flavoring • caramel • citric acid • corn syrup • FD&C red#40 • glycerin • menthol • methylparaben • propylene glycol • polyparaben • purified water • sodium citrate • sucrose

COLD, COUGH, ALLERGY PRODUCTS — continued

	Product & Manufacturer	Dosage Form	Decongestant	Antihistamine
AL LA SL PE	Dorcol Children's Cough Syrup Sandoz Pharm.	syrup	pseudoephedrine hydrochloride, 15mg/5ml	
AL LA PE	Dorcol Children's Decongestant Liquid Sandoz Pharm.	liquid	pseudoephedrine hydrochloride, 15mg/5ml	
AL LA SL PE	Dorcol Children's Liquid Cold Formula Sandoz Pharm.	liquid	pseudoephedrine hydrochloride, 15mg/5ml	chlorpheniramine maleate, 1mg/5ml
GL	Dristan Allergy Whitehall	caplet	pseudoephedrine hydrochloride, 60mg	brompheniramine maleate, 4mg
AF GL	Dristan Cold and Flu Whitehall	powder	pseudoephedrine hydrochloride, 60mg	chlorpheniramine maleate, 4mg
AF GL SO	Dristan Cold, Multi-Symptom Whitehall	tablet	phenylephrine hydrochloride, 5mg	chlorpheniramine maleate, 2mg
AF GL	Dristan Cold, Multi-Symptom Maximum Strength Whitehall	caplet	pseudoephedrine hydrochloride, 30mg	brompheniramine, 2mg
AF GL	Dristan Cold, No Drowsiness Whitehall	caplet	pseudoephedrine, 30mg	
AF GL	Dristan Juice Mix-In Whitehall	powder	pseudoephedrine hydrochloride, 60mg	
AF GL SO	Dristan Sinus Whitehall	caplet	pseudoephedrine hydrochloride, 30mg	
AL	Drixoral Schering-Plough	syrup	pseudoephedrine sulfate, 30mg/5ml	brompheniramine maleate, 2mg/5ml
	Drixoral Cold and Allergy, Sustained Action Schering-Plough	timed-release tablet	pseudoephedrine sulfate, 120mg	dexbrompheniramine maleate, 6mg
AF	Drixoral Cold and Flu & Sinus, Extended Release Schering-Plough	timed-release tablet	pseudoephedrine sulfate, 60mg	dexbrompheniramine maleate, 3mg
	Drixoral Non-Drowsy Formula, Extended Release Schering-Plough	timed-release tablet	pseudoephedrine sulfate, 120mg	
AL PU	Efidac/24 CIBA Consumer	tablet	pseudoephedrine hydrochloride, 240mg	
SO	Emagrin Forte Otis Clapp	tablet	phenylephrine hydrochloride	
	Excedrin Sinus Bristol-Myers	caplet • tablet	pseudoephedrine hydrochloride, 30mg	
	Extra Action Cough Syrup, Guaifenesin-DM Rugby	syrup		
GL	Fedahist Schwarz Pharma	tablet	pseudoephedrine hydrochloride, 60mg	chlorpheniramine maleate, 4mg
AL LA	Fedahist Decongestant Schwarz Pharma	syrup	pseudoephedrine hydrochloride, 30mg/5ml	chlorpheniramine maleate, 2mg/5ml

COLD, COUGH, ALLERGY PRODUCTS — continued

Analgesic	Expectorant	Cough Suppressant	Other Ingredients
	guaifenesin, 50mg/5ml	dextromethorphan hydrobromide, 5mg/5ml	benzoic acid • flavors • purified water • sodium hydroxide • sucrose • red#40 • tartaric acid • blue#1 • edetate disodium • glycerin • propylene glycol
			sorbitol • benzoic acid • edetate disodium • flavors • purified water • sodium hydroxide • sucrose • yellow #6 • yellow #10
			sorbitol • sucrose • benzoic acid • blue #1 • flavors • purified water • red #40 • yellow #10
acetaminophen, 500mg		dextromethorphan hydrobromide, 20mg	
acetaminophen, 325mg			
acetaminophen, 500mg			
acetaminophen, 500mg			
acetaminophen, 500mg		dextromethorphan hydrobromide, 20mg	
ibuprofen, 200mg			
acetaminophen, 500mg			
			cellulose • cellulose acetate • FD&C blue#1 • hydroxypropyl methylcellulose • hydroxypropyl cellulose • polysorbate 80 • povidone • sodium chloride • titanium dioxide
acetaminophen	guaifenesin		caffeine
acetaminophen, 500mg			
	guaifenesin, 100mg/5ml	dextromethorphan hydrobromide, 10mg/5ml	citric acid • FD&C red#40 • flavors • glucose • glycerin • corn syrup • saccharin sodium • sodium benzoate • water
			lactose • colloidal silicon dioxide • magnesium stearate • microcrystalline cellulose • stearic acid • talc
			saccharin • sorbitol • sucrose • grape flavor

COLD, COUGH, ALLERGY PRODUCTS — continued

	Product & Manufacturer	Dosage Form	Decongestant	Antihistamine
AL LA SU	Fedahist Expectorant Schwarz Pharma	liquid	pseudoephedrine hydrochloride, 30mg/5ml	
AL LA SU PE	Fedahist Expectorant Pediatric Schwarz Pharma	drops	pseudoephedrine hydrochloride, 7.5mg/ml	
SO	Fendol Buffington	tablet	phenylephrine hydrochloride	
AF	Flu, Cold and Cough Medicine Goldline	individual packet	pseudoephedrine hydrochloride, 60mg	chlorpheniramine maleate, 4mg
	Formula 44 Cough Mixture Procter & Gamble	liquid		
AL PE	Formula 44 Pediatric Cough Medicine Procter & Gamble	liquid		
	Formula 44D Decongestant Cough Mixture Procter & Gamble	liquid	pseudoephedrine hydrochloride, 20mg/5ml	
	Formula 44M Multisymptom Cough and Cold Medicine Procter & Gamble	liquid	pseudoephedrine hydrochloride, 15mg/5ml	chlorpheniramine maleate, 1mg/5ml
AL PE	Formula 44d Pediatric Cough and Decongestant Medicine Procter & Gamble	liquid	pseudoephedrine hydrochloride, 30mg/15ml	
	Formula 44e Cough and Expectorant Medicine Procter & Gamble	liquid		
AL PE	Formula 44e Pediatric Cough and Expectorant Medicine Procter & Gamble	liquid		
AL PE	Formula 44m Pediatric Multisymptom Cough & Cold Medicine Procter & Gamble	liquid	pseudoephedrine hydrochloride, 30mg/15ml	chlorpheniramine maleate, 2mg/15ml
	GG-Cen Central	capsule		
	Genac Goldline	tablet	pseudoephedrine hydrochloride, 60mg	triprolidine hydrochloride, 2.5mg
AF	Genahist Goldline	capsule		diphenhydramine hydrochloride, 25mg
	Genahist Goldline	elixir		diphenhydramine hydrochloride, 12.5mg/5ml
	Genamin Goldline	syrup	phenylpropanolamine hydrochloride, 12.5mg/5ml	chlorpheniramine maleate, 2mg/5ml
	Genaphed Goldline	tablet	pseudoephedrine hydrochloride, 30mg	

COLD, COUGH, ALLERGY PRODUCTS — continued

Analgesic	Expectorant	Cough Suppressant	Other Ingredients
	guaifenesin, 200mg/5ml		saccharin • sorbitol • fruit flavor
	guaifenesin, 40mg/ml		saccharin • sorbitol • fruit flavor
salicylamide • acetaminophen	guaifenesin		caffeine
acetaminophen, 500mg		dextromethorphan hydrobromide, 20mg	yellow #6
		dextromethorphan hydrobromide, 15mg/5ml	alcohol, 10% • sugar • caramel • carboxymethylcellulose sodium • citric acid • FD&C red#40 • flavor • propylene glycol • purified water • sodium citrate
		dextromethorphan hydrobromide, 15mg/15ml	carboxymethylcellulose sodium • cellulose • citric acid • FD&C red#40 • flavor • glycerin • polysorbate 80 • potassium sorbate • propylene glycol • purified water • sodium citrate • sorbitol
		dextromethorphan hydrobromide, 10mg/5ml	alcohol, 10% • saccharin sodium • citric acid • FD&C red#40 • flavor • glycerin • propylene glycol • purified water • sodium citrate • sucrose
acetaminophen, 125mg/5ml		dextromethorphan hydrobromide, 7.5mg/5ml	alcohol, 20% • saccharin sodium • citric acid • FD&C blue#1 • FD&C red#40 • flavor • glycerin • purified water • sodium benzoate • sodium citrate • sucrose
		dextromethorphan hydrobromide, 15mg/15ml	carboxymethylcellulose sodium • cellulose • citric acid • FD&C red#40 • flavor • glycerin • polysorbate 80 • potassium sorbate • propylene glycol • purified water • sodium citrate • sorbitol • sucrose
	guaifenesin, 200mg/15ml	dextromethorphan hydrobromide, 20mg/15ml	alcohol, 10% • citric acid • FD&C blue#1 • FD&C red#40 • flavor • glycerin • propylene glycol • purified water • saccharin sodium • sodium citrate • sucrose
	guaifenesin, 100mg/15ml	dextromethorphan hydrobromide, 10mg/15ml	carboxymethylcellulose sodium • cellulose • citric acid • FD&C red#40 • flavor • glycerin • polysorbate 80 • potassium sorbate • propylene glycol • purified water • sodium citrate • sorbitol • sucrose
		dextromethorphan hydrobromide, 15mg/15ml	carboxymethylcellulose sodium • cellulose • citric acid • FD&C red#40 • flavor • glycerin • polysorbate 80 • potassium sorbate • propylene glycol • purified water • sodium citrate • sorbitol • sucrose
	guaifenesin, 200mg		
			alcohol, 14%

COLD, COUGH, ALLERGY PRODUCTS — continued

	Product & Manufacturer	Dosage Form	Decongestant	Antihistamine
	Genatap Goldline	elixir	phenylpropanolamine hydrochloride, 12.5mg/5ml	brompheniramine maleate, 2mg/5ml
	Genatuss Goldline	syrup		
	Gencold Goldline	capsule	phenylpropanolamine hydrochloride, 75mg	chlorpheniramine maleate, 8mg
AF	**Gendecon** Goldline	tablet	phenylephrine hydrochloride, 5mg	chlorpheniramine maleate, 2mg
	Genex Goldline	capsule	phenylpropanolamine hydrochloride, 18mg	
	Genite Goldline	liquid	pseudoephedrine hydrochloride, 10mg/5ml	doxylamine succinate, 1.25mg/5ml
	Genatuss DM Goldline	syrup		
	Guaifenesin Syrup USP Muro	syrup		
AF GL PU	**Histatab Plus** Century	tablet	phenylephrine hydrochloride, 5mg	chlorpheniramine maleate, 2mg
	Hydramine Cough Goldline	syrup		diphenhydramine hydrochloride, 12.5mg/5ml
AF GL PU SO	**Hytuss** Hyrex	tablet		
AF GL PU SO	**Hytuss 2X** Hyrex	capsule		
AF GL PU SO	**Isoclor** CIBA Consumer	tablet	pseudoephedrine hydrochloride, 60mg	chlorpheniramine maleate, 4mg
AF GL PU SO	**Isoclor Timesules** CIBA Consumer	timed-release capsule	pseudoephedrine hydrochloride, 120mg	chlorpheniramine maleate, 8mg
AF GL PU	**Medi-Flu** Parke-Davis	caplet	pseudoephedrine hydrochloride, 30mg	chlorpheniramine maleate, 2mg
LA PR SL	**Medi-Flu** Parke-Davis	liquid	pseudoephedrine hydrochloride, 60mg/30ml	chlorpheniramine maleate, 4mg/30ml
AF GL PU	**Medi-Flu Without Drowsiness** Parke-Davis	caplet	pseudoephedrine hydrochloride, 30mg	
AF GL PU SO	**ND-Gesic** Hyrex	tablet	phenylephrine hydrochloride, 5mg	pyrilamine maleate, 12.5mg • chlorpheniramine maleate, 2mg
LA SL	**Naldecon DX Adult Liquid** Apothecon	liquid	phenylpropanolamine hydrochloride, 12.5mg/5ml	
LA SL PE	**Naldecon DX Children's Syrup** Apothecon	syrup	phenylpropanolamine hydrochloride, 6.25mg/5ml	

COLD, COUGH, ALLERGY PRODUCTS — continued			
Analgesic	Expectorant	Cough Suppressant	Other Ingredients
			alcohol, 2.3% • saccharin • sorbitol • grape flavor
	guaifenesin, 100mg/5ml		alcohol, 3.5%
acetaminophen, 325mg			
acetaminophen, 325mg			
acetaminophen, 167mg/5ml		dextromethorphan hydrobromide, 5mg/5ml	alcohol, 25% • tartrazine
	guaifenesin, 100mg/5ml	dextromethorphan hydrobromide, 15mg/5ml	alcohol, 1.4% • sucrose • saccharin • glucose
	guaifenesin, 100mg/5ml		sucrose • glucose • sorbitol • citric acid • tartaric acid • saccharin sodium • methylparaben • propylparaben • FD&C red#40 • FD&C yellow#6 • alcohol • flavorings • purified water
			alcohol, 5%
	guaifenesin, 100mg		
	guaifenesin, 200mg		
			colloidal silicon dioxide • microcrystalline cellulose • starch • stearic acid
			castor wax • ethylcellulose • gelatin • mineral oil • silicone oil • sugar spheres • white petrolatum
acetaminophen, 500mg		dextromethorphan hydrobromide, 15mg	
acetaminophen, 1000mg/30ml		dextromethorphan, 30mg/30ml	alcohol, 20% • sodium citrate
acetaminophen, 500mg		dextromethorphan hydrobromide, 15mg	
acetaminophen, 300mg			
	guaifenesin, 200mg/5ml	dextromethorphan hydrobromide, 10mg/5ml	
	guaifenesin, 100mg/5ml	dextromethorphan hydrobromide, 5mg/5ml	

COLD, COUGH, ALLERGY PRODUCTS — continued

	Product & Manufacturer	Dosage Form	Decongestant	Antihistamine
LA SU PE	Naldecon DX Pediatric Drops Apothecon	drops	phenylpropanolamine hydrochloride, 6.25mg/ml	
LA SL PE	Naldecon EX Children's Syrup Apothecon	syrup	phenylpropanolamine hydrochloride, 6.25mg/5ml	
AL LA SU SL GE	Naldecon Senior DX Apothecon	liquid		
AL LA SU SL GE	Naldecon Senior EX Apothecon	liquid		
AL	Night Time Cold Medicine Goldline	liquid	pseudoephedrine hydrochloride, 60mg/oz	doxylamine succinate, 7.5mg/oz
	Nolahist Carnrick	tablet		phenindamine tartrate, 25mg
	Novahistine SmithKline Beecham	elixir	phenylephrine hydrochloride, 5mg/5ml	chlorpheniramine maleate, 2mg/5ml
	Novahistine DH SmithKline Beecham	liquid	pseudoephedrine hydrochloride, 30mg/5ml	chlorpheniramine maleate, 2mg/5ml
	Novahistine DMX SmithKline Beecham	syrup	pseudoephedrine hydrochloride, 30mg/5ml	
	Novahistine Expectorant SmithKline Beecham	liquid	pseudoephedrine hydrochloride, 30mg/5ml	
	NyQuil Adult Nighttime Cold/Flu Medicine, Cherry Flavor Procter & Gamble	liquid	pseudoephedrine hydrochloride, 60mg/30ml	doxylamine succinate, 12.5mg/30ml
	NyQuil Adult Nighttime Cold/Flu Medicine, Original Formula Procter & Gamble	liquid	pseudoephedrine hydrochloride, 60mg/30ml	doxylamine succinate, 12.5mg/30ml
AL PE	NyQuil Children's Allergy/Head Cold Medicine Procter & Gamble	liquid	pseudoephedrine hydrochloride, 30mg/15ml	chlorpheniramine maleate, 2mg/15ml
AL PE	NyQuil Children's Cold/Cough Medicine Procter & Gamble	liquid	pseudoephedrine hydrochloride, 30mg/15ml	chlorpheniramine maleate, 2mg/15ml
AL AF	NyQuil LiquiCaps Adult Nighttime Cold/Flu Medicine Procter & Gamble	capsule	pseudoephedrine hydrochloride, 30mg/capsule	doxylamine succinate, 6.25mg/capsule
SO	Nycoff Dover	tablet		
	Nytcold Cough & Cold Medicine Rugby	liquid	pseudoephedrine hydrochloride, 60mg/oz	doxylamine succinate, 7.5mg/oz
SO	Oranyl Otis Clapp	tablet	pseudoephedrine hydrochloride, 30mg	
SO	Oranyl Plus Otis Clapp	tablet	pseudoephedrine hydrochloride, 30mg	
AF	Ornex Menley & James	caplet	pseudoephedrine hydrochloride, 30mg	

COLD, COUGH, ALLERGY PRODUCTS — continued

Analgesic	Expectorant	Cough Suppressant	Other Ingredients
	guaifenesin, 50mg/ml	dextromethorphan hydrobromide, 5mg/ml	
	guaifenesin, 100mg/5ml		
	guaifenesin, 200mg/5ml	dextromethorphan hydrobromide, 10mg/5ml	citric acid • FD&C red#40 • FD&C blue#1 • natural and artificial flavor • polyethylene glycol • saccharin sodium • sodium benzoate • sodium citrate • sorbitol solution • purified water
	guaifenesin, 200mg/5ml		citric acid • FD&C blue#1 • FD&C red#40 • natural and artifical flavor • polyethylene glycol • saccharin sodium • sodium benzoate • sodium citrate • sorbitol solution • purified water
acetaminophen, 1000mg/oz		dextromethorphan hydrobromide, 30mg/oz	
			alcohol, 5% • sorbitol
		codeine phosphate, 10mg/5ml[a]	alcohol, 5% • sugar • saccharin • sorbitol
	guaifenesin, 100mg/5ml	dextromethorphan hydrobromide, 10mg/5ml	alcohol, 10% • saccharin • sorbitol
	guaifenesin, 100mg/5ml	codeine phosphate, 10mg/5ml[a]	alcohol, 7.5% • saccharin • sorbitol • invert sugar
acetaminophen, 1000mg/30ml		dextromethorphan hydrobromide, 30mg/30ml	alcohol, 25% • citric acid • FD&C blue#1 • FD&C red#40 • flavor • glycerin • purified water • sodium citrate • saccharin sodium • sucrose
acetaminophen, 1000mg/30ml		dextromethorphan hydrobromide, 30mg/30ml	alcohol, 25% • citric acid • FD&C blue#1 • flavor • glycerin • purified water • sodium benzoate • sodium citrate • sucrose • FD&C yellow#5 (tartrazine)
			citric acid • FD&C blue#1 • FD&C red#40 • flavor • methylparaben • potassium sorbate • propylene glycol • purified water • sodium citrate • sorbitol • sucrose
		dextromethorphan hydrobromide, 15mg/15ml	citric acid • FD&C red#40 • flavor • potassium sorbate • propylene glycol • purified water • sodium citrate • sucrose
acetaminophen, 250mg/capsule		dextromethorphan hydrobromide, 10mg/capsule	D&C yellow#10 • FD&C blue#1 • gelatin • glycerin • polyethylene glycol • povidone • propylene glycol • purified water • may contain edible ink
		dextromethorphan hydrobromide	
acetaminophen, 1000mg/oz		dextromethorphan hydrobromide, 30mg/oz	alcohol, 25% • citric acid • color • FD&C yellow#6 • flavor • glucose • methylparaben • propylparaben • purified water • saccharin • sodium citrate • sucrose
acetaminophen, 500mg			
acetaminophen, 325mg			FD&C blue#1 • microcrystalline cellulose • povidone • starch

COLD, COUGH, ALLERGY PRODUCTS — continued

	Product & Manufacturer	Dosage Form	Decongestant	Antihistamine
AF	Ornex Maximum Strength Menley & James	caplet	pseudoephedrine hydrochloride, 30mg	
AF	Ornex Severe Cold Menley & James	caplet	pseudoephedrine hydrochloride, 30mg	
	Orthoxicol Roberts Pharm.	liquid	phenylpropanolamine hydrochloride, 25mg	chlorpheniramine maleate, 4mg
AF GL PU SO PE	PediaCare Cold-Allergy Chewable Tablets For Ages 6 to 12 McNeil	chewable tablet	pseudoephedrine hydrochloride, 15mg	chlorpheniramine maleate, 1mg
AF GL PU SO PE	PediaCare Cough-Cold Chewable Tablets For Ages 6 to 12 McNeil	chewable tablet	pseudoephedrine hydrochloride, 15mg	chlorpheniramine maleate, 1mg
AL LA SL PE	PediaCare Cough-Cold Formula Liquid McNeil	liquid	pseudoephedrine hydrochloride, 15mg/5ml	chlorpheniramine maleate, 1mg/5ml
AL LA SL PE	PediaCare Infants' Decongestant Drops McNeil	drops	pseudoephedrine hydrochloride, 7.5mg/0.8ml	
AL LA SU SL PE	PediaCare Night Rest Cough-Cold Formula McNeil	liquid	pseudoephedrine hydrochloride, 15mg/5ml	chlorpheniramine maleate, 1mg/5ml
LA SL GE	Pertussin AM Blairex	liquid	pseudoephedrine hydrochloride, 60mg/15ml	
AL LA SL PE	Pertussin CS Blairex	liquid		
AL LA SL GE	Pertussin ES Blairex	liquid		
LA SL GE	Pertussin PM Blairex	liquid	pseudoephedrine hydrochloride, 60mg/oz	doxylamine succinate, 7.5mg/oz
	Phenapap Sinus Headache & Congestion Without Drowsiness Rugby	tablet	pseudoephedrine hydrochloride, 30mg	
	Phenylgesic Goldline	tablet		phenyltoloxamine citrate, 30mg
	Pinex Alvin Last	syrup		
	Pinex Concentrate Alvin Last	syrup		
	Primatuss 4 Cough Mixture Rugby	liquid		chlorpheniramine maleate, 4mg/10ml

COLD, COUGH, ALLERGY PRODUCTS — continued

Analgesic	Expectorant	Cough Suppressant	Other Ingredients
acetaminophen, 500mg			microcrystalline cellulose • povidone • starch
acetaminophen, 500mg		dextromethorphan hydrobromide, 15mg	FD&C yellow#6 • D&C yellow#10 • microcrystalline cellulose • povidone • starch
		dextromethorphan hydrobromide, 20mg	alcohol, 8% • glycerin • methylparaben • propylene glycol • propylparaben • sodium chloride • sorbitol solution
			aspartame • cellulose • citric acid • corn starch • flavors • mannitol • colloidal silicon dioxide • stearic acid • red #7
		dextromethorphan hydrobromide, 5mg	aspartame • cellulose • citric acid • flavors • magnesium stearate • magnesium trisilicate • mannitol • starch • red #7
		dextromethorphan hydrobromide, 5mg/5ml	citric acid • corn syrup • cherry flavors • glycerin • propylene glycol • sodium benzoate • sodium carboxymethylcellulose • sorbitol • purified water • red #40
			benzoic acid • citric acid • flavors • glycerin • polyethylene glycol • propylene glycol • purified water • sodium benzoate • sorbitol • sucrose • red #40
		dextromethorphan hydrobromide, 7.5mg/5ml	citric acid • corn syrup • cherry flavors • glycerin • propylene glycol • sodium benzoate • sodium carboxymethylcellulose • sorbitol • purified water • red #40
	guaifenesin, 200mg/15ml	dextromethorphan, 20mg/15ml	alcohol, 10% • citric acid • colors • flavor • propylene glycol • purified water • sodium benzoate • sodium citrate • sodium saccharin • sucrose
		dextromethorphan, 7mg/10ml	citric acid • colors • flavor • sorbic acid • sorbitol • sucrose • water
		dextromethorphan, 30mg/10ml	caramel • carboxymethylcellulose sodium • citric acid • D&C red#33 • flavor • sorbic acid • sorbitol • sugar • water
acetaminophen, 1000mg/oz		dextromethorphan hydrobromide, 30mg/oz	citric acid • FD&C blue#1 • FD&C red#40 • flavor • glycerin • purified water • sodium citrate • sodium saccharin • sucrose
acetaminophen, 325mg			microcrystalline cellulose • stearic acid • amorphous fumed silica • powdered cellulose • FD&C red#27 • FD&C red#40
acetaminophen, 325mg			
		dextromethorphan hydrobromide, 7.5mg/5ml	sucrose • purified water • glycerin • caramel • honey • flavor
		dextromethorphan hydrobromide, 7.5mg/5ml (when diluted to 16fl.oz.)	alcohol, 16% (3% when diluted) • purified water • sucrose • glycerin • honey • flavor • caramel • sodium hydroxide
		dextromethorphan hydrobromide, 30mg/10ml	alcohol, 10% • caramel • citric acid • flavor • methylparaben • propylene glycol • purified water • sodium benzoate • sodium citrate • sorbitol solution • sucrose

COLD, COUGH, ALLERGY PRODUCTS — continued

	Product & Manufacturer	Dosage Form	Decongestant	Antihistamine
	Primatuss 4D Cough Mixture Rugby	liquid	pseudoephedrine hydrochloride, 60mg/15ml	
	Propagest Carnrick	tablet	phenylpropanolamine hydrochloride, 25mg	
AF	**Pyrroxate** Roberts Pharm.	capsule	phenylpropanolamine hydrochloride, 25mg	chlorpheniramine maleate, 4mg
	Quelidrine Cough Abbott	syrup	phenylephrine hydrochloride 5mg/5ml • ephedrine hydrochloride, 5mg/5ml	chlorpheniramine maleate, 2mg/5ml
	Queltuss Forest	tablet		
AL	**REM** Alvin Last	liquid		
	Robitussin A.H. Robins	syrup		
	Robitussin CF A.H. Robins	syrup	phenylpropanolamine hydrochloride, 12.5mg/5ml	
	Robitussin DM A.H. Robins	syrup		
	Robitussin Maximum Strength Cough A.H. Robins	liquid		
	Robitussin Maximum Strength Cough & Cold A.H. Robins	liquid	pseudoephedrine hydrochloride, 30mg/5ml	
	Robitussin Night Relief A.H. Robins	liquid	pseudoephedrine hydrochloride, 60mg/30ml	pyrilamine maleate, 50mg/30ml
	Robitussin PE A.H. Robins	syrup	pseudoephedrine hydrochloride, 30mg/5ml	
PE	**Robitussin Pediatric Cough** A.H. Robins	liquid		
PE	**Robitussin Pediatric Cough & Cold** A.H. Robins	liquid	pseudoephedrine hydrochloride, 15mg/5ml	
AL SU	**Silexin** Otis Clapp	syrup		
SO	**Silexin** Otis Clapp	tablet		
AF GL PU SO	**Sinarest** CIBA Consumer	tablet	pseudoephedrine hydrochloride, 30mg	chlorpheniramine maleate, 2mg
AF GL PU	**Sinarest Extra Strength** CIBA Consumer	tablet	pseudoephedrine hydrochloride, 30mg	chlorpheniramine maleate, 2mg

COLD, COUGH, ALLERGY PRODUCTS — continued

Analgesic	Expectorant	Cough Suppressant	Other Ingredients
	guaifenesin, 200mg/15ml	dextromethorphan hydrobromide, 30mg/15ml	alcohol, 10% • citric acid • color • corn syrup • flavor • methylparaben • propylene glycol • purified water • sodium benzoate • sodium citrate • sorbitol solution • sucrose
acetaminophen, 500mg			benzyl alcohol • butylparaben • erythrosine sodium • gelatin • glycerin • magnesium stearate • methylparaben • propylparaben • sodium lauryl sulfate • sodium propionate • starch • talc
	ammonium chloride, 40mg/5ml • ipecac fluid extract, 0.005ml/5ml	dextromethorphan hydrobromide, 10mg/5ml	alcohol, 2% • sucrose • D&C red#33 • glycerin • liquid glucose • magnesium carbonate • methylparaben • propylparaben • tolu balsam tincture • water • artificial flavors
	guaifenesin, 100mg/5ml	dextromethorphan hydrobromide, 15mg/5ml	alcohol, 1.4%
	citric acid • sodium citrate	dextromethorphan hydrobromide, 5mg/5ml	corn syrup • sucrose • glycerin • purified water • caramel • sodium chloride • sodium benzoate • eucalyptol • licorice • anise oil • disodium EDTA
	guaifenesin, 100mg/5ml		alcohol, 3.5%
	guaifenesin, 100mg/5ml	dextromethorphan hydrobromide, 10mg/5ml	alcohol, 4.75% • saccharin • sorbitol
	guaifenesin, 100mg/5ml	dextromethorphan hydrobromide, 10mg/5ml	saccharin
		dextromethorphan hydrobromide, 15mg/5ml	alcohol, 1.4% • saccharin
		dextromethorphan hydrobromide, 15mg/5ml	alcohol, 1.4% • saccharin
acetaminophen, 650mg/30ml		dextromethorphan hydrobromide, 30mg/30ml	saccharin • sorbitol
	guaifenesin, 100mg/5ml		alcohol, 1.4% • saccharin
		dextromethorphan hydrobromide, 7.5mg/5ml	sorbitol • saccharin
		dextromethorphan hydrobromide, 7.5mg/5ml	sorbitol • saccharin
	guaifenesin	dextromethorphan hydrobromide	
		dextromethorphan hydrobromide	benzocaine
acetaminophen, 325mg			magnesium stearate • microcrystalline cellulose • povidone • pregelatinized starch • yellow #6 lake • yellow #10 lake
acetaminophen, 500mg			magnesium stearate • microcrystalline cellulose • povidone • pregelatinized starch • sodium starch glyconate • yellow#6 lake • yellow#10 lake

COLD, COUGH, ALLERGY PRODUCTS — continued

	Product & Manufacturer	Dosage Form	Decongestant	Antihistamine
AF GL PU	Sinarest No-Drowsiness CIBA Consumer	tablet	pseudoephedrine hydrochloride, 30mg	
GL PR PU	Sine-Aid Maximum Strength McNeil	caplet	pseudoephedrine hydrochloride, 30mg	
AF GL PU	Sine-Aid Maximum Strength McNeil	gelcap	pseudoephedrine hydrochloride, 30mg	
AF GL PU	Sine-Aid Maximum Strength McNeil	tablet	pseudoephedrine hydrochloride, 30mg	
	Sine-Off Maximum Strength Allergy/Sinus SmithKline Beecham	caplet	pseudoephedrine hydrochloride, 30mg	chlorpheniramine maleate, 2mg
	Sine-Off Maximum Strength No Drowsiness Formula SmithKline Beecham	caplet	pseudoephedrine hydrochloride, 30mg	
	Sine-Off Sinus Medicine SmithKline Beecham	tablet	phenylpropanolamine hydrochloride, 12.5mg	chlorpheniramine maleate, 2mg
	Singlet SmithKline Beecham	tablet	pseudoephedrine hydrochloride, 60mg	chlorpheniramine maleate, 4mg
	Sinulin Carnrick	tablet	phenylpropanolamine hydrochloride, 25mg	chlorpheniramine maleate, 4mg
	Sinustop Pro Murdock	capsule	pseudoephedrine hydrochloride, 60mg	
AF GL PU	Sinutab Parke-Davis	tablet	pseudoephedrine hydrochloride, 30mg	
AF GL PU	Sinutab Maximum Strength Parke-Davis	caplet • tablet	pseudoephedrine hydrochloride, 30mg	chlorpheniramine maleate, 2mg
AF GL PU	Sinutab Maximum Strength Without Drowsiness Parke-Davis	tablet • caplet	pseudoephedrine hydrochloride, 30mg	
AF PE	St. Joseph Cold Tablets For Children Schering-Plough	chewable tablet	phenylpropanolamine hydrochloride, 3.125mg	
AL PE	St. Joseph Cough Suppressant For Children Schering-Plough	syrup		
	Suda-Tussin-DM Reese Chemical	liquid	pseudoephedrine hydrochloride	
AF	Sudafed Burroughs Wellcome	tablet	pseudoephedrine hydrochloride, 30mg	
AF	Sudafed Burroughs Wellcome	tablet	pseudoephedrine hydrochloride, 60mg	
AF GL GE	Sudafed 12 Hour Burroughs Wellcome	tablet	pseudoephedrine sulfate, 120mg	

COLD, COUGH, ALLERGY PRODUCTS — continued

Analgesic	Expectorant	Cough Suppressant	Other Ingredients
acetaminophen, 500mg			magnesium stearate • microcrystalline cellulose • povidone • pregelatinized starch • sodium starch glycolate
acetaminophen, 500mg			cellulose • corn starch • hydroxypropyl methylcellulose • magnesium stearate • polyethylene glycol • sodium starch glycolate • titanium dioxide • blue #1 • red #40
acetaminophen, 500mg			benzyl alcohol • butylparaben • castor oil • cellulose • cornstarch • edetate calcium disodium • gelatin • hydroxypropyl methylcellulose • iron oxide black • magnesium stearate • methylparaben • propylparaben • sodium lauryl sulfate • sodium propionate • sodium starch glycolate • titanium dioxide • FD&C red#40
acetaminophen, 500mg			cellulose • corn starch • magnesium stearate • sodium starch glycolate
acetaminophen, 500mg			
acetaminophen, 500mg			
aspirin, 325mg			
acetaminophen, 650mg			
acetaminophen, 650mg			
			echinacea purpurea herb • golden seal root • ginger root
acetaminophen, 325mg			
acetaminophen, 500mg			
acetaminophen, 500mg			
acetaminophen, 80mg			
		dextromethorphan hydrobromide, 7.5mg/5ml	
	guaifenesin	dextromethorphan	
			lactose • sugar

COLD, COUGH, ALLERGY PRODUCTS — continued

	Product & Manufacturer	Dosage Form	Decongestant	Antihistamine
AF GL SO GE	Sudafed 12 Hour Caplet, Extended Release Burroughs Wellcome	timed-release caplet	pseudoephedrine hydrochloride, 120mg	
AL LA SL PE	Sudafed Children's Burroughs Wellcome	liquid	pseudoephedrine hydrochloride, 30mg/5ml	
LA	Sudafed Cough Burroughs Wellcome	syrup	pseudoephedrine hydrochloride, 15mg/5ml	
AF GL GE	Sudafed Maximum Strength Severe Cold Formula Burroughs Wellcome	tablet	pseudoephedrine hydrochloride, 30mg	
AL LA SL PE	Sudafed Plus Burroughs Wellcome	syrup	pseudoephedrine hydrochloride, 30mg/5ml	chlorpheniramine maleate, 2mg/5ml
AF GE	Sudafed Plus Burroughs Wellcome	tablet	pseudoephedrine hydrochloride, 60mg	chlorpheniramine maleate, 4mg
AF GL GE	Sudafed Severe Cold Formula Burroughs Wellcome	caplet	pseudoephedrine hydrochloride, 30mg	
AF GL GE	Sudafed Sinus Burroughs Wellcome	caplet • tablet	pseudoephedrine hydrochloride, 30mg	
SO	Sudanyl Dover	tablet	pseudoephedrine hydrochloride, 30mg	
AF GL PU SO	Tavist-1 Antihistamine Sandoz Pharm.	tablet		clemastine fumarate, 1.34mg
AF GL PU SO	Tavist-D Antihistamine/ Nasal Decongestant Sandoz Pharm.	tablet	phenylpropanolamine hydrochloride, 75mg	clemastine fumasate, 1.34mg
	Teldrin SmithKline Beecham	timed-release capsule		chlorpheniramine maleate, 12mg
AF GL PU	TheraFlu Maximum Strength NightTime Sandoz Pharm.	individual packet	pseudoephedrine hydrochloride, 60mg	chlorpheniramine maleate, 4mg
AF GL PU	TheraFlu; Flu and Cold Medicine Sandoz Pharm.	individual packet	pseudoephedrine hydrochloride, 60mg	chlorpheniramine maleate, 4mg
AF GL PU	TheraFlu; Flu, Cold and Cough Medicine Sandoz Pharm.	individual packet	pseudoephedrine hydrochloride, 60mg	chlorpheniramine maleate, 4mg
	Theracof Reese Chemical	liquid	phenylpropanolamine	pyrilamine maleate
SU PE GE	Tolu-Sed DM Scherer	liquid		

COLD, COUGH, ALLERGY PRODUCTS — continued

Analgesic	Expectorant	Cough Suppressant	Other Ingredients
	guaifenesin, 100mg/5ml	dextromethorphan hydrobromide, 5mg/5ml	alcohol, 2.4%
acetaminophen, 500mg		dextromethorphan hydrobromide, 15mg	
			sucrose
			lactose
acetaminophen, 500mg		dextromethorphan hydrobromide, 15mg	
acetaminophen, 500mg			
			lactose • povidone • starch • talc • stearic acid
			colloidal silicon dioxide • yellow #10 • dibasic calcium phosphate dihydrate • lactose • magnesium stearate • methylcellulose • polyethylene glycol • povidone • starch • synthetic polymers • titanium dioxide
			benzyl alcohol • cetylpyridinium chloride • ethylcellulose • colors • gelatin • hydrogenated castor oil • silicon dioxide • sodium lauryl sulfate • starch • sucrose
acetaminophen, 1000mg		dextromethorphan hydrobromide, 30mg	ascorbic acid • citric acid • natural lemon flavors • maltol • pregelatinized starch • silicon dioxide • sodium citrate • sucrose • titanium dioxide • tribasic calcium phosphate • yellow#6 • yellow#10
acetaminophen, 650mg			natural lemon flavors • sucrose • ascorbic acid • citric acid • sodium citrate • titanium dioxide • tribasic calcium phosphate • pregelatinized starch • yellow #6 • yellow #10
acetaminophen, 650mg		dextromethorphan hydrobromide, 20mg	natural lemon flavors • sucrose • ascorbic acid • citric acid • sodium citrate • titanium dioxide • tribasic calcium phosphate • pregelatinized starch • yellow #6 • yellow #10
acetaminophen		dextromethorphan	
	guaifenesin, 100mg/5ml	dextromethorphan hydrobromide, 10mg/5ml	alcohol, 10%

COLD, COUGH, ALLERGY PRODUCTS — continued

Product & Manufacturer	Dosage Form	Decongestant	Antihistamine
AF GL PU SO **Triaminic Allergy Tablets** Sandoz Pharm.	tablet	phenylpropanolamine hydrochloride, 25mg	chlorpheniramine maleate, 4mg
AF GL PU PE **Triaminic Chewables** Sandoz Pharm.	chewable tablet	phenylpropanolamine hydrochloride, 6.25mg	chlorpheniramine maleate, 0.5mg
AF GL PU SO **Triaminic Cold Tablets** Sandoz Pharm.	tablet	phenylpropanolamine hydrochloride, 12.5mg	chlorpheniramine maleate, 2mg
AL LA SL **Triaminic Expectorant** Sandoz Pharm.	liquid	phenylpropanolamine hydrochloride, 12.5mg/10ml	
AL LA SL PE **Triaminic Nite Light** Sandoz Pharm.	liquid	pseudoephedrine hydrochloride, 15mg/5ml	chlorpheniramine maleate, 1mg/10ml
AL LA SL **Triaminic Syrup** Sandoz Pharm.	syrup	phenylpropanolamine hydrochloride, 12.5mg/10ml	chlorpheniramine maleate, 2mg/10ml
AF GL PU SO **Triaminic-12 Tablets** Sandoz Pharm.	timed-release tablet	phenylpropanolamine hydrochloride, 75mg	chlorpheniramine maleate, 12mg
AL LA SL **Triaminic-DM Syrup** Sandoz Pharm.	timed-release liquid	phenylpropanolamine hydrochloride, 12.5mg/10ml	
AF GL PU **Triaminicin Tablets** Sandoz Pharm.	tablet	phenylpropanolamine hydrochloride, 25mg	chlorpheniramine maleate, 4mg
AF GL PU SO **Triaminicol Multi-Symptom Cold Tablets** Sandoz Pharm.	tablet	phenypropanolamine hydrochloride, 12.5mg	chlorpheniramine maleate, 2mg
AL LA SL **Triaminicol Multi-Symptom Relief** Sandoz Pharm.	liquid	phenylpropanolamine hydrochloride, 12.5mg/10ml	chlorpheniramine maleate, 2mg/10ml
LA SU SL PE **Trind** Mead Johnson Nutrit'l	liquid	phenylpropanolamine hydrochloride, 12.5mg/5ml	chlorpheniramine maleate, 2mg/5ml
LA SU SL PE **Trind-DM** Mead Johnson Nutrit'l	liquid	phenylpropanolamine hydrochloride, 12.5mg/5ml	chlorpheniramine maleate, 2mg/5ml
Triphenyl Rugby	syrup	phenylpropanolamine hydrochloride, 12.5mg/5ml	chlorpheniramine maleate, 2mg/5ml
Triphenyl Expectorant Rugby	liquid	phenylpropanolamine hydrochloride, 12.5mg/5ml	

COLD, COUGH, ALLERGY PRODUCTS — continued

Analgesic	Expectorant	Cough Suppressant	Other Ingredients
			calcium stearate • calcium sulfate • colloidal silicon dioxide • methylcellulose • methylparaben • microcrystalline cellulose • polyethylene glycol • povidone • pregelatinized starch • titanium dioxide • yellow #10
			saccharin sodium sucrose • calcium stearate • citric acid • flavors • magnesium trisilicate • mannitol • microcrystalline cellulose • yellow #6 • yellow #10
			saccharin • calcium stearate • colloidal silicon dioxide • flavor • lactose • methylcellulose • methylcellulose • methylparaben • microcrystalline cellulose • polyethylene glycol • povidone • pregelatinized starch • red #40 • titanium dioxide • yellow #6
	guaifenesin, 100mg/10ml		saccharin • sorbitol • sucrose • benzoic acid • edetate disodium • flavors • purified water • saccharin sodium • sodium hydroxide • yellow #6 • yellow #10
		dextromethorphan hydrobromide, 7.5mg/10ml	sorbitol • sucrose • benzoic acid • blue #1 • citric acid • flavors • propylene glycol • purified water • red #33 • dibasic sodium phosphate
			sorbitol • sucrose • benzoic acid • edetate disodium • flavors • purified water • sodium hydroxide • yellow #6
			carnauba wax • colloidal silicon dioxide • lactose • methylcellulose • polyethylene glycol • povidone • red #30 • stearic acid • titanium dioxide • yellow #6
		dextromethorphan hydrobromide, 10mg/10ml	sorbitol • sucrose • benzoic acid • blue #1 • flavors • propylene glycol • purified water • red #40 • sodium chloride
acetaminophen, 650mg			colloidal silicon dioxide • croscarmellose sodium • hydroxypropyl cellulose • lactose • magnesium stearate • methylcellulose • methylparaben • polyethylene glycol • povidone • pregelatinized starch • red #40 • titanium dioxide • yellow #10
		dextromethorphan hydrobromide, 10mg	calcium stearate • colloidal silicon dioxide • lactose • methylcellulose • methylparaben • microcrystalline cellulose • polyethylene glycol • povidone • pregelatinized starch • red #40 • titanium dioxide
		dextromethorphan hydrobromide, 10mg/10ml	sorbitol • sucrose • benzoic acid • flavors • propylene glycol • purified water • red #40 • saccharin sodium • sodium chloride
			alcohol, 5% • sorbitol • orange flavor
		dextromethorphan hydrobromide, 7.5mg/5ml	alcohol, 5% • sorbitol • fruit flavor
	guaifenesin, 100mg/5ml		alcohol, 5%

COLD, COUGH, ALLERGY PRODUCTS — continued

	Product & Manufacturer	Dosage Form	Decongestant	Antihistamine
LA PR SU SL	Tuss Kote Parnell	solution		diphenhydramine, 25mg/5ml
AF GL PU SO	Tuss-DM Hyrex	tablet		
	Tussar-2 Rhone-Poulenc Rorer	syrup	pseudoephedrine hydrochloride, 30mg/5ml	
AL	Tussar-DM (Alcohol Free) Rhone-Poulenc Rorer	syrup	pseudoephedrine hydrochloride USP, 30mg	chlorpheniramine maleate USP, 2mg
SU	Tussar-SF (Sugar Free) Rhone-Poulenc Rorer	syrup	pseudoephedrine hydrochloride, 30mg/5ml	
	Tusscidin Syrup H.R. Cenci	liquid		
AF GL PU	Tylenol Allergy Sinus Maximum Strength McNeil	caplet	pseudoephedrine hydrochloride, 30mg	chlorpheniramine maleate, 2mg
AF GL PU	Tylenol Allergy Sinus Maximum Strength Gelcaps McNeil	gelcap	pseudoephedrine hydrochloride, 30mg	chlorpheniramine maleate, 2mg
AL LA SL PE	Tylenol Children's Cold Multi-Symptom Liquid McNeil	liquid	pseudoephedrine hydrochloride, 15mg/5ml	chlorpheniramine maleate, 1mg/5ml
AL LA SL PE	Tylenol Children's Cold Multi-Symptom Plus Cough Liquid McNeil	liquid	pseudoephedrine hydrochloride, 15mg/5ml	chlorpheniramine maleate, 1mg/5ml
AF GL PU	Tylenol Cold Effervescent McNeil	effervescent tablet	phenylpropanolamine hydrochloride, 12.5mg	chlorpheniramine maleate, 2mg
LA SL	Tylenol Cold Night Time Liquid McNeil	liquid	pseudoephedrine hydrochloride, 60mg/30ml	diphenhydramine hydrochloride, 50mg/30ml
AF GL PU	Tylenol Cold No Drowsiness Formula McNeil	caplet	pseudoephedrine hydrochloride, 30mg	
AF GL PU	Tylenol Cold No Drowsiness Formula McNeil	gelcap	pseudoephedrine hydrochloride, 30mg	
AF GL PU	Tylenol Cold and Flu Hot Medication McNeil	individual packet	pseudoephedrine hydrochloride, 60mg/packet	chlorpheniramine maleate, 4mg/packet

COLD, COUGH, ALLERGY PRODUCTS — continued

Analgesic	Expectorant	Cough Suppressant	Other Ingredients
			xylitol • sorbitol • yerba santa • citric acid • ascorbic acid • sodium benzoate • sodium saccharin
	guaifenesin, 200mg	dextromethorphan, 10mg	
	guaifenesin USP, 100mg/5ml	codeine phosphate USP, 10mg/5ml[a]	alcohol USP, 2.5%
		dextromethorphan hydrobromide USP, 15%	artificial flavor • citric acid • FD&C red#40 • glucose • glycerin • sodium citrate • sucrose
	guaifenesin USP, 100mg/5ml	codeine phosphate USP, 10mg/5ml[a]	alcohol USP, 2.5%
	guaifenesin, 100mg/5ml		
acetaminophen, 500mg			cellulose • hydroxypropyl cellulose • hydroxypropyl methylcellulose • magnesium stearate • polyethylene glycol • sodium starch glycolate • cornstarch • titanium dioxide • blue#1 • yellow#6 • yellow#10
acetaminophen, 500mg			benzyl alcohol • butylparaben • castor oil • cellulose • edetate calcium disodium • gelatin • hydroxypropyl methylcellulose • magnesium stearate • methylparaben • propylparaben • sodium lauryl sulfate • sodium propionate • sodium starch glycolate • cornstarch • titanium dioxide • blue #1 • blue #2 • yellow #10
acetaminophen, 160mg/5ml			benzoic acid • citric acid • grape flavors • glycerin • malic acid • polyethylene glycol • propylene glycol • sodium benzoate • sorbitol • sucrose • purified water • blue #1 • red #40
acetaminophen, 160mg/5cc		dextromethorphan hydrobromide, 5mg/5ml	citric acid • corn syrup • flavors • polyethylene glycol • propylene glycol • sodium benzoate • sodium carboxymethylcellulose • sorbitol • purified water • red #33 • red #40
acetaminophen, 325mg			citric acid • flavor • potassium benzoate • povidone • saccharin • sodium bicarbonate • sodium carbonate • sodium docusate • sorbitol
acetaminophen, 650mg/30ml			alcohol, 10% • citric acid • cherry flavors • glycerin • polyethylene glycol • purified water • sodium benzoate • sucrose • red #40 • red #33 • blue #1
acetaminophen, 325mg		dextromethorphan hydrobromide, 15mg	cellulose • glyceryl triacetate • hydroxypropyl methylcellulose • magnesium stearate • sodium starch glycolate • corn starch • titanium dioxide • blue #1 • yellow #10
acetaminophen, 325mg		dextromethorphan hydrobromide, 15mg	benzyl alcohol • butylparaben • castor oil • cellulose • corn starch • edetate calcium disodium • gelatin • hydroxypropyl methylcellulose • magnesium stearate • methylparaben • propylparaben • sodium propionate • sodium lauryl sulfate • sodium starch glycolate • titanium dioxide • red #40 • yellow #10
acetaminophen, 650mg/packet		dextromethorphan hydrobromide, 30mg/packet	aspartame • citric acid • corn starch • honey lemon flavors • sodium citrate • sucrose • red #40 • yellow #10

COLD, COUGH, ALLERGY PRODUCTS — continued

	Product & Manufacturer	Dosage Form	Decongestant	Antihistamine
AF GL PU	Tylenol Cold and Flu No Drowsiness Formula Hot Medication McNeil	individual packet	pseudoephedrine hydrochloride, 60mg/packet	
LA SL	Tylenol Cough Maximum Strength Medication McNeil	liquid		
LA SL	Tylenol Cough Maximum Strength With Decongestant McNeil	liquid	pseudoephedrine, hydrochloride, 60mg/20ml	
AF GL PU	Tylenol Multi-Symptom Cold Medication McNeil	caplet	pseudoephedrine hydrochloride, 30mg	chlorpheniramine maleate, 2mg
AF GL PU SO	Tylenol Multi-Symptom Cold Medication McNeil	tablet	pseudoephedrine hydrochloride, 30mg	chlorpheniramine maleate, 2mg
AF GL PU	Tylenol Sinus Maximum Strength McNeil	caplet	pseudoephedrine hydrochloride, 30mg	
AF GL PU	Tylenol Sinus Maximum Strength McNeil	gelcap	pseudoephedrine hydrochloride, 30mg	
AF GL PU	Tylenol Sinus Maximum Strength McNeil	tablet	pseudoephedrine hydrochloride, 30mg	
AF GL PU SO PE	Tylenol, Children's Cold Multi-Symptom McNeil	chewable tablet	pseudoephedrine hydrochloride, 7.5mg	chlorpheniramine maleate, 0.5mg
GL PU	Ursinus Inlay-Tabs Sandoz Pharm.	tablet	pseudoephedrine hydrochloride, 30mg	
SO	Valihist Otis Clapp	tablet	phenylephrine hydrochloride	chlorpheniramine maleate
	Vaporizer In A Bottle Air Wick Inhaler Columbia	nasal inhaler		
AF GL	Viro-Med Whitehall	tablet	pseudoephedrine hydrochloride, 30mg	chlorpheniramine maleate, 2mg

[a]Schedule V drug; nonprescription sale forbidden in some states.

COLD, COUGH, ALLERGY PRODUCTS — continued

Analgesic	Expectorant	Cough Suppressant	Other Ingredients
acetaminophen, 650mg/packet		dextromethorphan hydrobromide, 30mg/packet	aspartame • citric acid • corn starch • lemon flavors • sodium citrate • sucrose • red #40 • yellow #10
acetaminophen, 1000mg/20ml		dextromethorphan hydrobromide, 30mg/20ml	alcohol, 10% • citric acid • flavors • glycerin • polyethylene glycol • purified water • sodium benzoate • sodium carboxymethylcellulose • sodium saccharin • sorbitol • sucrose • red #33 • red #40
acetaminophen, 1000mg/20ml		dextromethorphan hydrobromide, 30mg/20ml	alcohol, 10% • citric acid • flavors • glycerin • polyethylene glycol • purified water • sodium benzoate • sodium carboxymethylcellulose • sodium saccharin • sorbitol • sucrose • red #33 • red #40 • blue #1
acetaminophen, 325mg		dextromethorphan hydrobromide, 15mg	cellulose • glyceryl triacetate • hydroxypropyl methylcellulose • magnesium stearate • sodium starch glycolate • corn starch • titanium dioxide • blue #1 • yellow #6 • yellow #10
acetaminophen, 325mg		dextromethorphan hydrobromide, 15mg	cellulose • corn starch • magnesium stearate • yellow #6 • yellow #10
acetaminophen, 500mg			cellulose • hydroxypropyl methylcellulose • magnesium stearate • polyethylene glycol • polysorbate 80 • sodium starch glycolate • cornstarch • titanium dioxide • blue #1 • red #40 • yellow #10
acetaminophen, 500mg			benzyl alcohol • butylparaben • castor oil • cellulose • cornstarch • edetate calcium disodium • gelatin • hydroxypropyl methylcellulose • iron oxide black • magnesium stearate • methylparaben • propylparaben • sodium lauryl sulfate • sodium propionate • sodium starch glycolate • titanium dioxide • blue#1 • yellow#10
acetaminophen, 500mg			cellulose • cornstarch • magnesium stearate • sodium starch glycolate • blue #1 • yellow #6 • yellow #10
acetaminophen, 80mg			aspartame • citric acid • ethylcellulose • grape flavors • magnesium stearate • mannitol • microcrystalline cellulose • pregelatinized cornstarch • blue #1 • red #7 • sucrose
aspirin, 325mg			calcium stearate • lactose • microcrystalline cellulose • pregelatinized starch • sodium starch • yellow #6 • yellow #10
acetaminophen			caffeine
			camphor, 3.6% • menthol, 0.55% • eucalyptus oil, 4.5% • isopropyl alcohol • propylene glycol • methyl salicylate • isobornyl acetate • oil of spike lavender • isoamyl acetate • oil of peppermint
acetaminophen, 500mg		dextromethorphan hydrobromide, 15mg	

TOPICAL DECONGESTANT PRODUCTS

Product & Manufacturer	Dosage Form	Sympathomimetic Agent	Preservative	Other Ingredients
4-Way Fast Acting, Menthol and Regular Bristol-Myers	nasal spray	phenylephrine hydrochloride, 0.5% • naphazoline hydrochloride, 0.05%	benzalkonium chloride, 0.04% • boric acid/sodium borate	pyrilamine maleate, 0.2%
4-Way Long Lasting Bristol-Myers	nasal spray	oxymetazoline hydrochloride, 0.05%	phenylmercuric acetate, 0.002%	
Adrenalin Chloride Parke-Davis	nasal drops	epinephrine hydrochloride, 0.1%	chlorobutanol • sodium bisulfite	
Afrin 12-Hour Schering-Plough	nasal drops • nasal pump • nasal spray	oxymetazoline hydrochloride, 0.05%	benzalkonium chloride • phenylmercuric acetate, 0.002%	sorbitol • glycine
Afrin 12-Hour Cherry Schering-Plough	nasal spray	oxymetazoline hydrochloride, 0.05%	benzalkonium chloride • phenylmercuric acetate	glycine • sorbitol
Afrin 12-Hour Menthol Schering-Plough	nasal spray	oxymetazoline hydrochloride, 0.05%	benzalkonium chloride • phenylmercuric acetate, 0.002%	camphor • eucalyptol • glycine • menthol • sorbitol • polysorbate 80
PE Afrin 12-Hour Pediatric Schering-Plough	nasal drops	oxymetazoline hydrochloride, 0.025%	benzalkonium chloride • phenylmercuric acetate, 0.002%	glycine • sorbitol
Alconefrin 12 PolyMedica	nasal drops	phenylephrine hydrochloride, 0.16%		
Alconefrin 25 PolyMedica	nasal drops • nasal spray	phenylephrine hydrochloride, 0.25%		
Alconefrin 50 PolyMedica	nasal drops	phenylephrine hydrochloride, 0.5%		
SL Allerest CIBA Consumer	nasal spray	oxymetazoline hydrochloride, 0.05%	benzalkonium chloride • disodium edetate	dibasic sodium phosphate • monobasic sodium phosphate • sodium chloride • purified water
Benzedrex Menley & James	nasal inhaler	propylhexedrine, 250mg		menthol • lavender oil
Benzedrex Menley & James	nasal spray	phenylephrine hydrochloride, 0.5%	benzalkonium chloride methylparaben	sodium chloride • sodium citrate
Benzedrex 12 HR Menley & James	nasal spray	oxymetazoline hydrochloride, 0.5%	benzalkonium chloride • phenylmercuric acetate	glycine • sorbitol solution
Cheracol Spray Nasal Pump Roberts Pharm.	nasal pump	oxymetazoline hydrochloride, 0.05%	phenylmercuric acetate, 0.02 mg/ml in an aqueous solution of benzalkonium chloride	glycine • sodium hydroxide • sorbitol • artificial cherry flavor • purified water
SL Dristan Whitehall	nasal spray	phenylephrine hydrochloride, 0.5%	benzalkonium chloride, 0.02% • thimerosal, 0.002%	pheniramine maleate, 0.2% • alcohol • eucalyptol • menthol • hydroxypropyl methylcellulose • sodium chloride • sodium phosphate • water
SL Dristan 12-Hour Whitehall	nasal spray	oxymetazoline hydrochloride, 0.05%	benzalkonium chloride, 0.02% • thimerosal, 0.002%	hydroxypropyl methylcellulose • potassium phosphate • sodium chloride • sodium phosphate • water
SL Dristan Menthol Whitehall	nasal spray	phenylephrine hydrochloride, 0.5%	benzalkonium chloride, 0.02% • thimerosal, 0.002%	pheniramine maleate, 0.2% • alcohol camphor • eucalyptol • menthol • methyl salicylate • hydroxypropyl methylcellulose • polysorbate 80 • sodium chloride • sodium phosphate • water
Duration Schering-Plough	nasal spray	oxymetazoline hydrochloride, 0.05%	phenylmercuric acetate, 0.002% • benzalkonium chloride	

TOPICAL DECONGESTANT PRODUCTS — continued

	Product & Manufacturer	Dosage Form	Sympathomimetic Agent	Preservative	Other Ingredients
	Genasal Goldline	nasal solution	oxymetazoline hydrochloride, 0.05%	phenylmercuric acetate	
SL	**NTZ Long Lasting** Sterling Health	nasal drops • nasal spray	oxymetazoline hydrochloride, 0.05%	benzalkonium chloride • phenylmercuric acetate, 0.002%	
SL	**Neo-Synephrine Extra** Sterling Health	nasal drops • nasal spray	phenylephrine hydrochloride, 1%	benzalkonium chloride • thimerosal, 0.001%	
SL	**Neo-Synephrine Maximum-12 Hour** Sterling Health	nasal pump • nasal spray	oxymetazoline hydrochloride, 0.05%	benzalkonium chloride • thimerosal, 0.001%	
SL	**Neo-Synephrine Mild** Sterling Health	nasal spray	phenylephrine hydrochloride, 0.25%	benzalkonium chloride • thimerosal, 0.001%	
PE	**Neo-Synephrine Pediatric** Sterling Health	nasal drops	phenylephrine hydrochloride, 0.125%	benzalkonium chloride • thimerosal, 0.001%	
SL	**Neo-Synephrine Regular** Sterling Health	nasal drops • nasal pump • nasal spray	phenylephrine hydrochloride, 0.5%	benzalkonium chloride thimerosal, 0.001%	
SL	**Otrivin** CIBA Consumer	nasal drops • nasal spray	xylometazoline hydrochloride, 0.1%	benzalkonium chloride, 1:5000 • disodium edetate	sodium phosphate monobasic • sodium chloride • sodium phosphate dibasic • purified water
SL PE	**Otrivin Pediatric** CIBA Consumer	nasal drops	xylometazoline hydrochloride, 0.05%	benzalkonium chloride, 1:5000 • disodium edetate	sodium phosphate monobasic • sodium chloride • sodium phosphate dibasic • purified water
	Oxymetazoline Hydrochloride Various Manufacturers	nasal spray	oxymetazoline hydrochloride, 0.05%		
	Phenylephrine Hydrochloride Various Manufacturers	nasal solution	phenylephrine hydrochloride, 0.25%; 1%		
SL	**Pretz-D** Parnell	nasal drops	ephedrine, 0.25%	phenylmercuric acetate	glycerine, 3% • citric acid • sodium citrate • sodium chloride • yerba santa
SL	**Privine** CIBA Consumer	nasal drops • nasal spray	naphazoline hydrochloride, 0.05%	benzalkonium chloride, 1:5000 • EDTA	sodium chloride • dibasic sodium phosphate • monobasic sodium phosphate • purified water
SL	**Rhinall** Scherer	nasal drops • nasal spray	phenylephrine hydrochloride, 0.25%	chlorobutanol • sodium bisulfite • benzalkonium chloride	sodium chloride • sorbitol • disodium EDTA • tween 80
SL	**Sinarest** CIBA Consumer	nasal spray	oxymetazoline hydrochloride, 0.05%	benzalkonium chloride • disodium edetate	dibasic sodium phosphate • monobasic sodium phosphate • sodium chloride • purified water
	Sinex Long Acting Procter & Gamble	nasal spray	oxymetazoline hydrochloride, 0.05%	benzalkonium chloride • chlorhexidine gluconate • disodium edetate	camphor • menthol • eucalyptol • potassium phosphate • purified water • sodium chloride • sodium phosphate • lyloxapol
	Sinex Regular Procter & Gamble	nasal spray	phenylephrine hydrochloride, 0.5%	thimerosal, 0.001%	menthol • eucalyptol • camphor • cetylpyridinium chloride • potassium phosphate • purified water • sodium chloride • sodium phosphate • lyloxapol

TOPICAL DECONGESTANT PRODUCTS — continued

Product & Manufacturer	Dosage Form	Sympathomimetic Agent	Preservative	Other Ingredients
Vapo Rub Procter & Gamble	ointment			menthol, 2.6% • camphor, 4.7% • eucalyptus oil, 1.2% • cedarleaf oil • mineral oil • nutmeg oil • petrolatum • spirits of turpentine • thymol
Vapo Steam Procter & Gamble	liquid			menthol, 3.2% • camphor, 6.2% • eucalyptus oil, 1.5% • cedarleaf oil • nutmeg oil • poloxamer 124 • polyoxyethylene dodecanol • silicone • specially denatured alcohol, 74%
Vicks Vapor Inhaler Procter & Gamble	nasal inhaler	levodesoxyephedrine, 50mg/inhaler		menthol • camphor • bornyl acetate • lavender oil
Xylometazoline Hydrochloride Various Manufacturers	nasal spray	xylometazoline hydrochloride, 0.1%		

MISCELLANEOUS NASAL PRODUCTS

Product & Manufacturer	Dosage Form	Preservative	Other Ingredients
Ayr B.F. Ascher	nasal drops	benzalkonium chloride • thimerosal	sodium chloride, 0.65%
Ayr B.F. Ascher	nasal spray	benzalkonium chloride • thimerosal	sodium chloride, 0.65%
PR SL Dey-Vial Sodium Chloride Solution Dey	nasal solution		sodium chloride, 0.9%
SL Dristan Saline Nasal Spray Whitehall	nasal spray	benzyl alcohol • benzalkonium chloride • disodium EDTA	water • sodium chloride • hydroxypropyl methyl cellulose • sodium phosphate • disodium phosphate
SL Efidac/24 CIBA Consumer	tablet		
SL HuMIST Saline Scherer	nasal spray	chlorobutanol	sodium chloride, 0.65% • disodium EDTA • sodium phosphate dibasic anhydrous • sodium phosphate monobasic
SL Nasal Moist Blairex	nasal solution	benzyl alcohol	sodium chloride, 0.65 %
SL Nasal Saline Nasal Moisturizer Sterling Health	nasal drops	benzalkonium chloride • thimerosal, 0.001%	sodium chloride, 0.65%
SL Nasal Saline Nasal Moisturizer Sterling Health	nasal spray	benzalkonium chloride • thimerosal, 0.001%	sodium chloride, 0.65%
PR SL Nebu-Sol Sodium Chloride Solution Dey	nasal pump		sodium chloride, 0.9%
PR Nichols Nasal Douche Powder Alvin Last	powder		sodium bicarbonate • sodium chloride • sodium borate • menthol • eucalyptol
SL Ocean Mist Fleming	nasal spray		benzyl alcohol • sodium chloride, 0.65%
SL Pretz Parnell	drops	phenylmercuric nitrate, ns	glycerin, 3% • citric acid • sodium citrate • sodium chloride • yerba santa
SL Pretz Parnell	nasal solution	phenylmercuric nitrate, ns	glycerin, 3% • citric acid • sodium citrate • sodium chloride • yerba santa
SL Pretz Parnell	spray	phenylmercuric nitrate, ns	glycerin, 3% • citric acid • sodium citrate • sodium chloride • yerba santa
Salinex Muro	nasal drops	EDTA • benzalkonium chloride	sodium chloride, 0.4%
PR SL Sodium Chloride Solution Dey	nasal solution		sodium chloride, 3%
PR SL Sodium Chloride Solution Dey	nasal solution		sodium chloride, 10%

LOZENGE PRODUCTS

Product & Manufacturer	Anesthetic[a]	Antibacterial Agent[a]	Cough Suppressant	Other Ingredients
Bi-Zets Reese Chemical	benzocaine, 15mg	cetylpyridinium chloride, 2mg		
Cepacol SmithKline Beecham	benzyl alcohol, 3%	cetylpyridinium chloride, 0.07%		sucrose
Cepacol Anesthetic SmithKline Beecham	benzocaine, 10mg	cetylpyridinium chloride, 0.07%		glucose • sucrose
Cepastat Cherry SmithKline Beecham		phenol, 14.5mg		antifoam emulsion • D&C red#33 • FD&C yellow#6 • flavor • gum crystal • menthol • saccharin sodium • sorbitol
Cepastat Extra Strength SmithKline Beecham		phenol, 29mg		antifoam emulsion • caramel • eucalyptus oil • gum crystal • mannitol • menthol • saccharin sodium • sorbitol
PE **Children's Chloraseptic Sore Throat Lozenges, grape** Procter & Gamble	benzocaine, 5mg			corn syrup • FD&C blue#1 • FD&C red#40 • flavor • sucrose
Chloraseptic Sore Throat Lozenges, cherry Procter & Gamble	benzocaine, 6mg • menthol, 10mg			corn syrup • FD&C blue#1 • FD&C red#40 • flavor • sucrose
Chloraseptic Sore Throat Lozenges, cool mint Procter & Gamble	benzocaine, 6mg • menthol, 10mg			corn syrup • FD&C blue#1 • flavor • sucrose
Chloraseptic Sore Throat Lozenges, menthol Procter & Gamble	benzocaine, 6mg • menthol, 10mg			corn syrup • FD&C yellow#10 • FD&C blue#1 • FD&C yellow#6 • flavor • sucrose
Conex Forest	benzocaine, 5mg	cetylpyridinium chloride, 0.5mg		methylparaben, 2mg • propylparaben, 0.5mg • sucrose, 738mg
SU **Cylex Sugar Free** Pharmakon	benzocaine, 15mg	cetylpyridinium hydrochloride, 5mg		sorbitol • cherry flavor
SU **Fisherman's Friend, extra strong formula** Lofthouse			menthol	sorbitol • natural licorice • magnesium stearate • eucalyptus oil • capsicum
SU **Fisherman's Friend, mint** Lofthouse			menthol	sorbitol • peppermint oil • magnesium stearate • aspartame
Fisherman's Friend, original extra strong Lofthouse			menthol	sugar • natural licorice • edible gums • eucalyptus oil • capsicum
Halls Menthol-Lyptus Warner-Lambert			menthol	eucalyptus oil • flavor
Halls Plus Center-Filled Drops Warner-Lambert			menthol	eucalyptus oil • flavor • citric acid
Halls Soothers, Center-Filled Drops Warner-Lambert			menthol	flavor • citric acid
Hold Menley & James			dextromethorphan hydrobromide, 5mg	corn syrup • sucrose • vegetable oil • flavors • FD&C blue#1 • FD&C red#40 • FD&C yellow#5 • FD&C yellow#10
Isodettes Sore Throat Lozenges Goody's		phenol, 40.6mg/oz		sugar • corn syrup, 40% • cherry flavor • red solution (FD&C #40 & #3), 3%
SU **Larynex** Dover	benzocaine			

LOZENGE PRODUCTS — continued

Product & Manufacturer	Anesthetic[a]	Antibacterial Agent[a]	Cough Suppressant	Other Ingredients
N'Ice Cough SmithKline Beecham			menthol, 5mg	
Robitussin Cough Calmers A.H. Robins			dextromethorphan hydrobromide, 7.5mg	sucrose
Sepo Otis Clapp	benzocaine			
Silexin Otis Clapp	benzocaine		dextromethorphan hydrobromide	
Spec-T Lozenge Sore Throat Anesthetic Squibb	benzocaine, 10mg			
Spec-T Lozenge Sore Throat/Decongestant Apothecon	benzocaine, 10mg			phenylephrine hydrochloride, 5mg • phenylpropanolamine hydrochloride, 10.5mg
Spec-T Lozenges Sore Throat/Cough Suppressant Squibb	benzocaine, 10mg		dextromethorphan hydrobromide, 10mg	
Sucrets Assorted SmithKline Beecham	dyclonine hydrochloride, 2mg			citric acid • corn syrup • colors • flavors • silicon dioxide • sucrose • tartaric acid
Sucrets Childrens Cherry Flavored Sore Throat SmithKline Beecham	dyclonine hydrochloride, 1.2mg			citric acid • corn syrup • silicon dioxide • sucrose • flavor
Sucrets Maximum Strength Sore Throat, Vapor Black Cherry SmithKline Beecham	dyclonine hydrochloride, 3mg			colors • corn syrup • flavor • menthol • silicon dioxide • sucrose • tartaric acid
Sucrets Maximum Strength Sore Throat, Wintergreen SmithKline Beecham	dyclonine hydrochloride, 3mg			citric acid • corn syrup • silicon dioxide • sucrose • flavor
Sucrets Original Mint SmithKline Beecham		hexylresorcinol, 2.4mg		colors • corn syrup • flavors • silicon dioxide • sucrose
Sucrets Vapor Lemon SmithKline Beecham	dyclonine hydrochloride, 2mg			citric acid • corn syrup • flavors • menthol • silicon dioxide • sucrose • color
Sucrets Wild Cherry SmithKline Beecham	dyclonine hydrochloride, 2mg			colors • corn syrup • flavor • silicon dioxide • sucrose • tartaric acid
Synthaloids Buffington	benzocaine			calcium-iodine complex
Tetra-Formula Reese Chemical	benzocaine, 15mg		dextromethorphan hydrobromide, 7.5mg	
Thorets Buffington	benzocaine			
Throat Discs SmithKline Beecham				sucrose • starch • acacia • glycyrrhiza extract • gum tragacanth • anethole • linseed • cubeb oleo resin • anise oil • peppermint oil • capsicum • mineral oil
Vicks Cough Drops Extra Strength, cherry Procter & Gamble			menthol, 10mg	corn syrup • FD&C blue#2 • FD&C red#40 • flavor • sucrose
Vicks Cough Drops Extra Strength, cool peppermint Procter & Gamble			menthol, 10mg	corn syrup • flavor • peppermint oil • sucrose

LOZENGE PRODUCTS — continued

Product & Manufacturer	Anesthetic[a]	Antibacterial Agent[a]	Cough Suppressant	Other Ingredients
Vicks Cough Drops Extra Strength, honey-lemon Procter & Gamble			menthol, 10mg	citric acid • corn syrup • D&C yellow#10 • FD&C yellow#6 • flavor • sucrose
Vicks Cough Drops Extra Strength, menthol Procter & Gamble			menthol, 8.4mg	corn syrup • FD&C blue#1 • flavor • sucrose
Vicks Cough Drops, cherry Procter & Gamble			menthol	citric acid • corn syrup • FD&C blue#1 • FD&C red#40 • flavor • sucrose
Vicks Cough Drops, menthol Procter & Gamble	benzyl alcohol		menthol	camphor • caramel • corn syrup • eucalyptus oil • flavor • sucrose • tolu balsam • thymol

[a] Phenol is both an anesthetic and an antibacterial agent.

ASTHMA INHALANT PRODUCTS

	Product & Manufacturer	Dosage Form	Epinephrine	Other Ingredients
	Adrenalin Chloride Parke-Davis	solution for nebulization	1:100 epinephrine hydrochloride	benzethonium chloride • sodium bisulfite
AL	**Asthma Haler** Menley & James	oral inhaler	0.16mg base/spray (0.3mg epinephrine bitartrate/spray)	cetylpyridinium chloride • propellants • sorbitan trioleate
AL	**Asthma Nefrin** Menley & James	solution for nebulization	2.25% base (as racemic epinephrine hydrochloride)	chlorobutanol, 0.5% • benzoic acid • potassium metabisulfite • sodium bisulfite • sodium chloride • propylene glycol
AL PR SU SL PE GE	**Broncho Saline** Blairex	solution for nebulization		sodium chloride, 0.9%
AL SU SL	**Bronitin Mist** Whitehall	oral inhaler	epinephrine base, 0.16mg/spray (0.3mg epinephrine bitartrate/spray)	fluorocarbons (propellant) • sorbitan trioleate
PR SO SU SL	**Bronkaid Mist** Sterling Health	oral inhaler	0.25mg base/spray	alcohol, 33%
	Bronkaid Mist Suspension Sterling Health	oral inhaler	0.16mg base/spray (0.3mg epinephrine bitartrate/spray)	
	Epinephrine Various Manufacturers	oral inhaler	0.2mg/spray	
	Micro NEFRIN Bird	solution for nebulization	2.25% base (as racemic epinephrine hydrochloride)	chlorobutanol, 0.5g
SU SL	**Primatene Mist** Whitehall	oral inhaler	epinephrine base, 0.22mg/spray	alcohol, 34% • fluorocarbons (propellant) • ascorbic acid • water
AL SU SL	**Primatene Mist Suspension** Whitehall	oral inhaler	epinephrine base, 0.16mg/spray (0.3mg epinephrine bitartrate/spray)	fluorocarbons (propellant) • sorbitan trioleate

ASTHMA ORAL COMBINATION PRODUCTS

	Product & Manufacturer	Dosage Form	Ephedrine	Theophylline	Other Ingredients[b]
	Amesec Whitby	capsule	25mg (as hydrochloride)	104mg	
	Azma Aid[a] Various Manufacturers	tablet	24mg (as hydrochloride)	118mg	phenobarbital, 8mg
GL PU SO	**Bronkaid** Sterling Health	tablet	24mg (as sulfate)	100mg	guaifenesin, 400mg
	Bronkolixir[a] Sanofi Winthrop	elixir	2.4mg/ml (as sulfate)	3mg/ml	guaifenesin, 10mg/ml • phenobarbital, 0.8mg/ml • alcohol, 19%
	Bronkotabs[a] Sanofi Winthrop	tablet	24mg (as sulfate)	100mg	guaifenesin, 100mg • phenobarbital, 8mg
	Ephedrine Sulfate Various Manufacturers	capsule	25mg; 50mg		
	Guaiphed[a] Various Manufacturers	elixir	2.4mg/ml (as sulfate)	3mg/ml	guaifenesin, 10mg/ml • phenobarbital, 0.8mg/ml
GL PU SO	**Primatene** Whitehall	tablet	24mg (as hydrochloride)	130mg (anhydrous)	
GL PU SO	**Primatene Dual Action Formula** Whitehall	tablet	12.5mg (as hydrochloride)	60mg (anhydrous)	guaifenesin, 100mg
	Tedrigen[a] Goldline	tablet	25mg (as hydrochloride)	125mg	phenobarbital, 8mg
	Theotal Major	tablet	25mg (as hydrochloride)	125mg	phenobarbital, 8mg • lactose

[a] Limited availability according to state laws.
[b] Flourocarbons are standard propellants for aerosol inhalers. Check product packaging for further information.

SLEEP AID PRODUCTS

	Product & Manufacturer	Dosage Form	Antihistamine	Other Ingredients
	Anacin P.M. Aspirin Free A.H. Robins	caplet	diphenhydramine hydrochloride, 25mg	acetaminophen, 500mg
	Compoz Medtech	tablet	diphenhydramine hydrochloride, 50mg	
	Compoz Gelcaps Medtech	gelcap	diphenhydramine, 25mg	
	Doan's P.M. Extra Strength CIBA Consumer	tablet	diphenhydramine hydrochloride, 25mg	magnesium salicylate, 500mg • carnauba wax • colloidal silicon dioxide • croscarmellose sodium • microcrystalline cellulose • magnesium stearate • Opadry blue • stearic acid • talc
	Excedrin P.M. Bristol-Myers	caplet • tablet	diphenhydramine citrate, 38mg	acetaminophen, 500mg
	Excedrin P.M. Bristol-Myers	liquid	diphenhydramine hydrochloride, 50mg/30ml	acetaminophen, 1000mg/30ml
AF PU	Nervine Nighttime Sleep-Aid Miles Incorporated	caplet	diphenhydramine hydrochloride, 25mg	calcium • phosphate dibasic • calcium sulfate • carboxymethylcellulose sodium • corn starch • magnesium stearate • microcrystalline cellulose
	Night-Time Sleep-Aid Goldline	tablet	doxylamine succinate, 25mg	
	Nytol Block	tablet	diphenhydramine hydrochloride, 25mg	cellulose • cornstarch • lactose • silica • stearic acid
	Nytol Maximum Strength Block	tablet	diphenhydramine hydrochloride, 50mg	cellulose • corn starch • lactose • silica • stearic acid • FD&C blue#1 aluminum lake
AF GL SO	Sleep-Eze 3 Whitehall	tablet	diphenhydramine hydrochloride, 25mg	
	Sleep-ettes-D Reese Chemical	caplet	diphenhydramine hydrochloride, 50mg	
AF GL PU SO	Sleepinal Capsules Thompson Medical	capsule	diphenhydramine hydrochloride, 50mg	lactose • magnesium stearate • talc, USP
AF PU	Sleepinal Medicated Nite Tea Thompson Medical	powder	diphenhydramine hydrochloride, 50mg	aspartame • citric acid • colloidal silicon dioxide • D&C yellow#10 • FD&C blue#1 • FD&C red#40 • flavor • lactose • polyethylene glycol • povidone • sodium chloride • sodium citrate
	Sominex SmithKline Beecham	caplet	diphenhydramine hydrochloride, 50mg	
	Sominex SmithKline Beecham	tablet	diphenhydramine hydrochloride, 25mg	
	Sominex Pain Relief Formula SmithKline Beecham	tablet	diphenhydramine hydrochloride, 25mg	acetaminophen, 500mg
AF CA SO SU	Tranquil Plus Alva-Amco	caplet	diphenhydramine hydrochloride, 25mg	acetaminophen, 250mg • magnesium salicylate, 250mg • magnesium carbonate • magnesium oxide • calcium carbonate

CHAPTER 10 Sleep Aids & Stimulants

SLEEP AID PRODUCTS — continued

Product & Manufacturer	Dosage Form	Antihistamine	Other Ingredients
AF GL PU **Tylenol Extra Strength PM** McNeil	caplet	diphenhydramine hydrochloride, 25mg	acetaminophen, 500mg • cellulose • citric acid • colloidal silicon dioxide • hydroxypropyl methylcellulose • magnesium stearate or stearic acid • polyethylene glycol • sodium starch glycolate • cornstarch • titanium dioxide • blue#1 • blue#2
AF GL PU **Tylenol Extra Strength PM** McNeil	gelcap	diphenhydramine hydrochloride, 25mg	acetaminophen, 500mg • benzyl alcohol • butylparaben • castor oil • cellulose • cornstarch • edetate calcium disodium • gelatin • hydroxypropyl methylcellulose • magnesium stearate • propylparaben • sodium lauryl sulfate • sodium citrate • sodium propionate • sodium starch glycolate • titanium dioxide • blue #1 • red #28
AF GL PU **Tylenol Extra Strength PM** McNeil	tablet	diphenhydramine hydrochloride, 25mg	acetaminophen, 500mg • cellulose • citric acid • colloidal silicon dioxide • magnesium stearate or stearic acid • sodium starch glycolate • cornstarch • blue#1
AF GL PU **Unisom Nighttime Sleep Aid** Pfizer	tablet	doxylamine succinate, 25mg	
AF GL PU SO **Unisom With Pain Relief** Pfizer	tablet	diphenhydramine, 50mg	acetaminophen, 650mg

STIMULANT PRODUCTS

Product Manufacturer	Dosage Form	Caffeine	Other Ingredients
PU **Caffedrine Caplets** SO Thompson Medical	caplet	200mg (time released)	calcium sulfate • lactose • ethylcellulose • povidone • isopropyl alcohol • stearic acid • magnesium stearate • methyl alcohol • hydroxypropyl methylcellulose • triacetin • FD&C yellow#6 aluminum lake • D&C yellow#10 aluminum lake • titanium dioxide • propylene glycol
PU **Caffedrine Capsules** Thompson Medical	capsule	200mg (time released)	D&C red#22 • D&C red#28 • D&C yellow#10 • FD&C blue#1 • FD&C red#3 • FD&C yellow#6 • gelatin • magnesium stearate • pharmaceutical glaze • povidone • silicon dioxide • starch • sucrose • talc • titanium dioxide
Caffeine Various Manufacturers	capsule	200mg; 250mg	
Caffeine Various Manufacturers	tablet	100mg	
GL **Enerjets Lozenges** PU Chilton SO	lozenge	75mg	sugar • flavoring
Keep Alert Reese Chemical	caplet	200mg	
No Doz Bristol-Myers	tablet	100mg	cornstarch • flavor • mannitol • microcrystalline cellulose • stearic acid • sucrose
No Doz Maximum Strength Caplets Bristol-Myers	caplet	200mg	benzoic acid • carnauba wax • cornstarch • color • flavor • hydroxypropyl methylcellulose • microcrystalline cellulose • propylene glycol • simethicane emulsion • stearic acid • sucrose • titanium dioxide • water
SO **Pep-Back Tablets** Alva-Amco	tablet	100mg	calcium carbonate
GL **Quick-Pep Tablets** PU Thompson Medical	tablet	150mg	dextrose, anhydrous • microcrystalline cellulose • sodium starch glycolate • colloidal silicon dioxide • FD&C yellow#6 aluminum lake • D&C yellow#10 aluminum lake • stearic acid • magnesium stearate • FD&C red#3 • starch • sucrose • talc
SO **Ultra Pep-Back Caplets** Alva-Amco	caplet	200mg	calcium carbonate
Vivarin SmithKline Beecham	caplet	200mg	dextrose, 150mg
Vivarin SmithKline Beecham	tablet	200mg	dextrose, 150mg

CHAPTER 10 Sleep Aids & Stimulants

ANTACID PRODUCTS

	Product & Manufacturer	Dosage Form	Calcium Carbonate	Aluminum Hydroxide	Magnesium Salts	Sodium Bicarbonate	Other Ingredients
SO	Alamag Goldline	suspension		dried gel equivalent =225mg/5ml	magnesium hydroxide, 200mg/5ml		
	Alenic Alka Rugby	suspension		6.3mg/ml	magnesium carbonate, 27.4mg/ml		sodium alginate • EDTA • saccharin • sorbitol
SO	Alenic Alka Improved Rugby	chewable tablet		80mg	magnesium trisilicate, 20mg	ns	butterscotch flavor
AF	Alka-Seltzer Miles Incorporated	effervescent tablet				958mg (sodium, 311mg)	citric acid, 832mg • potassium bicarbonate, 312mg
	Alka-Seltzer Extra Strength Miles Incorporated	effervescent tablet				1985mg (sodium, 588mg)	aspirin, 500mg • citric acid, 1000mg
	Alka-Seltzer Flavored, lemon-lime Miles Incorporated	effervescent tablet				1710mg (sodium, 506mg)	aspirin, 325mg • flavors • saccharin sodium
	Alka-Seltzer Original Miles Incorporated	effervescent tablet				1916mg (sodium, 567mg)	aspirin, 325mg • citric acid, 1000mg
	Alkets Roberts Pharm.	chewable tablet	500mg				dextrose • flavors • magnesium stearate • maltodextrin
	Alkets Extra Strength Roberts Pharm.	chewable tablet	750mg				dextrose • flavors • magnesium stearate • maltodextrin
	Almacone Rugby	chewable tablet		200mg	magnesium hydroxide, 200mg		simethicone, 20mg • peppermint flavor
SO	Almacone Rugby	suspension		40mg/ml	magnesium hydroxide, 40mg/ml		simethicone, 4mg/ml • peppermint flavor
	Almacone II Rugby	suspension		80mg/ml	magnesium hydroxide, 80mg/ml		simethicone, 8mg • saccharin • sorbitol
	Almora Forest	chewable tablet			magnesium gluconate, 500mg		
	Aluminum Hydroxide Gel Various Manufacturers	suspension		64mg/ml; 120mg/ml			
SU	Aluminum Hydroxide, Concentrated Roxane	suspension		135mg/ml (equivalent to dried gel USP)			sorbitol solution, 15%w/v • flavor
SO	Amitone Menley & James	chewable tablet	350mg				mint flavor • magnesium stearate • mineral oil • powdered peppermint • sodium phosphate (2mg sodium) • starch • stearic acid • sucrose • talc • elemental calcium, 140mg

ANTACID PRODUCTS — continued

Product & Manufacturer	Dosage Form	Calcium Carbonate	Aluminum Hydroxide	Magnesium Salts	Sodium Bicarbonate	Other Ingredients
SO **Banacid** SU Buffington	chewable tablet		ns	magnesium hydroxide • magnesium trisilicate		
Bell/Ans C.S. Dent	chewable tablet				520mg (sodium, 144mg)	wintergreen, ginger flavor • acacia • charcoal • cornstarch • gelatin • potato starch • propylene glycol • sucrose • cream mint flavor
GL **Bromo-Seltzer** PU Warner-Lambert	granular effervescent				2781mg	acetaminophen, 325mg • citric acid, 2224mg
Calcium Carbonate Various Manufacturers	chewable tablet	250mg; 500mg; 650mg; 1250mg;				
GL **Calglycine** SO Rugby SU	chewable tablet	420mg				glycine, 150mg • spearmint flavor
PU **Chooz** SO Schering-Plough	gum	500mg				
Citrocarbonate Roberts Pharm.	granular effervescent	sodium citrate hydrous, 1.19g			2.34g	citric acid anhydrous • calcium lactate pentahydrate • sodium chloride • monobasic sodium phosphate anhydrous • magnesium sulfate dried
Citrocarbonate Roberts Pharm.	powder			magnesium sulfate	sodium bicarbonate	sodium citrate • citric acid anhydrous • calcium lactate pentahydrate • sodium chloride • monobasic sodium phosphate anhydrous
LA **Di-Gel** SO Schering-Plough SL	liquid		40mg/ml	magnesium hydroxide, 40mg/ml		simethicone, 4mg/ml
GL **Di-Gel,** PU **Advanced** SO **Formula** Schering-Plough	chewable tablet	280mg		magnesium hydroxide, 128mg		simethicone, 20mg • mint or lemon/orange flavor
SO **Dicarbosil** BIRA	chewable tablet	500mg				peppermint oil
SO **Dimacid** SU Otis Clapp	chewable tablet	ns		magnesium carbonate, ns		fruit flavor
GL **Gas-X** PU Sandoz Pharm. SO	chewable tablet					simethicone, 80mg • dibasic and tribasic calcium phosphates • colloidal silicon dioxide • calcium silicate • microcrystalline cellulose • cherry or peppermint creme flavors • compressible sugar • talc
GL **Gas-X Extra** PU **Strength** SO Sandoz Pharm.	chewable tablet					simethicone, 125mg • dibasic and tribasic calcium phosphate • colloidal silicon dioxide • calcium silicate • microcrystalline cellulose • cherry or peppermint creme flavors • compressible sugar • talc • red #30 • yellow #10

ANTACID PRODUCTS — continued

	Product & Manufacturer	Dosage Form	Calcium Carbonate	Aluminum Hydroxide	Magnesium Salts	Sodium Bicarbonate	Other Ingredients
	Gaviscon SmithKline Beecham	chewable tablet		80mg	magnesium trisilicate, 20mg	70mg (sodium, 19mg)	alginic acid, 200mg
	Gaviscon Cool Mint Flavor SmithKline Beecham	suspension		9.5mg/ml	magnesium carbonate, 35.8mg/ml		sodium alginate, 27.2mg/ml
	Gaviscon ESR SmithKline Beecham	chewable tablet		160mg	magnesium carbonate, 105mg		alginic acid, 200mg
	Gaviscon ESRF SmithKline Beecham	suspension		50.8mg/ml	magnesium carbonate, 47.5mg/ml		sodium alginate, 20mg/ml
	Gaviscon-2 SmithKline Beecham	chewable tablet		160mg	magnesium trisilicate, 40mg	140mg (sodium, 36.8mg)	alginic acid, 400mg
GL PU SO	Gelusil Parke-Davis	chewable tablet		200mg	magnesium hydroxide, 200mg		simethicone, 25mg • magnesium stearate • mannitol • sorbitol • sugar
LA PR SL	Gelusil Parke-Davis	liquid		40mg/ml	magnesium hydroxide, 40mg/ml		simethicone, 5mg/ml • citric acid • hydroxypropyl methylcellulose • sodium carboxymethyl cellulose • sodium saccharin • sorbitol solution • xanthan gum
LA SO	Kudrox Schwarz Pharma	suspension		100mg/ml	hydroxide, 90mg/ml		simethicone, 8mg/ml
SO	Losopan Goldline	suspension					magaldrate, 540mg/5ml
SO	Losopan Plus Goldline	suspension					magaldrate, 540mg/5ml • simethicone, 20mg/5ml
	Lowsium Rugby	suspension					magaldrate, 108mg/ml
	Lowsium Plus Rugby	suspension					magaldrate, 108mg/ml • simethicone, 8mg/ml
SU	Maalox Caplets Rhone-Poulenc Rorer	caplet	1000mg				corn starch • croscarmellose • magnesium stearate • sodium lauryl sulfate
SU	Maalox HRF Rhone-Poulenc Rorer	chewable tablet		aluminum hydroxide-magnesium carbonate co-dried gel, 180mg • magnesium carbonate, 160mg	see aluminum hydroxide column		compressible sugar • cornstarch • D&C yellow#10 • FD&C blue#2 • flavors • magnesium alginate • magnesium stearate • potassium bicarbonate
	Maalox HRF Rhone-Poulenc Rorer	suspension		aluminum hydroxide-magnesium carbonate co-dried gel, 280mg • magnesium carbonate USP, 350mg/10ml	see aluminum hydroxide column		calcium carbonate • calcium saccharin • FD&C blue#1 • FD&C yellow#5 (tartrazine) • mint flavor • magnesium alginate • methyl and propylparabens • potassium bicarbonate • sorbitol

ANTACID PRODUCTS — continued

	Product & Manufacturer	Dosage Form	Calcium Carbonate	Aluminum Hydroxide	Magnesium Salts	Sodium Bicarbonate	Other Ingredients
GL PU SO SU	**Mag-Ox 400** Blaine	chewable tablet			magnesium oxide, 400mg (elemental magnesium, 241.3mg or 19.86mEq)		
	Magnesia And Alumina Oral Suspension Roxane	suspension		44mg/ml	magnesium hydroxide, 40mg/ml		sorbitol, 15% • peppermint
	Milk Of Magnesia Various Manufacturers	chewable tablet			magnesium hydroxide, 325mg/tablet		
	Milk Of Magnesia Various Manufacturers	liquid			magnesium hydroxide, 78mg/ml		
SO	**Mylagen II** Goldline	liquid		dried gel equivalent =400mg/5ml	magnesium hydroxide, 400mg/5ml		simethicone, 40mg/5ml
SO	**Mylanta** Johnson&Johnson Merck	chewable tablet		200mg	magnesium hydroxide, 200mg		simethicone, 20mg
SO	**Mylanta** Johnson&Johnson Merck	suspension		40mg/ml	magnesium hydroxide, 40mg/ml		simethicone, 4mg/ml
	Mylanta Double Strength Johnson&Johnson Merck	chewable tablet		400mg	magnesium hydroxide, 400mg		simethicone, 40mg
SO	**Mylanta Double Strength** Johnson&Johnson Merck	suspension		80mg/ml	magnesium hydroxide, 80mg/ml		simethicone, 8mg/ml
	Mylanta Gas Johnson&Johnson Merck	chewable tablet					simethicone, 40mg
	Mylanta Gas Johnson&Johnson Merck	chewable tablet					simethicone, 80mg
	Mylanta Gas Maximum Strength Johnson&Johnson Merck	chewable tablet					simethicone, 125mg
	Mylanta Gelcaps Johnson&Johnson Merck	gelcap	311mg		magnesium carbonate, 232mg		
	Mylicon Johnson&Johnson Merck	drops					simethicone, 40mg/0.6ml
SO SU	**Neutralin** Dover	chewable tablet	ns		magnesium dioxide		
LA SO SL	**Percy Medicine** Merrick	liquid					bismuth subnitrate, 95.9mg/ml • calcium hydroxide, 2.19mg/ml • potassium carbonate, 0.56mg/ml • water • ethyl alcohol, 5% • glycerin • gum arabic • rhubarb fluid extract • sugar • flavors • natural color

ANTACID PRODUCTS — continued

	Product & Manufacturer	Dosage Form	Calcium Carbonate	Aluminum Hydroxide	Magnesium Salts	Sodium Bicarbonate	Other Ingredients
	Phillips' Milk Of Magnesia Sterling Health	chewable tablet			magnesium hydroxide, 311mg		
	Phillips' Milk Of Magnesia, mint or cherry Sterling Health	suspension			magnesium hydroxide, 80mg/ml		mint or cherry flavor
LA SO SU SL	**Riopan** Whitehall	suspension					magaldrate, 108mg/ml • mint flavor
GL PU SO	**Riopan Plus** Whitehall	chewable tablet					magaldrate, 480mg/tablet • simethicone, 20mg/tablet • mint flavor
LA SO SU SL	**Riopan Plus** Whitehall	suspension					simethicone, 8mg/ml • magaldrate, 108mg/ml • mint flavor
LA SO SU SL	**Riopan Plus 2 Mint or Cherry Flavor** Whitehall	suspension					magaldrate, 216mg/ml • simethicone, 8mg/ml • mint or cherry flavor
GL PU SO	**Riopan Plus 2 Mint or Cherry-Vanilla Flavor** Whitehall	chewable tablet					magaldrate, 1080mg/tablet • simethicone, 20mg/tablet • mint or cherry-vanilla flavor
GL PU	**Rolaids** Warner-Lambert	chewable tablet					dihydroxy-aluminum sodium carbonate, 334mg (sodium, 53mg) • peppermint, spearmint, or wintergreen flavor
GL PU SO	**Rolaids Calcium Rich** Warner-Lambert	chewable tablet	1000mg				simethicone, 25mg • peppermint, spearmint, or wintergreen flavor
GL PU SO	**Rolaids Sodium Free** Warner-Lambert	chewable tablet	550mg				cherry, strawberry, lemon-lime, orange, or peppermint flavor
	Rulox Rugby	suspension		45mg/ml	magnesium hydroxide, 40mg/ml		
	Rulox #1 Rugby	chewable tablet		200mg	magnesium hydroxide, 200mg		mint flavor
	Rulox #2 Rugby	chewable tablet		400mg	magnesium hydroxide, 400mg		sorbitol • mint flavor
	Rulox Plus Rugby	chewable tablet		200mg	magnesium hydroxide, 200mg		simethicone, 25mg • lemon flavor and cherry flavor
	Rulox Plus Rugby	suspension		100mg/ml	magnesium hydroxide, 90mg/ml		simethicone, 8mg/ml
SO	**Simaal 2 Gel** Schein	liquid		80mg/ml	magnesium hydroxide, 80mg/ml		simethicone, 8mg/ml • butylparaben • carboxymethylcellulose sodium • hydroxypropyl methylcellulose • microcrystalline cellulose • potassium citrate • propylparaben • purified water • sodium saccharin • sorbitol

ANTACID PRODUCTS — continued

Product & Manufacturer	Dosage Form	Calcium Carbonate	Aluminum Hydroxide	Magnesium Salts	Sodium Bicarbonate	Other Ingredients
SO **Simaal Gel** Schein	liquid		40mg/ml	magnesium hydroxide, 40mg/ml		simethicone, 4mg/ml • sorbitol • butylparaben • carboxymethylcellulose • microcrystalline cellulose • propylparaben • purified water • sodium saccharin
Soda Mint Various Manufacturers	chewable tablet				325mg	
Sodium Bicarbonate Various Manufacturers	chewable tablet				325mg; 650mg	
SO **Tempo Drops** Thompson Medical	chewable tablet	414mg	133mg	magnesium hydroxide, 81mg		simethicone, 20mg
SO **Titralac Antacid** SU 3M	chewable tablet	420mg				glycine, 150mg • saccharin starch • magnesium stearate • spearmint flavor
SO **Titralac Extra** SU **Strength Antacid** 3M	chewable tablet	750mg				glycine • magnesium stearate • saccharin • spearmint oil • starch
SO **Titralac Plus** SU **Liquid Antacid** 3M	liquid	100mg/ml				simethicone, 4mg/ml • saccharin • spearmint flavor
SO **Titralac Plus** SU **Tablets** 3M	chewable tablet	420mg				simethicone, 21mg • glycine • magnesium stearate • saccharin • spearmint oil • starch • may also contain croscarmellose sodium
Tums SmithKline Beecham	chewable tablet	500mg				original and assorted flavors
Tums Anti-gas/ Antacid SmithKline Beecham	chewable tablet	500mg				simethicone, 20mg • adipic acid • corn syrup • colors • flavors • microcrystalline cellulose • mineral oil • sodium polyphosphate • starch • sucrose • talc • triglycerol monoleate
Tums E-X Extra Strength SmithKline Beecham	chewable tablet	750mg				wintergreen, peppermint, cherry, or fruit flavor
GL **Uro-Mag** PU Blaine SO SU	capsule			magnesium oxide, 140mg (elemental magnesium, 84.5mg or 6.93mEq)		
Win Gel Sterling Health	suspension		36mg/ml	magnesium oxide or hydroxide, 32mg/ml		mint flavor

ANTIEMETIC PRODUCTS

	Product & Manufacturer	Dosage Form	Active Ingredients	Other Ingredients
PU SU	**Bonine** Pfizer	chewable tablet	meclizine hydrochloride, 25mg	raspberry flavor • cornstarch • FD&C red#40 • lactose • magnesium stearate • purified siliceous earth • saccharin • talc
	Dimenhydrinate Various Manufacturers	tablet	dimenhydrinate, 50mg	
GL PU	**Dizmiss** JMI-Canton	chewable tablet	meclizine hydrochloride, 25mg	
	Dramamine Upjohn	chewable tablet	dimenhydrinate, 50mg	aspartame • citric acid • FD&C yellow#5 (tartrazine) • flavor • magnesium stearate • methacrylic acid copolymer • sorbitol
SU	**Dramamine** Upjohn	tablet	dimenhydrinate, 50mg	acacia • carboxymethylcellulose sodium • cornstarch • magnesium stearate • sodium sulfate
SU	**Dramamine II** Upjohn	tablet	meclizine hydrochloride, 25mg	colloidal silicon dioxide • cornstarch • lactose • D&C yellow#10 aluminum lake • microcrystalline cellulose • magnesium stearate
	Marezine Burroughs Wellcome	tablet	cyclizine hydrochloride, 50mg	
	Meclizine HCl Various Manufacturers	tablet	meclizine hydrochloride, 25mg	
	Meclizine HCl Various Manufacturers	tablet	meclizine hydrochloride, 12.5mg	
	Meclizine HCl Chewable Various Manufacturers	chewable tablet	meclizine hydrochloride, 25mg	
	Triptone Caplets Del	caplet	dimenhydrinate, 50mg	

ANTIDIARRHEAL PRODUCTS

	Product Manufacturer	Dosage Form	Adsorbent	Other Active Ingredients	Inactive Ingredients
LA SL	Aromatic Compound Furst-McNess	liquid		extracts of blackberry, rhubarb, and ginger	caramel color • cinnamic aldehyde • glycerin • oils of anise and clove • sodium benzoate • sugar • water
SO	Diarrest Dover	tablet	activated attapulgite		
	Diasorb Columbia	liquid	activated nonfibrous attapulgite, 750mg/5ml		
	Diasorb Columbia	tablet	activated nonfibrous attapulgite, 750mg		
SO	Diatrol Otis Clapp	tablet	activated attapulgite		
	Domagel A.H. Robins	chewable tablet	activated attapulgite, 600mg		
	Imodium Janssen	capsule		loperamide hydrochloride, 2mg	lactose
	Imodium A-D McNeil	liquid		loperamide hydrochloride, 1mg/5ml	alcohol, 5.25% • cherry or licorice flavor
	Imodium A-D McNeil	tablet		loperamide hydrochloride, 2mg/tablet	lactose
LA SU SL	K-C Century	suspension	kaolin 5.2g/30ml • pectin, 260mg/30ml • bismuth subcarbonate, 260mg/30ml		
LA SU SL	Kao-Spen Century	suspension	kaolin, 5.2g/30ml • pectin, 260mg/30ml		
SU SL	Kaolin Pectin Suspension Roxane	suspension	kaolin, 190mg/ml • pectin, 4.34mg/ml	carboxymethylcellulose sodium, 0.4%	glycerin, 1.75% • lime/mint flavor • saccharin • sodium, 0.025%
PU SO	Kaopectate Upjohn	caplet	attapulgite, 750mg		croscarmellose sodium • hydroxypropyl cellulose • hydroxypropyl methylcellulose • methylparaben • pectin • propylene glycol • propylparaben • sucrose • titanium dioxide • zinc stearate
PU SO PE	Kaopectate Children's Chewable Tablets Upjohn	chewable tablet	attapulgite, 300mg		cornstarch • D&C red#27 lake • D&C red#30 lake • dextrins • dextrose • flavor • magnesium stearate • sucrose • titanium dioxide
LA SO SL PE	Kaopectate Children's Liquid Upjohn	liquid	attapulgite, 300mg/7.5ml		FD&C red#40 • flavors • glucono-delta-lactone • magnesium aluminum silicate • methylparaben • sorbic acid • sucrose • titanium dioxide • xanthan gum • purified water

ANTIDIARRHEAL PRODUCTS — continued

	Product Manufacturer	Dosage Form	Adsorbent	Other Active Ingredients	Inactive Ingredients
LA SO SL	Kaopectate Concentrated Upjohn	liquid	attapulgite, 600mg/15ml		flavors • glucono-delta-lactone • magnesium aluminum silicate • methylparaben • sorbic acid • sucrose • titanium dioxide • xanthan gum • purified water
PU	Kaopectate II Upjohn	caplet		loperamide hydrochloride, 2mg	cornstarch • lactose • magnesium stearate • microcrystalline cellulose
	Kapectolin Goldline	suspension	kaolin, 90gr/10ml	pectin, 2gr/10ml	
SU	Loperamide Hydrochloride Solution Roxane	solution		loperamide hydrochloride, 1mg/5ml	propylene glycol • methylparaben • propylparaben • sodium saccharin • glycerin • flavoring
	Parepectolin Rhone-Poulenc Rorer	suspension	attapulgite, 600mg		glucono-delta-lactone • magnesium aluminum silicate • methylparaben • sorbic acid • sucrose • titanium dioxide • xanthan gum • flavor
	Pepto Diarrhea Control Caplets Procter & Gamble	caplet		loperamide hydrochloride, 2mg/caplet	lactose • cornstarch • microcrystalline cellulose • magnesium stearate
LA	Pepto Diarrhea Control Liquid Procter & Gamble	liquid		loperamide hydrochloride, 1mg/tsp	citric acid • alcohol, 5.25% • cherry flavor • methylparaben • propylparaben • water • glycerin
SO	Pepto-Bismol Cherry Tablets Procter & Gamble	tablet		bismuth subsalicylate, 262.39mg	calcium carbonate • adipic acid • mannitol • magnesium stearate • povidone • D&C red #27 aluminum lake • FD&C red #40 aluminum lake • saccharin sodium • talc
	Pepto-Bismol Maximum Strength Liquid Procter & Gamble	liquid		bismuth subsalicylate, 1050mg/30ml	benzoic acid • flavor • magnesium aluminum silicate • methylcellulose • D&C red #22 • D&C red #28 • saccharin sodium • salicylic acid • sodium salicylate • sorbic acid • water
	Pepto-Bismol Original Formula Liquid Procter & Gamble	liquid		bismuth subsalicylate, 525mg/30ml	water • methylcellulose • magnesium aluminum silicate • flavor • saccharin sodium • benzoic acid • sorbic acid • D&C red#22 • D&C red#28 • salicylic acid • sodium salicylate
SO	Pepto-Bismol Original Tablets Procter & Gamble	tablet		bismuth subsalicylate, 262.39mg	calcium carbonate • flavor • magnesium stearate • mannitol • povidone • D&C red #27 aluminum lake • saccharin sodium • talc

ANTIDIARRHEAL PRODUCTS — continued

	Product Manufacturer	Dosage Form	Adsorbent	Other Active Ingredients	Inactive Ingredients
LA SO SL	**Percy Medicine** Merrick	liquid	bismuth subnitrate, 959mg/10ml	calcium hydroxide, 21.9mg/10ml • potassium carbonate, 5.6mg/10ml	distilled water • ethyl alcohol, 5% • glycerin • gum arabic • rhubarb fluid extract • sugar • flavors • natural color
GL PU	**Rheaban** Pfizer	caplet	activated attapulgite, 750mg		carnauba wax • croscarmellose sodium • D&C yellow#10 aluminum lake • D&C blue#1 aluminum lake • hydroxypropyl cellulose • hydroxypropyl methylcellulose • methylparaben • pectin • pharmaceutical glaze • propylene glycol • propylparaben • sucrose • titanium dioxide • zinc stearate

ANTHELMINTIC PRODUCTS

Product & Manufacturer	Dosage Form	Active Ingredients	Inactive Ingredients
LA **Antiminth** SL Pfizer	suspension	pyrantel, 250mg/5ml (as pamoate)	caramel-currant flavor • citric acid • glycerin • lecithin • magnesium aluminum silicate • polysorbate • povidone • simethicone emulsion • sodium benzoate • sorbitol solution
Pin-x Effcon	liquid	pyrantel, 250mg/5ml (as pamoate)	ns
Reese's Pinworm Reese Chemical	caplet	pyrantel, 180mg (the equivalent to 62.5mg pyrantel base)	ns
Reese's Pinworm Reese Chemical	liquid	pyrantel, 250mg/5ml (as pamoate)	sucrose • glycerin • methylcellulose • sodium chloride • flavor • sodium saccharin • methylparaben • preservative

LAXATIVE PRODUCTS

Product & Manufacturer	Dosage Form	Stimulant	Bulk	Emollient/Lubricant	Other Laxatives	Other Ingredients
AL **Adlerika** SU Alvin Last	liquid				magnesium sulfate, 33%	purified water • methyl salicylate • fennel seed • licorice • sodium benzoate • glycerin • cascara extract • tragacanth gum • anise oil • ginger oil • cinnamal • caramel
LA **Agoral** SU Parke-Davis SL	emulsion	phenolphthalein, 0.2g	agar • tragacanth • acacia	mineral oil, 4.2g		benzoic acid • egg albumin • glycerin • sodium, 0.98mEq/15ml • citric acid • flavor
GL **Alophen** PU Parke-Davis SO	tablet	phenophthalein, 60mg				
Bisacodyl Various Manufacturers	suppository • tablet	bisacodyl, 10mg and 5mg				
Black Draught Chattem Consumer	granule	senna equivalent, 660mg				sucrose, 54.6%
Black Draught Chattem Consumer	syrup	casanthranol, 90mg/tbs				sucrose, 54.6% • tartrazine • alcohol, 5%
Caroid Laxative Mentholatum	tablet	cascara sagrada extract, 50mg • phenophthalein, 32.4mg				acacia • beeswax • calcium carbonate • carnauba • dicalcium phosphate dihydrate • gelatin • iron oxide • lactose • magnesium stearate • microcrystalline cellulose • silica • sodium lauryl sulfate • stearic acid • sucrose
SO **Carter's** GE **Laxative** Carter-Wallace	tablet	bisacodyl, 5mg				acacia • carnauba • gelatin • lac • magnesium stearate • polyvinyl acetate phthalate • starch • stearic acid • sucrose • talc • titanium dioxide • white wax
Cascara Sagrada Various Manufacturers	various	cascara sagrada, 325mg; 450mg				
Cascara Sagrada Aromatic Fluid Various Manufacturers	liquid	cascara sagrada				alcohol, 18%

LAXATIVE PRODUCTS — continued

Product & Manufacturer	Dosage Form	Stimulant	Bulk	Emollient/Lubricant	Other Laxatives	Other Ingredients
Castor Oil Various Manufacturers	liquid	castor oil				
GL PU SU Ceo-Two Beutlich	suppository					sodium bicarbonate • potassium bitartrate
Citrate Of Magnesia Various Manufacturers	solution				magnesium citrate	
Citrucel SmithKline Beecham	powder		methylcellulose, 2g/tbs			flavor • sodium, 3mg
GL Colace Capsules Mead Johnson Nutrit'l	capsule			docusate sodium, 50mg or 100mg		
LA SL Colace Liquid Mead Johnson Nutrit'l	liquid			docusate sodium, 10mg/ml		
LA SL Colace Syrup Mead Johnson Nutrit'l	syrup			docusate sodium, 20mg/5ml		
Colax Rugby	tablet	phenophthalein, 65mg		docusate sodium, 100mg		
Correctol Schering-Plough	tablet	yellow phenolphthalein, 65mg		docusate sodium, 100mg		sodium, 0.34mEq
Correctol Extra Gentle Schering-Plough	capsule			docusate sodium, 100mg/capsule		
DC 240 Goldline	capsule			docusate calcium, 240mg		
Dialose Johnson&Johnson Merck	tablet			docusate sodium, 100mg/tablet		
Dialose Plus Johnson&Johnson Merck	tablet	yellow phenophthalein, 65mg/tablet		docusate sodium, 100mg/tablet		
Docusate Calcium Various Manufacturers	capsule			docusate calcium, 240mg		
Docusate Potassium with Casanthranol Various Manufacturers	capsule	casanthranol, 30mg		docusate calcium, 100mg		
Docusate Sodium Roxane	syrup			docusate sodium, 3.33mg/ml; 4mg/ml		sodium, 0.06mEq/ml • propylene glycol 20% • sucrose, 55% • methylparaben • propylparaben

LAXATIVE PRODUCTS — continued

	Product & Manufacturer	Dosage Form	Stimulant	Bulk	Emollient/ Lubricant	Other Laxatives	Other Ingredients
	Docusate Sodium Various Manufacturers	various			docusate sodium, 50mg, 100mg & 250mg		
	Docusate Sodium with Casanthranol Various Manufacturers	capsule	casanthranol, 30mg		docusate sodium, 100mg		
	Docusate Sodium with Casanthranol Various Manufacturers	syrup	casanthranol, 2mg/ml		docusate sodium, 4mg/ml		
LA SO SU	**Doxidan** Upjohn	liqui-gel	yellow phenolphthalein, 65mg		docusate calcium, 60mg		alcohol up to 1.5% • corn oil • FD&C blue #1 • FD&C red #40 • gelatin • glycerin • hydrogenated vegetable oil • lecithin • parabens • sorbitol • titanium dioxide • vegetable shortening • yellow wax
LA SO SL	**Dr. Caldwell Senna Laxative** Gebauer	liquid	senna, 33.3mg/ ml				alcohol, 4.9%
	Dulcolax CIBA Consumer	suppository	bisacodyl, 10mg				hydrogenated vegetable oil
	Dulcolax CIBA Consumer	tablet	bisacodyl, 5mg				
	Effersyllium Johnson&Johnson Merck	powder		psyllium hydrocolloid, 3g/ tsp			sodium <5mg/tsp • sucrose • flavor
SU	**Emulsoil** Paddock	liquid	castor oil, 95%				flavor
	Epsom Salt Various Manufacturers	granule				magnesium sulfate, 40mEq/ 5mg	
GL PU SU	**Espotabs** Combe	tablet	yellow phenolphthalein, 97.2mg				
	Evac-Q-Kwik Savage	liquid				magnesium citrate, 300ml	sodium, 0.84mEq/ dose • carbon dioxide • citric acid • FD&C red #4 • cherry flavor • potassium citrate • water
	Evac-Q-Kwik Savage	suppository	bisacodyl, 10mg				sodium, trace

LAXATIVE PRODUCTS — continued

Product & Manufacturer	Dosage Form	Stimulant	Bulk	Emollient/Lubricant	Other Laxatives	Other Ingredients
Evac-Q-Kwik Savage	tablet	phenolphthalein, 130mg				sodium, trace • acacia • calcium carbonate • calcium sulfate • cornstarch • dibasic calcium phosphate • FD&C red #40 • lactose • magnesium stearate • polyvinylpyrrolidone • shellac • sodium benzoate • talc • titanium dioxide • water • white wax
GL PU GE Evac-U-Gen Walker	chewable tablet	yellow phenolphthalein, 97.2mg				sodium, 0.004mEq
GL PU SO Ex-Lax Chocolate Laxative Tablets Sandoz Pharm.	tablet	yellow phenolphthalein, 90mg				cocoa • confectioner's sugar • hydrogenated palm kernel oil • lecithin • nonfat dry milk • vanillin
GL PU Ex-Lax Extra Gentle Sandoz Pharm.	tablet	yellow phenolphthalein, 65mg		docusate sodium, 75mg • acacia		croscarmellose sodium • dibasic calcium phosphate • colloidal silicon dioxide • magnesium stearate • microcrystalline cellulose • red #7 • stearic acid • sucrose • talc • titanium dioxide
GL PU SU Ex-Lax Gentle Nature, Natural Laxative Sandoz Pharm.	tablet	sennosides A & B, 20mg				alginic acid • calcium phosphate dibasic • magnesium stearate • microcrystalline cellulose • silicon dioxide • sodium lauryl sulfate • starch • stearic acid
GL PU Ex-Lax Maximum Relief Formula Sandoz Pharm.	tablet	yellow phenolphthalein, 135mg		acacia		alginic acid • blue #1 • carnauba wax • colloidal silicon dioxide • dibasic calcium phosphate • magnesium stearate • microcrystalline cellulose • povidone sodium benzoate • sodium lauryl sulfate • starch • stearic acid • sucrose • talc • titanium dioxide

LAXATIVE PRODUCTS — continued

Product & Manufacturer	Dosage Form	Stimulant	Bulk	Emollient/Lubricant	Other Laxatives	Other Ingredients
GL PU **Ex-Lax Regular Strength** Sandoz Pharm.	tablet	yellow phenolphthalein, 90mg		acacia		alginic acid • carnauba wax • colloidal silicon dioxide • dibasic calcium phosphate • iron oxides • magnesium stearate • microcrystalline cellulose • sodium benzoate • sodium lauryl sulfate • starch • stearic acid • sucrose • talc • titanium dioxide
Feen-A-Mint Schering-Plough	gum	yellow phenolphthalein, 97.2mg				flavor
Feen-A-Mint Schering-Plough	tablet	yellow phenolphthalein, 65mg		docusate sodium, 100mg		flavor
Feen-A-Mint Pills Schering-Plough	tablet	yellow phenolphthalein, 65mg		docusate sodium, 100mg		sodium, 0.34mEq
Femilax G & W	tablet	phenolphthalein, 65mg		docusate sodium, 100mg		
GL PU SO **FiberCon** Lederle	tablet		calcium polycarbophil, 625mg			calcium carbonate • caramel • crospovidone • hydroxypropyl methylcellulose • magnesium stearate • microcrystalline cellulose • povidone • silica gel
GL PU SO SU **Fiberall** CIBA Consumer	tablet		calcium polycarbophil, 1250mg			crospovidone • dextrose • flavors • magnesium stearate • yellow #10 aluminum lake
PU SU **Fiberall, Natural** CIBA Consumer	powder		psyllium hydrophilic mucilloid, 3.4g			citric acid • flavor • wheat bran • polysorbate 60
PU **Fiberall, Oatmeal Raisin Or Fruit & Nut** CIBA Consumer	wafer		psyllium hydrophilic mucilloid, 3.4g			wheat bran
AL LA PR SO SU SL PE **Fleet Babylax** C.B. Fleet	liquid				glycerin	
Fleet Bagenema with Soap Packet C.B. Fleet	enema				liquid castile soap, 10ml	

LAXATIVE PRODUCTS — continued

	Product & Manufacturer	Dosage Form	Stimulant	Bulk	Emollient/ Lubricant	Other Laxatives	Other Ingredients
	Fleet Bisacodyl Enema C.B. Fleet	enema	bisacodyl, 10mg				
PU	Fleet Laxative Tablets C.B. Fleet	tablet	bisacodyl, 5mg				
	Fleet Mineral Oil Enema C.B. Fleet	enema			mineral oil, 133ml		
	Fleet Prep Kit 1 C.B. Fleet	liquid • tablet • suppository	bisacodyl, 5mg (tablet) • bisacodyl, 10mg (suppository)			monobasic sodium phosphate, 0.48g/ml • dibasic sodium phosphate, 0.18g/ml	sodium, 550mg/ 5ml • flavor
	Fleet Prep Kit 3 C.B. Fleet	liquid • tablet • enema	bisacodyl, 5mg (tablet) • bisacodyl, 10mg (enema)			monobasic sodium phosphate, 0.48g/ml • dibasic sodium phosphate, 0.18g/ml	sodium, 550mg/ 5ml • flavor
	Fleet Prep Kit 4 C.B. Fleet	emulsion • tablet • suppository	castor oil, 67% (emulsion) • bisacodyl, 5mg (tablet) • bisacodyl, 10mg (suppository)				
	Fleet Prep Kit 5 C.B. Fleet	emulsion • tablet • enema	castor oil, 67% (emulsion) • bisacodyl, 5mg (tablet)			liquid castile soap, 10ml (enema)	
	Fleet Ready-to-Use Enema C.B. Fleet	enema				monobasic sodium phosphate, 19g • dibasic sodium phosphate, 7g	sodium, 4.4g/118ml
PE	Fleet Ready-to-Use Enema for Children C.B. Fleet	enema				monobasic sodium phosphate, 9.5g • dibasic sodium phosphate, 3.5g	sodium, 2.2g/59ml
LA SL PE	Fletcher's Castoria Mentholatum	liquid	senna concentrate, 33.3mg/ml				alcohol, 3.5% • flavor • glycerin • sucrose • water
SL PE	Fletcher's Children's Laxative Cherry Flavor Mentholatum	liquid	yellow phenolphthalein, 0.3%				citric acid • FD&C red#40 • flavor • glycerin • magnesium aluminum silicate • methylparaben • sodium benzoate • sucrose • water • xanthan gum

LAXATIVE PRODUCTS — continued

	Product & Manufacturer	Dosage Form	Stimulant	Bulk	Emollient/ Lubricant	Other Laxatives	Other Ingredients
SO SU	Garfields Tea Alvin Last	cut plant	senna, 610mg/ 1/2tsp	psyllium seed husks • buckthorn bark			mixed botanicals
	GenFiber Goldline	powder		psyllium hydrophilic mucilloid, 3.4gm/ 7gm			dextrose
	Genasoft Goldline	capsule			docusate sodium, 100mg		
	Genasoft Plus Goldline	capsule	casanthranol, 30mg		docusate sodium, 100mg		
	Glycerin Various Manufacturers	suppository				glycerin	sodium stearate
SU	Haleys M-O Sterling Health	emulsion			mineral oil, 25%	magnesium hydroxide, 6%	
SU	Herb-Lax Shaklee	tablet	senna leaf powder, 300-600mg/ dose				8 botanicals
SU	Hydrocil Instant Solvay	powder		psyllium, 95%			povidone
SO SU	Innerclean Herbal Alvin Last	cut plant • tablet	senna leaves	psyllium seed husks • buckthorn bark			anise seed • fennel seed
SO	Kasof Roberts Pharm.	capsule			docusate potassium, 240mg		gelatin • glycerin • methylparaben • polyethylene glycol • propylparaben • purified water • red#40 • blue#1 • sorbitol • yellow#10
SO	Kellogg's Tasteless Castor Oil BIRA	liquid		castor oil, 100%			
AL LA SU SL	Kondremul CIBA Consumer	emulsion			mineral oil, 55%		
	LBC-LAX Murdock	capsule	cascara sagrada				barberry root bark • ginger root • golden seal root • cramp bark • red raspberry leaves • fennel seed • turkey rhubarb root • cayenne pepper fruit
	Lax-Pills G & W	tablet	phenolphthalein, 90mg				
AL LA PR SU SL	Liqui-Doss Ferndale	emulsion			mineral oil		

LAXATIVE PRODUCTS — continued

	Product & Manufacturer	Dosage Form	Stimulant	Bulk	Emollient/ Lubricant	Other Laxatives	Other Ingredients
GL PU SO SU	Mag-Ox 400 Blaine	tablet				magnesium oxide, 400mg (elemental magnesium, 241.3mg or 19.86mEq)	
	Metamucil Fiber Wafers, Apple Crisp Flavor Procter & Gamble	wafer		psyllium hydrophilic mucilloid, 3.4g/2 wafers			ascorbic acid • brown sugar • cinnamon • corn oil • flavors • fructose • lecithin • modified food starch • molasses • oat hull fiber • sodium bicarbonate • sucrose • water • wheat flour
SU	Metamucil Orig. Text., Effervescent/ Sugar Free/ Lemon-Lime Procter & Gamble	individual packet		psyllium hydrophilic fiber, 3.4g/packet			aspartame • calcium carbonate • citric acid • flavoring • potassium bicarbonate • silicon dioxide • sodium bicarbonate
	Metamucil Orig. Texture, Orange Procter & Gamble	powder		psyllium hydrophilic mucilloid, 3.4g/ tbs			citric acid • FD&C yellow #6 • flavoring • sucrose • sodium, 4mg/tsp
	Metamucil Orig. Texture, Original Flavor Procter & Gamble	powder		psyllium hydrophilic mucilloid, 3.4g/ tsp			dextrose • sodium, 3mg/tsp
SO	Metamucil Smooth Texture, Citrus Procter & Gamble	individual packet		psyllium hydrophilic mucilloid, 3.4g/ packet			citric acid • D&C yellow #10 • FD&C yellow #6 • flavoring • sucrose
	Metamucil Smooth Texture, Sugar Free, Regular Flavor Procter & Gamble	powder		psyllium hydrophilic mucilloid, 3.4g/ tsp			citric acid, 1% • magnesium sulfate • maltodextrin
	Milk Of Magnesia Various Manufacturers	liquid				magnesium hydroxide, 80mEq magnesium/ 30ml	
SU	Milk Of Magnesia Roxane	suspension				magnesium hydroxide, 0.078g/ml	sodium, 0.03mEq/ 15ml • citric acid • methylparaben • propylparaben
	Milk Of Magnesia, Concentrated Roxane	suspension				magnesium hydroxide, 0.233g/ml	glycerin • sorbitol, 29% • sugar, 8% • lemon • sodium, 0.09mEq/ml

LAXATIVE PRODUCTS — continued

Product & Manufacturer	Dosage Form	Stimulant	Bulk	Emollient/ Lubricant	Other Laxatives	Other Ingredients
SU **Milk Of Magnesia-Cascara Suspension, Concentrated** Roxane	suspension	cascara sagrada (equiv. to 5ml fluidextract)			magnesium hydroxide, 0.078g/ml	sodium, 0.12mEq/15ml • sorbitol • alcohol • methylparaben • propylparaben
LA **Milkinol** SO Schwarz SU Pharma	emulsion			mineral oil		butylated hydroxyanisole • emulsifier • color • flavor
Mineral Oil Various Manufacturers	liquid			mineral oil		
Modane Savage	tablet	phenolphthalein, 130mg				acacia • calcium carbonate • calcium sulfate • cornstarch • dibasic calcium phosphate • FD&C red #40 aluminum lake • lactose • magnesium stearate • povidone • shellac • sodium benzoate • sucrose • talc • titanium dioxide • water • white wax
Modane Plus Savage	tablet	phenolphthalein, 60mg		docusate sodium, 100mg		acacia • calcium carbonate • calcium sulfate • croscarmellose sodium • FD&C yellow #6 aluminum lake • magnesium stearate • microcrystalline cellulose • povidone • shellac • silica gel • sodium benzoate • sucrose • talc • titanium dioxide • water • carnauba wax
Modane Soft Savage	capsule			docusate sodium, 100mg		sodium, 0.27mEq/dose • gelatin • glycerin • methylparaben • polyethylene glycol 400 • propylene glycol • propylparaben • sorbitol • water
Natural Vegetable Various Manufacturers	powder		psyllium mucilloid, 3.4g			sodium, <10mg • dextrose
Nature's Remedy SmithKline Beecham	enema				sodium biphosphate, 19g • sodium phosphate, 7g (sodium, 4.4g per deL dose)	

LAXATIVE PRODUCTS — continued

Product & Manufacturer	Dosage Form	Stimulant	Bulk	Emollient/ Lubricant	Other Laxatives	Other Ingredients
Nature's Remedy SmithKline Beecham	tablet	aloe, 100mg • cascara sagrada, 150mg				
Nature's Remedy, Mineral Oil Enema SmithKline Beecham	enema			mineral oil, 118ml/dose		
GL Naturlax PU Sunlax SO Citrus Cenci Powder	powder		psyllium hydrophilic mucilloid, 3.4g/dose			citric acid • D&C yellow #10 • FD&C yellow #5 • flavor • sucrose
GL Naturlax PU Sunlax SO Orange SU Sugar Free Cenci Powder	powder		psyllium hydrophilic mucilloid, 3.4g/dose			aspartame • citric acid • FD&C yellow #6 • D&C yellow #10 • flavor • maltodextrin
Perdiem Rhone-Poulenc Rorer	granule	senna, 0.74g/tsp (cassia pod concentrate)	psyllium, 3.25g/tsp			sodium, 1.8mg • potassium, 35.5mg • acacia • iron oxides • natural flavors • paraffin • sucrose • talc
Perdiem Fiber Rhone-Poulenc Rorer	granule		psyllium, 4.03g/tsp			sodium, 1.8mg • potassium, 36.1mg • acacia • iron oxides • natural flavors • paraffin • sucrose • talc • titanium dioxide
GL Peri-Colace Capsules Mead Johnson Nutri'l	capsule	casanthranol, 30mg		docusate sodium, 100mg		
LA Peri-Colace SL Syrup Mead Johnson Nutri'l	syrup	casanthranol, 30mg		docusate sodium, 60mg		
Peri-Dos Goldline	capsule	casanthranol, 30mg		docusate sodium, 100mg		
Phillips' Laxative Gelcaps Sterling Health	capsule	phenolphthalein, 90mg		docusate sodium, 83mg		
Phillips' Milk Of Magnesia, mint or cherry Sterling Health	suspension				magnesium hydroxide, 80mg/ml	cherry or mint flavor
Phillips' Milk of Magnesia Sterling Health	tablet				magnesium hydroxide, 311mg	peppermint oil, 1.166mg • sodium, 0.13mEq

LAXATIVE PRODUCTS — continued

Product & Manufacturer	Dosage Form	Stimulant	Bulk	Emollient/Lubricant	Other Laxatives	Other Ingredients
Phospho-soda Buffered Oral Saline Unflavored & Ginger-Lemon C.B. Fleet	liquid				monobasic sodium phosphate, 0.48g/ml • dibasic sodium phosphate, 0.18g/ml	sodium, 550mg/5ml • flavor
Purge Evacuant Fleming	liquid	castor oil, 95%				
Reguloid, Natural Rugby	powder		psyllium hydrophilic mucilloid, 3.4g			dextrose
Reguloid, Orange Rugby	powder		psyllium hydrophillic mucilloid, 3.4g			sucrose, 70% • flavor
Sani-Supp G & W	suppository				glycerin	sodium stearate
Senexon Rugby	tablet	senna concentrate, 187mg				
Senna-Gen Goldline	tablet	senna concentrate, 217mg				
Senokot Purdue Frederick	suppository	senna concentrate, 652mg				
Senokot Purdue Frederick	syrup	senna concentrate, 8.8mg sennosides/tsp				alcohol, 7%
Senokot Purdue Frederick	tablet	senna concentrate, 8.6mg sennosides/tablet				sodium, 0.007mEq/dose
Senokot-S Purdue Frederick	tablet	senna concentrate, 8.6mg sennosides/tablet		docusate sodium, 50mg		sodium, 0.15mEq
Senokot-X-Tra Purdue Frederick	tablet	senna concentrate, 17mg sennosides/tablet				sodium, 0.014mEq/dose
Senolax Schein	tablet	senna concentrate, 187mg				dicalcium phosphate • microcrystalline cellulose • magnesium stearate • colloidal silica
Serutan Menley & James	granule		psyllium hydrophillic mucilloid, 2.5mg			saccharin sodium, <0.1g • sucrose • flavor
Serutan Menley & James	powder		psyllium hydrophillic mucilloid, 3.4g			dextrose • flavors • wheat germ • sodium, <0.1g
Siblin Parke-Davis	granule		psyllium seed husks, 2.5g			sucrose, 2.4g

LAXATIVE PRODUCTS — continued

	Product & Manufacturer	Dosage Form	Stimulant	Bulk	Emollient/ Lubricant	Other Laxatives	Other Ingredients
SO SU	**Surfak** **240mg** Upjohn	liqui-gel			docusate calcium, 240mg		alcohol up to 3% • corn oil • FD&C blue #1 • FD&C red #40 • gelatin • glycerin • parabens • sorbitol
AL LA PR SO SU SL	**Therac Plus** JMI-Canton	enema			docusate sodium, 283mg	glycerin	benzocaine, 20mg • PEG-400
AL LA PR SU SL	**Therevac-SB** JMI-Canton	enema			docusate sodium, 283mg	glycerin	PEG-400
SU	**Unilax** B.F. Ascher	capsule	yellow phenolphthalein, 130mg		docusate sodium, 230mg		
GL PU SO SU	**Uro-Mag** Blaine	capsule				magnesium oxide, 140mg (elemental magnesium, 84.5mg or 6.93mEq)	
GL PU SO	**V-Lax** Century	powder		psyllium hydrophilic mucilloid, 50%			dextrose, 50%
	Woman's Gentle Laxative Goldline	tablet	yellow phenolphthalein, 65mg		docusate sodium, 100mg		

INSULIN PREPARATIONS PRODUCTS

Product & Manufacturer	Species Source[a]	Onset (hrs.)	Peak (hrs.)	Duration (hrs.)	pH[b]	Preservative	Purity ppm of Proinsulin	Stability at Room Temp. (mos.)	Zinc (mg/100 U)	Protein (mg/100 U)
Rapid Acting										
Humulin R (Regular Human Insulin) Eli Lilly	h	0.5	2-4	6-8	n	metacresol	<10	30 days	0.01-0.04	ns
Novolin R (Regular, Human Insulin Injection) Novo Nordisk	h	0.5	2.5-5	6-8	n	metacresol	<1	24		ns
Novolin R Penfill (Regular, Human Insulin Injection) Novo Nordisk	h	0.5	2.5-5	6-8	n	metacresol	<1	30 days		ns
Regular (Insulin Injection, Beef) Novo Nordisk	b	0.5	2.5-5	8	n	phenol	<10	24		ns
Regular (Purified Pork Insulin Injection) Novo Nordisk	p	0.5	2.5-5	8	n	phenol	<1	24		ns
Regular Iletin I Eli Lilly	b • p	0.5	2-4	6-8	n	metacresol	<10	30 days	0.01-0.04	ns
Regular Iletin II (Purified Pork) Eli Lilly	p	0.5	2-4	6-8	n	metacresol	<10	30 days	0.01-0.04	ns
Semilente (Prompt Insulin Zinc Suspension, Beef) Novo Nordisk	b	1.5	5-10	16	n	methylparaben	<10	24	0.15	none
Velosulin (Purified Pork Insulin) Novo Nordisk	p	0.5	1-3	8	7.3	metacresol, 0.3%	<1	18	0.01-0.04	ns
Velosulin Human (Insulin Injection, semi-synthetic) Novo Nordisk	h	0.5	1-3	8	7.3	metacresol, 0.3%	<1	18	0.01-0.04	ns
Intermediate Acting										
Humulin L (Lente Human Insulin Zinc Suspension) Eli Lilly	h	1-3	6-12	18-24	n	methylparaben	<10	30 days	0.12-0.25	none
Humulin N (NPH Human Insulin Isophane Suspension) Eli Lilly	h	1-2	6-12	18-24	n	phenol • metacresol	<10	30 days	0.01-0.04	0.3-0.5
Insulatard NPH (Isophane Purified Pork Insulin Suspension) Novo Nordisk	p	1.5	4-12	24	7.3	metacresol, 0.15% • phenol, 0.06%	<1	20	0.01-0.04	protamine, 0.32-0.36

INSULIN PREPARATIONS PRODUCTS — continued

Product & Manufacturer	Species Source[a]	Onset (hrs.)	Peak (hrs.)	Duration (hrs.)	pH[b]	Preservative	Purity ppm of Proinsulin	Stability at Room Temp. (mos.)	Zinc (mg/ 100 U)	Protein (mg/ 100 U)
Insulatard NPH Human (Insulin Isophane Susp., semi-synth.) Novo Nordisk	h	1.5	4-12	24	n	phenol • metacresol	<1	24	0.02	protamine, 0.35
Lente (Insulin Zinc Suspension, Beef) Novo Nordisk	b	2.5	7-15	24	n	methylparaben	<10	24	0.15	ns
Lente (Purified Pork Insulin Zinc Suspension) Novo Nordisk	p	2.5	7-15	22	n	methylparaben	<1	24	0.15	ns
Lente Iletin I (Insulin Zinc Suspension) Eli Lilly	b • p	1-3	6-12	18-36	n	methylparaben	<10	30 days	0.12-0.25	none
Lente Iletin II (Insulin Zinc Suspension, Purified Pork) Eli Lilly	p	1-3	6-12	18-36	n	methylparaben	<10	30 days	0.12-0.25	none
Novolin L (Lente Human Insulin Zinc Suspension) Novo Nordisk	h	2.5	7-15	22	n	methylparaben	<1	24	0.15	ns
Novolin N (NPH, Human Insulin Isophane Suspension) Novo Nordisk	h	1.5	4-12	24	n	phenol • metacresol	<1	24	0.02	protamine, 0.35
Novolin N Penfill (NPH, Human Insulin Isophane Suspension) Novo Nordisk	h	1.5	4-12	24	n	phenol • metacresol	<1	7 days in use	0.02	protamine, 0.35
NPH (Isophane Insulin Suspension, Beef) Novo Nordisk	b	1.5	4-12	24	n	phenol • metacresol	<10	24	0.02	protamine, 0.43
NPH (Purified Pork Isophane Insulin) Novo Nordisk	p	1.5	4-12	24	n	phenol • metacresol	<1	24	0.02	protamine, 0.35
NPH Iletin I (Isophane Insulin Suspension) Eli Lilly	b • p	1-2	6-12	18-36	n	phenol • metacresol	<10	30 days	0.01-0.04	protamine, 0.3-0.5
NPH Iletin II (Isophane Insulin Suspension, Purified Pork) Eli Lilly	p	1-2	6-12	18-36	n	phenol • metacresol	<10	30 days	0.01-0.04	protamine, 0.3-0.5

INSULIN PREPARATIONS PRODUCTS — continued

Product & Manufacturer	Species Source[a]	Onset (hrs.)	Peak (hrs.)	Duration (hrs.)	pH[b]	Preservative	Purity ppm of Proinsulin	Stability at Room Temp. (mos.)	Zinc (mg/ 100 U)	Protein (mg/ 100 U)
Mixed (Intermediate/Rapid Acting)										
Humulin 50/50 (50% NPH Isophane Susp., 50% Regular Inj.) Eli Lilly	h	within 1hr	within 4hrs	up to 24hrs		phenol metacresol	<10	30 days	0.01-0.04	protamine, 0.270
Humulin 70/30 (70% NPH Isophane Susp., 30% Regular Inj.) Eli Lilly	h	within 1hr	within 4hrs	up to 24hrs		phenol metacresol	<10	30 days	0.01-0.04	protamine, 0.270
Mixtard (70% Isophane Pur. Pork Susp. & 30% Pur. Pork Inj.) Novo Nordisk	p	0.5	4-8	24	7.3	metacresol, 0.15% • phenol, 0.06%	<1	20	0.01-0.04	protamine, 0.22-0.25
Mixtard Hum. 70/30 (70% Hu. Iso. Sus./30% Hu. Inj.,sem-syn) Novo Nordisk	h	0.5	2-12	24	n	phenol • metacresol	<1	24	0.02	protamine, 0.25
Novolin 70/30 Penfill (70% NPH Hum. Susp./30% Regular Inj.) Novo Nordisk	h	0.5	2-12	24	n	phenol • metacresol	<1	7 days	0.02	protamine, 0.25
Novolin 70/30 (70% NPH, Hum. Iso. Susp./ 30% Reg., Hum. Inj.) Novo Nordisk	h	0.5	2-12	24	n	phenol • metacresol	<1	24	0.02	protamine, 0.25
Long Acting										
Humulin U (Ultralente Human Insulin Extended Zinc Susp.) Eli Lilly	h	4-6	8-20	24-28	n	methylparaben	<10	30 days	0.12-0.25	ns
Ultralente (Extended Insulin Zinc Suspension, Beef) Novo Nordisk	b	4	10-30	36	n	methylparaben	<10	24	0.15	none

[a] b=beef, p=pork, h=human insulin derived through recombinant DNA biotechnology. Insulins with a combination of beef and pork contain 70% beef and 30% pork.
[b] n=neutral

INSULIN SYRINGES AND RELATED PRODUCTS

Product & Manufacturer	Comments
Alcohol Swabs And Alcohol Wipes Becton Dickinson	70% isopropyl alcohol for single use unit dose of alcohol swabs • more expensive but good for travel
Autojector Ulster Scientific	spring-loaded plastic syringe holder positioned over skin • press device against site, push button to insert needle and deliver insulin simultaneously • increases injection-site alternatives
Automatic Injector Becton Dickinson	spring-loaded plastic syringe holder positioned over skin • to insert needle, press button • increases injection-site alternatives
Count-a-dose Jordan	syringe-filling device • empty syringe secured in easy-to-locate platform • slide moves syringe plunger to control insulin intake • click wheel activates slide to ensure accurate dosage (in 1- or 2-unit increments depending on model used) • "click" heard and felt as wheel is rotated • holds 1 or 2 bottles of insulin for mixed doses
Holdease Meditec	needle guide and syringe/vial holder • unit holds syringe and insulin together in easy-to-handle unit while user fills syringe
Inject-Ease Palco	spring-loaded plastic syringe holder positioned over skin • to insert needle, press button • includes plunger cap to pre-load syringes
Injectomatic Kendall-Futuro	spring-loaded metal syringe holder positioned over skin • press device against selected site to insert needle • increases injection-site alternatives
Instaject Jordan	combination syringe injector and blood lancet device • button-activated • self-contained as injector • lancet adaptor only
Insul-eze Palco	device holds syringe and insulin bottle while dosage is drawn • magnifies syringe calibration for full length of syringe • design allows device to sit firmly on any flat surface (in vertical or horizontal position) • works with all types of insulin bottles
Insulgage Meditec	permanent, precalibrated device; purchased according to dose (from 2 to 85 units) • dose marked in Inkprint, raised numbers, Braille and raised numbers, or Braille • two gauges can be used for mixed dosages
Insulin Needle Guide Amer. Fdn. for Blind	guide fits over vial cap • funnel-shaped opening guides needle into rubber seal of vial
Insulin Syringe, Single Use Lo-Dose Becton Dickinson	0.5cc with 28 gauge or 29 gauge 1/2" needle • 30/package and 100/package • cannot change needle size • used for patients taking less than 50 units of U-100 insulin • larger print of calibration allows more accurate dosing • can be used up to 3 times
Insulin-Aid Seabee	plexiglass device • magnetically attaches to a metal surface and holds any insulin bottle inverted • makes it easier to withdraw insulin into syringe • enables user to use both hands to draw insulin into syringe
Isopropyl Alcohol, 91% Various Manufacturers	used for sterilizing needles and syringes and for cleansing skin before injections • safer to use with insulin than rubbing alcohol because it is not denatured and has less water
Load-Matic Palco	allows person to load syringes by touch alone • aligns needle with bottle top, loads syringe by separate ten- or single-unit increments • holds any size insulin bottle • after setting the desired dosage it can be used repeatedly without further adjustment
Magni-Guide Becton Dickinson	syringe is slipped into curved channel of Magni-Guide • at opposite end, insulin vial is snapped into collar • guide magnifies entire scale 2 times
Monoject Ultra Comfort Insulin Syringe, 28 Gauge Kendall	28 gauge • 1/2 or 1cc • 30 or 100 count • for U-100 insulin • packaged in individual, tamper-evident sterile peel packs • bold numbers • zero dead space design • flat plunger tips • permanently attached needles • advanced laser-welded needles • improved lubricants

INSULIN SYRINGES AND RELATED PRODUCTS — continued

Product & Manufacturer	Comments
Monoject Ultra Comfort Insulin Syringe, 29 Gauge Kendall	29 gauge • 3/10, 1/2, or 1cc • 30 or 100 count • for U-100 insulin • packaged in individual, tamper-evident, sterile peel packs • bold numbers • zero dead space design • flat plunger tips • permanently attached needles • advanced laser-welded needles • improved lubricant
NovoPen Insulin Delivery Device Novo Nordisk	one device/package • designed to resemble a fountain pen • uses a replaceable, 1.5ml cartridge of Novolin human insulin • delivers 2 or more units by push-button • made of nickel- and chromium-plated brass • 6" long, 7 oz. in weight • standard deviation for a dose is 0.1 units
Novolin 70/30 Prefilled Novo Nordisk	lightweight, prefilled disposable syringe • 14cm long • weighs less than 1/2oz • designed for multi-dose usage • delivers 2-58 units of insulin in 2-unit increments • each syringe prefilled with 150 units of Novolin 70/30 human insulin • syringe is disposable once emptied • for use with PenNeedle disposable needle
PenNeedle Disposable Needle Novo Nordisk	disposable needles • 100/box • beveled needletip • siliconized throughout its length • ensures minimal friction with skin • 27 gauge • 1/2 inch (12.5mm) long • for single use only • disposable needles specifically designed for use with NovoNordisk insulin delivery systems • protective outer cap, smooth plastic needle cap, and a protective tab • should not be used if protective tab is missing or damaged
Self Contained Insulin Syringe Becton Dickinson	1cc with 28 gauge 1/2" needle in U-40 and U-100 • 1cc with 27 gauge 1/2" needle • 1cc, 1/2cc, and 3/10cc with 29 gauge 1/2" needle in U-100 • no dead space • excellent for travel • more expensive than reusable but sterile and convenient • less pain with 27 1/2 gauge • can be reused up to 3 times
Syringe Support Amer. Fdn. for Blind	syringe loading device allows user to both align needle with bottle top and set dosage levels based on the number of full turns of a thumb screw with a raised ridge • one full turn of the screw equals 2 units • uses Lilly insulin bottles
Yale 0.35cc Special Insulin Syringe Becton Dickinson	0.35cc, calibrated up to 35 units • available for patients using small doses of U-100 insulin

BLOOD SUGAR–ELEVATING PRODUCTS

Product & Manufacturer	Comments
B-D Glucose Tablets Becton Dickinson	glucose, 5g • for the treatment of hypoglycemia
DEX4 Glucose Tablets Can-Am	orange-, lemon-, raspberry- or grape-flavored • carbohydrate, 4g/tablet
DextroEnergy Glucose Tablets Can-Am	lemon-, orange-, raspberry- or black currant-flavored • carbohydrate, 3g/tablet
Dextrosol Energy Chewable Tablets (CPC United Kingdom)	variety of flavors • 25 cal • dextrose, 6g • vitamin C • used to treat hypoglycemia
DextroTabs British-Amer. Medical	lime- and orange-flavored • carbohydrate, 1.6g/tablet
Glutose Tablets Paddock	oral glucose • 5g/tablet • used to treat insulin reaction (hypoglycemia)
Glutose Gel Paddock	oral glucose (40% dextrose solution) • used to treat insulin reaction (hypoglycemia) before unconsciousness occurs
Insta-Glucose Liquid ICN	convenient plastic tube of carbohydrate gel • for use by diabetics to treat hypoglycemic symptoms • cherry flavor • one unit dose tube contains 24g carbohydrate
Monojel Glucose Gel Kendall-Futuro	orange gel used to relieve hypoglycemia • each package contains 4-25g doses of 40% glucose (dextrose USP) in foil wrapped pouches

DIABETES MONITORING PRODUCTS

Product Manufacturer	Product Form	Biological Fluid Tested	Active Ingredients
Acetest Miles Incorporated	tablet	urine • blood	nitroprusside-glycine • buffer
Albustix Miles Incorporated	strip	urine	tetrabromphenol blue • buffer
Bili-Labstix Miles Incorporated	stick	urine	see Multistix 10 SG
Chemstrip 10 With SG Boehringer Mannheim	strip	urine	specific gravity: EGTA • ethyleneglycol-bis (aminoethylether) tetraacetic acid • bromthymol blue • leukocytes: indoxylcarbonic acid ester • diazonium salt • nitrite: 3-hydroxy-1,2,3,4-tetrahydro-7,8-benzoquinoline • sulfanilamide • pH: bromthymol blue • methyl red • phenolphthalein • protein: tetrachlorophenol-tetrabromosulfophthalein • glucose: tetramethylbenzidine • glucose oxidase • peroxidase • ketones: sodium nitroferricyanide • glycine • urobilinogen: 4-methoxybenzene-diazonium-tetrafluoroborate • bilirubin: 2, 6-dichlorobenzene-diazonium-tetrafluoroborate • blood: tetramethylbenzidine • 2,5-dimethyl-2,5-dihydroperoxthexane
Chemstrip 2GP Boehringer Mannheim	strip	urine	glucose: tetramethylbenzidine • glucose oxidase • peroxidase • protein: tetrachlorophenol • tetrabromosulfophthalein
Chemstrip 8 Boehringer Mannheim	strip	urine	glucose oxidase • peroxidase • o-tolidine • sodium nitroferricyanide
Chemstrip 9 Boehringer Mannheim	strip	urine	see Chemstrip 10 With SG
Chemstrip bG Boehringer Mannheim	strip	blood	glucose oxidase • peroxidase • o-tolidine • tetramethylbenzidine
Chemstrip G Boehringer Mannheim	strip	urine	glucose oxidase • peroxidase • o-tolidine
Chemstrip GK Boehringer Mannheim	strip	urine	glucose: glucose oxidase • peroxidase • ketones: sodium nitroferricyanide
Chemstrip K Boehringer Mannheim	strip	urine	sodium nitroferricyanide • glycine
Chemstrip uG Boehringer Mannheim	strip	urine	glucose oxidase (aspergillus niger) • peroxidase (horseradish) • tetramethylbenzidine
Chemstrip uGK Boehringer Mannheim	strip	urine	glucose: see Chemstrip uG • ketones: see Chemstrip K
Clinistix Miles Incorporated	strip	urine	glucose oxidase • peroxide o-tolidine
Clinitest Miles Incorporated	tablet, 2 drops or 5 drops	urine	copper reduction
Combistix Miles Incorporated	strip	urine	see Hema-Combistix
Dextrostix Miles Incorporated	strip	blood	see Clinistix
Diastix Miles Incorporated	strip	urine	glucose oxidase • peroxidase • potassium iodide • chromogen
Glucometer Elite Test Strips Miles Incorporated	strip	blood	glucose oxidase

DIABETES MONITORING PRODUCTS — continued

Indication Of Product Deterioration	Time Needed to Evaluate (seconds)	Drug Interference	Comments[a]
tan-to-brown discoloration or darkening	30	some false (+)	tests for ketones • requires dropper and clean, white paper
discoloration or darkening of reagent area	60	some false (+) • some masking of color development	tests for protein • match strip to color blocks
see Multistix 10 SG	see Multistix 10 SG	see Multistix 10 SG	tests for glucose, protein, pH, blood, ketones, & bilirubin
discoloration of test area	60 (dip & read)	phenazopyridine • mesna	tests for specific gravity, leukocytes, nitrite, pH, protein, glucose, ketones, urobilinogen, bilirubin, & blood
discoloration of test area	60 (dip & read)	phenazopyridine	tests for glucose & protein
discoloration of test area	1-60 (dip & read)	no false (+) for glucose	tests for glucose, protein, pH, blood, ketones, bilirubin, urobilinogen & leukocytes
see Chemstrip 10 With SG	see Chemstrip 10 With SG	see Chemstrip 10 With SG	tests for leukocytes, nitrite, pH, protein, glucose, ketones, urobilinogen, bilirubin, & blood
darkening of test area	120-180	no false (+) • possibly some false (-)	tests for glucose • requires drop of blood on both zones of the test strip • requires cotton ball to wipe off blood after 60 seconds
discoloration of test area	60	no false (+) • possibly some false (-)	tests for glucose • convenient for type II diabetics • not quantitative
discoloration of test area	60	ketones: false (+) possible but rare • glucose: no false (+), some false (-) possible	tests for glucose & ketones
discoloration of test area	60 (dip & read)	mesna	tests for ketones
discoloration of test area	60 (dip & read)		tests for glucose
discoloration of test area	60 (dip & read)	mesna	tests for glucose & ketones
tan or dark test area	10	no false (+) • some false (-) (levodopa, ascorbic acid, aspirin)	tests for glucose • convenient for type II diabetics • not quantitative
deep blue tablet	15	false (+) in presence of reducing agents • no false (-)	tests for glucose • most reliable at high glucose levels • use for "sliding scale" • use for type I • requires water dropper and test tube
see Hema-Combistix	see Hema-Combistix	see Hema-Combistix	tests for glucose, protein, & pH
test area does not resemble "0" on color chart	60	no false (+) • some false (-)	tests for glucose • useful in screening • accurate if read by dextrometer • can use to correlate blood and urine levels
variation from light blue or "neg" on color chart	30	no false (+) • some complete false (-) (levodopa, ascorbic acid, aspirin)	tests for glucose • under-reading possible at high glucose levels • for use by both type I and type II
	60		test for glucose

DIABETES MONITORING PRODUCTS — continued

Product Manufacturer	Product Form	Biological Fluid Tested	Active Ingredients
Glucostix Miles Incorporated	strip	blood	glucose oxidase • peroxidase • ortho-tolidine dihydrochloride
Hema-Combistix Miles Incorporated	strip	urine	pH: methyl red • bromthymol blue • protein: tetrabromphenol blue • buffer • glucose: glucose oxidase • peroxidase • potassium iodide • buffer • blood: disopropylbenzene dihydroperoxide • 5,5'-tetramethylbenzidine • buffer
Keto-Diastix Miles Incorporated	strip	urine	glucose oxidase • nitroprusside
Ketostix Miles Incorporated	strip	urine	nitroprusside
Labstix Miles Incorporated	strip	urine	glucose oxidase • nitroprusside
Multistix Miles Incorporated	strip	urine	see Multistix 10 SG
Multistix 10 SG Miles Incorporated	strip	urine	glucose: glucose oxidase • peroxidase • potassium iodide • buffer • bilirubin: 2,4-dichloroaniline diazonium salt • buffer • ketone: sodium nitroprusside • buffer • specific gravity: bromthymol blue • poly (methyl vinyl ether/maleic anhydride) • sodium hydroxide • blood: disopropylbenzene dihydroperoxide • 5.5'-tetramethylbenzidine • buffer • pH: methyl red • bromthymol blue • protein: tetrabromphenol blue • buffer • urobilinogen: p-diethylaminobenzaldehyde • nitrite: p-arsanilic acid • 1,2,3, 4-tetrahydrobenzo(h)-quinolin-3-ol • buffer • leukocytes: derivatized pyrrole amino acid ester • diazonium salt • buffer
Multistix 2 Miles Incorporated	stick	urine	see Multistix 10 SG
Multistix 7 Miles Incorporated	stick	urine	see Multistix 10 SG
Multistix 8 SG Miles Incorporated	stick	urine	see Multistix 10 SG
Multistix 9 Miles Incorporated	stick	urine	see Multistix 10 SG
Multistix 9 SG Miles Incorporated	stick	urine	see Multistix 10 SG
Multistix SG Miles Incorporated	stick	urine	see Multistix 10 SG
N-Multistix Miles Incorporated	strip	urine	see Multistix 10 SG
N-Multistix SG Miles Incorporated	stick	urine	see Multistix 10 SG
Tes-Tape (Glucose Enzymatic Test Strip) Eli Lilly	strip	urine	glucose oxidase • peroxidase • o-tolidine • yellow dye
Tracer bG Reagent Boehringer Mannheim	strip	blood	

[a] Protect all products from light, heat, & moisture.

DIABETES MONITORING PRODUCTS — continued

Indication Of Product Deterioration	Time Needed to Evaluate (seconds)	Drug Interference	Comments[a]
discoloration or darkening of reagent area	30-90	some slightly lower results	tests for glucose
discoloration or darkening of test area	proper read time is critical for optimal results • glucose: 30 • blood: 60 • protein & pH: up to 120	no false (+) for glucose • some false (+) • some false (-) • color may be masked	tests for glucose, pH, protein, & blood
glucose area green; ketone area darkened	15-30	no false (+) for glucose • some false (-)	tests for glucose and ketones
tan or brown	15	false (+) possible but rare (levodopa)	tests for acetoacetic acid • useful in determining whether or not a diabetic is developing ketoacidosis
discoloration of test area	30-60 (dip and read)	no false (+) for glucose • some false (-)	tests for blood, pH, glucose, ketones & protein
see Multistix 10 SG	see Multistix 10 SG	see Multistix 10 SG	tests for glucose, protein, pH, bilirubin, & urobiligin
discoloration or darkening of test area	proper read time is critical for optimal results • glucose & bilirubin: 30 • ketone: 40 • specific gravity: 45 • urobilinogen, blood & nitrite: 60 • leukocytes: 120 • pH & protein: up to 120	no false (+) for glucose • some false (+) • some false (-) • color may be masked	test for glucose, bilirubin, ketones, specific gravity, blood, pH, protein, urobilinogen, nitrite, & leukocytes
see Multistix 10 SG	see Multistix 10 SG	see Multistix 10 SG	tests for nitrite & leukocytes
see Multistix 10 SG	see Multistix 10 SG	see Multistix 10 SG	tests for glucose, protein, pH, blood, ketones, nitrite, & leukocytes
see Multistix 10 SG	see Multistix 10 SG	see Multistix 10 SG	tests for glucose, protein, pH, blood, ketones, nitrite, leukocytes, & specific gravity
see Multistix 10 SG	see Multistix 10 SG	see Multistix 10 SG	tests for glucose, protein, pH, blood, ketones, bilirubin, urobilinogen, & nitrite
see Multistix 10 SG	see Multistix 10 SG	see Multistix 10 SG	tests for glucose, protein, pH, blood, ketones, bilirubin, nitrite, & specific gravity
see Multistix 10 SG	see Multistix 10 SG	see Multistix 10 SG	tests for glucose, protein, pH, blood, ketones, bilirubin, urobilinogen, leukocytes, & specific gravity
see Multistix 10 SG	see Multistix 10 SG	see Multistix 10 SG	tests for glucose, protein, pH, blood, ketones, bilirubin, & nitrite
see Multistix 10 SG	see Multistix 10 SG	see Multistix 10 SG	tests for glucose, protein, pH, blood, ketones, bilirubin, urobilinogen, nitrite, & specific gravity
brown color or doesn't resemble "O" on test with distilled water	50	no false (+) • some partial false (-) (levodopa, ascorbic acid, aspirin)	convenient for home and travel • accuracy adequate if all 3+ read as 4+ • not as quantitative as Diastix or Clinitest
			tests for glucose

MISCELLANEOUS DIABETES PRODUCTS

Product & Manufacturer	Comments
Auto-Lancet Palco	comes with 1 regular and 1 deep tip guard, 2 lancets, case • guard screws on • 5-year warranty
Autolet Lite Clinisafe Ulsters Scientific	professional lancet device for clinically safer blood sampling • ejection of both unilet lancet and platform after each use at a push of a button • separate depth platforms for patient comfort and optimum blood volume
B-D Autolance Becton Dickinson	one-piece construction • automatic, precisely controlled skin penetration • for use only with 23 gauge B-D Micro-Fine Lancets (5 starter B-D Micro-Fine Lancets included)
Clinilog Miles Incorporated	a diary to record date, urine sugars, urine acetone and remarks • glossary of terms • diet information
Dialet Home Diagnostics	pen-shaped • comes with one regular, one deep tip • for safety, blue dot appears when device is armed
Glucolet Automatic Device Ames	comes with 10 Unilet Lancing lancets, one opaque regular puncture endcap • multilingual instruction insert
Glucometer Elite Diabetes Care System Miles Incorporated	battery powered, technique-independent monitor • digital display • built-in timer • uses Glucometer Elite test strips
Glucometer III Miles Incorporated	battery powered reflectance photometer • digital display • built-in timer • used with Gluco Film reagents
Hypolet Auto Lancet Device British-Amer. Medical	pen-shaped • clear guard for adults • colored guard for children
Medi-Let Medicore	kit includes device • comes with 20 platforms, two depths, and 10 lancets • patented lancet ejector arm • uses all lancets except B-D Autolance
MediSense Lancing Device MediSense	lightweight, ultra TLC lancets • provides controlled depth penetration • 5-year warranty • pen-shaped
Monolets Kendall-Futuro	a plastic-covered lance that is used with the Monojector or by itself to assist diabetic patients in getting a drop of blood for blood glucose self-monitoring • monolets are the original "universal fit" lancet
Penlet II Automatic Blood Sampling Device LifeScan	pen-shaped • "hands-off" lancet removal system to minimize possibility of accidental lancet "sticks" • comes with LifeScan lancets and two different caps to control the depth of penetration
Urine Specimen Jars Various Manufacturers	pharmacists should keep available for diabetic patients and encourage patients to take urine specimens when seeing their physicians

FOOD SUPPLEMENT PRODUCTS

	Product & Manufacturer	Dosage Form	Calories (per ml)	Protein[a] (g)	Carbohydrate[a] (g)	Fat[a] (g)	Vitamins, Minerals	Comments[e]
	Alitra Q Ross	individual packet	1	15.8/packet	49.5/packet	4.65/packet	various [b,c,d] • glutamine, 21.3/1500calories • arginine • carnitine • taurine	elemental nutrition with glutamine • 5 servings = 100% vitamin RDA • 300calories/packet
CO GL LA PU SU	**Casec** Mead Johnson Nutrit'l	powder	3.7/g	88/100g		2/100g		calcium caseinate
CO LA	**CitriSource** Sandoz Nutrition	liquid	0.76	37	150	0	various [b,c,d]	
CO GL LA	**Citrotein** Sandoz Nutrition	powder	0.66	41	122	1.6	various [b,c,d]	
LA	**Compleat Modified Formula** Sandoz Nutrition	liquid	1.07	43/L	140/L	37/L	various [b,c,d]	
	Compleat Regular Formula Sandoz Nutrition	liquid	1.07	43/L	130/L	43/L	various [b,c,d]	milk base
CO LA SU	**Criticare HN** Mead Johnson Nutrit'l	liquid	1.06	38/L	222/L	5.3/L	various [b]	
	Egg Nog Sandoz Nutrition	powder	1.2	62.3/L	154/L	37.5/L	various [b]	prepare with whole milk
LA	**Ensure** Ross	liquid	1.06	8.8/8fl oz	34.3/8fl oz	8.8/8fl oz	various [b,c,d]	
GL LA	**Ensure** Ross	powder	1.06	8.8/8fl oz	34.3/8fl oz	8.8/8fl oz	various [b,c,d]	
LA	**Ensure HN** Ross	liquid	1.06	10.5/8fl oz	33.4/8fl oz	8.4/8fl oz	various [b,c,d]	high nitrogen
LA	**Ensure Plus** Ross	liquid	1.5	13.0/8fl oz	47.3/8fl oz	12.6/8fl oz	various [b,c,d]	high calorie
LA	**Ensure Plus HN** Ross	liquid	1.5	14.8/8fl oz	47.3/8fl oz	11.8/8fl oz	various [b,c,d] • l-carnitine, 0.038g/8fl oz • taurine, 0.038g/8fl oz	high nitrogen • high calorie
GL	**Ensure Pudding** Ross	pudding	250	6.8/5oz	34.0/5oz	9.7/5oz	various [b,c,d]	complete RDA
LA	**Ensure w/Fiber** Ross	liquid	1.1	9.4/8fl oz	38.3/8fl oz	8.8/8fl oz	various [b,c,d]	3.4g dietary fiber/8fl oz
LA SU	**Fibersource** Sandoz Nutrition	liquid	1.2	43	170	41	various [b,c,d]	contains fiber
LA SU	**Fibersource HN** Sandoz Nutrition	liquid	1.2	53	160	41	various [b,c,d]	contains fiber
LA	**Forta Drink** Ross	powder	85/0.8 oz mix	5/0.8 oz mix	15/0.8 oz mix	<1/0.8 oz mix	various [b,c,d]	lactose free
	Forta Shake Ross	powder	140/1.4 oz mix	9/1.4 oz mix	26/1.4 oz mix	<1/1.4 oz mix	various [b,c,d]	milk base
	Frozen Nutritious Pudding Sandoz Nutrition	pudding	1.67	60/L	233/L	53/L	various [b]	
	Glucerna Ross	liquid	1	9.9/8fl oz	22.2/8fl oz	13.2/8fl oz	various [b,c,d]	for patients with abnormal glucose tolerance • high fiber • RDA
	Health Shake Sandoz Nutrition	liquid	1.58	50.9/L	271/L	33.9/L	various [b,c]	
LA	**High Protein Broth** Sandoz Nutrition	powder	0.67	39/L	122/L	2.3/L		prepare with water

FOOD SUPPLEMENT PRODUCTS — continued

	Product & Manufacturer	Dosage Form	Calories (per ml)	Protein[a] (g)	Carbo-hydrate[a] (g)	Fat[a] (g)	Vitamins, Minerals	Comments[e]
LA	High Protein Gelatin Sandoz Nutrition	powder	1.2	99.6/L	215.8/L	3.32/L		prepare with water
LA SU	Impact Sandoz Nutrition	liquid	1	56	130	28	various [b,c,d]	contains RNA, arginine & fish oil
LA SU	Impact with Fiber Sandoz Nutrition	liquid	1	56	140	28	various [b,c,d]	contains RNA, arginine & fish oil • contains soluble & insoluble fiber
	Instant Breakfast Sandoz Nutrition	liquid	1.04	50/L	137.6/L	33.4/L	various [b]	
	Instant Breakfast Sandoz Nutrition	powder	1.2	63	156	38	various [b]	prepare with whole milk
	Introlite Ross	liquid	0.53	22.2/liter	70.5/liter	18.4/liter	various [b,c,d]	for introductory tube feeding • 700 calories = 100% USRDA
CO LA SU	Isocal Mead Johnson Nutrit'l	liquid	1.06	34/L	135/L	44/L	various [b,c]	
CO LA SU	Isocal HCN Mead Johnson Nutrit'l	liquid	2	75/L	200/L	102/L	various [b,c]	
CO LA	Isocal HN Mead Johnson Nutrit'l	liquid	1.06	44/L	123/L	45/L	various [b,c]	
LA SU	Isosource Sandoz Nutrition	liquid	1.2	43	170	41	various [b,c,d]	
LA SU	Isosource HN Sandoz Nutrition	liquid	1.2	53	160	41	various [b,c,d]	
GL LA	Isotein HN Sandoz Nutrition	powder	1.19	68/L	160/L	34/L	various [b,c,d]	
LA	Jevity Ross	liquid	1.06	10.5/8fl oz	35.9/8fl oz	8.7/8fl oz	various [b,c,d] • l-carnitine, 0.027g/8fl oz • taurine, 0.027g/8fl oz	added fiber • high nitrogen
CO LA	Lipisorb Mead Johnson Nutrit'l	liquid	1.35	57/L	161/L	57/L	various [b,c]	
CO GL LA PU	Lipisorb Mead Johnson Nutrit'l	powder	5.39/g	16.5/100g	54/100g	23/100g	various [b]	
CO GL PU SU	Lonalac Mead Johnson Nutrit'l	powder	1.01	53.7/L	75.5/L	55.7/L	various [b,c]	milk base • low sodium
CO LA SU	MCT Oil Mead Johnson Nutrit'l	oil	8.3/g			100/100g		
GL	Meritene Sandoz Nutrition	powder	1.06	69	120	34	various [b,c,d]	milk base
	Milk Shake Sandoz Nutrition	powder	1.58	50.9/L	271/L	33.9/L	various [b]	prepare with whole milk
	Milk Shake Plus Sandoz Nutrition	powder	1.2	63/L	156/L	38/L	various [b]	prepare with whole milk
CO GL LA PU SU	Moducal Mead Johnson Nutrit'l	powder	3.8/g		95/100g			maltodextrin
LA	Nepro Ross	liquid	2	16.6/8fl oz	51.1/8fl oz	22.7/8fl oz	various [b,c,d] • l-carnitine, 0.062g/8fl oz • taurine, 0.062g/8fl oz	for dialyzed patients with renal failure
	Nutritious Pudding Sandoz Nutrition	powder	1.67	60/L	233/L	53.4/L	various [b]	prepare with whole milk

FOOD SUPPLEMENT PRODUCTS — continued

	Product & Manufacturer	Dosage Form	Calories (per ml)	Protein[a] (g)	Carbo-hydrate[a] (g)	Fat[a](g)	Vitamins, Minerals	Comments[e]
LA	Osmolite Ross	liquid	1.06	8.8/8fl oz	34.3/8fl oz	9.1/8fl oz	various [b,c,d] • l-carnitine, 0.019g/8fl oz • taurine, 0.019g/8fl oz	isotonic
LA	Osmolite HN Ross	liquid	1.06	10.5/8fl oz	33.4/8fl oz	8.7/8fl oz	various [b,c,d] • l-carnitine, 0.027g/8fl oz • taurine, 0.027g/8fl oz	high nitrogen • isotonic
LA PE	PediaSure Ross	liquid	1	7.1/8fl oz	26/8fl oz	11.8/8fl oz	various [b,c,d] • l-carnitine, 0.004g/8fl oz • taurine, 0.017g/8fl oz	for children 1-6 years old • 1000ml =100% RDA
	Perative Ross	liquid	1.3	15.8/8fl oz	42.0/8fl oz	8.8/8fl oz	various [b,c,d] • l-carnitine, 0.031g/8fl oz • taurine, 0.031g/8fl oz	for management of metabolically stressed patients • 1500 calories=100% USRDA
GL PU SO	Peridin-C Beutlich	tablet					ascorbic acid • hesperidin complex • hesperidin methyl • chalcone	
LA	Polycose Ross	liquid	2		50g/100ml			glucose polymers to supply carbohydrate calories
LA	Polycose Ross	powder	2		50g/100ml			glucose polymers to supply carbohydrate calories
CO GL LA	Precision High Nitrogen Diet Sandoz Nutrition	powder	1.05	44	216	1.3	various [b,c,d]	
CO GL LA	Precision Isotonic Diet Sandoz Nutrition	powder	1	29	144	30	various [b,c,d]	
CO GL LA	Precision LR Diet Sandoz Nutrition	powder	1.6	26	248	1.6	various [b,c,d]	
	Pro Mod Ross	powder	28/6.6g (scoop)	5/6.6g (scoop)	<0.67g/6.6g (scoop)	<0.6g/6.6g (scoop)		protein supplement
LA	Promote Ross	liquid	1	14.8/8fl oz	30.8/8fl oz	6.2/8fl oz	various [b,c,d] • l-carnitine, 0.029g/8fl oz • taurine, 0.029g/8fl oz	high protein
LA	Pulmocare Ross	liquid	1.5	14.8/8fl oz	25/8fl oz	21.8/8fl oz	various [b,c,d]	for pulmonary patients
CO LA	Resource Sandoz Nutrition	liquid	1.06	37	140	37	various [b,c,d]	
CO GL LA	Resource Crystals Sandoz Nutrition	powder	1.06	37	140	37	various [b,c,d]	
CO LA	Resource Plus Sandoz Nutrition	liquid	1.5	55	200	53	various [b,c,d]	
	Resource Shake Sandoz Nutrition	liquid	1.5	50.9/L	254/L	33.9/L	various [b]	<1g of lactose/serving
GL LA SU	Stresstein Sandoz Nutrition	powder	1.21	70/L	170/L	28/L	various [b,c,d]	for severe metabolic stress and trauma
	Suplena Ross	liquid	2	7.1/8fl oz	60.6/8fl oz	22.7/8fl oz	various [b,c,d] • l-carnitine, 0.038g/8fl oz • taurine, 0.038g/8fl oz	for dietary management of renal patients prone to uremia • 1900 calories=100% USRDA
CO LA	Sustacal Mead Johnson Nutrit'l	liquid	1.01	61/L	140/L	23/L	various [b]	

FOOD SUPPLEMENT PRODUCTS — continued

	Product & Manufacturer	Dosage Form	Calories (per ml)	Protein[a] (g)	Carbo-hydrate[a] (g)	Fat[a](g)	Vitamins, Minerals	Comments[e]
CO GL PU	**Sustacal** Mead Johnson Nutrit'l	pudding	1.7/g	6.8/5oz	32/5oz	9.5/5oz	various [b]	milk base
CO GL LA PU	**Sustacal** Mead Johnson Nutrit'l	powder	1.1	79/L	180/L	2.6/L	various [b]	mix with skim milk
CO LA	**Sustacal 8.8** Mead Johnson Nutrit'l	liquid	1.06	37/L	148/L	35/L	various [b]	
CO LA	**Sustacal HC** Mead Johnson Nutrit'l	liquid	1.5	61/L	190/L	58/L	various [b]	
CO LA	**Sustacal with Fiber** Mead Johnson Nutrit'l	liquid	1.06	46/L	140/L	35/L	various [b]	
GL PU	**Sustagen** Mead Johnson Nutrit'l	powder	1.8	115/L	317/L	16.8/L	various [b]	milk base
CO GL LA SU	**Tolerex** Sandoz Nutrition	powder	1	21	230	1.5	various [b,c,d]	elemental diet containing 100% free amino acids
CO LA	**TraumaCal** Mead Johnson Nutrit'l	liquid	1.5	83/L	145/L	68/L	various [b]	
LA	**Two Cal HN** Ross	liquid	2	19.8/8fl oz	51.4/8fl oz	21.5/8fl oz	various [b,c,d]	high calorie • high nitrogen
CO LA	**Ultracal** Mead Johnson Nutrit'l	liquid	1.06	44/L	123/L	45/L	various [b,c]	
LA	**Vital High Nitrogen** Ross	individual packet	1	12.5/packet	55.4/packet	3.25/packet	various [b,c,d]	for patients with limited digestion, absorption • 300 calories/packet
CO GL LA SU	**Vivonex T.E.N.** Sandoz Nutrition	powder	1	38	210	2.8	various [b,c,d]	high nitrogen elemental diet containing 100% free amino acids enriched with glutamine

[a] Unless otherwise specified, content given in grams per liter. Powder products must be added to liquid as package directs.
[b] Includes vitamins A, D, E, ascorbic acid, thiamine, riboflavin, niacin, pyridoxine hydrochloride, cyanocobalamin, and/or various other substances having vitamin activity.
[c] Includes iron, calcium, phosphorus, iodine, magnesium, copper, zinc, potassium, sodium, manganese, chromium, selenium, and/or molybdenum.
[d] Includes choline, biotin, inositol, and/or folic acid.
[e] All products are for enteral use only.

IRON PRODUCTS

Product & Manufacturer	Iron (elemental)	Vitamins & Nutrients	Other Ingredients
Albee C-800 Plus Iron Tablets A.H. Robins	27mg (as ferrous fumarate)	E, 45 IU • B_1, 15mg • B_2, 17mg • B_6, 25mg • B_{12}, 12mcg • C, 800mg • folic acid, 0.4mg • niacin, 100mg • pantothenic acid, 25mg	
Femiron Multivitamins and Iron Menley & James	20mg (as ferrous fumarate)		alginic acid • calcium phosphate • FD&C red#40 • starch
Feosol Capsules SmithKline Beecham	50mg (as ferrous sulfate)		
Feosol Elixir SmithKline Beecham	44mg/5ml (as ferrous sulfate)		alcohol, 5%
Feosol Tablets SmithKline Beecham	65mg (as ferrous sulfate)		
Feostat Chewable Tablets Forest	33mg (as ferrous fumarate)		flavor
Feostat Drops Forest	15mg/0.6ml (as ferrous fumarate)		flavor
Feostat Suspension Forest	33mg/5ml (as ferrous fumarate)		flavor
GL PU SU **Fer-In-Sol Iron Capsules** Mead Johnson Nutrit'l	60mg (as ferrous sulfate)		
LA SL PE **Fer-In-Sol Iron Drops** Mead Johnson Nutrit'l	15mg/0.6ml (as ferrous sulfate)		alcohol, 0.2%
LA SL PE **Fer-In-Sol Iron Syrup** Mead Johnson Nutrit'l	18mg/5ml (as ferrous sulfate)		alcohol, 5%
Fergon Tablets Sterling Health	36mg (as ferrous gluconate)		
Fero-Grad-500 Tablets Abbott	105mg (as ferrous sulfate)	sodium ascorbate, 500mg	cellulosic polymers • D&C red#7 • FD&C blue#1 • magnesium stearate • methyl acrylate-methyl methacrylate copolymers • polyethylene glycol • povidone • pregelatinized starch (contains cornstarch) • propylene glycol • talc • titanium dioxide • vanillin
Fero-Gradumet Tablets Abbott	105mg (as ferrous sulfate)		castor oil • cellulosic polymers • FD&C red#40 • FD&C yellow#6 • magnesium stearate • methyl acrylate-methyl methacrylate copolymers • polyethylene glycol • povidone • propylene glycol • titanium dioxide • vanillin
Ferra-TD Capsules Goldline	50mg (as ferrous sulfate)		
GL PU SU **Ferro-Sequels Tablets** Lederle	50mg (as ferrous fumarate)		docusate sodium, 100mg
Ferrous Fumarate Tablets Various Manufacturers	106mg (as ferrous fumarate)		
Ferrous Gluconate Capsules Various Manufacturers	38mg (as ferrous gluconate)		
Ferrous Gluconate Tablets Various Manufacturers	35mg (as ferrous gluconate)		

IRON PRODUCTS — continued

	Product & Manufacturer	Iron (elemental)	Vitamins & Nutrients	Other Ingredients
	Ferrous Sulfate Capsules Various Manufacturers	30mg; 50mg (as ferrous sulfate)		
	Ferrous Sulfate Elixir Various Manufacturers	44mg/5ml (as ferrous sulfate)		
	Ferrous Sulfate Tablets Various Manufacturers	60mg; 65mg (as ferrous sulfate)		
	Generet-500 Tablets Goldline	105mg (as ferrous sulfate)	B_1, 6mg • B_2, 6mg • B_6, 5mg • B_{12}, 25mcg • niacin, 30mg • pantothenic acid, 10mg • sodium ascorbate, 500mg	
	Geriot Tablets Goldline	50mg (as ferrous sulfate)	B_1, 5mg • B_2, 5mg • B_6, 0.5mg • B_{12}, 3mcg • niacin, 30mg • pantothenic acid, 2mg • sodium ascorbate, 75mg	
GL PU	**Hytinic Capsules** Hyrex	150mg (as polysaccharide-iron complex)		sodium, 0.2mEq
LA SU SL	**Hytinic Injections** Hyrex	ferrous gluconate, 25mg/ml	cyanocobolamin, 15mcg • liver, 1mcg • riboflavin, 0.75mg • calcium • pantothenate, 1.25mg • niacinamide, 50mg • citric acid, 8.2mg	• sodium citrate, 11.8mg • procaine 2% • benzyl • alcohol 2% • sodium hydroxide
	Iberet Liquid Abbott	78.75mg/15ml (as ferrous sulfate)	B_1, 4.5mg/15ml • B_2, 4.5mg/15ml • B_6, 3.75mg/15ml • B_{12}, 18.75mcg/15ml • C, 112.5mg/15ml • niacinamide, 22.5mg/15ml • dexpanethol, 7.5mg/15ml	sorbitol • parabens • alcohol, 1% • raspberry/mint flavor • water
	Iberet Filmtabs Abbott	105mg (as ferrous sulfate)	B_1, 6mg • B_2, 6mg • B_6, 5mg • B_{12}, 25mcg • sodium ascorbate, 150mg • niacinamide, 30mg • calcium pantothenate, 10mg	albumen • castor oil • cellulosic polymers • cornstarch • FD&C red#40 • FD&C yellow#6 • iron oxide • magnesium stearate • methyl acrylate-methyl methacrylate copolymers • polyethylene glycol • povidone • stearic acid • talc • titanium dioxide • vanillin
	Iberet-500 Liquid Abbott	78.75mg/15ml (as ferrous sulfate)	B_1, 4.5mg/15ml • B_2, 4.5mg/15ml • B6, 3.75mg/15ml • B_{12}, 18.75mcg/15ml • C, 375mg/15ml • niacinamide, 22.5mg/15ml • dexpanethol, 7.5mg/15ml	sorbitol • parabens • citrus flavor • glycerin • propylene glycol • sodium bicarbonate • sucrose • water
	Iberet-500 Filmtabs Abbott	105mg (as ferrous sulfate)	B_1, 6mg • B_2, 6mg • B_6, 5mg • B_{12}, 25mcg • sodium ascorbate, 500mg • niacinamide, 30mg • calcium pantothenate, 10mg	castor oil • cellulose polymers • cornstarch • FD&C red#40 • FD&C yellow#6 • magnesium stearate methyl acrylate-methyl methacrylate copolymers • polyethylene glycol • propylene glycol • povidone • stearic acid • talc • titanium dioxide • vanillin
LA SO SL	**Incremin With Iron Syrup** Lederle	30mg/5ml (as ferric pyrophosphate)	B_1, 10mg/5ml • B_6, 5mg/5ml • B_{12}, 75mcg/5ml	l-lysin, 300mg/5ml • sorbitol • alcohol, 0.75% • cherry flavor
	Iron Plus Caplets Goldline	50mg (as ferrous fumarate)		docusate sodium, 100mg
	Irospan Capsules Fielding	60mg	ascorbic acid, 150mg	
SU	**Irospan Tablets** Fielding	60mg	ascorbic acid, 150mg	
	Mol-Iron Tablets Schering-Plough	39mg (as ferrous sulfate)		
GL PU SO SU	**Nephro-Fer Tablets** R&D Laboratories	115mg (from fumarate)		whey • ac-di-sol • starch • silica • stearic acid

IRON PRODUCTS — continued

	Product & Manufacturer	Iron (elemental)	Vitamins & Nutrients	Other Ingredients
SU	Niferex Elixir Central	20mg/ml (as polysaccharide-iron complex)		alcohol, 10%
	Niferex Tablets Central	50mg (as polysaccharide-iron complex)		
	Niferex With Vitamin C Tablets Central	50mg (as polysaccharide-iron complex)	sodium ascorbate, 168.75mg • ascorbic acid, 100mg	
	Niferex-150 Capsules Central	150mg (as polysaccharide-iron complex)		
	Rogenic Tablets Forest	60mg (as ferrous fumarate, ferrous sulfate, and ferrous gluconate)	B_6, 6mg • B_{12}, 25mcg • C, 100mg	desiccated liver, 25mg
	Simron Capsules SmithKline Beecham	10mg (as ferrous gluconate)		polysorbate 20, 400mg • FD&C red#40 • flavor • gelatin • glycerin • methylparaben • polyethylene glycol 8000 • propylparaben • simethicone • titanium dioxide • water
GL PU SO SU	Slow Fe Tablets CIBA Consumer	50mg (as ferrous sulfate)		
GL PU SO SU	Stresstabs 600 With Iron Lederle	27mg (as ferrous fumarate)	E, 30 IU • B_1, 10mg • B_2, 10mg • B_6, 5mg • B_{12}, 12mcg • C, 500mg • folic acid, 0.4mg • biotin, 45mcg • niacin, 100mg • pantothenic acid, 20mg	
	Surbex-750 With Iron Filmtabs Abbott	27mg (as ferrous sulfate)	E, 30 IU • B_1, 15mg • B_2, 15mg • B_6, 25mg • B_{12}, 12mcg • C, 750mg • folic acid, 0.4mg • niacinamide, 100mg • calcium pantothenate, 20mg	cellulosic polymers • colloidal silicon dioxide • FD&C red#3 • cornstarch • iron oxide • magnesium stearate • microcrystalline cellulose • polyethylene glycol • povidone • vanillin
SU	Theragran Stress Formula Tablets Bristol-Myers	27mg (as ferrous fumarate)	E, 30 IU • B_1, 15mg • B_2, 15mg • B_6, 25mg • B_{12}, 12mcg • C, 600mg • folic acid, 0.4mg • biotin, 45mcg • niacin, 100mg • pantothenic acid, 20mg	
AL	Troph-Iron Liquid Menley & James	20mg/5ml (as ferric pyrophosphate)	B_1, 10mg/5ml • B_{12}, 25mcg/5ml	saccharin • parabens • cherry flavor • FD&C red#40
	Vitron-C Tablets CIBA Consumer	66mg (as ferrous fumarate)	ascorbic acid, 125mg	colloidal silicon dioxide • flavor • glycine • hydroxypropyl methylcellulose • iron oxides • magnesium stearate • microcrystalline cellulose • polyethylene glycol • polysorbate 80 • povidone • saccharin sodium • talc • titanium dioxide
GL PU SO SU	Vitron-C Plus Tablets CIBA Consumer	132mg (as ferrous fumarate)	ascorbic acid, 250mg	castor oil • colloidal silicon dioxide • FD&C blue#1 lake • FD&C red#40 • FD&C yellow#6 lake • hydroxypropyl cellulose • hydroxypropyl methylcellulose • lactose anhydrous • polyethylene gylcol • povidone • pregelatinized starch • propylene glycol • shellac • stearic acid • titanium dioxide

CALCIUM PRODUCTS

	Product & Manufacturer	Dosage Form	Calcium	Vitamin D	Other Ingredients
	Calcarb 600 Various Manufacturers	tablet	600mg		
	Calcarb 600 + D Various Manufacturers	tablet	600mg	125 IU	
GL PU SO	**Calci-Chew** R&D Laboratories	chewable tablet	500mg (from carbonate)		sugar • cherry flavor • citric acid • stearic acid • silica • magnesium stearate
GL PU SO SU	**Calci-Mix** R&D Laboratories	capsule	500mg (from carbonate)		talc
	Calcium Various Manufacturers	tablet	600mg		
SO SU	**Calcium 600** Schein	tablet	600mg (from carbonate)		gelatin • microcrystalline cellulose • hydroxypropyl methylcellulose • stearic acid • magnesium stearate • cellulose gum • sodium lauryl sulfate • polyethylene glycol • mineral oil • titanium dioxide • polysorbitol • artificial color (blue#2, red#40, yellow#6)
	Calcium Carbonate Various Manufacturers	tablet	260mg and 500mg (from carbonate)		
SU	**Calcium Carbonate** Roxane	suspension	500mg/5ml (from carbonate)		sorbitol • propylene glycol • methylparaben • propylparaben • flavoring • sodium hypochlorite • water • xanthan gum
	Calcium Gluconate Various Manufacturers	tablet	45mg; 58.5mg; 87.75mg; 90mg (all from gluconate)		
	Calcium Lactate Various Manufacturers	tablet	42.25mg; 84.5mg (from lactate)		
SU	**Calcium Oyster Shell** Schein	tablet	500mg		oyster shell • cellulose • hydroxypropyl methylcellulose • hydroxypropyl cellulose • crospovidone • silica • polyethylene glycol • stearic acid • magnesium stearate • pharmaceutical glaze
SO SU	**Calcium With Vitamin D** Schein	tablet	600mg (as calcium carbonate)	125 IU	gelatin • microcrystalline cellulose • hydroxypropyl methylcellulose • stearic acid • magnesium stearate • cellulose gum • sodium lauryl sulfate • polyethylene glycol • mineral oil • titanium dioxide • polysorbitol • artificial color (blue#2, red#40, yellow#6)
	Calcium plus Vitamin D Various Manufacturers	tablet	600mg	125 IU	
SU	**Calel-D** Rhone-Poulenc Rorer	chewable tablet	500mg/tablet	200 IU/tablet	cornstarch • croscarmellose sodium • hydroxypropyl methylcellulose • propylene glycol • calcium stearate

CALCIUM PRODUCTS — continued

	Product & Manufacturer	Dosage Form	Calcium	Vitamin D	Other Ingredients
GL PU SO SU	**Caltrate** Lederle	tablet	600mg (from carbonate)		
GL PU SO SU	**Caltrate 600 + D** Lederle	tablet	600mg (from carbonate)	125 IU	
GL PU SO SU	**Caltrate 600 + Iron** Lederle	tablet	600mg (from carbonate)	125 IU	iron, 18mg
	Caltro Geneva	tablet	250mg	125 IU	
	Dical-D Abbott	tablet	117mg	133 IU	phosphorus, 90mg • microcrystalline cellulose • sodium starch glycolate • cornstarch • hydrogenated vegetable oil wax • magnesium stearate • talc
	Dical-D Abbott	wafer	464mg	200 IU	phosphorus, 0.18g • sucrose • dextrose • talc • stearic acid • mineral oil • salt • natural and artificial flavorings
GL PU SU	**Florical** Mericon	capsule	145.6mg (from carbonate)		sodium flouride, 8.3mg
SO SU GE	**Gerimed** Fielding	tablet	carbonate, 200mg • phosphate (dibasic), 600mg	400 IU	vitamin A, 5000 IU • vitamin E, 30 IU • vitamin C, 120mg • niacinamide, 25mg • zinc, 15mg • vitamin B_1 (thiamine), 3mg • vitamin B_2 (riboflavin), 3mg • vitamin B_6 (pyridoxine), 2mg • vitamin B_{12}, 6mcg
GL PU SO SU	**Nephro-Calci** R&D Laboratories	tablet	600mg (from carbonate)		sodium starch glycolate • stearic acid • magnesium stearate
	Os-Cal 250 + D SmithKline Beecham	tablet	250mg	125 IU	
	Os-Cal 500 SmithKline Beecham	chewable tablet	500mg (from carbonate)		
	Os-Cal 500 + D SmithKline Beecham	tablet	500mg	125 IU	
	Os-Cal Forte SmithKline Beecham	tablet	250mg	125 USP units	vitamin A (palmitate) • thiamine mononitrate • riboflavin • pyridoxine hydrochloride • ascorbic acid di-alpha tocopherol acetate • niacinamide • iron • magnesium • manganese • zinc
	Os-Cal Plus SmithKline Beecham	tablet	elemental calcium, 250mg	125 USP units	vitamin A • vitamin C • vitamin B_2 • vitamin B_1 • vitamin B_6 • niacinamide • iron • zinc • manganese
	Oyst-Cal 500 Goldline	tablet	500mg (from carbonate)		
	Oyst-Cal D Various Manufacturers	tablet	500mg	125 IU	
	Oyst-Cal-D Goldline	tablet	250mg	125 IU	tartrazine

CALCIUM PRODUCTS — continued

Product & Manufacturer	Dosage Form	Calcium	Vitamin D	Other Ingredients
Oyster Shell Calcium Various Manufacturers	tablet	1250mg		
Oyster Shell Calcium + Vitamin D Reese Chemical	tablet	1200mg	250 USP units	
Oyster Shell Calcium Plus Vitamin D Various Manufacturers	tablet	500mg	125 IU	
GL SU **Posture** Whitehall	tablet	600mg (as phosphate)		
GL SU **Posture D** Whitehall	tablet	600mg (as phosphate)	125 IU	

MULTIPLE VITAMIN PRODUCTS

Product & Manufacturer	Vitamin A (IU)	Vitamin D (IU)	Vitamin E (IU)	Ascorbic Acid (C) (mg)	Thiamine (B$_1$) (mg)	Riboflavin (B$_2$) (mg)	Niacin (mg)
A.C.N. Tablets Person & Covey	25000			250			25
Albee C-800 Plus Iron Tablets A.H. Robins			45	800	15	17	100
Albee C-800 Tablets A.H. Robins			45	800	15	17	100
Albee with C Caplets A.H. Robins				300	15	10.2	50
Antioxidant Murdock	beta carotene, 15000 • fish liver oil, 5000			500			
Arbon Forest	5000	400	30	60	1.5	1.7	20
Avail Menley & James	5000	400	30	90	2.25	2.55	20
Bee-T-Vites Tablets Rugby				300	15	10	niacinamide, 100mg
Bee-Zee Tablets Rugby			45mg	600	15	10.2	100
GL **Beelith** PU **Tablets** SO Beach Pharm. SU							
Beminal-500 Tablets Whitehall				500	25	12.5	
SU **Bugs Bunny** PE **Complete** Miles Incorporated	5000 (as acetate and beta carotene)	400	30	60	1.5	1.7	20

MULTIPLE VITAMIN PRODUCTS — continued								
Pyridoxine Hydrochloride (B$_6$)(mg)	Cyanocobalamin (B$_{12}$)(mcg)	Folic Acid (mg)	Pantothenic Acid (mg)	Iron (mg)	Calcium (mg)	Phosphorous (mg)	Magnesium (mg)	Other Ingredients
25	12	0.4	25	27				
25	12		25					
5			10					saccharin • lactose
								zinc, 30mg • selenium, 200mcg • copper, 3mg • manganese, 5mg
2	6	0.4	22	18	100	80	100	copper, 2mg • zinc, 15mg • iodine, 150mcg
3	9	0.4		18	400		100	chromium • iodine • selenium • zinc, 22.5mg
5	4		20					
10	6		25					zinc, 22.5mg
20							600	
10	5							niacinamide, 100mg • calcium pantothenate, 20mg
2	6	0.4	10	18 (elemental)	100	100	20	sorbitol • sodium ascorbate • gelatin • stearic acid • natural flavors • starch • citric acid • annatto-carmine-grape skin extract colors • carrageenan • glycine • hydrogenated vegetable oil • zinc, 15mg • stearic acid glyceride • palmitic acid glyceride • malic acid • silica • xylitol • aspartame • copper, 2mg • monoammonium glycyrrhizinate • potassium iodide • biotin, 40mcg

MULTIPLE VITAMIN PRODUCTS — continued

	Product & Manufacturer	Vitamin A (IU)	Vitamin D (IU)	Vitamin E (IU)	Ascorbic Acid (C) (mg)	Thiamine (B_1) (mg)	Riboflavin (B_2) (mg)	Niacin (mg)
SU PE	**Bugs Bunny Plus Iron** Miles Incorporated	2500 (as acetate and beta carotene)	400	15	60	1.05	1.2	13.5
SU PE	**Bugs Bunny Vitamins** Miles Incorporated	2500 (as acetate and beta carotene)	400	15	60	1.05	1.2	13.5
SU PE	**Bugs Bunny with Extra C** Miles Incorporated	2500 (as acetate and beta carotene)	400	15	250	1.05	1.2	13.5
GL PU SO	**Centrum** Lederle	5000	400	30	60	1.5	17	20
	Centrum Jr. Plus Iron Chewable Tablets Lederle	5000	400	30	60	1.5	1.7	20
GL PU SO SU GE	**Centrum Silver Gel-Tabs** Lederle	6000 (as acetate and beta carotene)	400	45	60	1.5	1.7	niacinamide, 20mg

MULTIPLE VITAMIN PRODUCTS — continued

Pyridoxine Hydrochloride (B$_6$)(mg)	Cyanocobalamin (B$_{12}$)(mcg)	Folic Acid (mg)	Pantothenic Acid (mg)	Iron (mg)	Calcium (mg)	Phosphorous (mg)	Magnesium (mg)	Other Ingredients
1.05	4.5	0.3		15 (elemental)				sorbitol • sodium ascorbate • starch • stearic acid • natural flavors • gelatin • citric acid • magnesium stearate • annatto-carmine-grape skin extract colors • stearic acid glyceride • palmitic acid glyceride • malic acid • xylitol • aspartame • silica • monoammonium glycyrrhizinate
1.05	4.5	0.3						sorbitol • sodium ascorbate • starch • stearic acid • natural flavors • gelatin • citric acid • magnesium stearate • annatto-carmine-grape skin extract colors • stearic acid glyceride • palmitic acid glyceride • malic acid • xylitol • aspartame • silica • monoammonium glycyrrhizinate
1.05	4.5	0.3						sorbitol • sodium ascorbate • starch • stearic acid • natural flavors • gelatin • magnesium stearate • annatto-carmine-grape skin extract colors • stearic acid glyceride • palmitic acid glyceride • xylitol • aspartame • silica • malic acid • monoammonium glycyrrhizinate
2	6	0.4	10	18	162	109	100	biotin, 30mcg • iodine, 150mcg • copper, 2mg • zinc, 15mg • manganese, 2.5mg • potassium 40mg • chloride, 36.3mg • chromium, 25mcg • molybdenum, 25mcg • selenium, 20mcg • vitamin K, 25mcg • nickel, 5m
2	6	0.4	10	18	ns	ns	ns	chromium • copper • iodine • manganese • molybdenum • zinc, 15mg • biotin, 45mcg • vitamin K, 10mcg
3	25	0.2	10	9	200	48	100	vitamin K, 10mcg • copper, 2mg • iodine, 150mcg • zinc, 15mg • chloride, 72mg • chromium, 100mcg • manganese, 2.5mg • molybdenum, 25mcg • nickel, 5mcg • potassium, 80mg • selenium, 25mcg • silicon, 10mcg • vanadium, 10mcg

MULTIPLE VITAMIN PRODUCTS — continued

	Product & Manufacturer	Vitamin A (IU)	Vitamin D (IU)	Vitamin E (IU)	Ascorbic Acid (C) (mg)	Thiamine (B₁) (mg)	Riboflavin (B₂) (mg)	Niacin (mg)
	Cerovite Jr. Tablets Rugby	5000	400	15	60	1.5	1.7	20
SO SU	**Certagen** Goldline	5000	400	30	60	1.5	1.7	naicinamide, 20
	Cod Liver Oil Concentrate Schering-Plough	10000	400					
	Cod Liver Oil Concentrate With Vitamin C Schering-Plough	4000	200		50			
	Daily-Vite With Iron & Minerals Rugby	5000	400	30	60	1.5	1.7	20
	Dayalets Filmtabs Abbott	5000	400	30	60	1.5	1.7	20
SU	**Daylets Plus Iron Filmtabs** Abbott	5000	400	30	60	1.5	1.7	20
	Decagen Tablets Goldline	9000	400	30mg	90	10	10	20
GL PU SO SU PE	**Ecee Plus** Edwards			200	100			
	Femiron Multivitamins and Iron Menley & James	5000	400	15	60	1.5	1.7	20
GL PU SO SU	**Filibon** Lederle	5000	400	30mg	60	1.5	1.7	20

MULTIPLE VITAMIN PRODUCTS — continued

Pyridoxine Hydrochloride (B_6)(mg)	Cyanocobalamin (B_{12})(mcg)	Folic Acid (mg)	Pantothenic Acid (mg)	Iron (mg)	Calcium (mg)	Phosphorous (mg)	Magnesium (mg)	Other Ingredients
2	6	0.4	10	18			ns	copper • iodine • zinc • biotin, 45mcg
2	6	0.4	10	18	162	125	100	biotin, 30mcg • copper • zinc • iodine • manganese • potassium • chloride • chromium • molybdenum • selenium • nickel • tin • silicon • vanadium • boron
2	6	0.4	10	18	ns	ns	ns	chlorine • chromium • copper • iodine • potassium • manganese • molybdenum • selenium • zinc, 15mg • biotin, 30mcg • vitamin K, 50mcg
2	6	0.4						cellulose • hydroxypropyl methylcellulose • povidone • hydroxyl methylcellulose • magnesium stearate • FD&C red#40 • silicon dioxide • FD&C yellow#6 • vanillin
2	6	0.4		18				methylcellulose • hydroxypropyl methylcellulose • povidone • hydroxypropyl cellulose • FD&C yellow#6 • magnesium stearate • silicon dioxide • FD&C blue#2 • vanillin • titanium dioxide
5	10	0.4	20	30	ns	ns	ns	chromium • copper • iodine • potassium • manganese • molybdenum • selenium • zinc, 15mg • vitamin K, 25mcg • biotin, 45mcg
							70	zinc sulfate, 80mg
2	6	0.4	10	20				FD&C red #40 • FD&C blue #2 • calcium carbonate • microcrystalline cellulose • starch
2	6	0.4		18	125		100	iodine, 150mcg

MULTIPLE VITAMIN PRODUCTS — continued

Product & Manufacturer	Vitamin A (IU)	Vitamin D (IU)	Vitamin E (IU)	Ascorbic Acid (C) (mg)	Thiamine (B_1) (mg)	Riboflavin (B_2) (mg)	Niacin (mg)
Flintstones Complete Miles Incorporated	5000 (as acetate and beta carotene)	400	30	60	1.5	1.7	20
PE **Flintstones Plus Extra C** Miles Incorporated	2500 (as acetate and beta carotene)	400	15	250	1.05	1.2	13.5
PE **Flintstones Plus Iron** Miles Incorporated	2500 (as acetate and beta carotene)	400	15	60	1.05	1.2	13.5
PE **Flintstones Vitamins** Miles Incorporated	2500 (as acetate and beta carotene)	400	15	60	1.05	1.2	13.5
Fruity Chews Goldline	2500 (with beta carotene)	400	15mg	60	1.05	1.2	13.5
Fruity Chews With Iron Goldline	2500 (with beta carotene)	400	15mg	60	1.05	1.2	13.5
Garfield Complete Vitamins with Minerals Menley & James	5000	400	30	60	1.5	1.7	20
Garfield Vitamins Plus Extra C Menley & James	2500	400	15	250	1.05	1.2	13.5
Garfield Vitamins Plus Iron Menley & James	2500	400	15	60	1.05	1.2	13.5

MULTIPLE VITAMIN PRODUCTS — continued

Pyridoxine Hydrochloride (B$_6$)(mg)	Cyanocobalamin (B$_{12}$)(mcg)	Folic Acid (mg)	Pantothenic Acid (mg)	Iron (mg)	Calcium (mg)	Phosphorous (mg)	Magnesium (mg)	Other Ingredients
2	6	0.4	10	18 (elemental)	100	100	20	sorbitol • sodium ascorbate • gelatin • stearic acid • starch • carrageenan • hydrogenated vegetable oil • zinc, 15mg • artificial flavors including fruit acids • yellow#6 • stearic acid glyceride • palmitic acid glyceride • silica • xylitol • aspartame • copper, 2mg • monoammonium glycyrrhizinate • potassium • iodine, 150mcg • biotin
1.05	4.5	0.3						sucrose • sodium ascorbate • fructose • microcrystalline food grade cellulose • stearic acid • gelatin • magnesium stearate • malto dextrins • artificial flavors including fruit acids • starch • yellow#6 • stearic acid glyceride • palmitic acid glyceride • lactose
1.05	4.5	0.3		15 (elemental)				sucrose • sodium ascorbate • stearic acid • gelatin • artificial flavors including fruit acids • malto dextrins • magnesium stearate • yellow#6 • stearic acid glyceride • palmitic acid glyceride
1.05	4.5	0.3						sucrose • sodium ascorbate • stearic acid • gelatin • malto dextrins • artificial flavors including fruit acids • magnesium stearate • yellow#6 • stearic acid glyceride • palmitic acid glyceride
1.05	4.5	0.3						
1.05	4.5	0.3		15				zinc, 8mg • copper, 0.8mg
2	6	0.4	10	18	100	100	20	copper • iodine • zinc, 15mg • biotin, 40mcg • FD&C red#40 • FD&C blue#2 • FD&C yellow#6 • calcium phosphate • sorbitol • aspartame • flavors
1.05	4.5	0.3						FD&C red#40 • FD&C yellow#6 • FD&C blue#2 • FD&C blue#1 • sucrose • talc • flavors
1.05	4.5	0.3		15				FD&C red#40 • FD&C yellow#6 • FD&C blue#2 • FD&C blue#1 • sucrose • talc • flavors

MULTIPLE VITAMIN PRODUCTS — continued

	Product & Manufacturer	Vitamin A (IU)	Vitamin D (IU)	Vitamin E (IU)	Ascorbic Acid (C) (mg)	Thiamine (B_1) (mg)	Riboflavin (B_2) (mg)	Niacin (mg)
	Garfield Vitamins, Regular Menley & James	2500	400	15	60	1.05	1.2	13.5
	Gen-Bee with C Goldline				300	15	10.2	50
	Generix-T Goldline	10000	400	5.5	150	15	10	100
SO SU GE	**Gerimed** Fielding	5000	400	30	120	3	3	25
LA SL GE	**Geriplex-FS** Parke-Davis					0.2/5ml	0.28/5ml	2.5/5ml
GL PU SU GE	**Geriplex-FS Kapseals** Parke-Davis	5000		5mg	50	5	5	15
	Geritol SmithKline Beecham					2.5/15ml	2.5/15ml	50/15ml
	Geritol Complete SmithKline Beecham	6000	400	30	60	1.5	1.7	20
	Geritol Extend SmithKline Beecham	3333	200	15	60	1.2	1.4	15
GL PU SO SU	**Gevral T** Lederle	5000	400	45	90	2.25	2.6	30
SO SU	**Herpetrol** Alva-Amco	313		3.75	15		4	
	Lipovite Rugby					1	1	niacinamide, 10mg
PU SU	**Mucoplex** ICN						1.5	
	Multilex Rugby	10000	400	5.5	100	10	5	niacinamide, 30mg
	Multilex T & M Rugby	10000	400	5.5	150	15	10	niacinamide, 100mg

MULTIPLE VITAMIN PRODUCTS — continued

Pyridoxine Hydrochloride (B_6)(mg)	Cyanocobalamin (B_{12})(mcg)	Folic Acid (mg)	Pantothenic Acid (mg)	Iron (mg)	Calcium (mg)	Phosphorous (mg)	Magnesium (mg)	Other Ingredients
1.05	4.5	0.3						FD&C red#40 • FD&C yellow#6 • FD&C blue#2 • FD&C blue#1 • sucrose • talc • flavors
5			10					
2	7.5		10	15			ns	copper • iodine • manganese • zinc, 1.5mg
2	6				200 (carbonate)	600 (calcium phosphate diabasic)		zinc, 15mg
0.17/5ml	0.83/5ml				2.5/5ml			alcohol, 18% • sorbitol • saccharin
	2			6	59			zinc, 0.5mg • cholin, 20mg • copper • manganese • docusate sodium, 100mg • aspergillus oryzea • enzymes, 162.5mg
0.5/15ml	0.75/15ml		2/15ml	50/15ml				methionine, 25mg/oz • choline bitartrate, 50mg/15ml
2	6	0.4	10	50	162	125	100	vitamin K, 25mcg • biotin, 45mcg • iodine, 150mcg • copper, 2mg • manganese, 2.5mg • potassium, 37.5mg • chloride, 34mg • chromium, 15mcg • molybdenum, 15mcg • selenium, 15mcg • zinc, 15mg • nickel, 5mcg • silicon, 80mcg • tin, 10mcg • vanadium, 10mcg
2	2	0.2		10	130	100	35	vitamin K, 80mcg • zinc, 15mg • selenium, 70mcg • iodine, 150mcg
3	9	0.4		27	162	125	100	iodine, 225mcg • copper, 1.5mg • zinc, 22.5mg
				19 (as sulfate)				lysine hydrochloride, 315mg • zinc, 2mg (as oxide)
1	5		5					choline bitartrate, 334mg
	5							liver fraction A, 375mg • liver fraction 2, 375mg
1.7	3		10	15			5	copper • iodine • manganese • zinc, 1.5mg
2	7.5		10	15			5	copper • iodine • manganese • zinc

CHAPTER 17 Nutritional

MULTIPLE VITAMIN PRODUCTS — continued

Product & Manufacturer	Vitamin A (IU)	Vitamin D (IU)	Vitamin E (IU)	Ascorbic Acid (C) (mg)	Thiamine (B_1) (mg)	Riboflavin (B_2) (mg)	Niacin (mg)
GL **Myadec** PR Parke-Davis SO SU	9000	400	30mg	90	10	20	20
GL **Natabec** PU **Kapseals** SO Parke-Davis SU	4000	400		50	3	2	10
Natalins Mead Johnson Nutrit'l	4000	400	15	70	1.5	1.6	17
SU **Nestabs** Fielding	5000	400	30	120	3	3	20
Niferex Daily Central	5000 (as acetate)	400	30 (as dl-alpha tocopheryl)	60	1.5	1.7	niacinamide, 20mg
GL **OcuCaps** PU Akorn SU	5000		200	400			
One-A-Day Essential Miles Incorporated	5000 (as acetate and beta carotene)	400	30	60	1.5	1.7	20

MULTIPLE VITAMIN PRODUCTS — continued

Pyridoxine Hydrochloride (B_6)(mg)	Cyanocobalamin (B_{12})(mcg)	Folic Acid (mg)	Pantothenic Acid (mg)	Iron (mg)	Calcium (mg)	Phosphorous (mg)	Magnesium (mg)	Other Ingredients
5	10	0.4	20	30	70	54	100	vitamin K, 25mcg • biotin, 45mcg • chromium • copper • iodine • potassium • manganese • molybdenum • selenium • zinc, 15mg
3	5			30	240			
2.6	2.5	0.5		30	200		100	sodium ascorbate • povidone • microcrystalline cellulose • dl-alpha-tocopheryl acetate • acacia • zinc, 15mg • polacrilin potassium • beta-carotene • hydroxypropyl methylcellulose • polyethylene glycol • cholecalciferol • magnesium stearate • hydroxypropyl cellulose • copper, 1.5mg • silicon dioxide
3	8	0.8	110	500		iodine, 150mcg • zinc, 15mg		
2	6	0.4	10	18 (as polysaccharide complex)	259 (as calcium carbonate and dicalcium phosphate)	5.4 (as dicalcium phosphate)	100 (as magnesium oxide)	biotin, 0.3mg • iodine, 150mcg (as potassium iodine) • manganese, 5mg (as manganese sulfate) • zinc, 15mg (as zinc sulfate) • copper, 2mg (as copper sulfate)
								zinc, 40mg • l-glutathione, 5mg • sodium pyrurate, 3mg • copper, 2mg • selenium, 40mcg
2	6	0.4	10					calcium carbonate • gelatin • starch • calcium silicate • calcium pantothenate • hydroxypropyl methylcellulose • artificial color • hydroxypropylcellulose • magnesium stearate • sodium hexametaphosphate • lecithin

MULTIPLE VITAMIN PRODUCTS — continued

	Product & Manufacturer	Vitamin A (IU)	Vitamin D (IU)	Vitamin E (IU)	Ascorbic Acid (C) (mg)	Thiamine (B_1) (mg)	Riboflavin (B_2) (mg)	Niacin (mg)
SU	**One-A-Day Maximum Formula** Miles Incorporated	5000 (as acetate and beta carotene)	400	30	60	1.5	1.7	20
SU	**One-A-Day Plus Extra C** Miles Incorporated	5000 (as acetate and beta carotene)	400	30	300	1.5	1.7	20
SU	**One-A-Day Stressgard** Miles Incorporated	5000 (as acetate and beta carotene)	400	30	600	15	10	100
SU	**One-A-Day Women's** Miles Incorporated	5000 (as acetate and beta carotene)	400	30	60	1.5	1.7	20
	One-Tablet Daily With Minerals Goldline	6500 (with beta carotene)	400	30	60	1.5	1.7	20
	One-Tablet-Daily Goldline	5000	400	30	60	1.5	1.7	20

MULTIPLE VITAMIN PRODUCTS — continued

Pyridox-ine Hydro-chloride (B_6)(mg)	Cyanoco-balamin (B_{12})(mcg)	Folic Acid (mg)	Panto-thenic Acid (mg)	Iron (mg)	Calcium (mg)	Phos-phorous (mg)	Magne-sium (mg)	Other Ingredients
2	6	0.4	10	18 (elemental)	130	100	100	cellulose • potassium, 37.5mg • chloride, 34mg • gelatin • starch • zinc, 15mg • citric acid • hydroxypropyl methylcellulose • selenium, 10mcg • artificial color • polyvinylpyrrolidone • hydroxypropylcellulose • manganese, 2.5mg • silica • copper, 2mg • chromium, 10mcg • molybdenum, 10mcg • potassium, 37.5mg • iodine, 150mcg • sodium hexametaphosphate • biotin, 30mcg • lecithin
2	6	0.4	10					calcium carbonate • gelatin • starch • cellulose • calcium silicate • calcium pantothenate • hydroxypropyl methylcellulose • FD&C yellow#6 • hydroxypropylcellulose • magnesium stearate • sodium hexametaphosphate • lecithin
5	12	0.4	20	18 (elemental)				calcium carbonate • starch • gelatin • calcium silicate • cellulose • hydroxypropyl methylcellulose • calcium pantothenate • zinc, 15mg • FD&C yellow#6 • hydroxypropylcellulose • magnesium stearate • copper, 2mg • lecithin • sodium hexametaphosphate
2	6	0.4	10	27 (elemental)	450 (elemental)			acacia • gelatin • cellulose • hydroxypropyl methylcellulose • zinc, 15mg • modified cellulose gum • magnesium stearate • FD&C yellow#5 • FD&C yellow#6 • hydroxypropylcellulose • starch • lecithin • sodium hexametaphosphate
2	6	0.4	10	18	130	100	100	biotin, 30mcg • iodine • copper • zinc • chromium • selenium • molybdenum • manganese • potassium • chloride
2	6	0.4	10					

MULTIPLE VITAMIN PRODUCTS — continued

Product & Manufacturer	Vitamin A (IU)	Vitamin D (IU)	Vitamin E (IU)	Ascorbic Acid (C) (mg)	Thiamine (B_1) (mg)	Riboflavin (B_2) (mg)	Niacin (mg)
Optilets-500 Filmtabs Abbott	5000	400	30	500	15	10	niacinamide, 100mg
Optilets-M-500 Filmtabs Abbott	5000	400	30	500	15	10	niacinamide, 100mg
Os-Cal Forte SmithKline Beecham	1668	125	0.8	50	1.7	1.7	niacinamide, 15mg
Os-Cal Plus SmithKline Beecham	1666	125		33	0.5	0.66	3.3
SU **Osteogard** Alva-Amco		100				7.5	
GL **Poly-Vi-Sol** PU **Chewable** PE **Vitamins** Mead Johnson Nutrit'l	2500	400	15	60	1.05	1.2	13.5
AL **Poly-Vi-Sol** LA **Vitamin** SU **Drops** SL Mead Johnson PE Nutrit'l	1500/ml	400/ml	5/ml	35/ml	0.5/ml	0.6/ml	8/ml
GL **Poly-Vi-Sol** PU **with Iron** PE **Chewable Vitamins and Minerals** Mead Johnson Nutrit'l	2500	400	15mg	60	1.05	1.2	13.5
AL **Poly-Vi-Sol** LA **with Iron** SU **Vitamin** SL **Drops** PE Mead Johnson Nutrit'l	1500/ml	400/ml	5/ml	35/ml	0.5/ml	0.6/ml	8/ml
AL **Poly-Vita** LA **Drops** SO H.R. Cenci SU SL PE	1500/ml	400/ml	5/ml	35/ml	0.5/ml	0.6/ml	8/ml
Polyvitamin With Iron Rugby	1500/ml	400/ml	5mg/ml	35/ml	0.5/ml	0.6/ml	8/ml

MULTIPLE VITAMIN PRODUCTS — continued

Pyridoxine Hydrochloride (B₆)(mg)	Cyanocobalamin (B₁₂)(mcg)	Folic Acid (mg)	Pantothenic Acid (mg)	Iron (mg)	Calcium (mg)	Phosphorous (mg)	Magnesium (mg)	Other Ingredients
5	12		20 (as calcium pantothenate)					cellulosic polymers • cornstarch • D&C yellow#10 • FD&C yellow#6 • iron oxide • polyethylene glycol • povidone • stearic acid • talc • titanium dioxide • vanillin
5	12		20 (as calcium pantothenate)	20			80	copper, 2mg • iodine, 0.15mg • manganese, 1mg • zinc, 1.5mg • polyethylene glycol • propylene glycol • povidone • cellulosic polymers • colloidal silicon dioxide • cornstarch • D&C red#7 • FD&C blue#1 • titanium dioxide • iron oxide • magnesium stearate • microcrystalline cellulose • sorbic acid
2				5	250		1.6	manganese, 0.3mg • zinc, 0.5mg
0.5				16.6	250			manganese • zinc, 0.75mg
					500 (as carbonate)			
1.05	4.5	0.3						sucrose • flavor
0.4/ml	2/ml							flavor
1.05	4.5	0.3		12				copper, 0.8mg • zinc, 8mg
0.4/ml				10/ml				
0.4/ml	2/ml							polysorbate 80 • glycerin • methylparaben • propylparaben • FD&C red#40 • D&C yellow#10 • flavor • purified water
0.4/ml				10/ml				

MULTIPLE VITAMIN PRODUCTS — continued

	Product & Manufacturer	Vitamin A (IU)	Vitamin D (IU)	Vitamin E (IU)	Ascorbic Acid (C) (mg)	Thiamine (B_1) (mg)	Riboflavin (B_2) (mg)	Niacin (mg)
	Prenatal-S Goldline	4000	400	11	100	1.5	1.7	18
	Prenavite Rugby	8000	400	30	60	1.7	2	20
GL SO SU	**Preventamine Multivitamin Mineral Complex (Iron-free)** Murdock	fish liver oil, 10000 • beta carotene, 15000	100	400	1200	50	50	75
GL SO SU	**Preventamins Multivitamin Mineral Complex (with Iron)** Murdock	fish liver oil, 10000 • beta carotene, 15000	100	400	1200	50	50	75
SO	**Pro-Pep** Alva-Amco	375	30	2.16	5	0.17	0.12	1.375
	Ru-Lets 500 Rugby	10000	400	30	500	15	10	niacinamide, 100mg
	Secran B Vitamin Supplement Scherer					10/tsp		10/tsp
GL PU PE	**Sesame Street Complete Vitamins and Minerals** McNeil	2250 (as acetate) • 500 (as beta carotene)	200	10	40	0.75	0.85	10
GL PU PE	**Sesame Street Vitamins Plus Extra C** McNeil	2250 (as acetate) • 500 (as beta carotene)	200	10	80	0.75	0.85	10

MULTIPLE VITAMIN PRODUCTS — continued

Pyridox-ine Hydrochloride (B_6)(mg)	Cyanoco-balamin (B_{12})(mcg)	Folic Acid (mg)	Panto-thenic Acid (mg)	Iron (mg)	Calcium (mg)	Phos-phorous (mg)	Magne-sium (mg)	Other Ingredients
2.6	4	0.8		60	200			zinc, 25mg
4	8	0.8		60	200		100	iodine, 150mcg
50	100	0.8	150		500		500	vitamin K, 60mcg • niacinamide, 150mg • boron, 3mg • biotin, 300mcg • choline, 100mg • potassium, 99mg • copper, 2mg • zinc, 20mg • manganese, 10mg • iodine, 150mcg • chromium, 200mcg • selenium, 200mcg • molybdenum, 100mcg • vanadium, 25mcg • PABA, 50mg • inositol, 100mg • quercetin, 100mg • hesperidin, 100mg • rutin, 50mg
50	100	0.8	150	20	500		500	vitamin K, 60mcg • niacinamide, 150mg • boron, 3mg • biotin, 300mcg • choline, 100mg • potassium, 99mg • copper, 2mg • zinc, 20mg • manganese, 10mg • iodine, 150mcg • chromium, 200mcg • selenium, 200mcg • molybdenum, 100mcg • vanadium, 25mcg • PABA, 50mg • inositol, 100mg • quercetin, 100mg • hesperidin, 100mg • rutin, 50mg
0.17	0.5	0.03	0.78	1.2				zinc, 1mg • copper, 0.14mg • iodine, 9mcg • biotin, 23mcg • dextrose • maltodextrin • sorbitol
5	12		20					
	25/tsp							alcohol, 17% • sodium citrate • sugar • glycerin • sherry wine conc. • FD&C red#40
0.7	3	0.2	5	10	80		20	iodine, 75mcg • zinc, 8mg • copper, 1mg • sucrose • talc • natural flavors and coloring • glycerides of stearic and palmitic acids • gelatin • silicon dioxide • magnesium stearate • starch • lactose • citric acid • dicalcium phosphate
0.7	3	0.2	5					sucrose • talc • natural flavors • glycerides of stearic and palmitic acids • gelatin • silicon dioxide • magnesium stearate • starch • natural coloring • lactose • citric acid • dicalcium phosphate

MULTIPLE VITAMIN PRODUCTS — continued

Product & Manufacturer	Vitamin A (IU)	Vitamin D (IU)	Vitamin E (IU)	Ascorbic Acid (C) (mg)	Thiamine (B_1) (mg)	Riboflavin (B_2) (mg)	Niacin (mg)
GL PU PE **Sesame Street Vitamins Plus Iron** McNeil	2250 (as acetate) • 500 (as beta carotene)	200	10	40	0.75	0.85	10
Sigtab-M Roberts Pharm.	6000	400	45		mononitrate, 5mg	5	niacinamide, 25mg
Sigtabs Roberts Pharm.	acetate, 5000	400	acetate, 15		mononitrate, 10.3	10	100
Simron Plus SmithKline Beecham				50			
Stress Formula Goldline			30	500	15	10	niacinamide, 100
Stress Formula With Zinc Goldline			30	500	15	10	niacinamide, 100
GL PU SO SU **Stresstabs 600 Plus Zinc** Lederle			30mg	500	10	10	100
GL PU SO SU **Stresstabs Advanced Formula** Lederle			30mg	500	10	10	100
Stuart Prenatal Stuart	4000	400	11mg	100	1.5	1.7	18

MULTIPLE VITAMIN PRODUCTS — continued									
Pyridox-ine Hydro-chloride (B$_6$)(mg)	Cyanoco-balamin (B$_{12}$)(mcg)	Folic Acid (mg)	Panto-thenic Acid (mg)	Iron (mg)	Calcium (mg)	Phos-phorous (mg)	Magne-sium (mg)	Other Ingredients
0.7	3	0.2	5	10				sucrose • talc • natural flavors • glycerides of stearic and palmitic acids • gelatin • silicon dioxide • magnesium stearate • starch • natural coloring • lactose • citric acid • dicalcium phosphate
pyroxidine, 3mg	18	0.4	0.015	18	200	150	100	vitamin K$_1$, 25mcg • biotin, 45mcg • copper, 2mg • zinc, 15mg • iodine, 150mcg • manganese sulfate, 5mg • potassium chloride, 40mg • chloride, 36.3mg • selenium, 25mcg • molybdenum, 25mcg • chromium, 25mcg • nickel, 5mcg • tin, 10mcg • vanadium, 19mcg • silicon, 2mcg • boron, 150mcg • microcrystalline cellulose • stearic acid • croscarmellose sodium • magnesium stearate • hydroxypropyl methylcellulose • propylene glycol
6	18	0.4	20					sucrose • calcium sulfate • niacinamide • calcium pantothenate • gelatin • povidone • lacca • magnesium stearate • silica • sodium benzoate • polyethylene glycol • cholecalciferol • carnauba wax • cyanocobalamin • sesame seed oil • titanium dioxide
1	3.33	0.1		10				
5	12	0.4	20					biotin, 45mcg
5	12	0.4	20					biotin, 45mcg • copper • zinc, 23.9mg
5	12	0.4	20					zinc, 23.9mg • copper, 3mg • biotin, 45mcg
5	12	0.4	20					biotin, 45mcg
2.6	4		0.8	60	200			dl-alpha tocopheryl acetate • zinc, 25mg • cholecalciferol cyanocobalamin • croscarmellose sodium • hydroxypropyl methylcellulose • microcrystalline cellulose • pregelatinized starch • red iron oxide • titanium dioxide

MULTIPLE VITAMIN PRODUCTS — continued

Product & Manufacturer	Vitamin A (IU)	Vitamin D (IU)	Vitamin E (IU)	Ascorbic Acid (C) (mg)	Thiamine (B$_1$) (mg)	Riboflavin (B$_2$) (mg)	Niacin (mg)
GL Sunkist PU Multis SO Complete SU CIBA Consumer	5000	400	30	60	1.5	1.7	niacinamide, 20mg
GL Sunkist PU Multis Plus C SO CIBA SU Consumer	2500	400	15	250	1.05	1.2	niacinamide, 13.5mg
GL Sunkist PU Multis Plus SO Iron SU CIBA Consumer	2500	400	15	60	1.05	1.2	niacinamide, 13.5mg
GL Sunkist PU Multis SO Regular SU CIBA Consumer	2500	400	15	60	1.05	1.2	niacinamide, 13.5mg
Super 28 Formula Reese Chemical	10000	400	15	75	4	5	
Super Vikaps Reese Chemical	10000	400	15		10	10	
Surbex Filmtabs Abbott					6	6	niacinamide, 30mg
Surbex With C Abbott				250	6	6	niacinamide, 30mg
Surbex-750 With Iron Abbott			30	750	15	15	niacinamide, 100mg
Surbex-750 With Zinc Abbott			30	750	15	15	100

MULTIPLE VITAMIN PRODUCTS — continued

Pyridoxine Hydrochloride (B₆)(mg)	Cyanocobalamin (B₁₂)(mcg)	Folic Acid (mg)	Pantothenic Acid (mg)	Iron (mg)	Calcium (mg)	Phosphorous (mg)	Magnesium (mg)	Other Ingredients
2	6	0.4	10	18	100	78	20	biotin, 40mcg • vitamin K₁, 10mcg • iodine, 150mcg • zinc, 10mg • manganese, 1mg • copper, 2mg
1.05	4.5	0.3						vitamin K₁, 5mcg
1.05	4.5	0.3		15				vitamin K₁, 5mcg
1.05	4.5	0.3						vitamin K₁, 5mcg
5			4			50		
5	5	0.4	20					
2.5	5		10 (as calcium pantothenate)					cellulosic polymers • cornstarch • D&C yellow#10 • dibasic calcium phosphate • FD&C yellow#6 • magnesium stearate • polyethylene glycol • povidone • propylene glycol • stearic acid • titanium dioxide • vanillin
2.5	5		10 (as calcium pantothenate)					cellulosic polymers • cornstarch • D&C yellow#10 • FD&C yellow#6 • lactose • magnesium stearate • polyethylene glycol • microcrystalline cellulose • povidone • propylene glycol • titanium dioxide • vanillin
25	12	0.4	20 (as calcium pantothenate)	27				cellulosic polymers • colloidal silicon dioxide • FD&C red#3 • cornstarch • iron oxide • magnesium stearate • microcrystalline cellulose • polyethylene glycol • povidone • vanillin
20	12	0.4	20					zinc, 22.5mg • cellulose • povidone • talc • magnesium stearate • titanium dioxide • polyethylene glycol • colloidal silicon dioxide • vanillin • iron oxide

MULTIPLE VITAMIN PRODUCTS — continued

Product & Manufacturer	Vitamin A (IU)	Vitamin D (IU)	Vitamin E (IU)	Ascorbic Acid (C) (mg)	Thiamine (B_1) (mg)	Riboflavin (B_2) (mg)	Niacin (mg)
Surbex-T Abbott				500	15	10	niacinamide, 100mg
Surbu-Gen-T Goldline				500	15	10	100
Thera-Combex H-P Kapseals Warner-Lambert				500	25	15	100
Theragenerix Goldline	5000 (with beta carotene)	400	30mg	90	3	3.4	30
Theragenerix-M Goldline	5000 (with beta carotene)	400	30mg	90	3	3.4	30
Theragran High Potency Multivitamin Bristol-Myers	5000 (as acetate and beta carotene)	400	30mg	90	3	3.4	20
Theragran High Potency Multivitamin Liquid Bristol-Myers	5000/5ml	400/5ml		200/5ml	10/5ml	10/5ml	100/5ml
Theragran Stress Formula Bristol-Myers			30	600	15	15	100
Theragran-M High Potency Vitamins with Minerals Bristol-Myers	5000	400	30	90	3	3.4	20
Therems Rugby	5000	400	30mg	120	3	3.4	30
Therems-M Rugby	5000	400	30	90	3	3.4	20
Thex Forte Medtech				500	25	15	100
Tri-Vi-Sol Vitamins A,D +C Drops Mead Johnson Nutrit'l	1500/ml	400/ml		35/ml			

MULTIPLE VITAMIN PRODUCTS — continued								
Pyridox-ine Hydro-chloride (B$_6$)(mg)	Cyanoco-balamin (B$_{12}$)(mcg)	Folic Acid (mg)	Panto-thenic Acid (mg)	Iron (mg)	Calcium (mg)	Phos-phorous (mg)	Magne-sium (mg)	Other Ingredients
5	10		20 (as calcium pantothenate)					cellulosic polymers • cornstarch • D&C yellow#10 • FD&C yellow#6 • magnesium stearate • microcrystalline cellulose • polyethylene glycol • povidone • stearic acid • titanium dioxide • vanillin
5	10		20					
10	5		20					
3	9	0.4	10					biotin, 30mcg
3	9	0.4	10	27	40	31	100	biotin, 30mcg • chlorine • chromium • copper • iodine • potassium • manganese • molybdenum • selenium • zinc, 15mg
3	9	0.4	10					biotin, 30mcg • sucrose
4.1/5ml	5/5ml		21.4/5ml					sugar
25	12	0.4	20	27				biotin, 45mcg
3	9	0.4	10	27	40	31	100	chlorine, 7.5mg • chromium, 15mcg • copper, 2mg • iodine, 150mcg • potassium, 7.5mg • manganese, 5mg • molybdenum, 15mcg • selenium, 10mcg • zinc, 15mg • biotin, 30mcg
3	9	0.4	10					biotin, 15mcg • beta carotene, 1250 IU
3	9	0.4	10	27			ns	chlorine • chromium • copper • iodine • potassium • manganese • molybdenum • selenium • zinc, 15mg • biotin, 15mcg
5			10					

MULTIPLE VITAMIN PRODUCTS — continued

	Product & Manufacturer	Vitamin A (IU)	Vitamin D (IU)	Vitamin E (IU)	Ascorbic Acid (C) (mg)	Thiamine (B$_1$) (mg)	Riboflavin (B$_2$) (mg)	Niacin (mg)
AL LA SU SL PE	Tri-Vi-Sol With Iron Vitamin A,D +C Drops Mead Johnson Nutrit'l	1500/ml	400/ml		35/ml			
AL LA SO SU SL PE	Tri-Vita Drops H.R. Cenci	1500/ml	400/ml		35/ml			
AL	Trophite Menley & James					10/5ml		
	Unicap Upjohn	5000	400	15	60	1.5	1.7	20
	Unicap Jr. Upjohn	5000	400	15	60	1.5	1.7	20
	Unicap M Upjohn	5000	400	30	60	1.5	1.7	20
	Unicap Plus Iron Upjohn	5000	400	30	60	1.5	1.7	20
	Unicap Senior Upjohn	5000	200	15	60	1.2	1.4	16
	Unicap Softgel Capsules Upjohn	5000	400	30	60	1.5	1.7	20
	Unicap T Upjohn	5000	400	30mg	500	10	10	100
	Unicomplex M Rugby	5000	400	30	60	1.5	1.7	20
	Unicomplex T & M Rugby	5000	400	30	500	10	10	100
LA SU PE	Vi-Daylin ADC Vitamins Ross	1500/ml	400/ml		35/ml			
LA SU PE	Vi-Daylin ADC Vitamins Plus Iron Ross	1500/ml	400/ml		35/ml			
LA SU PE	Vi-Daylin Multi-Vitamin Drops Ross	1500/ml	400/ml	4.13mg/ml (5 IU)	35/ml	0.5/ml	0.6/ml	8/ml

MULTIPLE VITAMIN PRODUCTS — continued								
Pyridox- ine Hydro- chloride (B$_6$)(mg)	Cyanoco- balamin (B$_{12}$)(mcg)	Folic Acid (mg)	Panto- thenic Acid (mg)	Iron (mg)	Calcium (mg)	Phos- phorous (mg)	Magne- sium (mg)	Other Ingredients
				10/ml				
								polysorbate 80 • glycerin • methylparaben • propylparaben • FD&C red#40 • D&C yellow#10 • flavor • purified water
	25/5ml							FD&C blue #1 • D&C red #33 • D&C yellow #6 • dextrose • glycerin • parabens
2	6	0.4						tartrazine
2	6	0.4						sucrose • mannitol • flavor
2	6	0.4	10	18	60	45		tartrazine • copper, 2mg • iodine, 150mcg • potassium, 5mg • manganese, 1mg • zinc, 15mg
2	6	0.4	10	22.5	100			sucrose
2.2	3	0.4	10	10	100	77	30	copper, 2mg • iodine, 150mcg • potassium, 5mg • manganese, 1mg • zinc, 15mg
2	6	0.4						tartrazine
6	18	0.4	25	18				tartrazine • copper, 2mg • iodine, 150mcg • potassium, 5mg • manganese, 1mg • selenium, 10mcg • zinc, 15mg
2	6	0.4	10	18	60	45		copper • iodine • potassium • manganese • zinc
6	4	0.4	25	18	ns		ns	copper • iodine • potassium • manganese
								flavor • propylene glycol • polysorbate 80 • glycerin • water
				10/ml				flavor • glycerin • water • polysorbate 80
0.4/ml	1.5/ml							alcohol, < 0.5% • flavor • glycerin • water

MULTIPLE VITAMIN PRODUCTS — continued

	Product & Manufacturer	Vitamin A (IU)	Vitamin D (IU)	Vitamin E (IU)	Ascorbic Acid (C) (mg)	Thiamine (B_1) (mg)	Riboflavin (B_2) (mg)	Niacin (mg)
LA	Vi-Daylin Multi-Vitamin Liquid Ross	2500/5ml	400/5ml	11mg/5ml (15 IU)	60/5ml	1.05/5ml	1.2/5ml	13.5/5ml
LA SU PE	Vi-Daylin Multi-Vitamin Plus Iron Drops Ross	1500/ml	400/ml	4.1mg/ml (5 IU)	35/ml	0.5/ml	0.6/ml	8/ml
GL PE	Vi-Daylin Multi-Vitamin Plus Iron Chewable Tablets Ross	2500	400	15	60	1.05	1.2	13.5
GL PE	Vi-Daylin Multivitamin Ross	2500	400	15	60	1.05	1.2	13.5
LA	Vi-Daylin Plus Iron Ross	2500/5ml	400/5ml	11mg/5ml (15 IU)	60/5ml	1.05/5ml	1.2/5ml	13.5/5ml
	Vigortol Rugby					2.5/15ml	1.25/15ml	25/15ml
	Viogen-C Goldline				300	20	10	100
	Vita Bee C-800 Rugby			45	800	15	17	100
	Vita-Bee With C Rugby				300	15	10.2	50
	Vita-Kaps Abbott	5000	400		50	3	2.5	20
SU	Vita-Lea Shaklee	5000/dose	400/dose	30/dose	90/dose	2.1/dose	2.4/dose	20/dose
	Vita-Lea For Children Shaklee	2000/dose	400/dose	10/dose	60/dose	1.1/dose	1.2/dose	14/dose
	Vital B-50 Goldline					50	50	50
	Z-Bec A.H. Robins			45	600	15	10.2	100
	Z-Gen Goldline			45mg	600	15	10.2	100
PU SO SU	Ze Caps Everett			200				
PU SO SU	Ze Caps Plus Everett	beta carotene, 5000		200				
	Zymacap Roberts Pharm.	palmitate, 5000	400	acetate, 15	90	mononitrate, 2.25	2.6	30

MULTIPLE VITAMIN PRODUCTS — continued

Pyridox-ine Hydro-chloride (B_6)(mg)	Cyanoco-balamin (B_{12})(mcg)	Folic Acid (mg)	Panto-thenic Acid (mg)	Iron (mg)	Calcium (mg)	Phos-phorous (mg)	Magne-sium (mg)	Other Ingredients
1.05/5ml	4.5/5ml							alcohol, < 0.5% • glucose • sucrose • flavor
0.4/ml				10/ml				alcohol, < 0.5% • flavor • glycerin • water
1.05	4.5	0.3		12				sucrose • flavor • dextrins • mannitol
1.05	4.5	0.3						sucrose • flavor • dextrins
1.05/5ml	4.5/5ml			10/5ml				alcohol, < 0.5% • flavor • glucose • sucrose
0.5/15ml	0.5/15ml		5/15ml	75/15ml			ns	zinc, 1mg/15ml • choline, 50mg/15ml • inositol, 50mg/15ml • iodine • potassium • manganese • alcohol, 18%
5			20				50	tartrazine • zinc, 50mg
25	12		25					
5			10					tartrazine
1	3							
2/dose	9/dose	0.4/dose	10/dose	18/dose	600/dose	450/dose	200/dose	biotin, 300mcg • iodine, 150mcg • copper, 2mg • zinc, 15mg
1.6/dose	3/dose	0.32/dose	4/dose	10.8/dose	130/dose	100mg/dose	60/dose	biotin, 105mcg • iodine, 15mcg • copper, 0.2mg • zinc, 1.5mg
50	50	0.1	50					d-biotin, 50mcg • PABA, 50mg • choline bitartrate, 50mg • inositol, 50mg • bromelain, 20mg
10	6		25					zinc, 22.5mg
10	6		25					zinc, 22.5mg
								zinc gluconate, 75mg (yields 9.6mg elemental zinc)
								zinc gluconate, 75mg • selenium, 50mcg
3	9	0.4	15		pantothenate, ns			soybean oil • gelatin • glycerin • niacinamide • lecithin • corn oil • titanium dioxide • ethyl vanillin • cholecalciferol

FORMULA PRODUCTS FOR INFANTS AND CHILDREN

Product[a] & Manufacturer	Dosage Form	Kcal per oz[b]	Protein Type	Protein g/L	Carbohydrate Type	Carbohydrate g/L	Fat Type	Fat g/L
Human Breast Milk, Mature — Mother	liquid	21	casein, 40% • whey, 60%	9	lactose	68	human milk fat	40
Cow Milk, Whole — Cows Various	liquid	20	casein, 80% • whey, 20%	31	lactose	49	cow milk fat	38
Milk-based Formulas								
Carnation Follow-Up — Carnation	ready-to-feed • concentrate • powder	20	nonfat milk	18	lactose • corn syrup	89.2	palm olein • soy • coconut • high oleic safflower oils	27.7
Enfamil — Mead Johnson Nutrit'l	ready-to-feed • concentrate • powder	20	nonfat milk, whey-predominant	15	lactose	70	palm olein • soy oil • coconut oil • high-oleic sunflower oil	38
Enfamil with Iron — Mead Johnson Nutrit'l	ready-to-feed • concentrate • powder	20	nonfat milk, whey-predominant	15	lactose	70	palm olein • soy oil • coconut oil • high-oleic sunflower oil	38
Gerber Baby Formula Low Iron — Gerber	ready-to-feed • concentrate • powder	20	nonfat milk • casein-predominant	14.9	lactose	71.9	palm olein • soy oil • coconut oil • high oleic sunflower oil	37
Gerber Baby Formula with Iron — Gerber	ready-to-feed • concentrate • powder	20	nonfat milk • casein-predominant	14.9	lactose	71.9	palm olein • soy oil • coconut oil • high oleic sunflower oil	37
LA Lactofree — Mead Johnson Nutrit'l	ready-to-feed • concentrate • powder	20	nonfat milk • casein-predominant	15	glucose polymers	70	palm olein • soy oil • coconut oil • high oleic sunflower oil	37
Similac — Ross	ready-to-feed • concentrate • powder	20	nonfat milk, casein-predominant	14.5	lactose	72.3	soy oil • coconut oil	36.5
Similac With Iron — Ross	ready-to-feed • powder • concentrate	20	nonfat milk, casein-predominant	14.5	lactose	72.3	soy oil • coconut oil	36.5
Soy-based Therapeutic Formulas								
Gerber Baby Formula with Soy — Gerber	ready-to-feed • concentrate • powder	20	soy protein isolate	20.3	corn syrup • sucrose	67.6	palm olein • soy oil • coconut oil • high oleic sunflower oil	35.9
I Soyalac — Nutricia	powder	20	soy protein isolate	21	sucrose • potato maltodextrin	67.7	soy oil	37.2
I Soyalac — Nutricia	ready-to-feed • concentrate	20	soy protein isolate	21	sucrose • tapioca dextrin	67.7	soy oil	37.2
LA Isomil — Ross	ready-to-feed • powder • concentrate	20	soy protein isolate • L-methionine	18	corn syrup • sucrose	68.3	soy oil • coconut oil	36.9
LA SU Isomil SF — Ross	ready-to-feed • concentrate	20	soy protein isolate • L-methionine	18	glucose polymers	68.3	soy oil • coconut oil	36.9

FORMULA PRODUCTS FOR INFANTS AND CHILDREN — continued

Sodium mEq/L	Potassium mEq/L	Calcium mg/L	Phosphorus mg/L	Ca:P Ratio	Iron mg/L	Osmolality mOsm/kg	Renal Solute Load mOsm/L	Comments[c]
7	13	340	150	2.3:1	0.5	300	93	
21	39	1200	920	1.3:1	0.5	288	308	
11.5	23.4	912.6	609	1.5:1	13	326	122	for infants 6-12 months old eating solid foods
8	18.7	530	360	1.47:1	3.4	300	134	
8	18.7	530	360	1.47:1	12.7	300	134	
9.65	18.7	507.36	391.09	1.30:1	3.38	320	135.2	
9.65	18.7	507.36	391.09	1.30:1	12.16	320	135.2	
8.8	19	554	372	1.5:1	12	200	136	milk-based
8	18.1	493	380	1.3:1	1.5	300	96.3	
8	18.1	493	380	1.3:1	12	300	96.3	
13.79	20.06	634.2	496.79	1.28:1	12.16	230	182.5	
12.4	20.3	690	426.2	1.62:1	12.85	220	132	
12.4	20.3	690	426.2	1.62:1	12.85	270	132	
13	18.7	710	510	1.4:1	12	280	115.6	
13	18.7	710	510	1.4:1	12	180	115.6	

FORMULA PRODUCTS FOR INFANTS AND CHILDREN — continued

Product[a] & Manufacturer	Dosage Form	Kcal per oz[b]	Protein Type	Protein g/L	Carbo-hydrate Type	Carbo-hydrate g/L	Fat Type	Fat g/L
ProSobee Mead Johnson Nutrit'l	ready-to-feed • concentrate • powder	20	soy protein isolate • L-methionine	20	corn syrup solids	68	palm olein • soy oil • coconut oil • high-oleic sunflower oil	36
LA SU **RCF** Ross	concentrate	12 (diluted 1:1 with water, no carbohydrates added)	soy protein isolate • L-methionine	20	selected by physician	0.04	soy oil • coconut oil	36
LA **Soyalac** Nutricia	ready-to-feed • powder • concentrate	20	soy protein solids	21	sucrose • corn syrup solids • soybean carbohydrate	67.7	soy oil	37.2

Other Therapeutic Formulas

Product[a] & Manufacturer	Dosage Form	Kcal per oz[b]	Protein Type	Protein g/L	Carbo-hydrate Type	Carbo-hydrate g/L	Fat Type	Fat g/L
LA **Alimentum** Ross	ready-to-feed	20	casein hydrolysate supplemented with L-cystine, L-tyrosine, and L-tryptophan	18.6	sucrose • modified tapioca starch	68.9	medium chain triglycerides • safflower oil • soy oil	37.5
Carnation Good Start[d] Carnation	ready-to-feed • concentrate • powder	20	enzymatically hydrolized reduced minerals • whey	16	lactose • maltodextrin	74.4	palm olein • soy • coconut • high oleic safflower oils	34.5
Nutramigen Mead Johnson Nutrit'l	ready-to-feed • concentrate • powder	20	casein hydrolysate supplemented with L-cystine, L-tyrosine, and L-tryptophan	19	corn syrup solids • modified corn starch	91	corn oil • soy oil	27
LA **Portagen** Mead Johnson Nutrit'l	powder	20	sodium caseinate	24	corn syrup solids • sucrose	78	medium chain triglyceride oil • corn oil	32
Pregestimil Mead Johnson Nutrit'l	powder	20	casein hydrolysate supplemented with L-cystine, L-tyrosine, and L-tryptophan	19	corn syrup solids • modified cornstarch • dextrose	69	medium chain triglycerides • corn oil • soy oil • high-oleic safflower oil	38
3232A Mead Johnson Nutrit'l	powder	20	casein hydrolysate	19	modified tapioca starch	28.6	medium chain triglyceride oil • corn oil	28

Formulas for Premature Infants

Product[a] & Manufacturer	Dosage Form	Kcal per oz[b]	Protein Type	Protein g/L	Carbo-hydrate Type	Carbo-hydrate g/L	Fat Type	Fat g/L
Enfamil Premature Formula Mead Johnson Nutrit'l	ready-to-feed • nursette bottle	24	nonfat milk, whey-predominant	24	corn syrup solids • lactose	90	medium chain triglycerides • soy oil • coconut oil	41

FORMULA PRODUCTS FOR INFANTS AND CHILDREN — continued

Sodium mEq/L	Potassium mEq/L	Calcium mg/L	Phosphorus mg/L	Ca:P Ratio	Iron mg/L	Osmolality mOsm/kg	Renal Solute Load mOsm/L	Comments[c]
10.4	21	640	500	1.27:1	12.8	200	178	
13	18.7	700	500	1.4:1	1.5	74	123.6	carbohydrate-free base • carbohydrate must be added before feeding
12.9	20.3	636	phosphorus, 372mg/L	1.71:1	12.8	240	130	
13	20.5	710	510	1.4:1	12	370	123.2	for protein sensitivity or allergy, pancreatic insufficiency, and intractable diarrhea
7	17	433	243	1.8:1	10	265	99.3	
13.9	18.9	640	430	1.49:1	12.8	320	172	for severe diarrhea, protein sensitivity & food allergies
16	21.6	630	473	1.33:1	12.8	230	200	for malabsorption problems and pancreatic insufficiency • higher amounts of vitamins added
11.7	18.9	640	430	1.49:1	12.8	320	169	for fat malabsorption, severe diarrhea, GI immaturity, and protein intolerance
12.6	19	635	426	1.5:1	12.7	[e]	170	for disaccharidase deficiencies, impaired glucose transport and intractable diarrhea • carbohydrate must be added before feeding
13.9	21	1340	670	2:1	2	310	210	

FORMULA PRODUCTS FOR INFANTS AND CHILDREN — continued

Product[a] & Manufacturer	Dosage Form	Kcal per oz[b]	Protein Type	Protein g/L	Carbo-hydrate Type	Carbo-hydrate g/L	Fat Type	Fat g/L
Enfamil Premature Formula Mead Johnson Nutrit'l	ready-to-feed • nursette bottle	20	nonfat milk, whey-predominant	20	corn syrup solids • lactose	75	medium chain triglycerides • soy oil • coconut oil	35
Enfamil Premature Formula with Iron Mead Johnson Nutrit'l	ready-to-feed • nursette bottle	24	nonfat milk, whey-predominant	24	corn syrup solids • lactose	90	medium chain triglycerides • soy oil • coconut oil	41
Enfamil Premature Formula with Iron Mead Johnson Nutrit'l	ready-to-feed • nursette bottle	20	nonfat milk, whey-predominant	20	corn syrup solids • lactose	75	medium chain triglycerides • soy oil • coconut oil	35
Similac PM 60/40 Ross	ready-to-feed	20	whey protein • sodium caseinate	15.8	lactose	69	soy oil • coconut oil	37.6
Similac Special Care 20 Ross	ready-to-feed	20	nonfat milk, whey-predominant	18.3	lactose • glucose polymer	71.7	medium chain triglycerides • soy oil • coconut oil	36.7
Similac Special Care 24 Ross	ready-to-feed	24	nonfat milk, whey-predominant	22	lactose • glucose polymer	86.1	medium chain triglycerides • soy oil • coconut oil	44.1
Similac Special Care 24 With Iron Ross	ready-to-feed	24	nonfat milk, whey-predominant	22	lactose • glucose polymer	86.1	medium chain triglycerides • soy oil • coconut oil	44.1
Miscellaneous Products								
PediaSure Ross	ready-to-feed	30	low lactose whey protein • sodium caseinate	30	hydrolyzed corn starch • sucrose	110	high oleic safflower & soy oils • medium chain triglycerides	50
PediaSure with Fiber Ross	ready-to-feed	30	low lactose whey protein • sodium caseinate	30	hydrolyzed corn starch • sucrose • soy fiber	114	high oleic safflower and soy oils • medium chain triglycerides	50
Enfamil Human Milk Fortifier[f] Mead Johnson Nutrit'l	powder	14	whey protein • sodium caseinate		corn syrup solids • lactose	2.7	—	<0.1
Similac Natural Care Ross	ready-to-feed	24	nonfat milk, whey-predominant	22	lactose • glucose polymer	86.1	medium chain triglycerides • soy oil • coconut oil	44.1

[a]Refer to the text of Chapter 13, "Antidiarrheal Products," for information on fluid and electrolyte replacement products.
[b]Unless otherwise noted, calorie content and other nutritional information is given as ready-to-feed formula or when appropriately prepared for infant consumption.
[c]Formulas contain appropriate range of vitamins, minerals, and trace elements unless noted in "Comments" section.
[d]Listed as a therapeutic formula because it is a whey hydrolyzed formula but is intended for feeding full-term infants.
[e]Osmolality not determined by manufacturer.
[f]Values are listed for 4 packets of fortifier only, *before* mixing with breast milk.

FORMULA PRODUCTS FOR INFANTS AND CHILDREN — continued

Sodium mEq/L	Potassium mEq/L	Calcium mg/L	Phosphorus mg/L	Ca:P Ratio	Iron mg/L	Osmolality mOsm/kg	Renal Solute Load mOsm/L	Comments[c]
11.7	17.9	1120	560	2:1	1.7	260	176	
13.9	21	1340	670	2:1	14.6	310	210	
11.7	17.9	1120	560	2:1	12.2	260	176	
7	14.8	380	190	2:1	1.5	280	96.3	low in sodium, potassium, and minerals
12.6	22.3	1220	610	2:1	2.5	235	123.6	
15.2	26.9	1460	730	2:1	3	280	148.7	
15.2	26.9	1460	730	2:1	15	280	148.7	
16.5	33.5	970	800	1.2:1	14	310	198.5	liquid nutrition for children 1-6 years of age • tube or oral feeding
16.5	33.5	970	800	1.2:1	14	345	198.5	liquid nutrition for children 1-6 years of age • tube or oral feeding
0.3	0.4	90	45	2:1	–	120	–	values are listed for 4 packets of fortifier only • adequate vitamins, minerals, and trace elements only when added to breast milk
15.2	26.9	1710	850	2:1	3	280	148.7	may use alone or add to breast milk

Appetite Suppressant Product Table

APPETITE SUPPRESSANT PRODUCTS

	Product & Manufacturer	Phenylpropanolamine Hydrochloride	Other Ingredients
GL PU SO SU	Acutrim 16 Hour Steady Control CIBA Consumer	75mg	cellulose acetate • hydroxypropyl methylcellulose • stearic acid
GL PU SO SU	Acutrim II Maximum Strength CIBA Consumer	75mg	cellulose acetate •FD&C yellow#10 • FD&C blue#1 • FD&C yellow#6 •hydroxypropyl methylcellulose • povidone • propylene glycol • stearic acid • titanium dioxide
GL PU SO SU	Acutrim Late Day CIBA Consumer	75mg	cellulose acetate • FD&C yellow #6 • hydroxypropyl methylcellulose • isopropyl alcohol • propylene glycol • riboflavin • stearic acid • titanium dioxide
PU	Appedrine Caplets Thompson Medical	25mg	vitamin A, 1667 IU • vitamin D, 133 IU • thiamine, 1mg • riboflavin, 1mg • pyridoxine hydrochloride, 0.33mg • vitamin E, 10 IU • folic acid, 0.13mg • vitamin B_1, 0.5mg • vitamin B_2, ns
PU	Control Capsules Thompson Medical	75mg	D&C yellow#10 • FD&C yellow#6 • methanol • DI water • shellac • polyvinyl pyrolidone • magnesium stearate • talc • pharmaceutical glaze
PU SO	Dexatrim Caffeine Free Maximum Strength Caplets Thompson Medical	75mg	calcium sulfate • lactose • stearic acid • ethyl cellulose • isopropyl alcohol • magnesium stearate • D&C yellow#10 aluminum lake • FD&C yellow#6 aluminum lake • hydroxypropyl methylcellulose • iron oxide • polyethylene glycol • propylene glycol • titanium dioxide
PU SO SU	Dexatrim Caffeine Free Maximum Strength with Vitamin C Thompson Medical	75mg	ascorbic acid, 180mg • croscarmellose sodium • ethylcellulose • FD&C blue#1 aluminum lake • FD&C red#40 aluminum lake • FD&C yellow#6 aluminum lake • hydroxypropyl methylcellulose • lactose • magnesium stearate • polyethylene glycol • polysorbate 80 • stearic acid • titanium dioxide
PU SO	Dexatrim Maximum Strength Caffeine Free Capsules Thompson Medical	75mg	gelatin • pharmaceutical glaze • povidone • sucrose • talc • D&C yellow#10 • FD&C yellow#6 • magnesium stearate • FD&C yellow#6 aluminum lake • methanol
PU SO SU	Dexatrim Maximum Strength Extended Duration Thompson Medical	75mg	calcium sulfate • D&C yellow#10 aluminum lake • ethylcellulose • FD&C yellow#6 aluminum lake • hydroxypropyl methylcellulose • iron oxide • magnesium stearate • propylene glycol • povidone • stearic acid • titanium dioxide • triacetin
PU SO	Dexatrim Plus Vitamin C, Maximum Strength Thompson Medical	75mg	ascorbic acid, 180mg • pharmaceutical glaze • povidone • FD&C red#3 • FD&C red#40 • FD&C yellow#6 • methanol • talc • magnesium stearate • sucrose
PU SO	Dexatrim Regular Strength Capsules Thompson Medical	50mg	gelatin • pharmaceutical glaze • povidone • sucrose • talc • D&C yellow#10 • FD&C yellow#6 • magnesium stearate • FD&C red#3 • FD&C red#40 • methanol
	Just One Per Day Reese Chemical	75mg	calcium carbonate • maltodextrin M150 • ethylcellulose • calcium sulfate • magnesium stearate • titanium dioxide • polyethylene glycol 8000 • FD&C yellow#6 • shellac • talc • plasdone • propylene glycol
	Super Odrinex Fox	25mg	
SO SU	Thinz Back-To-Nature Alva-Amco	75mg	
SO	Thinz-Span Alva-Amco	75mg	

ARTIFICIAL TEAR PRODUCTS

	Product & Manufacturer	Viscosity Agent	Preservative	pH	Other Ingredients
	Adsorbotear Alcon	hydroxyethylcellulose, 0.42% • povidone, 1.67%	thimerosal, 0.004%	7.1-7.6	
PU	**Akwa Tears Drops** Akorn	polyvinyl alcohol	benzalkonium chloride, 0.01%	5.21	sodium chloride • edetate disodium • potassium chloride
PR PU	**Akwa Tears Ointment** Akorn			5.21	white petrolatum • mineral oil • anhydrous lanolin
PR PU	**Cellufresh** Allergan, Inc.	carboxymethylcellulose, 0.5%		ns	calcium chloride • magnesium chloride • potassium chloride • sodium lactate • may contain hydrochloric acid or sodium hydroxide to adjust pH
PR PU	**Celluvisc** Allergan, Inc.	carboxymethylcellulose sodium, 1%		ns	calcium chloride • potassium chloride • sodium chloride • sodium lactate
	Comfort Tears Liquid Pilkington Barnes Hind	hydroxyethylcellulose	benzalkonium chloride, 0.005% • edetate disodium, 0.02%	ns	sodium chloride
	Comfort Tears Drops Pilkington Barnes Hind	hydroxyethylcellulose • polyvinyl alcohol	benzalkonium chloride, 0.005% • edetate disodium, 0.02%	ns	
	Dry Eye Therapy Bausch & Lomb	glycerin, 0.3%		ns	calcium chloride • magnesium chloride • potassium chloride • sodium chloride • sodium citrate • sodium phosphate • zinc chloride
	Duolube Bausch & Lomb	white petrolatum, 80% • mineral oil, 20%		ns	
PR	**Hypotears PF Drops** Iolab	polyvinyl alcohol, 1%		ns	polyethylene glycol 400 • dextrose • edetate disodium • purified water
	Hypotears Drops Iolab	polyvinyl alcohol, 1%	benzalkonium chloride, 0.01%	6.6	
PR	**Hypotears Ointment** Iolab			ns	white petrolatum • light mineral oil
	Isopto Alkaline Alcon	hydroxypropyl methylcellulose, 1%	benzalkonium chloride, 0.01%	6.0-7.8	
	Isopto Plain Alcon	hydroxypropyl methylcellulose, 0.5%	benzalkonium chloride, 0.01%	6.0-7.8	
	Isopto Tears Alcon	hydroxypropyl methylcellulose, 0.05%	benzalkonium chloride, 0.01%	6.0-7.8	
PU	**Just Tears** Blairex	hydroxypropyl methylcellulose	benzalkonium chloride, 0.01% • edetate disodium, 0.025%	ns	sodium chloride • potassium chloride • sodium borate • boric acid
PU	**Lacril** Allergan, Inc.	hydroxypropyl methylcellulose, 0.5% • gelatin a, 0.01%	chlorobutanol, 0.5%	ns	calcium chloride • dextrose • magnesium chloride • polysorbate 80 • potassium chloride • purified water • sodium acetate • sodium borate • sodium chloride • sodium citrate • may contain acetic acid to adjust pH

ARTIFICIAL TEAR PRODUCTS — continued

	Product & Manufacturer	Viscosity Agent	Preservative	pH	Other Ingredients
PU	Liquifilm Forte Allergan, Inc.	polyvinyl alcohol, 3%	thimerosal, 0.002%	ns	edate disodium • mono- and dibasic sodium phosphate • purified water • sodium chloride • may contain hydrochloric acid or sodium hydroxide to adjust pH
PU	Liquifilm Tears Drops Allergan, Inc.	polyvinyl alcohol, 1.4%	chlorobutanol, 0.5%	ns	sodium chloride • purified water • may contain hydrochloric acid or sodium hydroxide to adjust pH
	Moisture Drops Bausch & Lomb	hydroxypropyl methylcellulose, 0.5% • dextran 70, 0.1% • glycerin, 0.2%	benzalkonium chloride, 0.01% • edetate disodium	ns	sodium chloride • potassium chloride • sodium borate • boric acid
PU	Murine Eye Lubricant Ross	polyvinyl alcohol, 1.4% • povidone, 0.6%	benzalkonium chloride • edetate disodium	ns	dextrose • potassium chloride • sodium bicarbonate • sodium chloride • sodium citrate • sodium phosphate • purified water
	Murocel Bausch & Lomb	methylcellulose, 1%		ns	propylene glycol • sodium chloride • boric acid • parabens
PR PU	Refresh Allergan, Inc.	polyvinyl alcohol, 1.4% • povidone, 0.6%		ns	sodium chloride • purified water • may contain hydrochloric acid or sodium hydroxide to adjust pH
	Tear Gard Medtech	hydroxyethylcellulose	edetate disodium, 0.1%	ns	sorbic acid, 0.25%
	Teargen II Goldline	hydroxypropyl methylcellulose, 0.3% • dextran, 0.1%	benzalkonium chloride, 0.01%	ns	
	Tearisol Iolab	hydroxypropyl methylcellulose, 0.5%	benzalkonium chloride, 0.01%	7.5	boric acid • potassium chloride • sodium carbonate
	Tears Naturale Alcon	hydroxypropyl methylcellulose, 0.3% • dextran 70, 0.1%	benzalkonium chloride, 0.01% • edetate disodium, 0.05%	6.6-7.8	
	Tears Naturale & Free Alcon	hydroxypropyl methylcellulose, 0.3% • dextran 70, 0.1%		6.0-8.0	
	Tears Naturale II Alcon	hydroxypropyl methylcellulose, 0.3% • dextran 70, 0.1%	polyquad, 0.0001%	6.5-8.0	potassium chloride • sodium chloride • polyquaternium-1, 0.001%
PU	Tears Plus Allergan, Inc.	polyvinyl alcohol, 1.4% • povidone, 0.6%	chlorobutanol, 0.5%	ns	purified water • sodium chloride • may contain hydrochloric acid or sodium hydroxide to adjust pH
PU	Tears Renewed Akorn	hydroxypropyl methylcellulose • dextran 70	benzalkonium chloride, 0.01%	6.7-7.3	sodium chloride • potassium chloride • edetate disodium • hydrochloric acid and/or sodium hydroxide
	Ultra Tears Alcon	hydroxypropyl methylcellulose, 1%	benzalkonium chloride, 0.01%	6.0-7.8	

OPHTHALMIC DECONGESTANT PRODUCTS

Product Manufacturer	Viscosity Agent	Vasoconstrictor	Preservative	Buffer	pH	Other Ingredients
PU **A K-Nefrin** Akorn	hydroxyethylcellulose, 0.5%	phenylephrine hydrochloride, 0.12%	benzalkonium chloride, 0.01% • EDTA		6.2-6.8	sodium chloride • edetate disodium • sodium phosphate monobasic • sodium phosphate dibasic • purified water
Allerest Eye Drops CIBA Consumer		naphazoline hydrochloride, 0.012%	benzalkonium chloride • EDTA	boric acid • sodium borate	ns	
Allergy Drops Bausch & Lomb	polyethylene glycol 300, 0.2%	naphazoline hydrochloride, 0.012%	benzalkonium chloride, 0.01% • edetate disodium		ns	boric acid • sodium borate • sodium chloride
Allergy Drops Maximum Strength Bausch & Lomb	hydroxypropyl methylcellulose, 0.5%	naphazoline hydrochloride, 0.03%	benzalkonium chloride, 0.01% • edetate disodium		ns	boric acid • sodium borate • sodium chloride
PU **Clear Eyes ACR** Ross	glycerin, 0.2%	naphazoline hydrochloride, 0.012%	benzalkonium chloride • edetate disodium	boric acid • sodium borate	ns	zinc sulfate, 0.25% • purified water
PU **Clear Eyes Lubricating Eye Redness Reliever** Ross	glycerin, 0.2%	naphazoline hydrochloride, 0.012%	benzalkonium chloride • edetate disodium	boric acid • sodium borate	ns	purified water
Comfort Eye Drops Pilkington Barnes Hind	hydroxyethylcellulose • polyvinyl alcohol	naphazoline hydrochloride, 0.03%	benzalkonium chloride, 0.005% • edetate disodium, 0.02%	mono- and dibasic sodium phosphate	ns	sodium chloride
Degest 2 Pilkington Barnes Hind	hydroxyethylcellulose	naphazoline hydrochloride, 0.012%	benzalkonium chloride, 0.0067% • edetate disodium, 0.02%	sodium citrate	ns	povidone
Estivin II Alcon	hydroxypropyl methylcellulose, 0.3% • dextrin 70, 0.1%	naphazoline hydrochloride, 0.012%	benzalkonium chloride, 0.01%		5.5-6.5	
Isopto-Frin Alcon	hydroxypropyl methylcellulose, 0.5%	phenylephrine hydrochloride, 0.12%	benzalkonium chloride, 0.01%	sodium citrate • sodium phosphate • sodium biphosphate	7.3	
PU **Murine Plus Lubricating Eye Redness Reliever** Ross	polyvinyl alcohol, 1.4% • povidone, 0.6%	tetrahydrozoline hydrochloride, 0.05%	benzalkonium chloride • edetate disodium		ns	dextrose potassium chloride • purified water • sodium bicarbonate • sodium chloride • sodium citrate • sodium phosphate

OPHTHALMIC DECONGESTANT PRODUCTS — continued

	Product & Manufacturer	Viscosity Agent	Vasoconstrictor	Preservative	Buffer	pH	Other Ingredients
	Naphcon Alcon		naphazoline hydrochloride, 0.012%	benzalkonium chloride, 0.01%		ns	
	Ocu Clear Schering-Plough		oxymetazoline hydrochloride, 0.025%	benzalkonium chloride, 0.01% • EDTA		ns	
PU	Prefrin Liquifilm Allergan, Inc.	polyvinyl alcohol, 1.4%	phenylephrine hydrochloride, 0.12%	benzalkonium chloride, 0.005%	mono- and dibasic sodium phosphate	ns	purified water • sodium acetate • sodium thiosulfate • may have hydrochloric acid or sodium hydroxide to adjust pH
PR PU	Relief Allergan, Inc.	polyvinyl alcohol, 1.4%	phenylephrine hydrochloride, 0.12%		mono- and dibasic sodium phosphate	ns	purified water • sodium acetate • sodium thiosulfate • may have hydrochloric acid and/or sodium chloride to adjust pH
	Soothe Alcon	povidone	tetrahydrozoline hydrochloride, 0.05%	benzalkonium chloride, 0.004% • EDTA, 0.1%		ns	
	Tetrahydrozoline Hydrochloride Various Manufacturers		tetrahydrozoline hydrochloride, 0.05%			ns	
	Vaso Clear Iolab	polyvinyl alcohol	naphazoline hydrochloride, 0.02%	benzalkonium chloride, 0.01% • EDTA		ns	PEG-8000
	Vaso Clear A Iolab	polyvinyl alcohol, 0.25%	naphazoline hydrochloride, 0.02%	benzalkonium chloride, 0.005% • EDTA		ns	zinc sulfate, 0.25% • PEG-8000, ns
PU	Visine Pfizer		tetrahydrozoline hydrochloride, 0.05%	benzalkonium chloride, 0.01% • EDTA, 0.1%	boric acid • sodium borate	ns	sodium chloride
PU	Visine A.C. Pfizer		tetrahydrozoline hydrochloride, 0.05%	benzalkonium chloride, 0.01% • EDTA, 0.1%	boric acid • sodium citrate	ns	zinc sulfate, 0.25% • sodium chloride
PU	Visine Extra Pfizer		tetrahydrozoline hydrochloride, 0.05%	benzalkonium chloride, 0.013% • EDTA, 0.1%	boric acid • sodium borate	ns	polyethylene glycol-400, 1% • sodium chloride
PU	Visine L.R. Pfizer		oxymetazoline hydrochloride, 0.025%	benzalkonium chloride, 0.01% • EDTA, 0.10%	boric acid • sodium borate	ns	sodium chloride
	Zincfrin Alcon		phenylephrine hydrochloride, 0.12%	benzalkonium chloride, 0.01%		ns	zinc sulfate, 0.25%

EYE WASH PRODUCTS

Product & Manufacturer	Buffer	pH	Preservative	Other Ingredients
Blinx Pilkington Barnes Hind	sodium phosphate	ns	benzalkonium chloride, 0.005% • disodium edetate, 0.02%	sodium and potassium chlorides
Dacriose Iolab	sodium phosphate	ns	benzalkonium chloride, 0.01% • edetate disodium, 0.3%	potassium chloride • sodium chloride
Enuclene[a] Alcon		ns	benzalkonium chloride, 0.02%	tyloxapol, 0.25%
Eye Wash Bausch & Lomb	borate buffer		sorbic acid, 0.1% • EDTA, 0.025%	sodium chloride
Eye-Scrub[b] CooperVision		ns		PEG-200 glyceryl monotallowate • disodium laureth sulfosuccinate • cocoamido propyl amine oxide • PEG-78 glyceryl monococoate • benzyl alcohol • EDTA
Eye-Stream Alcon	sodium acetate, 0.39% • sodium citrate, 0.17%	6.5-7.5	benzalkonium chloride, 0.13%	calcium chloride, 0.048% • magnesium chloride, 0.03% • potassium chloride, 0.075% • sodium chloride, 0.64% • sodium hydroxide and/or hydrochloric acid
Lauro Eye Wash Otis Clapp	sodium phosphate	7	edetate disodium • benzalkonium chloride	sodium chloride
Lavoptik Eye Wash Lavoptik	sodium phosphate	7	edetate sodium • benzalkonium chloride, 0.005%	sodium chloride, 0.49%
PR Lid Wipes - SPF[b] PU Akorn	sodium dihydrogen phosphate • sodium hydroxide	ns		PEG-200 glyceryl monotallowate • PEG-80 glyceryl monococoate • laureth-23 • cocoamido propyl amine oxide • sodium chloride • glycerin
OCuSOFT[b] Cynacon/OCuSOFT		ns		PEG-80 sorbitan laurate • sodium trideceth sulfate • PEG-150 distearate • cocoamido propyl hydroxysultaine • lauroamphocarboxyglycinate • sodium laureth-13 carboxylate • PEG-15 tallow polyamine • quaternium-15
OcuClenz[b] Storz/Lederle		ns		disodium oleamido PEG-2 sulfosuccinate • cocoamphodiacetate • poloxamer 185 • poloxamer 188 • methylparaben • propylparaben • citric acid • EDTA
Trisol Eye Wash Buffington	sodium phosphate	7	edetate disodium • benzalkonium chloride	sodium chloride

[a] For artificial eyes.
[b] Eyelid scrub only—not for use in the eye.

HARD AND RIGID GAS-PERMEABLE LENS PRODUCTS

Product & Manufacturer	Suggested Use	Viscosity Agent	Preservative	Other Ingredients
Adapettes Alcon	rewetting	adsorbobase • povidone	EDTA, 0.1% • sorbic acid, 0.2%	
Adapt Alcon	wetting • rewetting	adsorbobase • hydroxyethylcellulose	thimerosal, 0.004% • EDTA, 0.1%	
PR PU **Blairex Hard Contact Lens Cleaner** Blairex	cleaning			surfactants
Boston Advance Cleaner[b] Polymer Technology	cleaning			alkyl ether sulfate • ethoxylated alkyl phenol • triquaternary cocoa-based phospholipid • silica gel
Boston Advance Conditioning Solution[b] Polymer Technology	wetting • soaking • disinfection	hydroxyethylcellulose • polyvinyl alcohol • cationic cellulose derivatives	polyaminopropyl biguanide • EDTA	
Boston Cleaner[b] Polymer Technology	cleaning			alkyl ether sulfate • silica gel
Boston Conditioning Solution[b] Polymer Technology	wetting • soaking • disinfection	hydroxyethylcellulose • polyvinyl alcohol • cationic cellulose derivatives	chlorhexidine gluconate • EDTA	
Boston Rewetting Drops[b] Polymer Technology	lubricating • rewetting	hydroxyethylcellulose • polyvinyl alcohol • cationic cellulose derivatives	chlorhexidine gluconate • EDTA	
Clean-N-Soak Allergan Optical	cleaning • soaking		phenylmercuric nitrate, 0.004%	cleaning agent
Clens Alcon	cleaning		benzalkonium chloride, 0.02% • EDTA, 0.1%	cleaning agents
Comfortcare GP Daily Cleaner Liquid[b] Pilkington Barnes Hind	cleaning	hydroxyethylcellulose	potassium sorbate, 0.13% • edetate disodium, 2%	polyoxyethylene • polyoxypropylene block polymer • tris (hydroxymethyl) amino methane
Comfortcare GP Daily Cleaner Suspension[b] Pilkington Barnes Hind	cleaning			sodium lauryl ether sulfate • boric acid • silica • sodium chloride • glyceryl polyethylene glycol stearate • polyoxyalkylene dimethylsiloxane
Comfortcare GP Dual Action Daily Cleaner[a, b] Pilkington Barnes Hind	cleaner			subtilisin • poloxamer 338 • potassium carbonate • citric acid • sodium benzoate • povidone
Comfortcare GP Wetting & Soaking Solution[b] Pilkington Barnes Hind	wetting • disinfection • storage	hydroxyethylcellulose • polyvinyl alcohol • povidone	chlorhexidine gluconate, 0.005% • edetate disodium, 0.02%	octylphenoxy (oxyethylene) ethanol • propylene glycol • sodium chloride
Concentrated Cleaner[b] Bausch & Lomb	cleaning			sodium chloride • sulfate surfactant
Gas Permeable Comfort Drops[b] Pilkington Barnes Hind	rewetting • lubricating	hydroxyethylcellulose	potassium sorbate, 0.13% • edetate disodium, 0.1%	octylphenoxy (oxyethylene) ethanol • sodium chloride
LC-65 Daily Contact Lens Cleaner Allergan Optical	cleaning		thimerosal, 0.001% • EDTA	cleaning agent

HARD AND RIGID GAS-PERMEABLE LENS PRODUCTS — continued

Product & Manufacturer	Suggested Use	Viscosity Agent	Preservative	Other Ingredients
Lens Lubricant Bausch & Lomb	rewetting • lubricating	povidone	thimerosal, 0.004% • EDTA, 0.1%	polyoxyethylene
Liquifilm Wetting Solution Allergan Optical	wetting	hydroxypropyl methylcellulose • polyvinyl alcohol	benzalkonium chloride, 0.004% • EDTA	sodium chloride • potassium chloride
Opti-Clean Alcon	cleaning		thimerosal, 0.004% • EDTA, 0.1%	polymeric cleaning beads • polysorbate 21
Opti-Clean II Alcon	cleaning	hydroxyethylcellulose	EDTA, 0.1% • polyquaternium-1, 0.01%	cleaning agent • polysorbate 21
Opti-Zyme Enzymatic[b] Alcon	weekly protein cleaning			pancreatin
Pro Free/GP Weekly Enzymatic Cleaner[a, b] Allergan Optical	weekly protein cleaning		edetate disodium	sodium chloride • sodium carbonate • sodium borate • papain
Resolve/GP Daily Cleaner[b] Allergan Optical	cleaning			fatty acid amide • sodium lauryl sulfate • hexylene glycol • alkyl ether sulfate • surfactants • cocoamphocarboxyglycinate
SLC Ocular Pharm.	cleaning		sorbic acid, 0.1% • EDTA, 0.1%	cleaning agent
SWS Ocular Pharm.	soaking • wetting	polyvinyl alcohol • hydroxyethylcellulose	benzalkonium chloride, 0.01% • EDTA, 0.025%	sodium chloride • potassium chloride
Soaclens Alcon	soaking • wetting		thimerosal, 0.004% • EDTA, 0.1%	buffers • wetting agents
Titan Pilkington Barnes Hind	cleaning	hydroxyethylcellulose	potassium sorbate, 0.13% • edetate disodium, 2.0%	polyoxyethylene • polyoxypropylene block polymer • tris (hydroxymethyl) amino methane
Total All-In-One Contact Lens Solution Allergan Optical	cleaning • soaking • wetting	polyvinyl alcohol	benzalkonium chloride • EDTA	
Wet & Soak Rewetting Drops[b] Allergan Optical	rewetting • lubricating		WSCP, 0.0060%	borate • hydroxyethylcellulose
Wet-N-Soak Plus Wetting And Soaking[b] Allergan Optical	wetting • soaking	polyvinyl alcohol	benzalkonium chloride, 0.003% • EDTA	
Wetting & Soaking Solution[b] Bausch & Lomb	rinsing • disinfection • storage		chlorhexidine gluconate, 0.006% • EDTA, 0.05%	polyvinyl alcohol • hydroxyethyl cellulose
Wetting And Soaking Solution[b] Pilkington Barnes Hind	soaking • wetting	polyvinyl alcohol • povidone • hydroxyethylcellulose	benzalkonium chloride, 0.005% • edetate disodium, 0.1%	
Wetting Solution Pilkington Barnes Hind	wetting	polyvinyl alcohol	benzalkonium chloride, 0.004% • edetate disodium, 0.02%	

[a]Tablet; must be dissolved in water.
[b]For rigid gas-permeable lenses.

Soft Lens Product Table

SOFT LENS PRODUCTS

Product & Manufacturer	Suggested Use	Viscosity Agent	Preservative	Other Ingredients
Surface Active Cleaners				
Ciba Vision Cleaner CIBA Vision	cleaning	cocoamphocarboxyglycinate	sorbic acid, 0.1% • EDTA, 0.2%	sodium lauryl sulfate • hexylene glycol
Daily Cleaner Bausch & Lomb	cleaning	hydroxyethylcellulose • polyvinyl alcohol	thimerosal, 0.004% • EDTA, 0.2%	tyloxapol • sodium phosphate • sodium chloride
DURAcare Blairex	cleaning		thimerosal, 0.004% • edetate disodium, 0.001%	nonionic detergents
DURAcare II Blairex	cleaning		sorbic acid, 0.1% • edetate disodium, 0.25%	block copolymers of ethylene and propylene oxide • octoyplhenoxy polyethoxyethanol
Lens Plus Daily Cleaner Allergan Optical	cleaner	cocoamphocarboxyglycinate	EDTA	sodium lauryl sulfate • hexylene glycol • sodium chloride • sodium phosphate
Mira Flow Extra Strength CIBA Vision	cleaning			isopropyl alcohol, 20% • poloxamer 407 • amphoteric 10
Opti-Clean Alcon	cleaning		thimerosal, 0.004% • EDTA, 0.1%	tween 21
Opti-Clean II Alcon	cleaning	hydroxyethylcellulose	EDTA, 0.1% • polyquaternium-1, 0.019%	polysorbate 21 • cleaning agent
Pliagel Wesley-Jessen	cleaning		sorbic acid, 0.25% • EDTA, 0.5%	sodium chloride • potassium chloride • poloxamer 407
Preflex For Sensitive Eyes Alcon	cleaning	hydroxyethylcellulose • polyvinyl alcohol	EDTA, 0.2% • sorbic acid, 0.2%	sodium chloride • sodium phosphate • tyloxapol
Sensitive Eyes Daily Bausch & Lomb	cleaning	hydroxypropyl methylcellulose	sorbic acid, 0.25% • EDTA, 0.5%	sodium chloride • borate buffer • surfactant
Sensitive Eyes Saline/Cleaning Solution Bausch & Lomb	cleaning		sorbic acid • EDTA	sodium chloride • borate buffer • surfactant
Soft Mate Daily Cleaning For Sensitive Eyes Pilkington Barnes Hind	cleaning	hydroxyethylcellulose	potassium sorbate, 0.13% • edetate disodium, 0.2%	sodium chloride • octylphen (oxyethylene) ethanol
Soft Mate Hands Off Daily Cleaner Pilkington Barnes Hind	cleaning	hydroxyethylcellulose	potassium sorbate, 0.13% • edetate disodium, 0.20%	sodium chloride • octylphen (oxyethylene) ethanol
Enzymatic Cleaners				
Allergan Enzymatic Contact Lens Cleaner Allergan Optical	weekly protein cleaning		EDTA	sodium chloride • papain • sodium carbonate • sodium borate
Opti-Zyme Enzymatic Alcon	weekly protein cleaning			pancreatin
ReNu Effervescent Enzymatic Bausch & Lomb	weekly protein cleaning			subtilisin PEG • sodium carbonate • sodium chloride • tartaric acid
ReNu Thermal Enzymatic Bausch & Lomb	weekly protein cleaning			subtilisin PEG • sodium carbonate • sodium chloride • boric acid
Sensitive Eyes Effervescent Enzymatic Bausch & Lomb	weekly protein cleaning			subtilisin PEG • sodium carbonate • sodium chloride • tartaric acid

SOFT LENS PRODUCTS — continued

Product & Manufacturer	Suggested Use	Viscosity Agent	Preservative	Other Ingredients
Ultrazyme Enzymatic Cleaner Allergan Optical	weekly protein cleaning			subtilisin A • effervescing agents • buffers

Chemical Disinfection Products

Product & Manufacturer	Suggested Use	Viscosity Agent	Preservative	Other Ingredients
Allergan Hydrocare Cleaning & Disinfecting Solution Allergan Optical	chemical disinfection	polysorbate 80	thimerosal, 0.002% • hydrochloric acid • tris (2-hydroxyethyl) tallow ammonium chloride, 0.013% • bis (2-hydroxyethyl) tallow ammonium chloride	sodium bicarbonate • propylene glycol • sodium phosphate • soluble polyhema
Disinfecting Solution Bausch & Lomb	rinsing • chemical disinfection • storing		thimerosal, 0.001% • chlorhexidine gluconate, 0.005% • EDTA, 0.1%	sodium chloride • sodium borate • boric acid
Flex-Care Alcon	rinsing • chemical disinfection		chlorhexidine gluconate, 0.005% • EDTA, 0.1%	sodium chloride • sodium borate • boric acid
Opti-Free Alcon	rinsing • chemical disinfection • storing		EDTA, 0.05% • polyquaternium-1, 0.001%	citrate buffer • sodium chloride
ReNu Multi-Purpose Solution Bausch & Lomb	rinsing • chemical disinfection • storing • cleaning		EDTA	sodium chloride • sodium borate • boric acid • poloxamine • polyaminopropyl biguanide, 0.00005%
Soft Mate Disinfecting Solution Pilkington Barnes Hind	rinsing • chemical disinfection • storing	povidone	chlorhexidine gluconate, 0.005% • edetate disodium, 0.1%	octylphen (oxyethylene) ethanol • sodium chloride

Hydrogen Peroxide Disinfection Products

Product & Manufacturer	Suggested Use	Viscosity Agent	Preservative	Other Ingredients
Aosept CIBA Vision	disinfecting • neutralizing			hydrogen peroxide, 3% • sodium chloride, 0.85% • sodium stannate • phosphate buffers • stabilized with phosphoric acid
Lens Plus Oxysept 2 Rinse and Neutralizer Allergan Optical	rinsing • neutralizing			catalase • sodium chloride • mono- & dibasic sodium phosphates
Lensept CIBA Vision	disinfecting • neutralizing		sorbic acid (rinse & neutralizer) • EDTA (rinse & neutralizer)	disinfecting solution: hydrogen peroxide, 3% • sodium stannate • sodium nitrate • phosphate buffers • rinse & neutralizer: bovine catalase • sodium chloride • sodium borate decahydrate • boric acid
Mira Sept Wesley-Jessen	disinfecting • neutralizing		EDTA (rinse & neutralizer)	disinfecting solution: hydrogen peroxide, 3% • sodium stannate • sodium nitrate • rinse & neutralizer: sodium pyruvate • sodium chloride • sodium borate • boric acid
Oxysept 1 Disinfecting Solution Allergan Optical	disinfection			hydrogen peroxide, 3% • sodium stannate • sodium nitrate • phosphate buffers

SOFT LENS PRODUCTS — continued

Product & Manufacturer	Suggested Use	Viscosity Agent	Preservative	Other Ingredients
Oxysept 2 Neutralizing Tablets Allergan Optical	neutralizing			catalase • buffering and tableting agents
Soft Mate Consept-1 Pilkington Barnes Hind	cleaning • disinfection			hydrogen peroxide, 3% • polyoxyl 40 stearate • sodium stannate • sodium nitrate • phosphate buffer
Soft Mate Consept-2 Pilkington Barnes Hind	rinsing • neutralizing			sodium thiosulfate, 0.5% • borate buffer
Ultracare Disinfectanta/Neutralizer System[a] Allergan Optical	disinfecting • neutralizing			hydrogen peroxide, 3% • sodium stannate • sodium nitrate • phosphates • purified water

Rewetting Products

Product & Manufacturer	Suggested Use	Viscosity Agent	Preservative	Other Ingredients
Adapettes For Sensitive Eyes Alcon	lubricating • rewetting	povidone	EDTA, 0.1% • sorbic acid, 0.2%	polymers
Lens Drops CIBA Vision	rewetting • lubricating		sorbic acid, 0.15% • EDTA, 0.2%	sodium chloride • borate buffer • carbamide • poloxamer 407
Lens Lubricant Bausch & Lomb	rewetting • lubricating	povidone	thimerosal, 0.004% • EDTA, 0.1%	polyoxyethylene
Lens Plus Rewetting Drops Allergan Optical	rewetting			sodium chloride • boric acid
Opti-Free Rewetting Drops Alcon	moistens eyes and lenses		polyquaternium-1, 0.01%	citric acid • sodium citrate • sodium chloride
Opti-Tears Alcon	rewetting • lubricating	hydroxypropyl methylcellulose	EDTA, 0.1% • polyquaternium-1, 0.001%	dextran • sodium chloride • potassium chloride
ReNu Rewetting Drops Bausch & Lomb	rewetting		sorbic acid, 0.15% • EDTA	borate buffer
Sensitive Eyes Drops Bausch & Lomb	rewetting		sorbic acid, 0.1% • EDTA	borate buffer
Soft Mate Comfort Drops Pilkington Barnes Hind	rewetting • lubricating	hydroxyethylcellulose	potassium sorbate, 0.13% • edetate disodium, 0.10%	octylphen (oxyethylene) ethanol • sodium chloride • borate buffer
Sterile Lens Lubricant Blairex	rewetting • lubricating	hydroxypropyl methylcellulose	sorbic acid, 0.25% • edetate disodium, 0.1%	borate buffer • sodium chloride • glycerin

Saline Products

Product & Manufacturer	Suggested Use	Viscosity Agent	Preservative	Other Ingredients
Alcon Saline ESE Alcon	storage • heat disinfection		sorbic acid, 0.125% • edetate disodium, 0.1%	sodium borate • boric acid • sodium chloride
Allergan Hydrocare Preserved Saline Solution Allergan Optical	rinsing • thermal disinfection • storing		thimerosal, 0.001% • edetate disodium, 0.01%	sodium hexametaphosphate • sodium chloride • boric acid • sodium borate • sodium hydroxide
PR Blairex Steril Saline Solution Blairex	rinsing • thermal disinfection • storage			sodium chloride, 0.9% • boric acid • sodium borate
Ciba Vision Saline CIBA Vision	rinsing • thermal disinfection • storing			sodium chloride • boric acid

SOFT LENS PRODUCTS — continued

Product & Manufacturer	Suggested Use	Viscosity Agent	Preservative	Other Ingredients
Lens Plus Sterile Saline Solution Allergan Optical	rinsing • thermal disinfection • storing			sodium chloride • boric acid
Opti-Soft Alcon	rinsing • thermal disinfection • storing		EDTA, 0.1% • polyquaternium-1, 0.001%	sodium chloride • borate buffer
Preserved Saline Solution Bausch & Lomb	rinsing • thermal disinfection • storing		thimerosal, 0.001% • EDTA	boric acid • sodium chloride
ReNu Saline Bausch & Lomb	rinsing • thermal disinfection • storing • enzyme diluent		EDTA • polyaminopropyl biguanide, 0.00003%	sodium chloride • boric acid
Sensitive Eyes Plus Saline Bausch & Lomb	rinsing • thermal disinfection • enzyme diluent		polyaminopropyl biguanide, 0.00003%	sodium chloride • potassium chloride
Sensitive Eyes Saline Solution Bausch & Lomb	rinsing • thermal disinfection • storing		sorbic acid, 0.1% • EDTA	sodium chloride • borate buffer
Sensitive Eyes Saline Spray Bausch & Lomb	rinsing • thermal disinfection • storing • enzyme diluent			sodium chloride • boric acid • sodium borate
Soft Mate Saline for Sensitive Eyes Pilkington Barnes Hind	rinsing • storing • thermal disinfection		potassium sorbate, 0.13% • edetate disodium, 0.025%	sodium chloride • borate buffer
Soft Mate Saline Solution Pilkington Barnes Hind	rinsing • thermal disinfection • storing		potassium sorbate, 0.13% • edetate disodium, 0.025%	sodium chloride • borate buffer
Soft Mate Saline Spray Pilkington Barnes Hind	rinsing • thermal disinfection • storing			sodium chloride • borate buffer
Softwear Saline CIBA Vision	rinsing			sodium chloride • sodium borate • boric acid • sodium perborate

[a]Disinfects and neutralizes in one step.

OTIC PRODUCTS

Product & Manufacturer	Ingredients
Auraphene-B Reese Chemical	carbamide peroxide, 6.5%
Aurinol Ear Drops Various Manufacturers	chloroxylenol • acetic acid • benzalkonium chloride • glycerin
Auro Ear Drops Del	carbamide peroxide, 6.5%
Auro-Dri Del	boric acid, 2.75% • isopropyl alcohol
Debrox Drops SmithKline Beecham	carbamide peroxide, 6.5% • glycerin • propylene glycol
E.R.O. Scherer	carbamide peroxide, 6.5% • anhydrous glycerin
Ear Wax Removal System Bausch & Lomb	carbamide peroxide, 6.5% in an anhydrous glycerine vehicle
Ear-Dry Scherer	boric acid, 2.75% • isopropyl alcohol
Earsol Parnell	alcohol, 44% • propylene glycol • benzylbenzoate • fragrance
Mollifene Ear Drops Pfeiffer	anhydrous glycerin • carbamide peroxide, 6.5% • propylene glycol • sodium stannate
Murine Ear Wax Removal System And Ear Drops Ross	carbamide peroxide, 6.5% • alcohol, 6.3% • glycerin • polysorbate 20
Swim-Ear E. Fougera	isopropyl alcohol, 95% • anhydrous glycerin, 5%

DENTIFRICE PRODUCTS

Product & Manufacturer	ADA Approved[a]	Abrasive Ingredient	Therapeutic Ingredient	Foaming Agent	Other Ingredients[b]
Aim Anti Tartar Gel Formula with fluoride Chesebrough-Pond's		hydrated silica	sodium monofluorophosphate	sodium lauryl sulfate	sorbitol • polyols • glycerin • alcohol • flavor • cellulose gum • sodium saccharin • sodium benzoate • zinc citrate trihydrate • color
Aim Baking Soda Gel with fluoride Chesebrough-Pond's		hydrated silica	sodium monofluorophosphate	sodium lauryl sulfate	sorbitol • polyols • glycerin • alcohol • flavor • cellulose gum • sodium saccharin • sodium benzoate • zinc citrate trihydrate • sodium bicarbonate
Aim Regular Strength Gel with fluoride Chesebrough-Pond's		hydrated silica	sodium monofluorophosphate	sodium lauryl sulfate	sorbitol • polyols • glycerin • alcohol • flavor • cellulose gum • sodium saccharin • sodium benzoate • blue#1 • yellow#10
Aqua-Fresh Tartar Control, paste SmithKline Beecham	Yes	hydrated silica	sodium fluoride, 0.221%	sodium lauryl sulfate	tetrapotassium pyrophosphate • tetrasodium pyrophosphate • sorbitol • glycerin • PEG-8 • flavor • xanthan gum • sodium saccharin • sodium benzoate • D&C red#30 lake • FD&C blue#1 • D&C yellow#10
Aqua-Fresh Triple Protection, paste SmithKline Beecham	Yes	hydrated silica • calcium carbonate	sodium monofluorophosphate	sodium lauryl sulfate	PEG-8 • sorbitol • cellulose gum • sodium benzoate • titanium dioxide • calcium • carrageenan • flavor • sodium saccharin
PE Aqua-Fresh for Kids, paste SmithKline Beecham	Yes	hydrated silica • calcium carbonate	sodium monofluorophosphate	sodium lauryl sulfate	sorbitol • water • glycerin • PEG-8 • titanium dioxide • cellulose gum • flavor • mineral oil • sodium saccharin • calcium carrageenan • colors
SU Arm & Hammer Dental Care Gel with Fluoride Church & Dwight		hydrated silica • sodium bicarbonate		sodium lauryl sulfate	sorbitol • glycerin • water • PEG-8 • flavor blend • cellulose gum • sodium lauryl sarcosinate • sodium saccharin • FD&C blue#1 • D&C yellow#1
Caffree Anti-Stain Fluoride Toothpaste Block	Yes		sodium monofluorophosphate	sodium lauryl sulfate	water • diatomaceous earth • glycerin • sorbitol • aluminum silicate • titanium dioxide • hydroxyethylcellulose • flavor • sodium saccharin • methylparaben • propylparaben
Close-Up Anti-Plaque Gel Chesebrough-Pond's		hydrated silica	stannous fluoride	sodium lauryl sulfate	sorbitol • PEG-32 • alcohol • flavor • zinc citrate trihydrate • cellulose gum • sodium saccharin • sodium benzoate • sodium hydroxide • color
Close-Up Fluoride, gel & paste Chesebrough-Pond's		hydrated silica	sodium monofluorophosphate	sodium lauryl sulfate	sorbitol • polyols • glycerin • alcohol • flavor • cellulose gum • sodium saccharin • sodium benzoate • color (gel)
Close-Up Tartar Control Gel Chesebrough-Pond's		hydrated silica	sodium monofluorophosphate	sodium lauryl sulfate	sorbitol • polyols • glycerin • zinc citrate trihydrate • alcohol • flavor • cellulose gum • sodium saccharin • sodium benzoate • color
Colgate Baking Soda, paste Colgate-Palmolive		hydrated silica	sodium fluoride, 0.243%	sodium lauryl sulfate	glycerin • sodium bicarbonate • cellulose gum • flavor • sodium saccharin • titanium dioxide
PE Colgate Junior, gel Colgate-Palmolive	Yes	hydrated silica	sodium fluoride, 0.243%	sodium lauryl sulfate	sorbitol • PEG-12 • sodium benzoate • flavor • tetrasodium pyrophosphate • cellulose gum • sodium saccharin • mica • glycerin • titanium dioxide • FD&C blue#1 • D&C yellow#10
Colgate Tartar Control, gel Colgate-Palmolive	Yes	hydrated silica	sodium fluoride, 0.243%	sodium lauryl sulfate	sorbitol • glycerin • PEG-12 • tetrasodium pyrophosphate • PVM/MA copolymer • cellulose gum • flavor • sodium hydroxide • sodium saccharin • FD&C blue#1
Colgate Winterfresh Gel Colgate-Palmolive	Yes	hydrated silica	sodium fluoride, 0.243%	sodium lauryl sulfate	sorbitol • glycerin • PEG-12 • flavor • tetrasodium pyrophosphate • cellulose gum • sodium saccharin • FD&C blue#1

DENTIFRICE PRODUCTS — continued

	Product & Manufacturer	ADA Approved[a]	Abrasive Ingredient	Therapeutic Ingredient	Foaming Agent	Other Ingredients[b]
	Colgate, paste Colgate-Palmolive	Yes	dicalcium phosphate dihydrate	sodium monofluorophosphate, 0.76%	sodium lauryl sulfate	glycerin • cellulose gum • sodium benzoate • tetrasodium pyrophosphate • sodium saccharin • flavor
	Crest Baking Soda Mint Paste Procter & Gamble	Yes	hydrated silica	sodium fluoride	sodium lauryl sulfate	sorbitol • water • sodium bicarbonate • glycerin • flavor • cellulose gum • sodium saccharin • titanium dioxide
	Crest Cavity Fighting Toothpaste (Regular & Mint) Procter & Gamble	Yes	hydrated silica	sodium fluoride	sodium lauryl sulfate	sorbitol • water • flavor • sodium phosphate • xanthan gum • carbomer 956 • titanium dioxide • FD&C blue#1
	Crest Cavity Fighting Gel Procter & Gamble	Yes	hydrated silica	sodium fluoride	sodium lauryl sulfate	sorbitol • water • trisodium phosphate • sodium phosphate • xanthan gum • sodium saccharin • carbomer 956 • FD&C blue#1 • flavor
	Crest Tartar Control Gel Procter & Gamble	Yes	hydrated silica	sodium fluoride	sodium lauryl sulfate	water • sorbitol • glycerin • tetrapotassium pyrophosphate • PEG-6 • disodium pyrophosphate • tetrasodium pyrophosphate • flavor • xanthan gum • sodium saccharin • carbomer 956 • FD&C blue#1 (Fresh Mint & Smooth Mint) • FD&C yellow#5 (Smooth Mint)
PE	**Crest for Kids Sparkle Blue Gel, Bubblegum Flavor** Procter & Gamble	Yes	hydrated silica	sodium fluoride	sodium alkyl sulfate	sodium saccharin • sorbitol • trisodium phosphate • bubblegum flavor • xanthan gum • carbomer 956 • titanium dioxide • water
	Denquel Sensitive Teeth Toothpaste Procter & Gamble	Yes	hydrated silica • calcium	potassium nitrate, 5% carbonate	sodium lauryl sulfate	water • sorbitol • glycerin • xanthan gum • flavor • sodium saccharin • carbomer 956
	Dentagard, paste Colgate-Palmolive	Yes	hydrated silica	sodium monofluorophosphate, 0.76%	sodium lauryl sulfate	sorbitol • glycerin • PEG-12 • flavor • sodium benzoate • titanium dioxide • cellulose gum • sodium saccharin • FD&C red#40
	Gleem Toothpaste Procter & Gamble		hydrated silica	sodium fluoride	sodium lauryl sulfate	sorbitol • water • trisodium phosphate • flavor • xanthan gum • sodium saccharin • carbomer 956 • titanium dioxide
	Interplak Toothpaste with Fluoride Bausch & Lomb		hydrated silica	sodium fluoride	sodium lauryl sulfate	purified water • poloxamer 407 • sorbitol • glycerin • flavor • dibasic sodium phosphate • sodium saccharin • monobasic sodium phosphate • sodium benzoate • FD&C color • D&C yellow#10
SU	**Mouth Kote Toothpaste** Parnell		calcium carbonate	sodium fluoride	sodium lauryl sulfate	yerba santa
	Pearl Drops Baking Soda Whitening Toothpaste Fluor.-Tartar Carter-Wallace		sodium bicarbonate • hydrated silica	sodium fluoride	sodium lauryl sulfate	sorbitol • glycerin • tetrapotassium pyrophosphate • tetrasodium pyrophosphate • PEG-12 • titanium dioxide • flavor • sodium saccharin • cellulose gum
	Pearl Drops Extra Strength Whitening Toothpaste w/ Flouride Carter-Wallace		hydrated silica • calcium pyrophosphate • dicalcium phosphate	sodium monofluorophosphate	sodium lauryl sulfate	sorbitol • glycerin • PEG-12 • flavor • titanium dioxide • cellulose gum • trisodium phosphate • sodium phosphate • sodium saccharin
	Pearl Drops Whitening Gel Fluor.-Tartar Carter-Wallace		hydrated silica	sodium fluoride	sodium lauryl sulfate	sorbitol • glycerin • tetrapotassium pyrophosphate • tetrasodium pyrophosphate • PEG-12 • flavor • cellulose gum • sodium saccharin • FD&C blue#1 • FD&C yellow#10

Dentifrice Product Table

DENTIFRICE PRODUCTS — continued

	Product & Manufacturer	ADA Approved[a]	Abrasive Ingredient	Therapeutic Ingredient	Foaming Agent	Other Ingredients[b]
	Pearl Drops Whitening Toothpolish w/ Fluoride, paste Carter-Wallace		aluminum hydroxide • hydrated silica	sodium monofluorophosphate	sodium lauryl sulfate	sorbitol • glycerin • PEG-12 • flavor • titanium dioxide • cellulose gum • trisodium phosphate • sodium phosphate • sodium saccharin
	Pepsodent Baking Soda Gel Chesebrough-Pond's		hydrated silica	sodium fluoride	sodium lauryl sulfate	sorbitol • sodium bicarbonate • PEG-32 • alcohol • flavor • cellulose gum • sodium saccharin • titanium dioxide
	Pepsodent Fluoride Toothpaste Chesebrough-Pond's		hydrated silica	sodium monofluorophosphate	sodium lauryl sulfate	sorbitol • polyols • glycerin • alcohol • flavor • titanium dioxide • cellulose gum • sodium saccharin • sodium benzoate
SU	PeriGel Oral Care System, paste Zila		sodium bicarbonate	sodium fluoride	hydrogen peroxide	
	Promise Toothpaste, Sensitive Teeth & Cavity Prevention Block	Yes	hydrated silica	sodium monofluorophosphate • potassium nitrate	sodium lauryl sulfate	water • dicalcium phosphate dihydrate • glycerin • sorbitol • dicalcium phosphate • hydroxyethylcellulose • flavor • sodium saccharin • methylparaben • propylparaben • D&C yellow#10 • FD&C blue#1
	Protect, gel John O. Butler	provisional		dibasic sodium citrate, 2% (in a pleuronic gel)		
	Rembrandt Whitening Toothpaste, mint Den-Mat			sodium monofluorophosphate, 0.76%	sodium lauryl sulfate	dicalcium phosphate dihydrate • water • glycerin • sorbitol • alumina • papain • sodium citrate • flavor • sodium carrageenan • sodium saccharin • methylparaben • citric acid • FD&C blue#1
SU	Revelation, powder Alvin Last		calcium carbonate		vegetable soap powder	methyl salicylate • menthol
SU	Sensodyne Toothpaste, Sensitive Teeth/ Cavity Prev. Dentco	Yes	silica	potassium nitrate • sodium monofluorophosphate	sodium lauryl sulfate	water • dicalcium phosphate dihydrate • glycerin • sorbitol • dicalcium phosphate • hydroxyethylcellulose • flavor • sodium saccharin • methylparaben • propylparaben • D&C yellow#10 • FD&C blue#1
	Sensodyne-SC Toothpaste for Sensitive Teeth Dentco	Yes	silica	strontium chloride hexahydrate, 10%		water • diatomaceous earth • glycerin • sorbitol • sodium methyl cocoyl taurate • hydroxyethylcellulose • flavor • titanium dioxide • guar gum • PEG-40 • stearate • sodium saccharin • methylparaben • propylparaben • D&C red#28
	Tom's Natural Baking Soda Toothpaste with fluoride Tom's of Maine		calcium carbonate • sodium bicarbonate	sodium monofluorophosphate	sodium lauryl sulfate	glycerin • carrageenan • xylitol • peppermint oil
PE	Tom's Natural Toothpaste for Children, with fluoride Tom's of Maine		calcium carbonate • hydrated silica	sodium monofluorophosphate	sodium lauryl sulfate	glycerin • fruit extracts • carrageenan
	Tom's Natural Toothpaste with propolis and myrrh Tom's of Maine		calcium carbonate		sodium lauryl sulfate	glycerin • carrageenan • spearmint and peppermint oil • propolis and myrrh (astringent and gum stimulant)
	Topol, gel & paste Dep	Yes	hydrated silica	sodium monofluorophosphate	sodium lauryl sulfate	sorbitol • glycerin • PEG-6 • flavor • xanthan gum • titanium dioxide (paste only) • sodium saccharin • methylparaben • propylparaben • zirconium silicate

DENTIFRICE PRODUCTS — continued

	Product & Manufacturer	ADA Approved[a]	Abrasive Ingredient	Therapeutic Ingredient	Foaming Agent	Other Ingredients[b]
	Ultra Brite, gel Colgate-Palmolive	Yes	hydrated silica	sodium monofluorophosphate, 0.76%	sodium lauryl sulfate	sorbitol • PEG-12 • flavor • cellulose gum • sodium saccharin • glycerin • FD&C blue#1 • D&C red#33
	Ultra Brite, paste Colgate-Palmolive		hydrated silica alumina	sodium monofluorophosphate, 0.76%	sodium lauryl sulfate	glycerin • cellulose gum • sodium benzoate • titanium dioxide • sodium saccharin • flavor
SU	**Viadent Fluoride Gel** Colgate-Palmolive		hydrated silica	sodium monofluorophosphate • sanguinaria extract	sodium lauryl sulfate	sodium saccharin • zinc chloride • teaberry flavor
SU	**Viadent Fluoride, paste** Colgate-Palmolive		hydrated silica	sodium monofluorophosphate • sanguinaria extract	sodium lauryl sulfate	sorbitol • titanium dioxide • carboxymethylcellulose • flavor • sodium saccharin • citric acid • zinc chloride

[a] Carries American Dental Association (ADA) seal indicating safety & efficacy.
[b] Sodium bicarbonate can also be considered an abrasive.

ARTIFICIAL SALIVA PRODUCTS

Product & Manufacturer	Dosage Form	Ingredients
Moi-Stir 10[a] Kingswood	spray	sodium carboxymethyl cellulose • potassium chloride • dibasic sodium phosphate • parabens
Moi-Stir Mouth Moistening Spray Kingswood	spray	carboxymethylcellulose
Moi-Stir Oral Swabsticks[a] Kingswood	swab	carboxymethylcellulose
MouthKote Parnell	spray	water • xylitol • sorbitol • yerba santa • citric acid • flavor • ascorbic acid • sodium benzoate • sodium saccharin
Saliva Substitute[a] Roxane	spray	sorbitol • sodium carboxymethylcellulose • methylparaben
Salivart[a] Westport	aerosol	sodium carboxymethylcellulose, 1% • sorbitol, 3% • sodium chloride, 0.084% • potassium chloride, 0.120% • calcium chloride, 0.015% • magnesium chloride, 0.005% • dibasic potassium phosphate, 0.034% • nitrogen (as propellant)
Xero-Lube[a] Colgate-Palmolive	spray	phosphate and chloride salts • sodium fluoride • xylitol

[a] Carries American Dental Association (ADA) seal indicating safety & efficacy.

ORAL RINSE PRODUCTS

	Product & Manufacturer	ADA Approved[a]	Antiseptic	Other Ingredients
	Act J&J Consumer Products	Yes	alcohol, 6%	sodium fluoride, 0.05% • edetate calcium disodium • color • flavor • monobasic sodium phosphate • poloxamer 407 • polysorbate 80 • sodium benzoate • sodium saccharin • sorbitol
	Cepacol SmithKline Beecham		alcohol, 14% • cetylpyridinium chloride, 0.05%	edetate disodium • colors • flavors • glycerin • polysorbate 80 • saccharin • sodium B phosphate • sodium phosphate • water
	Cepacol Mint SmithKline Beecham		alcohol, 14.5% • cetylpyridinium chloride	colors • flavors • glucono delta-lactone • glycerin • poloxamer-407 • sodium saccharin • sodium gluconate • water
SU	Chloraseptic Mouthwash/Gargle Procter & Gamble		phenol, 1.4%	color • flavor • glycerin • saccharin sodium • menthol
	Chloraseptic Throat Spray Procter & Gamble		phenol, 1.4%	color • flavor • glycerin • saccharin sodium
	Clear Choice Bausch & Lomb		cetylpyridinium chloride	glycerin • sodium phosphate • poloxamer 338 • flavor • sodium saccharin • domiphen bromide
	Fluorigard Anti-Cavity Fluoride Rinse[c] Colgate-Palmolive	Yes		sodium fluoride, 0.05%
	Gly-Oxide[b] SmithKline Beecham		carbamide peroxide, 10%	citric acid • flavor • glycerin • propylene glycol • sodium stannate
	Isodettes Spray Goody's		phenol, 1.4%	sodium hydroxide, 0.0047% • propylene glycol, 10% • artificial & natural eucalyptus flavor, 0.02% • artificial & natural wild cherry flavor, 0.5% • FD&C red#40, 0.015% • water
	Lavoris Dep		alcohol	glycerin • citric acid • poloxamer 407 • saccharin • clove oil • polysorbate 80 • zinc chloride • zinc oxide • sodium hydroxide • flavor • color
SU	Listerine Warner-Lambert	Yes	alcohol, 26.9%	menthol • methyl salicylate • eucalyptol • thymol
SU	Listerine Coolmint Warner-Lambert	Yes	alcohol, 21.6%	menthol • methyl salicylate • eucalyptol • thymol • anetmole
SU	Listermint With Fluoride Warner-Lambert		alcohol, 6.65%	zinc chloride • sodium fluoride, 0.02% • glycerin • poloxamer 407 • sodium lauryl sulfate • sodium citrate • flavor • sodium saccharin • citric acid • D&C yellow#10 • FD&C green#3
SU	Peroxyl Mouthrinse[b] Colgate-Palmolive		hydrogen peroxide, 1.5% • alcohol, 6%	mint flavor
SU	Plax Original Flavor & Softmint Pfizer			sodium lauryl sulfate • water • glycerin • alcohol, 7.5% • sodium benzoate • sodium bicarbonate • allantoin • polysorbate 20 • sodium salicylate • sodium borate • saccharin (Original) • flavor • xanthan gum • red#40 (Original) • FD&C blue #1 (Softmint) • FD&C yellow #5 (Softmint)
	Scope Original Mint Procter & Gamble		cetylpyridinium chloride • domiphen bromide • SD alcohol 38-F, 18.9%	purified water • glycerin • sodium saccharin • sodium benzoate • flavor • benzoic acid • FD&C blue#1 • FD&C yellow#5 (tartrazine)
	Scope Peppermint Procter & Gamble		cetylpyridinium chloride • domiphen bromide • SD alcohol 38-F, 16.6%	purified water • glycerin • sodium saccharin • sodium benzoate • flavor • benzoic acid • FD&C blue#1
	Sucrets Maximum Strength Throat Spray (Cherry) SmithKline Beecham		alcohol, 12%	dyclonine hydrochloride, 0.1% • dibasic sodium phosphate • cherry flavor • glycerin • monobasic sodium phosphate • phosphoric acid • potassium sorbate • colors • sorbitol • water
	Sucrets Maximum Strength Throat Spray (Mint) SmithKline Beecham		alcohol, 10%	dyclonine hydrochloride, 0.1% • chlorobutanol • dibasic sodium phosphate • glycerin • monobasic sodium phosphate • mint flavor • phosphoric acid • potassium sorbate • sorbitol • water • color
SU	Viadent Oral Rinse Colgate-Palmolive		alcohol, 10%	sanguinaria extract • glycerin • polysorbate 80 • flavor • sodium saccharin • poloxamer 237 • citric acid • zinc chloride, 0.2%

[a]Carries American Dental Association (ADA) seal indicating safety & efficacy.
[b]Oral debriding agent/wound cleanser.
[c]Topical flouride rinse.

DENTURE CLEANSER PRODUCTS

Product & Manufacturer	Dosage Form	Ingredients
Complete[a] Procter & Gamble	paste	glycerin • sorbitol solution • calcium carbonate • silicon dioxide • sodium CMC • sodium lauryl sulfate • sodium saccharin • methylparaben • propylparaben • magnesium aluminum silicate • ethanol • flavors • 3-Hexene-1-01 • ethylene brassylate • artificial rose oil
Denalan Whitehall	ns	sodium percarbonate, 30% • sodium tripolyphosphate • sodium sulfate • sodium lauryl sulfate • flavor
Denclenz Liquid Denture Cleaner Sandoz Pharm.	liquid	hydrochloric acid and detergents in a brush/bottle applicator
Dentu-Creme Denture Toothpaste Block	paste	dicalcium phosphate dihydrate • propylene glycol • calcium carbonate • silica • sodium lauryl sulfate • glycerin • hydroxyethylcellulose • flavor • magnesium aluminum silicate • sodium saccharin • parabens
Divi-Dent Denture Cleanser Block	ns	sorbitol • triethanolamine lauryl sulfate • silica • trisodium EDTA
Efferdent, 2 Layer Warner-Lambert	tablet	sodium bicarbonate • sodium carbonate • citric acid • potassium monopersulfate • sodium perborate monohydrate • sodium lauryl sulfoacetate • flavor
Efferdent[a] Warner-Lambert	tablet	potassium monopersulfate • sodium perborate monohydrate • sodium carbonate • sodium lauryl sulfoacetate • sodium bicarbonate • citric acid • magnesium stearate • flavor
Effervescent Denture Tablets Rexall	tablet	sodium bicarbonate • citric acid • sodium perborate • sodium acid pyrophosphate • sodium benzoate • trisodium phosphate • sodium lauryl sulfate • poloxamer 188 • sorbitol • silica • peppermint oil
Extar Denture Cleanser Extar	ns	sodium polymetaphosphate • sodium saccharin • parabens • peppermint • sodium phosphate • sequestrene • lactose
K.I.K. K.I.K. Co.	ns	sodium perborate, 25% • trisodium phosphate, 75%
Kleenite Procter & Gamble	granule	anhydrous trisodium phosphate • monohydrate sodium perborate • dendritic sodium chloride • color • peppermint flavor • sodium lauryl sulfate • ACL-60
Polident Block	tablet	potassium monopersulfate • sodium perborate monohydrate • sodium carbonate • surfactant • chelating agents • proteolytic enzyme • sodium bicarbonate • citric acid • fragrance
Polident Denture Cleanser Block	powder	sodium perborate monohydrate • potassium monopersulfate • sodium carbonate • sodium acid pyrophosphate • surfactant • sodium bicarbonate • fragrance
Rembrandt Daily Denture Renewal Gel Den-Mat	gel	citroxain
Smokers' Polident Denture Cleanser Block	tablet	sodium carbonate • potassium monopersulfate • citric acid • sodium bicarbonate • sodium perborate monohydrate • surfactant • chelating agent • proteolytic enzyme • fragrance

[a]Carries American Dental Association (ADA) seal indicating safety & efficacy.

DENTURE ADHESIVE PRODUCTS

Product & Manufacturer	Dosage Form	Ingredients
Dentlock Medtech	powder	karaya gum
Effergrip Denture Adhesive Cream Warner-Lambert	cream	carboxymethylcellulose sodium, 24.6% • calcium sodium mixed salt of methyl vinyl ether-maleic anhydride, 29.6%
Ezo Denture Cushions Medtech	pad	paraffin wax • cotton
Fasteeth Procter & Gamble	powder	calcium/zinc poly (vinyl methyl ether maleate) • sodium carboxymethylcellulose • cornstarch • silicon oil • peppermint oil, rectified
Fasteeth Extra Hold Procter & Gamble	powder	calcium/zinc poly (vinyl methyl ether maleate) • sodium carboxymethylcellulose • silicon dioxide • peppermint oil, rectified
Firmdent[a] Moyco	cream	karaya gum • sodium borate • peppermint flavor
Fixodent Procter & Gamble	cream	calcium/zinc poly (vinyl methyl ether maleate) • sodium carboxymethylcellulose • mineral oil • petrolatum • silicon dioxide • color
Fixodent Fresh Procter & Gamble	cream	calcium/zinc poly (vinyl methyl ether maleate) • sodium carboxymethylcellulose • mineral oil • petrolatum • silicon dioxide • color • peppermint flavor • methyl lactate • menthol
Orafix SmithKline Beecham	cream	karaya gum, 51% • petrolatum, 30% • mineral oil, 13% • peppermint oil, 0.08%
Orafix Special[a] SmithKline Beecham	cream	gantrez MS 955 • sodium carboxymethylcellulose Type 7H4XF • povidone K-90 • white petrolatum • mineral oil, heavy • isopropyl palmitate • isopropyl myristate • flavors • colors
Poli-Grip Block	ns	karaya gum, 51% • petrolatum, 36.7% • liquid petrolatum, 9.4% • magnesium oxide, 2.7% • propylparaben • flavor
Polident Dentu-Grip Block	cream	carboxymethylcellulose gum, 49% • ethylene oxide polymer, 21% • flavor, 0.4%
Rigident Carter-Wallace	powder	acacia gum • karaya gum • sodium borate
Rigident[a] Carter-Wallace	cream	carboxymethylcellulose sodium • calcium sodium salts of methyl vinyl ether maleic anhydride copolymer • petrolatum • mineral oil • talc • flavor • propylparaben • D&C red#27 aluminum lake • D&C red #30 talc lake
Super Poli-Grip Block	liquid	carboxymethylcellulose sodium • ethylene oxide polymer • petrolatum • mineral oil • flavor • propylparaben
Super Poli-Grip Block	powder	calcium sodium methyl vinyl ether-maleic anhydride copolymer • carboxymethylcellulose sodium • flavor
Wernet's Cream Block	cream	carboxymethylcellulose gum, 32% • petrolatum, 42% • mineral oil, 12% • ethylene oxide polymer, 13% • propylparaben, 0.05% • flavor, 0.5%
Wernet's Powder Block	powder	karaya gum, 94.6% • water-soluble ethylene oxide polymer, 5% • flavor, 0.4%

[a] Carries American Dental Association (ADA) seal indicating safety & efficacy.

MOUTH PAIN, COLD SORE, CANKER SORE PRODUCTS

Product & Manufacturer	Anesthetic/ Analgesic	Other Ingredients
AL **Amosan, powder** SU Oral-B		sodium peroxyborate monohydrate • sodium bitartrate • saccharin • peppermint, menthol and vanilla flavors
AL **Anbesol Gel, Baby, grape** SU **and original**[a] PE Whitehall	benzocaine, 7.5%	viscous water-soluble base without alcohol
SU **Anbesol Maximum Strength, gel** Whitehall	benzocaine, 20%	alcohol, 60%, viscous water-soluble base
SU **Anbesol Maximum Strength, liquid** Whitehall	benzocaine, 20%	alcohol, 60%
SU **Anbesol, gel** Whitehall	benzocaine, 6.3%	phenol, 0.5% • alcohol, 70% • viscous water-soluble base
SU **Anbesol, liquid** Whitehall	benzocaine, 6.3%	phenol, 0.5% • alcohol, 70% • povidone-iodine • camphor • glycerin • menthol • potassium iodide
Benzodent Analgesic Denture Ointment Procter & Gamble	benzocaine, 20%	
Betadine Mouthwash/Gargle Purdue Frederick		povidone-iodine, 0.5% • alcohol, 8.8%
SU **Blistex Lip Ointment** Blistex	camphor, 0.5% • menthol, 0.6% • phenol, 0.5%	allantoin, 1%
Campho-Phenique Gel Sterling Health	phenol, 4.7%	camphor, 10.8%
Campho-Phenique Liquid Sterling Health	phenol, 4.7%	camphor, 10.8%
Dent-Zel-Ite Oral Mucosal Analgesic, liquid Alvin Last	benzocaine, 5%	alcohol, 81% • camphor • wintergreen • glycerin
Dent-Zel-Ite Temporary Dental Filling, liquid Alvin Last	alcohol, 55%	sandarac gum • camphor • methyl salicylate
Dent-Zel-Ite Toothache Relief Drops Alvin Last	eugenol, 85%	alcohol, 13.5% • camphor • wintergreen
Dentapaine, ointment Reese Chemical	benzocaine, 20%	glycerin • oil of clove • sodium saccharin • methylparaben • polyethylene glycol-400 • polyethylene glycol-4000 • water
Dents 3 In 1 Toothache Relief, gel/gum/drops C.S. Dent	eugenol (drops, gum) • benzocaine (gel, gum)	alcohol, 54% (drops) • chlorobutanol anhydrous, 0.09% (drops)
Dents Toothache Drops C.S. Dent	eugenol	alcohol, 54% • chlorobutanol, 0.09% • propylene glycol • FD&C red#40
Dents Toothache Gum C.S. Dent	benzocaine • eugenol	petrolatum • cotton and wax base • beeswax • FD&C red#40 aluminum lake
Double-Action Kit, drops/ tablets C.S. Dent	eugenol, 7.5%	denatured alcohol, 54% • chlorobutanol, 0.09% • acetaminophen, 325mg/tablet
SU **Dr. Hand's Teething Gel** PE Medtech	clove oil	hamamelis water • alcohol, 10%
SU **Dr. Hands Teething Lotion** PE Medtech	oil of cloves	hamamelis water • alcohol, 11%
AL **Herpecin-L** SU Campbell		allantoin • padimate O • titanium dioxide
AL **Hurricaine, aerosol** SU Beutlich	benzocaine	polyethylene glycol • saccharin • flavoring
AL **Hurricaine, gel** SU Beutlich	benzocaine	polyethylene glycol • saccharin • flavoring
AL **Hurricaine, liquid** SU Beutlich	benzocaine	polyethylene glycol • saccharin • flavoring

MOUTH PAIN, COLD SORE, CANKER SORE PRODUCTS — continued

	Product & Manufacturer	Anesthetic/ Analgesic	Other Ingredients
SU	Kank-A Liquid Professional Strength[a] Blistex	benzocaine, 20%	cetylpyridinium chloride, 0.1% • ethylcellulose • benzoin tincture compound
	Kank-A Mouth Sore Medication[a] Blistex	benzocaine, 20%	SD alcohol 38B, 24.7% • cetylpyridinium chloride, 0.5% • aspartame • benzyl alcohol • castor oil • ethylcellulose • film formers • natural flavors • propylene glycol • purified water • tannic acid • tetrasodium EDTA
AL SU	Lip Medex, ointment Blistex	camphor, 1.0% • menthol, 0.5% • phenol, 0.5%	petrolatum, 73.7%
	Lotion-Jel C.S. Dent	benzocaine	distilled water • methylparaben • propylparaben • propylene glycol • carbopol 934-P • methyl salicylate • FD&C red#40 • 2.2' iminodiethanol
SU	Mouth Kote-OR, solution Parnell	benzyl alcohol, 1%	water • sorbitol • sodium chloride • yerba santa • flavor • poloxamer 407 • menthol • sodium saccharin • cetylpyridinium chloride • disodium EDTA
SU	Mouth Kote-PR, ointment Parnell	diphenhydramine, 1.25% • benzyl alcohol, 3.5%	PEG 8 • cellulose gum • PEG 75 • poloxamer 407 • yerba santa • flavor
SU	Mouth Kote-PR, solution Parnell	diphenhydramine, 1.25% • benzyl alcohol, 1.0%	water • cetylpyridinium chloride • disodium EDTA • flavor • sodium benzoate • sodium hydroxide • sodium saccharin • yerba santa
	Numzident Gel-Adult Strength Goody's	benzocaine, 10%	PEG 400, 47.86% • glycerin (96%), 30.0% • PEG 3350, 10% • sodium saccharin, 1.0% • cherry vanilla flavor, 0.4% • purified water, 0.75%
	Numzit Cold Sore Lotion Goody's	benzoin resinoid, 2.6%	SDA alcohol, 52.1% • camphor powder, 7% • polysorbate 80, 2.1% • castor oil, 9.984% • aluminum chloride, 0.2% • lavendar oil, 0.0184% • water, 21%
	Numzit Teething Gel Goody's	benzocaine, 7.5%	PEG-400, 66.2% • PEG-3350, 26.1% • sodium saccharin, 0.036% • clove oil, 0.09% • peppermint oil, 0.018% • purified water, 0.056%
	Numzit Teething Lotion Goody's	benzocaine, 0.2%	alcohol, 12.1% • glycerin, 2% • kelgin MV, 0.5% • sodium saccharin, 0.02% • methylparaben, 0.1% • FD&C red#40, 0.1% • FD&C blue#1, 0.009%
AL SU	Orabase Baby, gel Colgate-Palmolive	benzocaine, 7.5%	glycerin
AL SU	Orabase Lip Healer, cream Colgate-Palmolive	benzocaine, 5%	allantoin, 1% • menthol, 0.5%
AL SU	Orabase Plain, cream Colgate-Palmolive		pectin • gelatin • carboxymethylcellulose sodium • polyethylene • mineral oil
AL SU	Orabase-B with Benzocaine, cream Colgate-Palmolive	benzocaine, 20%	pectin • carboxymethylcellulose sodium • polyethylene • mineral oil • guar gum
	Orabase-B with Benzocaine, paste[a] Colgate-Palmolive	benzocaine, 20%	plasticized hydrocarbon gel • guar • carboxymethylcellulose • tragacanth • pectin • preservatives • flavors
	Orajel Del	benzocaine, 10%	saccharin
	Orajel Denture Del	benzocaine, 10% • eugenol	saccharin
	Orajel Maximum Strength Del	benzocaine, 20%	clove oil • flavor • polyethylene glycols • sodium saccharin • sorbic acid
	Orajel Mouth-Aid Del	benzocaine, 20%	benzalkonium chloride, 0.12% • zinc chloride, 0.1% • allantoin • flavor • polyethylene glycols • propyl gallate • propylene glycol • sodium saccharin • sorbic acid
	Orajel, Baby Del	benzocaine, 7.5%	FD&C red#40 • flavor • glycerin • polyethylene glycols • sodium saccharin • sorbic acid • sorbitol
	Orajel, Baby Nighttime Formula Del	benzocaine, 10%	FD&C red#40 • flavor • glycerin • polyethylene glycols • sodium saccharin • sorbic acid • sorbitol
SU	Peroxyl Mouthrinse Colgate-Palmolive		hydrogen peroxide, 1.5% • mint flavor • alcohol, 6%

MOUTH PAIN, COLD SORE, CANKER SORE PRODUCTS — continued

Product & Manufacturer	Anesthetic/ Analgesic	Other Ingredients
SU Peroxyl Oral Spot Treatment Gel Colgate-Palmolive		hydrogen peroxide, 1.5% • mint flavor
Stopzit, cream Goody's	sucrose octaacetate, 5% w/v	isopropyl alcohol • butyl acetate • ethylcellulose • SD alcohol
Tanac Roll-On, lotion Del	benzocaine, 5%	tannic acid, 6% • benzalkonium chloride, 0.125% • saccharin
Tanac Stick Del	benzocaine, 7.5%	tannic acid, 6% • benzalkonium chloride, 0.125% • allantoin, 0.2% • octyl dimethyl PABA, 0.75% • saccharin
Tanac, liquid Del	benzocaine, 10%	tannic acid, 6% • benzalkonium chloride, 0.125% • saccharin
SU ZilaDent, gel Zila	benzocaine	hydroxypropyl cellulose filmformer
SU Zilactin Medicated Gel Zila		tannic acid • hydroxypropyl cellulose filmformer
SU Zilactin-L Liquid Zila	lidocaine	

[a] Carries American Dental Association (ADA) seal indicating safety & efficacy.

OSTOMY PRODUCTS

Product & Manufacturer	Ingredients
Adhesive Disk Products	
HoliHesive Skin Barrier Blanket Hollister	gelatin • pectin • carboxymethylcellulose sodium • polyisobutylene
HoliSeal Skin Barrier Blanket Hollister	gelatin • pectin • polyisobutylene
Pre-Cut Adhesive Supports Smith & Nephew	rubber-based adhesive
Seal-Tite Gaskets Smith & Nephew	rubber-based adhesive
Cement Products	
Mastisol Ferndale	gum mastic
Skin-Bond Cement Smith & Nephew	natural rubber • hexane
Skin-Bond Cement (Nonflammable) Smith & Nephew	natural rubber • trichloroethane
Skin-Hesive Cement Smith & Nephew	natural rubber • petroleum solvent
Solvent Products	
Cleaning Solvent Nu-Hope	mineral spirits
Detachol Ferndale	paraffin hydrocarbons
Uni-Solve Adhesive Remover Smith & Nephew	1, 1, 1-trichloroethane • naptha
Universal Remover Hollister	organic solvents • silicone oil • ethyl alcohol
Appliance Deodorizer Products	
Banish II Liquid Deodorant Smith & Nephew	zinc ricinoleate
Odo-Way Appliance Deodorant Tablets Smith & Nephew	chlorine-producing tablets
Oxychinol Ferndale	potassium oxyquinoline sulfate
Super Banish Appliance Deodorant Smith & Nephew	silver nitrate • ethylene thiourea
Uri-Kleen Deodorizing Detergent Smith & Nephew	phosphoric acid
Internal Deodorizer Products	
Charcocaps Requa	activated charcoal, 260mg
Derifil Tablets Rystan	chlorophyllin copper complex, 100mg
Devrom Chewable Tablets Parthenon	bismuth subgallate
Skin Protective Products	
Karaya Gum Various Manufacturers	karaya gum powder

OSTOMY PRODUCTS — continued

Product & Manufacturer	Ingredients
Moisture Barrier Skin Ointment Hollister	petrolatum • propylparaben • BHA • vitamins A, D, E
Premium Skin Barrier Hollister	gelatin • pectin • carboxymethylcellulose sodium • polyisobutylene
Refined Karaya Gum Powder Smith & Nephew	karaya gum powder
Skin Conditioning Creme Hollister	aloe juice • isopropyl palmitate • isopropyl myristate • isopropyl stearate • vitamins
Skin Gel Hollister	glycerin • allantoin • isopropyl alcohol • film-formers • plasticizers
Skin-Prep Protective Dressing Smith & Nephew	poly MVE/MA n-butyl monoester
Tincture of Benzoin Various Manufacturers	tincture of benzoin
Uni-Care Lotion Smith & Nephew	allantoin • dimethicone • isopropyl palmitate • aloe vera gel
Uni-Derm Protective Moisturizer Smith & Nephew	anhydrous lanolin • petrolatum • isopropyl palmitate
Uni-Salve Ointment Smith & Nephew	petrolatum • casein

SPERMICIDE PRODUCTS

Product & Manufacturer	Dosage Form	Spermicide	Other Ingredients
Conceptrol Ortho	suppository	nonoxynol-9, 8.34%	lauroamphodiacetate • sodium trideceth sulfate • polyethylene glycol 1000 • polyethylene glycol 1450 • povidone
Conceptrol Disposable Ortho	gel	nonoxynol-9, 4%	
Conceptrol Gel Ortho	gel	nonoxynol-9, 4%	cellulose gum • lactic acid • methylparaben • povidone • propylene glycol • purified water • sorbic acid • sorbitol solution
Delfen Ortho	foam	nonoxynol-9, 12.5%	
Emko Foam Schering-Plough	foam	nonoxynol-9, 8%	
Encare Thompson Medical	suppository	nonoxynol-9, 100mg	polyethylene glycol • tartaric acid • sodium citrate • sodium bicarbonate
Gynol II ES Ortho	jelly	nonoxynol-9, 3%	lactic acid • methylparaben • povidone • propylene glycol • purified water • sodium carboxymethylcellulose • sorbic acid • sorbitol solution
Gynol II[a] Ortho	jelly	nonoxynol-9, 2%	
Koromex Schmid	foam	nonoxynol-9, 12.5%	
Koromex Crystal Clear[a] Schmid	gel	nonoxynol-9, 3%	boric acid • cellulose gum • propylene glycol • simethicone • sorbitol • water • pH, 4.5
Koromex Jelly[a] Schmid	jelly	nonoxynol-9, 3%	boric acid • cellulose gum • propylene glycol • simethicone • sorbitol • water • fragrance • soluble starch
Koromex[a] Schmid	cream	octoxynol, 3%	
Ortho-Creme Ortho	cream	nonoxynol-9, 2%	benzoic acid • castor oil • cetyl alcohol • fragrance • glacial acetic acid • methylparaben • potassium hydroxide • propylene glycol • propylparaben • purified water • cellulose gum • sodium lauryl sulfate • sorbic acid • stearic acid • trolamine
Ortho-Gynol[a] Ortho	jelly	otoxynol-9, 1%	boric acid • castor oil • fragrance • glacial acetic acid • methylparaben • potassium hydroxide • propylene glycol • purified water • sorbic acid • sodium carboxymethylcellulose
Ramses Schmid	jelly	nonoxynol-9, 5%	
Semicid Inserts Whitehall	suppository	nonoxynol-9, 100mg	benzethonium chloride • citric acid • D&C red#21 lake • D&C red#33 lake • methylparaben • polyethylene glycol • water
Shur-Seal Milex Products	jelly	nonoxynol-9, 2%	water • propylene glycol • methylcellulose • methylparaben • simethicone • boric acid • pH adjusted to 4 • citric acid
Today Sponge Whitehall	sponge	nonoxynol-9, 1000mg	benzoic acid • citric acid • sodium dihydrogen citrate • sodium metabisulfite • sorbic acid • water • polyurethane foam sponge
Vaginal Contraceptive Film (VCF) Apothecus	film square	nonoxynol-9, 20%	glycerin • polyvinyl alcohol

[a] For use with a diaphram.

CONDOM PRODUCTS

Product & Manufacturer	Material[a]	Spermicide	Comments
Excita Extra Schmid	latex	nonoxynol-9, 8%	ribbed • lubricated • reservoir end
Excita Fiesta Schmid	latex	No	lubricated with assorted colors
Fourex Schmid	animal membrane[a]	nonoxynol-9, 7%	
Gold Circle Safetex	latex	No	reservoir
Mentor Carter-Wallace	latex	No	adhesive seal • applicator hood • reservoir end • packaged with silicone lubricant
Mentor Plus Carter-Wallace	latex	Yes	reservoir end • adhesive seal and applicator hood • packaged with silicone spermicidal lubricant
Naturalamb Carter-Wallace	lamb cecum[a]	No	packaged with water-based lubricant
Naturalamb with spermicide Carter-Wallace	lamb cecum[a]	Yes	packaged with water-based spermicidal lubricant
Ramses Extra Strength Schmid	latex	nonoxynol-9, 8%	reservoir end • spermicidal lubricant
Ramses Sensitol Lubricated Schmid	latex	No	sensitol lubricated • reservoir end
Ramses Ultra Thin Schmid	latex	nonoxynol-9, 8%	spermicidal lubricant • reservoir end
Saxon Safetex	latex	nonoxynol-9, 6.6%	spermicidal lubricant
Saxon Safetex	latex	No	lubricated • reservoir end
Sheik Elite Schmid	latex	nonoxynol-9, 8%	spermicidal lubricant
Sheik Super Thin Schmid	latex	No	lubricated • 36% thinner
Sheik Super Thin with spermicide Schmid	latex	nonoxynol-9, 8%	spermicidal lubricant • 36% thinner
Touch Schmid	latex	nonoxynol-9, 8%	ribbed • spermicidal lubricant • reservoir end
Touch Schmid	latex	No	ribbed • lubricated • reservoir end
Trojan Extra Strength with spermicide Carter-Wallace	latex	Yes	reservoir end • packaged with silicone spermicidal lubricant
Trojan Magnum with spermicide Carter-Wallace	latex	Yes	larger sized • reservoir end • packaged with silicone spermicide lubricant
Trojan Naturalube Ribbed Carter-Wallace	latex	No	reservoir end • contoured shape • ribbed/textured • packaged with water-based lubricant
Trojan Plus Carter-Wallace	latex	No	reservoir end • contoured shape • colored • packaged with silicone lubricant
Trojan Plus 2 Carter-Wallace	latex	Yes	reservoir end • contoured shape • packaged with water-based spermicidal lubricant
Trojan Very Sensitive Carter-Wallace	latex	No	contour shape • reservoir end • packaged with silicone lubricant
Trojan Very Thin with spermicide Carter-Wallace	latex	Yes	receptacle end • packaged with silicone spermicide lubricant

CONDOM PRODUCTS — continued

Product & Manufacturer	Material[a]	Spermicide	Comments
Trojan-Enz Large with spermicide Carter-Wallace	latex	Yes	larger sized • reservoir end • packaged with water-based spermicidal lubricant
Trojan-Enz with spermicidal lubricant Carter-Wallace	latex	Yes	reservoir end • packaged with water-based spermicidal lubricant
Trojans Carter-Wallace	latex	No	plain end • packaged dry

[a] Animal membrane condoms are more porous than latex ones and may allow transmission of the AIDS virus.

HEMORRHOIDAL PRODUCTS

Product & Manufacturer	Dosage Form	Anesthetic	Antiseptic	Astringent	Protectant	Other Ingredients
A-Caine Rectal A.V.P.	ointment	diperodon hydrochloride, 0.25%		zinc oxide, 5% • bismuth subcarbonate, 0.2%	cod liver oil and petrolatum base	phenylephrine hydrochloride, 0.25% • pyrilamine maleate, 0.1%
Americaine Hemorrhoidal Ointment CIBA Consumer	ointment	benzocaine, 20%				benzethonium chloride, 0.1% • polyethylene glycol 300 • polyethylene glycol 3350
Anusert G & W	suppository				hard fat, 88.7%	phenylephrine, 0.25%
Anusol Parke-Davis	ointment	pramoxine hydrochloride, 1%		zinc oxide, 12.5% • balsam nicaragua, 3.0%		polyethylene wax • mineral oil
Anusol Parke-Davis	suppository			phenylephrine hydrochloride, 0.25%	vegetable oil base	
Anusol Ointment 1% Hydrocortisone Parke-Davis	ointment				white petrolatum	hydrocortisone, 1% • mineral oil • multiwax • sorbitan sesquioleate • preservative
BiCozene Sandoz Pharm.	cream	benzocaine, 6%			cream base	resorcinol, 1.67%
Calmol 4 Suppositories Mentholatum	suppository			bismuth subgallate • zinc oxide, 10%	cocoa butter, 80%	glyceryl stearate • methylparaben • propylparaben
Fleet Relief Medicated Hemorrhoidal Ointment C.B. Fleet	ointment			zinc oxide	white petrolatum • mineral oil	
Formulation R G & W	cream				shark liver oil, 3%	live yeast cell derivative • phenylmercuric nitrate, 1:10,000
Formulation R G & W	ointment				shark liver oil, 3%	live yeast cell derivative • phenylmercuric nitrate, 1:10,000
Gentz Wipes Roxane	pad	pramoxine hydrochloride, 1%	cetylpyridinium chloride, 0.05%	hamamelis water, 50% • aluminum chlorhydroxy allantoinate, 0.2%	propylene glycol, 10%	fragrance
Hem-Prep G & W	ointment			zinc oxide, 11%	petrolatum, 89%	phenylephrine, 0.25%
Hem-Prep G & W	suppository			zinc oxide, 11%	hard fat, 89%	phenylephrine, 0.25%
Hemet Hemorrhoidal Halsey	suppository	benzocaine		zinc oxide • bismuth subgallate • balsam peru	vegetable oil base	
Hemet Rectal Halsey	ointment	diperodon hydrochloride, 0.25%		bismuth subcarbonate, 0.2% • zinc oxide, 5%	cod liver oil • petrolatum	pyrilamine maleate, 0.1% • phenylephrine hydrochloride, 0.25%
Lanacane Creme Combe	cream	benzocaine, 6%	benzethonium chloride, 0.1%		water-washable base	
Medicone Rectal Medicone	ointment	benzocaine, 2%	menthol, 0.4%	zinc oxide, 10% • balsam peru, 1.26%	castor oil, 1.26% • petrolatum-lanolin, 83.6%	hydroxyquinoline sulfate, 0.5%

HEMORRHOIDAL PRODUCTS — continued

Product & Manufacturer	Dosage Form	Anesthetic	Antiseptic	Astringent	Protectant	Other Ingredients
Medicone Rectal Medicone	suppository	benzocaine, 130mg	hydroxyquinoline sulfate, 16mg • menthol, 9mg	zinc oxide, 195mg • balsam peru, 65mg	vegetable and petrolatum oil base	
Mediconet Medicone	wipe		benzalkonium chloride, 0.02%	hamamelis water, 50%	ethoxylated lanolin, 0.5% • glycerin, 10%	methylparaben, 0.15%
Non-Steroid Procto Foam Reed & Carnrick	foam	pramoxine hydrochloride, 1%			mineral oil	
Nupercainal CIBA Consumer	ointment	dibucaine, 1%			lanolin • white petrolatum • light mineral oil	acetone • sodium bisulfite
Nupercainal Suppositories CIBA Consumer	suppository			zinc oxide	cocoa butter	acetone sodium bisulfite • bismuth subgallate
Pazo Bristol-Myers	ointment		camphor, 2%	zinc oxide, 5%	lanolin, 5%	ephedrine sulfate, 0.24% • petrolatum
Pazo Bristol-Myers	suppository			zinc, oxide, 5%		ephedrine sulfate, 0.24% • hydrogenated vegetable oil
Pontocaine Sterling Health	cream	tetracaine hydrochloride (equivalent to 1% base)				methylparaben • sodium bisulfite
Pontocaine Sterling Health	ointment	tetracaine base, 5%	menthol, 0.5%		white petrolatum • white wax	
Preparation H Whitehall	cream				shark liver oil, 3% in a base of petrolatum	live yeast cell derivative (supplying 2000 units of skin respiratory factor/oz)
Preparation H Whitehall	ointment				shark liver oil, 3% in a base of petrolatum	live yeast cell derivative (supplying 2000 units of skin respiratory factor/oz)
Preparation H Whitehall	suppository				shark liver oil, 3% in a base of cocoa butter	live yeast cell derivative (supplying 2000 units of skin respiratory factor/oz)
Preparation H Cleansing Tissues Whitehall	wipe					purified water • propylene glycol • phenoxyethanol • methylparaben • propylparaben • butylparaben • citric acid
Primaderm-B Arrow Medical	ointment	benzocaine		zinc oxide	cod liver oil • petrolatum-lanolin base	
Prompt Relief Hemorrhoidal Ointment Goldline	ointment				shark liver oil, 3%	live yeast derivative, 2000 units/oz

HEMORRHOIDAL PRODUCTS — continued

Product & Manufacturer	Dosage Form	Anesthetic	Antiseptic	Astringent	Protectant	Other Ingredients
Prompt Relief Hemorrhoidal Suppositories Goldline					shark liver oil, 3%	live yeast cell derivative, 2000 units/oz
Rectagene Medicated Pfeiffer	ointment	benzocaine, 3%		bismuth subgallate, 1% • zinc oxide, 1.5%	polyethylene glycol base	phenylephrine hydrochloride, 0.2% • pyrilamine maleate • cetalkonium chloride
Tronolane Ross	cream	pramoxine hydrochloride, 1%				beeswax • cetyl alcohol • cetyl esters wax • glycerin • methylparaben • propylparaben • sodium lauryl sulfate • zinc oxide
Tronolane Ross	suppository			zinc oxide, 5%	hard fat, 95%	
Tucks Parke-Davis	cream			hamamelis water, 52%		cetyl alcohol, 8%
Tucks Parke-Davis	pad			hamamelis water, 50%	glycerin, 10%	aloe vera gel, 0.1%
Vaseline Pure Petroleum Jelly Chesebrough-Pond's	ointment				white petrolatum, 100%	
Wyanoid Relief Factor Wyeth-Ayerst	suppository		boric acid	zinc oxide • bismuth subcarbonate • bismuth oxyiodide • balsam peru	cocoa butter • beeswax	belladonna extract, 15mg • ephedrine sulfate, 3mg

PERSONAL CARE PRODUCTS

Product[a] & Manufacturer	Antimicrobial	Local Anesthetic/ Antipruritic/Counterirritant	Hydrocortisone	Other Ingredients
Abscents Gordon				sodium potassium • aluminosilicate
Acu-Dyne Douche Acme United	povidone-iodine			
Acu-Dyne Skin Cleanser Acme United	available iodine, 0.75%			
Betadine Antiseptic Lubricating Gel Purdue Frederick	povidone-iodine, 10%			
Betadine Medicated Douche Purdue Frederick	povidone-iodine, 10%			
Betadine Medicated Premixed Disposable Douche Purdue Frederick	povidone-iodine, 0.30%			
Betadine Medicated Vaginal Gel Purdue Frederick	povidone-iodine, 10%			
Betadine Vaginal Suppository Purdue Frederick	povidone-iodine, 10%			
Cortef Feminine Itch Cream Upjohn			acetate equivalent to hydrocortisone, 0.5%	aloe vera • cetyl palmitate • glyceryl stearate • polyethylene glycol • stearamidoethyl diethylamine • parabens • purifed water
Gyne-Moistrin Vaginal Moisturizing Gel Schering-Plough				polyglycerylmethacrylate • water • propylene glycol • methylparaben • propylparaben
Gyne-cort Combe			0.5%	
Gyne-cort Extra Strength 10 Combe			1%	
H-R Lubricating Jelly Carter-Wallace				propylene glycol • hydroxypropyl methylcellulose • carbomer 934P • propylparaben • methylparaben • sodium hydroxide
Massengill Baking Soda Disposable Douche SmithKline Beecham				sodium bicarbonate

PERSONAL CARE PRODUCTS — continued

Product[a] & Manufacturer	Antimicrobial	Local Anesthetic/ Antipruritic/Counterirritant	Hydrocortisone	Other Ingredients
Massengill Disposable Douche Mountain Breeze Scent SmithKline Beecham	cetylpyridinium chloride • diazolidinyl urea			EDTA • SD alcohol 40 • lactic acid • octoxynol-9 • fragrance • colors
Massengill Douche Powder Floral & Unscented SmithKline Beecham		methyl salicylate • phenol • thymol • menthol • eucalyptus oil		ammonium alum • sodium chloride • PEG-8
Massengill Medicated Disposable Douche SmithKline Beecham	povidone-iodine, 0.3%			
Massengill Medicated Towlette SmithKline Beecham	diazolidinyl urea		0.5%	DMDM hydantoin • isopropyl myristate • methylparaben • propylparaben • polysorbate 60 • propylene glycol • sorbitan stearate • steareth-2 • steareth 21 • water
Massengill Vinegar & Water Disposable Douche Extra Mild SmithKline Beecham				vinegar
Norforms Fresh Flowers C.B. Fleet	benzethonium chloride			PEG-18 • PEG-32 • PEG-20 stearate • fragrance • methylparaben • lactic acid
Norforms, Unscented C.B. Fleet	benzethonium chloride			PEG-18 • PEG-32 • PEG-20 stearate • methylparaben • lactic acid
PMC Douche Thomas & Thompson	boric acid, 82%	thymol, 0.3% • phenol, 0.2% • menthol		ammonium aluminum sulfate, 16% • eucalyptus oil • peppermint oil
Personal Lubricant Ortho				glycerin • propylene glycol • sodium carboxymethylcellulose • sodium alginate • sorbic acid • methylparaben
Preparation H Cleansing Tissues Whitehall				purified water • propylene glycol • phenoxyethanol • methylparaben • polyparaben • butylparaben • citric acid
Replens Parke-Davis				sorbic acid • carbomer 934P • polycarbophil • glycerin • mineral oil • hydrogenated palm oil glyceride

PERSONAL CARE PRODUCTS — continued

Product[a] & Manufacturer	Antimicrobial	Local Anesthetic/ Antipruritic/Counterirritant	Hydrocortisone	Other Ingredients
Summers Eve Fresh Scent Douche C.B. Fleet				citric acid • sodium benzoate • purified water • fragrances
Summers Eve Herbal & White Flowers Scent C.B. Fleet				octoxynol-9 • citric acid • sodium benzoate • disodium EDTA • fragrance • water
Summers Eve Medicated Douche C.B. Fleet	povidone-iodine, 0.3% (when mixed)			purified water • citric acid
Summers Eve Post-Menstrual Douche C.B. Fleet				sodium lauryl sulfate • monobasic sodium & dibasic sodium phosphates • sodium chloride • disodium EDTA • methylparaben • propylparaben • water
Summers Eve Vinegar & Water Disposable Douche C.B. Fleet				vinegar • water • benzoic acid
Today Personal Lubricant Whitehall				carbomer 940 • chlorohexidine gluconate • hydroxypropyl methylcellulose • propylene glycol • sodium hydroxide • water
Trichotine Reed & Carnrick				sodium borate • aromatics • sodium lauryl sulfate • alcohol, 8%
Trichotine Reed & Carnrick				sodium perborate • aromatics • sodium lauryl sulfate • sodium chloride
Trimo-San Vaginal Jelly Milex Products				glycerine • carbomer • sodium citrate • citric acid • methylparaben • simethicone • lilac perfume • oxyquinoline sulfate, 0.025% • sodium lauryl sulfate • triethanolamine
Tucks Parke-Davis				aloe vera gel • preservative • hammamelis water, 50% • glycerin, 10%
Vagisil Combe		benzocaine, 5%		resorcinol, 2%

[a] Vaginal anti-infective products are covered in Chapter 28, "Topical Anti-Infectives."

TOPICAL ANTI-INFECTIVE PRODUCTS

Product & Manufacturer	Antiseptic	Antifungal Agent	Antibiotic	Other Ingredients
ACU-Dyne Ointment & Solution Acme United	available iodine, 1%			
Achromycin Lederle			tetracycline hydrochloride, 3%	
Aftate For Jock Itch Aerosol Schering-Plough		tolnaftate, 1%		alcohol, 14%
Aftate For Jock Itch Gel Schering-Plough		tolnaftate, 1%		
Aftate For Jock Itch Powder Schering-Plough		tolnaftate, 1%		talc
B.F.I. Powder Menley & James	bismuth formic iodide, 16%			bismuth subgallate • boric acid • eucalyptol • menthol • potassium alum • thymol • zinc phenylsulfonate
Baciguent Roberts Pharm.			bacitracin, 500units/g	white petroleum • mineral oil
Bacitracin Zinc USP E. Fougera			bacitracin zinc, 500units/g	white petrolatum base
Bacitracin Zinc-Neomycin Polymyxin E. Fougera			bacitracin zinc, 400units/g • neomycin sulfate, 5mg/g • polymyxin B sulfate, 5000units/g	white petrolatum base
Bacitracin Zinc-Polymyxin B Sulfate E. Fougera			bacitracin zinc, 500units/g • polymyxin B sulfate, 10000units/g	white petrolatum base
Benza Century	benzalkonium chloride, 1:750			
Benzalkonium Chloride Various Manufacturers	benzalkonium chloride, 17%			
Betadine Ointment & Douche Purdue Frederick	povidone-iodine, 10%			
Betadine First Aid Cream & Spray Purdue Frederick	povidone-iodine, 5%			
Breezee Mist Pedinol	aluminum chlorhydrate	undecylenic acid		menthol
Campho-Phenique Sterling Health	phenol, 4.7%			camphor, 10.8%
Clioquinol Various Manufacturers		clioquinol, 3%		
Clomycin Roberts Pharm.	lidocaine, 40mg/g	polymyxin B sulfate, 5000units/g	bacitracin, 500units/g • neomycin sulfate, 3.5mg/g	yellow petrolatum • anhydrous lanolin • mineral oil
Clorpacin WCS-90 Guardian	available chlorine, 3-4%			
Cruex Powder CIBA Consumer		calcium undecylenate, 10%		

TOPICAL ANTI-INFECTIVE PRODUCTS — continued

Product & Manufacturer	Antiseptic	Antifungal Agent	Antibiotic	Other Ingredients
Cruex Medicated Cream CIBA Consumer		total undecylenate, 20% (as undecylenic acid and zinc undecylenate)		
Cruex Spray Powder CIBA Consumer		total undecylenate, 19% (as undecylenic acid and zinc undecylenate)		
Dakins Century	sodium hypochlorite, 0.5%			
Dakins 1/2 Strength Century	sodium hypochlorite, 0.25%			
Decylenes Rugby		undecylenic acid • zinc undecylenate		
Desenex Cream, Powder & Ointment CIBA Consumer		total undecylenate, 25% (as undecylenic acid and zinc undecylenate)		
Desenex Antifungal Foam CIBA Consumer		undecylenic acid, 10%		isopropyl alcohol
Efodine E. Fougera	available iodine, 1%			
FemCare Cream Schering-Plough		clotrimazole, 1%		
FemCare Tablets Schering-Plough		clotrimazole, 100mg		
FungiCure Alva-Amco		undecylenic acid, 10%		salicylic acid, 5% • isopropyl alcohol, 70% • aloe vera gel • vitamin E
Genaspor Goldline		tolnaftate, 1%		
Gentian Violet Various Manufacturers		gentian violet, 1% or 2%		
Gyne-Lotrimin Cream Schering-Plough		clotrimazole, 1%		benzyl alcohol • cetearyl alcohol • cetyl esters wax • octyl-dodecanol • polysorbate 60 • purified water • sorbitan monostearate
Gyne-Lotrimin Tablets Schering-Plough		clotrimazole, 100mg		cornstarch • lactose • magnesium stearate • povidone
Hibiclens Liquid & Sponge Brush Stuart	chlorhexidine gluconate, 4%			
Hibistat Stuart	chlorhexidine gluconate, 0.5%			
Iodex Regular Medtech	iodine, 4.7%			oleic acid
Iodex-P Medtech	povidone-iodine, 10%			
Iodine Tincture Various Manufacturers	iodine, 2% • sodium iodide, 2.4%			alcohol, 47%

TOPICAL ANTI-INFECTIVE PRODUCTS — continued

Product & Manufacturer	Antiseptic	Antifungal Agent	Antibiotic	Other Ingredients
Iodine Tincture, Strong Various Manufacturers	iodine, 7% • potassium iodide, 5%			alcohol, 83%
Iodine Topical Various Manufacturers	iodine, 2% • sodium iodide, 2.4%			
Iodine, Strong Various Manufacturers	iodine, 2% • potassium iodide, 10%			
Lagol Oil Alvin Last	8-hydroxyquinoline, 0.0377%			mineral oil • cottonseed oil • fragrance
Lanabiotic Ointment Combe			polymyxin B sulfate, 10,000units/g • bacitracin, 500units/g • neomycin sulfate, 5mg/g	
Lotrimin AF Cream Schering-Plough		clotrimazole, 1%		
Lotrimin AF Lotion Schering-Plough		clotrimazole, 1%		cetearyl alcohol • cetyl esters wax • octyldodecanol • polysorbate • sodium biphosphate dibasic • sorbitan monostearate • water • benzyl alcohol, 1%
Lotrimin AF Solution Schering-Plough		clotrimazole, 1%		
Lotrimin Jock Itch Schering-Plough		clotrimazole, 1%		
Lubraseptic Jelly Guardian	o-phenylphenol, 0.1% • p-tert-pentylphenol, 0.02% • phenylmercuric nitrate, 0.007%			
Medi-Quik Triple Antibiotic Ointment Mentholatum			bacitracin, 500units/g • neomycin sulfate, 3.5mg/g • polymyxin B sulfate, 5000units/g	mineral oil • petrolatum
Mercurochrome Various Manufacturers	merbromin, 2%			
Mersol Century	thimerosal, 1:1000			alcohol, 52.5%
Micatin Cream & Spray Ortho		miconazole nitrate, 2%		
Monistat 7 Cream Ortho		miconazole nitrate, 2%		benzoic acid • BHA • mineral oil • peglicol 5 oleate • pegoxyol 7 stearate • purified water
Monistat 7 Suppository Ortho		miconazole nitrate, 100mg/suppository		hydrogenated vegetable oil base
Myciguent Roberts Pharm.			neomycin sulfate, 3.5mg/g	anhydrous lanolin • mineral oil • white petroleum

TOPICAL ANTI-INFECTIVE PRODUCTS — continued

Product & Manufacturer	Antiseptic	Antifungal Agent	Antibiotic	Other Ingredients
Mycitracin Upjohn			polymyxin B sulfate, 5000units/g • bacitracin, 500units/g • neomycin sulfate equivalent to 3.5mg/g neomycin	
Mycitracin Plus Upjohn			bacitracin • neomycin sulfate • polymyxin B sulfate • lidocaine	
N.B.P. Forest			polymyxin B sulfate, 5000units/g • bacitracin, 500units/g • neomycin sulfate, 5mg/g	
NP-27 Aerosol Thompson Medical		tolnaftate, 1%		alcohol, 14.9%
NP-27 Solution & Cream Thompson Medical		tolnaftate, 1%		
Neomycin Various Manufacturers			neomycin sulfate, 3.5mg/g	
Neosporin Cream Burroughs Wellcome			polymyxin B sulfate, 10,000units/g • neomycin base, 3.5mg/g	methylparaben, 0.25% • mineral oil • emulsifying wax • propylene glycol • polyoxyethylene polyoxypropelene compound • white petrolatum • purified water
Neosporin Ointment Burroughs Wellcome			polymyxin B sulfate, 5000units/g • bacitracin zinc, 400units/g • neomycin base, 3.5mg/g	white petrolatum
Neosporin Plus Maximum Strength Cream Burroughs Wellcome			polymyxin B sulfate, 10000units/g • neomycin base, 3.5mg/g	lidocaine, 40mg/g • methylparaben, 0.25% • emulsifying wax • mineral oil • poloxamer 188 • purified water • white petrolatum
Neosporin Plus Maximum Strength Ointment Burroughs Wellcome			polymyxin B sulfate, 10,000units/g • bacitracin zinc, 500units/g • neomycin base, 3.5mg/g	lidocaine, 40mg/g • white petrolatum
New Skin Liquid Bandage Medtech	8-hydroxyquinoline, 1%			clove oil, 1% • proxylin (collodion), 98%
Obtundia Cream Otis Clapp	metacresol-camphor complex			
Obtundia First Aid Spray Otis Clapp	metacresol-camphor complex			
Polydine Ointment & Solution Century	povidone-iodine			
Polysporin Ointment Burroughs Wellcome			polymyxin B sulfate, 10,000 units/g • bacitracin zinc, 500 units/g	white petrolatum
Polysporin Powder Burroughs Wellcome			polymyxin B sulfate, 10,000 units/g • bacitracin zinc, 500 units/g	lactose

TOPICAL ANTI-INFECTIVE PRODUCTS — continued

Product & Manufacturer	Antiseptic	Antifungal Agent	Antibiotic	Other Ingredients
Povidone-Iodine Various Manufacturers	povidone-iodine, 10%			
ST 37 Menley & James	hexylresorcinol, 0.1%			glycerin • propylene glycol • citric acid • edetate disodium • sodium bisulfite • sodium citrate
Salicylic Acid & Sulfur Soap Stiefel				salicylic acid, 3% • sulfur, 10%
Salicylic Acid Soap Stiefel				salicylic acid, 2%
Thimerosal Spray Various Manufacturers	thimerosal, 1:1000			alcohol, 72%
Thimerosal Tincture Various Manufacturers	thimerosal, 1:1000			alcohol, 50%
Tinactin, Various Forms Schering-Plough		tolnaftate, 1%		
Ting Aerosol Powder CIBA Consumer		tolnaftate, 1%		alcohol, 14% • talc
Ting, Various Forms CIBA Consumer		tolnaftate, 1%		
Tolnaftate Cream & Solution Goldline		tolnaftate, 1%		
Tribiotic Plus Thompson Medical			bacitracin, 600units/g • neomycin sulfate, 3.85mg/g • polymyxin B sulfate, 5500units/g	lidocaine, 40mg/g • petrolatum • lanolin anhydrous • light mineral oil
Triple Antibiotic Rugby			polymyxin B sulfate, 5000units/g • bacitracin, 400units/g • neomycin base, 3.5mg/g	white petrolatum base
Zeasorb-A F Stiefel		miconazole nitrate, 2%		talc

ACNE PRODUCTS

Product & Manufacturer	Dosage Form	Benzoyl Peroxide	Sulfur	Resorcinol/Salicylic Acid	Other Ingredients
Acne-10 Goldline	lotion	10%			
Acne-5 Goldline	lotion	5%			
Acne-Aid Stiefel	cleansing bar				surfactant blend, 6.3%
Acnomel Menley & James	cream		8%	resorcinol, 2%	alcohol, 11% • bentonite • titanium dioxide
BUF-PUF Acne Cleansing Bar 3M	cleansing bar			salicylic acid, 2%	titanium dioxide • pentasodium pentetate • sodium cocoate • sodium tallowate • tetrasodium etidronate • triethanolamine • vitamin E acetate • water
Benoxyl 10 Stiefel	lotion	10%			
Benoxyl 5 Stiefel	lotion	5%			
Bensulfoid ECR Pharm.	cream		8% (colloidal)	resorcinol, 2%	alcohol, 10% • zinc oxide, 6% • thymol, 0.5%
Brasivol Stiefel	abrasive				aluminum oxide particles in a surfactant cleansing base • sodium lauryl sulfate
Brasivol Base Stiefel	liquid				surfactant base with neutral soaps and polyoxyethylene lauryl ether
Clear By Design SmithKline Beecham	gel	2.5%			carbomer 940 • dioctyl sodium sulfosuccinate • sodium hydroxide • EDTA
Clearasil Adult Care Procter & Gamble	cream • stick		3%	resorcinol, 2%	alcohol, 10%
Clearasil Adult Care Procter & Gamble	cream • stick		8%	resorcinol, 2%	alcohol, 10%
Clearasil Antibacterial Soap Procter & Gamble	cleansing bar				triclosan, 0.75%
Clearasil Benzoyl Peroxide Procter & Gamble	cream • lotion	10%			
Clearasil Clearstick Maximum & Sensitive Procter & Gamble	liquid			salicylic acid, 2.0%	
Clearasil Clearstick Regular Procter & Gamble	liquid			salicylic acid, 1.25%	
Clearasil Double Clear Pads Maximum Strength Procter & Gamble	pad			salicylic acid, 2%	alcohol, 40%
Clearasil Double Clear Pads Regular Strength Procter & Gamble	pad			salicylic acid, 1.25%	alcohol, 40%
Clearasil Medicated Astringent Procter & Gamble	liquid			salicylic acid, 0.5%	alcohol, 43%
Fostex 10% BPO Bristol-Myers	cleansing bar	10%			urea • dextrin • sodium lauryl sulfoacetate • boric acid • disodium EDTA • lactic acid
Fostex 10% BPO Bristol-Myers	gel	10%			

ACNE PRODUCTS — continued

Product & Manufacturer	Dosage Form	Benzoyl Peroxide	Sulfur	Resorcinol/ Salicylic Acid	Other Ingredients
Fostex 10% BPO Wash Bristol-Myers	liquid	10%			
Fostex Medicated Bristol-Myers	cleansing bar			salicylic acid, 2%	boric acid • sodium • urea • dextrin • sodium lauryl sulfoacetate • cake gel • sodium dioctyl sulfosuccinate • lactic acid • triton X-200 • disodium EDTA • ocher
Fostex Medicated Cleansing Bristol-Myers	cream			salicylic acid, 2%	triton X-200 • liquid sodium dodecyltenzene sulfonate • water for production • poloxamer 188 • sodium dioctyl sulfosuccinate • stearyl alcohol C-20 • methocel A4M • modified foodstarch • sodium chloride • perfume • EDTA • color
Fostril Westwood-Squibb	lotion		2%		laureth-4 • zinc oxide • talc • PEG-40 stearate • magnesium • aluminum silicate • PEG-8 stearate • bentonite • iron oxides • methylcellulose • methylparaben • citric acid • EDTA • fragrance • quaternium-15 • simethicone
Listerex Scrub, Golden & Herbal Warner-Lambert	lotion			salicylic acid, 2%	polyethylene granules • surface-active cleansers
Loroxide Dermik	lotion	5.5%			tinted base
Neutrogena Acne Mask Neutrogena	mask	5%			
Neutrogena Oil-Free Acne Wash Neutrogena	liqui-gel			salicylic acid, 2%	
Noxzema Clear-Ups Acne Medicated Maximum Strength Procter & Gamble	lotion	10%			
Noxzema Clear-Ups Medicated Maximum Strength Procter & Gamble	pad			salicylic acid, 2%	alcohol, 64%
Noxzema Clear-Ups Medicated Regular Strength Procter & Gamble	pad			salicylic acid, 0.5%	alcohol, 63%
Oxy Clean Medicated Cleanser & Pads SmithKline Beecham	liquid • pad			salicylic acid, 0.5%	alcohol, 40% • citric acid • menthol • sodium lauryl sulfate
Oxy Maximum Strength Medicated Pad SmithKline Beecham	pad			salicylic acid, 2%	alcohol, 50% • citric acid • menthol • sodium lauryl sulfate
Oxy Medicated Soap SmithKline Beecham	cleansing bar				triclosan, 1.0% • bentonite • cocoa MPH odipropionate • fragrance • glycerin • iron oxides • magnesium silicate • sodium chloride • sodium borohydride • sodium cocoate • sodium tallowate • talc • tetrasodium EDTA • titanium dioxide • trisodium HEDTA • water

ACNE PRODUCTS — continued

Product & Manufacturer	Dosage Form	Benzoyl Peroxide	Sulfur	Resorcinol/ Salicylic Acid	Other Ingredients
Oxy Night Watch Maximum Strength SmithKline Beecham	lotion			salicylic acid, 2%	cetyl alcohol • disodium EDTA • methylparaben • propylene glycol • propylparaben • silica • sodium lauryl sulfate • stearyl alcohol • water
Oxy Res: Don't Medicated Face Wash SmithKline Beecham	lotion				triclosan, 0.6% • cocamidopropyl betaine • diazolidinyl urea • sodium cocoyl isethionate • sodium laureth sulfate • water
Oxy-10 Daily Face Wash SmithKline Beecham	liquid	10%			citric acid • cocamidopropyl betaine • diazolidinyl urea • methylparaben • propylparaben • sodium citrate • sodium cocoyl isethionate • sodium laureth sulfate sarcosinate • water • xanthan gum
Oxy-5 Vanishing Sensitive Skin SmithKline Beecham	lotion	5%			
Pan Oxyl Bar 10 Stiefel	cleansing bar	10%			mild surfactant base
Pan Oxyl Bar 5 Stiefel	cleansing bar	5%			mild surfactant base
Pernox Westwood-Squibb	lotion		2%	salicylic acid, 1.5%	polyethylene granules • sodium octoxynol-2 • ethane sulfonate • sodium dodecylbenzene sulfonate • fragrance • docusate sodium • modified starch • magnesium aluminum • silicate • methylcellulose • EDTA
Pernox Lemon & Regular Westwood-Squibb	abrasive		2%	salicylic acid, 1.5%	polyethylene granules • sodium octoxynol-2 • ethane sulfonate • sodium dodecylbenzene sulfonate • poloxamer 184 • docusate sodium • methylcellulose • foodstarch • fragrance • EDTA • D&C yellow#10 • FD&C blue #1 (Regular)
Propa pH Acne Medication Cleansing Pads Sensitive Skin Del	pad			salicylic acid, 0.5%	aloe • alcohol, 25%
Propa pH Acne Medication Cream Del	cream			salicylic acid, 2%	
Rezamid Acne Lotion Summers	liquid		5%	resorcinol, 2%	
SalAc Cleanser GenDerm	liquid			salicylic acid, 2%	
Salicylic Acid & Sulfur Soap Stiefel	cleansing bar		10% (precipitated)	salicylic acid, 3%	
Salicylic Acid Soap Stiefel	cleansing bar			salicylic acid, 3.5%	
Sastid Plain Therapeutic Shampoo & Wash Stiefel	liquid		1.6%	salicylic acid, 1.6%	surfactant base
Sastid Soap Stiefel	cleansing bar		10%	salicylic acid, 3%	

ACNE PRODUCTS — continued

Product & Manufacturer	Dosage Form	Benzoyl Peroxide	Sulfur	Resorcinol/ Salicylic Acid	Other Ingredients
Sebasorb Summers	liquid			salicylic acid, 2%	attapulgite, 10% • polysorbate 80
Stri-Dex Antibacterial Cleansing Bar Sterling Health	cleansing bar				triclosan, 1%
Stri-Dex Antibacterial Cleansing Bar with Glycerin Sterling Health	cleansing bar				triclosan, 1% • glycerin
Stri-Dex Clear Gel Sterling Health	gel			salicylic acid, 2.0%	glycerin • SD alcohol, 9.3%
Stri-Dex Dual & Single Textured Pads Maximum Strength Sterling Health	liquid			salicylic acid, 2%	SD alcohol, 44%
Stri-Dex Dual Textured Pads Regular Strength Sterling Health	liquid			salicylic acid, 0.5%	SD alcohol, 28%
Stri-Dex Maximum Strength Medicated Sterling Health	pad			salicylic acid, 2%	ammonium xylenesulfonate • sodium dodecylbenzene sulfonate • fragrance • simethicone emulsion • sodium carbonate • citric acid • alcohol, 44%
Stri-Dex Medicated Sterling Health	pad			salicylic acid, 0.5%	dodecylbenzene sulfonate • sodium xylene sulfonate • fragrance • citric acid • alcohol, 28%
Stri-Dex Super Scrub Pads Sterling Health	liquid			salicylic acid, 2%	SD alcohol, 54%
Sulfur Soap Stiefel	cleansing bar		10% (precipitated)		
Sulray Alvin Last	cleansing bar		5%		sulfur, 5% in a fragrance free natural soap base • also contains aloe vera • trisodium HEDTA
Sulray Alvin Last	cream		3%		sulfurated lime (calcium) solution • zinc sulfate • aloe vera gel • glyceryl, stearate, and laureth-23 • PEG-8 stearate • glycerin • silica • methylparaben • propylparaben
Tyrosum Liquid & Packets Summers	liquid • swab				alcohol, 50% • acetone, 10% • polysorbate 80, 2%
Vanoxide Dermik	lotion	5%			
Xerac Alcohol Gel Person & Covey	gel		4%		alcohol, 44%
Xerac BP10 Person & Covey	gel	10%			laureth-4
Xerac BP5 Person & Covey	gel	5%			laureth-4

Dermatitis and Psoriasis Product Table

DERMATITIS AND PSORIASIS PRODUCTS

Product & Manufacturer	Dosage Form	Hydro-cortisone	Keratolytic	Tar Product	Other Ingredients
Ammoniated Mercury Various Manufacturers	ointment				ammoniated mercury, 5%
Balnetar Westwood-Squibb	bath oil			coal tar, 2.5%	mineral oil • lanolin oil • PEG-4-dilaurate • laureth 4 • fragrance • docusate sodium
CaldeCORT CIBA Consumer	spray	1%			
CaldeCORT Light CIBA Consumer	cream	0.5%			aloe vera gel • isopropyl myristate • methylparaben • polysorbate 60 • propylparaben • sorbitan monostearate • sorbitol solution • stearic acid
CaldeCORT Maximum Strength CIBA Consumer	cream	1%			isopropyl myristate • methyparaben • polysorbate 60 • propylparaben • purified water • sorbitan monostearate • sorbitol solution • stearic acid
Cetaphil Owen/Galderma	bar				sodium cocoyl isethionate • stearic acid • sodium tallowate
Cetaphil Owen/Galderma	liquid				cetyl and stearyl alcohol • propylene glycol • sodium lauryl sulfate • parabens
Clocort Roberts Pharm.	cream	10mg			glycerin • glyceryl stearate • mineral oil • methylparaben • polysorbate 60 • propylparaben • sorbitan stearate • purified water • aloe vera gel
Coal Tar Various Manufacturers	solution			coal tar, 20%	
Cortaid Upjohn	lotion	0.5%			butylparaben • cetyl palmitate • glyceryl monostearate • methylparaben • polysorbate 80 • propylene glycol • stearamidoethyl diethylamine • purified water
Cortaid Upjohn	spray	0.5%			alcohol • glycerin • methylparaben • purified water
Cortaid with Aloe Upjohn	cream	0.5%			aloe • butylparaben • cetyl palmitate • glyceryl stearate • methylparaben • propylethylene glycol • stearamidoethyl diethylamine • purified water
Cortaid, Maximum Strength Upjohn	cream	1%			butylparaben • cetyl alcohol • glycerin • methylparaben • sodium lauryl sulfate • stearic acid • stearyl alcohol • purified water • white petrolatum
Cortaid, Maximum Strength Upjohn	ointment	1%			butylparaben • cholesterol • methylparaben • microcrystalline wax • mineral oil • white petrolatum

DERMATITIS AND PSORIASIS PRODUCTS — continued

Product & Manufacturer	Dosage Form	Hydro-cortisone	Keratolytic	Tar Product	Other Ingredients
Cortisone-10 Cream Thompson Medical	cream	1%			aluminum sulfate • calcium acetate • cetearyl alcohol • glycerin • light mineral oil • methylparaben • propylparaben • potato dextrin • sodium lauryl sulfate • water • white petrolatum • white wax
Cortisone-10 Ointment Thompson Medical	ointment	1%			white petrolatum
Cortizone-5 Cream Thompson Medical	cream	0.5%			aluminum sulfate • calcium acetate • cetearyl alcohol • glycerin • light mineral oil • methylparaben • propylparaben • potato dextrin • sodium lauryl sulfate • water • white petrolatum • white wax
Cortizone-5 Ointment Thompson Medical	ointment	0.5%			white petrolatum
Cutar Summers	emulsion			coal tar, 1.5%	
Denorex with Conditioners Whitehall	shampoo			coal tar solution, 9% (equivalent to 1.8% coal tar)	
Denorex, Extra Strength Whitehall	shampoo			coal tar solution, 12.5% (equivalent to 2.5% coal tar)	
Denorex, Regular Formula and Mountain Fresh Scent Whitehall	shampoo			coal tar solution, 9% (equivalent to 1.8% coal tar)	
Dermolate Schering-Plough	cream	0.5%			
Doak Tar Lotion Doak	lotion			tar distillate, 5%	doak oil, 10%
Dr. Gordshells Salve Thomas & Thompson	ointment			rosin	lard • tallow • beeswax • elder flowers • bayberry • sassafras oil • benzoic acid
Estar Westwood-Squibb	gel			coal tar, 5%	alcohol, 15.6% • alanine • benzyl alcohol • carbomer 940 • glycereth-7 cocoanate • laureth-4 • polysorbate 80 • simethicone • sorbitol
Hydrocortisone Various Manufacturers	cream	0.5%; 1%			
Hydrocortisone Various Manufacturers	lotion	0.5%; 1%			
Hydrocortisone Cream 0.5% Goldline	cream	0.5%			

DERMATITIS AND PSORIASIS PRODUCTS — continued

Product & Manufacturer	Dosage Form	Hydro-cortisone	Keratolytic	Tar Product	Other Ingredients
Hydrocortisone Maximum Strength Cream 1% Goldline	cream	1%			
Hytone Dermik	cream • lotion • ointment	0.5%			
Ionil T Owen/Galderma	shampoo			coal tar solution, 4.25%	polyoxyethylene ethers • benzalkonium chloride • alcohol • isopropyl alcohol • EDTA
Ionil T Plus Owen/Galderma	shampoo			tar distillate, 2%	sodium laureth sulfate • lauramide DEA • quaternium-22 • laureth-23 • talloweth-60 myristyl glycol • TEA lauryl sulfate • glycol distearate • laureth-4 • TEA-abietoyl hydrolyzed collagen • DMDM hydantoin • EDTA • fragrance • FD&C blue#1 • Ext D&C yellow#7
Kericort HC Cream 1% Bristol-Myers	cream	1%			citric acid, anhydrous • sodium citrate • methylparaben • sorbic acid • polyoxyl 40 stearate • glyceryl stearate • white wax • stearyl alcohol • isopropyl myristate • cetyl alcohol • sorbitan monostearate • polysorbate 60 • propylparaben • propylene glycol
Lanacort Combe	cream	0.5%			
Lanacort 10 Combe	cream	1%			
Lanacort 10 Combe	ointment	1%			
Lavatar Doak	bath oil			tar distillate, 25%	
Neutrogena T/Derm Neutrogena	body oil			Neutar, 5% (coal tar, 1.2%)	emollient oil base
Neutrogena T/Gel Neutrogena	shampoo			Neutar, 2% (coal tar, 0.5%)	shampoo base
Neutrogena T/Gel Conditioner Neutrogena	conditioner			Neutar, 2% (coal tar, 0.5%)	conditioner base
Neutrogena T/Sal Neutrogena	shampoo		salicylic acid, 2%		shampoo base
Oxipor VHC Whitehall	lotion			coal tar solution, 25% (equivalent to 5% coal tar)	alcohol, 81% • citric acid • PEG-8 • water
P&S Plus Baker Cummins	gel			coal tar solution, 8% • tar product (crude coal tar, 1.6%)	
PROSAL Summers	liquid		salicylic acid, 3%		

DERMATITIS AND PSORIASIS PRODUCTS — continued

Product & Manufacturer	Dosage Form	Hydro-cortisone	Keratolytic	Tar Product	Other Ingredients
Panscol Baker Cummins	lotion		salicylic acid, 3%		
Panscol Baker Cummins	ointment		salicylic acid, 3%		
Pentrax GenDerm	shampoo			coal tar extract, 8.75% (equivalent to coal tar, 4.3%)	detergents
Pentrax Gold GenDerm	shampoo			equivalent to crude coal tar, 2%	detergents
Polytar Stiefel	cleansing bar			polytar, 1%	
Polytar Stiefel	shampoo			polytar, 2.5%	conditioners
Poslam Psoriasis Ointment Alvin Last	ointment		sulfur, 5% • salicylic acid, 2%		petrolatum • cornstarch • lanolin • zinc oxide • ozokerite • phenol • menthol • fragrance • talc • iron oxides
Preparation H Hydrocortisone 1% Anti-Itch Cream Whitehall	cream	1%			various
PsoriNail Summers	liquid			LCD, 2.5% (equivalent to coal tar, 0.5%)	
Psorigel Owen/Galderma	gel			coal tar solution, 8.8%	alcohol • laureth-4 • fragrance • propylene glycol • hydroxyethylcellulose
Sebutone Westwood-Squibb	shampoo		sulfur, 1.5% • salicylic acid, 1.5%	tar, 0.5%	sodium dodecyl • benzene sulfonate • sodium octoxynol-2-ethane sulfonate • PEG-6 lauramide • sodium dioctyl sulfosuccinate • titanium dioxide • sodium chloride • PEG-90M • fragrance • lanolin oil • EDTA • FD&C blue#1 • D&C yellow#10
Tarpaste Doak	paste			tar distillate, 5%	zinc oxide
Tarsum Shampoo/Gel Summers	shampoo			coal tar solution, 10%	
Tersa-Tar Doak Tar Shampoo Doak	shampoo			tar distillate, 3%	
X-Seb T Pearl Baker Cummins	shampoo			coal tar solution, 10% • crude coal tar, 2%	
Zetar Dermik	shampoo			whole colloidal coal tar, 1%	chloroxylenol, 0.5%

DRY SKIN PRODUCTS

Product & Manufacturer	Dosage Form	Keratin Softener	Humectant	Other Ingredients
ACID Mantle Creme Acid pH Sandoz Pharm.	cream		glycerin	aluminum acetate • aluminum sulfate • calcium acetate • cetearyl alcohol • light mineral oil • methylparaben • purified water • sodium lauryl sulfate • synthetic beeswax • white petrolatum • white potato dextrin • citric acid • ammonium hydroxide
Aloe Grande Creme Gordon	cream		aloe	vitamin E, 1500 IU/oz • vitamin A, 100,000 IU/oz
Alpha Keri Bristol-Myers	bar		glycerin	sodium tallowate • sodium cocoate • mineral oil • PEG-75 • titanium dioxide • lanolin oil • sodium chloride • BHT • EDTA • color • fragrance
Alpha Keri Bristol-Myers	gel			TEA lauryl sulfate • lauramide DEA • linoleamide DEA • hydrolyzed animal protein • ethylene glycol monostearate • methyl cellulose • sodium chloride • perfume • citric acid • DM DM hydantoin • polyquaternium-10 • methylparaben • propylene glycol • propylparaben • tetrasodium EDTA
Alpha Keri Bristol-Myers	oil			mineral oil • lanolin oil • PEG-4-dilaurate • benzophenone-3 • fragrance • color
Alpha Keri Bristol-Myers	spray			mineral oil • lanolin oil • alcohol • PPG-15 stearyl ether • C12-15 alcohols benzoate • PEG-4-dilaurate • polysorbate 85 • fragrance
Aqua A Baker Cummins	cream			water • caprylic/capric triglyceride • methyl gluceth-10 • glyceryl stearate squalane • mineral oil • PPG-20 methyl glucose ether distearate • dimethicone • stearic acid • PEG-50 stearate • retinyl palmitate • sodium hyaluronate • lecithin • sodium polyglutamate • magnesium aluminum silicate • carbomer 934 • dichlorobenzyl alcohol • cetyl alcohol • BHT • diazolidinyl urea • xanthan gum • menthol • sodium hydroxide • tetrasodium EDTA
Aqua Care Menley & James	cream	urea, 10%	glycerin	cetyl esters • DEA-oleath-3 • phosphate • petrolatum • triethanolamine • carbomer • lanolin oil • mineral oil/lanolin alcohol • benzyl alcohol • fragrance
Aqua Care Menley & James	lotion	urea, 10%		mineral oil • petrolatum • propylene glycol stearate • sorbitan stearate • cetyl alcohol • lactic acid • magnesium aluminum silicate • sodium lauryl sulfate • parabens
Aquaderm Baker Cummins	lotion			water • caprylic/capric triglyceride • methyl gluceth-10 • glyceryl stearate • dimethicone • petrolatum • mineral oil • ether distearate • stearic acid • sodium hyaluronate • lecithin • sodium polyglutamate • magnesium aluminum silicate • carbomer 934 • dichlorobenzyl alcohol • cetyl alcohol • BHT • diazolidinyl urea • xanthan gum • menthol • tetrasodium EDTA • sodium hydroxide
Aveeno Bath Treatment Moisturizing Formula/Dry, Itchy Skin S.C. Johnson Wax	powder			colloidal oatmeal, 43% • mineral oil • calcium silicate • laureth-4
Aveeno Bath Treatment Soothing Formula/Itchy Irritated Skin S.C. Johnson Wax	powder			colloidal oatmeal, 100%
Aveeno Cleansing Bar Combination Skin S.C. Johnson Wax	cleansing bar	petrolatum	glycerin	colloidal oatmeal, 51% • sodium cocoyl isethionate • lactic acid • sodium lactate • magnesium aluminum silicate • potassium sorbate • titanium dioxide • PEG-14M

DRY SKIN PRODUCTS — continued

Product & Manufacturer	Dosage Form	Keratin Softener	Humectant	Other Ingredients
Aveeno Cleansing Bar Dry Skin S.C. Johnson Wax	cleansing bar		glycerin	colloidal oatmeal, 51% • sodium cocoyl isethionate • vegetable oil (hydrogenated) • vegetable shortening • PEG-75 • lauramide DEA • lactic acid • sodium lactate • sorbic acid • titanium dioxide
Aveeno Moisturizing Cream & Lotion S.C. Johnson Wax	cream • lotion	petrolatum	glycerin	colloidal oatmeal, 1% • distearyldimonium chloride • isopropyl palmitate • cetyl alcohol • dimethicone • sodium chloride • benzyl alcohol
Aveeno Shower & Bath Oil S.C. Johnson Wax	bath oil			colloidal oatmeal, 4% • mineral oil • laureth-4 • benzaldehyde • quaternium-18 hectorite • phenylcarbinol • silica
Candermyl Owen/Galderma	cream		glycerin	oleic/palmitoleic triglycerides • polyamidoacid • sodium lactate methylsilanol • propylene glycol • polyglyceryl-3 • hexadecylether • cholesterol
Catrix Savage	cream	imidazolidinyl urea	glycerin	octyl methoxycinnamate, 7.5% • menthyl anthranilate, 3.5% • catrix • purified water • sesame oil • cetearyl alcohol • ceteareth-20 • stearyl stearate • caprylic/capric triglyceride • glycereth-7 • dimethicone • magnesium aluminum silicate • xanthan gum • tocopheryl linoleate • alanin • glycine • magnesium aspartate • urea • saccharide hydrolyzate • butylene glycol • trisodium EDTA • disodium phosphate • phosphoric acid buffer • sorbic acid • methylparaben • propylparaben • butylparaben • phenoxyethanol • orange oil • cardamon oil • titanium dioxide
Catrix Lip Saver Savage	stick			ethylhexyl p-methoxycinnamate, 7.0% • oxybenzone, 3.0% • allantoin, 1.0% • catrix • mineral oil • castor oil • petrolatum • octyl palmitate • paraffin • carnauba wax • beeswax • caprylic/capric triglyceride • vitamin E • lemon extract • propylparaben
Catrix with Sunscreen Savage	cream	imidazolidinyl urea	glycerin	octyl methoxycinnamate, 7.5% • menthyl anthranilate, 3.5% • catrix • purified water • sesame oil • cetearyl alcohol • ceteareth-20 • stearyl stearate • caprylic/capric triglyceride • glycereth-7 • dimethicone • magnesium aluminum silicate • xanthan gum • tocopheryl linoleate • alanin • glycine • magnesium aspartate • urea • saccharide hydrolyzate • butylene glycol • trisodium EDTA • disodium phosphate • phosphoric acid buffer • sorbic acid • methylparaben • propylparaben • butylparaben • phenoxyethanol • orange oil • cardamon oil • titanium dioxide
Cetaphil Owen/Galderma	bar			sodium cocoyl isethionate • stearic acid • sodium tallowate
Cetaphil Owen/Galderma	liquid			cetyl and stearyl alcohol • propylene glycol • sodium lauryl sulfate
Clocream Roberts Pharm.	cream			cetylpalmitate • vitamin A palmitate • cottonseed oil • glycerin • glyceryl monostearate • methylparaben • mineral oil • potassium stearate • propylparaben • sodium citrate • vitamins A & D • cholecalciferol • fragrance • purified water
Complex 15 Face & Hand & Body Cream Schering-Plough	cream		glycerin • lecithin	
Complex 15 Hand & Body Lotion Schering-Plough	lotion		glycerin • lecithin	
Corn Huskers Warner-Lambert	lotion		glycerin, 8%	SD alcohol 40 • algin • tea-oleoyl sarcosinate • methylparaben • guar gum • calcium sulfate • calcium chloride • tea-fumarate • tea-borate

DRY SKIN PRODUCTS — continued

Product & Manufacturer	Dosage Form	Keratin Softener	Humectant	Other Ingredients
Correction Cream Wash Savage	cream	diazolidinyl urea	glycerin	water • glycol stearate • isopropyl myristate • lanolin ester • stearyl alcohol • petrolatum • octoxynol-9 • propylene glycol • lecithin • methylparaben • lemon extract • sodium dehydroacetate • propylparaben
Curel Moisturizing S.C. Johnson Wax	cream • lotion	petrolatum	glycerin	quaternium-5 • isopropyl palmitate • 1-hexadecanol • dimethicone • parabens • sodium chloride
Cutemol Summers	cream			liquid petrolatum • acetylated lanolin • lanolin alcohols extract • isopropyl myristate wax • allantoin • sorbitan sesquioleate
DML Forte Person & Covey	cream		glycerin	petrolatum • PPG-2 • myristyl ether propionate • glyceryl stearate • simethicone • benzyl alcohol • silica • EDTA • sodium carbomer 1342
DermKote Parnell	lotion		glycerin	dimethicone, 1% • mineral oil • yerba santa • cetyl alcohol • glyceryl stearate • isopropyl myristate • PEG-40 stearate • squalane • stearic acid • diazolidinyl urea • lecithin • PEG-12 oleate • propylene glycol • benzoic acid • quaternized acetamide MEA • BHT • retinyl palmitate • tocopheryl acetate
Emollia Gordon	lotion			mineral oil • cetyl alcohol • propylene glycol • white wax • sodium lauryl sulfate • oleic acid • parabens
Gordo-Vite E Gordon	cream			vitamin E, 50mg/g
Gordon's Vite A Gordon	cream			vitamin A, 100,000 IU/oz
Gormel Gordon	cream	urea, 20%		
Hydrisinol Pedinol	lotion			sulfonated hydrogenated castor oil • hydrogenated vegetable oil
Keri Facial Soap Bristol-Myers	cleansing bar		glycerin	sodium tallowate • sodium cocoate • mineral oil • octyl hydroxystearate • fragrance • titanium dioxide • PEG-75 • lanolin oil • dioctyl sodium sulfosuccinate • PEG-4 dilaurate • propylparaben • PEG-40-stearate • glycerol monostearate/PEG-100-stearate
Keri Lotion Bristol-Myers	lotion			mineral oil • propylene glycol • glyceryl stearate • PEG-40 stearate • PEG-100 stearate • PEG-4-dilaurate • laureth-4 • lanolin oil • parabens • carbomer 934 • fragrance • quaternium-15 • sodium dioctyl sulfosuccinate
Keri Silky Smooth Bristol-Myers	lotion		glycerin	petrolatum • dimethicone • steareth-2 • cetyl alcohol • benzyl alcohol • laureth-23 • carbomer 934 • magnesium aluminum silicate • fragrance • quaternium 15 • sodium hydroxide • tocopheryl linoleate • BHT • disodium EDTA
Keri Silky-Fragrance Free Bristol-Myers	lotion		glycerin	petrolatum • dimethicone 200 • steareth-2 • cetyl alcohol • benzyl alcohol • laureth-23 • tocopheryl linoleate • carbomer 934 • BHT • disodium EDTA • sodium hydroxide • quaternium-15 • magnesium aluminum silicate
Lacti-Care Stiefel	lotion		lactic acid • sodium PCA	mineral oil • isopropyl palmitate • stearyl alcohol ceteareth-20 • sodium hydroxide • glyceryl stearate • PEG-100 stearate • myristyl lactate • cetyl alcohol • carbomer 940 • imidazolidinyl urea • dehydratoacetic acid
Lazer Creme Pedinol	cream			vitamin E, 3500 U/oz • vitamin A, 100,000 U/oz
Lowila Cake Westwood-Squibb	cleansing bar	urea	lactic acid	dextrin • sodium lauryl sulfoacetate • boric acid • sorbitol • mineral oil • PEG-14M • dioctyl sodium sulfosuccinate • cellulose gum • fragrance
Lubriderm Warner-Lambert	cream		glycerin	mineral oil • petrolatum • glyceryl stearate • PEG-100 stearate • hydrogenated polyisobutene • lanolin • lanolin alcohol • lanolin oil • cetyl alcohol • sorbitan laurate • fragrance • parabens • quaternium-15
Lubriderm Lubath Warner-Lambert	bath oil			mineral oil • PPG-15 stearyl ether • oleth-2 • nonoxynol-5

DRY SKIN PRODUCTS — continued

Product & Manufacturer	Dosage Form	Keratin Softener	Humectant	Other Ingredients
Lubriderm, Unscented Warner-Lambert	lotion			mineral oil • petroleum • sorbitol • lanolin • lanolin alcohol • stearic acid • triethanolamine • cetyl alcohol • parabens • sodium chloride
Mammol Abbott	ointment			bismuth subnitrate, 40% • castor oil, 30% • anhydrous lanolin, 22% • ceresin wax, 7% • peruvian balsam, 1%
Moisturel Cream Westwood-Squibb	cream		glycerin	petrolatum • PG dioctanoate • cetyl alcohol • steareth-2 • dimethicone • PVP/hexadecene copolymer • laureth-23 • magnesium aluminum silicate • diazolidinyl urea • carbomer 934 • sodium hydroxide • kathon CG
Moisturel Lotion Westwood-Squibb	lotion		glycerin	petrolatum • dimethicone • steareth-2 • cetyl alcohol • benzyl alcohol • laureth-23 • carbomer 934 • magnesium aluminum silicate • quaternium-15 • sodium hydroxide
Moisturel Sensitive Skin Westwood-Squibb	lotion			sodium laureth sulfate & laureth 6 carboxylic acid & disodium laureth sulfosuccinate • methyl gluceth 20 • cocamidopropyl betaine • diazolidinyl urea • kathon CG
Nephro-Derm R&D Laboratories	cream			water • eucerin • petrolatum • glyceril stearate • mineral oil • paraffin wax • tween • camphor • menthol • methylparaben • propylparaben • vitamin B_{12}
Neutrogena Body Lotion (FF) Neutrogena	lotion			purified water • isopropyl myristate • butylene glycol • glyceryl stearate • PEG-100 stearate • cetyl alcohol • carbomer • triethanolamine • diazolidinyl urea • methylparaben • ethylparaben • propylparaben • tetrasodium EDTA
Neutrogena Body Oil (FF) Neutrogena	body oil			isopropyl myristate • sesame oil • PEG-40 sorbitan peroleate • parabens
Neutrogena Norwegian Formula Emulsion (FF) Neutrogena	emulsion		glycerin, 25%	
Neutrogena Norwegian Formula Hand Cream (FF) Neutrogena	cream		glycerin, 41%	
Nivea Bath Silk Beiersdorf	cleansing bar		glycerin • aloe	sodium tallowate/sodium cocoate • fragrance • petrolatum • titanium dioxide • sodium chloride • octyldodecanol • macadamia nut oil • extract • sodium thiosulfate • triple purified water • lanolin alcohol • pentasodium pentetate • tetrasodium etidronate • BHT • beeswax
Nivea Creme Ultra Moisturizing Beiersdorf	cream		glycerin	water • mineral oil • petrolatum • isohexadecane • microcrystalline wax • lanolin • alcohol • paraffin • panthenol • magnesium sulfate • decyl oleate • octyldodecanol • aluminum stearate • fragrance • methylchloroisothiazolinone • methylisothiazolinone • citric acid • magnesium stearate
Nutraderm Owen/Galderma	bath oil			bath oil • mineral oil • lanolin oil • PEG-4 dilaurate • benzophenone-3 • butylparaben
Nutraderm Owen/Galderma	cream			mineral oil • sorbitan stearate • stearyl alcohol • sodium lauryl sulfate • cetyl alcohol • parabens • fragrance
Nutraderm Owen/Galderma	lotion			mineral oil • sorbitan stearate • stearyl and cetyl alcohol • carbomer 940
Nutraderm 30 Owen/Galderma	lotion		lactic acid • malic acid • sodium PCA • glycerin	petrolatum • cetearyl alcohol • ceteareth-20 • dimethicone • C10-30 cholesterol/lanosterol esters • cyclomethicone • cetyl alcohol • sodium lactate • cetyl lactate • C12-C15 alcohols lactate • xanthan gum • sodium hydroxide • parabens • diazolidinyl urea • fragrance
Nutraplus Owen/Galderma	cream	urea, 10%		glyceryl stearate • propylene glycol • mineral oil • parabens

DRY SKIN PRODUCTS — continued

Product & Manufacturer	Dosage Form	Keratin Softener	Humectant	Other Ingredients
Nutraplus Owen/Galderma	lotion	urea, 10%		glyceryl stearate • acetylated lanolin alcohol • isopropyl palmitate • stearic acid • petrolatum • parabens • carbomer 940
Oilatum Soap Stiefel	cleansing bar			polyunsaturated vegetable oil, 7.5%
Panscol Baker Cummins	lotion			salicylic acid, 3% • phenol, 0.5%
Pedi-Bath Pedinol	salts			colloidal sulfur • sodium bicarbonate • pine needle oil
Pedi-Vit-A Pedinol	cream			vitamin A, 100,000 IU/30mg
Pen-Kera B.F. Ascher	cream	urea	glycerin	octoyl palmitate • mineral oil • lanolin alcohol • polysorbate 60 • sorbitan stearate • carbomer 940 • triethanolamine • wheat germ glycerides • diazolidinyl urea • polyamino sugar condensate • dehydroacetic acid
Plexolan Moisturizing Cream Alvin Last	ointment			petrolatum • lanolin, 15.5% • mineral oil • ozokerite • PEG-400-distearate • fragrance • zinc oxide • methylparaben
Polysorb Hydrate E. Fougera	cream			sorbitan sesquioleate • wax & petrolatum base
Pretty Feet & Hands Menley & James	lotion			paraffin • magnesium aluminum silicate • palmitic acid • stearic acid • triethanolamine • methylparaben • propylparaben • fragrance
Pro-Cute Ferndale	cream		glycerin	water • stearic acid • cetyl alcohol • ceraphyl 230 • forlan-LM • deltyl prime • trolamine • silicone • povidone • dowicil 200 • perfume
Pro-Cute Ferndale	lotion		glycerin	cetyl alcohol • stearic acid • forlan-LM • deltyl prime • ceraphyl 230 • silicone • triethanolamine • povidone • sorbic acid • dowicil 200 • menthol
Purpose Dry Skin Ortho	cream		lactic acid	mineral oil • petrolatum • almond oil • propylene glycol • glyceryl stearate • sodium lactate • steareth-20 • cetyl alcohol • cetyl esters wax • steareth-2 • xanthan gum • sorbic acid
Sardo Schering-Plough	bath oil			mineral oil • isopropyl palmitate
Sardoettes Schering-Plough	wipe			mineral oil • isopropyl palmitate
Sarna Stiefel	lotion			0.5% each of camphor and menthol in an emollient base
Shepards Dermik	cream • lotion		glycerin	sesame oil • SD alcohol 40-B • stearic acid • propylene glycol • ethoxydiglycol • triethanolamine • glyceryl stearate • cetyl alcohol • simethicone • parabens • vegetable oil • monoglyceride citrate • BHT • citric acid
Shepards Skin Dermik	cream	urea	glycerin	glyceryl stearate • ethoxydiglycol • propylene glycol • stearic acid • isopropyl myristate • cetyl alcohol • lecithin • parabens
Silk Solution Thompson Medical	lotion			dimethicone, 2.0% • cetyl alcohol • cyclomethicone • dimethiconol • dioctyl adipate • glycerin • methyldibromoglutaronitrile • phenoxyethanol • stearic acid • triethanolamine • water
Therapeutic Bath Lotion Goldline	lotion			mineral oil • lanolin oil • glyceryl stearate • PEG-100 stearate • propylene glycol • PEG-40 stearate • laureth-4 • PEG-4 dilaurate • methylparaben • carbomer 934 • propylparaben • quaternium-15 • trolamine • dioctyl sodium sulfosuccinate
Therapeutic Bath Oil Goldline	bath oil	mineral oil • lanolin oil		PEG-4-dilaurate • benzophenone-3
Ultra Derm Baker Cummins	bath oil			mineral oil • lanolin oil • octoxynol-3

DRY SKIN PRODUCTS — continued

Product & Manufacturer	Dosage Form	Keratin Softener	Humectant	Other Ingredients
Ultra Derm Baker Cummins	lotion		glycerin	mineral oil • petrolatum • lanolin oil • glyceryl stearate • propylene glycol • PEG-50-stearate • propylene glycol stearate se • cetyl alcohol • sorbitan laurate • potassium sorbate • phosphoric acid • tetrasodium EDTA
Ultra Mide Moisturizer Baker Cummins	lotion	urea, 25%		
Ureacin-10 Pedinol	lotion	urea, 10%		vegetable oil base
Ureacin-20 Pedinol	cream	urea, 20%		vegetable oil base
Wibi Owen/ Galderma	lotion		glycerin	SD alcohol 40 • PEG-4 • PEG-6-32 • stearate • glycol stearate • carbomer 940 • PEG-75 • methylparaben • triethanolamine • menthol • fragrance

DANDRUFF AND SEBORRHEA PRODUCTS

Product & Manufacturer	Dosage Form	Keratolytic	Cytostatic Agent	Other Ingredients
Anti-Dandruff Brylcreem SmithKline Beecham	cream		pyrithione zinc, 1%	mineral oil • propylene glycol • paraffin wax • excipients • water • trilaneth-4 phosphate • petrolatum • poloxamer 284 • triethanolamine • carbomer 940 • fragrance
DHS Tar Person & Covey	shampoo			coal tar, 0.5%
DHS Zinc Person & Covey	shampoo		pyrithione zinc, 2%	
Denorex Medicated Shampoo Extra Strength with Conditioners Whitehall	shampoo			coal tar solution, 12.5% (equivalent to 2.5% coal tar) • chloroxylenol • citric acid • cocodimonium • hydrolyzed protein • FD&C red#40 • fragrance • glycol distearate • hydroxypropyl methylcellulose • lauramide DEA • menthol • PEG-27 lanolin • polyquaternium-6 • TEA-lauryl sulfate • water • alcohol, 10.4%
Denorex Medicated Shampoo with Conditioners Whitehall	shampoo			coal tar solution, 9% (equivalent to 1.8% coal tar) • chloroxylenol • citric acid • fragrance • hydroxypropyl methylcellulose • lauramide DEA • menthol • PEG-27 lanolin • polyquaternium-11 • TEA-lauryl sulfate • water • alcohol, 7.5%
Denorex Medicated Shampoo, Extra Strength Whitehall	shampoo			coal tar solution, 12.5% (equivalent to 2.5% coal tar) • chloroxylenol • FD&C red#40 • fragrance • glycol distearate • hydroxypropyl methylcellulose • lauramide DEA • menthol • TEA-lauryl sulfate • water • alcohol, 10.4%
Denorex Medicated Shampoo, Regular Formula Whitehall	shampoo			coal tar solution, 9% (equivalent to 1.8% coal tar) • chloroxylenol • lauramide DEA • menthol • stearic acid • TEA-lauryl sulfate • water • alcohol, 7.5%
Diasporal Cream Doak	cream	colloidal sulfur, 3% • salicylic acid, 2%		isopropyl alcohol in solidified base
Doctar Savage	shampoo			stantar, 2% (equivalent to 0.5% coal tar) • demineralized water • sodium laureth sulfate • TEA-lauryl sulfate • cocamidopropyl betaine • PEG-30 glyceryl stearate • polysorbate 80 • cocamidopropylamine oxide • cocamide DEA • fragrance
Head & Shoulders Dandruff Shampoo Procter & Gamble	shampoo		pyrithione zinc, 1%	shampoo base of anionic surfactants • conditioning ingredients

DANDRUFF AND SEBORRHEA PRODUCTS — continued

Product & Manufacturer	Dosage Form	Keratolytic	Cytostatic Agent	Other Ingredients
Head & Shoulders Intensive Treatment Procter & Gamble	shampoo		selenium sulfide, 1.0%	shampoo base of anionic surfactants • conditioners
Ionil Owen/Galderma	shampoo	salicylic acid, 2%		polyoxyethylene ethers • benzalkonium chloride • alcohol • tetrasodium edetate
Ionil Plus Owen/Galderma	shampoo	salicylic acid, 2%		sodium laureth sulfate • lauramide DEA • quaternium-22 • talloweth-60 • myristyl glycol • laureth-23 • TEA lauryl sulfate • glycol distearate • laureth-4 • TEA abietoyl hydrolyzed collagen • DMDM hydantoin • tetrasodium EDTA • sodium hydroxide • fragrance • FD&C blue#1
Ionil T Owen/Galderma	shampoo			coal tar solution, 5% • benzalkonium chloride, 0.2% • polyoxyethylene ethers • isopropyl alcohol, 4% • alcohol, 12%
Metasep MiLance	shampoo			parachlorometaxylenol, 2% • isopropyl alcohol, 9%
Meted GenDerm	shampoo	sulfur, 3% • salicylic acid, 2%		detergents
Neutrogena T/Gel Neutrogena	shampoo			Neutar, 2% (0.5% coal tar) • coal tar extract, 2%
Neutrogena T/Gel Conditioner Neutrogena	conditioner			Neutar, 2% (0.5% coal tar) • conditioner base
Neutrogena T/Sal Neutrogena	shampoo	salicylic acid, 2%		
P&S Baker Cummins	liquid			phenol • mineral oil • glycerin
P&S Baker Cummins	shampoo	salicylic acid, 2%		
Pentrax GenDerm	shampoo			equivalent to coal tar, 4.3% • detergents • conditioning agent
Pentrax Gold GenDerm	shampoo			equivalent to coal tar, 2% • detergents
Polytar Stiefel	shampoo			polytar, 2.5% • conditioners
Sebaquin Summers	shampoo			clioquinol, 3%
Sebex-T Rugby	shampoo	colloidal sulfur, 2% • salicylic acid, 2%		coal tar solution, 5%
Sebucare Westwood-Squibb	lotion	salicylic acid, 1.8%		laureth-4, 4.5% • alcohol, 61% • PEG-40 • butyl ether • dihydroabietyl alcohol • fragrance

DANDRUFF AND SEBORRHEA PRODUCTS — continued

Product & Manufacturer	Dosage Form	Keratolytic	Cytostatic Agent	Other Ingredients
Sebulex Conditioning With Protein Westwood-Squibb	shampoo	salicylic acid, 2% • sulfur, 2%		sodium octoxynol-3 sulfonate • sodium lauryl sulfate • lauramide DEA • acetaminde MEA • amphoteric-2 • hydrolyzed animal protein • magnesium aluminum silicate • propylene glycol • methylcellulose • PEG-14M • fragrance • disodium EDTA • FD&C blue#1 • D&C yellow#10 • dioctyl sodium sulfosuccinate
Sebulex Medicated Westwood-Squibb	shampoo	sulfur, 2% • salicylic acid, 2%		sodium octoxynol-2 ethane sulfonate • sodium dodecyl benzene sulfonate • PEG-6 lauramide • sodium dioctyl sulfosuccinate • PEG-14M • fragrance • EDTA • FD&C blue#1 • D&C yellow#10
Sebulon Westwood-Squibb	shampoo		pyrithione zinc, 2%	acetamide MEA • benzyl alcohol • cocamide DEA • D&C green#5 • disodium oleamido PEG-2 sulfosuccinate • FD&C green#3 • fragrance • guar gum • magnesium aluminum silicate • TEA lauryl sulfate
Sebutone Westwood-Squibb	shampoo	sulfur, 1.5% • salicylic acid, 1.5%		coal tar, 0.5% • sodium dodecyl benzene sulfonate • sodium octoxynol-2-ethane sulfonate • PEG-6 lauramide • sodium dioctyl sulfosuccinate • titanium dioxide • sodium chloride • PEG-90M • fragrance • lanolin oil • EDTA • FD&C blue#1 • D&C yellow#10
Selenium Sulfide Various Manufacturers	lotion • shampoo		selenium sulfide, 1%	
Selsun Blue Ross	shampoo		selenium sulfide, 1%	surfactants
Selsun Gold for Women Ross	shampoo		selenium sulfide, 1%	surfactants • conditioners
Sulray Alvin Last	cleansing bar	sulfur, 5%		fragrance free natural soap base • aloe vera • trisodium HEDTA
Sulray Alvin Last	cream	sulfur, 3%		sulfurated lime solution • zinc sulfate • water • glyceryl stearate • laureth-23 • PEG-8 stearate • glycerin • silica • parabens
Sulray Alvin Last	shampoo	sulfur, 2%		aloe vera gel • sodium lauryl sulfate • lauramide DEA • glycol stearate • methylparaben • propylparaben • citric acid
Tarsum Summers	shampoo			coal tar solution, 10%

DANDRUFF AND SEBORRHEA PRODUCTS — continued

Product & Manufacturer	Dosage Form	Keratolytic	Cytostatic Agent	Other Ingredients
Tegrin Extra Conditioning Formula Reedco	shampoo			coal tar solution, 7% (equivalent to 1.1% coal tar) • water • sodium lauryl sulfate • ammonium lauryl sulfate • alcohol, 7% • glycol stearate • sodium laureth sulfate • hexylene glycol • lauramide DEA • fragrance • hydroxypropyl methylcellulose • citric acid • guar hydroxypropyltrimonium chloride • methylparaben • propylparaben • FD&C blue#1
Tegrin Fresh Herbal Reedco	shampoo			soal tar solution, 7% • sodium lauryl sulfate • water • alcohol, 6.4% • glycol stearate • sodium laureth sulfate • hexylene glycol • cocamide DEA • fragrance • hydroxypropyl methylcellulose • citric acid • methylparaben • propylparaben • FD&C blue#1
X-Seb Baker Cummins	shampoo		pyrithione zinc, 1%	
X-Seb Plus Baker Cummins	shampoo		pyrithione zinc, 1%	
X-Seb T Baker Cummins	shampoo			coal tar solution, 10% • crude coal tar, 2%
X-Seb T Plus Baker Cummins	shampoo			coal tar solution, 10% • crude coal tar, 2%
ZNP Bar Stiefel	cleansing bar		pyrithione zinc, 2%	
Zetar Rhone-Poulenc Rorer	shampoo			whole colloidal coal tar, 1% • chloroxylenol, 0.5%
Zincon Lederle	shampoo		pyrithione zinc, 1%	surfactants

DIAPER RASH AND PRICKLY HEAT PRODUCTS

Product & Manufacturer	Dosage Form	Protectant	Powdered Agent	Antimicrobial	Other Ingredients
Ammens Medicated Powder Original Fragrance Bristol-Myers	powder	zinc oxide, 9.1%	talc • cornstarch		PPG methyl glucose ether • 8-hydroxyquinoline • 8-hydroxyquinoline sulfate • isostearic acid • fragrance
Ammens Medicated Powder Shower Fresh Scent Bristol-Myers	powder	zinc oxide, 9.1%	talc • cornstarch		fragrance • PPG-20 methyl glucose ether • isostearic acid • fragrance
Bagbalm Dairy	ointment	petrolatum		8-hydroxyquinoline sulfate, 0.3%	lanolin
Borofax Burroughs Wellcome	ointment			boric acid, 5%	lanolin
Calamine Goldline	lotion	zinc oxide, 8%			calamine, 8%
Caldesene Medicated Ointment CIBA Consumer	ointment	white petrolatum • zinc oxide			
Caldesene Medicated Powder CIBA Consumer	powder		talc	calcium undecyclenate, 10%	fragrance
Comfortine Dermik	ointment	zinc oxide, 12%			lanolin • vitamins A & D
DML Forte Person & Covey	cream				petrolatum • PPG-2 • myristyl ether propionate • glyceryl stearate • glycerin • simethicone • benzyl alcohol • silica • EDTA • sodium carbomer 1342
Desitin Pfizer	ointment	zinc oxide, 40%	talc		cod liver oil • petrolatum • lanolin
Diaparene Baby Powder L & F Products	powder		cornstarch		aloe • chamomile • evening primrose
Diaparene Diaper Rash Ointment L & F Products	ointment	zinc oxide			water-repellent base
Dyprotex Blistex	pad	micronized zinc oxide, 40% • dimethicone, 2.5% • petrolatum, 31.1%	zinc stearate		cod liver oil • aloe extract
Flanders Buttocks Ointment Flanders	ointment	zinc oxide			peruvian balsam • castor oil • boric acid, 1.25%
Panthoderm JMI-Canton	lotion				dexpanthenol, 2% • water-miscible base
Plexolan Lanolin Cream Alvin Last	cream	zinc oxide • petrolatum			water • lanolin, 15.5% • mineral oil • ozokerite • PEG-400 distearate • fragrance • methylparaben
Spectro-Jel Recsei	gel			cetylpyridinium chloride, 0.1%	glycol-polysiloxane, 1% • isopropyl alcohol, 5% • methylcellulose, 1.5%
Triple Paste Summers	ointment	white petrolatum, 52%			

External Analgesic Product Table

EXTERNAL ANALGESIC PRODUCTS

Product & Manufacturer	Dosage Form	Counterirritant	Other Ingredients
Absorbine Extra Strength W.F. Young	liquid	menthol, 4%	acetone • chloroxylenol
Absorbine Power Gel W.F. Young	gel	menthol, 4%	SD alcohol 40B
Absorbine, Jr. Liniment W.F. Young	liquid	menthol, 1.27%	acetone • chloroxylenol
Analgesic Balm Various Manufacturers	ointment	methyl salicylate • menthol	
Arthritis Hot Cream Thompson Medical	cream	menthol, 10% • methyl salicylate, 15%	methylparaben • glyceryl monostearate • lanolin • triethanolamine • citric acid • propylene glycol • stearic acid • water
Aspercreme Thompson Medical	cream		trolamine salicylate, 10% • cetyl alcohol • stearic acid • mineral oil • propylparaben • water • methylparaben • glycerin • potassium phosphate monobasic
Aspercreme Lotion Thompson Medical	lotion		trolamine salicylate, 10% • glyceryl monostearate • stearic acid • lanolin • cetyl alcohol • isopropyl palmitate • propylparaben • methylparaben • propylene glycol • sodium lauryl sulfate • potassium phosphate • water • fragrance
Avalgesic Various Manufacturers	lotion	methyl salicylate • menthol • camphor • methyl nicotinate • capsicum oleoresin	dipropylene glycol salicylate • oil of cassia • ginger oleoresin
Banalg Arthritic Pain Reliever Forest	lotion	methyl salicylate, 14% • menthol, 3%	greaseless base
Banalg Muscle Pain Reliever Forest	lotion	menthol, 1% • methyl salicylate, 4.9% • camphor, 2%	greaseless base
Bangesic Various Manufacturers	liniment	methyl salicylate • camphor • menthol • eucalyptus oil	greaseless base
Bee-Balm Ointment Ferndale	ointment	methyl salicylate • menthol	
Ben-Gay Arthritis Extra Strength Rub Pfizer	ointment	methyl salicylate, 30% • menthol, 8%	greaseless nonstaining emulsion base
Ben-Gay Daytime Pain Relieving Gel Pfizer	gel	menthol, 2.5%	hydroalcoholic gel base
Ben-Gay Original Formula Pain Relieving Rub Pfizer	ointment	methyl salicylate, 18.3% • menthol, 16%	oleaginous base
Ben-Gay Regular Strength Pain Relieving Rub Pfizer	cream	methyl salicylate, 15% • menthol, 10%	greaseless nonstaining emulsion base
Ben-Gay Ultra Strength, Pain Relieving Rub Pfizer	cream	methyl salicylate, 30% • menthol, 10% • camphor, 4%	greaseless nonstaining emulsion base
Ben-Gay Vanishing Scent Formula, Sports and Exercise Rub Pfizer	gel	menthol, 3%	smooth opaque light blue gel

EXTERNAL ANALGESIC PRODUCTS — continued

Product & Manufacturer	Dosage Form	Counterirritant	Other Ingredients
Betuline Ferndale	lotion	methyl salicylate • camphor • menthol	peppermint oil • water soluble base
Campho-Phenique Cold Sore Gel Sterling Health	gel	phenol, 4.7% • camphor, 10.8%	light mineral oil
Campho-Phenique Liquid Sterling Health	liquid	phenol, 4.7% • camphor, 10.8%	light mineral oil
Campho-Phenique Triple Antibiotic Plus Pain Reliever Sterling Health	ointment		bacitracin zinc, 500units/g • neomycin sulfate, 5mg/g • polymixin B sulfate, 5000units/g • lidocaine hydrochloride, 40mg/g
Deep-Down BIRA	ns	methyl salicylate, 15% • methyl nicotinate, 0.7% • menthol, 5% • camphor, 0.5%	
Dencorub Alvin Last	cream	methyl salicylate, 15% • camphor, 3.19% • menthol, 1.25%	purified water • stearic acid • beeswax • paraffin • glycol stearate • petrolatum • glycerin • mineral oil • triethanolamine • lanolin • eucalyptus oil • isobornyl acetate
Dencorub Alvin Last	liquid	capsicum oleoresin (as capsaicin, 0.025%)	purified water • quince seed • benzoic acid • disodium EDTA • algin • mullein extract • myrrh extract • valerian
DermaFlex Topical Anesthetic Gel Coating Zila	gel		hydroxypropyl cellulose film-former • lidocaine
Epi-Derm Pedinol	ns	methyl salicylate • menthol	propylene glycol • isopropyl alcohol
Eucalyptamint Muscle Pain Relief CIBA Consumer	cream	menthol, 8%	eucalyptus oil • fragrance • propylene glycol • SD 3A alcohol • triethanolamine • tween 80 • water
Eucalyptamint Ointment CIBA Consumer	ointment	menthol, 15%	lanolin • eucalyptus oil
Exocaine Medicated Rub Del	ns	methyl salicylate, 25%	
Exocaine Plus Rub Del	ns	methyl salicylate, 30%	
Flex-all Pain Relieving Gel Chattem Consumer	gel	menthol, 7% • methyl salicylate	alcohol • allantoin • aloe vera gel • boric acid • carbomer 940 • diazolidinyl urea • eucalyptus oil • glycerin • iodine • methylparaben • peppermint oil • polysorbate 60 • potassium iodide • propylene glycol • propylparaben • thyme oil • triethanolamine • water
Heet Whitehall	liniment	methyl salicylate, 15% • capsicum oleoresin (as capsaicin, 0.025%) • camphor, 3.6%	alcohol, 70% • acetone
Heet Whitehall	spray	methyl salicylate, 25% • menthol, 3% • camphor, 3% • methyl nicotinate, 1%	isopropyl alcohol • isobutane and propane as propellants
Icy Hot Extra Strength Long-Lasting Balm Pain Reliever Chattem Consumer	ointment	methyl salicylate, 29% • menthol, 7.6%	paraffin • white petrolatum

EXTERNAL ANALGESIC PRODUCTS — continued

Product & Manufacturer	Dosage Form	Counterirritant	Other Ingredients
Mentholatum Deep Heating Arthritis Formula Mentholatum	cream	methyl salicylate, 30% • menthol, 8%	glyceryl stearate • sodium lauryl sulfate • isoceteth-20 • poloxamer 407 • quaternium-15 • sorbitan stearate • water
Mentholatum Deep Heating Lotion Mentholatum	lotion	methyl salicylate, 20% • menthol, 6%	carbomer 941 • lanolin oil • mineral oil • polysorbate 60 • sorbitan stearate • trolamine • water
Mentholatum Deep Heating Rub Mentholatum	cream	methyl salicylate, 12.7% • menthol, 5.8%	chloroxylenol • fragrance • glyceryl stearate • sodium lauryl sulfate • lanolin • water
Mentholatum Ointment Mentholatum	ointment	camphor, 9% • natural menthol, 1.3%	fragrance • petrolatum • titanium dioxide
Minit-Rub Bristol-Myers	cream	methyl salicylate, 15% • menthol, 3.5% • camphor, 2.3%	lanolin • calcium benzoate • polysorbate 20 • sodium alginate • sorbitol • methylchloroisothiazoline/methylisothiazoline
Musterole Deep Strength Schering-Plough	ointment	methyl salicylate, 30% • menthol, 3% • methyl nicotinate, 0.5%	
Musterole Regular & Extra Strength Schering-Plough	ointment	camphor, 5% • menthol, 3%	
Myoflex CIBA Consumer	cream		trolamine salicylate, 10% • greaseless base
Panalgesic ECR Pharm.	cream	methyl salicylate, 35% • menthol, 4%	greaseless base
Panalgesic Gold ECR Pharm.	liniment	methyl salicylate, 55% • camphor, 3% • menthol, 1.25%	emollient oils, 19% • alcohol, 22%
Sloan's Liniment C.B. Fleet	liniment	capsaicin, 0.025% (from oleoresin capsicum) • turpentine oil, 47%	
Sportscreme Thompson Medical	cream		triethanolamine salicylate, 10% • cetyl alcohol • FD&C blue#1 • FD&C yellow#5 • fragrance • glycerin • methylparaben • mineral oil • potassium phosphate monobasic • propylparaben • stearic acid • water
Sportscreme Lotion Thompson Medical	lotion		triethanolamine salicylate, 10% • cetyl alcohol • fragrance • glyceryl monostearate • isopropyl palmitate • lanolin anhydrous • methylparaben • potassium phosphate monobasic • propylene glycol • propylparaben • sodium lauryl sulfate • stearic acid • water
Sports Spray Extra Strength Mentholatum	spray	methyl salicylate, 35% • menthol, 10% • camphor, 5%	alcohol, 58% • isobutane
Stimurub Otis Clapp	ointment	menthol • methyl salicylate • capsicum oleoresin	
Therapeutic Mineral Ice Bristol-Myers	gel	menthol, 2.2%	isopropyl alcohol • carbomer • ammonium hydroxide • thymol • magnesium sulfate • sodium hydroxide • cupric sulfate • color
Therapeutic Mineral Ice, Exercise Formula Bristol-Myers	gel	menthol, 4.4%	isopropyl alcohol • carbomer • ammonium hydroxide • fragrance • thymol • magnesium sulfate • sodium hydroxide • cupric sulfate • color

EXTERNAL ANALGESIC PRODUCTS — continued

Product & Manufacturer	Dosage Form	Counterirritant	Other Ingredients
Therapeutic Mineral Ice, Plus Moisturizer Bristol-Myers	gel	menthol, 4.4%	isopropyl alcohol • petrolatum • carbomer • ammonium hydroxide • fragrance • thymol • polysorbate 20 • magnesium sulfate • sodium hydroxide • cupric sulfate • color
Wonder Ice Pedinol	gel	menthol	
Zostrix GenDerm	cream	capsaicin, 0.025%	benzyl alcohol • cetyl alcohol • glyceryl monostearate • isopropyl myristate • polyoxyethylene stearate blend • sorbitol solution • petrolatum • water
Zostrix-HP GenDerm	cream	capsaicin, 0.075%	benzyl alcohol • cetyl alcohol • glyceryl monostearate • isopropyl myristate • polyoxyethylene stearate blend • sorbitol solution • petrolatum • water

BURN AND SUNBURN PRODUCTS

Product & Manufacturer	Dosage Form	Anesthetic	Antimicrobial	Other Ingredients
A and D Schering-Plough	ointment			vitamins A & D • lanolin • petrolatum
Ahhh Sunburn Therapy Tender	gel	lidocaine hydrochloride, 0.5%		aloe vera gel, 95% • fragrance, 0.5%
Ahhh Sunburn Therapy Tender	spray	lidocaine hydrochloride, 0.5%		aloe vera gel, 95% • fragrance, 0.5%
Americaine First Aid Ointment CIBA Consumer	ointment	benzocaine, 20%		benzethonium chloride, 0.1% • PEG 300 • PEG 3350
Americaine Topical Anesthetic Spray CIBA Consumer	aerosol	benzocaine, 20%		butane • isobutane • PEG 200 • propane
Aveeno Bath Treatment Moisturizing Formula Rydelle	powder			colloidal oatmeal, 43% • mineral oil
Aveeno Bath Treatment Soothing Formula Rydelle	powder			colloidal oatmeal, 100%
Benzocaine Various Manufacturers	cream	benzocaine, 5%		
Bicozene External Analgesic Creme Sandoz Pharm.	cream	benzocaine, 6%		resorcinol, 1.67% • castor oil • chlorothymol • ethanolamine stearates • glycerine • glyceryl stearates • parachloromet axylenol • polysorbate 80 • sodium stearate • triglycerol • perfume
Boric Acid Various Manufacturers	ointment			boric acid, 10%
Borofax Burroughs Wellcome	ointment			lanolin • zinc oxide • white petrolatum • mineral oil • perfume
Burntame Otis Clapp	spray	benzocaine, 20%	8-hydroxyquinoline	
Butesin Picrate Abbott	ointment	butamben picrate, 1%		anhydrous lanolin • ceresin wax • mineral oil • mixed triglycerides • parabens • potassium chloride • sodium borate • white wax
Clocream Roberts Pharm.	cream			vitamins A & D
Comfortine Dermik	ointment			vitamins A & D • zinc oxide, 12% • lanolin
DML Forte Person & Covey	cream			petrolatum • PPG-2 • myristyl ether propionate • glyceryl stearate • glycerin • simethicone • benzyl alcohol • silica • EDTA • sodium carbomer 1342
Dermoplast Whitehall	lotion	benzocaine, 8%		menthol, 0.5% • aloe vera oil • carbomer 934P • ceteth-16 • glycerin • glycerol stearate • laneth-16 (lanolin) • methylparaben • oleth-16 • propylparaben • simethicone • steareth-16 • triethanolamine • water

BURN AND SUNBURN PRODUCTS — continued

Product & Manufacturer	Dosage Form	Anesthetic	Antimicrobial	Other Ingredients
Dermoplast Whitehall	spray	benzocaine, 20%		menthol, 0.5% • acetylated lanolin alcohol • aloe vera oil • butane • cetyl acetate • hydrofluorocarbon • methylparaben • PEG-8 laurate • polysorbate 85
Desitin Pfizer	ointment			vitamins A & D • zinc oxide, 40% • talc • lanolin • petrolatum
Dibucaine Various Manufacturers	ointment	dibucaine, 1%		
Family Medic Tender	liquid	lidocaine hydrochloride, 2.5%	benzalkonium chloride, 0.13%	aloe vera gel, 94.88% • fragrance, 0.05%
Family Medic Tender	spray	lidocaine hydrochloride, 2.5%	benzalkonium chloride, 0.13%	aloe vera gel, 94.88% • fragrance, 0.05%
Foille Medicated First Aid Blistex	aerosol	benzocaine, 5%	chloroxylenol, 0.6%	benzyl alcohol
Foille Medicated First Aid Blistex	ointment	benzocaine, 5%	chloroxylenol, 0.1%	
Foille Plus Blistex	aerosol	benzocaine, 5%	chloroxylenol, 0.6%	water-washable base
Foille Plus Blistex	cream	benzocaine, 5%	chloroxylenol, 0.4%	water-washable base
Gordo-Vite E Gordon	cream			vitamin E, 50mg/g
Lagol Alvin Last	ointment	benzocaine, 5%		petrolatum • cornstarch • allantoin
Lanacane Combe	aerosol	benzocaine, 20%	benzethonium chloride, 0.1%	
Medi-Quik First Aid Spray Mentholatum	spray	lidocaine, 2%	benzalkonium chloride, 0.13%	camphor, 0.2% • benzyl alcohol • BHA • isobutane • isopropyl palmitate • methyl gluceth-20 sesquistearate • methyl glucose sesquistearate • phosphoric acid • polyglyceryl-6 distearate • water
Obtundia Otis Clapp	cream		metacresol	
Obtundia Otis Clapp	spray		metacresol-camphor complex	aromatic oils
Panthoderm JMI-Canton	cream			dexpanthenol, 2% • water-miscible base
Pramegel GenDerm	gel	pramoxine hydrochloride, 1% • menthol, 0.5%		benzyl alcohol • carbomer 940 • methyl gluceth-20 • SD alcohol 40 • sodium hydroxide • water
Prax Ferndale	cream	pramoxine hydrochloride, 1%		hydrophilic base
Prax Ferndale	lotion	pramoxine hydrochloride, 1%		hydrophilic base
Solarcaine Schering-Plough	cream	benzocaine	triclosan	menthol • camphor
Solarcaine Schering-Plough	lotion	benzocaine	triclosan	menthol • camphor
Solarcaine Spray Schering-Plough	spray	benzocaine	triclosan	SD alcohol, 35%

BURN AND SUNBURN PRODUCTS — continued

Product & Manufacturer	Dosage Form	Anesthetic	Antimicrobial	Other Ingredients
Tronothane HCl Abbott	cream	pramoxine hydrochloride, 1%		cetyl alcohol • glycerin • sodium lauryl sulfate • methylparaben • propylparaben • cetyl esters • wax
Unguentine Mentholatum	ointment		phenol, 1%	eucalyptus oil • oleostearine • petrolatum • thyme oil • zinc oxide
Unguentine Plus Mentholatum	cream	lidocaine hydrochloride, 2%	chloroxylenol, 2% • phenol, 0.5%	fragrance • glyceryl stearate • isoceteth-20 • isopropyl palmitate • methylparaben • mineral oil • poloxomer 407 • propylparaben • quaternium-15 • sorbitan stearate • tetrasodium EDTA • water
Vitamin E Various Manufacturers	cream			vitamin E
Vitamin E Various Manufacturers	liquid			vitamin E
Vitamin E Various Manufacturers	oil			vitamin E
Vitamins A & D Various Manufacturers	ointment			vitamins A & D
Xylocaine Astra	ointment	lidocaine, 2.5%		polyethylene glycols • propylene glycol
Zinc Oxide Various Manufacturers	ointment			zinc oxide, 20%
Zinc Oxide Various Manufacturers	paste			zinc oxide, 25% • starch, 25%

SUNSCREEN AND SUNTAN PRODUCTS

Product & Manufacturer	SPF Value	Sunscreen Agent	Other Ingredients
405 Solar Cream Doak	15	PABA	titanium dioxide[a]
A-Fil Cream GenDerm	8-15	menthyl anthranilate, 5% • titanium dioxide, 5%	
Aquaderm Sunscreen Moisturizer SPF15 Baker Cummins	15		octyl methoxycinnamate, 7.5% • oxybenzone, 6%
Bain de Soleil All Day Six Hour Waterproof Sunfilter Procter & Gamble	4 • 8	2-ethylhexyl 2-cyano-3, 3-diphenylacrylate • ethylhexyl p-methoxycinnamate • titanium dioxide	water • pvp/eicosene copolymer • isohexadecane • butylene glycol • dimethicone • cyclomethicone • panthenol • triethanolamine • cetyl palmitate • glyceryl tribehenate • stearoxytrimethyl silane • stearyl alcohol • tocopheryl acetate • DEA cetyl phosphate • carbomer • acrylates/C 10-30 • alkyl acrylate crosspolymer • disodium EDTA • DMDM hydantoin • iodopropynyl butyl carbamate
Bain de Soleil All Day Waterproof Sunblock Procter & Gamble	15 • 30	ethylhexyl p-methoxycinnamate • 2-ethylhexyl 2-cyano-3, 3-diphenylacrylate • oxybenzone • titanium dioxide	water • pvp/eicosene copolymer • isohexadecane • butylene glycol • dimethicone • cyclomethicone • panthenol • triethanolamine • cetyl palmitate • glyceryl tribehenate • stearoxytrimethyl silane • stearyl alcohol • tocopheryl acetate • DEA cetyl phosphate • carbomer • acrylates/C 10-30 • alkyl acrylate crosspolymer • disodium EDTA • DMDM hydantoin • iodopropynyl butyl carbamate
Bain de Soleil All Day for Kids Procter & Gamble	30	ethylhexyl p-methoxycinnamate • 2-ethylhexyl 2-cyano-3, 3-diphenylacrylate • oxybenzone • titanium dioxide	water • pvp/eicosene copolymer • isohexadecane • butylene glycol • dimethicone • cyclomethicone • panthenol • triethanolamine • cetyl palmitate • glyceryl tribehenate • stearoxytrimethyl silane • stearyl alcohol • tocopheryl acetate • DEA cetyl phosphate • carbomer • acrylates/C 10-30 • alkyl acrylate crosspolymer • disodium EDTA • DMDM hydantoin • iodopropynyl butyl carbamate
Blistex Lip Balm Blistex	10	padimate O, 6.6% • oxybenzone, 2.5%	dimethicone, 2%
Bull Frog Sunblock Chattem Consumer	18	benzophenone-3-octocrylene • octyl methoxycinnamate	aloe • extract • beeswax • cyclomethicone • fragrance • isostearyl alcohol • panthenol • silica • tocopheryl acetate
Chap Stick Sunblock 15 A.H. Robins	15	padimate O, 7% • oxybenzone, 3%	petrolatum, 44%
Chap-Et Sun Ban 15 Lip Conditioner Stanback	15	padimate O, 7% • oxybenzone, 3%	petrolatum • isopropyl myristate • aloe vera oil • ceresin flavor
Coppertone Schering-Plough	4	ethylhexyl p-methoxycinnamate • oxybenzone	
Coppertone Kids Schering-Plough	15	octyl salicylate • homosalate • oxybenzone	
Coppertone Kids Sunblock Schering-Plough	15	ethylhexyl p-methoxycinnamate • oxybenzone • 2-ethylhexyl salicylate • homosalate	
Coppertone Kids Sunblock Schering-Plough	30	octocrylene • ethylhexyl p-methoxycinnamate • oxybenzone • 2-ethylhexyl salicylate	
Coppertone LipKote Sunblock Lip Balm Schering-Plough	15	ethylhexyl p-methoxycinnamate • oxybenzone	

SUNSCREEN AND SUNTAN PRODUCTS — continued

Product & Manufacturer	SPF Value	Sunscreen Agent	Other Ingredients
Coppertone Moisturizing Sunblock Lotion Schering-Plough	15	ethylhexyl p-methoxycinnamate • oxybenzone	
Coppertone Moisturizing Sunblock Lotion Schering-Plough	45	ethylhexyl p-methoxycinnamate • 2-ethylhexyl salicylate • octocrylene • oxybenzone	
Coppertone Moisturizing Sunscreen Schering-Plough	6 • 8	ethylhexyl p-methoxycinnamate • oxybenzone	
Coppertone Moisturizing Suntan Oil Schering-Plough	2	homosalate	
Coppertone Sport Schering-Plough	4 • 15	ethylhexyl p-methoxycinnamate • oxybenzone	
Coppertone Sunblock Schering-Plough	15	ethylhexyl p-methoxycinnamate • oxybenzone	
Coppertone Sunblock Schering-Plough	25 • 30	ethylhexyl p-methoxycinnamate • oxybenzone • 2-ethylhexyl salicylate • homosalate	
Coppertone Sunblock Schering-Plough	45	ethylhexyl p-methoxycinnamate • oxybenzone • 2-ethylhexyl salicylate	octocrylene[a]
Coppertone Sunless Tanning Extra Moisturizing Lotion[b] Schering-Plough	0		dihydroxyacetone
Coppertone Sunless Tanning Lotion[b] Schering-Plough	0		dihydroxyacetone
Coppertone Sunscreen Schering-Plough	6	ethylhexyl p-methoxycinnamate • oxybenzone	
Coppertone Tan Magnifier Suntan Gel Schering-Plough	4	2-phenylbenzimidazole-5-sulfonic acid	
Coppertone Tan Magnifier Suntan Oil Schering-Plough	2	triethanolamine salicylate	
Curel Everyday Sun Protection Lotion S.C. Johnson Wax	8	octyl methoxycinnamate • oxybenzone	glycerin • petrolatum • dimethicone • dodecyl-pentadecyl benzoate esters
Daily Conditioning Treatment For Lips (DCT) Blistex	15	padimate O, 7.5% • oxybenzone, 3.5%	petrolatum • cetyl alcohol • aloe vera • cocoa butter • vitamin E • vitamin A
Dermsol-30 Parnell	30	ethylhexyl p-methoxycinnamate, 7.5% • oxybenzone, 6.0% • 2-ethylhexyl salicylate, 5.0%	octyldodecyl neopentanoate • glycerin • TEA stearate • DEA cetyl phosphate • ceteth-25 • cetyl alcohol • laneth-25 • oleth-25 • steareth-25 • diazolidinyl urea • methylparaben • propylparaben • yerba santa • hyaluronic acid • hydrolyzed collagen • sodium PCA • carbomer
Faces Only Clear Sunscreen by Coppertone Schering-Plough	6	ethylhexyl p-methoxycinnamate • oxybenzone	
Faces Only Moisturizing Sunblock by Coppertone Schering-Plough	15	ethylhexyl p-methoxycinnamate • oxybenzone	

SUNSCREEN AND SUNTAN PRODUCTS — continued

Product & Manufacturer	SPF Value	Sunscreen Agent	Other Ingredients
Formula 405 Solar Lotion Doak	8	octyl methoxycinnamate • DEA methyloxycinnamate	
Formula 405 Solar Lotion Doak	15	octyl dimethyl PABA • benzophenone-3	
Hawaiian Tropic 15 Plus Sunblock Tanning Research	15	2-ethylhexyl p-methoxycinnamate • oxybenzone • menthyl anthranilate	
Hawaiian Tropic 30 Plus Sunblock Tanning Research	30	homosalate • octyl methoxycinnamate • benzophenone-3 • menthyl anthranilate • octyl salicylate	
Hawaiian Tropic Baby Faces Sunblock Tanning Research	25	2-ethylhexyl p-methoxycinnamate • oxybenzone • menthyl anthranilate • octyl salicylate	
Hawaiian Tropic Dark Tanning With Sunscreen Tanning Research	4	2-ethylhexyl p-methoxycinnamate • menthyl anthranilate	
Maxafil GenDerm	ns	menthyl anthranilate, 5% • cinoxate, 4%	
Mentholatum Lipbalm Mentholatum	14.7	padimate O, 8%	petrolatum, 18% • camphor • fragrance • lanolin • menthol • mineral oil • ozokerite
Neutrogena Chemical-Free Sunblocker SPF 17 Neutrogena	17	titanium dioxide	
Neutrogena Moisture Neutrogena	5	octyl methoxycinnamate	
Neutrogena Sunblock Neutrogena	15	octyl methoxycinnamate • octyl salicylate • menthyl anthranilate	
Neutrogena Sunblock Neutrogena	30	octocrylene • octyl methoxycinnamate • menthyl anthranilate	
Neutrogena Sunblock Neutrogena	8	octyl methoxycinnamate • menthyl anthranilate	
Neutrogena Sunblock Stick Neutrogena	25	octyl methoxycinnamate • benzophenone-3 • octyl salicylate	
Photoplex Broad Spectrum Sunscreen Lotion Allergan Herbert	15	avobenzone, 3% • padimate O, 7%	benzyl alcohol • carbomer 934P • cetyl esters wax • edetate disodium • glycerin • imidurea • light mineral oil • oleth-3 phosphate • purified water • stearyl alcohol • ceteareth-20 • white petrolatum • may contain sodium hydroxide or hydrochloric acid to adjust pH
PreSun 15 Moisturizing Bristol-Myers	15	octyl dimethyl PABA • benzophenone-3	carbomer 940 • cetyl alcohol • DEA cetyl phosphate • diazolidinyl urea • dimethicone • isopropyl myristate • isodecyl neopentantoate • kathon CG • PG dioctanoate • pvp/eicosene copolymer • stearic acid • petrolatum • triethanolamine • fragrance
PreSun 15 Sensitive Skin Bristol-Myers	15	octyl methoxycinnamate • benzophenone-3 • octyl salicylate	carbomer 940 • cetyl alcohol • DEA cetyl phosphate • diazolidinyl urea • dimethicone • isopropyl myristate • isodecyl neopentantoate • kathon CG • PG dioctanoate • pvp/eicosene copolymer • stearic acid • triethanolamine

SUNSCREEN AND SUNTAN PRODUCTS — continued

Product & Manufacturer	SPF Value	Sunscreen Agent	Other Ingredients
PreSun 29 Sensitive Skin Bristol-Myers	29	octyl methoxycinnamate • oxybenzone • octyl salicylate	carbomer 940 • cetyl alcohol • DEA cetyl phosphate • diazolidinyl urea • dimethicone • isopropyl myristate • isodecyl neopentantoate • kathon CG • PG dioctanoate • pvp/eicosene copolymer • stearic acid • triethanolamine
PreSun 15 Sunscreen Bristol-Myers	15	octyl dimethyl PABA • benzophenone-3 • octyl salicylate	cyclomethicone • SD alcohol • C12-15 alcohol benzoates • PG dioctanoate • pvp/hexadecene copolymer • dimethicone
PreSun 23 Bristol-Myers	23	octyl dimethyl PABA • octyl methoxycinnamate • benzophenone-3 • octyl salicylate	cyclomethicone • SD alcohol • C12-15 alcohol benzoate • PG dioctanoate • pvp/hexadecene copolymer
PreSun 25 Moisturizing Bristol-Myers	25	octyl methoxycinnamate • benzophenone-3 • octyl salicylate	• dimethicone • diazolidinyl urea • carbomer 940 • triethanolamine • kathon CG • petrolatum • ispropyl myristate • PG dioctanoate • isodecyl neopentanoate • DEA cetyl phosphate • pvp/eicosene copolymer • stearic acid • cetyl alcohol
PreSun for Kids Bristol-Myers	29	octyl methoxycinnamate • octyl salicylate • benzophenone-3	carbomer 940 • cetyl alcohol • DEA cetyl phosphate • diazolidinyl urea • dimethicone • isopropyl myristate • isodecyl neopentantoate • • kathon CG • PG dioctanoate • pvp/eicosene • stearic acid • triethanolamine
PreSun for Kids Bristol-Myers	23	octyl dimethyl PABA • octyl methoxycinnamate • benzophenone-3 • octyl salicylate	cyclomethicone • SD alcohol • C12-15 alcohol benzoate • PG dioctanoate • pvp/hexadecene copolymer
PreSun 15 Active Bristol-Myers	15	benzophenone-3 • octyl methoxycinnamate • octyl salicylate	SD alcohol • PPG-15 stearyl ether • acrylates/t-octylpropenamide • hydroxypropylcellulose
Q.T. Quick Tanning Suntan by Coppertone Schering-Plough	2	ethylhexyl p-methoxycinnamate	dihydroxyacetone
Shade Sunblock Stick Schering-Plough	30	ethylhexyl p-methoxycinnamate • 2-ethylhexyl salicylate • oxybenzone • homosalate	
Shade Sunblock Schering-Plough	45	ethylhexyl p-methoxycinnamate • 2-ethylhexyl salicylate • oxybenzone • octocrylene	
Shade Sunblock Lotion Schering-Plough	30	ethylhexyl p-methoxycinnamate • 2-ethylhexyl salicylate • oxybenzone • homosalate	
Shade Sunblock Oil-Free Schering-Plough	15	ethylhexyl p-methoxycinnamate • octyl salicylate • oxybenzone	SD alcohol 40, 75%v/v
Shade Sunblock Oil-Free Schering-Plough	25	ethylhexyl p-methoxycinnamate • octyl salicylate • homosalate • oxybenzone	SD alcohol 40, 74%v/v
Shade UVAGuard Schering-Plough	15	octyl methoxycinnamate, 7.5% • avobenzone, 3% • oxybenzone, 3%	
Softsense Skin Essentials Everyday UV Protectant S.C. Johnson Wax	8	octyl methoxycinnamate • oxybenzone	glycerin • petrolatum • C12-15 alkyl benzoates • vitamin E • dimethicone
Solbar PF 15 Person & Covey	15	octyl methoxycinnamate, 7.5% • oxybenzone, 5%	

SUNSCREEN AND SUNTAN PRODUCTS — continued

Product & Manufacturer	SPF Value	Sunscreen Agent	Other Ingredients
Solbar PF Cream PABA Free Waterproof Person & Covey	50	octyl methoxycinnamate • oxybenzone	octocrylene[a]
Solbar PF Liquid PABA Free Person & Covey	15	octyl methoxycinnamate, 7.5% • oxybenzone, 6%	SD alcohol 40, 76%
Solbar Plus 15 Person & Covey	15	octyl dimethyl PABA, 6% • oxybenzone, 4% • dioxybenzone, 2%	
Stay Moist Moisturizing Lip Conditioner Stanback	15	padimate O, 7% • oxybenzone, 3%	petrolatum • ispropryl myristate • aloe vera oil • wax • flavor
Sundown Sunblock Johnson & Johnson Cons.	15	octyl methoxycinnamate • octyl salicylate • oxybenzone • titanium dioxide	BHT • C12-15 alcohol benzoate • carbomer • cetyl alcohol • DEA cetyl phosphate • dimethicone • dioctyl sodium sulfosuccinate • disodium EDTA • fragrance • glyceryl dilaurate • isopropyl isostearate • isopropyl PPG-2-isodecth-7 carboxylate • isostearic acid • propylene glycol • quaternium-15 • simethicone • tocopheryl acetate • water
Tropical Blend Dark Tanning Lotion Schering-Plough	4	ethylhexyl p-methoxycinnamate • oxybenzone	
Tropical Blend Dark Tanning Oil Schering-Plough	2	homosalate	
Tropical Blend Dark Tanning Oil Schering-Plough	4	padimate O • oxybenzone	
Tropical Blend Dry Oil Schering-Plough	2	homosalate	
Tropical Blend Sunless Tanning Clear Gel[b] Schering-Plough	0		dihydroxyacetone
Tropical Blend Tan Magnifier Schering-Plough	2	triethanolamine salicylate	
Tropical Tan Magnifier Schering-Plough	4	triethanolamine salicylate	
Water Babies Little Licks Sunblock Lip Balm by Coppertone Schering-Plough	30	ethylhexyl p-methoxycinnamate • oxybenzone • 2-ethylhexyl salicylate	
Water Babies SPF-15 Sunblock Schering-Plough	15	ethylhexyl p-methoxycinnamate • oxybenzone	
Water Babies SPF-30 Sunblock Schering-Plough	30	ethylhexyl p-methoxycinnamate • 2-ethylhexyl salicylate • oxybenzone • homosalate	
Water Babies SPF-45 Sunblock Schering-Plough	45	ethylhexyl p-methoxycinnamate • 2-ethylhexyl salicylate • oxybenzone • octocrylene	

[a] Also a sunscreen agent.
[b] "Sunless" tanning products; do not contain a sunscreen agent.

POISON IVY AND POISON OAK PRODUCTS

Product & Manufacturer	Dosage Form	Hydro-cortisone	Anesthetic	Antipruritic/ Antihistamine	Astringent	Other Ingredients
Aveeno Anti-Itch Cream & Lotion S.C. Johnson Wax	cream • lotion		pramoxine hydrochloride, 1%	camphor, 0.3%	calamine, 3%	glycerin • distearyldimonium chloride • petrolatum • oatmeal flour • isopropyl palmitate • 1-hexadecanol • dimethicone • sodium chloride
Aveeno Bath Treatment Moisturizing Formula Rydelle	powder					colloidal oatmeal, 43% • mineral oil • calcium silicate • laureth-4
Aveeno Bath Treatment Soothing Formula Rydelle	powder					colloidal oatmeal, 100%
Aveeno Moisturizing Cream & Lotion S.C. Johnson Wax	cream • lotion					colloidal oatmeal, 1% • glycerin • distearyldimonium chloride • petrolatum • isopropyl palmitate • cetyl alcohol • dimethicone • sodium chloride • benzyl alcohol
Benadryl Maximum Strength Anti-Itch Cream Parke-Davis	cream			diphenhydramine hydrochloride, 2%		zinc acetate, 0.1% • aloe vera • cetyl alcohol • dimidazole urea • methylparaben • polyethylene glycol monostearate 1000 • propylene glycol • propylparaben • purified water
Benadryl Maximum Strength Anti-Itch Spray Parke-Davis	spray			diphenhydramine hydrochloride, 2%		zinc acetate, 0.1% • alcohol, 71.3% • aloe vera • glycerin • povidone • tromethamine • purified water
Bluboro Allergan Herbert	powder					aluminum sulfate, 53.9% • calcium acetate, 43% • boric acid • blue #1
Caladryl Parke-Davis	lotion		pramoxine hydrochloride, 1%		calamine, 8%	propylene glycol • polysorbate 80 • alcohol, 2.2% • xanthan gum • hydroxypropyl methyl cellulose • preservative • camphor • fragrance
Caladryl Parke-Davis	spray			diphenhydramine hydrochloride, 1%	calamine, 8%	fragrance • camphor • alcohol

POISON IVY AND POISON OAK PRODUCTS — continued

Product & Manufacturer	Dosage Form	Hydro-cortisone	Anesthetic	Antipruritic/ Antihistamine	Astringent	Other Ingredients
Caladryl Clear Parke-Davis	lotion		pramoxine hydrochloride, 1%			alcohol, 2% • zinc acetate, 0.1% • sodium polysorbate • glycerin • methocel • fragrance • preservative • camphor • sodium citrate • citric acid
Calamine, Regular & Phenolated Various Manufacturers	lotion				calamine, 8% • zinc oxide, 8%	phenol, 1% (phenolate) • glycerin, 2% • bentonite magma • calcium hydroxide solution
CaldeCort CIBA Consumer	cream	1%				isopropyl myristate • methylparaben • polysorbate 60 • propylparaben • purified water • sorbitan monostearate • sorbitol solution • stearic acid
CaldeCort Light With Aloe CIBA Consumer	cream	0.5%				aloe vera gel • isopropyl myristate • methylparaben • polysorbate 60 • propylparaben • sorbitan monostearate • sorbitol solution • stearic acid • water
Cortaid Upjohn	lotion	0.5%				vanishing, greaseless base • parabens
Cortaid Upjohn	spray	0.5%			alcohol, 46%	glycerin • methylparaben • purified water
Cortaid with Aloe Upjohn	cream	0.5%				vanishing, greaseless base • aloe • parabens
Cortaid, Maximum Strength Upjohn	cream	1%				butylparaben • cetyl alcohol • glycerin • methylparaben • sodium lauryl sulfate • stearic acid • stearyl alcohol • purified water • white petrolatum
Cortaid, Maximum Strength Upjohn	ointment	1%				butylparaben • cholesterol • methylparaben • microcrystalline wax • mineral oil • white petrolatum

POISON IVY AND POISON OAK PRODUCTS — continued

Product & Manufacturer	Dosage Form	Hydro-cortisone	Anesthetic	Antipruritic/ Antihistamine	Astringent	Other Ingredients
Cortizone-10 Cream Thompson Medical	cream	1%				aluminum sulfate • calcium acetate • cetyl alcohol • glycerin • light mineral oil • methylparaben • propylparaben • potato dextrin • sodium lauryl sulfate • water • white petrolatum • white wax
Cortizone-5 & -10 Ointment Thompson Medical	ointment	0.5% • 1%				white petrolatum
Cortizone-5 Cream Thompson Medical	cream	0.5%				glycerin • mineral oil • white petrolatum • propylparaben • methylparaben • aluminum sulfate • calcium acetate • cetyl alcohol • potato dextrin • sodium lauryl sulfate • water • white wax
Cortizone-5 Cream For Kids Thompson Medical	cream	0.5%				aluminum sulfate • calcium acetate • cetyl alcohol • glycerin • light mineral oil • methylparaben • propylparaben • potato dextrin • sodium lauryl sulfate • water • white petrolatum • white wax • aloe
DermaFlex Topical Anesthetic Gel Coating Zila	gel		lidocaine		alcohol	hydroxypropyl cellulose film-former
Dermacort Solvay	cream	1%				benzyl • alcohol
Dermapax Recsei	spray			diphenhydramine hydrochloride, 0.5%		chlorobutanol, 1% • benzyl alcohol, 1% • isopropyl alcohol, 35%
Di-Delamine Del	gel • spray			tripelennamine hydrochloride, 0.5% • diphenhydramine hydrochloride, 1% • benzalkonium chloride, 0.12%		menthol, 0.1%

POISON IVY AND POISON OAK PRODUCTS — continued

Product & Manufacturer	Dosage Form	Hydro-cortisone	Anesthetic	Antipruritic/ Antihistamine	Astringent	Other Ingredients
FoilleCort Blistex	cream	0.5%				BHA • carbomer 934 • cetyl alcohol • fragrance • ispropyl palmitate • isopropyl myristate • ispropyl stearate • methylparaben • mineral oil • polysorbate 60 • propylparaben • purified water • stearic acid • sorbitan tristearate • triethanolamine
HC-DermaPax Recsei	spray	0.5%		diphenhydramine hydrochloride, 0.5%		benzyl alcohol, 1% isopropanol, 35%
Hydrocortisone Various Manufacturers	lotion • cream	0.25% • 0.05% • 1%				
Hytone Rhone-Poulenc Rorer	cream	1%				water washable base
Hytone Rhone-Poulenc Rorer	ointment	1%				emollient • mineral oil • white petrolatum base
Ivarest Blistex	cream		benzocaine, 5%	diphenhydramine hydrochloride, 2%	calamine, 14%	benzethonium chloride, 0.15% • hydroxyethylcellulose • lanolin oil • petrolatum • polysorbate 60 • propylene glycol • sorbitan stearate • fragrance • purified water • petrolatum • lanolin • alcohol • color
Ivarest Blistex	lotion		benzocaine, 5%		calamine, 14%	hydroxyethylcellulose • lanolin oil • petrolatum • polysorbate 60 • propylene glycol • sorbitan stearate • fragrance • purified water • mineral oil • lanolin • alcohol • color • chloroxylenol
Ivy Dry Cream Ivy Corp.	cream		benzocaine, 5mg/g • benzyl alcohol, 0.1ml/g	menthol, 4mg/g • camphor, 6mg/g	tannic acid, 80mg/g • zinc acetate, 20mg/g	methylparaben, 2.5mg/g • propylparaben, 0.3mg/g • isopropyl alcohol, 7.5% • cream base
Ivy Dry Liquid Ivy Corp.	liquid				tannic acid, 100mg/ml • zinc acetate, 20mg/ml	isopropyl alcohol, 12.5% • isopropyl alcohol, 12.5% • glycerin • acetic acid • parabens

POISON IVY AND POISON OAK PRODUCTS — continued

Product & Manufacturer	Dosage Form	Hydro-cortisone	Anesthetic	Antipruritic/ Antihistamine	Astringent	Other Ingredients
Ivy Super Dry Ivy Corp.	liquid		benzocaine, 5mg/ml	menthol, 2mg/ml • camphor, 4mg/ml	tannic acid, 100mg/ml • zinc acetate, 20mg/ml	benzyl alcohol, 0.1ml/ml • isopropyl alcohol, 35% • methylparaben, 0.01mg/ml • propylparaben, 0.1mg/ml • camphor • menthol • acetic acid
Ivy-Chex JMI-Canton	spray			methyl salicylate		benzalkonium chloride • SD alcohol, 89.5% • polyvinyl-pyrrolidone-vinylacetate copolymers
Kericort HC Cream 1% Bristol-Myers	cream	1%				citric acid, anhydrous • sodium citrate • methylparaben • sorbic acid • polyoxyl 40 stearate • glyceryl stearate • white wax • stearyl alcohol • isopropyl myristate • cetyl alcohol • sorbitan monostearate • polysorbate 60 • propylparaben • propylene glycol
Lanacane Combe	spray		benzocaine, 20%			benzethonium chloride
Lanacane Creme Combe	cream		benzocaine, 6%			benzethonium chloride
Lanacort 10 Combe	cream • ointment	1%				
Lanacort 5 Combe	cream	0.5%				aloe • parabens
Lanacort 5 Combe	ointment	0.5%				lanolin alcohols • aloe • petrolatum
Obtundia Calamine Cream Otis Clapp	cream				calamine • zinc oxide	cresol-camphor complex
PrameGel GenDerm	liquid		pramoxine hydrochloride, 1%	menthol, 0.5%		benzyl alcohol • carbomer 940 • methyl gluceth-20 • SD alcohol 40 • sodium hydroxide • water
Rhuli Cream S.C. Johnson Wax	cream		pramoxine hydrochloride, 1%	camphor, 0.3%	calamine, 3%	glycerin • distearyldimonium chloride • petrolatum • isopropyl palmitate • cetyl alcohol • dimethicone • sodium chloride

POISON IVY AND POISON OAK PRODUCTS — continued

Product & Manufacturer	Dosage Form	Hydro-cortisone	Anesthetic	Antipruritic/ Antihistamine	Astringent	Other Ingredients
Rhuli Gel S.C. Johnson Wax	gel			menthol, 0.3% • camphor, 0.3% • benzyl alcohol, 2%		SD alcohol, 23A, 31% • propylene glycol • carbomer 940 • triethanolamine • benzophenone-4 • EDTA
Rhuli Spray S.C. Johnson Wax	spray		benzocaine, 5%	camphor, 0.7%	calamine, 13.8%	benzyl alcohol • hydrated silica • isobutane • isopropyl alcohol, 70% • oleyl alcohol • sorbitan trioleate
Tronothane Hydrochloride Abbott	cream		pramoxine hydrochloride, 1%			cetyl alcohol • cetyl esters wax • glycerin • sodium lauryl sulfate • methylparaben • propylparaben
Vagisil Combe	cream		benzocaine, 5%	resorcinol, 2%		

INSECT STING AND BITE PRODUCTS

Product[a] & Manufacturer	Dosage Form	Primary Ingredients	Other Ingredients
After-Bite Tender	liquid • wipe	ammonium hydroxide, 3.6%	
Americaine First Aid Ointment CIBA Consumer	ointment	benzocaine, 20%	benzethonium chloride, PEG-300 • PEG-3350
Americaine Topical Anesthetic Spray CIBA Consumer	aerosol	benzocaine, 20%	butane • isobutane • PEG-200 • propane
Aveeno Anti-Itch Cream S.C. Johnson Wax	cream • lotion	pramoxine hydrochloride, 1% • calamine, 3% • camphor, 0.3%	glycerin • distearyldimonium chloride • petrolatum • oatmeal flour • isopropyl palmitate • 1-hexadecanol • dimethicone • sodium chloride
Bicozene External Analgesic Creme Sandoz Pharm.	cream	benzocaine, 6% • resorcinol, 1.67%	castor oil • chlorothymol • ethanolamine stearates • glycerine • glyceryl stearate • parachlorometaxylenol • polysorbate 80 • sodium stearate • triglycerol di-isostearate • perfume
Bluboro Allergan Herbert	powder		aluminum sulfate, 53.9% • calcium acetate, 43% • boric acid • blue #1
Caladryl Parke-Davis	spray	diphenhydramine hydrochloride, 1% • calamine, 8%	fragrance • camphor • alcohol
Chiggerex Scherer	ointment	benzocaine, 2%	camphor, 0.008% • olive oil, 0.008% • menthol, 0.005% • peppermint oil, 0.005% • methylparaben, 0.002% • clove oil, 0.002% • pegosperse 100, 12%
Chiggertox Scherer	liquid	isopropyl alcohol, 53% • benzocaine, 2.1%	benzyl benzoate, 21.4% • soft soap, 21.4%
Cortaid, Maximum Strength Upjohn	cream	hydrocortisone acetate (equivalent to hydrocortisone), 10mg (1%)	butylparaben • cetyl alcohol • glycerin • methylparaben • sodium lauryl sulfate • stearate acid • stearyl alcohol • purified water • white petrolatum
Cortaid, Maximum Strength Upjohn	ointment	hydrocortisone acetate (equivalent to hydrocortisone), 10mg (1%)	butylparaben • cholesterol • methylparaben • microcrystalline wax • mineral oil • white petrolatum
DermaFlex Topical Anesthetic Gel Coating Zila	gel	lidocaine	hydroxypropylcellulose film-former
Dermoplast Whitehall	lotion	benzocaine, 8% • menthol, 0.5%	aloe vera gel • carbomer 934P • ceteth-16 • glycerin • glyceryl stearate • laneth-16 (lanolin) • oleth-16 • methylparaben • propylparaben • simethicone • steareth-16 • triethanolamine • water
Dermoplast Whitehall	spray	benzocaine, 20% • menthol, 0.5%	acetylated lanolin alcohol • aloe vera oil • butane • cetyl acetate • hydrofluorocarbon • PEG-8 laurate • polysorbate 85 • methylparaben
Di-Delamine Double Antihistamine Del	gel • spray	tripelannamine hydrochloride, 0.5% • diphenhydramine hydrochloride, 1% • benzalkonium chloride, 0.12%	menthol, 0.1%
HC-DermaPax Recsei	spray	hydrocortisone, 0.5% • diphenhydramine hydrochloride, 0.5%	isopropanol, 35% • propylene glycol, 13% • benzyl alcohol, 1% • cetyl pyridinium chloride, 0.07%
Hydrocortisone Various Manufacturers	cream	hydrocortisone, 0.25%; 0.5%; 1%	
Hydrocortisone Cream 0.5% Goldline	cream	hydrocortisone, 0.5%	

INSECT STING AND BITE PRODUCTS — continued

Product[a] & Manufacturer	Dosage Form	Primary Ingredients	Other Ingredients
Hydrocortisone Maximum Strength Cream 1% Goldline	cream	hydrocortisone, 1%	
Itch-X B.F. Ascher	gel	benzyl alcohol, 10% • pramoxine hydrochloride, 1%	aloe vera gel
Kericort HC Cream 1% Bristol-Myers	cream	hydrocortisone, 1%	citric acid • anhydrous • sodium citrate • methylparaben • sorbic acid • polyoxyl 40 stearate • glyceryl stearate • white wax • stearyl alcohol • isopropyl myristate • cetyl alcohol • sorbitan monostearate • polysorbate 60 • propylparaben • propylene glycol
Lanacort 10 Combe	cream	hydrocortisone, 1%	
Lanacort 10 Combe	ointment	hydrocortisone, 1%	
Nupercainal CIBA Consumer	cream	dibucaine, 0.5%	acetone sodium bisulfite • glycerin • potassium hydroxide • stearic acid • fragrance • trolamine
Nupercainal CIBA Consumer	ointment	dibucaine, 1%	acetone sodium bisulfite • lanolin • light mineral oil • white petrolatum
Obtundia First Aid Otis Clapp	cream	metacresol-camphor complex	
Obtundia Surgical Dressing Otis Clapp	spray	metacresol-camphor complex	
PrameGel GenDerm	liquid	pramoxine hydrochloride, 1% • menthol, 0.5%	benzyl alcohol • carbomer 940 • methyl gluceth-20 • SD alcohol 40 • sodium hydroxide • water
Preparation H Hydrocortisone 1% Anti-Itch Cream Whitehall	cream	hydrocortisone, 1%	
Rhuli Cream S.C. Johnson Wax	cream	calamine, 3% • camphor, 0.3% • pramoxine hydrochloride, 1%	glycerin • distearyldimonium chloride • petrolatum • isopropyl palmitate • cetyl alcohol • dimethicone • sodium chloride
Rhuli Gel Rydelle	gel	benzyl alcohol, 2% • menthol, 0.3% • camphor, 0.3%	SD alcohol 23A, 31% • propylene glycol • carbomer 940 • triethanolamine • benzophenone-4 • EDTA
Rhuli Spray S.C. Johnson Wax	spray	calamine, 13.8% • benzocaine, 5% • camphor, 0.7%	benzyl alcohol • hydrated silica • isobutane • isopropyl alcohol, 70% (concentrate) • oleyl alcohol • sorbitan trioleate
Solarcaine Schering-Plough	aerosol	benzocaine, 20% • triclosan, 0.13%	isobutane SD alcohol 40, 35% w/w
Solarcaine Schering-Plough	cream	benzocaine • triclosan	
Solarcaine Schering-Plough	lotion	benzocaine • triclosan	
Xylocaine Astra	ointment	lidocaine, 2.5%	polyethylene glycols • propylene glycol

[a] See Poison Ivy and Poison Oak Product Table, Chapter 35, for additional hydrocortisone products.

PEDICULICIDE PRODUCTS

Product & Manufacturer	Dosage Form	Active Ingredients	Other Ingredients
A-200 Lice Control Spray SmithKline Beecham	spray	resmethrin, 0.500% • related compounds, 0.068%	
A-200 Pyrinate SmithKline Beecham	gel	pyrethrins, 0.33% • piperonyl butoxide, 4%	carbomer 940 • triisopropanolamine
A-200 Pyrinate SmithKline Beecham	shampoo	pyrethrins, 0.30% • piperonyl butoxide, 3%	benzyl alcohol • butyl stearate • mineral spirits • octoxynol 9 • oleic acid • oleoresin • parsley seed • petroleum distillate
Barc Del	liquid	pyrethrins, 0.18% • piperonyl butoxide, 2.2%	petroleum distillate, 5.52%
End-Lice Thompson Medical	liquid	pyrethrins, 0.3% • piperonyl butoxide, 3%	inert
Lice Treatment Goldline	liquid	pyrethrins, 0.3% • piperonyl butoxide technical, 3%	petroleum distillate
Lice-Enz Copley	foam	pyrethrins, 0.3% • piperonyl butoxide, 3%	
Licide Control Reese Chemical	spray	pyrethrins, 0.20% • piperonyl butoxide technical, 1%	inert, 98.8%
Licide Shampoo Reese Chemical	shampoo	pyrethrins, 0.3% • piperonyl butoxide technical, 3%	benzyl alcohol, 94.3%
Nix Burroughs Wellcome	cream rinse	permethrin, 1%	balsam canada • cetyl alcohol • citric acid • FD&C yellow#6 • fragrance • hydrolyzed animal protein • hydroxyethylcellulose • polyoxyethylene 10 cetyl ether • propylene glycol • stearalkonium chloride • isopropyl alcohol • methylparaben • propylparaben • imidiazolidinyl urea
Pronto Del	shampoo	pyrethrins, 0.33% • piperonyl butoxide, 4%	
R&C Shampoo Reed & Carnrick	shampoo	pyrethrins, 0.3% • piperonyl butoxide technical, 3%	C-13-14 isoparaffin • fragrance • isocetyl alcohol • isopropyl alcohol • lauramine oxide • laureth-4 • laureth-23 • petroleum distillate • TEA-lauryl sulfate • water
R&C Spray Reed & Carnrick	spray	3-phenoxybenzyl-2-2-dimethyl-3-cyclopropane carboxylate	inert, 99.6%
RID Pfizer	shampoo	pyrethrins, 0.33% • piperonyl butoxide, 4%	C13-C14 isoparaffin • fragrance • isopropyl alcohol • PEG-25 hydrogenated castor oil • water • xanthan gum
Triple X Carter-Wallace	shampoo	pyrethrins, 0.3% • piperonyl butoxide, 3%	petroleum distillate, 1.2% • benzyl alcohol, 2.4%

INSECT REPELLENT PRODUCTS

Product & Manufacturer	Dosage Form	Ingredients
Ben's Backyard Tender	lotion • pump	deet, 23%
Ben's Max Tender	lotion • pump	deet, 95%
Cutter Insect Repellent Miles Incorporated	aerosol	n-n-diethyl-m-toluamide, 21.85% • other isomers, 1.75% • inert ingredients, 77%
Muskol Maximum Strength Schering-Plough	pump	n-n-diethy-m-toluamide, 100%
Muskol Ultra Schering-Plough	aerosol	n-n-diethy-m-toluamide, 38% • other isomers, 2% • inert ingredients, 60%
Natrapel Tender	lotion	citronella oil, 10% • aloe vera gel, 89%
Natrapel Tender	pump	citronella oil, 10% • aloe vera gel, 89%
Off Deep Woods Formula S.C. Johnson Wax	aerosol	n-n-diethyl-meta-toluamide, 28.5% • other isomers, 1.5% • inert ingredients, 70%
Off Skintastic Insect Repellent S.C. Johnson Wax	lotion	n-n-diethyl-meta-toluamide, 7.125% • other isomers, 0.375% • inert ingredients, 92.5%
Off Spring Fresh S.C. Johnson Wax	aerosol	n-n-diethyl-m-toluamide, 14.25% • other isomers, 0.75% • inert ingredients, 85%

CALLUS, CORN, WART PRODUCTS

Product & Manufacturer	Dosage Form	Active Ingredients	Other Ingredients
Clear Away Plantar Wart Remover System Schering-Plough	disc	salicylic acid, 40%	
Clear Away Wart Remover System Schering-Plough	disc	salicylic acid, 40%	
Compound W Gel Wart Remover Whitehall	gel	salicylic acid, 17%	alcohol, 67.5% • camphor • castor oil • collodion • colloidal silicon dioxide • hydroxypropyl cellulose • hypophosphorous acid • polysorbate 80
Compound W Liquid Wart Remover Whitehall	liquid	salicylic acid, 17%	ether, 63.5% • alcohol, 21.2% • camphor • castor oil • collodion • ethylcellulose • hypophosphorous acid • menthol • polysorbate 80
Corn Fix Alvin Last	liquid	salicylic acid, 12%	collodion • alcohol, 33% • ether, 65.5%
Dr. Scholl's Callus Removers Schering-Plough	disc	salicylic acid, 40%	
Dr. Scholl's Corn Removers Schering-Plough	disc	salicylic acid, 40%	
Dr. Scholl's Ingrown Toenail Reliever Schering-Plough	liquid	tannic acid, 25% • chlorobutanol, 5%	isopropyl alcohol, 67%
Dr. Scholl's Liquid Corn Remover Schering-Plough	liquid	salicylic acid, 12.6% w/w	alcohol, 18% • ether, 55%
Dr. Scholl's Wart Remover Kit Schering-Plough	liquid	salicylic acid, 17% w/w	ether, 52% • alcohol, 17%
Dr. Scholl's Waterproof Corn Removers Schering-Plough	disc • pad	salicylic acid, 40% (disc)	
DuoFilm Schering-Plough	gel	salicylic acid, 17%	ether, 16.42%
DuoFilm Liquid Wart Remover Schering-Plough	liquid	salicylic acid, 17%	
DuoFilm Patch System Wart Remover Schering-Plough	disc	salicylic acid, 40%	
DuoPlant Schering-Plough	gel	salicylic acid, 17%	SD alcohol, 57.6%
DuoPlant Plantar Wart Remover for Feet Schering-Plough	gel	salicylic acid, 17%	
Freezone Solution Corn and Callus Remover Whitehall	liquid	salicylic acid, 13.6%	alcohol, 20.5% • ether, 64.8% • balsam oregon • castor oil • hypophosphorous acid • zinc chloride
Johnson's Foot Soap Combe	powder		borax • iodide • bran
Mosco Liquid Medtech	liquid	salicylic acid, 17%	flexible collodion • alcohol, 23%

CALLUS, CORN, WART PRODUCTS — continued

Product & Manufacturer	Dosage Form	Active Ingredients	Other Ingredients
Nail-A-Cain Medtech	liquid	benzocaine, 15% • tannic acid, 4%	isopropyl alcohol, 61% • diethyl ether, 20%
Occlusal HP GenDerm	liquid	salicylic acid, 17%	ethyl acetate • isopropyl alcohol • butyl acetate • polyvinyl butyral • dibutyl phthalate • acrylates copolymer • nitrocellulose
Off Ezy Wart Remover Kit Del	liquid	salicylic acid, 17%	flexible collodion
Sal-Plant Gel Pedinol	gel	salicylic acid, 17%	
Salactic Film Pedinol	liquid	salicylic acid, 17%	
Vergo gel Daywell	gel	salicylic acid, 17%	alcohol, 67.5% v/v • collodion • castor oil • camphor • colloidal silicone dioxide • polysorbate 80 • hydroxypropyl cellulose • hypophosphorous acid
Wart Fix Alvin Last	liquid	salicylic acid, 12%	collodion • alcohol, 33% • ether, 65.5%
Wart-Off Pfizer	liquid	salicylic acid, 17%	flexible collodion • alcohol • ether • propylene glycol dipelargonate

ATHLETE'S FOOT PRODUCTS

Product & Manufacturer	Dosage Form	Antifungal	Other Ingredients
Absorbine Antifungal Foot Cream & Powder W.F. Young	cream • powder	tolnaftate	methylparaben • propylparaben • diazolidinyl urea (powder)
Aftate Schering-Plough	aerosol	tolnaftate, 1%	BHT • propellants
Aftate Schering-Plough	gel	tolnaftate, 1%	propylene glycol • BHT
Aftate Schering-Plough	powder	tolnaftate, 1%	starch • talc
Antifungal Cream-Athlete's Foot Goldline	cream	miconazole nitrate, 2%	
Blis-To-Sol Chattem Consumer	liquid	undecylenic acid, 5%	
Blis-To-Sol Chattem Consumer	powder	zinc undecylenate, 10%	
Bluboro Allergan Herbert	powder		aluminum sulfate, 53.9% • calcium acetate, 43% • boric acid • blue #1
Buro-Sol Antiseptic Powder Doak	powder		aluminum acetate, 46.8% • sodium diacetate, 48.8% • benzethonium chloride, 4.4%
Clioquinol Various Manufacturers	cream • ointment	clioquinol, 3%	
Cruex CIBA Consumer	cream	total undecylenate, 20% as undecylenic acid and zinc undecylenate	anhydrous lanolin • fragrance • glycol stearate SE • methylparaben • PEG-6 stearate • PEG-8 laurate • propylparaben • sorbitol solution • stearic acid • trolamine • water • white petrolatum
Cruex CIBA Consumer	powder	calcium undecylenate, 10%	talc • colloidal silicon dioxide • fragrance • isopropyl myristate
Cruex Spray Powder CIBA Consumer	aerosol powder	total undecylenate, 19% as undecylenic acid and zinc undecylenate	fragrance • isobutane • isopropyl myristate • menthol • talc • trolamine
Desenex CIBA Consumer	cream	total undecylenate, 25% as undecylenic acid and zinc undecylenate	anhydrous lanolin • fragrance • glycol stearate SE • methylparaben • PEG-6 stearate • PEG-8 laurate • propylparaben • purified water • sorbitol solution • stearic acid • trolamine • white petrolatum
Desenex CIBA Consumer	powder	total undecylenate, 25% as undecylenic acid and zinc undecylenate	fragrance • talc
Desenex Antifungal CIBA Consumer	foam	undecylenic acid, 10%	isopropyl alcohol • emulsifying wax • fragrance • isobutane • purified water • sodium benzoate • trolamine
Desenex Spray Liquid CIBA Consumer	aerosol	tolnaftate, 1%	BHT • fragrance • isobutane • PEG-400 • SD alcohol 40-B
Dr. Scholl's Athletes Foot Schering-Plough	cream	tolnaftate, 1%	
Dr. Scholl's Athletes Foot Schering-Plough	powder	tolnaftate, 1%	talc • cornstarch
Dr. Scholl's Athletes Foot Spray Liquid Schering-Plough	aerosol	tolnaftate, 1%	SD alcohol, 36% • BHT • propellants
Dr. Scholl's Athletes Foot Spray Powder Schering-Plough	aerosol powder	tolnaftate, 1%	alcohol, 14% w/w (from SD alcohol 40) • BHT • propellants
Genaspor Goldline	cream	tolnaftate, 1%	

ATHLETE'S FOOT PRODUCTS — continued

Product & Manufacturer	Dosage Form	Antifungal	Other Ingredients
Lotrimin AF Cream & Solution Schering-Plough	cream • solution	clotrimazole, 1%	
Lotrimin Cream Schering-Plough	cream	clotrimazole, 1%	benzyl alcohol
Micatin Ortho	cream • powder • spray	miconazole nitrate, 2%	alcohol, 17% (spray)
Mycelex OTC Miles Incorporated	cream	clotrimazole, 1%	benzyl alcohol, 1% • cetosteryl alcohol • cetyl esters wax • polysorbate 60
Mycelex OTC Miles Incorporated	solution	clotrimazole, 1%	PEG-400
NP-27 Thompson Medical	aerosol powder	tolnaftate, 1%	talc • isobutane • isopropyl myristate • SD alcohol 40B, 14.6% w/w
NP-27 Thompson Medical	cream	tolnaftate, 1%	polyethylene glycol • carbopol • titanium dioxide • butylated hydroxytoluene • monoamylamine • propylene glycol
NP-27 Thompson Medical	powder	tolnaftate, 1%	talc • cornstarch
NP-27 Thompson Medical	solution	tolnaftate, 1%	polyethylene glycol • butylated hydroxytoluene • propylene glycol
Pedi-Pro Pedinol	powder	zinc undecylenate	deodorant • aluminum chlorhydroxide • menthol • formaldehyde
Podactin Reese Chemical	ointment • powder	tolnaftate, 1%	
Rid-Itch Thomas & Thompson	liquid	resorcinol, 1% • benzoic acid, 2% • chlorothymol, 1%	salicylic acid, 7% • boric acid, 5% • alcohol • glycerin
Tinactin Liquid Aerosol Schering-Plough	aerosol	tolnaftate, 1%	propellants • BHT
Tinactin Powder Schering-Plough	powder	tolnaftate, 1%	cornstarch • talc
Tinactin Powder Aerosol Schering-Plough	aerosol powder	tolnaftate, 1%	talc • propellants • BHT
Tinactin Solution Schering-Plough	solution	tolnaftate, 1%	PEG-400 • BHT
Ting CIBA Consumer	cream	tolnaftate, 1%	BHT • fragrance • PEG-400 • PEG-3350 • titanium dioxide
Ting Spray Liquid CIBA Consumer	spray	tolnaftate, 1%	BHT • fragrance • isobutane • PEG-400 • SD alcohol 40-B
Ting Spray Powder CIBA Consumer	spray powder	tolnaftate, 1%	BHT • fragrance • isobutane • PPG-12-buteth-16 • SD alcohol 40-B • talc
Tolnaftate Solution Goldline	solution	tolnaftate, 1%	
Tritin (Dr. Scholl's) Schering-Plough	aerosol powder	tolnaftate, 1%	BHT • propellants
Tritin (Dr. Scholl's) Schering-Plough	powder	tolnaftate, 1%	starch • talc
Undecylenic Acid Compound Various Manufacturers	ointment	undecylenic acid, 5% • zinc undecylenate, 20%	
Undelenic Tincture Gordon	liquid	undecylenic acid	isopropyl alcohol, 79% • chloroxylenol • propylene glycol • triethanolamine

Product Table Index

A
Acne Products, 836-839
Analgesic Products, External, 855-858
Analgesic Products, Internal, 644-656
Antacid Products, 716-721
Anthelmintic Products, 726
Antidiarrheal Products, 723-725
Antiemetic Products, 722
Anti-Infective Products, Topical, 831-835
Antipyretic Products, 657-665
Appetite Suppressant Products, 796
Artificial Saliva Products, 813
Artificial Tear Products, 797-798
Asthma Inhalant Products, 711
Asthma Oral Combination Products, 712
Athlete's Foot Products, 879-880

B
Blood Sugar-Elevating Products, 744, 745
Burn and Sunburn Products, 859-861

C
Calcium Products, 758-760
Callus, Corn, Wart Products, 877-878
Cold, Cough, Allergy Products, 670-703
Condom Products, 823-824

D
Dandruff and Seborrhea Products, 850-853
Decongestant Products, Topical, 704-706
Dentifrice Products, 809-812
Denture Adhesive Products, 816
Denture Cleanser Products, 815
Dermatitis and Psoriasis Products, 840-843
Diabetes Monitoring Products, 746-749
Diabetes Products, Miscellaneous, 750
Diaper Rash and Prickly Heat Products, 854
Dry Skin Products, 844-849

E
Electronic Oscillometric Blood Pressure Monitor Products, 639-640
External Analgesic Products, 855-858
Eye Wash Products, 801

F
Fecal Occult Blood Test Kits, 641
Food Supplement Products, 751-754
Formula Products for Infants and Children, 790-795

H
Hard and Rigid Gas-Permeable Lens Products, 802-803
Hemorrhoidal Products, 825-827

I
Insect Repellent Products, 876
Insect Sting and Bite Products, 873-874
Insulin Preparation Products, 739-741
Insulin Syringes and Related Products, 742-743
Internal Analgesic Products, 644-656
Iron Products, 755-757

L
Laxative Products, 727-738
Lens Products, Hard and Rigid Gas-Permeable, 802-803
Lens Products, Soft, 804-807
Lozenge Products, 708-710

M
Menstrual Products, 666-669
Miscellaneous Diabetes Products, 750
Miscellaneous Nasal Products, 707
Mouth Pain, Cold Sore, Canker Sore Products, 817-819
Multiple Vitamin Products, 762-789

N
Nasal Products, Miscellaneous, 707

O
Ophthalmic Decongestant Products, 799-800
Oral Rinse Products, 814
Ostomy Products, 820-821
Otic Products, 808
Ovulation Prediction Test Kits, 642

P
Pediculicide Products, 875
Personal Care Products, 828-830
Poison Ivy and Poison Oak Products, 867-872
Pregnancy Test Kits, 643

S
Saliva Products, Artificial, 813
Sleep Aid Products, 713-714
Soft Lens Products, 804-807
Spermicide Products, 822
Stimulant Products, 715
Sunscreen and Suntan Products, 862-866

T
Tear Products, Artificial, 797-798
Topical Anti-Infective Products, 831-835
Topical Decongestant, 704-706

V
Vitamin Products, Multiple, 762-789

General Index

Chapter titles are in color.

Major subject headings and product table titles are in black boldface.

Product trade names are in black italics. The designation "(text table)" means that the product appears in a chapter. Trade names that do not have this designation appear in the product tables. Some products appear in both places.

Subheadings are in black lightface.

A-200, 354
AAD
   See **Antibiotic-associated diarrhea**
A and D, 859
ABA
   See **Aminobenzoic acid**
Abrasives
   ophthalmic, 362-363
Abscents, 828
Abscesses
   anorectal, 470
   dental, 424
   periapical, 424
   pericoronal, 424
   periodontal, 424
   subperiosteal, 424
Absorbine Antifungal Foot Cream & Powder, 879
Absorbine Extra Strength, 855
Absorbine, Jr. Liniment, 855
Absorbine Power Gel, 855
Abuse of products
   definition, 5
   ipecac, 182, 185, 188-189
   laxatives, 230, 234
A-Caine Rectal, 825
Acanthamoeba, 378, 382, 384
Acanthamoeba keratitis, 384
Acculevel, 128
Accutane, 289, 518
Ace bandages, 632, 633
Acephen Suppositories, 644
Acesulfam, 346
Acesulfam potassium, 257
Aceta, 644, 657
Aceta-Gesic, 644, 670
Acetaminophen, 644, 657
Acetaminophen, 51, 95, 133, 420, 422, 428
   antipyretic activity, 71-72
   breast-feeding, 19, 58, 73, 74
   burn treatment, 571
   comparative efficacy, 60-61
   dosage, 72, 72 (text table), 83

dosage, children, 52 (text table), 72, 72 (text table)
   drug interactions, 55, 58, 62
   overdose, 58-59
   pregnancy, 18-19, 58, 73, 74
   use considerations, 58, 62, 71, 73
Acetaminophen Oral Solution USP, cherry, 644, 657
Acetaminophen Oral Solution USP, lime, 644, 657
Acetazolamide, 540
Acetest, 266, 746
Acetic acid, 622
   ear disorders, 399-400
Acetylsalicylic acid
   See **Aspirin**
Achilles tendinitis, 630-631
Achromycin, 266 (text table), 831
Acid denture cleansers, 426-427
ACID Mantle Creme Acid pH, 844
Acid-peptic disorders
   treatment, 150-161
A.C.N. Tablets, 762
Acne
   adult, 514
   classification, 514
   diet, 515, 519
   drug-induced, 515
   etiology, 511-514
   french fryers, 515
   inflammatory, 512, 514
   information sources, 520 (appendix)
   investigational therapy, 518
   nondrug treatment, 516
   pathogenesis, 513 (figure)
   pathophysiology, 511-514
   pomade, 515
   predisposing factors, 514-515
   self-treatment versus physician referral, 515-516
   steroid, 515
   sunlight treatment, 518-519
   systemic prescription products, 518
   terms, 512 (text table)
   topical prescription products, 517-518

topical products, 516-517
   treatment goals, 515-519
   UV radiation treatment, 518-519
Acne-5, 836
Acne-10, 836
Acne-Aid, 836
Acne cosmetica, 514-515
Acne mechanica, 516
Acne Products, 511-520
   formulation considerations, 519
   patient assessment, 511
   patient counseling, 511, 519
Acne product table, 836-839
Acne vulgaris, 289, 511, 516
Acnomel, 836
Acquired immunodeficiency syndrome, 58, 62, 213, 505
   AIDS-associated diarrhea, 206
   epidemiology, 463
   information resources, 467 (appendix)
   protection against, 455, 461
   See also **Human immunodeficiency virus**
Act, 419, 814
Actagen, 670
Actamin, 644, 657
Actamin Extra, 644, 657
Actamin Super, 644, 657
ACT for Kids, 419
Actifed, 670
Actifed Plus, 670
Actifed Sinus Daytime/Nighttime, 670
Actifed With Codeine, 670
Actinomyces viscosus, 418
Activated charcoal, 210
   comparative efficacy, 186
   compounds effectively bound by, 186 (text table)
   dosage, 185
   dosage, children, 185
   drug interactions, 185
   use considerations, 185-186
Active listening, 12
ACU-derm, 447 (text table)
Acu-Dyne Douche, 828
ACU-Dyne Ointment & Solution, 831

Acu-Dyne Skin Cleanser, 828
Acute aero-otitis media
   See **Barotrauma**
Acute atrophic candidiasis, 425
Acute erosive gastritis
   clinical presentation, 170
   complications, 170
   treatment, 170
Acute necrotizing ulcerative gingivitis
   etiology and pathophysiology, 416, 417
Acutrim 16 Hour Steady Control, 796
Acutrim II Maximum Strength, 796
Acutrim Late Day, 796
Adapettes, 802
Adapettes For Sensitive Eyes, 806
Adapt, 802
Adaptic, 447 (text table), 569
Addaprin, 644, 657, 666
Adlerika, 727
Adolescents
   acne, 511
   foot complaints, 610
   methyl salicylate, 556
   pregnancy risk, 453
   reproductive health counseling, 464
   Reye's syndrome, 96
   See also **Children**
Adrenalin Chloride, 704, 711
Adsorbents
   action, 210
   dosage, 210
   side effects, 210
   See also names of specific drugs in this class
Adsorbotear, 797
Advance, 643
Advance 2, 643
Advertising regulations, 36
Advil, 644, 657, 666
Advil Cold and Sinus, 670
Aerochamber, 130
Aerosols, 485-486
A-Fil Cream, 862
Afrin 12-Hour, 704
Afrin 12-Hour Cherry, 704
Afrin 12-Hour Menthol, 704

Aftate For Jock Itch Aerosol, 831
Aftate For Jock Itch Gel, 831
Aftate For Jock Itch Powder, 831
After-Bite, 873
Agoral, 727
Ahhh Sunburn Therapy, 859
AIDS
  See **Acquired immunodeficiency syndrome**
Aim Anti Tartar Gel Formula with fluoride, 809
Aim Baking Soda Gel with fluoride, 809
Aim Regular Strength Gel with fluoride, 809
AIRlens, 370 (text table)
Airstrip, 448 (text table)
A K-Nefrin, 799
Akwa Tears Drops, 797
Akwa Tears Ointment, 797
Alamag, 716
Albee C-800 Plus Iron Tablets, 755, 762
Albee C-800 Tablets, 762
Albee with C Caplets, 762
Albustix, 265, 746
Alcloxa, 475, 624
Alcohol, 530, 594
  disinfectant, 69
  mouthrinses, 415, 426, 428
  topical application, 71
Alcoholics
  folic acid deficiency, 294
  iron overload, 307
  nutrition, 285
  pellagra, 295
Alcohol Swabs And Alcohol Wipes, 742
Alcohol use
  diabetes, 257-258
  insomnia, 140
  metronidazole, 505
  oral health effects, 409, 421, 426
  peptic disorders, 150
  pregnancy, 19
  sleep, 140
  ulcers, 162
Alconefrin 12, 704
Alconefrin 25, 704
Alconefrin 50, 704
Alcon Saline ESE, 806
Aldioxa, 546
Aldomet, 266 (text table)
Alenic Alka, 716
Alenic Alka Improved, 716
Alginic acid, 154, 169, 176
Alimentum, 330, 792
Alitra Q, 751
Alkaline dermatitis, 441
Alkaline hypochlorite denture cleansers, 426
Alkaline peroxide denture cleansers, 426
Alkaline sulfides, 489
Alka-Seltzer, 56, 716
Alka-Seltzer Extra Strength, 644, 716
Alka-Seltzer Flavored, lemon-lime, 644, 716

Alka-Seltzer Plus Cold Medicine, 670
Alka-Seltzer Plus Maximum Strength Sinus Allergy Medicine, 670
Alka-Seltzer Plus Night-Time Cold Medicine, 670
Alkets, 716
Alkets Extra Strength, 716
Alkylamines, 100-101
Allantoin, 423, 529, 546
Aller-Chlor, 670
Allercreme, 593
Allerest, 670, 704
Allerest Children's, 670
Allerest Eye Drops, 799
Allerest Headache Strength, 644, 672
Allerest, No Drowsiness, 645, 672
Allerest Sinus Pain Formula, 645, 672
Allerfrim, 672
Allerfrim Nasal Decongestant & Antihistamine, 672
Allergan Enzymatic, 384
Allergan Enzymatic Contact Lens Cleaner, 804
Allergan Hydrocare, 385
Allergan Hydrocare Cleaning & Disinfecting Solution, 805
Allergan Hydrocare Preserved Saline Solution, 806
Allergic rhinitis
  adjunctive therapy, 110
  characteristics, 97 (text table)
  complications, 98
  conditions mimicking, 98
  duration of therapy, 114
  etiology, 96
  pathophysiology, 96-97
  patient considerations, 111-112
  pharmacologic agents, 99-104
  symptoms, 97-98, 111
  treatment, 98-99
Allergies
  atopic dermatitis, 524
  contact dermatitis, 499, 525-526, 580
  foods, 329
  insect stings, 601-603
  milk, 321-322, 329, 330
  phenolphthalein, 228
  photoallergy, 576
  poison ivy and poison oak, 589-595
Allergy Cold Tablets, 672
Allergy Drops, 799
Allergy Drops Maximum Strength, 799
Allergy Products, 99-104
  patient consultation, 112-113
  product considerations, 112
  product selection guidelines, 110-111
Allermed Maximum Strength, 672
Allyl isothiocyanate, 555-556

Aloe, 227
Aloe Grande Creme, 844
Aloin, 227
Alophen, 727
Alpha-hydroxy acids, 529
Alpha Keri, 844
Alpha-melanocyte-stimulating hormone, 583
Alpha-melanotropin, 583
Alphosyl, 566 (text table)
Alprazolam, 84
Alumina trihydrate, 413
Aluminum, 153, 154, 158
  infant formulas, 333
Aluminum acetate, 400, 529, 546, 547, 593, 595, 606
Aluminum chlorhydroxy allantoinate, 475
Aluminum chloride, 484, 485
Aluminum chlorohydrates, 484, 485
Aluminum hydroxide, 173, 189, 209, 530, 546
  phosphorus, 303
Aluminum Hydroxide, Concentrated, 716
Aluminum Hydroxide Gel, 716
Aluminum oxide, 415
Aluminum products, 441
Aluminum sulfate, 624
Aluminum zirconium chlorohydrates, 484
Aluminum zirconium salts, 485
Amantadine hydrochloride, 94
Ambenyl-D Decongestant Cough Formula, 672
Amebiasis, 204
Amenorrhea, 80
Americaine First Aid Ointment, 859, 873
Americaine Hemorrhoidal Ointment, 825
Americaine Topical Anesthetic Spray, 859, 873
Amesec, 712
Amin-Aid, 310
Aminobenzoic acid, 580
Aminoethanesulfonate
  See **Taurine**
Aminofen, 645, 657
Aminofen Max, 645, 657
Aminosalicylic acid, 110
Amitone, 716
Ammens Medicated Powder Original Fragrance, 854
Ammens Medicated Powder Shower Fresh Scent, 854
Ammonia, 544
Ammoniated Mercury, 840
Ammoniated mercury, 488
Ammonia vapor, 556
Ammonium chloride, 105
  dosage, 84
  side effects, 84
Ammonium hydroxide, 605
Amonidrin, 672
Amosan, powder, 817
Amphetamines, 110, 159

Amygdalin
  See **Laetrile**
Anacin, 645, 657
Anacin Aspirin Free, 645, 657
Anacin Maximum Strength, 645, 657
Anacin P.M. Aspirin, 713
Anacin P.M. Aspirin Free, 645, 657
Anal canal
  anatomy and physiology, 469-470
Anal crypts, 469
Anal fissure, 470
Anal fistula, 470
Analgesic adjuvants, 61, 62
Analgesic Balm, 855
Analgesics, 83, 95, 109-110, 112
  anorectal, 475
  breast-feeding, 19
  burns, 568 (text table), 571
  external, 546, 551, 604-605
  poisoning, 186
  topical, 422, 423, 428, 555
  See also **External Analgesic Products; Internal Analgesic Products**; *names of specific drugs in this class*
Anal hygiene, 476
Anaphylactic reactions
  insect stings, 600-601, 602-603
Anbesol, gel, 817
Anbesol Gel, Baby, grape and original, 817
Anbesol, liquid, 817
Anbesol Maximum Strength, gel, 817
Anbesol Maximum Strength, liquid, 817
Androgens, 18
Android fat distribution, 339
Anemia
  worm-induced, 217
Anesthetics
  anorectal, 475
  local, 473, 571, 594, 605
  oral, 109
  topical, 95, 422, 423, 428, 529
  See also *names of specific drugs in this class*
Angular cheilitis, 425
Anisakiasis
  symptoms, 217
  treatment, 217
Ankle sprains, 631
Anodynos, 645, 657
Anodynos Forte, 672
Anorectal antiseptics, 475
Anorectal diseases, 469, 470 (figure), 471-472
  drug dosage forms, 476
  patient consultation, 477-478
  treatment, 473-476, 476 (text table)
Anorectal disorders, 470-471
Answer Ovulation Test Kit, 642
Answer Plus, 643

General Index 885

Answer Plus 2, 643
Answer Quick & Simple 1-Step Pregnancy Test, 643
Antacid Products, 147-179
  patient assessment, 147, 175
  patient counseling, 147, 176
  product selection guidelines, 175-176
Antacid product table, 716-721
Antacids, 150-159, 441
  acid neutralization tests, 27
  action, 158
  adverse effects, 205-206
  breast-feeding, 19
  cholesterol-lowering effects, 173
  didanosine reconstitution, 173-174
  dosage, 189
  drug interactions, 156-157 (text table), 158-159, 189
  elderly persons, 174
  formulation, 154-155
  gastric pH, 158-159
  GI disorders, 161-173
  hangover, 173
  ingredients, 151-154
  overindulgence, 173
  palatability, 155
  phosphate-binding effects, 173
  potency, 155, 158
  pregnant women, 155, 174
  tablets, 155
  urine pH, 159
Anthelmintic product table, 726
Anthelmintic Products, 213-218
  patient assessment, 213
  patient counseling, 213
Anthralin, 539
Anthranilates, 580
Anthraquinones, 227, 230, 539
Antiadrenergic antihypertensives, 98
Antibacterials, 415
  insect stings and bites, 606-607
  oral, 109
Antibiotic-associated diarrhea, 205
Antibiotic ointments, 423, 547
Antibiotics, 445
  acne treatment, 518
  adverse effects, 188, 204-205, 409, 424, 425, 440, 441
  diaper rash, 544
  first-aid, 499
  infectious diarrhea prophylaxis, 207
  Jarisch-Herxheimer reaction, 68
  toxic shock syndrome, 87
Antibiotic sore mouth, 425
Anticancer drugs
  See **Antineoplastic agents**
Anticholinergic agents, 27, 101, 108, 109, 122, 124-125, 138-139
  acid-peptic disorders, 160
  adverse effects, 17, 424, 716

anorectal, 475
antihistamines, 111-112
efficacy, 210
mechanism of action, 210
oral antibacterials, 109
See also names of specific drugs in this class
Anticoagulants
  drug interactions, 55, 208
  pregnancy, 18
  See also names of specific drugs in this class
Anti-Dandruff Brylcreem, 850
Antidepressants
  adverse effects, 424
  poisoning, 185, 186
Antidiarrheal agents, 441
  breast-feeding, 19
Antidiarrheal Products, 199-211
  options, 209-210
  patient assessment, 199, 206-207
  patient counseling, 199
  selection guidelines, 210-211
Antidiarrheal product table, 723-725
Antidopaminergic drugs
  adverse effects, 206
  See also names of specific drugs in this class
Antiemetic Products, 181-198
  ingredients in nonprescription products, 189-190
  patient assessment, 181, 187-189
  patient counseling, 181
  pregnancy, 188
Antiemetic product table, 722
Antifungal Cream-Athlete's Foot, 879
Antifungals, 546, 621 (text table)
  side effects, 507
  skin infections, 502-503
  vaginal infections, 505-509, 508 (text table)
Antihistamines, 99-101, 100 (text table), 124, 128, 133, 218, 594
  adverse effects, 17, 424
  analgesic adjuvant effect, 61, 62
  anticholinergics, 111-112
  breast-feeding, 19
  drug interactions, 189
  insect bites, 605-606
  insect stings, 604
  motion sickness, 188
  pregnancy, 139, 189
  side effects, 99, 100-101, 189, 408-409
  sleep aid products, 137-139, 140
  topical, 525-526, 529
  See also names of specific drugs in this class
Antihypertensive drugs
  adverse effects, 206, 424
  drug interactions, 60
  See also names of specific drugs in this class

Anti-infectives
  acne treatment, 518
Anti-inflammatory agents, 122, 124, 530
  nonsteroidal, 80, 81, 133, 149, 150, 171
Antimicrobials, 485, 546, 547
  burns, 571-572
  deodorant sprays, 482
  douches, 481
  topical, 445
Antimicrobial soaps, 446
Antiminth, 215, 726
Antimotility drugs, 441
Antineoplastic agents, 576
  adverse effects, 181, 188, 205, 409
  pregnancy, 18
Antioxidant, 762
Antioxidants, 358
Antiperistaltic drugs
  contraindications, 208
  efficacy, 209
  side effects, 209
  See also names of specific drugs in this class
Antiperspirants, 483-486
  dosage forms, 485-486
  ingredients, 484-485
  labeling claims, 486
  patient assessment, 479
  patient counseling, 479
  use guidelines, 486
Antiplaque agents, 414
Antipruritics, 529, 594, 604-605
  anorectal, 475
Antipsychotic drugs
  adverse effects, 424
Antipyretic Drug Products, 65-75
  dosage, 72-73
  options, 71-72
  patient assessment, 65
  patient counseling, 65
  patient education, 73-74
  selection guidelines, 73
Antipyretic product table, 657-665
Antipyretics, 109-110, 112
Antipyrine, 400
Antiseptics, 446, 499-502, 594-595
  active ingredients, 500 (text table)
  anorectal, 475
  ophthalmic, 362
  topical, 547
Anti-Tuss, 672
Anti-Tuss DM, 672
Antitussives, 104, 107-109, 128
  dosages, 107 (text table)
  product selection, 104-105
  See also names of specific drugs in this class
Ants, 600, 601
ANUG
  See **Acute necrotizing ulcerative gingivitis**
A-Nuric, 666
Anusert, 825
Anusol, 825
Anusol Ointment 1% Hydrocortisone, 825

AO Sept, 382, 805
AO Soft, 372 (text table)
Aphrodisiacs, 27
Apomorphine
  emetic agent, 187
Appedrine Caplets, 796
Appetite suppressant product table, 796
Aqua A, 844
Aqua-Ban, 666
Aqua-Ban Plus, 666
Aqua Care, 844
Aquaderm, 844
Aquaderm Sunscreen Moisturizer SPF15, 862
Aqua-Fresh for Kids, paste, 809
Aqua-Fresh Tartar Control, paste, 809
Aqua-Fresh Triple Protection, paste, 809
Aquatar, 566 (text table)
Arachnids, 597-600
Arbon, 762
Aristocort, 593
A.R.M., 670
Arm & Hammer Dental Care, 414
Arm & Hammer Dental Care Gel with Fluoride, 809
Aromatic Compound, 723
Arthralgia
  epidemiology, 52
  etiology, 52
  treatment, 52
Arthriten, 645
Arthriten PM, 645
Arthritic pain, 553
Arthritis
  foot complaints, 610, 628
  See also **Rheumatoid arthritis**
Arthritis Hot Cream, 855
Arthritis Pain Formula, 645, 658
Arthritis Pain Formula Caplets, 666
Arthropan, 57
Arthropan Liquid, 645, 658
Artificial saliva product table, 813
Artificial sweeteners, 346
  See also **Sweeteners**
Artificial tear product table, 797-798
Artificial tear solutions, 358, 359, 415
Ascariasis
  See **Roundworms**
Ascaris lumbricoides, 216
Ascaris suum, 216
Ascorbic acid, 288
  adverse effects, 293
  common cold, 110, 292
  description, 292
  dose/RDA, 292-293
  drug interactions, 293
  indications, 292
Ascriptin AD, 658
Ascriptin Extra Strength, 658
Ascriptin Regular Strength, 658
Aspartame, 256, 257, 346, 414, 418
Aspercin, 645, 658
Aspercin Extra, 645, 658

Aspercreme, 855
Aspercreme Lotion, 855
Aspergillus, 393
Aspergum, 658
Aspergum, cherry and orange, 645
Aspermin, 645, 658
Aspermin Extra, 646, 658
Aspirin, 646, 658
Aspirin, 51, 52, 95, 133, 159, 420, 422, 459
  action, 52
  adverse effects, 53-55, 62, 67 (text table)
  antipyretic activity, 71-72
  breast-feeding, 19, 54, 73
  buffered, 56, 62
  burn treatment, 571
  comparative efficacy, 60-61
  dosage, 52-53, 72, 72 (text table), 83
  drug interactions, 55, 62
  enteric-coated, 56, 62
  gastrointestinal irritation, 53, 56, 62, 73
  heart attack prophylaxis, 56-57
  insect stings, 606
  overdose, 55-56
  pregnancy, 18-19, 54, 73
  Reye's syndrome, 53, 54-55, 62, 96
  sensitivity and methyl salicylate, 556
  use considerations, 53-55, 62, 73
  See also **Salicylates**
Aspirin, Buffered, 658
Aspirin, Children's, 658
Aspirin Enteric Coated, 646
Aspirtab, 646, 658
Aspirtab Max, 646, 658
Asteatotic eczema, 527
Astemizole, 101, 128
Asthma
  allergic rhinitis, 98
  cough, 105
  epidemiology, 118
  etiology, 118
  exercise-induced, 132
  nocturnal, 132
  pathology, 120 (figure)
  pathophysiology, 118-120
  peak flow, 121-122, 122 (text table), 132
  symptoms, 120
  treatment, 121, 122-132
Asthma Haler, 711
Asthma inhalant product table, 711
Asthma Nefrin, 711
Asthma oral combination product table, 712
Asthma Products, 117-134
  patient assessment, 117, 120-122
  patient counseling, 117
  patient education, 133
  selection guidelines, 132
Astringents, 415, 423, 474-475, 529, 595
  douches, 481
Athlete's foot, 497, 610
  diabetic patients, 628
  dosage forms, 624-625

  etiology, 617-618
  evaluation, 619
  pathophysiology, 618
  patient consultation, 625
  patient education, 625
  pharmacologic treatment, 620-625
  product selection guidelines, 625
  susceptibility, 618-619
  types, 618
Athlete's foot product table, 879-880
Atopic dermatitis, 523-524, 548-549
  sunlight, 577
  treatment, 524
Atropine, 109, 124-125
Atropine sulfate, 209
Attapulgite, 209, 210
  breast-feeding, 19
A-200 Lice Control Spray, 875
A-200 Pyrinate, 875
Aural drainage, 393
Auraphene-B, 808
Auricle
  anatomy, 390 (figure)
  disorders, 392-393
  interpretation of physical findings, 392 (text table)
Aurinol Ear Drops, 808
Auro-Dri, 808
Auro Ear Drops, 808
Autojector, 742
Auto-Lancet, 750
Autolet Lite Clinisafe, 750
Automatic Injector, 742
Avail, 762
Avalgesic, 855
Aveeno Anti-Itch Cream, 873
Aveeno Anti-Itch Cream & Lotion, 867
Aveeno Bath Treatment Moisturizing Formula, 859, 867
Aveeno Bath Treatment Moisturizing Formula/Dry, Itchy Skin, 844
Aveeno Bath Treatment Soothing Formula, 859, 867
Aveeno Bath Treatment Soothing Formula/Itchy Irritated Skin, 844
Aveeno Cleansing Bar Combination Skin, 844
Aveeno Cleansing Bar Dry Skin, 845
Aveeno Moisturizing Cream, 593
Aveeno Moisturizing Cream & Lotion, 845, 867
Aveeno Shower & Bath Oil, 845
Avobenzone, 582
Ayr, 707
Azelastine, 128
Azidothymidine
  See **Zidovudine**
Azma Aid, 712
Azmacort, 130
Azo-Standard, 646
Azothioprine, 515
AZT
  See **Zidovudine**
AZTECH, 384

Baby Anbesol Gel, 428
Baby bottle caries, 428
Baby Orajel Teething Pain Medicine, 428
Baciguent, 831
Bacillus cereus, 203
Bacitracin, 205
  dosage, 499
Bacitracin Zinc-Neomycin Polymyxin, 831
Bacitracin Zinc-Polymyxin B Sulfate, 831
Bacitracin Zinc USP, 831
Backache, 553
Backaid Pills, 646
Backaid PM Pills, 646
Back-Quell, 646
Bacterial skin infections
  treatment, 498-502
  types, 496-497
Bacterial vaginosis, 504, 505
Bacteroides, 480, 627
Bagbalm, 854
Bain de Soleil All Day for Kids, 862
Bain de Soleil All Day Six Hour Waterproof Sunfilter, 862
Bain de Soleil All Day Waterproof Sunblock, 862
Baking soda, 414, 415
Balnetar, 840
Banacid, 717
Banalg Arthritic Pain Reliever, 855
Banalg Muscle Pain Reliever, 855
Banesin, 646, 658
Bangesic, 855
Banish II Liquid Deodorant, 820
Barc, 875
Barnes Hind Daily Cleaner, 385
Barotrauma, 396
Barrier contraceptives, 86
  cervical cap, 453, 460
  condoms, 461-463
  diaphragm, 453, 460
  female condoms, 463
  sponge, 460-461, 464
Basal body temperature method of family planning, 457
Basal thermometry, 44
Bath oils, 527
Bausch & Lomb Sensitive Eyes Daily Cleaner, 384
Bayer Aspirin, Genuine, 646, 658
Bayer Aspirin, Maximum, 646, 659
Bayer Children's Aspirin, 646
Bayer Children's Chewable Aspirin, 659
Bayer Delayed Release Enteric Aspirin Adult Low Strength, 646

Bayer Delayed Release Enteric Aspirin Regular Strength, 646
Bayer Extended Release 8-Hour Aspirin, 647, 659
Bayer Plus Buffered Aspirin, 647, 659
Bayer Plus, Extra Strength Buffered Aspirin, 647, 659
Bayer Select Ibuprofen Pain Reliever/Fever Reducer, 647, 659
Bayer Select Maximum Strength Headache, 647
Bayer Select Maximum Strength Menstrual Multi-Symptom, 647, 666
Bayer Select Maximum Strength Night Time Pain Relief, 647
Bayer Select Maximum Strength Sinus Pain Relief Formula, 647
B-D Autolance, 750
B-D Glucose Tablets, 744
Bedbugs, 597
Bee-Balm Ointment, 855
Beechwood creosote, 106, 108
Beelith Tablets, 762
Bees, 600, 601
Beeswax, 421
Bee-T-Vites Tablets, 762
Bee-Zee Tablets, 762
Bell/Ans, 717
Beminal-500 Tablets, 762
Benadryl, 189, 254, 594, 672
Benadryl 25, 672
Benadryl Cold Nighttime Formula, 672
Benadryl Cold Tablet, 672
Benadryl Decongestant, 672
Benadryl Maximum Strength Anti-Itch Cream, 867
Benadryl Maximum Strength Anti-Itch Spray, 867
Bendectin, 189, 190
Benemide, 267 (text table)
Ben-Gay Arthritis Extra Strength Rub, 855
Ben-Gay Daytime Pain Relieving Gel, 855
Ben-Gay Original Formula Pain Relieving Rub, 855
Ben-Gay Regular Strength Pain Relieving Rub, 855
Ben-Gay Ultra Strength, Pain Relieving Rub, 855
Ben-Gay Vanishing Scent Formula, Sports and Exercise Rub, 855
Benoxyl 5, 836
Ben's Backyard, 876
Ben's Max, 876
Bensulfoid, 836
Benylin, 672
Benylin D Cough Syrup, 672
Benylin DM Pediatric Cough Syrup, 674
Benylin Expectorant, 674
Benza, 831
Benzalkonium Chloride, 831

Benzalkonium chloride, 358, 376-377, 502, 546, 594
Benzedrex, 704
Benzedrex 12 HR, 704
Benzethonium chloride, 358, 502, 546
Benzoate, 415
Benzocaine, 95, 345-346, 400, 423, 428, 529, 594, 605
Benzocaine, 859
Benzocaine
 anorectal, 473
 burns, 571
 oral lozenges, 109
Benzodent Analgesic Denture Ointment, 817
Benzoic acid, 415
 athlete's foot, 623
Benzoin preparations, 106
Benzoin tincture, 110, 422
Benzonatate, 108
Benzophenones, 580
Benzoyl peroxide, 516, 517
Benzyl alcohol, 109, 422
 anorectal, 473
Beriberi, 298
Beta$_2$ agonists, 122, 132
 side effects, 123-124
Beta blockers
 drug interactions, 60
Beta carotene, 288, 583
Betadine, 69, 482
Betadine Antiseptic Lubricating Gel, 828
Betadine First Aid Cream & Spray, 831
Betadine Medicated Douche, 828
Betadine Medicated Premixed Disposable Douche, 828
Betadine Medicated Vaginal Gel, 828
Betadine Mouthwash/Gargle, 817
Betadine Ointment & Douche, 831
Betadine Vaginal Suppository, 828
Betamethasone dipropionate, 593
Betamethasone valerate, 593
Bethanecol
 adverse effects, 206
Betuline, 856
B.F.I. Powder, 831
BiCozene, 825
BiCozene External Analgesic Creme, 859, 873
Bikini Condom, 463
Bili-Labstix, 746
Binding agents, 414
BioBrane II, 449 (text table)
Bioclusive, 437
Bioflavonoids, 298
Biotel/Diabetes Home Screening Test, 266
Biotin
 adverse effects, 299
 description, 298-299
 dose/RDA, 299
 drug interactions, 299
 indications, 299
 infant requirements, 318

Bisacodyl, 226, 227, 228-229, 229, 230
Bisacodyl, 727
Bismuth, 161
Bismuth salts, 190, 474
Bismuth subgallate, 485
Bismuth subnitrate, 530, 546
Bismuth subsalicylate, 190
 drug interactions, 208
 prophylactic dosage, 207-208
 Reye's syndrome, 190
Bi-Soft, 372 (text table)
Bi-Zets, 708
Black Draught, 727
Blairex Hard Contact Lens Cleaner, 802
Blairex Sterile Saline Solution, 806
Bleach denture cleansers, 426
Bleach tooth whiteners, 416
Bleeding
 anal, 472
 midcycle, 81
 uterine, 81
Blepharitis, 353, 354
 antiseptics, 362
Blindness
 diabetes, 238, 260-261
 night blindness, 288-289
Blind persons
 communicating with, 13
Blinx, 801
Blisters, 631
Blistex Lip Balm, 862
Blistex Lip Ointment, 817
Blis-To-Sol, 879
Blood glucose
 exercise, 254
 insulin, 238
 testing, 264-266
Blood pressure
 meters, 40
 monitoring, 39-42
Blood pressure monitor product table, 639-640
Blood sugar-elevating product table, 744
Blood tests
 diabetes, 264-267
 fecal occult, 42-43
Bluboro, 867, 873, 879
Body language, 13
Body odor, 483-484
Body surface area
 estimating, 209 (figure)
Body temperature
 basal body temperature family planning method, 457
 basal body temperature variations (figure), 457
 measurement, 69-70
 normal, 66
 thermoregulation, 65-66
 See also **Fever**
Boils
 auricle, 392
 external auditory canal, 393
 patient assessment, 397
Bonine, 189, 722
Boric Acid, 859
Boric acid, 362, 400, 546, 593
Borofax, 854, 859
Boston Advance Cleaner, 802

Boston Advance Conditioning, 380
Boston Advance Conditioning Solution, 802
Boston Cleaner, 802
Boston Conditioning Solution, 802
Boston Daily Cleaner, 379
Boston Equalens, 370, 370 (text table)
Boston Lenses, 370
Boston Lens II, 370 (text table)
Boston Reconditioning Drops, 380
Boston Rewetting Drops, 802
Boston RXD, 370 (text table)
B.Q. Cold, 672
Brasivol, 836
Brasivol Base, 836
Braun/Oral-B Plaque Remover, 412
Breast disease
 caffeine, 144
Breast-feeding, 313-314, 323-324
 acetaminophen, 58, 74
 antihistamines, 139
 aspirin, 54, 74
 asthma products, 132
 caffeine, 143-144
 contraceptive method, 458-459
 diaper rash, 543
 drug use, 19
 frequency of feedings, 335
 human immunodeficiency virus, 324
 human milk and cow milk comparison, 320-322
 human milk fortifiers, 331
 hyperbilirubinemia, 324
 ibuprofen, 60
 laxative use, 227, 230
 medications in breast milk, 324-325
 microwave oven warming of breast milk, 334-335
Breezee Mist, 831
Brethancer, 130
Brij, 530
Bromides, 515
Bromo-Seltzer, 647, 659, 717
Bromotap, 674
Brompheniramine, 19
Brompheniramine maleate, 99
Bronchitis, 89
Bronchodilator drugs, 123 (text table)
Broncho Saline, 711
Bronitin Mist, 711
Bronkaid, 712
Bronkaid Mist, 711
Bronkaid Mist Suspension, 711
Bronkolixir, 712
Bronkotabs, 712
Bron Kote, 674
Bruises, 552
Buffaprin, 647, 659
Buffaprin Extra, 647, 659
Buffasal, 647, 659
Buffasal Max, 647, 659
Buffered aluminum sulfate, 485

Bufferin AF Nite Time, 647, 659
Bufferin Arthritis Strength, Tri-Buffered, 659
Bufferin Arthritis, Tri-Buffered, 647
Bufferin Extra Strength, Tri-Buffered, 647, 659
Bufferin, Tri-Buffered, 648, 659
Buffers, 358
Buffinol, 648, 660
Buffinol Extra, 648, 660
Buf-Puf, 516
Buf-Puf Acne Cleansing Bar, 836
Bugs Bunny Complete, 762
Bugs Bunny Plus Iron, 764
Bugs Bunny Vitamins, 764
Bugs Bunny with Extra C, 764
Bulimia, 188-189
 See also **Eating disorders**
Bulimia nervosa, 230
Bulk-forming laxatives, 222-223, 230, 475
Bull Frog Sunblock, 862
Bunions, 612, 631
Burn and Sunburn Products, 563-573
 patient assessment, 563, 568-569
 patient counseling, 563
 product formulation, 572
 product selection, 572
 See also **Sunscreen and Suntan Products**
Burn and Sunburn products, 859-861
Burning
 anal, 472
Burns
 analgesics, 568 (text table), 571
 antimicrobials, 571-572
 categorization, 564-566, 565 (text table)
 chemical, 569
 cleansing, 569
 complications, 566-567
 counterirritants, 572
 depth, 564 (figure)
 dressings, 569
 electrical, 569
 establishing percentage of surface, 565 (figure)
 etiology, 563
 infection, 566-567
 local anesthetics, 571
 minor, 569-570
 outpatient treatment, 569-570
 pharmacologic agents, 570-572
 protectants, 568 (text table), 570-571
 thermal, 569
 topical hydrocortisone, 571, 572
 topical ingredients approved by FDA, 570 (text table)
 See also **Sunburn**
Burntame, 859

Burnt toast
  poisoning treatment, 186
Buro-Sol Antiseptic Powder, 879
Burow's solution, 400, 524, 526, 529, 593, 595, 624
Bursae, 552
Bursitis, 552-553
Butacaine, 422
Butacaine sulfate, 422
Butamben, 571
Butazolidin, 442 (text table)
Butesin Picrate, 859
Butoconazole, 505
Button Infuser, 250, 262
Butyrophenones, 68

C

Caffedrine Caplets, 715
Caffedrine Capsules, 715
Caffeine, 715
Caffeine
  adverse effects, 142-143
  analgesic adjuvant effect, 61, 62
  benign breast disease, 144
  breast-feeding, 19
  cardiovascular disease, 141
  central nervous system effects, 141, 141 (text table)
  content of beverages and foods, 140 (text table)
  diabetes, 258
  dosage, 84, 142
  drug interactions, 143
  fertility, 144
  laboratory test interferences, 143
  lactation, 143-144
  malignancy, 144
  neonates, 144
  patient education and counseling, 144
  physiologic effects, 141-142
  pregnancy, 19, 143-144
  side effects, 84
  therapeutic concerns, 143-144
  toxicity, 142-143
  warnings and precautions, 143
Caffeinism, 142-143
Caffree Anti-Stain Fluoride Toothpaste, 809
Caladryl, 867, 873
Caladryl Clear, 868
Calamine, 474-475, 606
Calamine, 854
Calamine lotion, 529, 546, 593
Calamine, Regular & Phenolated, 868
Calcarb 600, 758
Calcarb 600+D, 758
Calci-Chew, 758
Calciferol
  adverse effects, 290-291

  breast-fed full-term infants, 318-320
  chemicals, 290 (text table)
  deficiency diseases, 290
  description, 289-290
  dose/RDA, 290
  drug interactions, 290-291
  indications, 290
  infant formulas, 332-333
  infant requirements, 317
  preterm infant requirements, 320
Calci-Mix, 758
Calcium, 758
Calcium, 441
  adverse effects, 302
  description, 301
  dose/RDA, 301
  drug interactions, 302
  indications, 301
  infant requirements, 318
  preterm infant requirements, 320
Calcium 600, 758
Calcium Carbonate, 717, 758
Calcium carbonate, 152-153, 158, 189, 209, 413
Calcium Gluconate, 758
Calcium Lactate, 758
Calcium Oyster Shell, 758
Calcium plus Vitamin D, 758
Calcium polycarbophil, 223
Calcium product table, 758-760
Calcium pyrophosphate, 413
Calcium undecylenate, 546, 547, 548
Calcium With Vitamin D, 758
Calculus, 410-411, 414
CaldeCort, 840, 868
CaldeCort Light, 840
CaldeCort Light With Aloe, 868
CaldeCort Maximum Strength, 840
Caldesene Medicated Ointment, 854
Caldesene Medicated Powder, 854
Calel-D, 758
Calendar method of family planning, 455 (text table), 455-457
Calglycine, 717
Callus, corn, wart product table, 877-878
Calluses, 611-612, 613, 614 (figure)
  diabetic foot, 627-628
  evaluation, 614-615
  foot care products, 615 (text table)
  patient consultation, 617
  patient education, 617
  treatment, 615-617
  unapproved treatments, 616
Calmol 4 Suppositories, 825
Calm-X, 190
Caloric allowances, 339-340
Caltrate, 759
Caltrate 600 + D, 759
Caltrate 600 + Iron, 759
Caltro, 759
Cama Arthritis Pain Reliever, 660

Cama In-Lay, 660
Campho-Phenique, 831
Campho-Phenique Cold Sore Gel, 856
Campho-Phenique Gel, 817
Campho-Phenique Liquid, 817, 856
Campho-Phenique Triple Antibiotic Plus Pain Reliever, 856
Camphor, 400, 422, 423, 557, 594
  burns, 572
  cold products, 106, 108
  counterirritants, 474, 605
  hemorrhoids, 474, 475
Camphorated oil, 27
Camphor-containing ointments, 108
Campylobacter, 203
Campylobacter pylori, 149
Cancer
  artificial sweeteners, 346
  basal cell epithelioma, 578
  caffeine, 144
  colorectal, 42, 436
  keratoacanthoma, 578
  malignant melanoma, 578
  oral, 407, 409, 421
  premalignant actinic kertosis, 578
  skin, 538
  squamous cell carcinoma, 578
  sunscreens, 576
  UV radiation, 575
  See also **Antineoplastic agents**
Cancer chemotherapeutic agents
  See **Antineoplastic agents**
Candermyl, 845
Candida
  burns, 567
Candida albicans, 205, 424, 426, 498, 503, 504, 505, 544, 620
  vaginitis, 480-481
Candidiasis, 498, 504
  predisposing factors, 424, 425, 426, 505
  recurrent infections, 505
  symptoms, 424-425
  treatment, 425, 505-509
Canker sores
  epidemiology, 421
  etiology, 421-422
  pathophysiology, 422
  treatment, 422
Canned diet products, 346
Canthaxanthin, 583
Capsaicin, 558
Capsicum, 558
Caramiphen edisylate, 108
Carbamide, 528-529
Carbamide peroxide, 400-401, 416, 422, 423, 424
Carbetapentane citrate, 108
Carbohydrate metabolism, 238-239
Carbol-fuchsin solution, 620
Carbomer, 530
Carboxymethylcellulose, 185, 209

Carbuncles, 497
  treatment, 499
Cardiovascular disease, 360
  caffeine, 141
  diabetes, 256
Cardiovascular system
  caffeine, 141-142
Carnation Follow-Up, 790
Carnation Good Start, 792
Carnation Good Start H.A., 330
L-Carnitine
  adverse effects, 299
  description, 299
  dose/RDA, 299
  drug interactions, 299
  indications, 299
Caroid Laxative, 727
Carotenemia, 289
Carotenoids, 288
Carter's Laxative, 727
Casanthranol, 227
Cascara Sagrada, 727
Cascara sagrada, 227
Cascara Sagrada Aromatic Fluid, 727
Casec, 751
Casein hydrolysate-based infant formulas, 329-330
Castor Oil, 728
Castor oil, 226, 228
Cathartic colon, 227, 230
Cathartics, 185, 186
  adverse effects, 205
Catrix, 845
Catrix Lip Saver, 845
Catrix with Sunscreen, 845
Caustic ingestions, 187
Cellufresh, 359, 797
Celluvisc, 359, 797
Cenafed, 674
Cenafed Plus, 674
Central nervous system
  caffeine, 141, 141 (figure)
Central nervous system agents, 141
  See also *names of specific drugs in this class*
Centrum, 764
Centrum Jr. Plus Iron Chewable Tablets, 764
Centrum Silver Gel-Tabs, 764
Ceo-Two, 728
Cepacol, 708, 814
Cepacol Anesthetic, 708
Cepacol Mint, 814
Cepastat Cherry, 708
Cepastat Extra Strength, 708
Cephalosporins, 205
Cercarial dermatitis
  See **Swimmer's itch**
Cerovite Jr. Tablets, 766
Certagen, 766
Cerumen
  impacted, 394
Cerumen-softening products, 401-402
Cervical cap, 453, 460
Cervical mucus method of family planning, 457-458
  characteristics of cervical mucus through menstrual cycle, 458 (text table)
Cestodes
  See **Tapeworms**

Cetaphil, 524, 527, 840, 845
Cetirizine, 128
Cetyl alcohol, 530
Cetylpyridinium chloride, 415, 416
Chap-Et Sun Ban 15 Lip Conditioner, 862
Chap Stick Sunblock 15, 862
Charcoal, activated
 See **Activated charcoal**
Charcocaps, 820
Chemstrip 8, 746
Chemstrip 9, 746
Chemstrip 10 With SG, 746
Chemstrip bG, 746
Chemstrip G, 746
Chemstrip GK, 746
Chemstrip GP, 265
Chemstrip 2 GP, 746
Chemstrip K, 266, 746
Chemstrip uG, 746
Chemstrip uGK, 746
Cheracol D, 674
Cheracol Plus, 674
Cheracol Sinus, 674
Cheracol Sore Throat Spray, 674
Cheracol Spray Nasal Pump, 704
Chickenpox, 498
 Reye's syndrome, 96
Chiggerex, 873
Chiggers, 598
Chiggertox, 873
Children
 acetaminophen, 52 (text table), 62
 activated charcoal, 185
 allergic rhinitis, 98
 analgesics, 604
 antihistamines, 100, 101, 189, 606
 antitussives, 107-109
 aspirin, 52 (text table)
 asthma products, 130-131
 atopic dermatitis, 523-524
 benzocaine, 605
 body surface area, 209 (figure)
 body temperature, 66
 caffeine, 141
 capsicum preparations, 558
 colds, 91-92, 93
 common diseases, 18
 counterirritants, 555-556
 DEET, 607
 diarrhea, 203-204, 208-209
 dietary fat restriction, 322
 dosage considerations, 18
 expectorants, 104-107
 febrile seizures, 68-69, 71, 74
 fever, 65, 71
 fluoride, 428
 fluorine, 304
 furazolidone, 206
 guttate psoriasis, 534
 hay fever, 95
 heat stroke, 67
 hydrocortisone, 606
 ipecac, 185, 190
 iron poisoning, 307
 laxatives, 229
 lice, 354, 598
 loperamide, 209
 methyl nicotinate, 557
 methyl salicylate, 556
 motion sickness, 188
 nutrition, 285
 nutritional supplements, 311
 obesity, 341-342
 orthodontia, 428
 physiologic state, 17
 pinworms, 213
 polycarbophil, 210
 pyrantel pamoate, 215
 Reye's syndrome, 53, 54-55, 62, 96, 190
 sore throats, 95
 sunscreens, 585-586
 teething, 428
 temperature measurement, 70
 toothbrushes, 428
 topical decongestants, 103
 turpentine oil, 557
 vitamin A, 289
 vomiting, 188
 warts, 613
 zinc deficiency, 309
 See also **Infants**
Children's Chloraseptic Sore Throat Lozenges, grape, 708
Chlamydia, 459, 461, 463
Chloasma, 577
Chloraseptic Advanced Formula Sore Throat Gargle, cherry, 674
Chloraseptic Advanced Formula Sore Throat Spray, mint, 676
Chloraseptic Mouthwash/Gargle, 814
Chloraseptic Sore Throat Lozenges, cherry, 708
Chloraseptic Sore Throat Lozenges, cool mint, 708
Chloraseptic Sore Throat Lozenges, menthol, 708
Chloraseptic Sore Throat Spray Children's, grape, 676
Chloraseptic Throat Spray, 814
Chlorhexidine, 358, 376-377, 547, 548
Chlorhexidine gluconate, 501
Chlorobutanol, 358
Chloroform, 401
***p*-chloromercuriphenol**, 546
Chlorophyll, 485
Chlorophyllin copper complex, 485
Chlorophyllins, 423
Chlorothymol, 606
Chloroxylenol, 502, 546, 606, 623
Chlorpheniramine, 594
 breast-feeding, 19
Chlorpheniramine Maleate, 676
Chlorpheniramine maleate, 99, 100 (text table)
Chlorpheniramine Maleate, Extended Release, 676
Chlorpromazine
 hyperpigmentation, 486
Chlorpropamide, 247
Chlor-Rest, 674
Chlor-Trimeton Allergy, Sinus, Headache, 674
Chlor-Trimeton Allergy Syrup, 674
Chlor-Trimeton 12 Hour Allergy/Decongestant Tablets, 674
Chlor-Trimeton 12 Hour Allergy Tablets, 674
Chlor-Trimeton Non-Drowsy 4 Hour Tablets, 674
Cholecalciferol, 289, 546, 563
Cholesterol, 530
 antacid effects, 173
 lowering, 173
Cholestyramine, 205, 210
Choline
 adverse effects, 299
 description, 299
 dose/RDA, 299
 drug interactions, 299
 indications, 299
 infant requirements, 318
Cholinergic drugs
 adverse effects, 206
 See also names of specific drugs in this class
Choline salicylate, 57, 58
 See also **Salicylates**
Chooz, 717
Chromium
 adverse effects, 303
 description, 303
 dose/RDA, 303
 drug interactions, 303
 indications, 303
Chronic atrophic candidiasis, 425
Chronic fatigue syndrome, 95
Chronic nonerosive gastritis
 clinical presentation, 170
 complications, 170
 treatment, 171
Chronic otitis media, 396
Chrysophanic acid, 227
Cibasoft, 372 (text table)
Cibasoft soft colors, 372 (text table)
Cibathin, 372 (text table)
Cibathin soft colors, 372 (text table)
Ciba Vision Cleaner, 804
Ciba Vision Saline, 806
Cigarette smoking
 oral health effects, 409, 421, 425
 peptic disorder, 150
 during pregnancy, 19
 ulcers, 162
Cimetidine, 159, 168
Cinnamates, 580
Ciprofloxacin, 207
 dosage, 207
Cirrhosis
 selenium deficiency, 308
Citrate Of Magnesia, 728
Citrate salt, 415
CitriSource, 751
Citrocarbonate, 717
Citrotein, 310, 751
Citrucel, 728
Citrus bioflavinoids, 423
Cleaning Solvent, 820
Clean-N-Soak, 802
Cleansers, 527
Clearasil Adult Care, 836
Clearasil Antibacterial Soap, 836
Clearasil Benzoyl Peroxide, 836
Clearasil Clearstick Maximum & Sensitive, 836
Clearasil Clearstick Regular, 836
Clearasil Double Clear Pads Maximum Strength, 836
Clearasil Double Clear Pads Regular Strength, 836
Clearasil Medicated Astringent, 836
Clear Away Plantar Wart Remover System, 877
Clear Away Wart Remover System, 877
Clearblue Easy, 643
Clear By Design, 836
Clear Choice, 814
Clear Eyes ACR, 799
Clear Eyes Lubricating Eye Redness Reliever, 799
Clearplan Easy, 642
Clemastine
 reclassification, 23
Clemastine Fumarate Tablets, USP, 676
Clens, 802
Cleocin, 505
Clindamycin, 205, 505, 512, 518
Clinilog, 750
Clinistix, 293, 746
Clinitest, 265, 266, 293, 746
Clioquinol, 831, 879
Clioquinol, 503
 athlete's foot, 620
Clobetasol propionate, 540
Clocort, 840
Clocream, 845, 859
Clomycin, 831
Clorpacin WCS-90, 831
Closed-ended questions, 13
Close-Up Anti-Plaque Gel, 809
Close-Up Fluoride, gel & paste, 809
Close-Up Tartar Control Gel, 809
Clostridium difficile, 205, 206
Clostridium perfringens, 627
Clotrimazole, 503, 505, 548
 athlete's foot, 620-621
 reclassification, 23
Clove oil, 420, 605
Cluster headaches
 symptoms, 51
 treatment, 51
Coal Tar, 840
Coal tar products, 538, 540
 side effects, 538
Coast, 485
Cobalt, 303-304
Cocoa butter, 423, 546
Codeine, 107-108, 181
Codimal, 676
Codimal D.M., 676
Codimal P.H., 676

Cod liver oil, 108, 546
Cod Liver Oil Concentrate, 766
Cod Liver Oil Concentrate With Vitamin C, 766
Coitus interruptus
  contraception method, 453, 458
Colace Capsules, 728
Colace Liquid, 728
Colace Syrup, 728
Colax, 728
Colchicine
  adverse effects, 205
Cold, Cough, and Allergy Products, 89-115
  patient assessment, 89
  patient counseling, 89
Cold, cough, allergy product table, 670-702
Coldonyl, 676
Colds, 91-93
  adjunctive therapy, 110
  ascorbic acid, 110, 292
  complications, 93
  conditions mimicking, 93-95
  duration of therapy, 113, 114
  etiology, 92
  pathophysiology and symptoms, 92-93
  patient considerations, 111-112
  patient consultation, 112-113
  product considerations, 112
  product selection guidelines, 110-111
  symptoms, 111
  treatment, 95-96
Cold sores, 498, 577
  etiology, 422
  pathophysiology, 422-423
  treatment, 423
  treatment, nondrug, 423
Cold wraps, 633
Colgate Baking Soda, 414
Colgate Baking Soda, paste, 809
Colgate Junior, gel, 809
Colgate, paste, 810
Colgate Tartar Control, gel, 809
Colgate Winterfresh Gel, 809
Colic, 329
Collodion vehicles
  corn, callus, and wart treatment, 616
Colloidal oatmeal, 527, 546, 593
Colly-Seels, 437, 441
ColoCare, 42, 43, 641
Colon, 201
ColoScreen Self-Test, 42, 43
Colostomies
  ascending, 435 (figure), 436
  deodorants, 485
  descending and sigmoid, 435 (figure), 436
  irrigating sets, 438, 438 (figure)
  reasons for, 436
  temporary, 436
  transverse, 435 (figure), 436
  types, 434 (figure)
Colyte, 229
Combistix, 265, 746
Comfeel, 449 (text table)

Comfortcare GP Daily Cleaner Liquid, 802
Comfortcare GP Daily Cleaner Suspension, 802
Comfortcare GP Dual Action Daily Cleaner, 802
Comfortcare GP Wetting & Soaking Solution, 802
Comfort Eye Drops, 799
Comfortine, 854, 859
Comfort Tears Drops, 797
Comfort Tears Liquid, 797
Common cold
  See **Colds**
Communication
  listening techniques, 13
  nonverbal, 13
  between pharmacists and physician, 15
  physical barriers, 13
  principles, 12-13
  questioning techniques, 13
  special populations, 13
Compleat-B, 310
Compleat Modified Formula, 751
Compleat Regular Formula, 751
Complete, 427, 815
Complex 15 Face & Hand & Body Cream, 845
Complex 15 Hand & Body Lotion, 845
Compound W Gel Wart Remover, 877
Compound W Liquid Wart Remover, 877
Compoz, 713
Compoz Gelcaps, 713
Comtrex, 676
Comtrex Allergy-Sinus, 676
Comtrex Day/Night, 676
Comtrex Hot Flu Drink, 676
Comtrex Non-Drowsy, 676
Conceive, 642
Conceived, 643
Concentrated Cleaner, 802
Concentrated infant formulas, 331-332
  dilution, 333 (text table)
Conceptrol, 822
Conceptrol Disposable, 822
Conceptrol Gel, 822
CondomMate, 461, 462
Condom product table, 823-824
Condoms
  disadvantages, 462
  disease prevention, 461
  failure rate, 461
  female, 463
  latex sensitivity, 462-463
  lubricants, 461
  use guidelines, 462 (text table)
Condyloma acuminata, 470
Condyloma latumi, 470
Conex, 676, 708
Conex D.A., 676
Conex Plus, 676
Congespirin For Children, Aspirin Free, 660
Congespirin For Children, Aspirin-Free, 676

Congespirin For Children Chewable, 648
Congestac, 676
Conjunctivitis, 97, 353, 355-356
Constipation
  antacids, 174, 176
  associated disorders, 221 (text table)
  associated conditions, 221 (text table)
  causes, 219, 220 (text table)
  dietary issues, 222 (text table)
  diseases of the large intestine and, 222 (text table)
  hemorrhoids, 471
  symptoms, 222
  treatment, 222-234
  See also **Laxatives**
Consumers
  complaints, 3 (text table)
  education/sophistication, 4-5
  product safety, 6
  self-care attitudes and beliefs, 2-4
  See also **Patient assessment**; **Patient counseling**; **Patient education**
Contac Day & Night Allergy/Sinus, 678
Contac Day & Night Cold & Flu, 678
Contac JR, 678
Contac Maximum Strength 12 Hour, 678
Contac Severe Cold & Flu, 678
Contac Severe Cold & Flu Nighttime, 678
Contact dermatitis, 524-526
  allergic, 499, 525-526, 580
  irritant or sensitizing ingredients, 530
  sunlight, 577
  sunscreens, 585
  See also **Rhus dermatitis**
Contact lenses
  bifocal, 371
  care products, 376-385
  characteristics, 367-368, 369 (text table)
  chemical disinfection, 382-383, 383 (text table)
  cleaning, 377-379, 380-382, 384
  contraindications, 373
  corneal abrasions, 375
  corneal hypoxia and edema, 375
  cosmetics, 374-375
  demographics of wearers, 368 (figure)
  disinfecting, 382-383, 384
  disposable, 371
  drug interactions, 374, 374 (text table)
  elderly persons, 373
  enzymatic cleaners, 381 (text table), 381-382, 384
  extended-wear, 373, 387
  friction rubbing, 378
  hard, 369, 377 (figure), 377-379, 386
  hydraulic cleaning, 378

  indications, 372-373
  insertion, 379, 380, 385
  preservatives, 376-377
  problems, 373-376
  product formulation considerations, 376, 385
  product selection guidelines, 379, 380, 384
  removal, 379, 380, 385
  rewetting products, 379, 384
  rigid gas-permeable, 379-380, 380 (figure), 386
  rigid gas-permeable hard, 369-370
  saline solutions, 383-384
  soaking solutions, 378, 379
  soft, 370-372, 380-385, 381 (figure), 386-387
  solutions, 376-377
  spray cleaning, 378
  storage cases, 385
  subgroups, 371
  surface-active cleaners, 380-381, 384
  symptoms of problems, 375
  thermal disinfection, 382
  tinted, 371
  types, 368-372
  ultrasonic cleaning, 378
  wearing instructions, 385-387
  wetting solutions, 378, 379
Contact Lens Products, 367-388
  patient assessment, 367, 385-387
  patient counseling, 367, 385-387
Contac 12 Hour, 678
Contraceptive Methods and Products, 453-467
  choice, 455-464
  continuation rates, 454 (text table), 455
  effectiveness, 454 (text table), 455
  patient assessment, 453
  patient counseling, 453
  safety, 455
Contraceptives
  See **Barrier contraceptives**; **Oral contraceptives**; **Vaginal contraceptives**
Contraceptive sponge, 460-461, 464
Control Capsules, 796
Controlyte, 310
Cool Mint Listerine, 415
Cope, 648
Copper
  adverse effects, 304
  description, 304
  dose/RDA, 304
  drug interactions, 304
  false reduction reactions, 268 (text table)
  indications, 304
  infant requirements, 318
  molybdenum, 308
  substances that interfere with reduction test, 267 (text table)
Copper sulfate
  emetic agent, 186
Coppertone, 862

Coppertone Kids, 862
Coppertone Kids Sunblock, 862
Coppertone LipKote Sunblock Lip Balm, 862
Coppertone Moisturizing Sunblock Lotion, 863
Coppertone Moisturizing Sunscreen, 863
Coppertone Moisturizing Suntan Oil, 863
Coppertone Sport, 863
Coppertone Sunblock, 863
Coppertone Sunless Tanning Extra Moisturizing Lotion, 863
Coppertone Sunless Tanning Lotion, 863
Coppertone Sunscreen, 863
Coppertone Tan Magnifier Suntan Gel, 863
Coppertone Tan Magnifier Suntan Oil, 863
Coricidin, 678
Coricidin D, 678
Coricidin Demilets, 678
Coricidin Maximum Strength Sinus Headache, 678
Corneal edema, 356
Corn Fix, 877
Corn Huskers, 845
Corns, 611-612
 diabetic foot, 627-628
 evaluation, 614-615
 foot care products, 615 (text table)
 patient consultation, 617
 patient education, 617
 treatment, 615-617
 unapproved treatments, 616
Cornstarch, 546, 547
Correction Cream Wash, 846
Correctol, 728
Correctol Extra Gentle, 728
Cortaid, 840, 868
Cortaid, Maximum Strength, 840, 868, 873
Cortaid with Aloe, 840, 868
Cortef Feminine Itch Cream, 828
Corticosteroids, 97, 122, 124, 218
 acne, 515, 519
 adverse effects, 424
 calcium, 302
 peptic disorders, 150
 topical, 538-539, 593
 See also names of specific drugs in this class
Cortisone-5 Cream, 841
Cortisone-10 Cream, 841
Cortisone-5 Ointment, 841
Cortisone-10 Ointment, 841
Cortizone-5 Cream, 869
Cortizone-10 Cream, 869
Cortizone-5 Cream For Kids, 869
Cortizone-5 & -10 Ointment, 869
Cough preparations
 breast-feeding, 19
 Cough Products, 104-108
 patient assessment, 89
 patient counseling, 89

Coughs, 93
 product selection, 104-105
 reflex, 90-91
 treatment, 95, 104-108
Coumadin, 292
Count-a-Dose, 262, 742
Counterirritants, 551, 594
 action, 553-554
 burns, 572
 clinical considerations, 560
 combining, 559
 dosage forms, 559-560
 douches, 481
 hemorrhoids, 474
 insect stings and bites, 604, 605
 labelling, 560
 potencies, 555
 safety, 560
 of unproven effectiveness or safety, 558-560
Cow Milk, Whole, 790
Cresol, 530, 605, 606
Crest Baking Soda Mint Paste, 810
Crest Cavity Fighting Gel, 810
Crest Cavity Fighting Toothpaste (Regular & Mint), 810
Crest for Kids Sparkle Blue Gel, Bubblegum Flavor, 810
Crest Tartar Control Gel, 810
Crisco, 462
Criticare HN, 310, 751
Crohn's disease, 434
Cromolyn, 122, 132
 side effects, 124
Cruex, 879
Cruex Medicated Cream, 832
Cruex Powder, 831
Cruex Spray Powder, 832, 879
Cryptitis, 470
Cryptosporidium, 206
CSI, 384
CSI-T, 384
Curel Everyday Sun Protection Lotion, 863
Curel Moisturizing, 846
Cutar, 841
Cutemol, 846
Cutter Insect Repellent, 876
Cyanocobalamin
 adverse effects, 294
 description, 293
 dose/RDA, 294
 drug interactions, 294
 indications, 293-294
 supplements for infants, 319
Cyclizine, 189
 dosage, 189
 dosage, children, 189
Cyclomethycaine sulfate, 605
Cyclosporine, 540
Cylex Sugar Free, 708
Cyteine hydrochloride, 546
Cytomegalovirus, 545
Cytostatic agents, 536-537
Cytotoxic drugs
 adverse effects, 424, 445
 See also **Antineoplastic agents**

D

Dacriose, 801
Daily Cleaner, 804
Daily Conditioning Treatment For Lips (DCT), 863
Daily-Vite With Iron & Minerals, 766
Dairy Aid, 319
Dairy Ease, 210, 319
Dakins, 832
Dakins 1/2 Strength, 832
Dallergy-D, 678
Dandrolene, 515
Dandruff, 532
 features, 531 (text table)
 nonmonograph ingredients, 537 (text table)
 nonprescription ingredients, 536, 536 (text table)
 product selection guidelines, 540
Dandruff and seborrhea product table, 850-853
Danthron, 227
Dapa, 648, 660
Dapa-500, 660
Dapa, Extra Strength, 660
Dapa Extra Strength Capsules, 648
Dark corn syrup, 229
Dayalets Filmtabs, 766
Daylets Plus Iron Filmtabs, 766
DayQuil LiquiCaps, 678
DayQuil Liquid Non-Drowsy Cold/Flu Medicine, 678
Daytime sedatives, 27
DC 240, 728
Deaf or hearing impaired persons
 communicating with, 13
Debriding agents, 423
Debrisan Beads, 447 (text table)
Debrox Drops, 808
Decagen Tablets, 766
Decongestants, 16, 51, 132
 breast-feeding, 19
 dosages, 104 (text table)
 nasal, 95
 oral, 103-104, 104 (text table)
 topical, 101-103, 360-361
Decylenes, 832
Deep-Down, 856
DEET, 607
Defecation
 bleeding, 472
 process, 220-221
 See also **Feces**; **Stools**
Degenerative joint disease, 610
 epidemiology, 52
 etiology, 52
 pathophysiology, 52
 treatment, 52
 treatment, nondrug, 52
Degest 2, 799
Debist, 678

Dehydration, 66
 symptoms, 207
 treatment, 190, 208-209
Delfen, 822
Delsym, Extended Release, 680
Demazin, 680
Demulcents
 See **Artificial tear solutions**
Denalan, 815
Denclenz Liquid Denture Cleaner, 815
Dencorub, 856
Denorex, Extra Strength, 841
Denorex Medicated Shampoo, 566 (text table)
Denorex Medicated Shampoo, Extra Strength, 850
Denorex Medicated Shampoo Extra Strength with Conditioners, 850
Denorex Medicated Shampoo, Regular Formula, 850
Denorex Medicated Shampoo with Conditioners, 850
Denorex, Regular Formula and Mountain Fresh Scent, 841
Denorex with Conditioners, 841
Denquel, 421
Denquel Sensitive Teeth Toothpaste, 810
Dentagard, paste, 810
Denta 3 In 1 Toothache Relief, gel/gum/drops, 817
Dental abscesses
 etiology, 424
 symptoms, 424
 treatment, 424
 types, 424
Dental care, 259-260
 See also **Oral health problems**; **Teeth**
Dental caries
 etiology, 418
 infant formulas, 332
 pathophysiology, 418
 prevention, 418-420
Dental diseases
 See **Oral health problems**
Dental floss, 412-413
Dental fluorosis, 428
Dental specialty aids, 413
Dentapaine, ointment, 817
Dentifrice product table, 809-812
Dentifrices, 413-415
 children, 428
 desensitizing, 421
 fluoride, 419, 420 (text table)
Dentlock, 816
Dentopyogenic infections
 etiology, 424
 pathophysiology, 424
 symptoms, 424
 treatment, 424
 types, 424
Dento Spray, 412
Dents Toothache Drops, 817
Dents Toothache Gum, 817
Dentu-Creme Denture Toothpaste, 815
Denture adherents, 427
Denture adhesive product table, 816

Denture cleanser product table, 815
Denture cleansers, 426-427
Denture problems, 426-427
Denture reliners and cushions, 427
Denture stomatitis, 425, 426
Dent-Zel-Ite Oral Mucosal Analgesic, liquid, 817
Dent-Zel-Ite Temporary Dental Filling, liquid, 817
Dent-Zel-Ite Toothache Relief Drops, 817
Deodorants
 colostomies, 485
 dosage forms, 485-486
 feminine spray, 479, 482
 underarm, 479, 483-486
 use guidelines, 486
Depilation, 489
Depilatories, 479, 488-490
Derifil Tablets, 820
Dermacort, 869
DermaFlex Topical Anesthetic Gel Coating, 856, 869, 873
Dermapax, 869
Dermatitis, 568
 amount of medication needed, 530 (text table)
 causes, 522-523
 characteristics, 523 (text table)
 description, 522-523
 ear, 393
 eczema, 522, 568
 eyelid, 354
 ostomy-associated, 441
 treatment, 527-530
 types, 523-527
 See also **Diaper rash**; **Prickly heat**; **Rhus dermatitis**; **Seborrheic dermatitis**
Dermatitis and psoriasis product table, 840-843
Dermatologic Products, 521-541
 patient assessment, 521
 patient counseling, 521
 selection guidelines, 530-531, 540-541
Dermatologic terms, 522 (text table)
Dermatophytosis of the foot
 See **Athlete's foot**
DermKote, 846
Dermolate, 841
Dermoplast, 859, 860, 873
Dermsol-30, 863
Desenex, 879
Desenex Antifungal, 879
Desenex Antifungal Foam, 832
Desenex Cream, Powder & Ointment, 832
Desenex Spray Liquid, 879
Desitin, 546, 547, 854, 860
Desquamative external otitis
 See **External otitis**
Detachol, 820
Detergents
 ophthalmic, 362-363
Devrom Chewable Tablets, 820

Dexamethasone, 487
Dexatrim Caffeine Free Maximum Strength Caplets, 796
Dexatrim Caffeine Free Maximum Strength with Vitamin C, 796
Dexatrim Maximum Strength Caffeine Free Capsules, 796
Dexatrim Maximum Strength Extended Duration, 796
Dexatrim Plus Vitamin C, Maximum Strength, 796
Dexatrim Regular Strength Capsules, 796
DEX4 Glucose Tablets, 744
Dexpanthenol, 546
Dextranases, 414
DextroEnergy Glucose Tablets, 744
Dextromethorphan, 108
 breast-feeding, 19
Dextrose
 See **Glucose**
Dextrosol Energy Chewable Tablets, 744
Dextrostix, 746
DextroTabs, 744
Dey-Vial Sodium Chloride Solution, 707
DHS Tar, 850
DHS Tar Gel Shampoo, 566 (text table)
DHS Zinc, 850
DiaBeta, 248 (text table)
Diabetes, 189, 206, 237-238, 360
 alcohol, 257-258
 allergy and cold preparations, 111
 behavioral and psychosocial issues, 269, 273
 blood and urine testing, 264-267
 caffeine, 258
 carbohydrate metabolism, 238-239
 cardiovascular disease, 256
 complications, 242-243
 condition analysis form, 270-271 (figure)
 cost of care, 238
 dental care, 259-260
 detection programs, 274
 drugs of abuse that impair management, 260 (text table)
 drug therapy, 247-254
 etiology, 241-242
 eye care, 260-261
 foot care, 259, 627-628
 foot conditions, 610
 furuncles, 497
 general hygiene, 258-259
 glucose intolerance, 239 (text table)
 identification tags, 267
 information sources, 275-276 (appendix)
 injection aids for visually impaired, 262
 insulin-dependent, 241, 242 (figure)
 insulin infusion pumps, 263-264

 laxatives, 223, 230
 monitoring, 269
 nondrug therapy, 254-257
 noninsulin-dependent, 241, 242, 243 (figure)
 nonprescription products, 268-269
 obesity, 342
 preventing complications, 258-261
 product selection guidelines, 261-267
 record form, 272
 record keeping, 264-267
 screening, 245-246
 symptoms, 243-245
 syringes and needles, 261-262
 travel recommendations, 267-268
 treatment, 246-257
 type I, 238, 241, 242, 255-257
 type II, 239, 241, 242, 243 (figure), 247, 255-257
 vitamins and minerals, 258
 vomiting and diarrhea, 16
 See also **Diabetes mellitus**
Diabetes Care Products and Monitoring Devices, 237-281
 patient assessment, 237
 patient counseling, 237
 patient education, 273
 product selection guidelines, 261-267
Diabetes mellitus
 classification, 239-241
 complications, 244 (text table)
 diagnostic criteria, 246
 features, 240-241 (text table)
 foot complaints, 626-628
Diabetes monitoring product table, 746-748
Diabetic care center, 273-274
Diabinese, 248 (text table)
Dial, 485, 619
Dialet, 750
Dialose, 728
Dialose Plus, 728
Diaparene Baby Powder, 854
Diaparene Diaper Rash Ointment, 854
Diaper dermatitis
 See **Diaper rash**
Diaper rash
 complications, 544-545
 etiology, 543-544
 fungal infections, 544
 patient assessment, 543
 patient counseling, 543
 prevention, 548-549
 treatment, 502, 545-548
Diaper Rash and Prickly Heat Products, 543-550
 patient assessment, 543, 545
 patient counseling, 543
 selection guidelines, 549
Diaper rash and prickly heat product table, 854
Diapers
 changing frequency, 544, 548

 cloth and disposable comparison, 548-549
 diaper services, 548
 disposable, 548
 laundering, 548
Diaphragms, 453, 460
Diarrest, 723
Diarrhea, 230, 234
 acute, 202-206
 AIDS-associated, 206
 antacids, 153-154, 160-161, 174, 176
 children, 203-204
 chronic, 201 (text table), 206
 classification, 200 (text table), 201 (text table)
 drug-induced, 204-206
 electrolytes and water content, 200 (text table)
 etiology, 199, 201-202, 202 (figure)
 food-borne, 203
 food-induced, 203
 infant formulas, 332
 infectious, 204-205 (text table), 207-208
 mechanisms, 201-202
 nutritional supplements, 311
 patient assessment, 199, 206-207
 product selection guidelines, 210-211
 prophylaxis, 207
 protozoal, 204
 symptoms, 199
 travelers', 204-205 (text table), 207-208
 treatment, 16, 204-205 (text table), 207-210, 211
 viral, 203-204
Diasorb, 723
Diasporal Cream, 850
Diastix, 265, 746
Diatrol, 723
Dibasic sodium citrate, 421
Dibenzoylmethane, 582
Dibucaine, 860
Dibucaine, 423, 571, 594, 605
 anorectal, 473
Dicalcium phosphate, 413
Dical-D, 759
Dicarbosil, 717
Didanosine, 173-174
Di-Delamine, 869
Di-Delamine Double Antihistamine, 873
Diet
 acne, 515, 519
 diabetes, 255-257
Dietary fiber, 231-233 (text table)
Di-Gel, 717
Di-Gel, Advanced Formula, 717
Digestive enzymes, 210
Digestive system anatomy, 220 (figure)
Digestive tract
 anatomy, 434 (figure)
Digitalis
 adverse effects, 188
Digoxin
 drug interactions, 60
Dihydroxyacetone, 583
Dimacid, 717

Dimacol, 680
Dimenhydrinate, 722
Dimenhydrinate, 189
  dosage, 189
  dosage, children, 189
Dimetane, 680
Dimetane Decongestant, 680
Dimetapp, 680
Dimetapp Cold & Allergy, 680
Dimetapp Cold & Flu, 680
Dimetapp DM, 680
Dimetapp Extentabs, 680
Dimetapp 4-Hour Liqui-Gels, 680
Dimetapp Sinus, 680
Dimethicone, 546
Dioxybenzone, 580
Diperodon hydrochloride, 594
Diphenhist Antihistamine Captabs, 680
Diphenhist Cough Syrup, 680
Diphenhydramine, 189, 525, 529, 594, 606
  adverse effects, 138-139
  breast-feeding, 19
  dosage, 138, 189
  dosage, children, 189
  efficacy, 138
  toxicity, 138-139
Diphenhydramine hydrochloride, 99, 108
Diphenhydramine nitrate, 99
Diphenoxylate, 208
  efficacy, 209
  side effects, 209
Diphenylmethane stimulants, 227-228
Diprosone, 593
Disclosing agents, 413
Disinfectants, 69
Disinfecting Solution, 805
Disophrol, 680
Disophrol Chronotabs, Sustained Action, 680
Dithranol, 539
Diuretics, 84, 441
  drug interactions, 60
Diurex Long Acting Capsules, 666
Diurex MPR Tablets, 667
Diurex PMS Tablets, 667
Diurex Timed-Release Water Caplets, 667
Diurex Water Pills, 667
Diurex-2 Water Pills, 667
Diverticulitis, 436
Divi-Dent Denture Cleanser, 815
Dizmiss, 722
DJD
  See **Degenerative joint disease**
DML Forte, 846, 854, 859
DM Syrup, 678
DOAK Shampoo, 566 (text table)
Doak Tar Lotion, 841
Doan's Extra Strength, 648
Doan's Original, 648
Doan's P.M. Extra Strength, 648, 713

Doctar, 850
Docusate, 223, 226, 478, 481
Docusate Calcium, 728
Docusate Potassium with Casanthranol, 728
Docusate Sodium, 728, 729
Docusate Sodium with Casanthranol, 729
Domagel, 723
Domiphen bromide, 415, 416
Donnagel, 210
Dorcol Children's Cough Syrup, 682
Dorcol Children's Decongestant Liquid, 682
Dorcol Children's Liquid Cold Formula, 682
Double-Action Kit, drops/tablets, 817
Douches, 463
  administration, 482
  adverse effects, 482
  equipment, 482
  vaginal, 481-482
Dove, 527
Doxidan, 729
Doxycycline, 203, 512, 518
Doxylamine, 138, 141, 189
  adverse effects, 138-139
  toxicity, 138-139
Doxylamine succinate, 99
Dr. Caldwell Senna Laxative, 729
Dr. Gordshells Salve, 841
Dr. Hand's Teething Gel, 817
Dr. Hand's Teething Lotion, 817
Dr. Scholl's, 616
Dr. Scholl's Athletes Foot, 879
Dr. Scholl's Athletes Foot Spray Liquid, 879
Dr. Scholl's Athletes Foot Spray Powder, 879
Dr. Scholl's Callus Removers, 877
Dr. Scholl's Corn Removers, 877
Dr. Scholl's Ingrown Toenail Reliever, 877
Dr. Scholl's Liquid Corn Remover, 877
Dr. Scholl's Smooth Touch Pedi-spreads, 625
Dr. Scholl's Wart Remover Kit, 877
Dr. Scholl's Waterproof Corn Removers, 877
Dramamine, 189, 722
Dramamine II, 722
Drionic, 484
Dristan, 704
Dristan Allergy, 682
Dristan Cold and Flu, 682
Dristan Cold, Multi-Symptom, 682
Dristan Cold, Multi-Symptom Maximum Strength, 682
Dristan Cold, No Drowsiness, 682
Dristan Juice Mix-in, 682
Dristan Menthol, 704
Dristan Saline Nasal Spray, 707

Dristan Sinus, 682
Dristan 12-Hour, 704
Drixoral, 682
Drixoral Cold and Allergy, Sustained Action, 682
Drixoral Cold and Flu & Sinus, Extended Release, 682
Drixoral Non-Drowsy Formula, Extended Release, 682
Drug Efficacy Study Implementation, 24
Dry eye, 288, 356, 360
Dry Eye Therapy, 797
Dry skin, 526-527
  characteristics, 523 (text table)
  treatment, 527-530
Dry skin product table, 844-849
Drysol, 484
DUB
  See **Dysfunctional uterine bleeding**
Dulcolax, 729
Duodenal ulcers, 148 (figure), 149, 155 (text table), 161-164
  clinical presentation, 162
  complications, 162
  diagnosis, 162
  maintenance treatment, 164
  pathogenesis, 161-162
  treatment, 162-164
Duodenum
  See **Gastrointestinal system; Gastrointestinal tract**
DuoFilm, 877
DuoFilm Liquid Wart Remover, 877
DuoFilm Patch System Wart Remover, 877
Duolube, 797
DuoPlant, 877
DuoPlant Plantar Wart Remover for Feet, 877
DURAcare, 804
DURAcare II, 804
Duradyne, 648, 660
Dura-sil Front Surface Bifocal, 370 (text table)
DuraSoft, 372 (text table)
DuraSoft 3, 372 (text table)
Duration, 704
Dyclonine, 422, 529
Dyclonine hydrochloride
  anorectal, 473
Dymelor, 248 (text table)
Dyprotex, 854
Dysfunctional uterine bleeding, 81
Dysmenorrhea
  definition, 79-80
  patient assessment, 82-83
  symptoms, 59
  treatment, 59, 83-84
Dyspel, 648, 667
Dyspepsia
  nonulcer, 172-173

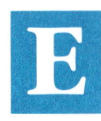

Earaches
  patient assessment, 389, 397
  patient counseling, 389
Ear conditions
  auricle, 391-393
  etiology, 390-391
  external auditory canal, 393-395
  middle ear, 395-396
  patient assessment, 389, 397-398
  patient counseling, 389
  self-treatment, 389
  symptoms, 391 (text table)
  treatment, 399-402
  See also **Hearing disorders**
Ear-Dry, 808
Early Detector, 42
Ear pain
  See **Earaches**
Ears
  anatomy and physiology, 390
Earsol, 808
Ear wax
  See **Cerumen**
Ear Wax Removal System, 808
Eating disorders
  ipecac abuse, 182, 185, 188-189
  laxative abuse, 230
  See also **Bulimia; Bulimia nervosa**
Ecee Plus, 766
Econazole nitrate, 625
Ecotrin Maximum Strength, 648, 660
Ecotrin Regular Strength, 648, 660
Ecthyma, 497
  treatment, 499
Eczema, 522, 568
Edentulism, 425
EDTA *See* **Ethylenediaminetetraacetic acid**
Efferdent, 427, 815
Efferdent, 2 Layer, 815
Efferdent paste, 427
Effergrip Denture Adhesive Cream, 816
Effersyllium, 729
Effervescent Denture Tablets, 815
Efidac/24, 682, 707
Efodine, 832
Egg Nog, 751
Elase, 448 (text table)
Elasto-Gel, 448 (text table)
Elderly persons
  antacids, 174
  antihistamines, 101
  asthma products, 130
  common diseases, 18
  contact lenses, 373
  denture repair kit, 427
  dentures, 426-427
  dosage considerations, 18

dry skin, 526-527
foot complaints, 610
heat stroke, 66-67
laxatives, 229-230
malnutrition, 286
nutrition, 285
osteomalacia, 290, 301
pellagra, 295
physiologic state, 17
prescription medications, 6
self-care, 5-6
sleep physiology, 136
thermoregulatory alterations, 67 (text table)
xerostomia, 425-426
Eldopaque, 487
Electric toothbrushes, 411-412
Electrolysis, 489
Electrolytes
in normal and diarrheal feces, 200 (text table)
replacement, 190, 208-209
Electronic oscillometric blood pressure monitor product table, 639-640
Elm bark, 108
Emagrin, 649, 660
Emagrin Forte, 682
Emesis
See **Vomiting**
Emetic and Antiemetic Products, 181-198
antiemetic options, 189-190
contraindications, 187
controversial areas, 187
patient assessment, 181, 187-189
patient counseling, 181
poisoning treatment, 184-187, 192-198 (appendix)
Emetrol, 190
Emko Foam, 822
Emollia, 846
Emollient laxatives, 223, 226, 230
Emollients, 527-528
deodorant sprays, 482
nonmedicated, 360
Empirin, 649, 660
EMS
See **Eosinophilia-myalgia syndrome**
Emulsifiers, 530
Emulsion stabilizers, 530
Emulsoil, 729
Encare, 822
Endemic nematode infections
See **Worm infections**
End-Lice, 875
Endocrine system
caffeine, 142
Enemas, 228-229, 229-230
Enerjets Lozenges, 715
Enfamil, 328, 331, 790
Enfamil Human Milk Fortifier, 331, 794
Enfamil Premature Formula, 792, 794
Enfamil Premature Formula with Iron, 794
Enfamil Preterm Formula, 331
Enfamil with Iron, 790
Ensure, 263, 310, 751
Ensure HN, 751

Ensure Plus, 310, 751
Ensure Plus HN, 751
Ensure Pudding, 751
Ensure w/Fiber, 751
Entamoeba histolytica, 204, 206
Enteral nutrition, 310
Enterobacter, 567
Enterobiasis
See **Pinworms**
Enterobius vermicularis, 213
Enterostomal therapy, 438, 440
Enuclene, 801
Enzymes, 414
Eosinophilia-myalgia syndrome, 139
Ephedrine, 103, 104, 125-126, 132
combination products, 129
diabetics, 269
dosage, 126
side effects, 126-127
Ephedrine Sulfate, 712
Ephedrine sulfate, 473-474
Epident, 412
Epi-Derm, 856
Epidermophyton, 497
Epidermophyton floccosum, 544, 617, 620, 621
EPIGARD, 449 (text table)
Epilady, 489
Epilation, 489
Epilepsy
prophylaxis, 69
Epinephrine, 711
Epinephrine, 132
combination products, 129
diabetics, 269
dosage, 125
Epinephrine hydrochloride, 473-474
insect stings, 604
Epsom Salt, 729
E.P.T. Stick, 643
Ergocalciferol, 289
E.R.O., 808
Erysipelas, 497
treatment, 499
Erythema multiforme, 577
Erythrodermic psoriasis, 534
Erythromycin, 205, 512, 518
Escherichia coli, 203, 627
Espotabs, 729
Essential fatty acids, 299-300
Essential oils, 414, 415
Estar, 566 (text table), 841
Estivin II, 799
Estrogen
acne treatment, 518
adverse effects, 188
female cycle, 43
ET
See **Enterostomal therapy**
Ethanedisulfonate, 108
Ethanol, 55, 500
Ethanolamines, 100, 137, 189
Ethionamide, 515
Ethylenediamines, 100
Ethylenediaminetetraacetic acid, 358, 377, 491

Ethylmorphine hydrochloride, 108
Etretinate, 539
Eucalyptamint Muscle Pain Relief, 856
Eucalyptamint Ointment, 856
Eucalyptol, 108, 414, 415
Eucalyptus oil, 106, 108, 558
Eugenol, 420, 422
Evac-Q-Kwik, 729, 730
Evac-U-Gen, 730
Evaporated milk infant formulas, 313
Evening primrose oil, 84
Excedrin AF Dual, 649, 660
Excedrin Caplets Aspirin Free, 649, 660
Excedrin Extra Strength, 649, 660
Excedrin IB, 649, 661, 667
Excedrin P.M., 649, 661, 713
Excedrin Sinus, 649, 682
Exceed, 310
Excita Extra, 823
Excita Fiesta, 823
Excoriation, 440
Exercise
amenorrhea, 80
asthma, 132
diabetes therapy, 254-255
for diabetics, 255 (text table)
foot problems, 630-633
pain related to, 551-552
patient education, 632-633
Ex-Lax Chocolate Laxative Tablets, 730
Ex-Lax Extra Gentle, 730
Ex-Lax Gentle Nature, Natural Laxative, 730
Ex-Lax Maximum Relief Formula, 730
Ex-Lax Regular Strength, 731
Exocaine Medicated Rub, 856
Exocaine Plus Rub, 856
Exostosis, 611
Expectorants, 95, 104-108, 106 (text table), 128
product selection, 104-105
See also names of specific drugs in this class
Extar Denture Cleanser, 815
Extenzyme, 384
External Analgesic Products, 551-562
patient assessment, 551, 554-561
patient counseling, 551
External analgesic product table, 855-858
External analgesics, 551, 604-605
External auditory canal
disorders, 393-395
External ear
anatomy, 390 (figure)
disorders, 392 (text table), 399
External otitis, 394-395
patient assessment, 397, 398 (text table)
Extra Action Cough Syrup, Guaifenesin-DM, 682
Extra-Strength Aim, 419
Eye disorders, 353-357

Eyedrops
self-administration, 359 (text table)
Eyelids, 351
anatomy, 352 (figure)
irritation, 354 (figure)
scrubs, 362-363, 363 (text table)
Eyes
anatomy and physiology, 351-357, 353 (figure)
artificial, 360
diabetic care, 260-261
drug formulations, 357-358
external, 351-352
internal, 352-353, 356-357
pharmacotherapy, 363-364
red, 355 (figure)
Eye-Scrub, 801
Eye-Stream, 801
Eye Wash, 801
Eye wash product table, 801
EZ-Detect, 42, 43, 641
Ezo Denture Cushions, 816

F

Faces Only Clear Sunscreen by Coppertone, 863
Faces Only Moisturizing Sunblock by Coppertone, 863
Fact Plus, 643
Family Medic, 860
Family planning
information sources, 466 (appendix)
See also **Contraceptive Methods and Products**; **Natural family planning**
Fasteeth, 816
Fasteeth Extra Hold, 816
Fat cells, 341
Faultless Instant Cold Pack, 633
FDA's Review of OTC Drugs, 21-37
Febrile seizures, 68-69, 71, 74
Fecal occult blood test kits, 42-43
Fecal occult blood test kits product table, 641
Feces
electrolytes and water content, 200 (text table)
medications that discolor, 442 (text table)
See also **Stools**
Fedahist, 682
Fedahist Decongestant, 682
Fedahist Expectorant, 684
Fedahist Expectorant Pediatric, 684
Federal Trade Commission
drug labeling study, 36
Feen-A-Mint, 731
Feen-A-Mint Pills, 731

General Index

Feet
- arthritis, 628
- complaints about, 609
- diabetic care, 259, 627-628
- exercise-induced problems, 630-633
- frostbite, 629-630
- general conditions, 609
- groups of patients with problems, 610
- orthotic devices, 609
- poor circulation, 628
- problems, 611-617
- running/jogging conditions, 609
- sole conditions, 614
- top conditions, 611 (figure)

Female condoms, 463
Femcaps, 667
FemCare Cream, 832
FemCare Tablets, 832
Femilax, 731

Feminine cleansing and deodorant products, 84, 479-483
- deodorant sprays, 482
- miscellaneous products, 482-483
- patient assessment, 479
- patient counseling, 479
- vaginal douches, 481-482

Feminine deodorant products
See **Feminine cleansing and deodorant products**

Feminine pads, 84-85
Femiron Multivitamins and Iron, 755, 766
Fendol, 684
Feosol, 266 (text table)
Feosol Capsules, 755
Feosol Elixir, 755
Feosol Tablets, 755
Feostat Chewable Tablets, 755
Feostat Drops, 755
Feostat Suspension, 755
Fergon Tablets, 755
Fer-In-Sol Iron Capsules, 755
Fer-In-Sol Iron Drops, 755
Fer-In-Sol Iron Syrup, 755
Fero-Grad-500 Tablets, 755
Fero-Gradumet Tablets, 755
Ferra-TD Capsules, 755
Ferro-Sequels Tablets, 755
Ferrous Fumarate Tablets, 755
Ferrous Gluconate Capsules, 755
Ferrous Gluconate Tablets, 755
Ferrous Sulfate Capsules, 756
Ferrous Sulfate Elixir, 756
Ferrous Sulfate Tablets, 756

Fertility
- caffeine, 144
- interval calculation, 455 (text table)

Fever, 93
- antipyretics/analgesics, 109-110
- common cold, 95-96
- complications, 68-69
- definition, 65
- drug-induced, 67 (text table), 67-68
- effects, 65
- etiology, 65, 66
- pathophysiology, 65-66
- patient assessment, 65
- patient education, 73-74
- perception, 65
- pharmacologic agents, 71-73
- product selection guidelines, 73
- symptoms, 65
- treatment, 65, 71
- treatment, nondrug, 71, 74

See also **Body temperature**
Feverall, 73
Feverall, Children's Suppositories, 661
Feverall, Infant's Suppositories, 661
Feverall, Junior Strength Suppositories, 661

Fever blisters
See **Cold sores**
Fiberall, 731
Fiberall, Natural, 731
Fiberall, Oatmeal Raisin Or Fruit & Nut, 731
FiberCon, 731
Fibersource, 751
Fibersource HN, 751
Filibon, 766
Firmdent, 816
First Response 1-Step Pregnancy Test, 643
First Response Ovulation Predictor Test, 642
First Response Pregnancy Test, 643
Fisherman's Friend, extra strong formula, 708
Fisherman's Friend, mint, 708
Fisherman's Friend, original extra strong, 708
Fish oil, 540
Fistula, 440
Fixodent, 816
Fixodent Fresh, 816
Flagyl, 204, 480, 505
Flanders Buttocks Ointment, 854
Flavoring agents, 414, 415, 426
Fleas, 597
Fleet Babylax, 731
Fleet Bagenema with Soap Packet, 731
Fleet Bisacodyl Enema, 732
Fleet DeteCAtest, 42
Fleet enemas, 228
Fleet Laxative Tablets, 732
Fleet Mineral Oil Enema, 732
Fleet Prep Kit 1, 732
Fleet Prep Kit 3, 732
Fleet Prep Kit 4, 732
Fleet Prep Kit 5, 732
Fleet Ready-to-Use Enema, 732
Fleet Ready-to-Use Enema for Children, 732
Fleet Relief Medicated Hemorrhoidal Ointment, 825
Fletcher's Castoria, 732
Fletcher's Children's Laxative Cherry Flavor, 732
Flex-all Pain Relieving Gel, 856
Flexcare, 385, 805
Flexural psoriasis, 534
Flintstones Complete, 768
Flintstones Plus Extra C, 768
Flintstones Plus Iron, 768
Flintstones Vitamins, 768
Florical, 759
Flu, 93
See also **Influenza**
Flu, Cold and Cough Medicine, 684
Fluconazole, 508
Flukes, 213, 217
Fluocinolone acetonide, 593
Fluoride, 414, 415, 416, 418-419
- breast-feeding, 19
- children, 428
- dosage, 320 (text table)
- elderly persons, 425
- public water supply, 419
- studies of fluoride dentifrices, 420 (text table)
- supplements for infants, 319-320

Fluoride gels, 420
Fluorigard, 419
Fluorigard Anti-Cavity Fluoride Rinse, 814
Fluorine
- adverse effects, 304-305
- description, 304
- dose/RDA, 304
Fluoroperm 92, 370 (text table)
Fluoroquinolones, 203, 205, 207
FoilleCort, 870
Foille Medicated First Aid, 860
Foille Plus, 860
Folacin
See **Folic acid**
Folic acid
- adverse effects, 295
- description, 294
- dose/RDA, 294-295
- drug interactions, 295
- indications, 294
- preterm infant requirements, 320

Folk remedies
- warts, 616
Folliculitis, 497
- treatment, 499
Food, Drug, and Cosmetic Act, 21
- amendments, 23-24
Food and Drug Administration
- labeling regulations, 7, 18
- OTC product review, 6, 21-37
Food supplement product table, 751-754
Foot Care Products, 609-634
- patient assessment, 609
- patient counseling, 609
- patient education and consultation, 625
Footwear
- athlete's foot, 625
- diabetic patients, 627
- exercise, 632
Foreign objects in the ear, 394
- patient assessment, 397

Formula 44 Cough Mixture, 684
Formula 44 Pediatric Cough Medicine, 684
Formula 44D Decongestant Cough Mixture, 684
Formula 44d Pediatric Cough and Decongestant Medicine, 684
Formula 44e Cough and Expectorant Medicine, 684
Formula 44e Pediatric Cough and Expectorant Medicine, 684
Formula 44M Multisymptom Cough and Cold Medicine, 684
Formula 44m Pediatric Multisymptom Cough & Cold Medicine, 684
Formula 405 Solar Lotion, 864
Formula for infants and children product table, 790-794
Formulation R, 825
Forta Drink, 751
Forta Shake, 751
Fortel, 642
Fostex 10% BPO, 836
Fostex 10% BPO Wash, 837
Fostex Medicated, 837
Fostex Medicated Cleansing, 837
Fostril, 837
Fourex, 823
405 Solar Cream, 862
4-Way Fast Acting, Menthol and Regular, 704
4-Way Long Lasting, 704
Fractured teeth, 421
Frangula, 227
Freckles, 486
Freezone Solution Corn and Callus Remover, 877
Fresh N' Brite, 427
Frostbite, 629-630
Frozen Nutritious Pudding, 751
Fructose, 190, 256-257, 346, 418
Fruity Chews, 768
Fruity Chews With Iron, 768
Fungal infections
- ear, 393
- skin, 497-498, 502-503, 533, 544
- treatment, 399
FungiCure, 832
Furazolidone, 206
Furuncles, 497
- treatment, 499

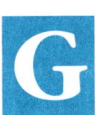

Gamma benzene hexachloride, 598
Gamma interferon, 540

Gardnerella vaginalis, 480, 504
Garfield Complete Vitamins with Minerals, 768
Garfields Tea, 733
Garfield Vitamins Plus Extra C, 768
Garfield Vitamins Plus Iron, 768
Garfield Vitamins, Regular, 770
Gargles, 109
Gas
 treatment, 190
Gas Permeable Comfort Drops, 802
Gastric acid, 147-149
 secretion, 149
Gastric lavage, 184, 185, 186, 187
Gastric mucosal barrier, 149
 factors disrupting, 149-150
Gastric ulcer, 148 (figure), 155 (text table)
 clinical presentation, 164
 complications, 165
 diagnosis, 165
 maintenance therapy, 165
 pathogenesis, 164
 treatment, 165
Gastrin, 148
Gastrinoma, 149
Gastritis, 169-170
 acute erosive, 170
 chronic nonerosive, 170-171
 treatment, 175
Gastrocolic reflex, 221
Gastroenteritis
 treatment, 208
Gastroesophageal reflux, 165, 189
 clinical presentation, 167
 complications, 167
 diagnosis, 167
 maintenance therapy, 169
 management, 168 (text table)
 pathogenesis, 166
 treatment, 167-169, 175
Gastrointestinal disease
 pathogenesis, 149-150
Gastrointestinal irritation
 aspirin, 53, 56, 62
Gastrointestinal system
 antacids, 161-173
 caffeine, 142
 disorders, 155 (text table)
Gastrointestinal tract
 bleeding, 42-43, 162
 pathophysiology, 221
 physiology, 147-149, 219-221
Gastrolyte, 190, 209
Gas-X, 717
Gas-X Extra Strength, 717
Gatorade, 190
Gaultheria oil, 556
Gaviscon, 718
Gaviscon-2, 718
Gaviscon Cool Mint Flavor, 718
Gaviscon ESR, 718
Gaviscon ESRF, 718
Gels, 559
Gelusil, 718
Gemnisyn, 649, 661

Genac, 684
Genahist, 684
Genamin, 684
Genapap, Children's Chewable, 649, 661
Genapap, Children's Elixir, 649, 661
Genapap Extra Strength, 649, 661
Genapap, Infants' Drops, 649, 661
Genaphed, 684
Genasal, 705
Genasoft, 733
Genasoft Plus, 733
Genaspor, 832, 879
Genatap, 686
Genatuss, 686
Genatuss DM, 686
Gen-Bee with C, 770
Gencold, 686
Gendecon, 686
Genebs, 649, 661
Genebs Extra Strength, 649, 661
Generalized juvenile periodontitis, 417
Generally recognized as safe and effective ingredients, 21, 344 (text table)
Generet-500 Tablets, 756
Generix-T, 770
Genex, 686
GenFiber, 733
Genital herpes, 498
Genite, 686
Genpril, 649, 661
Genprin, 649, 661
Gensan, 649, 661
Gentian Violet, 832
Gentian violet, 215
Gentz Wipes, 825
Gerber Baby Formula Low Iron, 790
Gerber Baby Formula with Iron, 790
Gerber Baby Formula with Soy, 790
Gerber Meat Base Formula, 310
GERD
 See **Gastroesophageal reflux**
Gerimed, 759, 770
Geriot Tablets, 756
Geriplex-FS, 770
Geriplex-FS Kapseals, 770
Geritol, 770
Geritol Complete, 770
Geritol Extend, 770
German measles, 94-95
Gevral T, 770
GG-Cen, 684
Ghostbusters Anti-Cavity Dental Rinse, 419
Giardia lamblia, 204, 206
Gingivitis, 259-260
 etiology and pathophysiology, 416-417
Glandosane Synthetic Saliva, 426
Glaucoma, 356-357
Gleem Toothpaste, 810

Glipizide
 drug interactions, 55
Glucerna, 751
Glucolet Automatic Device, 750
Glucometer Elite Diabetes Care System, 750
Glucometer Elite Test Strips, 746
Glucometer III, 750
Glucose, 190, 208
 blood, 238
 insulin, 250 (figure)
 intolerance, 239 (text table), 245
Glucose test
 false reactions, 267 (text table)
 substances that interfere with, 266 (text table)
Glucostix, 748
Glucotrol, 248 (text table)
Glue ear
 See **Chronic otitis media**
Glutaraldehyde, 485
Glutose Gel, 744
Glutose Tablets, 744
Glyburide
 drug interactions, 55
Glycerin, 401, 414, 474, 528, 546, 606
Glycerin, 733
Glycerin soaps, 527
Glycerin suppositories, 226, 229, 230
Glyceryl monostearate, 530
Glycine, 209
Glycopyrrolate, 124, 125
Glynase PresTab, 248 (text table)
Gly-Oxide, 416, 814
Gold Circle, 823
Golytely, 229
Gonorrhea, 459, 461, 463-464
Goody's Extra Strength, 649
Goody's Headache Powder, 649
Gordon's Vite A, 846
Gordo-Vite E, 846, 860
Gormel, 846
Gout, 245
Granuloma gluteale infantum, 545
GRASE
 See **Generally recognized as safe and effective ingredients**
Group therapy
 obesity, 347
Growth factors, 444, 445
 influencing wound healing, 443 (text table)
Guaifenesin, 105
 breast-feeding, 19
Guaifenesin Syrup USP, 686
Guaiphed, 712
Guanethidine
 adverse effects, 206
Guttate psoriasis, 534
Gynecoid fat distribution, 339
Gyne-cort, 828
Gyne-cort Extra Strength 10, 828

Gyne-Lotrimin Cream, 832
Gyne-Lotrimin Tablets, 832
Gyne-moistrin, 83
Gyne-Moistrin Vaginal Moisturizing Gel, 828
Gynol II, 822
Gynol II ES, 822

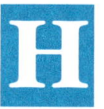

Habitrol, 630
Haemophilus **vaginitis**, 480
Hair
 hair grower/hair loss prevention, 27
 physiology, 490
Hair follicles, 494
Hair growth, 488
Hair removal methods, 488-490, 489 (text table)
Haleys M-O, 733
Halitosis
 etiology, 425
 treatment, 425
Halls Menthol-Lyptus, 708
Halls Plus Center-Filled Drops, 708
Halls Soothers, Center-Filled Drops, 708
Hallux valgus, 612 (figure)
Halobetasol, 540
Halogenated salicylanilides, 27
Haloperidol, 515
Haloprogin, 503, 547
Halothane, 515
Haltran Tablets, 667
Hamamelis **water**, 529, 606
Hand dermatitis, 526
Hangover, 173
H_2-antagonists
 acid-peptic disorders, 159
 gastroesophageal reflux, 169
 ulcers, 163
Hard and rigid gas-permeable lens product table, 802-803
Hawaiian Tropic Baby Faces Sunblock, 864
Hawaiian Tropic Dark Tanning With Sunscreen, 864
Hawaiian Tropic 15 Plus Sunblock, 864
Hawaiian Tropic 30 Plus Sunblock, 864
Hay fever, 89, 92, 95
HC-DermaPax, 870, 873
Headaches
 common cold, 95-96
 etiology, 50-51
 symptoms, 50-51
 treatment, 51
Head & Shoulders Dandruff Shampoo, 850
Head & Shoulders Intensive Treatment, 851
Health Shake, 751

General Index 897

Hearing disorders, 396-397
See also **Deaf or hearing impaired persons**; **Ear conditions**; **Hearing loss**
Hearing loss
  five minute hearing test, 403 (text table), 404
  obstructive, 396-397
  patient assessment, 389, 398
  patient counseling, 389
Heart attacks, 238
  aspirin prophylaxis, 56-57
Heartburn, 167, 175, 176
  treatment, 189, 190
Heart disease
  caffeine, 141
  fevers, 68
Heating pads, 554
Heat lamps, 554
Heat stroke, 66-67, 569
Heel pain, 631
Heet, 856
Helicobacter pylori, 149-150
  antacids, 151
  elderly persons, 174
  gastritis, 170-171
  nonulcer dyspepsia, 172-173
  ulcers, 161, 163, 164, 165
Helminthic infections
  See **Worm infections**
Hema-Combistix, 748
Hemagglutination inhibition reaction tests, 45
Hemet Hemorrhoidal, 825
Hemet Rectal, 825
Hemoccult Home Test, 42
Hemoccult Sensa, 641
Hemoccult II, 641
Hemorrhoidal Products, 469-478
  biopharmaceutical considerations, 477
  patient assessment, 469, 472-473
  patient considerations, 477
  patient counseling, 469
  product consideration, 477
  selection guidelines, 477
Hemorrhoidal product table, 825-827
Hemorrhoids
  antacids, 176
  etiology, 471
  external, 471
  internal, 471
  surgical treatments, 476
Hem-Prep, 825
Herb-Lax, 733
Herpecin-L, 817
Herpes
  contact lenses, 373
Herpes simplex, 464, 498, 545
Herpes simplex labialis, 422, 423, 577
Herpes simplex type 1 virus, 422, 423
Herpes simplex type 2 virus, 422, 423
Herpesvirus hominis, 498
Herpetiform diaper dermatitis, 545
Herpetrol, 770
Hexachlorophene, 546

Hexylresorcinol, 110, 422, 501-502
Hibiclens Liquid & Sponge Brush, 832
Hibistat, 832
High Protein Broth, 751
High Protein Gelatin, 752
Hirsutism, 488
Histamine dihydrochloride, 557
Histatab Plus, 686
HIV
  See **Human immunodeficiency virus**
Hold, 708
Holdease, 742
HoliHesive Skin Barrier Blanket, 820
HoliSeal Skin Barrier Blanket, 820
HolliHesive wafers, 437
Homatropine methylbromide, 209
Hookworm infection
  epidemiology, 216
  etiology, 216
  symptoms, 216-217
  treatment, 217
  See also **Worm infections**
Hordeolum, 353, 354
Horehound, 108
Hormones
  female cycle, 43-44
Hornets, 600, 601
Hot-water bottles, 554
H-R Lubricating Jelly, 828
Huggies, 548
Human Breast Milk, Mature, 790
Human immunodeficiency virus, 324, 509, 545
  contact lenses, 373
  diarrhea and, 206
  epidemiology, 463
  protection against, 455, 459, 461, 463
  transmission, 463
  treatment, 173
  See also **Acquired immunodeficiency syndrome**
Human milk fortifiers, 331
Humectants, 414, 415, 528
Humidification, 110
HuMIST Saline, 707
Humphrey's No. 11, 667
Humulin, 250
Humulin 50/50 (50% NPH Isophane Susp., 50% Regular Inj.), 741
Humulin 70/30 (70% NPH Isophane Susp., 30% Regular Inj.), 741
Humulin BR, 250, 251, 263
Humulin L (Lente Human Insulin Zinc Suspension), 739
Humulin N (NPH Human Insulin Isophane Suspension), 739
Humulin R (Regular Human Insulin), 739
Humulin U (Ultralente Human Insulin Extended Zinc Susp.), 741
Hurricaine, aerosol, 817

Hurricaine, gel, 817
Hurricaine, liquid, 817
Hydantoins
  pregnancy, 18
Hydragran, 447 (text table)
Hydra-Mat II, 378
Hydramine Cough, 686
Hydration, 632
Hydriotic acid, 105-106
Hydrisinol, 846
Hydrocarbon ingestion, 187
Hydrochloric acid, 426-427
Hydrocil Instant, 733
Hydrocortisone, 841, 870, 873
Hydrocortisone, 547, 604
  anorectal, 475
  children, 546
  dosage, 594
  insect bites, 606
  reclassification, 30-31
  side effects, 539
  topical, 530, 533, 538-539, 540, 546, 571, 572, 593, 594
  vaginal, 483
Hydrocortisone Cream 0.5%, 841, 873
Hydrocortisone Maximum Strength Cream 1%, 842, 874
Hydrocurve II, 372 (text table)
Hydrocurve II Toric, 372 (text table)
Hydrogen peroxide, 422, 423, 424, 501
Hydron Sero 4 Sof Blue, 372 (text table)
Hydrophilic colloid bulk laxatives, 222-223
Hydro Pik, 412
Hydroquinone, 487-488
Hydroxychloroquine
  hyperpigmentation, 486
Hydroxyquinoline, 547
8-hydroxyquinoline sulfate, 606-607
Hydroxyurea, 540
Hymenoptera, 600-601, 604
Hyoscyamine sulfate, 209
Hyperbilirubinemia, 324
Hypercalcemia, 302
Hyperglycemia, 269
  alcohol, 257
  diabetes mellitus, 239
  drugs that cause, 246 (text table)
  exercise, 254
  harmful effects, 241 (text table), 242, 243
Hyperhidrosis
  See **Wetness**
Hyperosmotic laxatives, 226
Hyperosmotics, 361-362
Hyperphosphatemia, 303
Hyperpigmentation
  syndromes, 486-487
  treatment, 487-488
Hyperplasia, 440-441
Hypersensitive teeth
  etiology, 421
  treatment, 421
Hypersensitivity reactions, 101, 354
  iodine, 106
  See also **Allergies**

Hypersensitization, 99
Hypertension, 39-40
  decongestants, 104
Hyperthermia
  etiology, 66
  symptoms, 66
  treatment, 67
Hypervitaminosis A, 289
Hypervitaminosis D, 291
Hypnotics, 135
  indications, 138
  pharmacokinetic and clinical properties, 138 (text table)
  poisoning, 186
  See also names of specific drugs in this class
Hypocalcemia, 301
Hypochlorite denture cleansers, 426
Hypoglycemia, 247, 269
  alcohol, 257
  drugs that cause, 246 (text table)
  exercise, 254-255
  psychologic changes, 245
  symptoms, 253
Hypoglycemic drugs
  drug interactions, 55
Hypoglycemics, 576
Hypolet Auto Lancet Device, 750
Hypomagnesemia, 302
Hyposensitization therapy
  allergic contact dermatitis, 592-593
Hypotears Drops, 797
Hypotears Ointment, 797
Hypotears PF Drops, 797
Hypothalamus, 43
Hytinic Capsules, 756
Hytinic Injections, 756
Hytone, 842, 870
Hytuss, 686
Hytuss 2X, 686

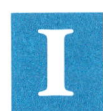

Iberet Filmtabs, 756
Iberet-500 Filmtabs, 756
Iberet Liquid, 756
Iberet-500 Liquid, 756
Ibufen-200, 649
Ibuprin Tablets, 650
Ibuprofen, 51, 52, 71, 95, 420, 422
  acne treatment, 518
  antipyretic activity, 71-72
  breast-feeding, 19, 60
  burn treatment, 571
  comparative efficacy, 60-61
  dosage, 59, 73 (text table), 83
  dosage, children, 73 (text table)
  drug interactions, 60, 62
  overdose, 60
  pregnancy, 60
  reclassification, 23, 33

side effects, 59-60, 62, 67 (text table), 83-84
use considerations, 59-60, 62, 72, 73
Ibuprofen-200, 650
Ice bags, 632-633
Ichthammol, 401, 572, 605
Ichthyosis vulgaris, 527
Icy Hot Extra Strength Long-Lasting Balm Pain Reliever, 856
Identification tags, 267
Ileostomy, 435 (figure), 485
components of an appliance, 439 (figure)
new procedures, 436
physical complications, 434
reasons for, 434
Illiterate persons
communicating with, 13
Imidazole, 360-361, 505, 507
Immunosuppressive drugs
adverse effects, 424
Immunotherapy
allergies, 99
Imodium, 207, 723
Imodium A-D, 207, 723
Impact, 752
Impact with Fiber, 752
Impetigo, 496-497
treatment, 499
Incremin With Iron Syrup, 756
Indigestion
patient assessment, 181, 187-189
treatment, 181, 188, 189
Indocin, 442 (text table)
Infalyte, 190
Infalyte Powder, 332
Infant Formula Act of 1980, 325
Infant Formula Products, 313-338
caloric density, 326
for children aged 1-6 years, 332
diarrhea, 332
dilution, 333 (text table)
formula preparation, 333-335, 334 (text table)
gastrointestinal problems, 332
for infants with metabolic diseases, 328 (text table), 331
microbiologic safety, 325-326
microwave oven warming, 334-335
milk-based, 328
milk-based with added whey protein, 328
nutritional deficiencies, 332-333
osmolality, 326
osmolarity, 326
patient assessment, 313
patient counseling, 313
renal solute load, 326, 328
selection guidelines, 335-336
therapeutic, 327 (text table), 328-332
tooth decay, 332

Infants
amino acid requirements, 316 (text table), 316-317
carbohydrate requirements, 316
diaper rash, 543-549
dietary allowances of nutrients, 314 (text table)
fat requirements, 317
feeding guidelines, 335, 335 (tables)
fluid requirements, 316
formulas, 313-336
growth, 315
nutritional recommendations, 315 (text table)
physiology, 314-315
preterm, 320, 331
prickly heat, 543-549
protein requirements, 316
recommended dietary allowances, 315
seborrhea capitis, 532
vitamin and mineral requirements, 317-318
vitamin and mineral supplements, 318-320
See also **Children**
Infection
ostomy-associated, 441
See also **Oral infections**; **Monilial infections**; **Worm infections**
Inflammation
anal, 472
Inflammatory papillary hyperplasia, 426
Influenza, 92, 93-94
Reye's syndrome, 96
symptoms, 94 (text table)
Infusaid, 264
Ingrown toenails
products, 621 (text table)
Inhal-Aid, 130
Inhalers
correct use, 129-130, 130 (text table), 133
In-Home Testing and Monitoring Products, 39-47
future, 46
patient counseling, 39, 41-42, 43, 44-46
Inject-Ease, 742
Injectomatic, 742
Innerclean Herbal, 733
Inositol, 300
infant requirements, 318
Insect bites
neutralizers, 605-606
reactions, 601
treatment, 603-607
types, 597-600
Insect repellent product table, 876
Insect repellents, 27, 607
Insect Sting and Bite Products, 597-608
patient assessment, 597
patient counseling, 597
selection guidelines, 607
Insect sting and bite product table, 873-874

Insect stings, 600-601
allergic reactions, 601-603
emergency kits, 603-604
preventive measures, 603
treatment, 603-607
Insomnia, 135
alcohol, 140
classification and assessment, 136-137
drugs that exacerbate, 136 (text table)
etiology, 137 (text table)
L-tryptophan, 139-140
InspirEase, 130
Insta-Glucose Liquid, 744
Instaject, 742
Instant Breakfast, 310, 752
Insulatard, 250
Insulatard NPH (Isophane Purified Pork Insulin Suspension), 739
Insulatard NPH Human (Insulin Isophane Susp., semi-synth.), 740
Insul-eze, 742
Insulgage, 742
Insulin, 238, 247-254
adverse reactions, 253-254
glucose and, 250 (figure)
infusion pumps, 263-264
injection, 252, 253 (figure)
injection sites, 252 (figure)
ketoacidosis, 248-249
preparations, 249-250
reaction, 267
regimens, 250-253
See also **Diabetes**; **Diabetes mellitus**
Insulin-Aid, 742
Insulin Dilution Fluid, 251
Insulin infusion pumps, 263-264
Insulin Needle Guide, 742
Insulin preparations product table, 739-741
Insulin syringes and related products table, 742-743
Insulin Syringe, Single Use Lo-Dose, 742
Intermetatarsal neuritis, 631
Internal Analgesic Products, 49-64
conditions responsive to, 50-52
options, 52-61
patient assessment, 49-50
patient counseling, 49
selection guidelines, 61-62
Internal analgesic product table, 644-656
Interplak Home Plaque Removal Instrument, 412
Interplak toothpaste, 412
Interplak Toothpaste with Fluoride, 810
Intestinal tract
physiology, 199-200
Intrauterine device, 453, 480
Introlite, 752
Iodex-P, 832
Iodex Regular, 832
Iodides, 105-106, 515
Iodinated glycerol, 105-106

Iodine, 501
adverse effects, 305
description, 305
dose/RDA, 305
drug interactions, 305
Iodine, Strong, 833
Iodine Tincture, 832
Iodine Tincture, Strong, 833
Iodine Topical, 833
Iodism, 305
Iodochlorhydroxyquin, 488
Iodophors, 501
Iodoquinol
dosage, 206
Ionil, 851
Ionil Plus, 851
Ionil T, 842, 851
Ionil T Plus, 566 (text table), 842
Ipecac, 106
abuse, 182, 185, 188-189
comparative efficacy, 185, 187
dosage, 184
drug interactions, 185
expired, 185
poisoning treatment, 182, 184-185, 187, 190
recommended procedure, 184-185
toxicity, 185
Ipratropium, 124, 125
Iron
adverse effects, 307
deficiency stages, 306
description, 305
dose/RDA, 306-307
drug interactions, 307
indications, 305-306
infant requirements, 318
preterm infant requirements, 320
supplements for infants, 319
Iron oxide, 595
Iron Plus Caplets, 756
Iron product table, 755-757
Iron supplements, 217, 319
Irospan Capsules, 756
Irospan Tablets, 756
Irrigants, 361
Irritant contact dermatitis, 525
Isocal, 752
Isocal HCN, 752
Isocal HN, 752
Isoclor, 686
Isoclor Timesules, 686
Isodettes Sort Throat Lozenges, 708
Isodettes Spray, 814
Isomil, 209, 328, 329, 790
Isomil SF, 329, 790
Isoniazid, 515
Isopropyl alcohol, 500-501
Isopropyl Alcohol, 91%, 742
Isopto Alkaline, 797
Isopto-Frin, 799
Isopto Plain, 797
Isopto Tears, 797
Isosource, 752
Isosource HN, 752
Isospora belli, 206
Isotein HN, 752
Isotretinoin, 514
acne treatment, 518

I-Soyalac, 329, 790
Itching
 anal, 471-472
 of the ear, 393
 See also **Dermatitis**; **Dry skin**; **Prickly heat**; **Rhus dermatitis**
Itch-X, 874
IUD
 See **Intrauterine device**
Ivarest, 870
Ivy-Chex, 871
Ivy Dry Cream, 870
Ivy Dry Liquid, 870
Ivy Super Dry, 871

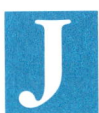

Jarisch-Herxheimer reaction, 68
Jejunal, 310
Jevity, 752
Jock itch, 497, 533, 620
Johnson's Foot Soap, 877
Joint pain, 555
 epidemiology, 52
 etiology, 52
 treatment, 52
Juniper tar, 474, 475
Just One Per Day, 796
Just Tears, 797

Kaltostat, 447 (text table)
Kank-A Liquid Professional Strength, 818
Kank-A Mouth Sore Medication, 818
Kaolin, 546
Kaolin-pectin
 breast-feeding, 19
Kaolin Pectin Suspension, 723
Kaopectate, 210, 723
Kaopectate Children's Chewable Tablets, 723
Kaopectate Children's Liquid, 723
Kaopectate Concentrated, 724
Kaopectate II, 724
Kao-Spen, 723
Kapectolin, 724
Karaya Gum, 820
Kasof, 733
Kawasaki syndrome, 545
K-C, 723
Keep Alert, 715
Kellogg's Tasteless Castor Oil, 733
Kenalog, 593
Keratin-softening agents, 528-529
Keratitis, 356

Keratolytic agents, 537-538
 anorectal, 475
Keratosis obturans, 393-394
Kericort HC Cream 1%, 842, 871, 874
Keri Facial Soap, 846
Keri Lotion, 83, 846
Keri Silky-Fragrance Free, 846
Keri Silky Smooth, 846
Ketoacidosis, 238, 239, 248-249
 testing, 266
Ketoconazole, 508, 518
Keto-Diastix, 748
Ketostix, 266, 748
Ketotifen, 128
K.I.K., 815
Klebsiella, 567, 627
Kleenite, 815
Kondremul, 733
Konsyl, 230
Koromex, 822
Koromex Crystal Clear, 822
Koromex Jelly, 822
Kudrox, 718
Kwashiorkor, 286
K-Y Jelly, 70, 83, 461, 462

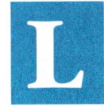

Labeling
 example, 35 (figure)
 FDA regulations, 7, 34, 36
 monographs, 22, 27
 NDMA guidelines, 7
Labstix, 748
Lacril, 797
Lactase enzymes, 210
Lactation
 See **Breast-feeding**
Lactational infertility, 458-459
Lacti-Care, 846
Lactobacillus, 480, 504, 505
Lactobacillus acidophilus, 209, 210, 423
Lactobacillus bulgaricus, 209, 210, 423
Lactobacillus casei, 418
***Lactobacillus* preparations**
 efficacy, 210
 side effects, 210
Lactofree, 790
Lactogest, 319
Lactose, 210, 418
Lactose intolerance, 203, 209, 210
Lactrase, 210
Lactulose, 230
Laetrile, 300
Lagol, 860
Lagol Oil, 833
Lanabiotic Ointment, 833
Lanacane, 860, 871
Lanacane Creme, 825, 871
Lanacort, 842
Lanacort 5, 871
Lanacort 10, 842, 871, 874

Lanolin, 528, 546
Lantiseptic Ointment, 547
Larynex, 708
Laryngitis, 89, 93
 treatment, 95-96
Lassar's paste, 529, 546, 547
Lauro Eye Wash, 801
LAVATAR, 566 (text table)
Lavatar, 842
Lavoptik Eye Wash, 801
Lavoris, 814
Laxative abuse, 206, 230, 234
Laxative Products, 219-236
 patient assessment, 219, 234
 patient counseling, 219, 235
 selection guidelines, 235
Laxative product table, 727-738
Laxatives, 441
 abuse, 206, 230, 234
 breast-feeding, 19
 bulk-forming, 222-223, 230, 475
 children, 229
 classification and properties, 224-225 (text table)
 dependence, 229
 dietary fiber, 231-233 (text table)
 dosage forms, 228-229
 dosages, 224-225 (text table)
 elderly persons, 229-230
 emollient, 223
 hyperosmotic, 226
 lubricant, 225-226
 pregnancy, 230
 saline, 226
 stimulants, 226-228
 See also **Constipation**
Lax-Pills, 733
Lazer Creme, 846
LBC-LAX, 733
LC-65 Daily Contact Lens Cleaner, 802
Lecithin, 299
Legatrin, 650
Lens Drops, 806
Lensept, 805
Lens Lubricant, 803, 806
Lens Plus Daily Cleaner, 804
Lens Plus Oxysept 2 Rinse and Neutralizer, 805
Lens Plus Rewetting Drops, 806
Lens Plus Sterile Saline Solution, 807
Lente (Insulin Zinc Suspension, Beef), 740
Lente (Purified Pork Insulin Zinc Suspension), 740
Lente Iletin I (Insulin Zinc Suspension), 740
Lente Iletin II (Insulin Zinc Suspension, Purified Pork), 740
Lentigines, 486
Levodesoxyephedrine, 103
Levulose
 See **Fructose**
Lice
 body, 599
 eyelid, 354
 head, 598
 pubic, 599
Lice-Enz, 875
Lice Treatment, 875

Licide Control, 875
Licide Shampoo, 875
Lidocaine
 anorectal, 473
 burn treatment, 571
Lid Wipes - SPF, 801
Lincomycin, 205
Lindane, 598
Liniments, 559
Linoleic acid, 299-300
 infant requirements, 317, 322
Linolenic acid, 299-300
Lipisorb, 752
Lip Medex, ointment, 818
Lipodystrophy, 254
Lipovite, 770
Lip protection, 585
Liquid dishwashing detergent
 emetic agent, 186
Liqui-Doss, 733
Liquid petrolatum, 225-226
Liquifilm Forte, 798
Liquifilm Tears Drops, 798
Liquifilm Wetting Solution, 803
Liquiprin Infants' Drops, 650, 661
Lisadimate, 580
Listening techniques, 13
Listerex Scrub, Golden & Herbal, 837
Listerine, 415
Listerine, 814
Listerine Coolmint, 814
Listermint With Fluoride, 814
Lithium, 515
 drug interactions, 60
Liver spots, 486
Live yeast cell derivative, 546
Load-Matic, 742
Local anesthetics, 594, 605
 anorectal, 473
 burns, 571
 side effects, 594
Localized juvenile periodontitis, 417
Lomotil, 208
Lonalac, 752
Loperamide
 dosage, 207, 209
 efficacy, 209
 reclassification, 23
 side effects, 209
Loperamide Hydrochloride Solution, 724
Loratidine, 128
Loroxide, 837
Losopan, 718
Losopan Plus, 718
Lotion-Jel, 818
Lotions, 559, 572
Lotrimin AF Cream, 833
Lotrimin AF Cream & Solution, 880
Lotrimin AF Lotion, 833
Lotrimin AF Solution, 833
Lotrimin Cream, 880
Lotrimin Jock Itch, 833
Low birthweight infants
 formulas, 331
Low-calorie balanced foods, 346
Lowila Cake, 846

Lowsium, 718
Lowsium Plus, 718
Low-sodium infant formulas, 331
Lozenge product table, 708-710
Lozenges, 109, 155
Lubrasceptic Jelly, 833
Lubricant laxatives, 225-226
Lubricants
  dosage, 83
  ophthalmic, 358-360
Lubriderm, 83, 846
Lubriderm Lubath, 846
Lubriderm, Unscented, 847
Lubrin, 462
Lugol's iodine solution, 501
Lumiscope Model 1081 Blood Pressure Monitor, 639
Lumiscope Model 1083 Blood Pressure Monitor, 639
Lumiscope Model 1091 Blood Pressure Monitor with Printer, 639
Lumiscope Model 1096 Blood Pressure Monitor with Printer, 639
Lupus erythematosus, 577
Lurline PMS Tablets, 650, 667
Luvs, 548
Lyme disease, 599-600
LYOfoam, 449 (text table)
LYOfoam "C" Odor Absorbent Dressing, 449 (text table)
L-lysine, 423
Lytren, 190, 332

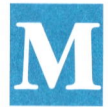

Maalox Caplets, 718
Maalox HRF, 718
Magaldrate, 154
Magnaprin, 650
Magnaprin Arthritis Strength, 650
Magnesia And Alumina Oral Suspension, 719
Magnesium, 153-154, 158, 441
  adverse effects, 302
  description, 302
  dose/RDA, 302
  drug interactions, 302
  indications, 302
  side effects, 205-206
Magnesium aluminum silicate, 530
Magnesium carbonate, 189
Magnesium hydroxide, 189
  breast-feeding, 19
Magnesium salicylate, 57
  See also **Salicylates**
Magnesium sulfate, 186, 226
Magni-Guide, 742
Mag-Ox 400, 719, 734
Malathion, 599
Malignancies
  caffeine, 144
  See also **Cancer**

Malignant neoplasm, 470-471
Malnutrition, 286
Malt soup extract, 223, 229
Mammol, 847
Manganese
  adverse effects, 308
  description, 307
  dose/RDA, 307
  drug interactions, 308
  indications, 307
  infant requirements, 318
Marasmus, 286
Marezine, 189, 722
Marshall Model 91 Automatic Inflation B.P. Monitor, 639
Marshall Model 94 Pressure Valve Preset B.P. Monitor, 639
Marshall Model 97 Measurement Print-out B.P. Monitor, 639
Marshall Model F-89 Finger Blood Pressure Monitor, 639
Massage, 554
Massengill Baking Soda Disposable Douche, 828
Massengill Disposable Douche Mountain Breeze Scent, 829
Massengill Douche Powder Floral & Unscented, 829
Massengill Medicated Disposable Douche, 829
Massengill Medicated Towelette, 829
Massengill Vinegar & Water Disposable Douch Extra Mild, 829
Mastisol, 820
Maxafil, 864
Maxair, 130
McNess Pain Tablets, 650
MCT Oil, 752
Measles, 94
Measurin, 56
Mebendazole
  dosage, 216, 217
  efficacy, 216
  pregnancy, 216
Meclizine, 189
  dosage, 189
Meclizine HCl, 722
Meclizine HCl Chewable, 722
MedicAlert identification bracelet, 267, 273
Medical Insulin Protector, 251
Medicone Rectal, 825, 826
Mediconet, 826
Medi-Flu, 686
Medi-Flu Without Drowsiness, 686
Medi-Let, 750
Medi-Quik First Aid Spray, 860
Medi-Quik Triple Antibiotic Ointment, 833
MediSense Lancing Device, 750
Medotar, 566 (text table)
Melanin, 486
Melanotropins, 583
Melasma, 486
Menadione, 291
Menadol Ibuprofen, USP, 650, 667
Menfegol-9, 459

Menorrhagia, 80-81
Menstrual cycle, 77-79, 79 (figure), 456 (figure)
  basal body temperature variations (figure), 457
  changing characteristics of cervical mucus, 458 (text table)
  iron loss, 306
Menstrual dysfunction, 79-82
  patient assessment, 83
Menstrual Products, 77-87
  patient assessment, 77, 82-83
  patient counseling, 77
Menstrual product table, 666-669
Menthol, 401, 415, 422, 423, 554, 594
  burn treatment, 572
  cold products, 106, 108
  counterirritant, 557
  hemorrhoids, 474, 475
  humidifier, 110
  insect bites, 605
Mentholatum Deep Heating Arthritis Formula, 857
Mentholatum Deep Heating Lotion, 857
Mentholatum Deep Heating Rub, 857
Mentholatum Lipbalm, 864
Mentholatum Ointment, 857
Menthol salicylate, 554
Menthylanthranilate, 580
Mentor, 823
Mentor Plus, 823
Merbromin, 501
Mercurial compounds, 501
Mercuric oxide, 362
Mercurochrome, 833
Meritene, 310, 752
Mersol, 833
Metaclopramide
  adverse effects, 206
Metamucil Fiber Wafers, Apple Crisp Flavor, 734
Metamucil Orig. Text., Effervescent/Sugar-Free/Lemon-Lime, 734
Metamucil Orig. Texture, Orange, 734
Metamucil Orig. Texture, Original Flavor, 734
Metamucil Smooth Texture, Citrus, 734
Metamucil Smooth Texture, Sugar Free, Regular Flavor, 734
Metaproterenol, 31-33
Metasep, 851
Meted, 851
Methacrylate, 427
Methotrexate, 539
  drug interactions, 55, 60, 62, 208
Methoxsalen, 539
Methylbenzethonium chloride, 502, 546
Methylcellulose, 530
Methyldopa
  adverse effects, 206
Methyl nicotinate, 557-558
Methylparaben, 358

Methylprednisolone, 593
Methyl salicylate, 415, 556, 605
Methylxanthine, 124, 141
Metrogel-Vaginal, 505
Metronidazole, 204, 206, 481, 505, 514
  dosage, 205, 206
Micatin, 880
Micatin Cream & Spray, 833
Miconazole, 503, 505
  reclassification, 23
  topical, 547
Miconazole nitrate, 620-621
Micronase, 248 (text table)
Micro NEFRIN, 711
Micropore, 263
Microporous cellulose, 546, 547
Microsporum, 497, 621
Midcycle bleeding, 81
Middle ear
  disorders, 395 (text table), 395-396
Midol For Cramps, Maximum Strength Caplets, 668
Midol IB, Cramp Relief Formula Caplets, 650, 668
Midol Menstrual, 668
Midol Menstrual, Maximum Strength Multisymptom Formula, 651, 668
Midol Menstrual, Regular Strength Multisymptom Formula, 651
Midol Multisymptom, 668
Midol PM, Nighttime Pain Reliever/Sleep Aid Caplets, 651, 668
Midol PMS Capsules, 651, 668
Midol Regular Strength, 668
Midol Teen, Multisymptom Formula Caplets, 651, 668
Midol 200, 667
Migraine headaches
  symptoms, 51
  treatment, 51
Migranol, 651
Miliaria rubra
  See **Prickly heat**
Milk
  allergic reaction, 321-322
  evaporated, 323
  goat milk, 323
  human milk and cow milk comparison, 320-322, 321 (text table)
  human milk fortifiers, 331
  reduced fat cow milk, 322
  renal solute loads, 323 (text table)
  whole cow milk, 322-323
  See also **Breast-feeding**; **Infant Formula Products**
Milk-alkali syndrome, 151-152
Milkinol, 735
Milk intolerance, 203, 209, 210
Milk of magnesia, 229
Milk Of Magnesia, 719, 734
Milk Of Magnesia-Cascara Suspension, Concentrated, 735

Milk Of Magnesia, Concentrated, 734
Milk Shake, 752
Milk Shake Plus, 752
Mineral Oil, 735
Mineral oil, 225-226, 229, 230, 546
Minerals, 300-303
  diabetes, 258
  recommended daily, 286 (text table)
  requirements for infants, 318
  supplements for infants, 318-320
  See also **Vitamins**
Minimal erythemal dose, 578
Minit-Rub, 857
Minocycline, 518
Mint Sensodyne, 421
Miraculin, 346
Mira Flow, 380, 384
Mira Flow Extra Strength, 804
Mira Sept, 805
Mirasoft, 385
Miscellaneous diabetes product table, 750
Miscellaneous nasal product table, 707
Misoprostol, 160-161
Mixtard (70% Isophane Pur. Pork Susp. & 30% Pur. Pork Inj.), 741
Mixtard Hum. 70/30 (70% Hu. Iso. Sus./30% Hu. Inj., sem-syn), 741
Mobigesic, 661
Modane, 735
Modane Plus, 735
Modane Soft, 735
Moducal, 310, 752
Moi-Stir 10, 813
Moi-Stir Mouth Moistener, 426
Moi-Stir Mouth Moistening Spray, 813
Moi-Stir Oral Swabsticks, 426, 813
Moisture Barrier Skin Ointment, 821
Moisture Drops, 798
Moisturel Cream, 847
Moisturel Lotion, 847
Moisturel Sensitive Skin, 847
Moisturizers, 527-528
Moleskin, 612
Mol-Iron Tablets, 756
Mollifene Ear Drops, 808
Molluscum contagiosum, 498
Molybdenum
  adverse effects, 308
  description, 308
  dose/RDA, 308
  drug interactions, 308
  indications, 308
Momentum, 651
Monellin, 346
Monilial infections, 258-259, 440
  diabetes, 244-245
Moniliasis
  See **Candidiasis**
Monistat 7 Cream, 833
Monistat 7 Suppository, 833

Monitoring Products, 39-47
  future, 46
  patient counseling, 39, 41-42
Monoamine oxidase inhibitors, 104, 139
Monobenzone, 487, 488
Monoclonal antibody tests, 45
Monographs, 22
  components, 25, 27
  nighttime sleep aid drug products, 26 (figure), 27
Monoject Ultra Comfort Insulin Syringe, 29 Gauge, 743
Monoject Ultra Comfort Insulin Syringe, 28 Gauge, 742
Monojel Glucose Gel, 744
Monolets, 750
Morning breath, 415, 425
Morning sickness, 181, 182, 188
Morphine, 181
Mosco Liquid, 877
Mosquitoes, 597
Motion sickness, 181
  children, 188
  etiology, 182
  symptoms, 188
  treatment, 188, 189, 190
Motrin IB, 651, 661
MouthKote, 813
Mouth Kote-OR, solution, 818
Mouth Kote-PR, ointment, 818
Mouth Kote-PR, solution, 818
Mouth Kote Toothpaste, 810
Mouth pain
  etiology, 408
  See also **Oral health problems**
Mouth pain, cold sore, canker sore product table, 817-819
Mouthrinses, 415-416
  children, 428
  fluoride, 419-420
Mouthwash, 109
MTX
  See **Methotrexate**
Mucoplex, 770
Mull-Soy, 310
Multilex, 770
Multilex T & M, 770
Multiple vitamin product table, 762-788
Multistix, 748
Multistix 2, 748
Multistix 7, 748
Multistix 9, 748
Multistix SG, 748
Multistix 8 SG, 748
Multistix 9 SG, 748
Multistix 10 SG, 748
Multivitamins
  ophthalmic, 363
Multivitamin therapy, 287-300
Murine Ear Wax Removal System And Ear Drops, 808
Murine Eye Lubricant, 798
Murine Plus Lubricating Eye Redness Reliever, 799
Murocel, 798

Muscle pain
  etiology, 51
  treatment, 51
Muscular pain
  etiology, 551-553
Muskol Maximum Strength, 876
Muskol Ultra, 876
Mustard plasters, 555
Mustard water
  emetic agent, 186
Musterole Deep Strength, 857
Musterole Regular & Extra Strength, 857
Myadec, 772
Myalgia
  etiology, 51
  treatment, 51
Mycelex OTC, 880
Myciguent, 833
Mycitracin, 423, 834
Mycitracin Plus, 834
Mycotic infections, 610
Mylagen II, 719
Mylanta, 719
Mylanta Double Strength, 719
Mylanta Gas, 719
Mylanta Gas Maximum Strength, 719
Mylanta Gelcaps, 719
Mylanta II, 155
Mylicon, 719
Myocardial infarct
  aspirin prophylaxis, 56-57
Myoflex, 857
Myrj, 530

Nail-A-Cain, 878
Nails, 495
  anatomical features, 495 (figure)
  psoriasis, 534
Naldecon DX Adult Liquid, 686
Naldecon DX Children's Syrup, 686
Naldecon DX Pediatric Drops, 688
Naldecon EX Children's Syrup, 688
Naldecon Senior DX, 688
Naldecon Senior EX, 688
Naloxone, 187
Naphazoline, 360, 361
Naphazoline hydrochloride, 103
Naphcon, 800
Nappies, 549
Narcolepsy, 136, 137
Narcotics
  adverse effects, 188
Nasal congestion, 92-93, 97
  treatment, 95, 112
Nasal drops, 102-103, 112-113
Nasal Moist, 707
Nasal Saline Nasal Moisturizer, 707

Nasal sprays, 101-102
Natabec Kapseals, 772
Natalins, 772
Natrapel, 876
Naturalamb, 823
Naturalamb with spermicide, 823
Natural family planning
  advantages, 459
  basal body temperature method, 457
  basal body temperature variations, 457 (figure)
  calendar method, 455-457
  cervical mucus characteristics through menstrual cycle, 458 (text table)
  cervical mucus method, 457-458
  coitus interruptus, 453, 458
  fertility interval calculation, 455 (text table)
  information sources, 466 (appendix)
  in-home ovulation prediction tests, 43-45, 459
  lactational infertility, 458-459
  pharmacist's role, 459
  risks, 459
  symptothermal method, 458
Natural Tin 03/04, 372 (text table)
Natural Vegetable, 735
Nature's Remedy, 735, 736
Nature's Remedy, Mineral Oil Enema, 736
Naturlax Sunlax Citrus, 736
Naturlax Sunlax Orange Sugar Free, 736
Nausea
  drug-induced, 188
  etiology, 183 (text table), 188-189
  patient assessment, 181, 187-189
  pregnancy, 181, 182, 188
  treatment, 189-190, 190
  See also **Vomiting**
Nausetrol, 190
N.B.P., 834
NDAs
  See **New drug applications**
ND-Gesic, 686
NDMA
  See **Nonprescription Drug Manufacturers Association**
Nebu-Sol Sodium Chloride Solution, 707
Nedocromil, 122
  side effects, 124
Needles, 261-262
Neferex Tablets, 757
Neomycin, 834
Neomycin, 205
  allergic reactions, 499
  dosage, 499
Neonates
  caffeine, 142, 144
  See also **Infants**
Neopap Suppositories, 651
Neosporin, 423
Neosporin Cream, 834
Neosporin Ointment, 834

Neosporin Plus Maximum Strength Cream, 834
Neosporin Plus Maximum Strength Ointment, 834
Neo-Synephrine Extra, 705
Neo-Synephrine Maximum-12 Hour, 705
Neo-Synephrine Mild, 705
Neo-Synephrine Pediatric, 705
Neo-Synephrine Regular, 705
Nephro-Calci, 759
Nephro-Derm, 847
Nephro-Fer Tablets, 756
Nephropathies
  drugs that may induce, 261 (text table)
Nepro, 752
Nervine Nighttime Sleep-Aid, 713
Nestabs, 772
Neuralgia
  etiology, 51
  symptoms, 51
  treatment, 51
Neurodermatitis, 391
Neuroleptic malignant syndrome, 68
Neuropathic pain, 49
Neuropathies
  drugs that could cause, 261 (text table)
Neuropeptides, 540
Neutralin, 719
Neutrogena, 524
Neutrogena Acne Mask, 837
Neutrogena Body Lotion (FF), 847
Neutrogena Body Oil (FF), 847
Neutrogena Chemical-Free Sunblocker SPF 17, 864
Neutrogena Moisture, 864
Neutrogena Norwegian Formula Emulsion (FF), 847
Neutrogena Norwegian Formula Hand Cream (FF), 847
Neutrogena Oil-Free Acne Wash, 837
Neutrogena Sunblock, 864
Neutrogena Sunblock Stick, 864
Neutrogena T/Derm, 842
Neutrogena T/Gel, 842, 851
Neutrogena T/Gel Conditioner, 842, 851
Neutrogena T/Sal, 842, 851
New drug applications, 21-22
New Skin, 631
New Skin Liquid Bandage, 834
Niacin
  adverse effects, 295-296
  description, 295
  dose/RDA, 295
  drug interactions, 295-296
Niacinamide, 296
N'Ice Cough, 709
Nichols Nasal Douche Powder, 707
Nickel, 308
Nicoderm, 630
Nicorette, 630
Nicotinic acid
  See **Niacin**
Nicotrol, 630

Niferex-150 Capsules, 757
Niferex Daily, 772
Niferex Elixir, 757
Niferex With Vitamin C Tablets, 757
Night blindness, 288-289
Night Time Cold Medicine, 688
Night-Time Sleep-Aid, 713
Nitromersol, 501
Nivea Bath Silk, 847
Nivea Creme Ultra Moisturizing, 847
Nix, 354, 875
N-Multistix, 748
N-Multistix SG, 748
Nocturnal asthma, 132
Nocturnal myoclonus, 136
No Doz, 715
No Doz Maximum Strength Caplets, 715
Nolahist, 688
Nonacetylated salicylates, 57-58
  See also **Salicylates**
Nonmonographs
  product categories, 27-28
Nonoxynol-9, 459, 460, 461, 463
Nonprescription Drug Manufacturers Association
  labeling guidelines, 7, 36
  self-medication decisions, 1
Nonprescription drugs
  approval process, 21-23
  definition, 2
  expenditures, 12 (figure)
  ingredient review product categories, 23 (text table)
  monograph provisions, 25-28
  reclassification from prescription drugs, 28, 29 (figure), 30-34
  regulatory approach to product approval, 22 (text table)
  review impact, 28
  review rulemaking process, 24 (figure), 24-25
  See also names of specific drugs and classes of drugs
Nonsteroidal anti-inflammatory drugs, 80, 81, 133, 149, 150
  gastropathy, 171
  See also **NSAID-induced ulcers**
Non-Steroidal Procto Foam, 826
Nonulcer dyspepsia
  clinical presentation, 172
  complications, 172
  pathogenesis, 172
  treatment, 172
Nonverbal communication, 13
Norfloxacin, 207
  dosage, 207
Norforms Fresh Flowers, 829
Norforms, Unscented, 829
Norplant, 480
NORPLANT (6 capsules), 454 (text table)

NORPLANT-2 (2 rods), 454 (text table)
Norwalk viruses, 203-204
Norwich Aspirin, 651, 661
Norwich Aspirin Caplets, 651, 662
Norwich Aspirin Enteric, Adult Low Strength, 652, 662
Norwich Aspirin Enteric Coated, 651, 662
Noscapine, 108
Not recognized as safe and effective ingredients, 21
Novahistine, 688
Novahistine DH, 688
Novahistine DMX, 688
Novahistine Expectorant, 688
Novolin, 250
Novolin L (Lente Human Insulin Zinc Suspension), 740
Novolin N (NPH, Human Insulin Isophane Suspension), 740
Novolin N Penfill (NPH, Human Insulin Isophane Suspension), 740
Novolin 70/30 (70% NPH, Hum. Iso. Susp./ 30% Reg., Hum. Inj.), 741
Novolin 70/30 Penfill (70% NPH Hum. Susp./30% Regular Inj.), 741
Novolin 70/30 Prefilled, 743
Novolin R Penfill (Regular, Human Insulin Injection), 739
Novolin R (Regular, Human Insulin Injection), 739
NovoPen Insulin Delivery Device, 743
Noxzema Clear-Ups Acne Medicated Maximum Strength, 837
Noxzema Clear-Ups Medicated Maximum Strength, 837
Noxzema Clear-Ups Medicated Regular Strength, 837
NPH (Isophane Insulin Suspension, Beef), 740
NPH (Purified Pork Isophane Insulin), 740
NPH Iletin I (Isophane Insulin Suspension), 740
NPH Iletin II (Isophane Insulin Suspension, Purified Pork), 740
NP-27, 880
NP-27 Aerosol, 834
NP-27 Solution & Cream, 834
NRASE
  See **Not recognized as safe and effective ingredients**
NSAID gastropathy, 171
NSAID-induced ulcers, 164
  antacid role, 172
  clinical presentation, 171
  complications, 171
  pathogenesis, 171
  prevention, 171-172
  treatment, 172
NSAIDs
  See **Nonsteroidal anti-inflammatory drugs**

NTZ Long Lasting, 705
Numzident Gel-Adult Strength, 818
Numzit Cold Sore Lotion, 818
Numzit Teething Gel, 818
Numzit Teething Lotion, 818
Nupercainal, 826, 874
Nupercainal Suppositories, 826
Nuprin, 652, 662, 668
Nursoy, 328, 329
Nutraderm, 847
Nutraderm 30, 847
Nutramigen, 310, 330, 792
Nutraplus, 847, 848
Nutritional assessment, 284-286
Nutritional Products, 283-311
  patient assessment, 283, 284-286
  patient counseling, 283
Nutritional supplements, 310-311, 311 (text table)
Nutritious Pudding, 752
Nycoff, 688
Nyctalopia
  See **Night blindness**
NyQuil, 140
NyQuil Adult Nighttime Cold/Flu Medicine, Cherry Flavor, 688
NyQuil Adult Nighttime Cold/Flu Medicine, Original Formula, 688
NyQuil Children's Allergy/Head Cold Medicine, 688
NyQuil Children's Cold/Cough Medicine, 688
NyQuil LiquiCaps Adult Nighttime Cold/Flu Medicine, 688
Nystatin, 505, 507, 547
Nystatin powder, 440, 441
Nytcold Cough & Cold, 688
Nytol, 713
Nytol Maximum Strength, 713

Oatmeal bath products, 527, 546, 593
Oatrim, 346-347
Obesity, 339-340
  adjunctive therapy, 347
  appetite control, 342
  caloric expenditure rates, 341 (text table)
  etiology, 340-342
  height and weight tables, 340 (text table)
  insulin, 239
  role in other conditions, 342-343
  symptoms, 343
  treatment, 343-347
  See also **Weight Control Products**
Obstructive hearing loss, 396-397

Obtundia, 860
Obtundia Calamine Cream, 871
Obtundia Cream, 834
Obtundia First Aid, 874
Obtundia First Aid Spray, 834
Obtundia Surgical Dressing, 874
Occlusal HP, 878
Ocean Mist, 707
Octocrylene, 580
Octoxynol-9, 459
Octyl salicylate, 582
OcuCaps, 772
Ocu Clear, 800
OcuClenz, 801
Ocular disorders, 353-357
  eyelid, 354
  internal eye, 356-357
  ocular surface, 354-356
Ocular pain
  etiology, 51
  symptoms, 51
  treatment, 51
Ocular pharmacotherapy
  history taking, 363-364
  self-administration of medication, 364
OCuSOFT, 801
Odor Attackers, 625
Odo-Way Appliance Deodorant Tablets, 820
Odrinil, 668
Off Deep Woods Formula, 876
Off Ezy Wart Remover Kit, 878
Off Skintastic Insect Repellent, 876
Off Spring Fresh, 876
Ofloxacin, 207
Oilatum Soap, 848
Ointments, 560, 572
  anorectal, 476
  bland, 360
  counterirritant, 556
  ophthalmic, 358, 360 (text table)
Oleaginous phenolic solutions, 501
Olestra, 347
Olive oil, 401
  insects in the ear, 394, 401
Omeprazole, 159-160, 163
Omni White & Brite, 416
Omron Model HEM-601 Wrist Blood Pressure Monitor, 639
Omron Model HEM-703CP Measurement Print-out B.P. Monitor, 639
Omron Model HEM-704C Self-Storage Blood Pressure Monitor, 639
Omron Model HEM-705CP Memory/Printout/Graph B.P. Monitor, 639
Omron Model HEM-706 Fuzzy Logic Blood Pressure Monitor, 639
Omron Model HEM-713C Automatic Inflation B.P. Monitor, 639
Omron Model HEM-815F Finger Blood Pressure Monitor, 640
One-A-Day Essential, 772

One-A-Day Maximum Formula, 774
One-A-Day Plus Extra C, 774
One-A-Day Stressgard, 774
One-A-Day Women's, 774
One-Tablet-Daily, 774
One-Tablet Daily With Minerals, 774
Open-ended questions, 13
Ophthalmic decongestant product table, 799-800
Ophthalmic drug formulations, 357-358
  preservatives used, 357 (text table), 357-358, 374
  vehicles, 357, 357 (text table), 374
Ophthalmic Products, 351-365
  antiseptics, 362
  artificial tears, 358, 359-360
  bland ointments, 360, 360 (text table)
  decongestants, 360-361
  detergents/abrasives, 362-363
  eyelid scrubs, 362-363, 363 (text table)
  hyperosmotics, 361-362
  imidazoles, 360-361
  irrigants, 361
  lubricants, 358-360
  major therapeutic categories, 358-363
  multivitamins, 363
  patient assessment, 351
  patient counseling, 351
  phenylephrine, 360, 361
  self-administration, 364
Opiate-derivatives
  efficacy, 209
  side effects, 209
Opiate-like agents
  action of, 209
  dependency, 209
  side effects, 209
Opiates
  action of, 209
  dependency, 209
  side effects, 209
Opium, 108
Opium tincture, 209
OpSite, 263, 437, 447 (text table)
Opti-Clean, 803, 804
OptiClean II, 384, 803, 804
Opti-Free, 384, 805
Opti-Free Rewetting Drops, 806
Optilets-500 Filmtabs, 776
Optilets-M-500 Filmtabs, 776
Optima Toric, 372 (text table)
Opti-Soft, 807
Opti-Tears, 806
Opti-Zyme, 803
Opti-Zyme Enzymatic, 804
Orabase, 422
Orabase Baby Analgesic Teething Gel, 428
Orabase Baby, gel, 818
Orabase-B with Benzocaine, cream, 818
Orabase-B with Benzocaine, paste, 818
Orabase Lip Healer, cream, 818

Orabase Plain, 422
Orabase Plain, cream, 818
Orafix, 816
Orafix Special, 816
Orajel, 818
Orajel, Baby, 818
Orajel, Baby Nighttime Formula, 818
Orajel Denture, 818
Orajel Maximum Strength, 818
Orajel Mouth-Aid, 818
Oral anesthetics
  anticholinergics, 109
Oral-B Indicator, 411
Oral-B Super Floss, 413
Oral cancer, 407, 409, 421
Oral contraceptives, 133
  acne, 515
  birth control pill, 453
  breast-feeding, 324
  menorrhagia, 81
  sunlight, 577
Oral health problems
  common problems, 410-425
  dental anatomy and physiology, 409-410
  epidemiology, 407-408
  patient assessment, 407, 408-409
  tooth anatomy, 410 (figure)
  value-added pharmacy services, 429
Oral Health Products, 407-431
  patient assessment, 407, 408-409
  patient counseling, 407, 408-409
  sales, 408
  value-added pharmacy services, 429
Oral hypoglycemic agents, 247
Oral infections
  candidiasis, 424-425
  dentopyogenic, 424
Oral irrigating devices, 412
Oral malodor
  See **Morning breath**
Oral mucosal injury or irritation
  etiology, 423
  treatment, 423-424
Oral mucosal lesions
  canker sores, 421-422
  cold sores, 421, 422-423
  minor oral mucosal injury or irritation, 423-424
  oral malignancies, 421
Oral rehydration solutions, 190, 208 (text table), 208-209
Oral rinse product table, 814
Oranyl, 688
Oranyl Plus, 688
Orex Saliva Substitute, 426
Organic fatty acids, 622
Orinase, 248 (text table)
Ornex, 652, 688
Ornex Maximum Strength, 652, 690
Ornex Severe Cold, 652, 690
Ornithobilharzia, 217

Orofacial pain
  fractured dentition and restorations, 421
  hypersensitive teeth, 421
  toothache, 420-421
Orphenadrine
  analgesic adjuvant effect, 61
Ortho-Creme, 822
Orthodontia, 428
Ortho-Gynol, 822
Ortho Personal Lubricant, 461
Orthotic devices, 609
Orthoxicol, 690
Os-Cal 250 + D, 759
Os-Cal 500, 759
Os-Cal 500 + D, 759
Os-Cal Forte, 759, 776
Os-Cal Plus, 759, 776
Osmolite, 310, 753
Osmolite HN, 753
Osteoarthritis
  See **Degenerative joint disease**
Osteogard, 776
Osteomalacia, 290, 301
Ostomies
  anatomy of digestive and urinary tracts, 434 (figure)
  colostomy, 433
  diet, 441
  ileostomy, 433, 434-436
  medication effects, 441-442, 442 (text table)
  medications that discolor feces, 442 (text table)
  physical complications, 433-434, 440-441
  psychologic complications, 440
  restorative proctocolectomy, 436
  surgery and care, 433
  types, 435 (figure)
  urostomy, 433
Ostomy and Wound Care Products, 433-451
  appliances and accessories, 437-438
  colostomy irrigation set, 438 (figure)
  fitting and application, 438
  major manufacturers, 450-451 (appendix)
  patient assessment, 433
  patient counseling, 433
  procedures for applying appliances, 439 (figure)
  wound care product selection guidelines, 446 (text table)
  wound management options, 447-449 (text table)
Ostomy product table, 820-821
Otic Products, 389-405
  patient assessment, 389
  patient counseling, 389
  See also **Ear conditions**
Otic product table, 808
Otitis media, 395-396
  chronic, 396
  patient assessment, 398, 398 (text table)
Otomycosis, 393
  patient assessment, 398

Otrivin, 705
Otrivin Pediatric, 705
Overeating, 181, 188
Overindulgence, 173
Over-the-counter products
See **FDA's Review of OTC Drugs**; **Nonprescription drugs**; *specific drugs by name*
OvuKIT, 642
Ovulation
test kit, 43-45, 459
Ovulation prediction test kits product table, 642
Ovulation prediction tests, 459
OvuQUICK, 642
Oxidases, 414
Oxidizing agents, 594
Oxipor VHC, 842
Oxy-5 Vanishing Sensitive Skin, 838
Oxy-10 Daily Face Wash, 838
Oxybenzone, 580, 582
Oxychinol, 820
Oxy Clean Medicated Cleanser & Pads, 837
Oxy Maximum Strength Medicated Pad, 837
Oxy Medicated Soap, 837
Oxymetazoline, 361
Oxymetazoline hydrochloride, 103
Oxy Night Watch Maximum Strength, 838
Oxyquinoline sodium propionate, 546
Oxyquinolone sulfate, 488
Oxy Res: Don't Medicated Face Wash, 838
Oxymetazoline Hydrochloride, 705
Oxysept 1 Disinfecting Solution, 805
Oxysept 2 Neutralizing Tablets, 806
Oyst-Cal 500, 759
Oyst-Cal D, 759
Oyst-Cal-D, 759
Oyster Shell Calcium, 760
Oyster Shell Calcium Plus Vitamin D, 760
Oyster Shell Calcium + Vitamin D, 760

PA1, 372 (text table)
P&S, 851
P&S Plus, 842
P-A-C, 652, 662
Padimate A, 580
Padimate O, 582
Pain
etiology, 49, 50 (figure)
gate-control theory, 551
overuse syndrome, 552
patient assessment, 49-50
perception, 49

referred, 49, 50 (figure)
skeletal muscle, 551-552
somatic, 49
treatment, 52-62
visceral, 49, 50 (figure)
See also specific types of pain
Pain-Eze +, 652, 662
Pain Reliever Tablets, 652
Pals, 485
Pamabrom
dosage, 84
Pampers, 548
Pamprin Maximum Pain Relief Caplets, 662, 668
Pamprin Multi-Symptom Formula, 662
Pamprin Multi-Symptom Formula Tablets, 668
Panadol Caplets, Maximum Strength, 652
Panadol Children's and Infants' Drops, 652, 662
Panadol Children's Chewable Tablets, 652, 662
Panadol Children's Liquid, 652, 662
Panadol Junior Strength, 652, 663
Panadol Maximum Strength, 653
Panadol, Maximum Strength, 662
Panalgesic, 857
Panalgesic Gold, 857
Panasonic Power Floss and Brush, 412
Pancreatitis
acute, 175
Pangamic acid, 300
Pan Oxyl Bar 5, 838
Pan Oxyl Bar 10, 838
Panscol, 843, 848
Panthoderm, 854, 860
Pantothenic acid
adverse effects, 296
description, 296
dose/RDA, 296
drug interactions, 296
indications, 296
Papain, 415, 481
Papaverine, 108
Papillomavirus, 612
Parabens, 530
Parachlorometaxylenol, 502
Paraperm EW, 370 (text table)
Parasitic infections
See **Worm infections**
Parasympathomimetic drugs
adverse effects, 206
See also names of specific drugs in this class
Paregoric, 209
Parepectolin, 724
Paronychia, 497
Patch testing
allergic contact dermatitis, 591-592
Patent medicines, 2
Patient assessment
acne products, 511
analgesic products, 49-50
antacid products, 147, 175
anthelmintic products, 213

antidiarrheal products, 199, 206-207
antiemetic products, 181, 187-189
antipyretic drug products, 65
asthma products, 117, 120-122
boils, 397
burn and sunburn products, 563, 568-569
cold products, 89
contact lens products, 367, 385-387
contraceptive methods and products, 453
cough products, 89
decongestants, 101
dermatologic products, 521
diabetes products, 237
diaper rash, 543
ear aches, 389, 397
ear conditions, 389, 397-398
emetic products, 181
external analgesic products, 551, 554-561
external otitis, 397, 398 (text table)
foreign objects in the ear, 397
hearing loss, 389, 398
hemorrhoidal products, 469, 472-473
infant formulas, 313
insect sting and bite products, 597
laxatives, 219, 234
menstrual products, 77, 82-83
monitoring products, in-home, 39
nutritional products, 283-286
ophthalmic products, 351
oral health products, 407, 408-409
ostomy and wound care products, 433
otic products, 389
otitis media, 398, 398 (text table)
otomycosis, 398
personal care products, 479
pharmaceutical care concept, 11
poison ivy products, 589, 591-592
poison oak products, 589, 591-592
prickly heat, 543
skin, 493
sleep aids, 135, 136-141, 142
sunscreen products, 575
suntan products, 575
testing products, in-home, 39
tinnitus, 389
topical anti-infective products, 493
weight control products, 339
Patient Assessment and Consultation, 11-20
Patient Consultation, 11-20
Patient consultation
allergic rhinitis, 112-113
anorectal disease, 477-478
colds, 112-113

Patient counseling
acne products, 511, 519
allergy products, 89
analgesic products, 49
antacid products, 147, 176
anthelmintic products, 213
antidiarrheal products, 199
antiemetic products, 181
antipyretic drug products, 65
asthma products, 117
blood pressure monitoring, 39, 41-42
burn and sunburn products, 563
burn products, 563
caffeine, 144
cold products, 89
contact lens products, 367, 385-387
contraceptive methods and products, 453
cough products, 89
decongestants, 101-102
dermatologic products, 521
diabetes products, 237
diaper rash, 543
earaches, 389
emetic products, 181
external analgesic products, 551
fecal occult blood test, 39, 43
hemorrhoidal products, 469
hypertension, 41-42
infant formulas, 313
insect sting and bite products, 597
laxatives, 219, 235
menstrual products, 77
nutritional products, 283
nutritional supplements, 311 (text table)
ophthalmic products, 351
oral health products, 407, 408-409
ostomy and wound care products, 433
otic products, 389
ovulation prediction, 39, 44-45
personal care products, 479
poison ivy products, 589
poison oak products, 589
pregnancy test, 39, 45-46
prickly heat, 543
as a professional function, 11-12
rhinitis, 111-113
sleep aids, 135
stimulant products, 144
sunburn products, 563
sunscreens, 575, 586-587
suntan products, 575, 586-587
testing products, 39
topical anti-infective products, 493
toxic shock syndrome, 86-87
urinary tract infections, 46
weight control products, 339
Patient education
asthma products, 133
athlete's foot, 625
caffeine, 144
calluses, 617
corns, 617

General Index 905

diabetes products, 247, 273
diabetic foot care, 627-628
diet therapy, 257
exercise issues, 632-633
fever, 73-74
inhaler use, 129-130, 133
self-treatment, 16-17
skin infections, 498
stimulant products, 144
sunscreens, 586-587
suntan products, 586-587
warts, 617
Patient interview
condition assessment, 15
history taking, 14-15
observed physical data, 15
patient-pharmacist consultation process, 14 (text table)
physician referral, 15-16
self-treatment advice, 16-17
Patient-pharmacist consultation process, 14 (text table)
Pazo, 826
PBZ, 594
Peak flow measurement, 121-122, 122 (text table), 132
Pearl Drops Baking Soda Whitening Toothpaste Fluor.-Tartar, 810
Pearl Drops Extra Strength Whitening Toothpaste w/ Fluoride, 810
Pearl Drops Whitening Gel Fluor.-Tartar, 810
Pearl Drops Whitening Toothpolish w/ Fluoride, paste, 811
Pectin, 210
PediaCare Cold-Allergy Chewable Tablets For Ages 6 to 12, 690
PediaCare Cough-Cold Chewable Tablets For Ages 6 to 12, 690
PediaCare Cough-Cold Formula Liquid, 690
PediaCare Infants' Decongestant Drops, 690
PediaCare Night Rest Cough-Cold Formula, 690
Pedialyte, 190, 209, 332
PediaSure, 332, 753, 794
PediaSure with Fiber, 332, 794
Pediatric Maintenance Solution, 190
Pedi-Bath, 848
Pediculicide product table, 875
Pediculicides, 354
Pediculosis, 598
Pedi-Pro, 880
Pedi-Vit-A, 848
Pellagra, 286, 295
Pelvic inflammatory disease, 482
Penicillins, 205
Pen-Kera, 848
Penlet II Automatic Blood Sampling Device, 750
PenNeedle Disposable Needle, 743
Pentrax, 843, 851

Pentrax Gold, 843, 851
Pep-Back, 715
Peppermint oil, 106, 108, 557, 605
Pepsodent Baking Soda Gel, 811
Pepsodent Fluoride Toothpaste, 811
Peptic ulcer disease, 161-165, 176
Pepto-Bismol, 161, 190, 207-208
Pepto-Bismol Cherry Tablets, 724
Pepto-Bismol Maximum Strength Liquid, 724
Pepto-Bismol Original Formula Liquid, 724
Pepto-Bismol Original Tablets, 724
Peptococcus, 627
Pepto Diarrhea Control Caplets, 724
Pepto Diarrhea Control Liquid, 724
Perative, 753
Perborates, 422, 424
Percogesic Coated Tablets, 653
Percy Medicine, 719, 725
Perdiem, 736
Perdiem Fiber, 736
Perfumes
deodorant spray, 482
Perianal area
anatomy and physiology, 469-470
itching, 215
Periapical abscess, 424
Periarticular pain
etiology, 51-52
patient assessment, 52
treatment, 52
Perichondritis, 392
Peri-Colace Capsules, 736
Peri-Colace Syrup, 736
Pericoronal abscess, 424
Peridin-C, 753
Peri-Dos, 736
PeriGel Oral Care System, paste, 811
Perimed, 424
Perio-aid, 413
Periodontal abscess, 424
Periodontal disease
etiology, 416-418
pathophysiology, 416-418
prevention, 418
Periodontitis
etiology, 417-418
pathophysiology, 417-418
periodontal abscess, 424
Permaflex Natural, 372 (text table)
Permalens, 372 (text table)
Permethrin
reclassification, 23
Permethrin cream rinse, 598
Pernox, 838
Pernox Lemon & Regular, 838
Peroxide products, 383 (text table)
Peroxides, 424
Peroxyl Mouthrinse, 814, 818

Peroxyl Oral Spot Treatment Gel, 819
Peroxyl Rinse, 424
Personal Care Products, 479-492
patient assessment, 479
patient counseling, 479
Personal care product table, 828-830
Personal Lubricant, 829
Perspiration, 483-484
treatment, 484-486
See also **Sweat glands**
Pertussin AM, 690
Pertussin CS, 690
Pertussin ES, 690
Pertussin PM, 690
Peruvian balsam oil, 546
Petrolatum, 423, 528, 546, 547
liquid, 225-226
pH
douches, 481
urine, 159
Pharmaceutical care concept, 11
Pharmacists
communication role with diabetics, 274
communication with physicians, 15
patient counseling as a professional function, 11-12
patient-pharmacist consultation process, 14 (text table)
patient's choice of, 11
role, 41-42, 112-113, 286-287
vitamin and mineral counseling, 286-287
Pharmacokinetics
caffeine, 142
diphenhydramine, 138
doxylamine, 138
Pharyngitis, 89, 93, 94 (text table)
streptococcal, 93, 109
treatment, 95, 109
Phenapap Sinus Headache & Congestion Without Drowsiness, 690
Phenindamine tartrate, 99
Pheniramine maleate, 99
Phenobarbital, 69, 128-129, 133, 185
combination products, 129
dosage, 129
side effects, 129
Phenol, 109, 415, 422, 423, 428, 546, 594, 605
in glycerin, 401
Phenolate sodium, 422, 428
Phenolic compounds, 414, 501, 622-623
Phenolphthalein, 227-228
Phenothiazines, 68, 459, 576
Phenylephrine, 104, 360, 361
breast-feeding, 19
diabetics, 269
Phenylephrine Hydrochloride, 705
Phenylephrine hydrochloride, 103, 473-474

Phenylgesic, 690
Phenylmercuric nitrate, 376
Phenylpropanolamine, 104, 343-345
breast-feeding, 19
diabetics, 269
side effects, 344-345
Phenyl salicylate, 209
Phenyltoloxamine
analgesic adjuvant effect, 61
Phenyltoloxamine citrate, 100
Phenytoin, 295, 515
Phillips' Laxative Gelcaps, 736
Phillips' Milk Of Magnesia, 720, 736
Phillips' Milk Of Magnesia, mint or cherry, 720, 736
pHisoHex, 619
Phosphate-binding antacids, 173
Phosphate salts, 226
Phospholipid products, 528
Phosphorated carbohydrate solution
dosage, 190
efficacy, 190
side effects, 190
Phosphorus
description, 302-303
dose/RDA, 303
indications, 303
infant requirements, 318
preterm infant requirements, 320
Phospho-soda Buffered Oral Saline Unflavored & Ginger-Lemon, 737
Photoallergy, 576
Photodermatoses, 577
Photoplex Broad Spectrum Sunscreen Lotion, 864
Photosensitivity
medications, 566-567 (text table)
sunscreens, 576-577
Photosensitization, 566-567 (text table), 568
Phybrex, 223
Physical barriers to communications, 13
Physician referral, 15-16
constipation, 234
diaper rash, 545
psoriasis, 535
rhus dermatitis, 593
Phytonadione, 291
PID
See **Pelvic inflammatory disease**
Pigmenting agents, 583
Pile pipe, 477
Pine tar, 107
Pinex, 690
Pinex Concentrate, 690
Pinworm neurosis, 215
Pinworms
differential diagnosis, 215
epidemiology, 213
etiology, 213-215
symptoms, 214
treatment, 215-216
Pin-X, 215, 726
Piritrexim, 540

Pityrosorum orbiculare, 498
Plak Trac, 412
Plantar fascitis, 631
Plaque
 disclosing agents, 413
 etiology, 410
 pathophysiology, 410
 plaque removal products, 411-416
 removal, 411
Plasters, 611, 616
Plax, 416
Plax Original Flavor & Softmint, 814
Plexolan Lanolin Cream, 854
Plexolan Moisturizing Cream, 848
Pliagel, 804
PMC Douche, 829
PMS
 See **Premenstrual syndrome**
Podactin, 880
Poison control centers, 192-198 (appendix)
Poisoning
 incidence, 182
 information for poison management, 182-184
 patient assessment, 181, 182-184
 symptoms, 183-184
 treatment, 184-187
Poison ivy, 590 (figure)
 See also **Rhus dermatitis**
Poison Ivy and Poison Oak Products, 589-596
 patient assessment, 589, 591-592
 patient counseling, 589
 selection guidelines, 595
Poison ivy and poison oak product table, 867-872
Poison oak, 590 (figure)
 See also **Rhus dermatitis**
Poison Oak Products, 589-596
 patient assessment, 589, 591-592
 patient counseling, 589
 selection guidelines, 595
Poison sumac, 591 (figure)
 See also **Rhus dermatitis**
Polident, 815
Polident Dentu-Grip, 816
Polident Denture Cleanser, 815
Poli-Grip, 816
Pollenosis
 See **Hay fever**
Polyaminopropyl biguanide, 377
Polycarbophil, 209
 dosage, 210
 dosage, children, 210
 efficacy, 210
 side effects, 210
Polycon II, 370 (text table)
Polycose, 753
Polydine Ointment & Solution, 834
Polymorphic light eruption, 577
Polymyxin B sulfate, 499

Polyoxyethylene lauryl ether, 530
Polyoxyethylene monostearate, 530
Polyoxyethylene sorbitan monolaurate, 530
Polyps, 471
Polyquaternium-1, 377
Polysorb Hydrate, 848
Polysporin Ointment, 834
Polysporin Powder, 834
Polytar, 843, 851
Poly-Vi-Sol Chewable Vitamins, 776
Poly-Vi-Sol Vitamin Drops, 776
Poly-Vi-Sol with Iron Chewable Vitamins and Minerals, 776
Poly-Vi-Sol with Iron Vitamin Drops, 776
Poly-Vita Drops, 776
Polyvitamin With Iron, 776
Pontocaine, 826
Portagen, 310, 330, 792
Poslam Psoriasis Ointment, 843
Posture, 760
Posture D, 760
Potassium guaiacolsulfonate, 106
Potassium nitrate, 421
Potassium permanganate, 593, 595
Potassium sorbate, 376
Povan, 442 (text table)
Povidone-Iodine, 835
Povidone-iodine, 482
Povodine, 445
Powders
 athlete's foot, 624-625
 deodorant, 486
 talc, 546, 547
Power Toothbrush, 412
PPA
 See **Phenylpropanolamine**
PrameGel, 871, 874
Pramegel, 860
Pramoxine
 burn treatment, 571
Pramoxine hydrochloride, 594
 anorectal, 473
Prax, 860
Precise, 643
Precision High Nitrogen Diet, 753
Precision Isotonic Diet, 753
Precision LR, 310
Precision LR Diet, 753
Pre-Cut Adhesive Supports, 820
Prednisone, 593
 acne, 519
Preemie SMA, 331
Preflex For Sensitive Eyes, 804
Prefrin Liquifilm, 800
Pregestimil, 330, 792
Pregnancy
 acetaminophen, 58, 74
 alcohol, 19
 antacids, 155, 174
 antihistamines, 139, 189
 aspirin, 54
 asthma products, 131-132
 caffeine, 143-144
 cigarette smoking, 19
 contact lenses, 373

 fetal risk from asthma medications, 131 (text table)
 folic acid deficiency, 294
 German measles, 94-95
 ibuprofen, 60
 iron loss, 306
 laxatives, 230
 mebendazole, 216
 nutrition, 286
 oral health effects, 429
 parasitic infections, 213
 pyrantel pamoate, 215, 216
 pyridoxine, 189-190
 self-treatment during, 19
 skin pigmentation, 486
 sunlight, 577
 teratogenicity of drugs, 18-19
 test kit, 45-46
 vaginal candidiasis, 504, 505, 508
 vitamin A, 289
 vitamin C, 293
 vomiting, 181, 188
 zinc, 309
 See also specific drugs by class or name
Pregnancy test kits product table, 643
Premature photoaging of skin, 577-578
Premenstrual syndrome, 81 (text table), 81-82
 patient assessment, 83
 treatment, 84
 vitamin B_{12}, 296
Premium Skin Barrier, 821
Premsyn PMS Caplets, 663, 669
Prenatal-S, 778
Prenavite, 778
Preparation H, 475, 826
Preparation H Cleansing Tissues, 826, 829
Preparation H Hydrocortisone 1% Anti-Itch Cream, 843, 874
Preservatives, 530
 ophthalmic, 357 (text table), 357-358, 374
Preserved Saline Solution, 807
PreSun 23, 865
PreSun 15 Active, 865
PreSun for Kids, 865
PreSun 15 Moisturizing, 864
PreSun 25 Moisturizing, 865
PreSun 15 Sensitive Skin, 864
PreSun 29 Sensitive Skin, 865
PreSun 15 Sunscreen, 865
Preterm infants
 formulas, 331
 vitamin and mineral supplements, 320
Pretty Feet & Hands, 848
Pretz, 707
Pretz-D, 705
Preventamine Multivitamin Mineral Complex (Iron-free), 778
Preventamins Multivitamin Mineral Complex (with Iron), 778
Prickly heat, 483, 545
 patient assessment, 543
 patient counseling, 543

 physical sunscreens, 582
 treatment, 545-548
Prickly Heat Products, 543-550
 patient assessment, 543
 patient counseling, 543
Primaderm-B, 826
Primatene, 712
Primatene Dual Action Formula, 712
Primatene Mist, 711
Primatene Mist Suspension, 711
Primatuss 4 Cough Mixture, 690
Primatuss 4D Cough Mixture, 692
Privine, 705
Probenecid
 drug interactions, 55, 208
Pro-Cute, 848
Pro-free/GP, 384
Pro Free/GP Weekly Enzymatic Cleaner, 803
Progestasert, 454 (text table)
Progesterone
 female cycle and, 43
Prolapse, 440
Promethazine
 reclassification, 33
Promise, 421
Promise Toothpaste, Sensitive Teeth & Cavity Prevention, 811
Pro Mod, 753
Promote, 753
Prompt Relief Hemorrhoidal Ointment, 826
Prompt Relief Hemorrhoidal Suppositories, 827
Pronto, 875
Propagest, 692
Propa pH Acne Medication Cleansing Pads Sensitive Skin, 838
Propa pH Acne Medication Cream, 838
Propellants
 deodorant sprays, 482
Pro-Pep, 778
Propionate, 540
Proprietary medicines
 definition, 2
Propylene glycol, 401, 528
Propylene glycol monostearate, 530
Propylhexedrine, 103
Propylparaben, 358
PROSAL, 842
ProSobee, 209, 328, 329, 792
Prostaglandins, 66, 80, 149
Prostat, 505
ProStep, 630
Protectants
 anorectal, 474
 burn, 568 (text table), 570-571
 skin, 529-530, 545, 546-547, 606
Protect, gel, 811
Protein hydrolysate, 546

Proteolytics
  douches, 481
Proteus, 205, 567, 627
Proteus mirabilis, 619
Proton pump inhibitors, 159-160
Protrusions
  anal, 472
Proxabrush, 413
Proxigel, 416
Pruritus
  athlete's foot, 619
  See also **Itching**
Pruritus ani, 472, 498
Pseudoephedrine, 104
  breast-feeding, 19
  diabetics, 269
Pseudomembranous colitis, 205, 210
Pseudomonas aeruginosa, 205, 496, 567, 619
Pseudovitamins, 298-300
Psoralens, 576
Psoriasis, 289, 533-536
  features, 531 (text table)
  nonmonograph ingredients, 537 (text table)
  nonprescription ingredients, 536, 536 (text table)
  pathophysiology, 534-535
  product selection guidelines, 540-541
  sunlight, 577
  treatment, 535-536
Psoriasis vulgaris, 534
Psoriatic arthritis, 533, 534
Psorigel, 843
PsoriNail, 843
Pteroylglutamic acid
  See **Folic acid**
Pulmocare, 310, 753
Pure Food and Drugs Act of 1906, 21
Purge Evacuant, 737
Purpose Dry Skin, 848
Pustular psoriasis, 534
PUVA therapy, 539
  dosage, 539
  side effects, 539
Py-Co-Prox, 413
Pyrantel pamoate, 213
  action of, 215
  dosage, 215, 217
  dosage, children, 215
  efficacy, 216
  pregnancy, 215, 216
  side effects, 215
  use guidelines, 215
Pyrethrins, 599
Pyridium, 442 (text table)
Pyridoxine, 189-190, 423
  adverse effects, 296-297
  description, 296
  dose/RDA, 296
  drug interactions, 296-297
Pyrilamine, 529, 594
Pyrilamine maleate, 99
Pyrithione zinc, 536-537
Pyrogens, 66
Pyrophosphates, 414, 415
Pyrosis
  See **Heartburn**
Pyrroxate, 692

Q.T. Quick Tanning Suntan by Coppertone, 865
Q-Test, 642, 643
Quaternary ammonium compounds, 414, 415, 502, 547, 594, 623
Quelidrine Cough, 692
Queltuss, 692
Questioning techniques, 13, 14
Quick-Pep Tablets, 715
Quinacrine, 204, 206
Quinidine, 159
  adverse effects, 205
Quinoline derivatives
  athlete's foot, 623-624

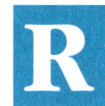

R&C Shampoo, 875
R&C Spray, 875
Racemethionine, 546
Radiation therapy
  adverse effects, 181, 424, 425
Ramses, 822
Ramses Extra Strength, 823
Ramses Sensitol Lubricated, 823
Ramses Ultra Thin, 823
Ranitidine, 540
RASE
  See **Recognized as safe and effective ingredients**
Raw fish, 217
RCF, 329, 792
RDA
  See **Recommended dietary allowances**
Reach Fluoride Dental Rinse, 419
Reality, 463
Reclassification of prescription drugs
  criteria, 28, 30
  examples, 30-33
  FDA guidelines, 29 (figure)
  future reclassifications, 33-34
  ingredient examples, 32 (text table)
  mechanisms, 30, 31 (figure)
Recognized as safe and effective ingredients, 21
Recommended dietary allowances, 283-284, 284-285 (text table)
  infants, 315
  labelling, 287 (text table)
Rectagene Medicated, 827
Rectum
  anatomy and physiology, 469-470

Red bugs
  See **Chiggers**
Red measles, 94
Reese's Pinworm, 215, 726
Referred pain, 49, 50 (figure)
Refined Karaya Gum Powder, 821
Reflex pathways, 553 (figure)
Refresh, 798
Regular (Insulin Injection, Beef), 739
Regular (Purified Pork Insulin Injection), 739
Regular Iletin I, 739
Regular Iletin II (Purified Pork), 739
Reguloid, Natural, 737
Reguloid, Orange, 737
Rehydralyte, 190, 209
Relief, 800
REM, 692
Rembrandt Daily Denture Renewal Gel, 815
Rembrandt Lighten Gel, 416
Rembrandt Whitening Toothpaste, 415
Rembrandt Whitening Toothpaste, mint, 811
Renal solute loads of milk and infant formulas, 323 (text table), 326, 328
Renal system, 142
ReNu, 384
ReNu Effervescent Enzymatic, 804
ReNu Multi-Purpose Solution, 805
ReNu Rewetting Drops, 806
ReNu Saline, 807
ReNu Thermal, 384
ReNu Thermal Enzymatic, 804
Replens, 83, 829
Reproductive cycle
  female, 43-44
Reserpine
  adverse effects, 206
Reserpine rhinitis, 98
Resol, 190, 209
Resolve/GP Daily Cleaner, 803
Resorcinol, 546, 623
  acne treatment, 516-517
Resorcinol monoacetate
  acne treatment, 516-517
Resource, 753
Resource Crystals, 753
Resource Plus, 753
Resource Shake, 753
Respiratory system
  caffeine, 142
Respiratory tract, 89-91
  anatomy, 90 (figure), 117-118, 119 (figure)
Restorative proctocolectomy, 436
Retin-A, 289, 517, 578
Retinoic acid, 288, 289, 487
Retinoids, 288, 578
  side effects, 539
Retinol, 288, 289
Retraction, 440
Revelation, powder, 811
Reye's syndrome, 96
  aspirin, 53, 54-55, 62

bismuth subsalicylate, 190
  methyl salicylate, 556
Rezamid Acne Lotion, 838
Rheaban, 725
Rheumatoid arthritis
  epidemiology, 52
  etiology, 52
  foot complaints, 614
  patient assessment, 52
  symptoms, 52
  treatment, 52
Rhinall, 705
Rhinitis, 89
  allergic, 89, 95, 96-110, 111-113
  characteristics, 97 (text table)
  medicamentosa, 98, 101
Rhinorrhea, 92, 97, 142
  cerebrospinal, 98
Rhubarb, 227
Rhuli Cream, 871, 874
Rhuli Gel, 872, 874
Rhuli Spray, 872, 874
Rhus dermatitis
  assessment, 591-592
  etiology, 589-591
  pharmacologic agents, 594-595
  symptoms, 591-592
  treatment, 592-594
Rhythm method of contraception, 455, 455 (text table)
Riboflavin, 303-304
  adverse effects, 297
  description, 297
  dose/RDA, 297
  drug interactions, 297
  indications, 297
Ricelyte, 190, 209, 332
Rickets, 290, 301, 318, 320
  infant formulas, 332
RID, 354, 875
Rid-Itch, 880
Rigident, 816
Ringworm, 497-498
Riopan, 720
Riopan Plus, 720
Riopan Plus 2 Mint or Cherry Flavor, 720
Riopan Plus 2 Mint or Cherry-Vanilla Flavor, 720
Robitussin, 692
Robitussin CF, 692
Robitussin Cough Calmers, 709
Robitussin DM, 692
Robitussin Maximum Strength Cough, 692
Robitussin Maximum Strength Cough & Cold, 692
Robitussin Night Relief, 692
Robitussin PE, 692
Robitussin Pediatric Cough, 692
Robitussin Pediatric Cough & Cold, 692
Rogenic Tablets, 757
Rolaids, 720
Rolaids Calcium Rich, 720
Rolaids Sodium Free, 720
Rosacea, 514, 515-516, 577
Rota-dent, 412
Rotahaler, 130

Rotaviruses, 203
Roundworms
  epidemiology, 216
  etiology, 216
  symptoms, 216
  treatment, 216
Rubefacients, 554
Rubella
  See **German measles**
Rubeola
  See **Measles**
Ru-Lets 500, 778
Rulox, 720
Rulox #1, 720
Rulox #2, 720
Rulox Plus, 720
Runner's bunion, 631
RX-56, 370 (text table)

S

Saccharin, 256, 346, 414, 418
  See also **Artificial sweeteners**; **Sweeteners**
Safeguard, 619
Safer sex practices, 464 (text table)
SalAc Cleanser, 838
Salactic Film, 878
Salicyl alcohol, 422
Salicylates, 159, 580
  absorption, 56
  action of, 52
  adverse effects, 53-55
  ascorbic acid, 110
  diabetes, 269
  dosage, 52-53
  dosage, children, 52 (text table)
  drug interactions, 55, 208
  nonacetylated, 57-58
  overdose, 55-56, 208
  Reye's syndrome, 53, 54-55, 62
  use considerations, 53-55, 62, 73
  See also **Aspirin**
Salicylic acid, 537-538, 540
  acne, 516, 517
  athlete's foot, 623
  corns, calluses, and warts, 615-616
  insect bites and stings, 607
Salicylic Acid Soap, 835, 838
Salicylic Acid & Sulfur Soap, 835, 838
Saline laxatives, 226, 230
Saline rinses, 422, 424
Saline solutions, 383-384
Salinex, 707
Saliva, artificial, 425-426
Salivart, 426, 813
Saliva Substitute, 426, 813
Salmonella, 203, 205
Sal-Plant Gel, 878
Salts of aluminum
  athlete's foot, 624
Salt water
  emetic agent, 186
  rinses, 422, 424

Sanguinarine, 414, 415
Sani-Supp, 737
Santy, 448 (text table)
Sarcoptes scabiei, 599
Sardo, 848
Sardoettes, 848
Sarna, 848
Sastid Plain Therapeutic Shampoo & Wash, 838
Sastid Soap, 838
Sauna, 110
Saxon, 823
Scabies, 599
Scope Original Mint, 814
Scope Peppermint, 814
Scopolamine
  efficacy, 190
  side effects, 190
  transdermal patch, 190
Scopolamine hydrobromide, 209
Scurvy, 286, 292, 293
Seal-Tite Gaskets, 820
Sebaceous glands, 494
Sebaquin, 851
Sebasorb, 839
Sebex-T, 851
Seborrhea
  features, 531 (text table)
Seborrheic dermatitis, 354, 532-533
  atopic dermatitis, 533
  nonmonograph ingredients, 537 (text table)
  nonprescription ingredients, 536, 536 (text table)
  tinea capitis, 533
  tinea cruris, 533
Sebucare, 851
Sebulex Conditioning With Protein, 852
Sebulex Medicated, 852
Sebulon, 852
Sebutone, 843, 852
Secran B Vitamin Supplement, 778
Sedatives, 68
  poisoning, 186
Seepage
  anal, 472
Seizures, 68-69, 71, 74
Selaquin, 487
Selegiline, 104
Selenium
  adverse effects, 308
  description, 308
  dose/RDA, 308
  drug interactions, 308
  indications, 308
Selenium Sulfide, 852
Selenium sulfide, 503, 537
Self-care
  advising patients on, 16-17
  consumer attitudes and beliefs, 2-4
  consumer complaints, 3 (text table)
  consumer education/sophistication, 4-5
  definition, 1
  demographics, 5-6
  drug labels, 7
  ear conditions, 389
  economic considerations, 6-7

  future of, 8
  health personnel availability, 6
  health service availability, 6
  illness experience model, 2 (text table)
  influencing factors, 4 (text table)
  nondrug, 16
  pharmacist's role, 7-8
  product availability, 6
  seeking professional health care factors, 5 (text table)
  self-medication, 1-2, 3 (text table), 4 (text table)
  sick-role options, 1
Self-Care Movement, 1-9
Self Contained Insulin Syringe, 743
Self-medication, 1-2
  influencing factors, 4 (text table)
  of laxatives during pregnancy, 230
  problem examples, 3 (text table)
Self-treatment
  See **Self-care**; **Self-medication**
Selsun Blue, 852
Selsun Gold for Women, 852
Semicid Inserts, 822
Semilente (Prompt Insulin Zinc Suspension, Beef), 739
Senexon, 737
Senna, 227, 229, 230
  breast-feeding, 19
Senna-Gen, 737
Senokot, 737
Senokot-S, 737
Senokot-X-Tra, 737
Senolax, 737
Sensitive Eyes Daily, 804
Sensitive Eyes Drops, 806
Sensitive Eyes Effervescent Enzymatic, 804
Sensitive Eyes Plus Saline, 807
Sensitive Eyes Saline/Cleaning Solution, 804
Sensitive Eyes Saline Solution, 807
Sensitive Eyes Saline Spray, 807
Sensodyne-SC Toothpaste for Sensitive Teeth, 811
Sensodyne Toothpaste, Sensitive Teeth/Cavity Prev., 811
Sepo, 709
Serotonin storm, 139-140
Serutan, 230, 737
Sesame Street Complete Vitamins and Minerals, 778
Sesame Street Vitamins Plus Extra C, 778
Sesame Street Vitamins Plus Iron, 780
Sexually transmitted diseases, 455, 459, 461, 463-464
  safer sex practices, 464 (text table)
  See also specific diseases
SF Metamucil, 230
Shade Sunblock, 865

Shade Sunblock Lotion, 865
Shade Sunblock Oil-Free, 865
Shade Sunblock Stick, 865
Shade UVAGuard, 865
Shampoos
  dandruff, 532
  lice, 598-599
  nonmedicated, 479, 490-491
  psoriasis, 540
Shark liver oil, 546
Sheik Elite, 823
Sheik Super Thin, 823
Sheik Super Thin with spermicide, 823
Shepards, 848
Shepards Skin, 848
Shigella, 203
Shingles, 498
Shin splints, 630
Shoes
  See **Footwear**
Shur-Seal, 822
Siblin, 737
Sick-role options, 1
Sigtab-M, 780
Sigtabs, 780
Sila Rx, 370 (text table)
Silexin, 692, 709
Silicates, 413
Silicon
  adverse effects, 308-309
  description, 308
  dose/RDA, 308
  drug interactions, 308-309
  indications, 308
Silk Solution, 848
Silsoft, 370 (text table)
Silver nitrate, 422
Silver protein, 362
Silver sulfadiazine, 445
Simaal Gel, 721
Simaal 2 Gel, 720
Simethicone, 309
  antacid products, 154
Similac, 328, 790
Similac Natural Care, 331, 794
Similac PM 60/40, 331, 794
Similac Special Care, 331
Similac Special Care 20, 794
Similac Special Care 24, 794
Similac Special Care 24 With Iron, 794
Similac With Iron, 790
Simplesse, 346
Simron Capsules, 757
Simron Plus, 780
Sinarest, 653, 692, 705
Sinarest Extra Strength, 692
Sinarest, No Drowsiness, 653
Sinarest No-Drowsiness, 694
Sine-Aid Maximum Strength, 694
Sine-Off Maximum Strength Allergy/Sinus, 694
Sine-Off Maximum Strength No Drowsiness Formula, 694
Sine-Off Sinus Medicine, 694
Sinex Long Acting, 705
Sinex Regular, 705
Singlet, 694
Sinulin, 694
Sinus headaches
  etiology, 51
  symptoms, 51
  treatment, 51

Sinusitis
  treatment, 16
Sinustop Pro, 694
Sinutab, 694
Sinutab Maximum Strength, 694
Sinutab Maximum Strength Without Drowsiness, 694
Sitz baths, 476, 478
Skelaxin, 267 (text table)
Skin
  anatomy and physiology, 563-564
  assessment, 493
  bacterial infections, 496-497, 498-502
  changes in body surface area with age, 564 (text table)
  components, 494-495
  cross section, 494 (figure)
  dermatologic terms, 522 (text table)
  fungal infections, 497-498, 502-503
  infants, 543
  medication-related photosensitivity, 566-567 (text table)
  normal, 493-494, 521
  percutaneous absorption, 495-496
  physiology, 521-522
  pigmentation, 486
  premature aging, 577-578
  skin types and recommended sunscreen products, 577 (text table)
  surface, 495
  viral infections, 498, 503
  See also **Dermatitis**; **Diaper rash**; **Prickly heat**; **Rhus dermatitis**; **Sunscreen and Suntan Products**
Skin barriers, 437
Skin-bleaching products, 479, 486-488
Skin-Bond Cement, 820
Skin-Bond Cement (Nonflammable), 820
Skin Conditioning Creme, 821
Skinfold measurements for obesity, 339
Skin Gel, 821
Skin-Hesive Cement, 820
Skin irritation
  ostomy-associated, 440-441
Skin-Prep Protective Dressing, 821
Skin protectants, 423, 529-530, 545, 546-547, 606
Skin protective dressings, 437
Skin wound cleansers, 446
Skin wound protectants, 446
SLC, 803
Sleep
  alcohol, 140
  physiology, 136
  principles of good hygiene, 137 (text table)

Sleep Aid and Stimulant Products, 135-146
  patient assessment, 135, 136-141, 142
  patient counseling, 135
Sleep aid product table, 713-714
Sleep aids, 135
  nighttime sleep aid drug products monograph, 27, 26 (figure)
Sleep apnea, 136, 137, 140
Sleep-ettes-D, 713
Sleep-Eze 3, 713
Sleepinal Capsules, 713
Sleepinal Medicated Nite Tea, 713
Sloan's Liniment, 857
Slow Fe Tablets, 757
SMA, 328, 331
Smokers' Polident Denture Cleanser, 815
Smoking
  See **Cigarette smoking**
Sneaker Snuffers, 625
Sneeze reflex, 91
Snuff
  oral health effects, 409, 421
Soaclens, 803
Soaks, 570
Socioeconomic factors
  self-medication, 6
Soda Mint, 721
Sodium
  antacid products, 154
Sodium benzoate, 416
Sodium Bicarbonate, 721
Sodium bicarbonate, 151-152, 423, 424, 485, 546
  burns, 569
Sodium borate plus fatty acid, 530
Sodium caseinate formulas, 330
Sodium chloride, 361-362
Sodium Chloride Solution, 707
Sodium citrate, 107
Sodium dodecyl benzenesulfonate, 414
Sodium edetate, 377
Sodium fluoride, 419
Sodium lauryl sulfate, 414, 416, 530
Sodium metaphosphate, 413
Sodium monofluorophosphate, 419
Sodium perborate monohydrate, 423, 424
Sodium saccharin, 414
Sodium Salicylate, 653, 663
Sodium salicylate, 57
  See also **Salicylates**
Sodium sulfide, 629
Sodium valproate, 69
Sof-Form 67, 372 (text table)
Soflens, 372 (text table)
Softcon, 372 (text table)
Soft lens product table, 804-807
Soft Mate Comfort Drops, 806
Soft Mate Concept-1, 806
Soft Mate Concept-2, 806
Soft Mate Daily Cleaning For Sensitive Eyes, 804

Soft Mate Disinfecting Solution, 805
Soft Mate Hands Off Daily Cleaner, 804
Soft Mate Saline for Sensitive Eyes, 807
Soft Mate Saline Solution, 807
Soft Mate Saline Spray, 807
Softmate I, 372 (text table)
Softmate II, 372 (text table)
Softsense Skin Essentials Everyday UV Protectant, 865
Softwear Saline, 807
Solarcaine, 860, 874
Solarcaine Spray, 860
Solbar PF 15, 865
Solbar PF Cream PABA Free Waterproof, 866
Solbar PF Liquid PABA Free, 866
Solbar Plus 15, 866
Sominex, 713
Sominex Pain Relief Formula, 653, 713
Soothe, 800
Sorbic acid, 376
Sorbitan monopalmitate, 530
Sorbitol, 256-257, 346, 414, 418, 426
Sorbsan, 447 (text table)
Soyalac, 209, 328, 329, 792
Soy-based infant formulas, 209
Soy-protein infant formulas, 328-329
Spacer devices, 130
Span, 530
Special Supplemental Food Program for Women, Infants, and Children, 313
Spec-T Lozenge Sore Throat Anesthetic, 709
Spec-T Lozenge Sore Throat/Decongestant, 709
Spec-T Lozenges Sore Throat/Cough Suppressant, 709
Spectro-Jel, 854
Spectrum Toric, 372 (text table)
Spermaceti, 530
Spermicide product table, 822
Spermicides
  advantages, 459
  contraceptive film, 460
  contraceptive sponge, 460-461, 464
  creams and jellies, 460
  disadvantages, 459
  effectiveness, 459
  foams, 460
  use during pregnancy, 19
  vaginal suppositories, 460
SPF
  See **Sun protection factor**
Sphygmomanometer
  aneroid, 40, 41 (figure)
  mercury, 40 (figure)
Spironolactone, 518
Sports
  See **Exercise**
Sportscreme, 857
Sportscreme Lotion, 857

Sports Spray Extra Strength, 857
Spotting
  See **Midcycle bleeding**
Sprains, 552
  ankle, 631
  bandages, 633
Sprays, 572
  deodorant, 479, 482
  nasal, 101-102
Spritz, 415
ST 37, 835
St. Joseph Aspirin-Free For Children And Infants, 663
St. Joseph Aspirin-Free Tablets For Children, 653
St. Joseph Cold Tablets For Children, 694
St. Joseph Cough Suppressant For Children, 694
St. Joseph Low Dose Adult Aspirin, 653, 663
Stanback AF Extra-Strength, 653
Stanback Powder, Original Formula, 653
Stannous, 414
Stannous fluoride, 419
Staphylococcus, 203, 480, 496, 497, 503
  burns, 567
Staphylococcus aureus, 205, 544-545, 627
Staphylococcus epidermidis, 627
Status epilepticus, 69
StayMoist Moisturizing Lip Conditioner, 866
Steam packs, 554
Stearyl alcohol, 530
Stenosis, 440
Sterile Lens Lubricant, 806
Sterilization, 453
Steroids
  side effects, 409, 445
  topical, 423
  See also **Corticosteroids**; **Hydrocortisone**
Stimi-U-Dent, 413
Stimulant laxatives, 230
  anthraquinone stimulants, 227
  castor oil, 228
  diphenylmethane stimulants, 227-228
Stimulant Products, 141-146
Stimulant product table, 715
Stimurub, 857
Stomach
  See **Gastrointestinal system**; **Gastrointestinal tract**
Stomach acidifiers, 27
Stomahesive wafers, 437
Stools
  in-home test, 42
  iron in, 307
  softeners, 223, 226, 441, 478
  See also **Feces**
Stopzit, cream, 819
Strains, 552
Streptococcus, 93, 480, 496, 497, 503, 627
  burns, 567

Streptococcus faecalis, 205
Streptococcus mutans, 418
Streptococcus pyogenes, 545
Stress Formula, 780
Stress Formula With Zinc, 780
Stress fractures, 630
Stresstabs Advanced Formula, 780
Stresstabs 600 Plus Zinc, 780
Stresstabs 600 With Iron, 757
Stresstein, 753
Stri-Dex Antibacterial Cleansing Bar, 839
Stri-Dex Antibacterial Cleansing Bar with Glycerin, 839
Stri-Dex Clear Gel, 839
Stri-Dex Dual & Single Textured Pads Maximum Strength, 839
Stri-Dex Dual Textured Pads Regular Strength, 839
Stri-Dex Maximum Strength Medicated, 839
Stri-Dex Medicated, 839
Stri-Dex Super Scrub Pads, 839
Stroke, 141
Stuart Prenatal, 780
Styes, 353
Subperiosteal abscesses, 424
Substance P, 558
Sucralfate, 158-159, 160, 163
Sucrets Assorted, 709
Sucrets Childrens Cherry Flavored Sore Throat, 709
Sucrets Maximum Strength Sore Throat, Vapor Black Cherry, 709
Sucrets Maximum Strength Sore Throat, Wintergreen, 709
Sucrets Maximum Strength Throat Spray (Cherry), 814
Sucrets Maximum Strength Throat Spray (Mint), 814
Sucrets Original Mint, 709
Sucrets Vapor Lemon, 709
Sucrets Wild Cherry, 709
Sucrose, 418
Sudafed, 694
Sudafed Children's, 696
Sudafed Cough, 696
Sudafed 12 Hour, 694
Sudafed 12 Hour Caplet, Extended Release, 696
Sudafed Maximum Strength Severe Cold Formula, 696
Sudafed Plus, 696
Sudafed Severe Cold Formula, 696
Sudafed Sinus, 696
Sudanyl, 696
Suda-Tussin-DM, 694
Sugar
  antacid products, 154
Sugar-free products
  diabetics, 268-269, 277-281 (appendix)
Sulfa drugs, 441
Sulfinpyrazone
  drug interactions, 55, 208
Sulfonamides, 207, 576

Sulfonylureas, 247, 248 (text table)
  drug interactions, 55
  See also names of specific drugs in this class
Sulfur, 538, 546
  acne treatment, 516-517
Sulfur Soap, 839
Sulisobenzone, 580
Sulray, 839, 852
Sultrin Triple Sulfa Cream, 505
Summers Eve Fresh Scent Douche, 830
Summers Eve Herbal & White Flowers Scent, 830
Summers Eve Medicated Douche, 830
Summers Eve Post-Menstrual Douche, 830
Summers Eve Vinegar & Water Disposable Douche, 830
Sunbeam Automatic Toothbrush, 412
Sunbeam Model 7650-10 Digital Blood Pressure Monitor, 640
Sunbeam Model 7655-10 Digital Finger B.P. Monitor, 640
Sunbeam Model 7656-10 Digital Finger B.P. Monitor, 640
Sunbeam Model 7657-10 Digital B.P. Monitor with Printer, 640
Sunburn, 567-568
  process, 576
  treatment, 569
Sunburn Products, 563-573
  patient assessment, 563, 568-569
  patient counseling, 563
  product formulation, 572
  product selection, 572
Sundown Sunblock, 866
Sunette, 257
Sunglasses, 584
Sunkist Multis Complete, 782
Sunkist Multis Plus C, 782
Sunkist Multis Plus Iron, 782
Sunkist Multis Regular, 782
Sunpak Aqua Floss Oral Irrigator, 412
Sun protection factor, 578-579, 584
Sunscreen and Suntan Products, 575-588
  application guidelines, 586-587
  patient assessment, 575
  patient counseling, 575, 586-587
  patient education, 586-587
  selection guidelines, 584-585
Sunscreen and suntan product table, 862-866
Sunscreens
  agents lacking safety and/or efficacy, 582 (text table)
  chemical, 580
  for children, 585-586
  efficacy, 578-579
  indications, 576-578
  lip protection, 585

  physical, 580, 582
  safe and effective, 581 (text table)
  skin types, 577 (text table)
  types, 579-580
  UVA sunscreens, 582
Suntan Products, 575-588
  application guidelines, 586-587
  patient assessment, 575
  patient counseling, 575, 586-587
  patient education, 586-587
  pigmenting agents, 583
  selection guidelines, 584-585
  sunglasses, 584
  tanning booths and beds, 583-584
  types, 582-583
Super Banish Appliance Deodorant, 820
Superchar, 185
Super 28 Formula, 782
Super Odrinex, 796
Super Poli-Grip, 816
Super Vikaps, 782
Suplena, 753
Suppositories, 228-229
  anorectal disease, 476
  vaginal, 460
Surbex Filmtabs, 782
Surbex-T, 784
Surbex With C, 782
Surbex-750 With Iron, 782
Surbex-750 With Iron Filmtabs, 757
Surbex-750 With Zinc, 782
Surbu-Gen-T, 784
Surfactants, 414, 415
  douches, 481
Surfak, 738
Surgery
  obesity, 347
Sushi, 217
Sustacal, 310, 753, 754
Sustacal 8.8, 754
Sustacal HC, 754
Sustacal Pudding, 310
Sustacal with Fiber, 754
Sustagen, 754
Sweat glands, 494-495
  anatomy and physiology, 483
  disorders, 483-484
Sweating
  ostomy-associated, 441
Sweet birch oil, 556
Sweeteners, 256-257, 414
Sweet oil
  See **Olive oil**
Sweet spirits of nitre, 27
Swim-Ear, 808
Swimmer's ear
  See **External otitis**
Swimmer's itch
  etiology, 217
  symptoms, 217-218
  treatment, 218
Switch drugs
  See **Reclassification of prescription drugs**
SWS, 803

Sympathomimetic amines, 95, 101, 103, 104
  diabetes, 269
  side effects, 103-104
  See also names of specific drugs in this class
Sympathomimetics
  patient considerations, 111
Symptothermal method of family planning, 458
Synabrom, 653
Synovitis
  etiology, 52
  symptoms, 52
  treatment, 52
Synthaloids, 709
Syphilis, 464
Syringes, 261-262
Syringe Support, 743
Systemic steroids, 539-540

T

Talc, 546, 547
Tampons, 84-85
  toxic shock syndrome, 85
Tan accelerators, 583
Tanac, liquid, 819
Tanac Roll-On, lotion, 819
Tanac Stick, 819
Tandearil, 442 (text table)
Tangent Streak, 370 (text table)
Tannic acid, 423, 485, 546, 595, 629
Tanning
  booths and beds, 583-584
  process, 576
Tapeworms, 213
Tarpaste, 843
Tarsum, 843, 852
Taurine, 300
Tavist-1 Antihistamine, 696
Tavist-D Antihistamine/Nasal Decongestant, 696
T/Derm Tar Emollient, 566 (text table)
Teaberry oil, 556
Tear Gard, 798
Teargen II, 798
Tearisol, 798
Tears Naturale, 798
Tears Naturale & Free, 798
Tears Naturale II, 798
Tears Plus, 798
Tears Renewed, 798
Tedral, 126, 129
  dosage, 127-128
Tedrigen, 712
Teeth
  anatomy and physiology, 409-410, 410 (figure)
  fractured, 421
  See also **Oral health problems**
Teething products, 428
Tegaderm, 263, 437
Tegrin Extra Conditioning Formula, 853

General Index 911

Tegrin Fresh Herbal, 853
Tegrin Shampoo, 566 (text table)
Teldrin, 696
Telfa, 447 (text table)
Temperature
  See **Body temperature**; **Fever**
Tempo Drops, 721
Tempra 1 Drops, 653, 663
Tempra 2 Syrup, 653, 663
Tempra 3 Chewable Tablets, 654, 663
Tempra 3 Chewable Tablets, Double Strength, 654, 663
Tender Care, 549
Tendinitis, 552
  achilles, 630-631
Tension headaches
  etiology, 51
  symptoms, 51
  treatment, 51
Teratogenicity of drugs, 18-19
Terconazole, 505
Terfenadine, 101, 128
Terpin hydrate, 106
Tersa-Tar Doak Tar Shampoo, 843
Tes-Tape, 265, 293
Tes-Tape (Glucose Enzymatic Test Strip), 748
Testing Products, 39-47
  future, 46
  patient counseling, 39, 43, 44-46
Test kits
  See **Testing Products**
Tetracaine
  anorectal, 473
  burns, 571
Tetracaine hydrochloride, 594
Tetracyclines, 205, 207, 499, 512, 514, 518, 576
  antacids, 158
  use in pregnancy, 18
Tetracyn, 266 (text table)
Tetra-Formula, 709
Tetrahydrozoline, 361
Tetrahydrozoline Hydrochloride, 800
T/Gel Therapeutic Shampoo, 566 (text table)
Thalidomide, 18
Thaumatin, 346
Theophylline, 122, 124, 133, 185
  adverse effects, 188
  children, 131
  combination products, 129
  dosage, 127 (text table), 127-128
  metabolic factors, 126 (text table)
  side effects, 128
Theotal, 712
Theracof, 696
Thera-Combex H-P Kapseals, 784
Therac Plus, 738
TheraFlu; Flu and Cold Medicine, 696
TheraFlu; Flu, Cold and Cough Medicine, 696

TheraFlu Maximum Strength NightTime, 696
Theragenerix, 784
Theragenerix-M, 784
Theragran High Potency Multivitamin, 784
Theragran High Potency Multivitamin Liquid, 784
Theragran-M High Potency Vitamins with Minerals, 784
Theragran Stress Formula, 784
Theragran Stress Formula Tablets, 757
Therapeutic Bath Lotion, 848
Therapeutic Bath Oil, 848
Therapeutic Mineral Ice, 857
Therapeutic Mineral Ice, Exercise Formula, 857
Therapeutic Mineral Ice, Plus Moisturizer, 858
Therems, 784
Therems-M, 784
Therevac-SB, 738
Thermogenesis, 341
Thermometers, 69
  basal, 44
  See also **Body temperature**
Thermoregulation, 563
Thex Forte, 784
Thiamine
  adverse effects, 298
  description, 297
  dose/RDA, 298
  drug interactions, 298
  indications, 297-298
  infant formulas, 332
Thiamine hydrochloride, 607
Thiazides, 576
Thimerosal, 358, 376, 501
Thimerosal Spray, 835
Thimerosal Tincture, 835
Thinz Back-To-Nature, 796
Thinz-Span, 796
Thioglycolates, 489
Thioxanthenes, 68
Thonzylamine hydrochloride, 99
Thorets, 709
3232A, 330, 792
Throat Discs, 709
Throat disorders
  See **Laryngitis**; **Pharyngitis**
Thrombosis, 472
Thrush, 424-425, 498, 544
Thymol, 108, 401, 414, 415
Thyroid hormones, 68
Tic douloureux
  See **Neuralgia**
Ticks, 599-600
  life cycle, 602 (figure)
Tin, 309
Tinactin Liquid Aerosol, 880
Tinactin Powder, 880
Tinactin Powder Aerosol, 880
Tinactin Solution, 880
Tinactin, Various Forms, 835
Tincture of Benzoin, 821
Tinea capitis, 497, 533
Tinea corporis, 497-498
Tinea cruris, 497, 533
Tinea pedis
  See **Athlete's foot**

Tinea versicolor, 498
Ting, 880
Ting Aerosol Powder, 835
Ting Spray Liquid, 880
Ting Spray Powder, 880
Ting, Various Forms, 835
Tinnitus, 397
  patient assessment, 389
  patient counseling, 389
Tioconazole, 505, 548
Titan, 803
Titanium dioxide, 415, 606
Titanium oxide, 582
Titralac Antacid, 721
Titralac Extra Strength Antacid, 721
Titralac Plus Liquid Antacid, 721
Titralac Plus Tablets, 721
Tobacco use
  oral health effects, 409, 421
Tocopherol
  adverse effects, 291
  description, 291
  dose/RDA, 291
  drug interactions, 291
  indications, 291
  infant formulas, 332
  infant requirements, 317
  preterm infant requirements, 320
Tocotrienols, 291
Today Personal Lubricant, 830
Today Sponge, 822
Toenails, 627
  fungus, 618, 619
  ingrown, 628-629
  loss, 631
  See also **Nails**
Tolazamide
  drug interactions, 55
Tolerex, 754
Tolinase, 248 (text table)
Tolnaftate, 503, 621-622
Tolnaftate Cream & Solution, 835
Tolnaftate Solution, 880
Tolu balsam, 107
Tolu-Sed DM, 696
Tom's Natural Baking Soda Toothpaste with fluoride, 811
Tom's Natural Toothpaste for Children, with fluoride, 811
Tom's Natural Toothpaste with propolis and myrrh, 811
Tonicity adjusters, 358, 374
Toothache
  treatment, 420-421
  See also **Dental caries**
Toothbrushes, 411-412
  pediatric, 428
Tooth decay
  See **Dental caries**
Toothlessness, 425
Tooth pain
  etiology, 408
  See also **Dental caries**; **Oral health problems**
Toothpaste, 413-415
  children, 428
  fluoride, 419, 420 (text table)
Tooth whiteners, 416
Topical analgesics, 555
Topical anesthetics, 529

Topical Anti-Infective Products, 493-510
  patient assessment, 493
  patient counseling, 493
Topical anti-infective product table, 831-835
Topical decongestant product table, 704-706
Topical decongestants
  dosage, 102 (text table)
  patient assessment, 101
  patient counseling, 101-102
  side effects, 101-103
Topical dyes, 583
Topical hormones, 27
Topol, gel & paste, 811
Total All-In-One Contact Lens Solution, 803
Touch, 823
Towelettes, 482-483
Toxicodendrol, 589
Toxic shock syndrome, 77, 85 (text table), 85-87, 461
  patient counseling, 86-87
Trace elements, 303
Tracer bG Reagent, 748
Tranquil Plus, 654, 713
TraumaCal, 754
Travelers' diarrhea, 204-205 (text table), 207-208
Travel recommendations to diabetics, 267-268
Trematodes
  See **Flukes**
Trench mouth, 417, 425
Tretinoin, 487, 578
  acne, 517-518
Triacetin, 622
Triaminic Allergy Tablets, 698
Triaminic Chewables, 698
Triaminic Cold Tablets, 698
Triaminic-DM Syrup, 698
Triaminic Expectorant, 698
Triaminic Nite Light, 698
Triaminic Syrup, 698
Triaminic-12 Tablets, 698
Triaminicin Tablets, 698
Triaminicol Multi-Symptom Cold Tablets, 698
Triaminicol Multi-Symptom Relief, 698
Tribiotic Plus, 835
Trichinosis, 213
Trichlorocarbanilide, 485
Trichobilharzia, 217
Trichomonas, 480, 481
Trichomonas vaginalis, 504
Trichomoniasis, 505
Trichophyton, 497
Trichophyton mentagrophytes, 617, 618, 620, 621
Trichophyton rubrum, 544, 617, 618, 620, 621
Trichotine, 830
Trichuris trichiura
  See **Whipworms**
Triclosan, 414, 485, 501, 546
Tricyclic antidepressants
  poisoning, 186
Triethanolamine plus fatty acid, 530
Triethanolamine salicylate, 558

912 General Index

Trigeminal neuralgia
See **Neuralgia**
Trimethadione, 515
Trimethanolamine, 605
Trimethoprim, 207, 295
Trimethoprim-sulfamethoxazole, 203, 205, 206, 207
acne, 518
Trimo-San Vaginal Jelly, 830
Trind, 698
Trind-DM, 698
Tri-Pain, 663
Tri-Pain Caplets, 654
Tripelennamine, 529, 594, 606
Triphenyl, 698
Triphenyl Expectorant, 698
Triple Antibiotic, 835
Triple Paste, 854
Triple X, 875
Triprolidine
breast-feeding, 19
Triprolidine hydrochloride, 99
Triptone Caplets, 722
Trisol Eye Wash, 801
Tritin (Dr. Scholl's), 880
Tri-Vi-Sol Vitamins A,D+C Drops, 784
Tri-Vi-Sol With Iron Vitamin A,D+C Drops, 786
Tri-Vita Drops, 786
Trojan-Enz Large with spermicide, 824
Trojan-Enz with spermicidal lubricant, 824
Trojan Extra Strength with spermicide, 823
Trojan Magnum with spermicide, 823
Trojan Naturalube Ribbed, 823
Trojan Plus, 823
Trojan Plus 2, 823
Trojans, 824
Trojan Very Sensitive, 823
Trojan Very Thin with spermicide, 823
Trolamine salicylate, 558-559
Tronolane, 827
Tronothane HCl, 861
Tronothane Hydrochloride, 872
Troph-Iron Liquid, 757
Trophite, 786
Tropical Blend Dark Tanning Lotion, 866
Tropical Blend Dark Tanning Oil, 866
Tropical Blend Dry Oil, 866
Tropical Blend Sunless Tanning Clear Gel, 866
Tropical Blend Tan Magnifier, 866
Tropical Tan Magnifier, 866
L-Tryptophan, 139-140
TSS
See **Toxic shock syndrome**
Tucks, 827, 830
Tums, 721
Tums Anti-gas/Antacid, 721
Tums E-X Extra Strength, 721

Turpentine oil, 107, 108, 556-557
Tussar-2, 700
Tussar-DM (Alcohol Free), 700
Tussar-SF (Sugar Free), 700
Tusscidin Syrup, 700
Tuss-DM, 700
Tuss Kote, 700
Tween, 530
12-Hour Cold Tablets, 670
Two Cal HN, 754
Tylenol Allergy Sinus Maximum Strength, 700
Tylenol Allergy Sinus Maximum Strength Gelcaps, 700
Tylenol, Children's Cold Multi-Symptom, 702
Tylenol Children's Cold Multi-Symptom Liquid, 700
Tylenol Children's Cold Multi-Symptom Plus Cough Liquid, 700
Tylenol Children's Elixir Cherry Flavor, 654, 663
Tylenol Children's Elixir Grape Flavor, 663
Tylenol Children's Fruit Flavor, 663
Tylenol Children's Grape Flavor, 664
Tylenol Children's Suspension Liquid, 654, 664
Tylenol Cold and Flu Hot Medication, 700
Tylenol Cold and Flu No Drowsiness Formula Hot Medication, 702
Tylenol Cold Effervescent, 700
Tylenol Cold Night Time Liquid, 700
Tylenol Cold No Drowsiness Formula, 700
Tylenol Cough Maximum Strength Medication, 702
Tylenol Cough Maximum Strength With Decongestant, 702
Tylenol Extra Strength Adult Liquid Pain Reliever, 654, 664
Tylenol Extra Strength Caplet, 654, 664
Tylenol Extra Strength Gelcap, 654, 664
Tylenol Extra Strength Headache Plus, 654
Tylenol Extra Strength PM, 655, 714
Tylenol Extra Strength Tablet, 655, 664
Tylenol Infants', 655, 664
Tylenol Infants' Suspension Drops, 655, 664
Tylenol Junior Strength Fruit Chewable Tablet, 665
Tylenol Junior Strength Grape Chewable Tablet, 655, 665
Tylenol Junior Strength Swallowable, 655, 665
Tylenol Multi-Symptom Cold Medication, 702
Tylenol Regular Strength Caplet, 655, 665

Tylenol Regular Strength Tablet, 665
Tylenol Sinus Maximum Strength, 702
Tympanic membrane perforation, 396
Type I diabetes, 241, 242
carbohydrate metabolism, 238
clinical manifestations, 242 (figure)
diet management, 255-257
Type II diabetes, 239, 241, 242
diet management, 255-257
drug therapy, 247
pathogenesis, 243 (figure)
Tyrosine, 583
Tyrosum Liquid & Packets, 839

U

Ulceration of the penile meatus, 545
Ulcerative colitis, 434
Ulcers
duodenal, 148 (figure), 149, 155 (text table), 161-164
gastric, 148 (figure), 155 (text table), 164, 165
NSAID-induced, 164, 171-172
symptoms, 175
ULTEC, 449 (text table)
Ultra Brite, gel, 812
Ultra Brite, paste, 812
Ultracal, 754
UltraCare, 383
Ultracare Disinfectanta/Neutralizer System, 806
Ultra Derm, 848, 849
Ultralente (Extended Insulin Zinc Suspension, Beef), 741
Ultra Mide Moisturizer, 849
Ultra Pampers, 548
Ultra Pep-Back Caplets, 715
Ultraprin, 655, 665, 669
Ultrasound, 540
Ultra Tears, 798
Ultraviolet radiation
measures of UVA protection, 578-579
psoriasis treatment, 538
skin and, 518-519, 563, 567, 568
UVA band, 576
UVB band, 575
UVC band, 575
See also **Sunscreens**
Ultrazyme Enzymatic Cleaner, 805
Undecylenic acid, 502-503
Undecylenic Acid Compound, 880
Undecylenic acid-zinc undecylenate, 622
Undelenic Tincture, 880
Unguentine, 861
Unguentine Plus, 861

Unibase, 258
Unicap, 786
Unicap Jr., 786
Unicap M, 786
Unicap Plus Iron, 786
Unicap Senior, 786
Unicap Softgel Capsules, 786
Unicap T, 786
Uni-Care Lotion, 821
Unicomplex M, 786
Unicomplex T & M, 786
Uni-Derm Protective Moisturizer, 821
Uniflex, 447 (text table)
Unilax, 738
Uni-Salve Ointment, 821
Uni-Solve Adhesive Remover, 820
Unisom Nighttime Sleep Aid, 714
Unisom With Pain Relief, 655, 714
Universal Remover, 820
Urea, 528-529
Ureacin-10, 849
Ureacin-20, 849
Uricosuric agents
drug interactions, 55
See also names of specific drugs in this class
Uri-Kleen Deodorizing Detergent, 820
Urinary diversions, 435 (figure), 437
continent urostomy, 437
Urinary ketones test, 266
Urinary tract
anatomy, 434 (figure)
infection tests, 46
Urine glucose tests, 293
Urine Specimen Jars, 750
Urine testing
diabetes, 264-267
disadvantages, 268 (text table)
Uristix, 265
Uro-Mag, 721, 738
Urostomies
See **Urinary diversions**
Ursinus Inlay-Tabs, 702
Urushiol, 589
Uterine bleeding, 81
Uveitis, 356
UV radiation
See **Ultraviolet radiation**

V

Vaginal Contraceptive Film (VCF), 822
Vaginal contraceptives
advantages, 459
contraceptive film, 460
creams and jellies, 460
disadvantages, 459
douches, 463
effectiveness, 459
foams, 460

General Index

sponge, 460-461, 464
suppositories, 460
use during pregnancy, 19
Vaginal dryness, 82
 patient assessment, 82
 treatment, 83
Vaginal infections, 503-504
 algorithm for patient management, 507 (figure)
 antifungal products and dosages, 506 (text table)
 causes, 504
 diagnosis, 504
 signs and symptoms, 504
Vaginal suppositories, 460
Vaginal tract
 pathology, 480-481
 physiology, 480, 504
Vaginex, 506
Vaginitis, 480-481
Vagisil, 506, 830, 872
Valihist, 702
Valisone, 593
Valorin, 655, 665
Valorin Extra, 655, 665
Valorin Super, 656, 665
Valprin, 656, 665, 669
Valproic acid
 drug interactions, 55
Vanadium, 309
Vancomycin
 dosage, 205
Vanoxide, 839
Vanquish Caplet, 656, 665
Vaporizer In A Bottle Air Wick Inhaler, 702
Vapo Rub, 706
Vapo Steam, 706
Varicella-zoster infections, 498
Vaseline, 83, 461, 462
Vaseline Intensive Care lotion, 461
Vaseline Pure Petroleum Jelly, 827
Vaso Clear, 800
Vaso Clear A, 800
Vasoconstrictors, 95, 473-474
 rhinitis, 98
Vegetarians
 infant formulas, 329
 vitamin supplements for infants, 319
Velosulin, 250, 251, 263
Velosulin (Purified Pork Insulin), 739
Velosulin Human (Insulin Injection, semi-synthetic), 739
Venereal warts, 464
Venom
 immunotherapy, 604
 insect, 601
Ventease, 130
Vergo gel, 878
Verin, 56
Vermox, 216
Verrucae
 See **Warts**

Verruca vulgaris
 See **Warts**, common
Viadent, 415-416
Viadent Fluoride Gel, 812
Viadent Fluoride, paste, 812
Viadent Oral Rinse, 814
Viasorb, 448 (text table)
Vicks Cough Drops, cherry, 709
Vicks Cough Drops Extra Strength, cherry, 709
Vicks Cough Drops Extra Strength, cool peppermint, 709
Vicks Cough Drops Extra Strength, honey-lemon, 709
Vicks Cough Drops Extra Strength, menthol, 709
Vicks Cough Drops, menthol, 709
Vicks Vapor Inhaler, 706
Vi-Daylin ADC Vitamins, 786
Vi-Daylin ADC Vitamins Plus Iron, 786
Vi-Daylin Multivitamin, 788
Vi-Daylin Multi-Vitamin Drops, 786
Vi-Daylin Multi-Vitamin Liquid, 788
Vi-Daylin Multi-Vitamin Plus Iron Chewable Tablets, 788
Vi-Daylin Multi-Vitamin Plus Iron Drops, 788
Vi-Daylin Plus Iron, 788
Videx, 173
Vigilon, 448 (text table)
Vigortol, 788
Vincent's stomatitis, 417
Vinegar
 See **Acetic acid**
Viogen-C, 788
Viral infections
 common cold, 92
 hot air nasal devices, 110
 Reye's syndrome, 96
 skin, 498, 503
Viro-Med, 702
Visine, 800
Visine A.C., 800
Visine Extra, 800
Visine L.R., 800
Vision
 diabetes and, 245
 See also **Blindness**;
 Ophthalmic Products
Vita Bee C-800, 788
Vita-Bee With C, 788
Vita-Kaps, 788
Vital B-50, 788
Vita-Lea, 788
Vita-Lea For Children, 788
Vital High Nitrogen, 754
Vitamin A, 363
 adverse effects, 289
 deficiency, 359
 description, 288
 diaper rash, 546
 dose/RDA, 289
 drug interactions, 289
 indications, 288-289
 infant requirements, 317
 supplements for infants, 319

Vitamin B_1
 See **Thiamine**
Vitamin B_2
 See **Riboflavin**
Vitamin B_6
 See **Pyridoxine**
Vitamin B_{12}
 See **Cyanocobalamin**
Vitamin B_{15}
 See **Pangamic acid**
Vitamin B_{17}
 See **Laetrile**
Vitamin C
 See **Ascorbic acid**
Vitamin D
 See **Calciferol**
Vitamin D_3, 540
Vitamin E, 861
Vitamin E
 See **Tocopherol**
Vitamin F
 See **Essential fatty acids**
Vitamin H
 See **Biotin**
Vitamin K
 adverse effects, 292
 description, 291-292
 dose/RDA, 292
 drug interactions, 292
 indications, 292
 infant formulas, 332
 infant requirements, 318
Vitamin-like compounds, 298-300
Vitamin P
 See **Bioflavonoids**
Vitamins
 breast-feeding and, 19
 deficiency stages, 288 (text table)
 diabetes, 258
 fat-soluble, 288-292
 multivitamins, 287-300, 363
 natural, 287-288
 populations at risk for deficiencies, 287
 recommended daily, 286 (text table)
 supplements for infants, 318-320, 319 (text table)
 water-soluble, 292-298
 See also specific vitamins by name
Vitamins A & D, 861
Vitron-C Plus Tablets, 757
Vitron-C Tablets, 757
Vivarin, 715
Vivonex, 310
Vivonex T.E.N., 754
V-Lax, 788
Volumatic, 130
Vomiting
 complications, 182
 contraindications to use, 187
 drug-induced, 188
 etiology, 181, 182, 183 (text table), 188-189
 inducing, 184-185, 186-187
 patient assessment, 181, 187-189
 pregnancy, 181, 182, 188

process, 181-182
treatment, 16, 189-190
von Zumbusch's type of psoriasis, 534

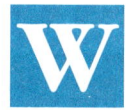

Warfarin
 drug interactions, 55
Wart Fix, 878
Wart-Off, 878
Warts, 612-614
 common, 613
 evaluation, 614-615
 flat, 613
 foot care products, 615 (text table)
 juvenile, 613
 mosaic, 613
 patient education and consultation, 617
 periungual and subungual, 613
 plantar, 613, 614 (figure)
 susceptibility, 613
 treatment, 615-617
 unapproved treatments, 616
 venereal, 464, 613
Wasps, 600, 601
Water Babies Little Licks Sunblock Lip Balm by Coppertone, 866
Water Babies SPF-15 Sunblock, 866
Water Babies SPF-30 Sunblock, 866
Water Babies SPF-45 Sunblock, 866
Water Pik, 260, 401
Water Pik Oral Irrigator, 412
Water Pik Powered Toothbrush, 412
Wax
 hair removal, 489
Weight Control Products, 339-349
 dosage forms, 347
 patient assessment, 339
 patient counseling, 339
 selection guidelines, 347-348
Weight loss
 diabetes, 244
Wernet's Cream, 816
Wernet's Powder, 816
Wernicke-Korsakoff syndrome, 297-298
Wetness
 sweat glands, 483
 treatment, 484-486
Wet-N-Soak Plus Wetting And Soaking, 803
Wet & Soak Rewetting Drops, 803
Wetting agents, 358, 378, 379
Wetting And Soaking Solution, 803
Wetting & Soaking Solution, 803
Wetting Solution, 803

Whey hydrolysate-based formulas, 330-331
Whipworms
 etiology, 217
 symptoms, 217
 treatment, 217
Whitfield's ointment, 623
Wibi, 849
WIC
 See **Special Supplemental Food Program for Women, Infants, and Children**
Wilson's disease, 304
Win Gel, 721
Wintergreen oil, 556
Winter itch
 See **Dry skin**
Witch hazel, 475, 529, 595, 606
Woman's Gentle Laxative, 738
Women
 obesity in postmenopausal, 343
 See also **Pregnancy**
Women's Choice, 463
Wonder Ice, 858
Worm infections, 214 (text table)
 anisakiasis, 217
 epidemiology, 213
 etiology, 213
 hookworms, 216-217
 pathophysiology, 213
 patient assessment, 213
 pinworms, 213-216
 pregnancy, 213
 roundworms, 216
 swimmer's itch, 217-218
 symptoms, 213
 treatment, 215-216, 217, 218
 treatment, nondrug, 216
 whipworms, 217
Wound Care Products, 433-451
 major manufacturers, 450-451 (appendix)
 options, 447-449 (text table)
 patient assessment, 433
 patient counseling, 433
 product selection guidelines, 446 (text table)
Wound cleansers, 446
Wound dressings, 445-446
 options, 447-449 (text table)
 product selection guidelines, 446 (text table)
Wound healing, 245
Wound-healing agents, 475
Wound protectants, 446
Wounds
 classification, 444
 deficient wound healing, 445
 growth factors influencing healing, 443 (text table)
 healing process, 444-445
 management, 444-446, 447-449 (text table)
 overview, 442-444
 treatment, 446
Wyanoid Relief Factor, 827
Wyanoids, 475

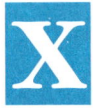

Xerac-AC, 484
Xerac Alcohol Gel, 839
Xerac BP5, 839
Xerac BP10, 839
Xeroflow, 569
Xero-Lube, 426, 813
Xerophthalmia
 See **Dry eye**
Xerosis
 See **Dry skin**
Xerostomia
 drug-induced, 425
 etiology, 425
 symptoms, 425
 treatment, 425-426
X-Seb, 853
X-Seb Plus, 853
X-Seb T, 853
X-Seb T Pearl, 843
X-Seb T Plus, 853
Xylitol, 346, 414, 418, 426
Xylocaine, 861, 874
Xylometazoline Hydrochloride, 706
Xylometazoline hydrochloride, 103

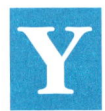

Yale 0.35cc Special Insulin Syringe, 743
Yeast infections
 See **Candidiasis**
Yellow jackets, 600, 601
Yersinia, 203

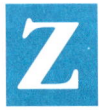

Z-Bec, 788
Zeasorb-A F, 835
Ze Caps, 788
Ze Caps Plus, 788
Zetar, 843, 853
Zetar Shampoo, 566 (text table)
Z-Gen, 788
Zidovudine
 drug interactions, 58
Zilactin-L Liquid, 819
Zilactin Medicated Gel, 819
ZilaDent, gel, 819
Zinc, 363, 414, 422
 adverse effects, 309
 description, 309
 dose/RDA, 309
 drug interactions, 309
 indications, 309
 infant requirements, 318
Zinc acetate, 546
Zinc bicarbonate, 546
Zinc chloride, 414, 415
Zinc citrate, 414, 415
Zincfrin, 800
Zincon, 853
Zinc Oxide, 861
Zinc oxide, 474-475, 485, 529, 546-547, 582, 593, 595, 606
Zinc phenolsulfonate, 209, 485
Zinc stearate, 547
Zinc sulfate, 362, 423, 516
 emetic agent, 186
Zinc undecylenate, 622
Zirconium aerosols, 27
ZNP Bar, 853
Zollinger-Ellison syndrome, 149, 159-160
Zorprin, 56
Zostrix, 858
Zostrix-HP, 858
Zymacap, 788

About the American Pharmaceutical Association

The American Pharmaceutical Association is the national professional society of pharmacists in the United States. Since its founding in 1852, APhA has been a leader in the professional and scientific advancement of pharmacy.

Services to Members

APhA works for members by offering a number of programs and services:
- Periodicals such as the official APhA journal, *American Pharmacy*, the timely *Pharmacy Today* newsletter, and the *Journal of Pharmaceutical Sciences*, recognized internationally as the authoritative monthly journal in the basic sciences.
- Reference books for pharmacists, such as the *Handbook of Nonprescription Drugs*, the *Drug Information Handbook*, the *Patient Counseling Handbook*, the *Geriatric Dosage Handbook*, and the *Pediatric Dosage Handbook*.
- An Annual Meeting that offers over 100 hours of educational sessions and exhibits the latest advancements in pharmaceutical technology.
- Testimony before Congress on issues of vital interest to the profession.

Membership

Active members must be licensed to practice pharmacy in the U.S. or hold a degree from an accredited school of pharmacy. Non-pharmacists with an interest in the mission of APhA and pharmacists licensed in other countries are **Associate members**. **Student membership** is available to any individual enrolled in a pre-pharmacy or pharmacy program at a university or college in the U.S.

For More Information...

about APhA's publications and services or about membership, contact:

> APhA-Membership Department
> 2215 Constitution Avenue, N.W.
> Washington, D.C. 20037-2985
> 800-237-APhA o FAX 202-783-2351

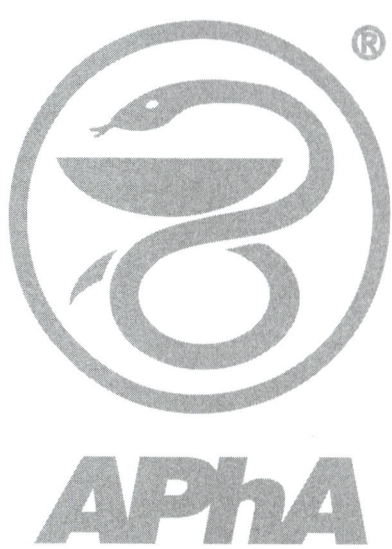

DATE DUE

GAYLORD   PRINTED IN U.S.A.